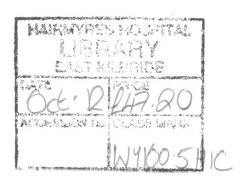

The Clinical Practice of Neurological and Neurosurgical Nursing

The Clinical Practice of Neurological and Neurosurgical Nursing

SIXTH EDITION

Joanne V. Hickey
PhD, RN, ACNP-BC, CNRN, FAAN, FCCM

Professor
The University of Texas Health Science Center
at Houston
School of Nursing
Houston, Texas

Wolters Kluwer | Lippincott Williams & Wilkins
Health

Philadelphia · Baltimore · New York · London
Buenos Aires · Hong Kong · Sydney · Tokyo

Senior Acquisitions Editor: Hilarie Surrena
Senior Managing Editor: Helen Kogut
Editorial Assistant: Brandi Spade
Senior Production Editor: Debra Schiff
Director of Nursing Production: Helen Ewan
Senior Managing Editor/Production: Erika Kors
Design Coordinator: Holly Reid McLaughlin
Cover Designer: Christine Jenny
Interior Designer: Marie Clifton
Manufacturing Coordinator: Karin Duffield
Production Services/Compositor: Aptara, Inc.

6th Edition

9 8 7 6 5 4 3 2

Printed in China

Library of Congress Cataloging-in-Publication Data

Hickey, Joanne V.
    The clinical practice of neurological and neurosurgical nursing / Joanne V. Hickey. —6th ed.
        p. ; cm.
    Includes bibliographical references and index.
    ISBN-13: 978-0-7817-9529-6
    ISBN-10: 0-7817-9529-X
1. Neurological nursing. I. Title. II. Title: Neurological and neurosurgical nursing.
    [DNLM: 1. Nervous System Diseases—nursing. 2. Neurosurgery—nursing. WY 160.5 H628c 2009]
    RC350.5.C55 2009
    616.8′04231—dc22

                                                                    2008039275

Care has been taken to confirm the accuracy of the information presented and to describe generally accepted practices. However, the authors, editors, and publisher are not responsible for errors or omissions or for any consequences from application of the information in this book and make no warranty, expressed or implied, with respect to the currency, completeness, or accuracy of the contents of the publication. Application of this information in a particular situation remains the professional responsibility of the practitioner; the clinical treatments described and recommended may not be considered absolute and universal recommendations.

The authors, editors, and publisher have exerted every effort to ensure that drug selection and dosage set forth in this text are in accordance with the current recommendations and practice at the time of publication. However, in view of ongoing research, changes in government regulations, and the constant flow of information relating to drug therapy and drug reactions, the reader is urged to check the package insert for each drug for any change in indications and dosage and for added warnings and precautions. This is particularly important when the recommended agent is a new or infrequently employed drug.

Some drugs and medical devices presented in this publication have Food and Drug Administration (FDA) clearance for limited use in restricted research settings. It is the responsibility of the health care provider to ascertain the FDA status of each drug or device planned for use in his or her clinical practice.

RRS1010

To neuroscience patients and their families who have lived the experience of neurological illness.

To the many nurses who compassionately and competently care for neuroscience patients, making a difference in the lives of patients and families, and serving communities locally, nationally, and internationally.

And as always . . . to my husband, Jim; daughter, Kathan; son, Christopher; and their families—who have given and continue to give my life meaning, direction, and purpose through their continued love and support. It is family that is the most precious of gifts and the substantive denominator of life. And to my grandchildren, Jenna, Matthew, Max, and Joanna, who are the wonderful and perfect gifts and links from the past to the future, and the joy of the present.

About the Author

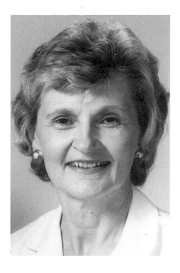

Currently, Dr. Hickey is Professor and the Director of the Doctor of Nursing Practice Program at the University of Texas Health Science Center at Houston School of Nursing. Dr. Hickey holds the Patricia L. Starck/PARTNERS Endowed Professorship in Nursing. She has focused her career on education, practice, research, and publications in the neurosciences and neuroscience patient populations. Dr. Hickey has been a faculty member in a number of schools of nursing. At Duke University, she developed and directed its first acute care nurse practitioner program. She has had clinical appointments at Massachusetts General Hospital in Boston, Massachusetts, and Duke University Medical Center in Durham, North Carolina, where she was Attending Nurse, Neuroscience Nursing. Her neuroscience research interests include cerebrovascular problems and increased intracranial pressure, and she was an American Foundation of Nursing Research Scholar in 1992 for research on preparing family caregivers for recovery from stroke.

The Clinical Practice of Neurological and Neurosurgical Nursing, now in its sixth edition, has received the *American Journal of Nursing* (AJN) Book of the Year Award and has been repeatedly cited by the Brandon and Hill listing of recommended books in nursing. The text has been translated into Japanese. Dr. Hickey serves on a number of editorial and advisory boards.

Dr. Hickey received her diploma in nursing from Roger Williams General Hospital School of Nursing in Providence, Rhode Island; her BSN from Boston College in Boston, Massachusetts; her MSN from the University of Rhode Island in Kingston, Rhode Island; her MA in counseling from Rhode Island College in Providence, Rhode Island; her PhD from the University of Texas in Austin, Texas; and her post-master's certificate as an acute care nurse practitioner from Duke University in Durham, North Carolina. She is certified in neuroscience nursing (CNRN) by the American Board of Neuroscience Nursing, and is board certified as an acute care nurse practitioner (APRN, BC) by the American Nurses Credentialing Center. She is a fellow in the American Academy of Nursing (FAAN) and a fellow in the American Academy of Critical Care Medicine (FCCM).

Dr. Hickey is a member of the American Nurses Association, the American Association of Neuroscience Nurses, and the Society of Critical Care Medicine. She serves or has served on a number of national boards and commissions, including the American Nurses Credentialing Center (ANCC) Board on Certification for Acute Care Nurse Practitioners (Chairperson 1995–1999), ANCC Commission on Certification (Chairperson 1999–2004), ANCC Board of Directors, and ANCC Institute of Credentialing Research (Chairperson 2004–present). She was the Scurlock Nurse Scholar at The Methodist Hospital in Houston, Texas. Dr. Hickey is a frequent national and international speaker and consultant on topics in neuroscience patient management, neuroscience nursing practice, and advanced practice nursing.

Contributors

The following individuals contributed to chapters in the sixth edition:

Kathryn Montgomery, MSN, RN, NP
Palliative Care Nurse Practitioner
St. Luke's Episcopal Hospital
Houston, TX
Chapter 3 • Ethical Perspectives and End-of-Life Care

Joseph Kanusky, MSN, RN, CRNA
Sugar Land, TX
Chapter 4 • Overview of Neuroanatomy and Neurophysiology

Theresa Dildy, RD, MS, LD, CNSD
Clinical Nutrition Manager
St. Luke's Episcopal Hospital
Houston, TX
Chapter 8 • Nutritional Support for Neuroscience Patients

Timothy F. Lassiter, PharmD, MBA
Clinical Pharmacist
Neuroscience Intensive Care Unit
Duke University Medical Center
Durham, NC
Chapter 12 • Pharmacologic Management of Neuroscience Patients

Amy I. Henkel, PharmD
Clinical Pharmacist
Duke University Medical Center
Durham, NC
Chapter 12 • Pharmacologic Management of Neuroscience Patients

DaiWai M. Olson, PhD, RN
Neuro Intensive Care
Duke University Medical Center,
Durham, NC
Chapter 13 • Intracranial Hypertension: Theory and Management of Increased Intracranial Pressure

Jamie Zoellner, MSN, RN, ACNP, BC
Nurse Practitioner
Duke University Medical Center,
Durham, NC
Chapter 14 • Management of Patients Undergoing Neurosurgical Procedures

Mary Bray Powers, BSN, RN, CNRN
Staff Nurse, Neuro Intensive Care Unit
The Methodist Hospital
Houston, TX
Chapter 15 • Nursing Management of Patients With a Depressed State of Consciousness

Susan Chioffi, MSN, RN, ACNP, BC
Neuroscience Nurse Practitioner
Duke University Medical Center
Durham, NC
Chapter 16 • Neuroscience Critical Care

Bettina C. Prator, MSN, RN, ACNP, BC
Nurse Practitioner
Tampa General Hospital
Tampa, FL
Chapter 17 • Craniocerebral Injuries

Andrea L. Strayer, MSN, RN, NP
Neuroscience Nurse Practitioner
University of Wisconsin, Department of Neurosurgery
Madison, WI
Chapter 19 • Back Pain and Spinal Disorders

Terri S. Armstrong, DSN, RN, APN
Associate Professor
MD Anderson Cancer Center and The University of Texas Health Science Center at Houston
School of Nursing
Houston, TX
Chapter 21 • Brain Tumors
Chapter 22 • Spinal Cord Tumors

Deidre A. Buckley, MS, RN, ANP-C
Nurse Practitioner, MGH Brain Aneurysm/AVM Center
Massachusetts General Hospital
Boston, MA
Chapter 23 • Cerebral Aneurysms
Chapter 24 • Arteriovenous Malformations and Other Cerebrovascular Anomalies

Ann Quinn Todd, RN, MSN, CNRN, FAHA
Director, Eddy Scurlock Stroke Center
The Methodist Hospital
Houston, TX
Chapter 25 • Stroke

Reviewers

Pat M. Bissonnet, LMSW
Advanced Practice Social Worker
St. Luke's Episcopal Hospital
Houston, Texas

Lauren Brandt, RN, MSN, CNS, CNRN
Director of Neurosciences
Brackenridge Hospital, Brain and Spine Center
Austin, Texas

Justin Calabrace, RN
Charge Nurse, Preceptor, Unit Board Chairman
Vanderbilt University Medical Center, Neuroscience
    ICU/Certified Stroke Center
Nashville, Tennessee

Theresa L. Dildy, MS, RD, LD
Clinical Nutrition Manager
St. Luke's Episcopal Hospital
Houston, Texas

Sylvia Dlugokinski-Plenz, RN, MS, CNRN
Nurse Case Manager
Roswell Park Cancer Institute
Buffalo, New York

Barbara Fitzsimmons, RN, MS, CNRN
Nurse Educator
Johns Hopkins Hospital, Department of Neuroscience Nursing
Baltimore, Maryland

Karen Gilbert, MS, ARNP, CNRN
Nurse Practitioner/Clinical Coordinator, Dartmouth Epilepsy
    Program
Dartmouth Hitchcock Medical Center
Lebanon, New Hampshire

Joseph Haymore, MS, RN, CNRN, CCRN, ACNP
Nurse Practitioner; Clinical Instructor
NeuroCare Associates; Georgetown University School of
    Nursing and Health Studies
Silver Spring, Maryland; Washington, DC

Matthew Hendell, MSN, CNRN, CPNP
Neurology Nurse Practitioner
Children's Hospital of Philadelphia
Philadelphia, Pennsylvania

Lynn Kennedy, MN, RN, CCRN
Assistant Professor of Nursing
Francis Marion University
Florence, South Carolina

Daisy Kumar, RN, CNN(c)
Pediatric Neurology Nurse Clinician
Children's Hospital Winnipeg Regional Health Authority
Winnipeg, Manitoba, Canada

Sera Nicosia, RN, BScN, MA, CNN(c), ARRN, ACNP
Acute Care Nurse Practitioner/Spinal Cord Injury Population
Hamilton Health Sciences
Hamilton, Ontario, Canada

Carol Ann Ottey, RN, MSN, CRRN, RNC
Faculty
Reading Hospital School of Nursing
Reading, Pennsylvania

Kimberly S. Priode, MSN, RN, CCRN
Nursing Instructor
Caldwell Community College
Hudson, North Carolina

Julia Retelski, BSN, RN, CNRN
Registered Nurse
Carolinas Medical Center
Charlotte, North Carolina

Marilyn M. Ricci, RN, MS, CNS, CNRN
Neuroscience CNS/Professor
Barrow Neurological Institute at St. Joseph's Hospital and
    Medical Center/Grand Canyon University College of Nursing
Phoenix, Arizona

Stephen Roberts, PhD, RN, CNRN, CCRN
Advanced Practice Nurse, Neurosurgery
Northwestern Memorial Hospital
Chicago, Illinois

Ingrid Scham, RN, CNN[C]
Pediatric Neurology Nurse
Children's Hospital, Health Sciences Center
Winnipeg, Manitoba, Canada

Alice Schuster, MSN, RN, APRN-BC, CNP
Nurse Practitioner, Neurosurgery
St. Joseph Healthcare
Clinton Township, Michigan

Karen A. Smith, RN, CNRN
Clinical Nurse IV
University of California Davis Medical Center
Department of Neurological Surgery
Sacramento, California

Renee Whitley, RN, ADN
Nurse Educator of Neurosurgical ICU
Carolinas Medical Center
Charlotte, North Carolina

Karena Wienands, RN
Registered Nurse
Mt. Sinai Hospital
New York, New York

Preface

With the sixth edition, we mark the 25th anniversary of publication of the first edition of *The Clinical Practice of Neurological and Neurosurgical Nursing*. Looking back over the many years, I have witnessed the phenomenal development of neurological and neurosurgical science, practice, and patient care. Since the first edition, neuroscience specialty practice has undergone a tremendous knowledge explosion and now includes understanding of neurophysiology and neuropathophysiology on molecular and genetic levels. The benefits based on this knowledge have remarkably influenced patient outcomes such as quality of life, higher functional status, and reduced morbidity and mortality. The content of the sixth edition reflects the extraordinary state of the science to which neuroscience patient care and practice has evolved.

As the nursing shortage deepens, many nurses who have not had specialty training in neuroscience patient care are assuming responsibility for patients with neurological problems. More than ever, nurses need the best-quality, up-to-date, patient-centered information reflecting evidence-based practice. I remain committed to the goals, purposes, scope, and intended audience of the text as discussed in the prefaces of all the other editions. This edition continues to focus on the care of *adult* neuroscience patients. It is intended to be a ready reference and reliable resource for practicing nurses in beginning and advanced practice roles, nursing students, nursing faculty, and other health professionals.

Together with patient safety, quality of care, and outcomes, evidence-based practice (EBP) continues to be the basis for the standard for care, clinical reasoning, and decision making for all health care professionals. Patient-centered care, which engages the patient's active participation in his or her own care, continues to shape processes of care. EBP challenges health care providers to rethink how they critically evaluate the enormous body of scientific knowledge and its application to patient care. Clinical expertise and judgment, along with patient preference, result in care that better meets the needs and expectations of patients. The continuing review of the processes of care and an increased emphasis on identifying potential system and provider error are changing the patient care environment by developing a culture of safety for patient care and practice. This sensitivity to safety is being used to redesign the processes of care including how health professionals practice as individuals and as members of interprofessional teams.

More care is being shifted from hospitals to community settings. Community-based care and home care for many neuroscience problems continue to grow. As technology becomes more compact, portable, and user friendly, more technology is being used in the home to support patient care and increasing the opportunity for home placement for patients previously destined for life-long institutional care. Concurrently, chronic health problems that require equally powerful but "low-tech" strategies, such as assessment and modification of risk factors, health promotion, disease prevention, and symptom-management strategies for optimal health and quality of life, are growing. The cornerstone of management is patient education for lifestyle changes and self-management. Empowerment of patients and families with knowledge and active decision-making roles regarding their own health care is a very effective cost saving and quality-promoting approach that needs to be developed and expanded.

The extensive revision of content in this edition reflects new knowledge and practice changes that have occurred since the last edition. It is sometimes difficult to determine what is still evolving and what are the established practices. It often depends on the setting of reference. Academic health care centers often provide a standard that might be considered "cutting edge" by community facilities. No new chapters have been added. Most chapters have undergone peer review; revisions are reflective of peer reviewers as well as development of evidence-based practice and best practice. More tables, charts, and figures have been added to clarify information. The addition of "Clinical Pearls" to most chapters is intended to highlight sage advice from practitioners to their peers. "Clinical Vignettes" have also been added to many chapters to illustrate points of clinical care and decision making.

With the enormous amount of new information published monthly, citations quickly become outdated, so lists of "other readings" has been eliminated. The references cited in each chapter support the treatment and management protocols presented in the chapter and are the most recent evidence-based practices and best practices. Websites are listed as resources for current information.

Nurses engaged in practice at different levels of acuity, including intensive care units, emergency departments, neuroscience specialty units, and other general units that provide care to neuroscience patients, should find this text a helpful and reliable reference. Throughout *The Clinical Practice of Neurological and Neurosurgical Nursing*, pathophysiology is correlated with nursing management to provide a rationale for care and to identify patient outcomes. Caring for patients with neurological problems and disabilities requires special knowledge and skills to support optimal functional level, quality of life, and patient outcomes. This book is written in an effort to respond to the diverse needs of the many committed nurses who provide compassionate, competent, quality care to patients and their families.

Joanne V. Hickey

Acknowledgments

The more things change the more they stay the same; that is what strikes me as I think about the work over the last 2 years. Writing is a demanding and all-consuming process that competes for time and creative energy with family, work, and professional commitments. Yet, somehow, major writing projects like *The Clinical Practice of Neurological and Neurosurgical Nursing,* sixth edition, are completed. It does not become easier as many people think; in some ways it is more challenging.

Many supportive and talented colleagues have sustained me during the writing of this book, and have challenged me to capture the complexity of clinical practice and patient care that is reflective of the practice arena. Patient-centered care is indeed the focus of this text, for patients and their families are the real teachers of what is critical to support a functional and acceptable quality of life. My thinking over the years about neuroscience patient care and neuroscience nursing practice has evolved from these interactions and the privilege of caring for neuroscience patients in a variety of settings with talented and committed health professionals. I am indebted to all of these numerous people who have touched my life.

This project would not have been completed without the support of my family, and especially my husband and best friend, Jim Hickey. It is he who sustained me through the many challenges faced in this enormous writing project and good-naturedly shared the major limitations placed on our life with the long evening and weekend writing schedule. Words cannot acknowledge how he enabled me to complete this work.

Finally, I would like to gratefully acknowledge and thank the contributors and the many reviewers who shared their expertise and thoughtful comments with me that strengthened the quality of the manuscript. They are listed elsewhere in this book.

Contents

Section 1

Neuroscience Nursing: Contemporary Practice

The State of the Science of Neuroscience Nursing Practice

Joanne V. Hickey

The current growth and development of the neurosciences is nothing short of phenomenal, and the translation and integration of the new scientific knowledge into practice is a formidable challenge for health professionals. To provide a context for appreciating contemporary neuroscience nursing practice, this chapter begins with a brief examination of the dynamic health care system in which neuroscience nurses practice.

THE STATE OF HEALTH CARE AND PRACTICE

While the 1990s was the era of reengineering, restructuring, and redesign in health care, the first decade of the 2000s is the era of quality, patient safety, and measurable patient outcomes. The imperative for evidence-based care grounded in a foundation of science and research is the goal of the health care agenda. The exponential growth of new knowledge coming from basic and clinical research has expanded the scientific basis for significant developments in all areas of practice including the neurosciences and neuroscience nursing. The impact of new knowledge on practice is evident in the striking strides made in neurology, neurosurgery, neuroradiology, neurogenetics, neuropharmacology, and neurorehabilitation balanced by the increased complexity of the knowledge required for clinical reasoning and decision making. New treatment options continue to raise questions about access, quality, cost, and ethical implications. Meanwhile, the knowledge explosion in the neurosciences and emerging subspecialties are encouraging many neuroscience nurses to become subspecialists in the care of specific neuroscience populations and to assume new roles as clinicians and advanced practice nurses. With the new roles come new levels of responsibility and accountability.

THE INFORMATION SOCIETY AND KNOWLEDGE WORKERS

For thousands of years mankind was engaged in the slow transformation from nomadic hunters-gatherers and warriors to communities of farmers dependent for survival on the soil, a strong extended family, and community networks during the agricultural revolution. During this era, the limited health care available was primarily home care provided by family members' home remedies, sometimes with the assistance of a lay midwife or poorly trained physician. This age was followed by the rise of the industrial revolution, which began in the 19th century and was well under way in the middle 1800s. Jobs shifted from the farms to the city factories, where a variety of industries manufactured products that the general population craved. The massive rural to urban shift brought with it the major societal change in family structure from an extended family to a nuclear family, creating radical social, political, economic, and health care delivery changes. Rampant communicable diseases and deplorable workplace conditions posed major health problems. Extended families were not available to care for sick family members, and health care shifted to hospitals. As the causes of common communicable diseases were understood, effective treatment options became available. People began to live longer and, as a result, chronic illness replaced acute and communicable disease as the prevalent health problem in the population.

Today we live in an information society, and the U.S. economy has shifted. White-collar workers outnumber blue-collar workers. A manufacturing economy is rapidly being replaced by an economy based on services and using information and knowledge. The workplace is becoming smaller as information businesses grow in importance and computer technology allows easy access to the information superhighways regardless of physical location. The emphasis in the Information Age is on knowledge work, knowledge-intense organizations, collaboration, and accountability.[1] Workers are generally classified as knowledge workers. This is an era that offers great opportunities for nursing, for patients, and for health care in general. With the promise comes the upheaval of rapid transition and transformational change. As knowledge workers in this recast health system where knowledge becomes outdated rapidly, nurses are subject to a high-intensity intellectual environment. The breadth of change experienced today signifies movement into a new era, an era that is still undefined.[2]

The fiber of the American culture is undergoing radical changes as the current political, economic, and societal

CHART 1-1	Trends Influencing the Health Care Delivery System

POLITICAL

Health policy
Power and lobbying (governmental and nongovernmental impact)
Impact of government regulations
   Demand for quality
   Measurement of outcomes
   Nongovernmental impact
   International perspective

ECONOMIC

Cost containment
Financing and reimbursement practice

DEMOGRAPHICS

Graying of America (more elderly with special needs of
   aging who are living longer)
Cultural diversity
Increase in chronic health problems across the lifespan

SOCIOLOGICAL

Consumer activism
Lifestyle changes
Quality of life expectations
Caregiver stress

TECHNOLOGICAL AND COMMUNICATIONS

Information technology integration into health care
Computers and the Internet for availability of information to
   anyone who has access to a computer and the Internet
Information superhighway

EXPLOSION OF SCIENTIFIC INFORMATION

Proliferation of scientific knowledge

structures that were erected to support an industrial economy are collapsing or being transformed to meet the needs of an information society. Concurrently, the health care industry is undergoing major transformation as it struggles to align itself with the needs and demands of contemporary society and a new evolving world paradigm. The only thing certain for the future of health care is change, like it or not.

TRENDS SHAPING HEALTH CARE DELIVERY

The complexity of the health care system is mind boggling. Powerful political, economic, demographic, sociological, technological, and health trends are shaping the health care delivery system as the nation endeavors to meet the growing health needs and expectations of its widely diverse population. These trends are summarized in Chart 1-1 and are discussed briefly to provide a framework for understanding their influence on the health care system. The overlapping nature of the trend categories speaks to the interrelatedness of trends, so that some of the discussion is overlapping. For efficiency, trends have been placed in the most logical category.

POLITICAL TRENDS AND REGULATIONS

The national political agenda reflects the multitude of political attitudes and processes that have tremendous impact on economic, demographic, sociological, and technological trends. Therefore, it is important to be aware of the importance of the political process in influencing societal trends.

The national mandate for comprehensive, affordable, quality health care for all Americans continues with the added caveat of safe care. The Institute of Medicine has published several important reports addressing quality and safety. *To Err Is Human: Building a Safer Health System*[3] shocked the nation with reports of 98,000 hospital deaths annually attributable to medical error. This report stimulated a wave of critical examination of how care is rendered, the work environment in health care facilities, and practice patterns that may lead to error. *Crossing the Quality Chasm: A New Health System for the 21st Century*[4] offers recommendations to improve the quality of health care through substantial changes in the health care system. *Health Professions Education: A Bridge to Quality*[5] addressed the need to prepare clinicians to meet both the needs of patients and the requirements of a changing health system. The new vision for all programs engaged in the clinical education of health professionals was summarized as follows[6]:

All health professionals should be educated to deliver patient-centered care as members of an interdisciplinary team, emphasizing evidence-based practice, quality improvement approaches, and informatics

The mandate for quality has stimulated a national dialogue about what is meant by quality and how it should be measured. Implicit in quality is safe care. As a result, a number of governmental and nongovernmental groups now collect data that are used for benchmarking against self, like cohorts, and national standards. It has also stimulated an examination of the health workforce, especially nurses and the work environment in which they practice. The interrelatedness of patient safety and the work environment of nurses has been addressed by the Institute of Medicine report entitled *Keeping Patients Safe: Transforming the Work Environment of Nurses*.[7] This report examined key elements of the work environment of nurses that have an impact on patient safety and provided recommendations for improvements in health care working conditions designed to increase patient safety. These recommendations are in various stages of consideration and implementation.

Finally, layers of federal and state regulatory agencies assume responsibility for multiple aspects of health care including eligibility and available services. For example, the Center for Medicare and Medicare Services (CMS) is a major federal agency that has authority and responsibility to regulate the Medicare and Medicaid programs. The CMS is the largest purchaser of health care in the United States. Through its rules and regulations the CMS has significant control on how practitioners provide care, as well as who can be reimbursed for professional services and at what level of reimbursement. These are important considerations that relate to the quality of care and safety of patients.

ECONOMIC TRENDS

Cost containment continues to be a driving force affecting all aspects of health care delivery. Maturing managed care markets, focused on cost containment, are developing integrated models of care with more community-based care to contain cost. Subacute units, home health care, hospice care, and various outpatient services are being expanded and justified based on cost savings. Another essential trend with cost-saving implications is reimbursement for preventive, health promotion, and rehabilitative services. Preventive and health promotion measures keep people healthy or identify problems in the early, less costly interventional stage. In addition, more rehabilitation programs are being developed that are designed to assist people to be as functional and as independent as possible, thus limiting disuse syndromes, disabilities, and other problems requiring more expensive care.

Fees for health care services in the United States are largely set by formulas promulgated by the federal and state governments such as the CMS and by third-party insurers. Employed individuals with health care benefits are often baffled by the array of health care plans and health care packages from which to choose. They are also being required by their employers to assume a greater portion of health care premiums. Some employers no longer offer health care insurance as a benefit of employment. Rather than hiring permanent employees, they now fill positions with temporary or part-time employees who are not given health care benefits.

DEMOGRAPHICS

There are two major demographic trends impacting on health care in the United States: the growing number of elderly, and the increasing cultural diversity associated with increased immigration.

The changing age profile of America will be the greatest force shaping health care for the next 40 years. The nation's baby boomers, those 76 million people born between 1946 and 1964, will drive the nation's health care consumption curve up steeply as they enter the age spectrum where the manifestations of chronic illness predominate. The demographic prediction of the 65 years and older population are telling for 2000, 2010, and 2030, respectively, as 35 million (12.4% of total population), 40 million (13%), and 71.5 million (19.7%).[8] Those 85 years of age and older are the fastest-growing segment of the population.

The graying of America is occurring not only because the absolute numbers entering these age groups are growing, but also because a larger percentage of people are surviving to older ages. Life expectancy has increased steadily for several decades, largely as a result of (1) improved economic conditions for older Americans, coupled with improved access to affordable, quality health care, at least for some; (2) strides made in the treatment of many diseases of older age, such as cancer and heart disease, which have extended life significantly; and (3) appreciation of the benefits of a healthy lifestyle, including diet, personal habits, exercise, and stress reduction. Nevertheless, with aging eventually comes an overall increase in chronic illnesses such as coronary heart disease, arthritis, chronic obstructive pulmonary disease, and Alzheimer's disease. The greatly increased prevalence of these diseases and others will impose an increased burden on the health care system and require a redirection of scarce societal resources toward these needs. Although management of chronic illness is causing a major shift in health care from acute to chronic care, with the projected number of elderly, the strain on the health care system is undetermined. Equity in distribution of health care resources for all segments of society will need to be addressed.

Related ethical decision making is likely to focus on the care provided for the growing number of chronically ill elderly who have a substantially decreased quality of life. It is well documented that the use of health care resources is highest during the last year of life and that these resources are often expended with little or no gain in quality or quantity of life. The underdevelopment of less costly community-based care and support services to assist the elderly and their families in managing their needs in their homes has led to utilization of the high-cost alternative, hospital care. Independent healthy elderly, on the other hand, need help with continued health promotion and preventive measures to keep them healthy and independent. There is a growing realization that the impending stress posed by the graying of America on the health care system has serious consequences for the future health of all sectors of the U.S. economy.

The second major demographic trend to shape health care in the 21st century is the greatly increased infusion of multiple ethnic and culturally diverse groups into the United States. This reality is changing the economics, process, and structure of health care delivery. The primary migration from Western Europe in the first half of the century has been replaced by an influx of people from Asia, Africa, and Central and South America. Smaller but growing numbers are coming from the Moslem countries of the Middle East and the newly configured countries of the former Soviet Union. A relatively small number come through the traditional and legal immigration channels.

Immigrant groups bring with them ethnic and cultural values that include belief-value systems about health and illness throughout the life cycle. Western medicine may be held suspect by members of these groups and may be rejected in favor of their own ethnic and folk medicine. Health care professionals must nevertheless understand and respect their cultural values and strive to develop cultural competence and implement programs that are culturally sensitive as well as effective. Education of both health care providers and health care recipients with the goal of easing the transition and blending of native and American cultures is necessary if mutual needs are to be addressed.

SOCIOLOGICAL TRENDS

Unlike temporary fads and fashions, deep-rooted trends in attitudes and values develop over generations in reaction to shared experiences on community, national, and global levels. They therefore have a tremendous impact on the ways in which people interact with societal institutions. Of the numerous sociological trends influencing society in general and the course of health care in particular, the following few are discussed briefly because of their relevance to practice: consumerism, lifestyle changes, quality of life, and family caregivers.

Consumerism

Individual values and attitudes toward health are formed, in part, by the information to which one is exposed. As more and more information has become widely available, consumers have become more active in choosing, evaluating, and criticizing the products and services available to them, including health care.

The Internet, television, and the print media are the principal sources of consumer health information. Computer technology and the Internet are growing in importance with all segments of society. For example, PubMed and on-line computer health bulletin boards are easily accessible by the public, and many people are using them to become informed about their health and medical problems. The quality of the information varies, and consumers are not always able to discern the accuracy and completeness of the information. As a result, more consumers are actively participating in making decisions about their health and health care options. They no longer follow recommendations of health providers without question or discussion of options. Consumers are also interested in complementary and alternative medicine (CAM) to augment their health care such as herbal therapy, homeopathic treatments, and relaxation therapies. The demand for information and involvement in decision making has created a new industry of educational material for the consumer.

Lifestyle Changes

Broad dissemination of information about the health implications of smoking, alcohol consumption, drug abuse, poor diet, overweight, sedentary practices, stress, and sexual practices has had an enormous impact on behavior. Counteractive lifestyle changes are decreasing disease frequency and severity. Failure to heed health promotion and disease prevention recommendations, however, continues to be a serious public health problem. For example, obesity, including childhood obesity, continues to increase. Smoking by adolescents continues to rise, while smoking in general has declined.[9] With so many serious chronic diseases associated with smoking and obesity, these are ominous trends. As women have become more engaged in high-stress occupations, negative lifestyle factors such as poor diet, infrequent exercise, and increased stress are afflicting them as grievously as they have been afflicting men. Positive lifestyle changes are also apparent. Exercise, weight control, low-fat and low-cholesterol diets, and stress reduction are all health promotion and disease prevention basics embraced by a growing number of Americans. The outcome of these conflicting trends on mortality and morbidity is unclear. Either way, their effects will be felt in practice settings.

Quality of Life

In many cases, technology now allows for extension of life indefinitely even though the quality of that life may be minimal or nonexistent. Some patients and family members have become more attuned to factoring quality of life into their decisions about health care and extraordinary means of maintaining life. New interest in end-of-life care is shedding new light on palliative care and decisions to control the intensity of care. Resolution of these issues, which are addressed in Chapter 3, has far-reaching implications for the future cost of health care, personal and clinical decision making, and the way health professionals practice.

Family Caregivers

The lay caregiver role is being assumed by an increasing number of family members who provide care in the home. Caring for someone with multiple problems and needs on a 24/7 basis is an overwhelming responsibility. Successful resuscitation of trauma victims and patients experiencing other acute neurological events has resulted in patients' surviving with multiple chronic deficits and conditions. Improved treatment options are leading to longer survival for patients with chronic neurological diseases, such as stroke, multiple sclerosis, and Parkinson's disease. Such patients have comprehensive needs that can place a tremendous burden on the family caregiver. Recognition of family caregiver stress and their needs has increased support services in the community for both patients and family caregivers. Effective strategies of support groups such as for cerebral trauma and Alzheimer's disease have focused attention and secured funds for the care of persons with neurological deficits. Many groups with worthwhile goals are competing for limited resources to fund programs for special patient populations. Great opportunities exist for neuroscience nurses to work with these groups to develop programs that address the special needs of patients and their family caregivers.

TECHNOLOGICAL TRENDS

The current information society is characterized by a proliferation of information about world, national, and local issues, all of which are rapidly disseminated to anyone able to read a newspaper, watch television, or access the Internet. Information technology is changing how we live, work, and learn. The Internet opens portals for the general population to detailed, specialized information on almost any subject, which previously would have required time-consuming dedicated research. Moreover, information is disseminated so rapidly that today's sensational product or treatment is already widely known by the time it is reported in conventional media. Even a casual observer cannot help but be amazed by the discoveries and new technologies that are emerging in almost every area of scientific study.

The areas impacted by the great technology explosion have been mentioned in previous sections. Diseases are being diagnosed at an earlier stage, new interventions are being developed for previously untreatable diseases (notably, genetically based diseases), less invasive interventions are emerging, and more precise and effective interventions with fewer complications and residual effects are becoming available for common medical problems. In response, medicine and nursing continue to become more specialized as the timeline and practice requirements to become expert in certain procedures and equipment extend. For example, in neurorehabilitation development of new, high-tech prosthetic devices, as well as the opportunity that new interventions offer for saving and restoring function, will have a profound effect on the quality of life of many patients who have sustained neurological trauma or who have chronic neurological diseases.

NATIONAL AGENDA FOR HEALTH

Primary care has become a central component of federal, state, local, and private initiatives to reorganize health care, highlighting preventive care as a component within the context of primary care. The Institute of Medicine (IOM) defines primary care as follows:[10]

> the provision of integrated, accessible health care services by clinicians who are accountable for addressing a large majority of personal health care needs, developing a sustained partnership with patients, and practicing in the context of family and community

As specialty practitioners, neuroscience nurses must be attuned to the holistic needs of patients by working collaboratively with primary care providers to achieve optimal outcomes across a seamless continuum of care.

Governmental, private, and professional organizations are forging new initiatives to influence the future direction of quality and safe health care for the nation through prevention, health promotion, and disease management initiatives. A few examples of the more ambitious and promising initiatives are *Healthy People 2010*[11] and *The Guide to Clinical Preventive Services, 2005*.[12] *Healthy People 2010* builds on the original *Healthy People 2000*,[13] and has as its two central goals

to increase quality and years of healthy life and to eliminate health disparities. Both components are committed to the single overarching purpose of promoting health and preventing illness, disability, and premature death. *Healthy People 2010* is organized around 467 objectives in 28 focus areas, and health improvement opportunities are outlined for the first decade of the 21st century. For the first time, a set of *leading health indicators* helps individuals and communities target desirable outcomes.

The Guide to Clinical Preventive Services, 2005, published by the Agency for Healthcare Research and Quality (AHRQ), is a compilation of abridged Task Force recommendations released from 2001 to 2004 and is useful as evidence-based preventive care recommendations at the point of patient care. Many consider the recommendations of the Task Force to be the "gold standard" for preventive services, recommendations developed by professional societies, coverage policies of many health plans and insurers, health care quality measures, and national health objectives. The recommendations are each linked to a letter grade that reflects the magnitude of the net benefit and the strength of the evidence supporting a specific preventive service. An "A" to "D" grading scale is used with "A" being strongly recommended and "D" being strongly recommended against. Neuroscience practitioners will find this book helpful as they assume more responsibility for preventive care. For example, specific information is included on modification of risk factors for stroke including management of hypertension and high cholesterol levels.

Health promotion and disease prevention are important aspects of every nurse's practice, neuroscience nurses included. From the intensive care unit (ICU) to community-based care, health promotion, risk assessment, and disease prevention strategies must be incorporated into practice regardless of setting. Primary prevention is the ultimate goal, but secondary and tertiary prevention are also necessary to provide optimal outcomes and quality of life for persons with health problems.

In summary, the health care system and how health care professionals practice continues to change significantly and rapidly and will have a major impact on both neuroscience patients and neuroscience nursing practice.

PROFESSIONAL NURSING AND NEUROSCIENCE SPECIALTY PRACTICE

Neuroscience nursing specialty practice builds on the foundation of professional nursing practice. The American Nurses Association (ANA) has developed and published *Nursing's Social Policy Statement*[14] and *Nursing: Scope & Standards of Practice*[15] that describe nursing's covenant with society and its unique contribution to society. Following the same format for *Nursing: Scope & Standards of Practice*, the American Association of Neuroscience Nurses (AANN), in collaboration with the ANA, has published the *Scope and Standards of Neuroscience Nursing Practice*,[16] but does not differentiate between general and advanced neuroscience practice nursing as the ANA publications have done.

The *Social Policy Statement*[14] notes that "the authority for the practice of nursing is based on a social contract that acknowledges the professional rights and responsibilities of nursing and includes mechanisms for public accountability." Further, it states that "nursing is the protection, promotion, and optimization of health and abilities, prevention of illness and injury, alleviation of suffering through the diagnosis and treatment of human response, and advocacy in the care of individuals, families, communities and populations." These statements provide the foundation for professional nursing practice by registered nurses. *Nursing: Scope & Standards of Practice*[15] outlines the expectations of the standards of professional nursing practice as boundaries from other health professionals and care providers. It also states that the profession of nursing has one scope of practice that encompasses the full range of nursing practice. The depth and breadth of scope in which individual registered nurses practice is dependent upon education, experience, role, and the population served. Scope is also contingent on legal authority given by the individual state regulatory laws that license and control authority to practice.

The *standards of practice* are defined as authoritative statements by which the nursing profession delineates the responsibilities for which its practitioners are held accountable. The six standards of practice describe the competencies required according to the critical thinking model known as the nursing process. The nine *standards of professional performance* describe competencies in professional roles that include quality, education, professional practice evaluation, collegiality, collaboration, ethics, research, resource utilization, and leadership. Both the standards of practice and the standards of professional performance include key indicators of measurable evidence of competency for each standard.

What is the relationship between the standards of practice, standards of professional performance, and clinical practice guidelines? Standards provide a broad framework for *nursing practice*. By comparison, clinical practice guidelines outline a *process of patient management* usually based on scientific evidence that has been developed through a deliberate review process of the scientific literature and expert opinion designed to provide quality care that leads to best patient outcomes. A synergistic relationship exists between the standards and clinical practice guidelines, which raise the bar on quality and the expectations of the professional nurse to deliver high-quality care.

Professional Practice and Specialization

Of the 2.8 million registered nurses (RNs) in the United States, most RNs are engaged in general practice roles, although many RNs work with a specialty patient population. Preparation for specialty patient population practice builds on the limited content offered in undergraduate programs, but generally occurs through continuing education courses and on-the-job training. Undergraduate nursing programs prepare generalists rather than specialists. Nurses usually assume the role of direct care providers as general duty staff nurses after undergraduate education.

Nurses educated at the graduate level as advanced practice nurses (APNs) are prepared to practice in an advanced practice model with substantial autonomy and independence within their scope of specialty practice. Specialization in practice can be based on general advanced practice roles (e.g., clinical nurse specialist, nurse practitioner, nurse anesthetist), specialty practice roles (e.g., acute care nurse practitioner or adult nurse practitioner), or subspecialization in a patient population (e.g., neuroscience patients, cardiovascular patients). Practice can be further delineated by a particular neuroscience practice focus such as traumatic brain injury, stroke, or Parkinson's disease. Differentiated nursing practice, within nursing and specifically neuroscience nursing practice, is evolving. The mandate for competency and quality care coupled with the knowledge explosion support differentiated and specialty practice for the foreseeable future. The current nursing shortage and the implications of an aging RN workforce will challenge models of differentiated practice, delegation of work to unlicensed personnel, and work environments.

Many APNs are assuming new roles in neuroscience practice as nurse practitioners and clinical nurse specialists. They are practicing in tertiary settings within Neuroscience ICUs, intermediate units, specialty clinics, rehabilitation programs, and community-based and home care programs. These nurses are assuming responsibility for diagnosing and prescribing treatment plans as they work in collaboration with physicians. Many chronic neurological problems can be well managed by APNs who combine a holistic nursing framework with a medical framework. Availability of medical residents in neuroscience practice is limited due to fewer choosing specialty practice and strict limitations of hours that they can work. An obvious source of high-level providers to meet patient care needs is APNs. However, there are few APNs trained in neuroscience specialty practice and very few programs to educate them in this specialty practice.

One way to demonstrate professional competency is through certification. Certification is a voluntary process by which professional nurses are recognized for a high level of competency in practice based on knowledge and clinical practice experience. The eligibility requirements (e.g., formal education, hours of practice) for a particular certification examination vary. The AANN provides a certification program in neuroscience nursing. Candidates must present evidence of years of neuroscience practice as a registered nurse to sit for the written examination. Upon successful completion of the examination, the nurse is designated as a certified neuroscience registered nurse (CNRN). The nurse can maintain ongoing certification by periodically taking the written examination or by providing evidence of clinical practice and continuing education credits. The AANN offers one examination for all registered nurses; there is not a special examination for advanced practice nurses. By 2007, there were approximately 2,350 CNRNs.[17]

Work Environments and Practice Models

Quality care is an expectation of professional practice. The IOM has defined quality as follows[5]:

the degree to which health services for individuals and populations increase the likelihood of desired health outcomes and are consistent with current professional knowledge

To provide quality care, a supportive work environment that includes respect for nursing within the institutional structure and administrative support for nursing must be in place. A number of studies have addressed the characteristics of work environments that contribute to quality care and nurse satisfaction.[18,19] It is vitally important that the research continues to examine the interaction of environment and nursing practice and its influence on safe quality care. Hospitals and now long-term facilities that meet high standards of nursing practice can be recognized for excellence by the Magnet Recognition Program of the American Nurses Credentialing Center. Designation as a magnet facility is recognition of *excellence in nursing care.* Characteristics of nursing practice found in all magnet facilities include nurse autonomy, nurse control of practice, and satisfying collaborative nurse–physician relationships.[20,21] These characteristics contribute to lower nurse turnover rates, greater patient satisfaction, improved patient outcomes, and overall high-quality patient care. More consumers and payers are becoming aware of the value of a magnet-designated facility.

Interdisciplinary Practice

The model of practice by which care is delivered is very important to quality. The IOM strongly recommends that all care must be patient-centered care that is evidence based and delivered by interdisciplinary practice teams. The preferred practice model of the 21st century is characterized by interdisciplinary teamwork, the hallmarks of which are mutual respect, collaboration, effective ongoing communications, mutual goals, shared decision making, and measurable outcomes. A distinction is made between multidisciplinary and interdisciplinary teams. A *multidisciplinary team* has *more than one discipline* in its membership. The core multidisciplinary team members often include the nurse, physician, case manager, respiratory therapist, pharmacist, nutritionist, physical therapist, speech therapist, occupational therapist, social worker, and chaplain, with other health care professionals included as needed. The hallmark of an *interdisciplinary team* is *collaborative interaction* between members of the different disciplines working together for mutual goals and outstanding outcomes. Such a model emphasizes joint responsibility in patient care management, with a shared decision-making process based on each practitioner's education and ability. The foundation of collaborative interdisciplinary practice is mutual respect for the contributions of each health professional to care and group dynamics that support shared leadership and responsibility for patient outcomes. Neuroscience nurses are members of interdisciplinary teams and contribute to the quality of patient care as direct-care staff nurses and advanced practice nurses.

Transformation of Care into Evidence-Based Practice

Practice, theory, and research, the familiar interrelated cornerstones of professional practice, imply that practice be based on scientific evidence forged from solid research. Of all the changes in the current professional practice environment, the transition to evidence-based practice is the most important and challenging. The demand for quality and the best patient outcomes have created the backdrop for professional accountability in the delivery of health care through evidence-based practice. In the early 1990s, the term **evidence-based practice** (EBP) emerged in the professional literature. Evidence-based practice is the conscientious use of current best evidence in making decisions about patient care.[22] EBP is an approach to practice and teaching that emphasizes knowledge of the evidence upon which practice is based and the strength of that evidence. The evidence includes scientific evidence from systematic reviews, randomized control trials, descriptive and correlational studies, and qualitative studies. It also includes personal expert opinion based on clinical experience and knowledge, opinions of expert thought leaders, and patient preference. The term **best practice** or **best practices** is used to describe nursing care that is based on the most current scientific information, expert opinion, and patient preference.

A deliberate process must be followed to engage in evidence-based practice that includes:

- Posing an answerable question
- Systematically searching for and identifying the most relevant evidence available to answer the question
- Critically reviewing and appraising the evidence and the strength of that evidence
- Integrating the evidence with one's clinical expertise, opinions of thought leaders, and patient preference for decision making
- Evaluating the outcome of the implemented practice decision

It is beyond the scope of this book to delve into the complex process of changing a care environment into an evidence-based practice culture. However, the complexity of the process and the development of EBP competencies in nursing staff as well as other health professionals have been grossly underestimated. The process is the equivalent of a culture transformation that requires a fundamental change in how nurses approach clinical practice and how they think. Yet, it is vitally important that an EBP care environment be established and maintained to support the mandates for quality, patient safety, and excellent patient outcomes. Nursing has supported research-based practice and encouraged nurses to critically evaluate research for utilization into practice. EBP is the final step in creating science-based practice that supports best practices. In addition to incorporating the existing scientifically based knowledge from research, EBP reaffirms the importance of clinical expertise and expert opinion in decision making. Obstacles for implementation of EBP must be addressed and overcome. In the near future, EBP capability will be available to all nurses at the point of care.

EBP and research comprise the perfect interrelated partnership for practice. As the evidence to answer clinical questions is critically evaluated, it often becomes evident that there is limited evidence available to answer the question or that the strength of the evidence is weak. This identifies gaps in knowledge and areas for the conduct of research. Research is the foundation for building a scientific knowledge base for practice and for the profession. The National Institute for Nursing Research (NINR) within the National Institutes of Health has been important in setting research priorities and supporting research efforts by nurses on a national level. A number of NINR research priorities focused on broad neuroscience problems are providing opportunities for neuroscience nurses to conduct research. Many other organizations also fund neuroscience research, making neuroscience practice a fertile area for both independent and collaborative research.

Application of Knowledge in Professional Practice

The intellectual demands required to practice nursing in a fast-paced technology- and knowledge-driven society are awesome. Nurses are surrounded by complex computer-driven technologies connected to exquisite databases. Patient assessment and treatment often involve interfacing with a computer. Sophisticated physiological monitoring systems provide an integration of waveforms and digital values from various physiological variables. Decision-making software recognizes deviations from set parameters and offers diagnostic and treatment suggestions. Along with the complexities of the practice environment are the complexities of patients who are sicker and older and who have multiple chronic comorbidities. The social and cultural diversity of patients influence expectations and acceptance of health care.

The need for nurses with well-developed critical thinking skills has never been more apparent than in the current health care system because critical thinking competencies drive nursing practice to EBP and directly influence the achievement of optimal patient outcomes. Nurses can be taught the principles of critical thinking in undergraduate programs and on through graduate and continuing education programs, but these skills are honed in clinical practice. They are also foundational for the development of EBP competencies.

The traditional approach to nursing practice has been the nursing process framework, which dates back to the early 1970s. The nursing process provides a systematic critical thinking and decision-making model that includes the five steps of assessment, analysis, planning, implementation, and evaluation. It is a logically organized scientific method of problem solving with the goal of identification of patient problems and prescription of appropriate nursing interventions followed by evaluation of outcome. It does not incorporate all of the cognitive and intuitive processes of the professional developmental model described by Benner in *From Novice to Expert.*[23] For APNs engaged in clinical practice, other more sophisticated models based on scientific problem solving are useful and are designed to include medical diagnosis and treatment decisions. For example, **clinical and diagnostic reasoning** models include all of the critical thinking and reasoning about patient care, management questions, and treatment decisions considered in providing care in clinical practice. Clinical reasoning skills provide the competencies to sustain effective lifelong practice in an ever-changing practice environment.

The Neuroscience Nurse: Present and Future

Neuroscience nursing specialty practice is set within the context of general professional nursing practice. Nurses

engaged in neuroscience nursing must be competent in general practice before engaging in specialty practice. Specialty practice builds on the knowledge of basic nursing science and then adds the in-depth knowledge and competencies required to provide specialized care to neuroscience patient populations. Staying current requires ongoing education in both areas to be able to provide evidence-based nursing that results in excellent outcomes. The shift to EBP is requiring nurses to think differently and also have computer and analytical skills to identify the best information for EBP and best practices. Building the repository of best practices for neuroscience nursing needs input from all neuroscience nurses who contribute information based on research, quality outcome practice changes, and other initiatives designed to improve patient outcomes. For example, fall risk assessment, prevention, and management programs cut across all clinical practice areas and patient populations.[24] However, what are the special risk assessment and prevention-management characteristics for neuroscience patients that need to be incorporated based on cognitive and functional deficits related to neurological illness? Such clinical situations require input and possible modification of practices from neuroscience nurses who are experts in caring for neuroscience patients. Patients expect that population-based care be translated to patient-centered care that is most appropriate for their special situation and needs.

Neuroscience-specific educational programs must be developed and shared nationally because there is a scarcity of such opportunities for nurses. Current neuroscience knowledge is critical as nurses forge new partnerships with other health care providers in new models of practice. Nurses must also be encouraged to become certified in neuroscience nursing practice to demonstrate a high level of knowledge and commitment to patient care.

This is the decade of quality, safety, and outcomes, all of which must be addressed as measurable outcomes that support better patient outcomes and thus care. The challenges to nursing are formidable, but nursing has always accepted the commitment of service to society as an earmark of a profession. Nurses, and especially neuroscience nurses, have unprecedented opportunities to shape the future of health care through quality initiatives that translate into best practice at the bedside. The breakthroughs in neuroscience knowledge and the genomic age promise that the rapidly changing treatment options available to patients will challenge the dimensions of practice and care. Neuroscience nurses must prepare for the increased and intense complexity of the future.

REFERENCES

1. Sorrells-Jones, J., & Weaver, D. (1999). Knowledge workers and knowledge-intense organizations, Part 1. *Journal of Nursing Administration, 29*(7/8), 12–18.
2. Covey, S. R. (2004). *The 8th habit: From effectiveness to greatness.* New York: Free Press.
3. Kohn, L. T., Corrigan, J. M., & Donaldson, M. S. (Eds.). (2000). *To err is human: Building a safer health system.* Washington, DC: National Academy Press.
4. Committee on Quality of Health Care in America Institute of Medicine. (2001). *Crossing the quality chasm: A new health system for the 21st century.* Washington, DC: National Academy Press.
5. Grenier, A. C., & Knebel, E. (Eds.). (2003). *Health professions education: A bridge to quality.* Washington, DC: National Academy Press.

6. Grenier, A. C., & Knebel, E. (Eds.). (2003). *Health professions education: A bridge to quality* (Executive Summary, pp. 3–4). Washington, DC: National Academy Press.

7. Page, A. (Ed.). (2004). *Keeping patients safe: Transforming the work environment of nurses.* Washington, DC: National Academy Press.

8. U.S. Census Bureau. (2005, April 21). Population division, interim state population projections. Retrieved June 20, 2006 from http://www.census.gov/ipc/www/usinterimproj.

9. U.S. Department of Health and Human Services. (2000). *Healthy people 2010* (pp. 7–8). Washington, DC: U.S. Government Printing Office.

10. Donaldson, M. S., Yordy, K. D., Lohr, K. N., & Vanselow, N. A. (Eds.). (1996). *Primary care: American's health in a new era.* Washington, DC: National Academy Press.

11. U.S. Department of Health and Human Services. (2000). *Healthy people 2010.* Washington, DC: U.S. Government Printing Office.

12. U.S. Preventive Services Task Force. (2004). *The guide to clinical preventive services, 2005.* Rockville, MD: Agency for Healthcare Research and Quality.

13. U.S. Department of Health and Human Services. (1990). *Healthy people 2000* (p. 6) (DHHS Publication No. PHS 91-50213). Washington, DC: U.S. Government Printing Office.

14. American Nurses Association. (2003). *Nursing's social policy statement* (2nd ed.). Washington, DC: Author.

15. American Nurses Association. (2004). *Nursing: Scope & standards of practice.* Washington, DC: Author.

16. American Association of Neuroscience Nurses (AANN) and American Nurses Association (ANA). (2002). *Scope and standards of neuroscience nursing practice.* Washington, DC: ANA.

17. Personal communication from Louise Miller, Executive Director of AANN, October 6, 2005.

18. Aiken, L. H., & Patrician, P. A. (2000). Measuring organization traits of hospitals: The revised nursing work index. *Nursing Research, 49*(3), 146–153.

19. Aiken, L. H., Clarke, S. P., Sloane, D. M., Sochalski, J., & Silber, J. H. (2002). Hospital nurse staffing and patient mortality, nurse burnout, and job dissatisfaction. *JAMA, 288*(16), 1987–1993.

20. Aiken, L. H., Havens, D. S., & Sloane, D. M. (2000). The magnet nursing services recognition program. *American Journal of Nursing, 111*(3), 26–35.

21. Havens, D. S., & Aiken, L. H. (1999). Shaping systems to promote desired outcomes. The magnet hospital model. *Journal of Nursing Administration, 29*(2), 14–20.

22. Sackett, D. L., Straus, S. E., Richardson, W. S., Rosenberg, W., & Hayes, R. B. (2000). *Evidence-based medicine: How to practice and teach EBM.* London: Churchill Livingstone.

23. Benner, P. (1985). *From novice to expert: Excellence and power in clinical nursing practice.* Menlo Park, CA: Addison-Wesley.

24. Poe, S. S., Cvach, M. M., Gartrell, D. G., Radzik, B. R., & Joy, T. I. (2005). An evidence-based approach to fall risk assessment, prevention, and management: Lessons learned. *Journal of Nursing Care Quality, 20*(2), 107–116.

RESOURCES

Published Material

DiCenso, A., Guyatt, G., & Ciliska, D. (2005). *Evidence-based nursing: A guide to clinical practice.* St. Louis: Mosby.

Malloch, K., & Porter-O'Grady, T. (Eds.). (2006). *Introduction to evidence-based practice in nursing and health care.* Sudbury, MA: Jones and Bartlett.

Melnyk, B. M., & Fineout-Overholt, E. (2005). *Evidence-based practice in nursing and healthcare: A guide to best practice.* Philadelphia: Lippincott Williams & Wilkins.

Websites

The following are but a few of the excellent websites for evidence-based practice guidelines. The reader should note that professional specialty organizations such as the American Association of Neuroscience Nurses and the American Association of Critical-Care Nurses as well as medical professional specialty organizations should be consulted for the latest evidence-based practice guidelines. The National Guideline Clearinghouse listed below includes a comprehensive list of all sites, making it easy to begin with this entry site.

Agency for Healthcare Research and Quality: http://www.ahrq.gov
The mission of the AHRQ includes both "translating research findings into better patient care and providing policy makers and other health care leaders with information needed to make critical health care decisions." The AHRQ sponsors many evidence-based practice centers and has published many clinical practice guidelines on major health problems.

National Guideline Clearinghouse: http://www.guideline.gov
Produced by the AHRQ, this site is "a comprehensive database of evidence-based clinical practice guidelines and related documents" intended for an audience of nurses, physicians, and other health care providers.

Cochrane Collaboration: http://cochrane.org
The Cochrane Collaboration provides current and accurate information and systematic reviews about randomized control trials and other interventional studies on a number of health care problems and diseases. It is an international nonprofit and independent organization dedicated to making accurate information available around the world.

Evidence-Based Nursing: http://ebn.bmjjournals.com
Jointly published by the British Medical Journal Publishing Group and the Royal College of Nursing Publishing Company, this journal scans 140 medical, specialist, and nursing journals to identify clinically important research for nurses. The abstract is structured and appears with a short expert review of the article for clinical relevance.

Joanna Briggs Institute for Evidence-Based Nursing and Midwifery: http://www.joannabriggs.edu.au
Based in Australia, the Joanna Briggs Institute provides a collaborative approach to the evaluation of evidence derived from a diverse range of sources, including experience, expertise, and all forms of research. It encourages translation, transfer, and utilization of the best practices available to be integrated into clinical care.

NHS Centre for Evidence-Based Medicine: http://www.cebm.net
The NHS Centre was established in Oxford, England, as the first of several centers around that country with the aim to promote evidence-based health care and provide support and resources.

Sarah Cole Hirsh Institution for Best Nursing Practices Based on Evidence: http://fpb.cwru.edu/HirshInstitute
From the Frances Payne Bolton School on Nursing at Case Western Reserve University, the institute offers evidence reviews for best nursing practices based on research evidence.

Care Settings and Transitions in Care

Joanne V. Hickey

This chapter briefly discusses health care settings from the perspective of the continuum of care and illness as it applies to neuroscience nursing practice. The configuration of a health care system to support varying intensity of care is driven by the needs of society and by economic and other resources allocated to support the system. All of these factors plus population-specific needs have an impact on neuroscience nursing practice.

HEALTH CARE FINANCING

A complex system of financing health care continues to evolve. The pace of health spending continues to grow, accounting for 16% of the gross domestic product. In the United States about 47 million Americans have no health insurance, and those with health insurance have a wide range of benefits from minimal to comprehensive and full-service coverage. Health insurance organizations, the "third party payers," have become the universal vehicles through which health care providers are paid. Health insurers have become powerful controllers and interpreters of services and reimbursement provided under the provisions of a contract. Control of services is intended to restrain cost and maintain quality of care. However, differences in opinion about application of cost-effective policies have created a discontinuity among the receivers, providers, and payers of health services.

Over the years, a trend of rising copayments by recipients of care is evident, and services previously covered in full now require a deductible resulting in more out-of-pocket expense for recipients. Despite these cost-sharing measures, it is questionable whether the current financing system can be sustained, particularly as a greater proportion of the population ages and becomes eligible for Medicare health benefits. Those without health care insurance and with limited financial assets receive some health care through Medicaid, the government program for the poor. Others without health insurance who do not qualify for Medicaid receive limited and sporadic care, often through hospital emergency departments with the cost transferred to the health insurance system.

What the future holds is uncertain. Many predict the imminent collapse of the current health care system, suggesting that the fundamental financing of health care will change with more control in the hands of the consumer. Rather than a prescribed health insurer, consumers will have health accounts that they will control. But how will consumers know what they need, how to assess quality and value, and where to access accurate and reliable information? How will the current nonconsumers be included? Will a national health voucher system be the answer? How will this be financed? What is certain is that the current health care system is seriously flawed—but the resolution is equally uncertain.

Managed Care

The term *managed care* refers to systems and techniques used to control the use of health care services including a review of medical necessity, incentives to use certain providers, and case management.[1] Managed care includes a body of clinical, financial, and organizational activities designed to ensure the provision of appropriate health care services in a cost-efficient manner. Managed care is a broad term and encompasses many different types of organizations, payment mechanisms, review mechanisms, and collaborations. In general, managed care is any system of health payment or delivery arrangements where the plan attempts to control or coordinate use of health services by its enrolled members in order to contain health expenditures, improve quality, or both.

Managed care systems are oriented toward measurable outcomes, cost containment, quality indicators, and patient satisfaction. As managed health care systems have developed and matured, the processes employed to achieve goals have also developed and include:

- Analyzing structures, processes, and outcomes of health care using sophisticated data management and information technology to determine best practices
- Developing and communicating practice guidelines for cost-effective quality outcomes that are evidence based
- Building networks of providers and models of care to improve coordination and continuity of cost-effective care
- Integrating processes for continuous quality improvement programs
- Facilitating access to health promotion and preventive services and early diagnosis and treatment

Managed care integrates the financing and delivery of health care through contracts with selected health care providers and facilities that provide comprehensive health care services to enrolled members of a health care plan. The provider network is an important feature distinguishing a managed care from a fee-for-service plan. Other characteristics of managed care plans are lower hospital use (both for admissions and length of stay), greater use of less costly procedures and tests, and greater emphasis on disease prevention and screening. Central components of a managed care environment include projected length of stay designation, use of case managers and care maps, and the requirement for approval before care is provided. Projected length of stay is guided by diagnostic related groups (DRGs) and insurer experience. Managed care relies heavily on case managers assigned to each patient to provide continuity of care through timely, coordinated care.

Continuity of care is a concept that describes the ideal result of goal-directed, well-coordinated care throughout a person's illness and across health care settings through involvement of all people involved in a person's health care including the person receiving the care. It is an expeditious process of providing uninterrupted, cohesive, continuous, seamless care that is maintained throughout the transition points of illness, including the transition from institutional care to community-based care or to the home.[2] It is interdisciplinary teams of health professionals working with the patient and family who provide continuity of care. *Coordination of care* implies that there is an active and effective coordinator (often the case manager or nurse) working with a health care team who is dedicated to providing coordinated, timely, and effective care. The case manager sees the "big picture" and helps team members identify short-term and long-term patient needs and key transition points in care to move the patient along the continuum of care through *appropriate and timely* use of resources and services. The coordinator must be able to communicate information to the appropriate stakeholders (e.g., patient, family, care providers) regarding specific needs with rationales and the expected measurable outcomes to be achieved. The person responsible and accountable for coordination must also be effective in follow-up to monitor the progression of activities and be able to identify when course modification or implementation of an alternative plan is necessary to achieve optimal outcomes.

Health care markets vary greatly across the United States, and many factors influence market penetration and maturity. As managed care markets mature, many smaller managed care organizations are being absorbed by a few large mega structure conglomerates, creating powerful integrated systems.

THE FOCUS OF HEALTH CARE

Much attention in health care has been on defining and ensuring quality. The Institute of Medicine (IOM) defines quality as "the degree to which health services for individuals and population increase the likelihood of desired health outcomes and are consistent with current professional knowledge."[3] Although this definition was first published in 1990, it is still the definition that is considered comprehensive and current. In the frequently cited 2001 report entitled *Crossing the Quality Chasm: A New Health System for the 21st Century*, the IOM set forth an expanded agenda for American health care quality by identifying six aims for improvement: safety, effectiveness, patient-centeredness, timeliness, efficiency, and equity.[4] All levels of health care are held to this standard.

In this section, health care is discussed from the perspectives of the focus of care. The three areas addressed include primary care, acute-critical care, and chronic care. Neurological patients may need different care settings with one injury or disease. Many patients move from one health care setting to another over the course of an illness.

Primary Care

The IOM defines primary care as follows: "the provision of integrated, accessible health care services by clinicians who are accountable for addressing a large majority of personal health care needs, developing a sustained partnership with patients, and practicing in the context of family and community."[4] This definition, although first published in 1996, continues to be the most respected definition. According to the IOM report, primary care is *comprehensive care*, that is, care of any and all health problems at a given stage of a person's life. It includes ongoing care of patients in various care settings, such as hospitals, nursing homes, clinicians' offices, community sites, schools, and homes.[5] The basic assumption is that primary care is the logical foundation of an effective health care system because primary care can address most health problems of the population. The diagnosis and treatment of some neurological problems will be managed exclusively by primary care physicians or collaboratively with neurologists and neurosurgeons who act as consultants. This positions the primary care physician as the gatekeeper for care, including referrals for specialty neurological care. Within the context of primary care, disease prevention, health promotion, and health maintenance are fundamental components.

Keeping people healthy through health promotion and disease prevention sets the course for a proactive health care system that provides for general and age-specific risk assessment, education of people about healthy lifestyles, and interventions designed to treat and control health problems. Risk assessment is the basis for tailoring an individualized plan of care. The new developing genomic age is adding new dimensions to risk assessment and interventions prior to the development of clinical signs and symptoms.[6] Genomics is also presenting new ethical issues about patient confidentiality and informed decision making.

When prevention is considered, three levels of prevention are generally recognized[7]:

- *Primary prevention:* any intervention that prevents a pathologic process from occurring. Examples include immunization or identification and control of risk factors, such as smoking, with the ultimate goal of preventing vascular disease such as stroke.
- *Secondary prevention:* interventions after a pathologic process has begun, but before symptoms occur. For example, a prescription for a statin drug ordered for a

patient with an elevated cholesterol level is designed to prevent coronary artery disease and stroke.

- *Tertiary prevention:* prevention of progressive disability or other complications in individuals with established disease. For example, community management of patients with Parkinson's disease or multiple sclerosis includes prevention of complications such as injury due to falls and decreased levels of mobility.

Health promotion and *health maintenance* are related terms that refer to the advocacy and provision of programs and strategies that have been demonstrated through research and practice to be beneficial in maintaining optimal health and preventing disease and disability. For instance, a low-fat diet, exercise, and sensible personal habits are essential for all people to live healthy and productive lives. Health promotion is every health professional's responsibility regardless of practice setting.

Primary care physicians are the gatekeepers for coordinating care and referring patients to other specialists. As primary care physicians become more involved in managing care of neurological patients, there will be an increased emphasis on maintaining and promoting health. This will be beneficial in preventing exacerbation of neurological conditions due to problems in other body systems and in preventing effects on other systems due to poorly managed neurological conditions. Primary care physicians and neuroscience health professionals are forging new collaborative partnerships. At the same time, neurological specialists will continue to assume oversight in coordinating and managing the care of patients with complex neurological problems, those requiring acute care management or hospitalization, and those needing long-term management of chronic illness. The neurological specialist assuming this role may be a physician, an advanced practice nurse, or a collaboration of both.

The efficient and economical movement of patients along the continuum of care remains focused on outcomes. The criteria for deciding when patients should be moved from one level of care to another will change based on new research findings related to knowledge of key indicators and transition points of diseases and illnesses. Transitions in care settings are occurring more rapidly, necessitating quick and efficient responses in health care services to provide transitional care and control costly delays in services.

Acute-Critical Care

One can view illness as a continuum of severity anchored by two distinct systems, acute-critical care at one end and chronic care at the other end. The purposes and underpinnings of the two systems are in sharp contrast to each other. *Acute-critical illness* is characterized by an abrupt onset of a disease process with the potential for single-system or multisystem complications. Treatment often takes days or weeks, and significant changes in condition can occur within hours or days. Patients require acute-critical care because they are physiologically unstable, are technologically dependent, are at high risk for complications, and/or require close monitoring. The vulnerability for complications is compounded by comorbidity and advancing age particularly in the elderly,

who are often living with multiple chronic health problems that increase the complexity of illness and need for care. In serious acute illness, care is usually provided within hospital settings where a wide variety of acute care services and cutting-edge treatment options are offered by multidisciplinary specialists working together in sophisticated high-tech environments to achieve a *cure* or the best outcomes for critically ill patients. In this physician-dominated model, the attending physician assumes the primary role of decision maker and directs the overall plan of care. Patients and families are included in decision making to the degree that it is possible, but the physician primarily maintains control over care. Acute care, and particularly critical care, is the most expensive care provided, and access is uneven depending on geographic location and health insurance of the recipient.

Chronic Care

Chronic illness is an irreversible condition characterized by an accumulation or latency of disease states or impairments that have an impact on a person's functional abilities and quality of life. Persons with chronic illness need supportive care and self-care management strategies to maintain function and prevent further disability.[7] Chronic illness tends to involve multiple, long-term diseases that span many years or a lifetime and follow an uncertain course. A major focus of management is stabilization of the disease, and may include palliation. Because *cure is usually not possible*, the goal of care is *adaptation,* that is, to learn to live with the illness in the least intrusive way and to maintain the highest functional level and quality of life for as long as possible. Care is provided mainly in a low-tech, community-based, primary care model with consultation from specialists as needed. The patient is the primary decision maker and coordinator of care, thus maintaining a high level of control. Emphasis in chronic illness management is on empowering the patient with knowledge through education and counseling to optimize self-management, adaptation, and symptom management.

How illness is viewed shapes care. A key transition point in illness comes when a patient moves from an acute care model to a chronic illness model, thus redefining the illness and needed care. The Corbin and Strauss[8] *chronic illness trajectory model* provides a comprehensive framework for understanding chronic illness and the roles of health care providers, the patient, and the family in management. This model is particularly helpful for elucidating the nurse's role in symptom management, rehabilitation, education, support, and advocacy for the patient–family dyad. The trajectory model is based on the fundamental idea that chronic illnesses have a course or trajectory that changes over time. The course can be optimally shaped and managed by an effective and collaborative partnership of the patient, family, and health care providers to support optimal outcomes. Although shaping may not change the direction of the illness, the course of the illness can be stabilized, and symptoms may be controlled and managed. The shaping process is complicated by the use of technology, which has a potential impact on the patient's personal identity, well-being, and activities of daily living.

The success of the United States' health care system in developing effective acute and critical care models has resulted in many people surviving acute episodes they might otherwise not have survived. These people survive with chronic health problems that must be managed for the remainder of their lives. The quality of their management directly influences their quality of life and that of their families. Both the acute-critical care and the chronic illness models are essential to meet the needs of modern society. The challenge remains to develop models that support seamless, cost-effective quality care as the patient moves from one level of care to another. Neurological patients require both acute-critical care and chronic illness care. For those persons who survive major neurological trauma, they survive with long-term chronic health problems that must be addressed. For others with neurological degenerative conditions, chronic illness management is the focus of care with acute care needs being required for periodic exacerbations that are quickly stabilized.

Institutional-Based Care Versus Community-Based Care

Health care is provided as either institutional-based care or community-based care. *Institutional-based care* is available at hospitals, nursing homes, and other facilities where patients stay until discharge to another type of institution, to a variety of community-based care options, or to their own homes. Within hospitals, specialty focused units have developed, such as chronically/critically ill units, ventilator-dependent units, stroke units, and collaborative care units. These units are designed to meet the needs of special patient populations efficiently and cost effectively.

Community-based care, available usually in the community where the patient resides, is provided in the home or at a site where the patient goes for care in his or her community as an outpatient and then returns home. Community-based care is generally less expensive than institutional care and is often preferred by and more convenient for the patient and family. The cost savings are particularly attractive to third-party payers. More and more high-tech care, traditionally provided only in institutions, is becoming available in the community. Home health care services, in particular, often provide infusion therapy, ventilation support therapy, rehabilitation, and other services traditionally associated with institutional care. The phenomenal growth of services in the community has led to corresponding complex organizational structures to support community-based care.

Although patients with neurological conditions have always been managed in the community, their number is greatly increasing and the interventions involved in their care are much more complex. Successful community-based management of a neuroscience patient with complex needs requires appropriate support and careful monitoring. An example is day-care programs that offer cognitive retraining programs for cognitively impaired adults, thus improving the client's quality of life and functional level. Another example is a weekly exercise program for persons with Parkinson's disease to improve muscle strength, balance, and disease management. High-tech care for neurological problems, such as ventilation support, is becoming increasingly available in the home but requires high-level support by appropriately skilled health professionals for it to be successful.

THE CONTINUUM OF HEALTH CARE SERVICES

A continuum is a coherent whole characterized by a progression of elements varying by degrees, and one that is anchored on each end by significantly different or opposite elements. This is true of the health care continuum anchored at one end by high-tech critical care and at the other end by a "no-tech" self-care focus. Between these two poles is an array of levels of care offered in traditional and nontraditional settings. Some are recent entrants; others are familiar terms that have been redefined, such as long-term care. New options, particularly in the subacute arena, are emerging, often in response to cost-containment mandates and unmet patient needs. The definition, focus, and intended recipients of the array of care options are indeed confusing, inexact, and changing. The assistance of the case manager or social worker is invaluable in helping to determine the best level of facility based on the patient's needs and resources.

Levels of Care

Definitions and interpretations relating to acute care, subacute care, long-term care, and supportive care are changing. Health care facilities are highly regulated by governmental agencies and accreditation bodies such as the Joint Commission. These regulatory mechanisms define services provided and reimbursement considerations. The regulations are complex and often change, creating confusion to both patients and providers. To make informed decisions about services offered and insurance coverage provided, each particular agency's policies must be investigated closely. See Table 2-1 for broad descriptions of major categories of care and examples of how they apply to neurological patients.

This section briefly addresses acute care, subacute care, long-term care, and other health care services. A number of texts provide comprehensive information about levels of care. The reader is directed to these resources for further discussion.

Acute Care Facilities

Acute care hospitals provide a wide range of acute care services for serious episodic illness and major surgical interventions from critical care to general care units. Acute care hospitals provide specialized personnel who use complex and sophisticated technical equipment to provide a wide range of acute care services and specialty care. Unlike chronic care, acute care is often necessary for only a short time.

A case can be made to include acute inpatient rehabilitation facilities in the category of acute care or subacute care. It has been placed in the acute care category based on author bias. *Acute inpatient rehabilitation facilities* provide comprehensive intensive rehabilitation programs designed to achieve a high level of independence and functional recovery. Admissions to acute inpatient rehabilitation facilities are

TABLE 2–1   MAJOR CATEGORIES OF CARE AND EXAMPLES OF CARE PROVIDED FOR PATIENTS WITH NEUROLOGICAL PROBLEMS

TYPE OF CARE	EXAMPLES OF CARE PROVIDED FOR PATIENTS WITH NEUROLOGICAL PROBLEMS
Acute-critical care is directed at acute episodic illness that requires a high-technology environment with a focus on physiologic stabilization and close monitoring to prevent complications. • The broad realm of acute care services is available along the acute care continuum for diagnostics and treatment of health problems delivered by highly trained professionals. • The acute care hospital may provide comprehensive services for a variety of health problems or may focus on specific conditions such as comprehensive cancer care. • Major acute care facilities are often affiliated with medical schools and research institutes.	• Specialized neuroscience intensive care units for life-threatening neurological conditions such as traumatic brain or spinal cord injuries, subarachnoid hemorrhage, hemorrhagic stroke, meningitis, encephalitis, and Guillain-Barré syndrome. • Continuation of acute care services on neurological step-down units such as stroke units or general neurological or neurosurgical units for patients who are relatively physiologically stable, but still need a significant amount of specialized care and evaluation.
Subacute care is a broad category of care services directed at assisting patients with recovery from illness through a broad spectrum of supportive and rehabilitation services. • Patients are generally physiologically stable or chronically ill (such as ventilator dependent). Many patients have multiple chronic conditions that need to be re-evaluated because of other conditions that may have caused well-controlled patients to have multisystem exacerbations of disease processes. • The subacute care category is viewed as transitional care in that the realm of services is directed at helping the patient achieve a higher level of function that will allow him or her to be independent or transition into a less intense level of care. • Supporting recovery through comprehensive rehabilitation is a major focus; this includes a strong commitment to patient education for disease management and self-care activities.	• This is a broad category of care services. • It includes skilled nursing care facilities (SNF) for patients who are not candidates for a comprehensive rehabilitation program but who need a significant amount of nursing care; these patients may be candidates for a comprehensive rehabilitation program in the future as their level of consciousness or other limiting factors improve. • Comprehensive in-patient rehabilitation programs are offered in a number of facilities with the goal of improving activities of daily living (ADLs), instrumental ADLs, and other functions related to achieve optimal independence. Patients with cerebrovascular conditions such as stroke, traumatic neurological injuries, and neurodegenerative conditions who have rehabilitation potential are appropriate candidates. The length of the program may vary from a few weeks to months. • Neurological patients may receive short-term care in other care settings to address physical, behavioral, or cognitive neurological deficits.
Long-term care (LTC) is a level of care in which persons who are dependent for ADLs and chronic illness management receive care. • As LTC facilities have evolved, some have focused on providing special services such as weaning ventilator-dependent patients from the ventilator. These LTC facilities are sometimes referred to as long-term acute care (LTAC) facilities. Once a patient is successfully weaned from the ventilator, there are more options available to the patient for rehabilitation. • Often patients in LTC facilities are frail elderly with multiple chronic health problems or younger patients with severe deficits resulting from catastrophic illness or injury who are unable to care for themselves. • Care is provided in a variety of clinical settings. • The goal of LTC facilities is supportive care to promote or maintain as much independence and quality of life as possible. • There is usually no single defining health condition for LTC admission; the key characteristics of the patient population in LTC facilities are chronicity and complete dependency for all aspects of care and survival.	• LTC facilities include a variety of health care services for patients with severe chronic neurological conditions that include major physical, behavioral, or cognitive deficits that preclude independence in living and self-care. • Patients with altered levels of consciousness who need complete physical care from stroke, traumatic neurological injuries, Parkinson's disease, and other neurodegenerative conditions are the recipients of LTC.
Other supportive care includes a variety of home health services designed to meet special needs of patients who have deficits in ADLs, managing chronic conditions, or other needs. • These services may be provided by persons without high-level professional skills or training for some aspects of needs. • Other services will require professional staff to provide care such as registered nurses, physical therapists, and others.	• There are a variety of special services available to persons with neurological conditions who have deficits in self-care or management of the health problems that are designed to avoid a more expensive level of care. • Examples of services provided include assistance with ADLs, medication administration, and management of feeding tubes. • Home health services are often critical in allowing a patient to return to his or her home environment because of support services available.

usually short term, often dictated by established criteria of the insurer. Inpatient rehabilitation facilities are limited. To optimize use of these scarce resources, patients are carefully screened for admission. Admission criteria to individual facilities generally includes the following[8]:

• Selected diagnoses (e.g., stroke, head trauma, spinal cord trauma, neurological disorders).
• The primary problem must include a recent functional loss (e.g., cognitive, mobility, bowel/bladder, communication dysfunctions) in a person previously independent.

- A physician must document the expected significant functional improvement to be achieved within a reasonable time frame.

Candidates must also meet other screening criteria that include being medically stable; possessing the mental ability to follow one- or two-step commands; and being able to withstand at least 3 hours of therapies, daily, five times per week. Therapy can consist of any combination of physical therapy (PT), occupational therapy (OT), speech therapy (ST), and cognitive therapy. Progress toward achieving stated goals is monitored closely. The patient may be discharged from the rehabilitation program for several reasons, including[9]:

- Achievement of stated goals
- Lack of progress toward stated goals after a reasonable trial period
- Onset of a severe complication necessitating transfer to an acute care setting
- Onset of a complication that requires discontinuation of the comprehensive rehabilitation program for more than 1 week

Transitional hospitals are acute care hospitals designed for medically stable patients with long-term care and rehabilitative needs that are too complex for skilled nursing facilities (SNF). They differ from traditional acute care hospitals in that they have fewer specialists and provide only basic diagnostic and surgical equipment. Major surgical interventions are not offered, although minor procedures such as tracheotomies and feeding tube placements are usually available. The nurse–patient staffing ratio is less than typically found in other acute care hospitals. Transitional hospitals admit medically stable patients with complex medication and treatment needs. Examples of patients admitted include ventilator-dependent patients, including those requiring weaning; patients needing extensive wound care; patients recovering from coma; and patients requiring cognitive or neurobehavioral rehabilitation.

Subacute Care Facilities

The classification of subacute care is the most confusing category of all health care facility categories with many subcategories of subacute care facilities evident. The National Association of Subacute/Post Acute Care offers the following definition[10]:

Subacute care is a comprehensive, cost-effective in-patient level of care for patients who:

- Have had an acute event resulting from injury, illness, or exacerbation of a disease process
- Have a determined course of treatment
- Though stable, require diagnostics or invasive procedures, but not intensive procedures requiring an acute level of care

The severity of the patient's condition requires:

- Active physician direction with frequent on-site visits
- Professional nursing care

- Significant ancillary services
- An outcomes-focused interdisciplinary approach utilizing a professional team
- Complex medical and/or rehabilitative care

Typically, short-term subacute care is designed to return patients to the community or transition them to a lower level of care.

The National Association of Subacute/Post Acute Care further defines *postacute care* as follows: postacute care (PAC) is designed to improve the transition from hospital to the community. PAC facilities provide services to patients needing additional support to assist them to recuperate following discharge from an acute hospital. The services include home nursing, personal care, childcare, allied health services, and home health care. PAC services also include (1) emergency department patients to prevent the need for admission to an acute care hospital, and (2) patients discharged from subacute services.[10] The objectives of PAC are:

- To provide additional postacute care services for individuals who require them
- To improve care planning for patients discharged from hospital
- To improve the links between hospitals and other health and community-care providers

Skilled nursing facilities (SNFs) include both free-standing and hospital-based units providing skilled nursing care. Most include rehabilitative services in addition to restorative nursing care. Patients may require maximum assistance with activities of daily living (ADLs) or bowel and bladder incontinence. Some SNFs admit patients with altered levels of consciousness from confusion/dementia to coma. There are eligibility criteria for admission and health insurance coverage. To be approved for payment, there must be a clear need for skilled licensed professional care on a daily basis. Examples of care provided include:

- Daily medication administration of parenteral medications or intravenous fluids
- Daily wound care requiring aseptic technique
- Enteral tube feeding and tube care including initial teaching and care
- Tracheostomy care including initial teaching and care
- Frequent monitoring and assessment by licensed personnel to prevent deterioration or complications
- Treatment of decubitus ulcers (i.e., grade 3 or lower) and severe skin conditions
- Early postoperative care and teaching of stomal care, Hickman catheters, and other tubes
- Physical therapy, occupational therapy, or speech therapy

Long-Term Care Facilities

Long-term care (LTC) facilities provide care for patients with functional deficits and health care needs serious enough that they are unable to care for themselves and have no one who is able to provide needed care. As the term implies, patients are placed in LTCs such as nursing homes for complete care that will probably be necessary for long periods of time or for the remainder of the person's life. The focus of care is to provide a broad spectrum of supportive care based on the needs of the patient. LTC facilities often have a special focus. For example, an LTC facility may focus on weaning ventilator-dependent patients who have been difficult to wean. Such a long-term *acute* care (LTAC) facility serves as a transition for a traumatic brain-injured patient who may spend the first 25 days at a facility to be weaned. The criteria for admission and the specific time limits before discharge are beyond the scope of this chapter. The case manager is the best resource to interpret the parameters of services for the patient.

Other Health Care Services

A number of special support services may be available to allow the patient to return home. Infusion therapy, supplemental oxygen therapy, and assistance with basic care are a few examples of services that may be offered.

Home health care agencies provide both skilled and unskilled services to patients in their homes. Services may include the use of technology (e.g., ventilator), therapy (PT, OT, oxygen), and skilled nursing care. A person who has lived independently before an acute episode of illness often prefers to return home, if possible. With the support of family and friends and with a few added services, this is often possible. A comprehensive medical and social assessment is needed to determine the feasibility of home care, stressing the adequacy of patient safety and support in the home. A very important component of this determination is an evaluation of the primary caregiver to be sure that he or she can safely care for the person at home.

Summary

Categories of care have been briefly reviewed through a discussion of the major components of the continuum for acute to chronic health care needs under broad headings. Demographers project large numbers of older people, many with chronic health problems, who will soon be requiring health care. The health care delivery system will continue to be challenged to provide options to meet the needs for cost-effective care while recognizing the concurrent and comparably important requirement for choice, maximal independence, and optimal quality of life.

TRANSITIONS IN CARE AND DISCHARGE PLANNING

A *transition* is a passage from one state, stage, or place to another; that is, it is a change. Passage suggests movement from one place to another, and the movement is along some path or trajectory. In health care, discharge planning and safe transfer to alternative levels of care are necessary to meet patient-centered health care needs. For many neurological patients, recovery from an acute episode does not mean return to pre-illness or preinjury states of health. Many neurological patients have unstable, complex needs that must be addressed to support optimal health through chronic illness

care. This may require a transition in level of care and the environment of care.

Whenever transition occurs, the goal is a smooth movement with bridges in place to facilitate the process and continuity of care. Smooth transition is made easier through coordination of care that anticipates potential problems, removes obstacles, addresses unmet needs, and prevents fragmentation. Coordinated care that prevents fragmentation is called *continuity of care*. Although a transition may represent some recovery, it often involves a move into an unknown environment and culture and can be unsettling to the patient and family. Transitions in care can occur among various facilities and levels of care. All require a coordinated approach to promote continuity.

Depending on the services available in a facility, a neuroscience patient may move from a high-acuity unit, such as an intensive care unit (ICU), to a lesser-acuity intermediate unit. The patient and family must be prepared for the transition through education, anticipatory guidance, and counseling. This includes a brief description of the new unit, the patient population, services available, visiting hours, care providers, and the ratio of nurses to patients. The ratio of nurses to patients in intermediate units is much lower than the 1:1 or 1:2 ratio common in ICUs, and patients and families need to be prepared for the decreased nursing intensity. Reassurance is needed that the transfer is a positive sign of recovery and that needed care will continue to be met by health professionals. A visit to the new unit to meet with a staff representative can alleviate anxiety.

If the patient is going to a special unit, such as one dedicated to rehabilitation or transitional care, the nurse should discuss the new unit's philosophy focus of care with the patient and family. In particular, the expected level of patient and family involvement should be addressed. For example, in a comprehensive rehabilitation program, the focus is on functional recovery and self-care to promote independence. Family members should be prepared to assist the patient with care after discharge. These skills must be taught and practiced in a supportive environment. Continuity of care for a transition within a facility or system is usually easier to coordinate because the system is the same, and there are usually procedures in place for transferring a patient. Transitions to other "outside" care environments can be more complex and require more coordination.

PLANNING FOR TRANSITIONS IN HEALTH CARE SETTINGS

Discharge planning is the vehicle through which the patient's unmet health care needs are met within the continuum of health care services. It is an activity required by health insurers, regulators, and accreditors of health care facilities.

Discharge planning is a logical, coordinated, multilevel process of decision making and other activities involving the patient, the family or significant other, and a team of multidisciplinary health professionals working together to facilitate a smooth, coordinated transition from one environment to another. The transitional environment may be an acute care facility, a chronic care or rehabilitation hospital, a nursing home, or the patient's home. The purpose of discharge planning is to assist the patient to make a smooth transition from one environment or level of care to another without sacrificing the progress that has already been achieved and to provide for other health care needs that are still unmet. Numerous studies have shown that hospitals and patients benefit from a smooth transition out of the hospital. Benefits cited include improved patient outcomes, increased patient and family satisfaction, decreased length of stay, decreased hospital readmission, enhanced cost effectiveness, decreased complications, and decreased mortality. There are many models of discharge planning. In most, the case managers assume major responsibility for facilitating the process.

DISCHARGE PLANNING FOR NEUROSCIENCE PATIENTS

The discharge planning process for neurologically impaired patients increases in complexity if cognitive or behavioral disabilities are present. Patient-centered discharge planning may involve patients with:

- Multitrauma (injury not only to the nervous system, but also to other body systems)
- Cerebral trauma or spinal cord injuries
- Neurological degenerative diseases (e.g., multiple sclerosis, amyotrophic lateral sclerosis, Parkinson's disease)
- Neurological deficits from infectious processes such as meningitis or encephalitis
- Nervous system neoplasms; and others

The specific needs of each patient must be comprehensively assessed and the discharge planning process individualized to provide the appropriate level of care for optimal outcomes. Although discharge planning may be organized differently for neurological patients than for patients with other problems, the steps in discharge planning are the same (Fig. 2-1). The steps, as with any process, are not compartmentalized; that is, simultaneous activities occur in multiple areas of the process. The case manager model assists in coordinating the discharge planning process, especially with the urgency to commence planning early caused by shorter hospital stays, which accelerates all patient-oriented activities. Discharge planning must begin upon admission to an acute care facility, and every health care provider involved in the care of the patient needs to participate. However, it is often the nurse who "pushes the envelope" to coordinate input and facilitate the process. A partnership between the nurse and the case manager is important to expedite the discharge planning. The patient often has several case managers representing different interests and who must interact to coordinate and support patient care choices and decisions. They include the hospital case manager, the payer (insurance company) case manager, and the community case manager who may work for a home care agency, a physician group, or a social service organization.

Assessment

Given that neuroscience patients are often cared for by a multidisciplinary team, they undergo various individual specialty-specific assessments. From the admission history and ongoing assessments collected by the nursing staff, data are available to begin predicting special needs, rehabilitative potential, and expected patient outcomes. When the patient is medically stable, deficits and needs can be validated, and the complete database for discharge planning refined.

Nurses often overlook the importance of resources and funding for patients past the acute care settings. Certain socioeconomic and health issues render some patients difficult to place in other levels of care and facilities. These

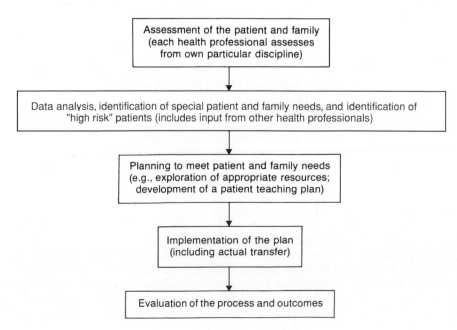

Figure 2-1 • Schematic representation of the steps involved in the discharge planning process.

patients include the uninsured, the homeless, drug abusers, patients with acquired immune deficiency syndrome (AIDS), and those with dysfunctional families or without families. For example, a patient admitted with a severe traumatic cerebral injury may also have a concurrent cocaine abuse problem. Planning must include provisions for special needs, such as drug abuse rehabilitation, as well as for the primary problem and deficits associated with the brain injury. Early identification of high-risk patients and those difficult to place is important so that the multiple issues related to their care can be addressed early and the case manager can be made aware of the complexity of the placement. Resolution of these problems often takes time and the efforts of the case manager. Before transfer, it may be necessary to submit an application for a Medicare or Medicaid number or undertake some other complicated process for health care coverage. These activities can take time and delay transfer.

Data Analysis and Planning

Health care professionals from each discipline analyze the database and provide their own specific input to consider the care provided by their discipline. This information is then brought to a multidisciplinary planning conference, and a problem list is generated. A plan of care is then developed based on the problem list that includes expected outcomes. The interdisciplinary care conferences are a common component of care units. Meetings usually occur on a scheduled basis from daily in the critical care setting to once or twice a week in less acute settings. It is an expeditious way to address the needs of patients and plan for moving the patient along the continuum to discharge. It is an excellent resource for outcome management.

Based on identification of short-term and long-term outcomes, planning, like the other steps in the discharge process, is ongoing and collaborative. Short-term outcomes are the steps that lead to achievement of long-term outcomes. Flexibility is the key to accommodating those changes likely to occur in the patient's condition. It is usually not possible to accurately predict the degree of recovery that can occur when the nervous system is injured. At times, the amount of improvement is a pleasant surprise. With other patients, hopes for improvement are not realized. Health care team members need to be prepared to alter the discharge plan based on changes in the patient's condition and a realistic appraisal of potential outcomes.

Collaborative interdisciplinary conferences with team members and with the patient and family are absolutely necessary for effective discharge planning. The plan should be documented in writing and updated as necessary. Remember to allow adequate time to complete all pretransfer activities, including patient and family teaching.

Implementation

Implementation of the discharge plan requires collaboration among many individuals working together to achieve mutual goals. Initially, the case manager, usually a nurse or social worker, contacts a potential transfer facility. Because space in subacute, rehabilitation, and long-term care facilities is limited, often a clinician from the transfer facility will visit the patient to evaluate whether the facility and its programs are suitable for the patient. The clinician assessing the patient must decide whether the patient is:

- An appropriate candidate for the facility or program and is ready for transfer
- An appropriate candidate but not ready for transfer requiring a re-evaluation to be scheduled in a few weeks
- An inappropriate candidate for transfer to the facility

After acceptance for transfer, it is helpful for the patient (alone or accompanied by a family member) or the family member, if the patient is not able to participate, to visit the facility to see the physical environment and to talk with staff members before transfer plans are formalized. After the transfer is formalized, patient information is shared with the receiving nursing staff and other health care providers to promote *seamless continuity of care*. This may be accomplished through a face-to-face meeting, telecommunications, or written referral forms. A physician from the transferring facility must communicate with the accepting physician to provide the necessary medical management information. For the homebound patient, timely arrangements, well in advance of discharge, should be made for provision of any necessary equipment or community agencies that will be providing services.

The patient and family need emotional and psychological preparation for the transfer. Transfer can be frightening to the patient who has been hospitalized for an extended period. Therefore, much reassurance is needed as the day approaches. Support groups in the community may be helpful to the patient or family. For example, the National Brain Injury Foundation has chapters throughout the country. Information about the purposes of such an organization and contact information should be provided to the patient and family. Printed materials and small group conferences with other patients and families may also be helpful. A discharge handbook or other form of printed material is especially useful because the patient or family member can read it at leisure and then ask questions as necessary.

As caregivers, health care professionals often experience mixed emotions about the discharge of a patient for whom they have cared. Many patients with neurological dysfunction are hospitalized for extended periods of time, with the result that strong bonds are forged between patients and caregivers. Health care professionals should recognize and deal with their own feelings of loss.

Evaluation

Evaluation is a critical component in any process. Health care providers should also evaluate the discharge planning process to identify any areas that need to be changed or improved for the future. This can be done during team conferences or through periodic reviews. Other foci of evaluation are patient and family satisfaction and benefit from treatment. Information about these topics can be collected at discharge or in a follow-up contact. The quality of the discharge planning system should be monitored through a hospital-wide CQI program. For an individual patient, the health team needs to know if the plan was effective.

Summary of Discharge Planning

In summary, discharge planning is a complex process of comprehensive assessment, problem solving, ongoing independent and collaborative professional activities, and effective communications directed at helping the patient make a smooth transition from one environment to another without loss of progress toward improved health already made. The new environment may be the home or an acute or subacute level of care that will continue to address unmet health care needs. Throughout the discharge planning process, health professionals work with the patient and family to achieve mutually accepted specific goals. Without comprehensive planning, there will be confusion, frustration, discouragement, and fragmentation of effort that will impede achievement of optimal rehabilitation outcomes for the patient.

REFERENCES

1. Glossary of terms in managed health care. Retrieved January 16, 2006, from http://pohly.com/terms_m.html
2. Continuity of care. The Merck manual of health and aging. Retrieved January 16, 2006, from http://www.merck.com/pubs/mmanual_ha/sec2/ch09/ch09a.html
3. Lohr, K. N. (Ed.). (1990). *Medicare: A strategy for quality assurance.* Washington, DC: National Academy Press.
4. Committee on Quality of Health Care in America, Institute of Medicine. (2001). *Crossing the quality chasm: A new health system for the 21st century.* Washington, DC: National Academy Press.
5. Donaldson, M., Yordy, K., Lohr, K. N., & Neal Vanselow, A. (Eds.). (1996). *Primary care: America's health in a new era.* Washington, DC: National Academy Press.
6. Guttmacher, A. E., & Collins, F. S. (2003). Welcome to the genomic era. *New England Journal of Medicine, 349*(10), 996–998.
7. U. S. Preventive Services Task Force. (2002). *Guide to clinical preventive services: Report of the U. S. Preventive Services Task Force* (3rd ed.). McLean, VA: International Medical Publishers.
8. Corbin, J., & Strauss, A. (1988). *Unending word and care: Managing chronic illness at home.* San Francisco: Jossey-Bass.
9. Powell, S. K. (2000). *Case management: A practical guide to success in managed care* (2nd ed.). Philadelphia: Lippincott Williams & Wilkins.
10. National Association of Subacute/Post Acute Care. Definition of subacute and post acute care. Retrieved January 14, 2006, from http://www.naspac.net/faq.asp

RESOURCES

Published Material

Betancourt, J. R., Green, A. R., Carrillo, J. E., & Park, E. R. (2005). Cultural competencies and health care disparities: Key perspectives and trends. *Health Affairs, 24*(2), 499–505.

Carr, D. D. (2005). The case manager's role in optimizing acute rehabilitation services. *Lippincott Case Management, 10*(4), 190–200.

Fuchs, V., & Emanuel, E. J. (2005). Health care reform: Why? What? When? *Health Affairs, 24*(6), 1399–1414.

Halm, M. A., Gagner, S., Goering, M., Sabo, J., Smith, M., & Zaccagnini, M. (2003). Interdisciplinary rounds: Impact on patients, families, and staff. *Clinical Nurse Specialist, 17*(3), 133–144.

Huber, D. (2005). *Disease management: A guide for case managers.* St. Louis, MO: Elsevier Saunders.

Kitchen, A., & Brook, J. (2005). Social work at the heart of the medical team. *Social Work Health Care, 40*(4), 1–18.

Kongstvedt, P. (2004). *Managed care: What it is and how it works* (2nd ed.). Sudbury, MA: Jones and Bartlett Publishers.

Lubkin, I. M., & Larsen, P. D. (2006). *Chronic illness. Impact and interventions* (6th ed.). Sudbury, MA: Jones and Bartlett Publishers.

Mullahy, C. M. (2004). *The case manager's handbook.* Sudbury, MA: Jones and Bartlett Publishers.

Naylor, M. D. (2002). Transitional care of older adults. *Annual Review of Nursing Research, 20,* 127–147.

Powell, S. K. (2000). *Advanced case management: Outcomes and beyond.* Philadelphia: Lippincott Williams & Wilkins.

San Antonio, P. M., & Rubinstein, R. L. (2004). Long-term care planning as a cultural system. *Journal of Aging Social Policy, 16*(2), 35–48.

Smith, C., Cowan, C., Sensenig, A., & Catlin, A. (2005). Health spending growth slows in 2003. *Health Affairs, 24*(1), 185–194.

Yamamoto, L., & Lucey, C. (2005). Case management "within the walls": A glimpse into the future. *Critical Care Nursing Quarterly, 28*(2), 162–178.

Ethical Perspectives and End-of-Life Care

Joanne V. Hickey and Kathryn Montgomery

The ethical dimensions of conduct in professional practice are especially compelling and complex in many situations faced by the neuroscience nurse. The primary focus of this chapter is clinical ethics and end-of-life care in neuroscience nursing practice. The Code of Ethics for Nurses with Interpretive Statements published by the American Association of Nurses provides a broad perspective of the standards of ethical conduct for nurses.[1] In addition, the International Council of Nurses (ICN) also provides the ICN Code of Ethics for Nurses.[2]

Clinical ethics is primarily concerned with the ethics of clinical practice and the ethical problems that arise in the care of patients. Judicial decisions that have influenced standards of practice are also included. The three main areas discussed in this chapter are (1) the basis for ethical and legal dimensions of practice, (2) a framework for ethical decision making, and (3) selected ethical issues common in neuroscience nursing practice, including end-of-life (EOL) care.

AN ETHICAL PERSPECTIVE OF NEUROSCIENCE PRACTICE

Unique ethical challenges are presented to neuroscience nurses by patients with neurological illnesses and impairments. These patients cross the lifespan, and frequently they experience damage to their personhood that compares with no other illness. Neuroscience nurses must be prepared to care for the young victim of trauma who is left with irreversible paralysis or in a persistent vegetative state, for the middle-aged adult who is newly diagnosed with a progressive neurological disease, and for the elderly person with dementia caused by multi-infarct small strokes. Recovery often does not mean a return to the pretrauma or pre-illness functional level. These patients may experience complete personality changes or, in other tragic cases, lose the ability to comprehend or communicate information. The ethical questions such as determining patient capacity in decision making or decisions about withholding or withdrawing treatments are similar in theory to other patients who are seriously ill. However, the *context* and *circumstances* surrounding neurologically compromised patients are unique. Before the advent of technology in medical practice, the failure of one or more body systems usually limited life well before cognitive capacity was affected. Now, technology is available to keep patients "alive" indefinitely. This includes

patients in a persistent vegetative state, in which the "organ of reason" is rendered permanently nonfunctional and the patient is unable to make informed-consent decisions.

Use of the term *ethical and legal* is avoided in this chapter to diminish confusion and to avoid the suggestion that ethics and legality are more synonymous than distinctly different. An **ethical perspective** addresses the *moral duties and obligations* to provide optimal care for patients and families. A **legal perspective** speaks to the *minimal standards of care set forth in the judicial system* to which health care providers must adhere. Simply relying on legal precedents does not necessarily imply that ethically grounded care is being provided. However, many issues, including decisions about withholding or withdrawing treatment or surrogate decision making, require addressing both the ethical dimensions and legal precedents for a comprehensive understanding of the complexity of clinical situations.

A generally recognized phenomenon in health care is the unprecedented development and rapid implementation of new technologies. The appropriate use of technology and its impact on human life are usually secondary, de facto considerations; the lag time between implementation of a new technology and recognition of its broader impact is often the foundation for the associated ethical dilemmas. In addition, sociocultural and economic factors including priorities for allocation of limited health care resources, consensus about self-determination, the cost-effective mandate, and the predominance of managed care environments impact on delivery of care.[3] The dynamics involved in this adjustment process are often addressed in the judicial system—the wrong institution to resolve ethical issues. As a result, there has been an uncomfortable uncertainty about the legalities surrounding many ethical issues, leaving the practitioner to sort them out at the bedside. The lack of clarity about how to proceed in ethical dilemmas and how to interpret personal wishes and laws has created further problems within the health care system.

ETHICS, MORALITY, AND LEGALITY

Ethics

Ethics, also called moral philosophy, involves systematizing, defending, and recommending concepts of right and wrong. Normative ethics, a subclass of ethics, addresses moral standards that regulate right and wrong conduct including the moral duty and obligation and the principles of conduct governing an individual or a group.[4] Ethics has also been defined as the inquiry into the nature of morality or moral acts and the search for the morally good life. Ethics dates back to the beginning of civilization, when mores and laws were developed to allow different groups of people to live together. Most ethical principles represent cultural and religious values of groups of people and, therefore, differ from culture to culture and from religion to religion. Even within cultures, some subcultures differ significantly in some aspects of their ethics and, therefore, in their standards of behavior.

When the concept of ethics is applied to professional practice, there are basic principles that govern how health care professionals practice within a culture. These principles are usually stated within a code, such as the *Code for Nurses*,[5] which explains to the public the guidelines that will govern how the professional nurse will practice.

Morality

Within the definition of ethics is the word *morality*. **Morality** addresses that which is regarded as right or wrong. The term encompasses three contexts: individual conscience; systems of principles and judgments, sometimes called moral values, shared within a cultural, religious, secular, professional, or philosophical community; and codes of behavior or conduct derived from these systems.[6] Morality also comprises the making of judgments about what is right in given circumstances and the guidance of one's conduct by reason.[7] It suggests doing what seems right while giving equal weight to the interests of each individual who will be affected by one's conduct. Six moral principles that are of particular importance in nursing practice are autonomy, beneficence, nonbeneficence, justice, fidelity, and dignity.[8]

- **Autonomy** is the act of self-governing, self-determining, or self-directing; it involves independence from the will of others, as well as the right to make and follow one's decisions. It is the right to refuse or choose their treatment (*Voluntas aegroti suprema lex*). The principle of autonomy affirms the nurse's duty to respect the decisions of the patient and the family and to assume the role of a patient/family advocate when necessary.
- **Beneficence** is the charge to do good. A practitioner should act in the best interest of the patient (*Salus aegroti suprema lex*).
- **Nonmaleficence** is the duty to prevent or avoid doing harm (*primum non nocere*).
- **Justice** is a concept involving the system of consequences that naturally derives from any action or choice.[9] It concerns the distribution of scarce health resources, and the decision of who gets what treatment. Justice includes fairness, correctness, and impartiality in the application of principles of rightness and of sound judgment. The nurse is obliged to treat patients fairly based on their needs and the situation. It suggests an obligation for nurses to distribute their time, expertise, and resources as fairly as possible among patients assigned to their care.
- **Fidelity** is the obligation to be truthful and to keep promises. This principle supports the practice of obtaining informed consent and being honest and genuine in interactions with the patient and family.
- **Dignity** is the right of the patient (and the person treating the patient) to be treated with respect.

Principles are guidelines and, as such, are not absolute in their application to situations. This is also true of moral and ethical principles. It is not uncommon to have more than one principle applicable to a situation simultaneously. Someone must determine which principle takes precedence in the given situation and why. These dilemmas are what make ethical decision making so difficult at times.

Legality

Legality refers to lawfulness or the obligations imposed by law to bind certain behaviors within a society. The professional nurse, licensed to practice in a particular state, is bound by the laws within that state. Each state has its own Nurse Practice Act that defines professional nursing practice within that state. In addition, there are other laws and legal decisions related to health care issues that set a precedent for practice within that state and, often, nationally. An example of a precedent-setting decision is the Karen Quinlan case.[10] In this well-known case, a young woman suffered unexplained apnea and did not receive immediate ventilatory support. She was subsequently placed on a ventilator and remained in a persistent vegetative state. In keeping with her prior stated wishes, the family allowed the ventilator to be removed so that she could die. Unexpectedly, she began to breathe spontaneously, and she lived in a persistent vegetative state for several years. This case established the precedent that a ventilator could be removed even when the consequence might be death. The fact that she lived for many years is related to the ongoing artificial feeding.

Laws and legal precedents related to health care matters may originate at the state or federal levels. The judicial system is divided into municipal, state, and federal courts. The right to appeal to a higher court is provided as a safeguard to protect individual and group rights. Some cases related to health care have reached the U.S. Supreme Court. Laws reflect the values and beliefs of society and thus are subject to review and to change. Although an act is legal, it may not seem moral to some individuals or groups. In a rapidly changing society such as that of the United States, challenges to current laws are common. With respect to health care issues, the changing and competing values and beliefs of a heterogeneous society, along with the unprecedented development of technology, account for the number of health-related issues referred to the courts.

FRAMEWORK FOR ETHICAL DECISION MAKING

Decision Making in General

Decision making includes distinct, logically organized steps that require choosing alternative courses of action. These steps include collecting relevant data, analyzing data, proposing alternative solutions, identifying the pros and cons of each alternative, and selecting the best alternative based on established criteria.

Ethical Decision Making

Ethical decision making is a dynamic process requiring reflection, discussion, and evaluation of outcomes. Like decision making in general, it should follow the same basic steps. Ethical decisions, as related to health care issues, can be unique in that they involve obligations, responsibilities, duties, rights, and values affecting life-and-death situations. Ethical decision making for the neurological patient often relates to end-of-life issues. The highly emotional nature of these issues often makes it difficult to separate feelings from facts. It is, therefore, of critical importance for decision makers to, as much as is possible, separate personal attitudes, beliefs, and feelings from the factual data that are relevant to the particular situation. While conscientious practice informs a nurse's personal ethical standard and sense of integrity, ethical decision making demands that the clinician remain objective: always aware of both professional and personal ethical standards, but also of emotional reactions.

Many ethical decisions require a multidisciplinary approach to provide a broad, comprehensive perspective of the issues at hand. Members of the interdisciplinary collaborative team must be knowledgeable about the fundamental principles of ethical decision making and end-of-life care to guide their analysis of complex cases. The unique input of each of the team members reflects his or her experience, knowledge, and collaborative role.

Collecting Relevant Data.

The database established by the physician related to the medical diagnosis and prognosis provides information necessary for the nurse's ethical decision-making process. Likewise, information collected by the nurse, as derived from periodic neurological examinations, preferences or responses expressed by the patient or family, and other sources, assists the physician. All information provides a current and updated database for ethical decision making. Data collected should include medical facts, medical goals of care, and patient goals of care or preferences for treatment. Determination of an accurate diagnosis and prognosis, made by the physician, is critical to the database. In cases of coma, a diagnosis detailing the type of brain damage and the likelihood of functional and/or cognitive recovery is important in planning care.

The most important information about goals of care comes from the patient if he or she is an adult and is mentally capable of making decisions. Consulting the patient in this regard recognizes the patient's right to autonomy and to define quality of life for himself or herself. If the patient decides to let family make important decisions, or is incapable as a result of coma, cognitive deficits, or other causes, then information regarding treatment preferences may be found in a living will or the expression of wishes made to the family or significant other while he or she was well. A surrogate decision maker may be necessary to represent the patient's wishes. The family's goals of care are also explored and established. Other data collected include information on state laws, hospital policies, and professional codes related to

the particular situation. In some situations, it may be necessary to seek advice from the institutional ethics committee or hospital attorney.

Analyzing Data.

Once data are collected, relevant data are analyzed. Using the moral principles of autonomy, beneficence, justice, and fidelity, consider the question, "What are the duties, rights, and responsibilities of all persons involved?"

Proposing Alternative Solutions.

Considering the diagnosis, evidence-based practice, prognosis, goals of care for the patient, laws, policies, and other relevant data, alternative actions are then identified.

Identifying the Risk–Benefit Ratio of Each Alternative.

The risks and benefits of each alternative action are weighed and considered on the basis of treatment preferences, potential outcomes (both desired and consequential), laws, and policies.

Selecting the Best Alternative Based on Established Criteria.

Finally, an alternative or action is selected on the basis of goals of care, acceptable ethical standards, laws, and policies, and with acceptance of the consequences and benefits of that action. The decision may be not to begin treatment at all but to proceed to palliative care. Physicians are not morally obliged to fulfill patients' requests for actions that they consider ethically objectionable, nor are they obliged to provide treatments that are not beneficial. Physicians have the right to be removed from the care of such patients, although they also have an obligation to arrange for another physician to care for the patient.[11] When clinicians are faced with difficult decisions or disagreements about the best course of action or treatment for a patient, a consultation may be requested from the institutional ethics committee. The purpose of an ethics committee is to review cases impartially and make recommendations. A statement, often written by the chairperson of the group, summarizes the recommendations of the committee as it relates to the *best interest* of the patient within the context of the situation. The criteria of the Joint Commission now require a formal mechanism to support ethical decision making.

Process of Ethical Decision Making

Ethical decision making, often centered around EOL issues, is an integral part of medical and nursing practice, regardless of the setting, and includes both the independent role and the collaborative role of professional practice. However, the responsibilities and participation of physicians and nurses in ethical decision making are dissimilar. While physicians primarily initiate and guide the decisions regarding EOL care, they are not always the ones to carry out the implementation of decisions. Also noted is physician reluctance to initiate EOL discussions,[12] thus leading to other stresses in ethical decision making. Reckling[13] commented on the nurses' passive roles in decisions to withhold or withdraw life-sustaining treatment, yet in the intensive care unit (ICU) setting nurses play a large role in communication about EOL issues.[14,15] The professional nurse in particular is well prepared to assume a proactive role in facilitating timely dialogue.[16]

There is need for increased research into and physician and nurse training related to ethical and EOL communication, decision making, and clinical care.

INDEPENDENT ROLE OF THE NURSE

The independent role of the nurse as it relates to ethical decision making at the end of life generally involves the following:

- Establishing a database, making nursing diagnoses, establishing expected outcomes, and developing a plan of care
- Orienting the family to the unit and unit policies (e.g., visiting hours, location of telephones and food services)
- Identifying a family spokesperson and scheduling timely updates regarding the patient's condition and progress
- Providing information about the patient's nursing care and response to care to other health providers
- Educating the patient and/or family about the disease process
- Determining whether the patient has designated a medical power of attorney or has any other advance directive, and if so, making sure copies are placed in the medical record
- Seeking information about the patient's or family's care preferences, including cultural and spiritual needs
- Managing pain appropriately to provide and maintain comfort
- Reassuring the family that the patient is receiving sensitive, compassionate care and that he or she is comfortable with adequate pain control
- Respecting the patient's/family's decisions regarding care
- Supporting the decision of the patient and/or family who do *not choose to begin treatment or who decide to withdraw from aggressive treatment*
- Assuming an advocacy role on behalf of the patient and/or family
- Facilitating communication between physicians and the patient/family related to understanding of disease processes and goals of care
- Supporting the patient and/or family in the grieving process
- Making appropriate referrals to clergy, psychiatric clinical nurse specialists, social workers, or other support resources as necessary
- Documenting the information and support and other interventions provided, and the patient's and/or family's responses
- Following up on how the family is coping (e.g., postcrisis, bereavement) in the home environment

INDEPENDENT ROLE OF THE PHYSICIAN

Both general and specific guidelines are provided for the physician who must make decisions about withdrawal of aggressive treatment for patients with severe, irreversible brain damage.[11] Care is never withdrawn but transitions from aggressive medical treatment to a comfort-oriented approach. However, these guidelines are applicable for any seriously ill patient and their loved ones:

General

- Communicate with the family
- Communicate with the staff
- Document decisions carefully
- Follow hospital by-laws

Specific

- Establish diagnosis
- Establish prognosis
- Identify the patient's preferences (determine if patient has advance directives or designated power of attorney or if he or she has ever expressed any desires about health care preferences)
- Identify the family's preference (desires for care)
- Choose level of treatment (describe risk–benefit of proposed treatment)
- Request oversight by the hospital ethics committee
- Refer to courts for judicial review

COLLABORATIVE ROLES

The **collaborative role** of the nurse and physician in ethical and end-of-life decision making is based on open, honest, and respectful communications and excellence in symptom management.[17] Ongoing communication with the patient and family is a shared responsibility, and is the foundation of ethical decision making at the end of life. This communication needs to be a priority both interprofessionally (between nurses and physicians and other health care team members) and between health care providers and the patient/family.[18] Nurses, who spend 8 to 12 hours at a time with patients and families, are uniquely situated to understand what information is needed to clarify medical issues, how the patient defines quality of life, and even what past experiences the patient or family have had in EOL issues. Open communication will elicit clinical outcomes that best meet decided upon goals of care for all involved. Once goals of care are clarified, both nurses and physicians participate in affirming patient or family choices in goals of care. Through the process of expert communications, nurses and doctors will also be able to collaborate in identifying and supporting the patient/family psychologically, spiritually, and emotionally.[19]

CLINICAL PEARLS: Language is crucial in end-of-life discussions. Words such as "nothing left to do" or "withdrawal of treatment" should not be used. To the layperson, these statements can be wildly misinterpreted. Be sure to explain what care will continue if a shift is made toward palliative care.

Frequent updates regarding the patient's condition and prognosis in a caring, gentle manner are necessary. Nurses should know what information has been provided to the family because clarification and reinforcement may be necessary. People in high-stress situations often do not absorb all of the information provided, and therefore may need repetition. Questions raised by the family with the nurse may need to be referred to the physician. The nurse is responsible for notifying the physician about family concerns and the possible need for a family meeting.

The steps of an ideal family meeting are well documented in the literature.[14,20,21] However, orchestrating and implementing ideal communication techniques in real-time patient care has proven more elusive, with physicians dominating family meetings rather than listening to family members' concerns and questions.[14,22]

While the attending physician usually leads a family meeting, the nurse should still be familiar in the essentials of conducting a family meeting to ensure the best possible quality of the meeting and to help prompt the physician if steps are missed.

The steps in conducting a family meeting include the following:

1. Why are you meeting?
   - Clarify conference goals with health care team members. What do you hope to accomplish? If other subspecialty physicians are involved, disagreements about patient care should be resolved *before* the meeting, not during it.
2. Where?
   - Private room away from distracting noises with seats available for all attending
3. Who?
   - Patient (if capable of participating)
   - Legal decision maker/health care power of attorney
   - Family members and social support
   - Hospital chaplain or family spiritual leader
   - Key health care professionals
4. Introduction and relationship building
   - Physician, nurse, and social worker are introduced to the family or representatives of the family, and the family or representatives of the family introduced to the health care providers.
   - Review goals of meeting; clarify if specific decisions need to be made.
   - Establish ground rules: each person will have a chance to ask questions and express views with no interruption. Establish legal decision maker. Describe importance of supportive care.
5. Determine what the patient/family already knows
   - Ask the family or family representatives to describe the patient as a person to get a sense of what kind of individual he or she is, his or her values, and any health care preferences (this builds trust and provides a context for discussion that is patient centered).
   - Ask the patients or family representatives to tell you their understanding of the current medical condition.
   - Ask each family member to speak.
   - Also ask about the past 1 to 6 months—what has changed in the patient's functional ability, weight, and quality of life?
6. Review medical status
   - Review what has happened and what is happening to the patient. Include prognosis and treatment options; this includes the best and worse outcome (often this information is not conveyed; to know that their loved one would live in a nursing home is NOT an acceptable option for many).

- Discuss issues in a way that is meaningful to the patient/family; acknowledge that prognosis is (often) uncertain; avoid euphemisms for the word *dying*.
- For decisions to withdraw aggressive medical interventions, reinforce that while medical treatments may stop, caring for the patient will continue; describe what the patient's natural death might be like as a result of discontinuing aggressive ineffective treatment and allowing a natural death.
- Ask the patient and each family member, in turn, if they have any questions about current status, plan, and prognosis.
- Defer discussion of decision making until the next step.
- Respond to emotional reactions.
7. Family discussion with a decisional patient
   - Ask patient, "What decision(s) are you considering?"
   - Ask each family member, "Do you have questions or concerns about the treatment plan? How can I (or other health care professionals) support the patient?"
8. Family discussion with a nondecisional patient
   - Ask each family member in turn, "What do you believe the patient would choose if he or she could speak for himself or herself?"
   - Ask each family member, "What do you think should be done?"
   - Ask the family if they would like you to leave the room to let them discuss alone.
   - If there is consensus, go to item 10; if no consensus, go to item 9.
9. When there is no consensus
   - Restate the goal: "What would the patient say if he or she could speak?"
   - Use time as an ally: schedule a follow-up conference the next day.
   - Try further discussion: "What values are your decisions based upon? How will the decision affect you and other family members?"
   - Identify other resources: minister/priest; other physicians; ethics committee to assist in making a decision.
10. Wrap-up
    - Summarize consensus, disagreements, decisions, and plan.
    - Caution against unexpected outcomes such as the patient living for several days; discussion of hospice care can be introduced.
    - Identify family spokesperson for ongoing communications.
    - Document in the chart who was present, what decisions were made, and follow-up plan.
    - Continuity: maintain contact with the family and medical team. Schedule follow-up meetings as needed.[20]

CLINICAL PEARLS: Professional interpreters should be used to translate. Family members may not feel comfortable talking about difficult or end-of-life issues; they may not be able to accurately translate medical jargon; or they may simply choose to protect the patient and not disclose information. In some cultures it is not acceptable to tell the patient. Determine what is culturally acceptable. If the patient is able to make decisions, determine if he or she wants to do so based on his or her culture.

For patients who are unable to participate in goals-of-care discussions and who do not have an advance directive, end-of-life decision making falls to family members. The evolution of how family members make difficult decisions on behalf of their loved one seems to occur in discrete phases.[23] First, information regarding the patient's disease state(s) is sought both formally through family meetings and informally by observing staff interactions or conversations. During this process trust is developed between the formal caregivers and family. Then, family members compare the reality of the patient's prognosis and quality life with what the patient would want, based on the patient's previously expressed values or statements. Families then acknowledge and accept the surrogate decision-maker role, and finally confront the question of continuing aggressive therapies versus seeking comfort care. Notably, this evolution requires much time and reflection, but ultimately provides the family with a legacy of "having done the right thing" and providing dignity and respect to their loved one.[21] Depending on the situation, the assistance of other professionals, such as clergy, social workers, palliative care specialists, or psychiatric or mental health professionals, and the ethics consultation team may be requested to provide support to the patient and family. Discussions with other collaborators can be very helpful in clarifying related issues, not only to the patient and family, but also to the health professionals involved.

Documentation

Written documentation of communications with the family and the decisions made is important to validate that the ethical and legal dimensions of care have been met. The written documentation of both the nurse and the physician helps to keep the professional staff aware of what has transpired in the decision-making process, what the goals of care are, and what issues need to be further addressed. The physician has the responsibility to provide data about the patient's condition and documentation of decisions for the plan of care. In special situations, such as with "do not resuscitate" (DNR) orders, hospital policy often dictates the frequency of documentation and specific data to be included.

DECISION-MAKING CAPACITY AND ADVANCE DIRECTIVES AND LIVING WILLS

Patient's Capacity to Make Decisions

Discussion about the appropriate use of "competency" has been raised. According to *Guidelines on the Termination of Life-Sustaining Treatment and the Care of the Dying,* the use of competence and incompetence should be restricted to situations in which a formal judicial determination has been made.[24] Under existing law, until such time as a judicial determination of incompetence has been made, individuals are presumed competent to manage their own affairs. The report goes on to promote the use of the notion of decision-making capacity.[24] **Decision-making capacity** refers to a patient's functional ability to make informed health care decisions in accordance with personal values. A person can be legally competent and nonetheless lack the capacity to make a particular treatment decision and vice versa.

Valid consent or refusal assumes adequacy of information provided, absence of coercion, and capacity to make decisions. The accepted standards in designating a patient's decision-making capacity were put forth in the President's Commission report on *Deciding to Forgo Life-Sustaining Treatment.*[25] The criteria include that the patient must be able to understand all information relevant to the decision; communicate with caregivers about the decision; and possess the ability to reason about relevant alternatives against a background of "reasonably stable personal values and life goals."

When cognitive abilities are compromised so that informed consent is no longer possible, the patient is not capable of making decisions. The health care team members then look to a designated family member or significant other as the surrogate to make decisions on behalf of the patient. The decisions made should be guided by the patient's previous expressions of wishes regarding treatment decisions (see discussion later of the substitute judgment standard) and an understanding of the patient's life goals, values, and beliefs and not those of the surrogate. Some states recognize living wills (discussed later in this chapter).

In neuroscience nursing practice, "the organ of reason" is often also the organ injured and/or impaired, so that cognitive function is often compromised. The nurse then becomes the patient's advocate to ensure that adequate care is provided within the context of the prior expressed wishes of the patient as best as they can be determined. There are times when the patient is admitted to a facility in a comatose state, and the nurse has no idea of what the wishes of the patient would be if he or she could convey them. As patient advocates, the health care team is obliged to seek this information as it has been expressed in the past to family members or is found in written documents.

Advance Directives and Living Wills

Advance directives are often misunderstood both by laypeople and health care professionals. Formalized **advance directives** are *written documents* signed by a competent person outlining the extent and form of care in the event of subsequent inability to participate in decision making. A **living will** is an advance directive invoked when the patient is incapable of participating in decision making, and specifies if life-sustaining treatments to postpone death should or should not be used in the event of a terminal and/or irreversible illness.[26] The living will is a provision under a state's "Natural Death Act" or "Terminal Care Document." The problem with a living will is that it often fails to provide the detailed instructions necessary for care and only applies when the patient is unable to communicate his or her wishes, and then only if death is imminent or would be imminent if life-prolonging measures would not be continued or pursued: it lacks the specifics to make decisions for many treatment options. Also, it does not automatically imply that the patient wishes to be designated DNR. A more useful directive is the *Durable Power of Attorney for Health Care* (DPAHC), and it is available for use in all states. The DPAHC permits adults to authorize a person to make surrogate medical decisions on his or her behalf if he or she becomes incapable of making decisions.[27]

Studies that have examined patients' advance preferences and the decisions that they or surrogates actually made over time found that treatment preferences are not stable and may change, especially when faced with serious illness.[28] This is important because providers must recognize that previous decisions may be revised because of changes in health status and the patient's definition of quality of life. Therefore, advance preferences should be reviewed with the patient with full recognition that decision making is a process and not an endpoint.[29]

The **Patient Self-Determination Act of 1990** supports proxy statutes specifically for health care. It also requires that health care providers elicit and clarify a patient's goals of care and treatment options. This information may be elicited through conversations with the patient or surrogate about the patient's beliefs, values, and life goals. States have different titles for their advance directives, living wills, and durable power of attorney documents.[30] The formalized designation of a surrogate decision maker for health care decisions is titled "Designation of a Health Care Power of Attorney" in some states and "Durable Power of Attorney for Health Care" in others. Nurses need to be familiar with the relevant documents and statutes in the state in which they practice. Medicare and Medicaid nursing home certification requires inpatient assessment to determine the status of advance directives and durable power of attorney in those settings. In the absence of any advance directives, the principles of nonmaleficence and best interest become operative.

CLINICAL PEARLS: The process of making an advance directive should ideally occur before a medical crisis occurs, to allow a patient and family to truly think about and discuss their feelings, values, and wishes. Inevitably an advance directive will not be able to guide families in the many discrete, nuanced medical decisions related to goals of care: one simply cannot prepare for every possible medical outcome. The process of making an advance directive should therefore really focus on values and the patient's definition of quality of life.

CLINICAL VIGNETTE: A 72-year-old Vietnamese male, Mr. NP, woke up at home out of a deep sleep with a severe headache; he quickly became obtunded. Upon admission to the emergency room, a stat computed tomography (CT) scan shows a subdural hematoma with a large area of infarction, and impending uncal herniation with midline shift. Emergency surgery followed to evacuate the hematoma, but 1 week postop the patient remains in a coma. On exam, Mr. NP is orally intubated and has a nasogastric (NG) tube for enteral feeding. He has a positive gag reflex and exhibits decerebrate posturing to painful stimuli, but is otherwise unresponsive. The prognosis is poor for any meaningful recovery, according to the physicians. The primary nurse suggests a palliative care (PC) consult.

The PC team assesses the patient and schedules a family meeting. The neurologist, primary nurse, and PC team meet with the family and a translator, as Mr. NP's wife and son speak Vietnamese as their primary language. The family reports that they understand the patient is very ill and that he has sustained a major stroke, and that the patient can't feel anything. They are, however, confused when they see the patient cough and turn his arms inward when he is suctioned. They wonder if this means the patient is "awake" or getting better. The neurologist, via the translator, describes the pathology of the hematoma, the resulting permanent brain damage, and how basic reflexes can remain intact. The physician explains that the options in care are to continue as is and place a tracheostomy and percutaneous endoscopic gastrostomy (PEG), or stop ventilation and artificial nutrition and institute total comfort care. The prognosis with each option is also outlined: months continuing with aggressive care, minutes to hours with comfort care.

The physicians ask the family what they think the patient would choose for himself. The patient's wife then produces a living will the patient made a few years prior. It states that the patient does not want advanced life support in the setting of a terminal or irreversible illness, but does not describe wishes pertaining to tracheostomy, feeding tubes, or whether he would want to be kept alive only to be in a coma. After describing code status and the option of designating the patient as DNR, the family unanimously agree on DNR status. The thought of not feeding the patient seemed particularly distressing. The neurologist and PC physicians explain that because of the severe brain damage sustained, the patient would not experience hunger or discomfort without artificial nutrition. The physicians explain that even without a PEG, gentle hydration can be given to ease any concerns about suffering. In addition, hydration could be harmful; the physician describes why this is true.

To help focus the family on the patient's wishes, the PC nurse prompts the family to describe the patient before he fell ill. After listening to the family describe Mr. NP, the PC nurse gently asked Mrs. NP, "Would your husband find meaning in his life if he could no longer fulfill any of those roles—engineer, grandfather, or coach?" Mrs. NP and her son both cry and quietly state that no, he would not be happy without the ability to do all those things he loved.

The PC physician offers, "I know this is a terrible, difficult decision to make for someone you love. I know you don't want your husband to die. But his body has already made the decision—he is dying. What we need to do now is figure out what is the best way to honor him, and take care of him during the end of his life."

The family asks what it would look like to take the breathing machine away. The PC nurse carefully describes the process, reviewing the normal changes that occur in a dying patient and how his comfort will be managed. The family seems reassured that they will be allowed to be present during the process, and are grateful to learn what to expect. Mr. NP's family agrees to pursue comfort care.

The primary nurse reviews the comfort care plan with the PC nurse, and Mr. NP is extubated that afternoon. The primary nurse and PC nurse remain at the bedside to comfort the family and answer questions. The family's pastor is present for spiritual support.

Two and a half hours postextubation the patient dies peacefully. Though acutely upset and grieving, the family communicates how grateful they are to all the nurses and doctors for taking care of Mr. NP, and for helping them through the difficult decision-making process.

With readily available technology, the question of appropriate use of technology is often raised. In making decisions about use of technology and other resources, the primary consideration is the expected outcomes of care—physiologically, functionally, and qualitatively—within a specified time frame rather than unqualified entitlement. Laws do not require physicians to provide treatment that is *medically futile* or ineffective. Some state laws include a futility clause about life-sustaining treatment decisions to clarify patients' rights and a mechanism to resolve dispute. The Texas Advance Directive Law of 1999[31] is such an example. Patients have the right to refuse treatment, but they do not have a right to demand and receive interventions that are judged by competent professionals to be of no benefit to them. The role of evidence-based medicine and best practice helps to determine ineffective treatment objectively in relationship to treatment goals and expected outcomes rather than subjective thinking. A second opinion and use of ethical consultation is helpful to resolve differences of opinion, especially when the patient or surrogate opinion is different from that of the physician.

END-OF-LIFE CARE

Nurses have always cared for the dying patient and the family across the continuum of care. But the clinical competencies and expertise that are required to care for the patient and family facing a life-threatening disease has not been a focus of attention for many reasons.[32] For nurses and other health care professionals, death is often viewed as a failure of medical care, as opposed to a natural part of the life cycle. For the general public and policy makers, it is an uncomfortable topic. The United States is a youth-oriented culture, where dying takes place primarily in an institutionalized setting after a long, chronic illness.[33] Thus, American society removes the death and dying experience to a remote location, under "controlled" circumstances. Inevitably, though, death becomes very personal: it is not something that only happens to others; it is something that we will all experience. After years of inattention, American society and American health care are re-examining how we approach dying and death and how we care for people at the end of life. In 1997, the Institute of Medicine published a report on improving care at the end of life with recommendations. This report reinforces the important ongoing work of nurses and how nurses have been addressing this understated problem.[34]

End-of-life care refers to the comprehensive aspects of care needed by patients and their families as they approach death.[35] Palliative care is an emerging medical and nursing specialty that addresses EOL issues comprehensively whether or not the patient is seeking life-prolonging therapies. According to the World Health Organization (WHO),

palliative care is "the active total care of patients whose disease is not responsive to curative treatment. Control of pain, of other symptoms, and of psychological, social, and spiritual problems is paramount. The goal of palliative care is achievement of the best quality of life for patients and their families"[36] while maximizing comfort and maintaining dignity.[37] Care is provided by an interdisciplinary team of health professionals. Other components of palliative care include maximizing quality of life (QOL); facilitating communications and setting goals of care; supporting roles/needs of the family; spiritual care, care for the actively dying patient, and postmortem care; issues of policy and ethics; and bereavement of family and staff.[38,39]

Often hospice care is confused with palliative care. While hospice and palliative care share the same philosophy—excellence in pain and symptom management, family care, and communication—hospice care is purely comfort care. Palliative care is often started while aggressive care is being sought; in hospice, only comfort measures are implemented. Nevertheless, hospice care remains an important resource for patients and families at the end of life and is available in the home and other settings.

It is apparent that the comprehensiveness of EOL care provides a broad framework for considering care needs for both patients and their families, education and research into clinical management of pain and other distressing symptoms, and the societal issues of policies and ethics.

CLINICAL PEARLS: In general, the earlier a palliative care consult is requested, the better. By instituting palliative care along with aggressive care, patients and families are better prepared to accomplish important tasks, such as preparing finances, making arrangements for children, saying goodbye, and finding closure emotionally and spiritually, as well as optimal symptom management.

SELECTED END-OF-LIFE ETHICAL ISSUES COMMON IN NEUROSCIENCE NURSING PRACTICE

Although many ethical decisions involve nurses on a daily basis, there are several challenging EOL issues often encountered in practice settings by neuroscience nurses. Those selected for discussion in this section include artificial hydration and nutrition, promotion of comfort, and relief of pain. Assisted suicide and euthanasia are briefly addressed. Decision making at the end of life is often complex, and there may be conflict around care issues both from care providers and family.[40,41] The nurse is often in the middle of these complex communications and decision-making processes.

End-of-Life Care Decisions: The Legal Precedent

Several court decisions have clearly addressed the deliberate discontinuation of life-sustaining treatment to allow for a natural death. Life-sustaining treatment can be legally removed from a patient with or without decision-making capacity. The following cases illustrate this right. In the landmark Quinlan decision of 1976, the court established the right for refusal of life-sustaining treatment by a guardian acting on behalf of a patient who was comatose and, therefore, incapable of making decisions.[42] The request to remove the ventilator was granted based on the irreversibility of her condition, as well as statements attributed to the patient prior to her illness that indicated an unwillingness to be maintained on life support indefinitely if there was no hope for quality of life. The *Satz v. Perlmutter* case pertains to a fully capable 73-year-old patient who depended on a ventilator as a result of amyotrophic lateral sclerosis.[43] He wanted the ventilator to be removed even though he knew death would result. The Florida court ruled that because Mr. Satz was a competent adult, he had a right to refuse life-sustaining treatment. The ventilator was discontinued, and he died within a short period of time.

In 1985, the New Jersey Supreme Court approved the removal of a feeding tube from Ms. Conroy, an elderly nursing home resident with profound dementia. The court ruled that a feeding tube is a medical device and intervention and may be accepted or rejected on behalf of an incompetent patient in the same way as other medical interventions.[44,45] The Brophy decision in 1986 was important in that his care was contested by New England Sinai Hospital. The Massachusetts Supreme Judicial Court allowed Mr. Brophy's family to transfer him to another facility. This act acknowledged the conscientious objection of the staff of New England Sinai Hospital.[46] In 1990, the U.S. Supreme Court heard the landmark Cruzan case. Nancy Cruzan was a young motor vehicle accident victim who was in a persistent vegetative state. The family wanted to discontinue the feeding tube. The Court affirmed the principle that a feeding tube is a medical device for artificial delivery of hydration and nutrition and is no different from other medical interventions that may be refused by or on behalf of patients.[47]

Finally, the Terri Schiavo case reaffirmed the protection of the central ethical tenet of patient autonomy, even when the patient has lost competence. Although much publicized, politicized, and debated, the case rigorously tested judiciary standards that ultimately supported the previously mentioned series of court decisions.[48] Professional organizations have published definitive position statements regarding life-sustaining treatment. In 1986, the Council of Ethical and Judicial Affairs of the American Medical Association published the "Statement on Withholding or Withdrawing Life Prolonging Medical Treatment," which stated that such treatment may be withheld from a patient in irreversible coma even when death is not imminent.[49] The Hastings Center, a highly respected source on ethical issues, published *Guidelines on the Termination of Life-Sustaining Treatment and the Care of the Dying.*[50] In these guidelines, life-sustaining treatment is defined as "any medical intervention, technology, procedure or medication that is administered to a patient in order to forestall the moment of death whether or not the treatment is intended to affect the underlying disease(s) or biological processes." The position paper of the American Academy of Neurology addressed persistent vegetative state and concluded that nutrition and

hydration provided through the enteral route is a medical therapy that can be discontinued.[51,52] The Society of Critical Care Medicine also has recommendations for EOL care.[53] Although these publications are not legal documents, they reflect evidence-based practice and the opinions of those prestigious organizations involved in ethical issues and the delivery of care. These guidelines provide guidance for clinical practice for all health care workers, and affirm the right to die as one that is highly personal, but also highly complex.

Artificial Hydration and Nutrition

Health care professionals and the general public have an easier time of understanding the ethical basis for forgoing ventilators in dying patients than forgoing *artificial hydration and nutrition* (AHN).[45] In this context, the term *artificial* refers to providing nutrition by medical devices designed to bypass the mouth through which food and water are normally consumed. Artificially delivered hydration and nutrition refers to water and nutrients provided either directly into the stomach or small intestines or indirectly into the vascular system. First, hydration and nutrition can be administered into the stomach by way of a nasogastric tube inserted through the nose or mouth, through a surgically inserted gastrostomy tube placed into the stomach or small intestines through the abdominal wall, or by way of a percutaneous endoscopic gastrostomy tube inserted into the stomach or jejunum endoscopically. Second, hydration and nutrition can be administered into the vascular system through a peripheral intravenous (IV) line or into larger vessels or right atria through a central venous catheter.

The American Nurses Association (ANA) published the "Position Statement on Forgoing Artificial Nutrition and Hydration" in 1992.[54] It affirms the principles set forth in the American Medical Association, Hastings Center, and American Academy of Neurology documents. Its central concept is recognition that artificially provided hydration and nutrition, like other interventions, may or may not be justified. As in all other interventions, the anticipated benefits must outweigh the anticipated burdens for the intervention to be justified.

The benefit–burden analysis of AHN reveals its complexities, and thus the need to individualize care for each patient and family considering this difficult choice. Therapeutically, AHN can be used to prolong life, prevent aspiration pneumonia, and maintain independence and physical functioning. It does not prevent aspiration of saliva or reflux of tube feeding. However, empirical evidence does not suggest that these goals are necessarily accomplished. Patients with end-stage, progressive diseases do not live longer when AHN is employed. Further, complications of AHN (infection, fluid overload) may even increase mortality. Finally, some patients may even have an increased risk of aspiration pneumonia when AHN is used.[37,55] The emotional implications of not providing AHN for families and often for caregivers alike are overwhelming. Caregivers often feel that patients will experience the sensation of hunger or starvation if AHN is not employed. In reality, when most patients are ill and at the end of life, they naturally become disinterested in food and experience profound anorexia, often developing nausea and vomiting when "forced" to eat either by mouth or by AHN. Xerostomia, defined as dry mouth, is a very common symptom for dying patients, but is not relieved by administration of AHN; rather, stringent oral care seems to best relieve this symptom.[37] On the other hand, for certain conditions like opioid toxicity or delirium secondary to dehydration, judicious use of parenteral fluids is sometimes recommended, even in the setting of hospice care.[55]

The ANA distinguishes between food and water taken by *mouth* from artificial nutrition and hydration. It also notes that assisting with feeding is a qualitative difference in taking oral nutrition and hydration and not a substantive one. The ANA statement supports the forgoing of tube feedings when there is questionable benefit. The statement also goes on to explain that "competent reflective adults are generally in the best position to evaluate various harms and benefits to themselves in the context of their own values, life projects and tolerance of pain" and that when patients are incapacitated, a surrogate, "preferably designated by the patient," should be relied on to make the decision on behalf of the patient.

Promotion of Comfort and Relief of Pain

Promotion of comfort and relief of pain can be viewed from the perspective of the dying patient and the perspective of acute pain. In 2003, the ANA published a "Position Statement on Pain Management and Control of Distressing Symptoms in Dying Patients."[56] It pointed out that when cure or prolongation of life in individuals with serious health problems is no longer possible, the focus of nursing care is on the individual's response to dying and palliative care. Promotion of comfort becomes the primary focus of nursing care. The overriding fear of many patients and families is severe, unrelenting pain during the dying process. Pain is commonly undertreated, and many patients experience inadequate pain control.[57] It is well recognized that severe pain can cause sleeplessness, loss of morale, fatigue, irritability, restlessness, withdrawal, and other serious problems in dying patients.[35,58,59] Further, a meta-analysis supports the concept of multiple symptoms "bundling" that forms a common pathway of symptoms at the end of life: pain, fatigue, and breathlessness have a prevalence rate of well over 50% in advanced cancer, acquired immune deficiency syndrome (AIDS), heart disease, chronic obstructive pulmonary disease, and renal disease.[60] Nurses play a key role in both assessment and control of pain and other distressing symptoms either by administering orders for pain or advocating on behalf of the patient for adequate pain and symptom management control when pharmacologic agents ordered are inadequate to keep the patient comfortable. The assessment and management of pain and other symptoms must be based on an understanding of pathophysiologic, emotional, and spiritual components as well as the knowledge of the particular disease. The ANA says the main goal of nursing intervention for a dying patient should be maximizing comfort through adequate management of pain and discomfort as is in keeping with the expressed desires of the patient. Further, toward that end, the patient should have whatever medication, in whatever dosage, and by whatever route is needed to control the level of pain as perceived by him or her.

CLINICAL PEARLS: End-of-life nursing care inevitably leads a nurse to confront personal beliefs, past losses, and one's own mortality. Take time to self-reflect on how dying patients and families affect you personally and professionally. Stringent self-care is often needed when patients and families demand so much energy and care.

Many nurses express concern about the patient's developing tolerance or addiction to analgesics and are fearful of "harming" the patient in that way. The ANA examined authoritative resources and addressed these concerns by stating that careful titration of pain medication is essential to promote comfort in dying patients. The proper dose is "the dose that is sufficient to reduce pain and suffering."[61] Tolerance to pain medications often develops in patients after repeated and prolonged use. Thus, both adults and children may require very high doses of medication to maintain adequate pain control.[62] These doses may exceed the usual recommended dosages of the particular drug for patients of similar age and weight. Regular dosing of pain medication has been shown to be more effective than PRN use.[63]

Demystifying the Fears of Addiction

The risk of addiction in a patient who requires long-term use of opioids is about the same as that for the general population. The hallmark of addiction is dysfunctional use, characterized by cravings and the need to use a drug for purposes other than pain relief. Tolerance is an expected physiologic response resulting from chronic use of many drugs, including opioids, that does not in and of itself reflect addiction or cause addiction. Tolerance is defined as the lessening of drug effect over time, requiring increasing doses to achieve the same physical effect. Physical dependence is also an expected physiologic response whereby abrupt cessation of the drug leads to a withdrawal syndrome. Opioids, steroids, beta-blockers, and many antidepressants cause physical dependence. As with the effect of tolerance, physical dependence does reflect or cause addiction. Finally, pseudoaddiction reflects behaviors of uncontrolled pain or fear of uncontrolled pain that are mislabeled and misinterpreted as addiction. The hallmark of pseudoaddiction is that once pain is relieved or once the patient trusts that future pain will be believed and treated, the "addictive" behaviors cease.[64] Clear understanding of these principles should help guide the nursing care of the patient in pain.

The ANA statement goes on to say that pain medications may have sedative or respiratory depressant side effects. This should not be an overriding consideration for dying patients so long as use of pain medication is consistent with the patient's wishes. Pain may continue even when a patient is unresponsive and at the end hours of life when respirations decrease. Pain relief should continue unless there is a reason to believe that the physiologic cause of pain is no longer present. Of particular interest is the following statement: "The increasing titration of medication to achieve adequate symptom control, even at the expense of maintaining life or hastening death secondarily, is ethically justified.

Nurses should not hesitate to use full and effective doses of pain mediation for the proper management of pain in the dying patient." Many clinicians feel ethically burdened by the thought that continuing to use opioid medications for a dying patient will actually hasten the patient's death. In fact, there is a lack of evidence supporting this fear.[65] Further, the rule of double effect provides ethical justification for the continued use of opioids in the dying patient. Four conditions define this doctrine[65,66]:

- The action itself must be morally good or neutral, regardless of the consequences. (The use of opioids to achieve pain and symptom relief in the dying patient is a "good act.")
- The clinician's intention must be for the good effect to occur, even if the bad effect is foreseen. (A nurse gives an opioid intending to relieve pain in a dying patient, but realizes that respiratory drive may be diminished to the point of cessation of breath.)
- The bad effect cannot be the means to achieve the good effect. (The patient does not need to die to have pain relieved.)
- The benefits of the good effect must outweigh the burdens of the bad effect. (Relieving pain in a dying patient is more beneficial than the minimal risk of hastening dying with opioid use.)

Spending 8 to 12 hours a day at the bedside, the nurse is best able to assess and monitor symptom management in the dying patient; control of pain and symptoms in the dying patient is a responsibility and an obligation of nurses.

The second focus of acute pain management is in a patient who is not necessarily classified as a "dying patient." Patients with severe headache related to subarachnoid hemorrhage, a brain tumor, stroke, intracranial bleed, or other causes are entitled to adequate pain control. Nurses worry about the reliability of the neurological assessment data if a patient is receiving an opioid analgesic for pain control. Specifically, concern is expressed about masking the level of consciousness (LOC), mental status, pupillary reflexes, and respiratory function. There is great reluctance to adequately manage pain and discomfort so that many patients are grossly undertreated or not treated at all. A patient may be holding his or her head with severe pain because the nurse is afraid to medicate him or her. Nurses need to consider the physiologic consequences (e.g., increased blood pressure or pulse, increased agitation) of inadequate pain management as well as central nervous system effects with the obligation to keep patients comfortable.

The Clinical Practice Guidelines (p. 29)[57] for acute pain address neurosurgical pain in the following way:

Patients undergoing surgery of the central nervous system frequently have neurological deficits that must be closely followed in the postoperative period. These patients may also receive drugs designed to reduce cerebral edema or prevent seizures. A major dilemma in this clinical setting is the need to carefully monitor critical neurological signs, such as pupillary reflexes and the level of consciousness (LOC), which may be affected by conventional opioid analgesics used for the relief of postoperative pain. Ideally, postoperative pain control should not interfere with

the ability to assess a patient's neurological status, particularly the LOC, or with assessment of motor and sensory function following spinal cord surgery. Therefore, the administration of opioids, benzodiazepines, and anxiolytics, in particular, is relatively contraindicated. However, the clinician must balance the need for analgesia with the requirement for appropriate neurological monitoring. The uncomplicated post-craniotomy patient typically has mild pain and is readily managed by a short period of parenteral medications followed by oral analgesics. Laminectomy and other spinal procedures usually are more painful than craniotomies. Ketorolac, a parenteral NSAID, may be considered in this setting because it has no effect on the LOC or pupillary reflexes. NSAIDs may be contraindicated in some postoperative settings when the risk of coagulopathy or hemorrhage is high, when the need to assess fever is important, when renal status is compromised, or when the degree of pain is higher than the analgesic ceiling of the agent. Furthermore, motor and sensory dysfunction associated with epidural local anesthetics (which are often co-administered with opioids) may obscure important neurological signs. Again remember to balance the need for adequate analgesia while minimizing the confounding central nervous system effects of analgesics and anesthetics.

From this cited information, it is evident that agents used for *acute* pain control must be weighed along with the effects on the central nervous system.

Assisted Suicide

The ANA defines assisted suicide as making a means of suicide (e.g., providing pills or a weapon) available to a patient with knowledge of the patient's intention to kill himself or herself.[67] People are not ethically obliged to accept life-sustaining treatment[68]: refusal of such treatment has been ruled legally acceptable in the courts. However, administration of drugs with the intent of causing death, even when requested by a mentally competent person, is considered an act of assisted suicide. When the primary intent of an act is to shorten or terminate life, this intent is considered to do harm, based on the ethical principle of nonmaleficence.[30] The Academy of Neurology has also published a position statement on assisted suicide.[69]

Assisting in a suicide is considered a criminal offense in all U.S. states except Oregon. In 1997, the U.S. Supreme Court, in a 9 to 0 decision, upheld the New York and Washington state laws that said physician-assisted suicide was a criminal offense.[70] The ANA, in a position statement, directs nurses not to support physician-assisted suicide and not to participate in voluntary active euthanasia.[71,72] Further, the Hospice and Palliative Care Nurses Association "Position Statement on Legalization of Assisted Suicide" opposes assisted suicide, but for nurses practicing in Oregon, leaves the choice to participate in this controversial action up to the individual.[73]

CLINICAL PEARLS: The patient who requests a health care team member to participate in assisted suicide or euthanasia needs expert palliative care. Most often this patient does not really wish to die, but is in such pain or discomfort physically, emotionally, or spiritually that he or she sees no other way out. Any such request should raise a red flag to consult the palliative care team, if available; chaplain or other spiritual support; or a psychiatrist or psychologist.

Euthanasia

Euthanasia, sometimes referred to as mercy killing, is the act of putting to death someone suffering from a painful and prolonged illness or injury. Euthanasia is a criminal offense in the United States. Euthanasia differs from assisted suicide. In euthanasia someone not only makes the means of death available, but also serves as the direct agent of death.[71] The acts of withholding or withdrawing treatments can be legally and ethically acceptable when a patient or family refuse undesired treatments or when treatments disproportionately cause suffering or burden. Further, actions that are intended to relieve suffering in the dying patient but risk hastening death are also legally and ethically acceptable.

Brain Death

Before engaging in a discussion about brain death, it is important to remind the nurse to consider organ donation as early as possible, preferably long before brain death is determined. For some unfortunate patients, the injury to the nervous system is so severe that the injuries are incompatible with life. Neuroscience nurses often are the first person to recognize a pattern that could lead to brain death. Potentially fatal brain injury (e.g., severe brain trauma, major stroke, severe subarachnoid hemorrhage), a Glasgow Coma Score of <5 or absence of two or more brainstem reflexes, being on a ventilator, or sustained intracranial pressure >30 mm Hg are triggers. The appropriate organ procurement organization (OPO) should be called as early as possible when organ donation is even a remote possibility. The OPO will assess each case to determine possible donation. It is the goal of the OPO to rule in as many people as possible for organ donation and, therefore, it is critical to contact the OPO so that they can be involved early to evaluate the patient and make necessary arrangements. For more information call 1-800-558-LIFE (5433).

In 1995 and then reaffirmed in 2003, the American Academy of Neurology published practice parameters for determining brain death in adults.[74] Brain death is a *clinical diagnosis* made by a physician. Brain death is defined as irreversible cessation of all functions of the entire brain, including the brainstem.[67, 75] Diagnosis of brain death is made based on fulfillment of strict, well-defined clinical criteria of irreversible coma, absence of cortical activity, absence of motor response to pain, loss of brainstem reflexes, and apnea. Ancillary diagnostic tests may be used to support the clinical diagnosis, but they are not strictly required to make the diagnosis. It is critical that the cause of the coma be investigated, and that a cause can be identified that is capable of causing irreversible apneic coma when there is no evidence of cerebral or brainstem function.[76]

Three Key Characteristics in Brain Death

The three key characteristics in brain death are coma or unresponsiveness, absence of brainstem reflexes, and apnea.[74]

- **Coma or unresponsiveness.** Definite clinical, neuroimaging, or cerebrospinal fluid evidence of an acute central nervous system catastrophic event compatible with death must be found. All reversible causes of coma must be *excluded* before a diagnosis of brain death can be made. Potentially reversible confounding factors of coma include hypothermia (core temperature below 32°C related to blunted brainstem reflexes); drug intoxication or poisoning; use of neuromuscular blocking agents; severe electrolyte imbalance; severe acid-base abnormalities; and severe metabolic or endocrine imbalance. If barbiturates have been used (e.g., barbiturate-induced coma), the diagnosis of brain death can still be made if the levels of drug are subtherapeutic. In addition, Wijdicks recommends that definite clinical, neuroimaging, or cerebrospinal fluid evidence of an acute central nervous system catastrophic event compatible with brain death must be found.[76]
- **Absence of brainstem reflexes.** Loss of brainstem function is incompatible with life. The brainstem reflexes that are assessed include pupillary reaction to light, corneal reflex, gag reflex, and oculovestibular reflex. All reflexes should be absent in brain death. There should not be a light response to a bright light introduced to the pupil. Most pupils are midposition (4 to 6 mm), although there may be variations from 4 to 9 mm, all of which are compatible with brain death. In addition, pupils may be round, ovoid, or irregularly shaped. The corneal reflex is tested with a wisp of cotton and should be absent. Observe for any grimacing in response to deep pain. The gag reflex is tested with a tongue blade. Along with an absent gag reflex, the cough reflex should also be absent. Ocular movements, as tested by head turning and caloric testing, are absent in brain death. (See Chap. 6 for a description of caloric testing and Chap. 7 for assessment of ocular movement, including precautions to be taken before testing.) Note that sedatives, aminoglycosides, tricyclic antidepressants, anticholinergics, anticonvulsants, and chemotherapeutic agents can diminish or completely abolish caloric response.[74,76] Loss of brainstem function also results in loss of breathing and vasomotor control, which results in apnea and hypotension.
- **Apnea.** In diagnosing brain death, demonstration of apnea to evaluate respiratory drive (brainstem function) is critical. Severe hypotension and cardiac arrhythmias (e.g., premature ventricular contractions, ventricular tachycardia) may occur during apnea testing, either spontaneously due to acidosis or related to inadequate precautions. Therefore, there are prerequisites recommended when testing for apnea: (1) core temperature is 36°C (97°F) or higher; (2) systolic blood pressure 90 mm Hg or more; (3) positive fluid balance in the past 6 hours; (4) arterial PCO_2 normalized between 35 and 45 mm Hg; and (5) arterial PO_2 200 mm Hg or more.[74,76,77]

Although there may be slight variations in institutional protocol for apnea testing, the following outlines a model apnea testing protocol for the physician to implement[74]:

- Preoxygenate with 100% FIO_2 for 30 minutes.
- Disconnect the patient from the ventilator (a PCO_2 rise of 3 to 6 mm Hg/min is estimated in the apneic patient).[78]

- Immediately on disconnection, place an oxygen cannula at the level of the carina and administer 100% oxygen at 9 to 12 L/min by tracheal cannula. Observe for respiratory movement of the chest/abdomen for 8 minutes (a respiration is defined as abdominal or chest movement that produces adequate tidal volume).

- After 10 minutes, draw arterial blood gases. If there is no respiratory movement and the PCO_2 is 60 mm Hg or higher, the clinical diagnosis of brain death is made. If the PCO_2 has not met the target level of 60 mm Hg or higher, apnea testing is repeated after a period of time and confirmatory testing may also be ordered. Note that the target PCO_2 may be higher in patients with chronic hypercapnia (e.g., severe chronic obstructive pulmonary disease, bronchiectasis, sleep apnea, morbid obesity) because the patient's PCO_2 baseline is higher. If chronic hypercapnia is suspected, additional noninvasive confirmatory tests are strongly recommended.[74,76]

Reflex Motor Activity

Spontaneous motor responses of spinal origin sometimes called the "Lazarus sign," observed as limb movements, may be seen in brain death.[79] Possible movements seen, especially in younger patients, can include any of the following: rapid flexion of the arms; raising of one or all of the limbs off of the bed; grasping movements; or jerking of one leg. In addition, multifocal vigorous myoclonus may be noted. Although unexpected, these movements are not purposeful and should not be interpreted as such.

Confirmatory Testing

As mentioned earlier, brain death is a *clinical diagnosis* made by a physician. In most instances, the clinical evaluation is conducted two times with an interval of hours (e.g., 6 to 8 hours) elapsing between examinations. Many hospitals have developed guidelines that often include a requirement of two independent clinical evaluations by two different physicians. Figure 3-1 provides a sample guideline. Confirmatory testing is not required to make the diagnosis of brain death in the United States. However, a physician may choose to include confirmatory tests for patients in whom specific components of the clinical evaluation cannot be reliably tested. Confirmatory tests that are accepted based on clinical experience and reliability include conventional angiography, blood-flow studies (e.g., technetium 99m), electroencephalography, and more recently, transcranial Doppler ultrasonography. Absence of blood flow and electrical activity of the brain are confirmatory findings of brain death. Wijdicks provides an excellent discussion of use, validity, and disadvantages of confirmatory tests and brain death.[76,80]

After brain death has been confirmed, the patient is pronounced brain dead and all treatment is stopped.[81] The time of death is when the second set of brain death clinical evaluations and possible confirmatory tests are met. The organs may be supported for a short period of time if organ harvest is planned.

Organ Procurement

One important result of declaring brain death is the possibility of organ donation. Although kidneys are the most common organs to be donated, other organs, such as the cornea, skin, bone, liver, and heart valves, may be given. When organ donation is considered, donor criteria must be strictly followed.[82] Donor criteria vary depending on the particular organ to be given, but criteria include a specified age range, no history of malignant neoplasms, absence of sepsis or transmittable diseases, and procurement of the organ as quickly as possible, but certainly within a few hours of death. In addition, the medical team involved in the declaration of brain death and the organ harvest team must be kept separate to avoid any special interests. After brain death has been declared and consent has been given for organ donation, the personnel of the organ donor program initiate management. The most common initial physiologic management issues are hypotension, diabetes insipidus, or both. Blood pressure, hydration, and ventilation are supported to provide adequate organ perfusion and oxygenation until surgery. Use of a ventilator, vasopressors, and inotropic drugs (e.g., dopamine, dobutamine) to maintain cardiac function and blood pressure, desmopressin to manage diabetes insipidus, and intravenous fluids is necessary to maintain organ perfusion.

The nurse conveys sensitivity and caring for the patient and family by keeping the patient clean and comfortable-looking.[83] Provisions must be made to support the family in their decision for or against organ donation. In addition, the family needs time and privacy to say their goodbyes to their loved one and to begin the bereavement process. Ideally, bereavement support that is developmentally appropriate for any children should be available. Organ donation requires collaboration among health providers to provide sensitive care.[84]

FOSTERING PROFESSIONAL GROWTH IN ETHICAL DECISION MAKING

Professional Development and Ethical Caring

Exploring the ethical dimensions of professional practice is necessary to understand the duties and obligations in providing care. It also may be uncomfortable because it forces us to examine fundamental and personal life–death issues and personal values as moral beings.[85] The Joint Commission Standards require a formal mechanism to assist in the resolution of ethical problems in patient care in all facilities. All clinicians are also encouraged to become familiar with the mechanisms that exist within their own institutions.

For those nurses engaged in neuroscience nursing, a number of ethical issues arise in everyday practice that can be sources of confusion and discomfort. Modern health care and technology create a complex intersection of culture, religion, politics, and science. It is important for the nurse to examine these situations, identify the type of problem that exists, identify the underlying ethical principles that have some impact on the situation, and sort out the components of

	DATE AND TIME OF EXAM	BODY TEMPERATURE	BLOOD ETHANOL (IF INDICATED)	TOXICOLOGY (IF INDICATED)
1 ST EXAM				
2 ND EXAM				

WRITE A "YES" OR "NO" RESPONSE TO EACH QUESTION	1 ST EXAM	2 ND EXAM
ABSENCE OF CEREBRAL FUNCTIONS IS THE PATIENT IN DEEP COMA, WITHOUT ANY SPONTANEOUS MOVEMENTS OR RESPONSE TO PAINFUL STIMULI ADMINISTERED OVER THE AREAS OF CRANIAL NERVE DISTRIBUTION (e.g., SUPRAORBITAL PRESSURE) AND WITHOUT DECORTICATE OR DECEREBRATE POSTURING? (SPINAL REFLEXES MAY BE PRESENT).		
ABSENCE OF BRAIN STEM FUNCTIONS—CRANIAL NERVE REFLEXES:		
1. ARE PUPILS FIXED TO LIGHT?		
2. ARE CORNEAL REFLEXES ABSENT?		
3. ARE OCULOCEPHALIC REFLEXES ABSENT?		
4. ARE COLD WATER OCULOVESTIBULAR REFLEXES ABSENT?		
5. ARE OROPHARYNGEAL RESPONSES ABSENT?		
6. ARE SPONTANEOUS RESPIRATIONS ABSENT?		
APNEA TEST 1. ARE SPONTANEOUS BREATHING MOVEMENTS ABSENT DURING APNEA TESTS?		
2. LIST $PaCO_2$ AT END OF APNEA TEST.		

NAMES AND SIGNATURE OF EXAMINING PHYSICIANS

	PHYSICIAN SIGNATURE	NAME PRINTED
1 ST EXAM	PHYSICIAN SIGNATURE	NAME PRINTED
	PHYSICIAN SIGNATURE	NAME PRINTED
2 ND EXAM	PHYSICIAN SIGNATURE	NAME PRINTED

CONFIRMATORY TEST(S) DATE, TIME, AND RESULTS OF ALL CONFIRMATORY TESTS

_____

_____

_____

CERTIFICATION OF DEATH BY NEUROLOGICAL CRITERIA

HAVING CONSIDERED THE ABOVE FINDINGS, WE HEREBY CERTIFY THE DEATH OF				
PATIENT NAME		DATE	TIME	☐ AM ☐ PM
PHYSICIAN SIGNATURE		NAME PRINTED		
PHYSICIAN SIGNATURE		NAME PRINTED		

Figure 3-1 • A sample checklist for determination of death by neurological criteria. The cause of coma must be established and sufficient to account for the loss of all brain function. Reversible conditions, such as drug sedation, metabolic disturbance, hypothermia (below 32.2°C), neuromuscular blockage, and shock, must be searched for and appropriately treated.

Two separate clinical examinations must be completed, the second no sooner than *6 hours after the first*. Each examination must be conducted by two physicians, independent of each other, who shall be licensed to practice medicine in the state. (Note that in this sample form, the institution requires two physicians to examine the patient each time.) The physicians may or may not choose to perform cold calorics.

the clinical situation to arrive at a sense of understanding that will guide clinical practice. Professional development in ethical care must be supported by departments of nursing and health care institutions in several ways; institutional ethics committees, ethics rounds, interdisciplinary ethical educational programs, palliative care services, and discussion groups are helpful in responding to individual patient situations and needs of health professionals.

Institutional Ethics Committee

All health care facilities have some form of an institutional ethics committee. Committee membership is multidisciplinary to represent multiple perspectives and expertise. Often, community representation is sought and may include an ethicist, an attorney, and a layperson. The committee's purposes include education, development of institutional guidelines and standards, concurrent case review, and retroactive case review. Many of the substantive issues center on neurological patients.

Ethics Rounds

Ethics rounds should be conducted on patient care units periodically to support ongoing staff education and to identify patient situations in need of ethical exploration. These rounds have a clinical focus and are usually directed by a group leader with an interest and background in ethics and clinical decision making. Particular patient situations can be reviewed to examine ethical components of care and the bases for decision making. Ethics rounds help to examine and clarify standards of care to address the ethical aspects of care and the rationale for those actions. Other resources can also be identified that may be helpful in resolving ethical matters when there is a need for assistance.

Ethics Educational Programs and Discussion Groups

Interprofessional educational programs with a focus in ethics are important to promote professional growth of the staff. They may be focused on the review of new guidelines or patient care situations. Ethics discussion groups are an informal method for discussion of topics of interest related to the ethical dimension of practice. The discussion may or may not address a currently active clinical situation in that facility. Cases reported in the press, recent legal opinions rendered, or the ethical dimensions of a new technology may be among the topics discussed. This forum provides the opportunity to consider a proactive approach to a potential problem. Other issues that may be addressed include clinical situations within the facility that were not adequately resolved in the past and that deserve a fresh review.

Application of the Ethical Dimension to Clinical Practice

Ethical and legal dimensions of nursing practice cut across all clinical areas of practice. Ethics and legality need to be rec-

ognized as separate, although often interacting, concerns.[86] For nurses practicing in neuroscience, the complexity of ethical practice is further compounded by the fact that the "organ of reason" is often impaired, thus raising questions about decision-making capability, autonomy, and best interest. Many of the clinical questions confronting the neuroscience nurse are life-and-death situations in which there are no second chances to undo previously made decisions. This places a tremendous burden of responsibility to do the "right thing." Some situations precipitate an ethical dilemma for the practitioner. It is, therefore, imperative to prepare oneself for this awesome responsibility through ongoing professional education and development.

REFERENCES

1. American Nurses Association. (2001). *Code ethics for nurses with interpretive statements*. Washington, DC: Author.
2. International Council of Nurses. (2006). *The ICN code of ethics for nurses*. Geneva, Switzerland: Author.
3. Riley, J. M., Mahoney, M. J., Fry, S. T., & Field, L. (1999). Factors related to adult patient decision making about withholding or withdrawing nutrition and/or hydration. *The Online Journal of Knowledge Synthesis for Nursing, 6*(3), 1–20.
4. The Internet Encyclopedia of Philosophy. *Ethics*. Retrieved June 24, 2006, from http://www.utm.edu/research/iep/e/ethics.htm
5. Pryor-McCann, J. M. (1990). Ethics in critical care nursing. *Critical Care Nursing Clinics of North America, 2*(1), 1–13.
6. Wikipedia. (2006). Morality. Retrieved June 24, 2006, from http://en.wikipedia.org/wiki/Morality
7. Rachels, J. (1986). *Elements of moral philosophy*. New York: Random House.
8. Wikipedia. (2006). Medical ethics. Retrieved June 24, 2006, from http://en.wikipedia.org/wiki/Medical_ethics
9. Wikipedia. (2006). Justice. Retrieved June 24, 2006, from http://en.wikipedia.org/wiki/Justice
10. *In re Karen Quinlan*, 70 N.J. 10, 335 A. 2d 647 (1976).
11. Ropper, A. H., Gress, D. R., Diringer, M. N., Green, D. M., Mayer, S. A., & Black, T. P. (2004). Ethical and legal aspects applicable to the neurological intensive care unit. In A. H. Ropper, D. R. Gress, M. N. Diringer, D. M. Green, S. A. Mayer, & T. P. Bleck (Eds.). *Neurological and neurosurgical intensive care* (4th ed., pp. 363–375). Philadelphia: Lippincott Williams & Wilkins.
12. SUPPORT Principal Investigators. (1995). A controlled trial to improve care of seriously ill hospitalized patients: The Study to Understand the Prognoses and Preferences for Outcomes and Risks of Treatment (SUPPORT). *Journal of the American Medical Association, 274*(20), 1591–1598.
13. Reckling, J. A. B. (1997). Who plays what role in decisions about withholding and withdrawing life-sustaining treatment? *Journal of Clinical Ethics, 8*(1), 30–45.
14. Curtis, J. R., Patrick, D. L., Shannon, S. E., Treece, P. D., Engelberg, R. A., and Rubenfeld, G. D. (2001). The family conference as a focus to improve communication about end-of-life care in the intensive care unit: Opportunities for improvement. *Critical Care Medicine, 29*(2), (Suppl.), 26–33.
15. Rushton, D. H., Williams, M. A., & Sabatier, K. H. (2002). The integration of palliative care and critical care: One vision, one voice. *Critical Care Nursing Clinics of North America, 14*, 133–140.
16. Terry, P. B., & Korzick, K. A. (1997). Thoughts about the end-of-life decision-making process. *The Journal of Clinical Ethics, 8*(1), 46–49.
17. Weissman, D. E. (2004). Decision making at a time of crisis near the end of life. *Journal of the American Medical Association, 292*(14), 1738–1743.

18. Fins, J. J., & Solomon, M. Z. (2001). Communications in intensive care settings: The challenge of futility disputes. *Critical Care Medicine, 29*(2), (Suppl.), N10–15.

19. Fetters, M. D., Churchill, L., & Danis, M. (2001). Conflict resolution at the end of life. *Critical Care Medicine, 29*(5), 921–925.

20. Ambuel, B., and Weissman, D. E. (2005). *Fast facts and concepts #16 moderating and end-of-life family conference* (2nd ed.). End-of-Life Palliative Education Resource Center. www.eperc.mcw.edu. Washington, DC.

21. Thelen, M. (2005). End-of-life decision making in intensive care. *Critical Care Nurse, 25*(6), 28–38.

22. Owens, D., & Flom, J. (2005). Integrating palliative and neurological critical care. *AACN Clinical Issues, 16*(4), 542–550.

23. Curtis, J. R., Patrick, D. L., Shannon, S. E., Treece, P. D., Engelberg, R. A., & Rubenfeld, G. D. (2001). The family conference as a focus to improve communications about end-of-life care in the intensive care unit: Opportunities for improvement. *Critical Care Medicine, 29*(2), (Suppl.), N26–33.

24. Hastings Center Report. (1987). *Guidelines on the termination of life-sustaining treatment and the care of the dying* (p. 131). Bloomington, IN: Indiana University Press.

25. President's Commission for the Study of Ethical Problems in Medicine and Biomedical and Behavioral Research. (1983). *Deciding to forego life-sustaining treatment: A report on the ethical, medical, and legal issues in treatment decisions* (p. 121). Washington, DC: U.S. Government Printing Office.

26. Hoffinan, N. (1992). Ethical considerations and quality of life. *Cardiovascular Clinics, 22*(2), 243–251.

27. Emanuel, E. J., & Emanuel, L. L. (1992). Proxy decision making for incompetent patients: An ethical and empirical analysis. *Journal of the American Medical Association, 267*(15), 2067–2071.

28. Lee, M. A., Smith, D. M., Fenn, D. S., & Ganzini, L. (1998). Do patients' treatment decisions match advanced statements of their preferences? *The Journal of Clinical Ethics, 9*(3), 258–262.

29. Kyba, F. C. N. (2000). End of life decisions: Legal and ethical quandaries. *Texas Nursing, 74*(3), 6–12.

30. Cranford, R. E. (1984). Termination of treatment in the persistent vegetative state. *Seminars in Neurology, 4,* 36–44.

31. Texas Health and Safety Code, Chapter 166. (1999). Advance directives. (Codification of S.B. 1260, An act pertaining to certain advance directives for medical treatment; providing administrative penalties.)

32. Winzelberg, G. S., Hanson, L. C., & Tulsky, J. A. (2005). Beyond autonomy: Diversifying end-of-life decision-making approaches to serve patient and families. *Journal of the American Geriatrics Society, 53,* 1046–1050.

33. Center for Disease Control and Prevention, National Center for Health Statistics. (2005). Table E: Deaths and percentage of total deaths for the 10 leading causes of death, by race: United States, 2002. *National Vital Statistics Reports, 53*(17), 9. http://www.cdc.gov/nchs/data/dvs/nvsr53_17tableE2002.pdf

34. Institute of Medicine. (1997). *Approaching death: Improving care at the end of life.* Washington, DC: National Academy of Sciences.

35. Matzo, M. L., & Sherman, D. W. (Eds.). (2001). *Palliative care nursing: Quality care to the end of life.* New York: Springer Publishing Company.

36. World Health Organization. (1990). *Cancer pain relief and palliative care.* Technical Report series 804. Geneva, Switzerland: Author.

37. Doyle, D., Hanks, G. W. C., & MacDonald, N. (1998). *Oxford textbook of palliative medicine* (2nd ed.). Oxford: Oxford University Press.

38. Ferrell, B., Virani, R., & Grant, M. (1999). Analysis of end-of-life content in nursing textbooks. *Oncology Nursing Forum, 26*(2), 869–876.

39. Mularski, R. A., Bascom, P., & Osborne, M. L. Educational agendas for interdisciplinary end-of-life curricula. *Critical Care Medicine, 29*(2), (Suppl.), N16–23.

40. Weissman, D. E. (2004). Decision making at a time of crisis near the end of life. *Journal of the American Medical Association, 292*(14), 1738–1743.

41. Black, A. L., & Arnold, R. M. (2005). Dealing with conflict in caring for the seriously ill: "It was just out of the question". *Journal of the American Medical Association, 293*(11), 1374–1381.

42. *In re Karen Quinlan,* 70 N.J. 10, 335 A. 2d 647 (1976).

43. *Satz v. Perlmutter,* 13 Sept. 1978. Florida District Court of Appeal, Fourth District. Southern Reporter, 2nd Series, 362:160–164.

44. *In re Conroy,* 486 A2d 1209 (N.J. 1985).

45. Price, D. M., & Murphy, P. A. (1994). Tube feeding and the ethics of caring. *Journal of Nursing Law, 1*(4), 53–59.

46. *Brophy v. New England Sinai Hospital, Inc.,* 497 N.E.2d 626 (Mass. 1986).

47. *Cruzan v. Director, Missouri Department of Health,* 497 U.S. 261 (1990).

48. Perry, J. E., Churchill, L. R., & Kirshner, H. S. (2005). The Terri Schiavo case: Legal, ethical and medical perspectives. *Annals of Internal Medicine, 143*(10), 744–748.

49. Corbett, T. E. (1986). Council on Ethical and Judicial Affairs, American Medical Association. Statement on withholding or withdrawing life prolonging treatment. *Journal of the American Medical Association, 256*(19), 1263.

50. The Hastings Center. (1987). *Guidelines on the termination of life-sustaining treatment and the care of the dying.* Briarcliff Manor, NY: Author.

51. American Academy of Neurology. (1989). Position of the American Academy of Neurology on certain aspects of the care and management of the persistent vegetative state patient. *Neurology, 39,* 125–126.

52. American Academy of Neurology. (1989). Guidelines on the vegetative state: Commentary on the American Academy of Neurology statement. *Neurology, 39,* 123–124.

53. Troug, R. D., Cist, A. F., Brackett, S. E., Burns, J. P., Curley, M. A., Danis, N., et al. (2001). Recommendations for end-of-life care in the intensive care unit: The Ethics Committee of the Society of Critical Care Medicine. *Critical Care Medicine, 29*(12), 2332–2348.

54. Committee on Ethics, American Nurses Association. (1992). Guidelines on withholding food and fluids from patients. *Nursing Outlook, 36,* 122–123, 148–150.

55. Wagner, B., Ersek, M., & Riddell, S. (2003). HPNA position statement: Artificial nutrition and hydration in end-of-life care. Retrieved July 6, 2006 from www.hpna.org

56. Committee on Ethics, American Nurses Association. (2003). Position statement on pain management and control of distressing symptoms in dying patients. Retrieved July 6, 2006 from http://www.nursingworld.org/readroom/position/ethics/etpain.htm

57. U. S. Department of Health and Human Services. (1994). *Management of cancer pain: Clinical practice guidelines, #9.* Rockville, MD: Author.

58. Amenta, M., & Bohnet, N. L. (Eds.). (1986). *Palliative care nursing.* Boston: Little, Brown.

59. Melzack, R. (1990). The tragedy of needless pain. *Scientific American, 262,* 27–33.

60. Solano, J. P., Gomes, B., & Higginson, I. J. (2006). A comparison of symptom prevalence in far advanced cancer, AIDS, heart disease, chronic obstructive pulmonary disease and renal disease. *Journal of Pain and Symptom Management, 31*(1), 58–69.

61. Dalton, J. A., & Fenerstein, M. (1988). Biobehavioral factors in cancer pain. *Pain, 33,* 137.

62. Kachoyenos, M. K., & Zollo, M. B. (1995). Ethics in pain management of infants and children. *Maternal Child Nursing, 20,* 142–147.

63. American Pain Society. (1993). *Principles of analgesic use in the treatment of acute pain and cancer pain* (3rd ed.). Skokie, IL: Author.

64. McCaffery, M., & Pasero, C. (1999). *Pain clinical manual* (2nd ed., p. 429). St. Louis, MO: Mosby.

65. Ersek, M., Wagner, B., Ferrell, B. R., Paice, J. A., & Scanlon, C. (2004). HPNA position statement: Providing opioids at the end of life. Retrieved July 6, 2006 from www.hpna.org

66. Huxtable, R. (2004). Get out of jail free? The doctrine of double effect English law. *Palliative Medicine, 18,* 62–68.

67. Guidelines for the determination of death: Report of the medical consultants on the diagnosis of brain death to the President's Commission for the Study of Ethical Problems in Medicine and Biomedical and Behavioral Research. (1981). *Journal of the American Medical Association, 246,* 2184–2186.

68. Beauchamp, T. L. (1996). Refusals of treatment and requests for death. *Kennedy Institute of Ethics Journal, 6*(4), 371–374.

69. The Ethics and Humanities Committee of the American Academy of Neurology. (1998). Assisted suicide, euthanasia, and the neurologist (position statement). *Neurology, 50,* 596–598.

70. Beder, J. (1998). Legalization of assisted suicide: A pilot study of gerontological nurses. *Journal of Gerontological Nursing, 23*(4), 14–20.

71. American Nurses Association. (1994). *Position statement on active euthanasia.* Washington, DC: Author.

72. American Nurses Association. (1996). Position statement on assisted suicide. In *Compendium of ANA position statements.* Washington, DC: Author.

73. HPNA position statement: Legalization of assisted suicide. (2001). Retrieved July 6, 2006 from www.hpna.org

74. Quality Standards Subcommittee of the American Academy of Neurology. (1995). Practice parameters for determining brain death in adults. *Neurology, 45,* 1012–1014 (reaffirmed October 18, 2003 on website).

75. Cantrill, S. V. (1997). Brain death. *Emergency Medicine Clinics of North America, 15*(3), 713–722.

76. Wijdicks, E. F. M. (2001). The diagnosis of brain death. *New England Journal of Medicine, 344*(16), 1215–1221.

77. Ropper, A. H., Kennedy, S. K., & Russell, L. (1981). Apnea testing in the diagnosis of brain death: Clinical and physiological observations. *Journal of Neurosurgery, 55,* 942–946.

78. Eger, E. I., & Severinghaus, J. W. (1961). The rate of rise of $PaCO_2$ in the apneic anesthetized patient. *Anesthesiology 22,* 419–425.

79. Ropper, A. H. (1984). Unusual spontaneous movements in brain-dead patients. *Neurology, 34,* 1012–1014.

80. Mayer, S. A., & Dossoff, S. B. (1999). Withdrawal of life support in the neurological intensive care unit. *Neurology, 52,* 1602–1609.

81. Cranford, R. E. (1989). The neurologist as ethics consultant and as a member of the institutional ethics committee. *Neurologic Clinics, 7*(4), 697–713.

82. Wood, K. E., Becker, B. N., McCartney, J. G., Alessandro, A. M., & Coursin, D. B. (2004). Care of the potential organ donor. *New England Journal of Medicine, 351*(26), 2730–2739.

83. Daly, B. J. (2006). End-of-life decision making, organ donation, and critical care nurses. *Critical Care Nurse, 26*(2), 78–86.

84. Shafer, T. J., Wagner, D., Chessare, J., Zampiello, F. A., & Perdue, J. (2006). Organ donation breakthrough collaborative: Increasing organ donation through system redesign. *Critical Care Nurse, 26*(2), 33–49.

85. Kaldjian, L. C., Weir, R. F., & Duffy, T. P. (2005). A clinician's approach to clinical ethical reasoning. *Journal of General Internal Medicine, 20*(3), 306–311.

86. Wocial, L. D. (1996). Achieving collaboration in ethical decision making: Strategies for nurses in clinical practice. *Dimensions of Critical Care Nursing, 15*(3), 150–159.

RESOURCES

Websites

American Nurses Association: http://www.nursingworld.org

End of Life/Palliative Education Resource Center: http://www.eperc.mcw.edu/ff_index.htm

Hospice and Palliative Nurses Association: http://www.hpna.org

The Joint Commission: http://thejointcommission.org

Last Acts: A national coalition to improve care and caring at the end of life: http://lastacts.org

National Consensus Project for Quality Palliative Care: http://www.nationalconsensusproject.org

Assessment and Evaluation of Neuroscience Patients

Overview of Neuroanatomy and Neurophysiology

Joanne V. Hickey and Joseph T. Kanusky

This chapter provides an overview of basic and essential neuroanatomy and neurophysiology as a quick reference to assist the reader in understanding the underlying principles of neurological function and dysfunction as a basis for nursing management. Further discussion of anatomy and physiology is included in many other chapters to enhance understanding. Neuroanatomy and neurophysiology texts should be consulted if more detail is desired.

EMBRYONIC DEVELOPMENT OF THE NERVOUS SYSTEM

The human brain is composed of about 100 billion cells. The nervous system is one of the first recognizable features in embryonic development. From a simple longitudinal invagination on the dorsal portion of the ectodermal layer, a neural groove and neural tube form at about 3 weeks. At the cranial end of the neural tube, rapid and unequal growth occurs, giving rise to the three primary vesicles of the brain: the prosencephalon, or forebrain; the mesencephalon, or midbrain; and the rhombencephalon, or hindbrain. Early in the second fetal month, these vesicles, in turn, become five cerebral areas: the telencephalon, or endbrain; the diencephalon, or between brain; the mesencephalon; the metencephalon, or afterbrain; and the myelencephalon, or spinal brain (Table 4-1). By 7 weeks, the brain and spinal cord are apparent. At 12 weeks, the brain is the size of a large pea.

Concurrently, cells of the neural tube form two types of cells: spongioblasts, which give rise to the neuroglia (glia) cells, and neuroblasts, which give rise to the nerve cells (neurons). Processes from the neuroblasts form the white matter of the brain. Some of these processes leave the brain and spinal cord to form the fibers of the cranial and ventral roots of the spinal nerves.

Throughout the prenatal period, there is further growth and refinement of the nervous system. All the neurons that a person will ever have are present at birth. These highly specialized cells do not have mitotic capacity and, therefore, are not replaceable. At birth, the brain is about one quarter the size of an adult brain. Abnormalities in neural tube development can result in spinal bifida, meningocele, or myelomeningocele.

CELLS OF THE NERVOUS SYSTEM

From the ectodermal layer, two types of cells develop: neurons and neuroglia cells. **Neurons** are the basic anatomic and functional unit of the nervous system. **Neuroglia cells** provide a variety of supportive functions for the neurons.

Neuroglia Cells

The term *glia* comes from a Greek word meaning "glue" or "holding together." In this regard, the glia cells provide structural support, nourishment, and protection for the neurons of the nervous system. There are 5 to 10 times more neuroglia cells than there are neurons. About 40% of the brain and spinal cord is composed of neuroglia cells.

From a clinical viewpoint, neuroglia cells are important because they can divide by mitosis and are the major source of primary tumors of the nervous system. In the central nervous system (CNS), glia is subdivided into four main types: astrocytes, oligodendrocytes, ependymal cells, and microglia. In the peripheral nervous system (PNS), Schwann cells form myelin sheaths.

Astrocytes have multiple processes extending from the cell body that give it a star-like appearance. Some astrocytic processes may terminate as swellings called *end-feet* on neurons and blood vessels. Functions attributed to astrocytes include providing nutrition for neurons, regulating synaptic connectivity, removing cellular debris, and controlling movement of molecules from blood to brain (part of the blood–brain barrier).

On microscopic examination, **oligodendrocytes** have few branching processes. Oligodendrocytes produce the myelin sheath of the axonal projections of neurons in the CNS. An individual cell can maintain the myelin sheaths of several axons.

Ciliated **ependyma cells** line the ventricular system and the choroid plexuses. They aid in the production of cerebrospinal fluid (CSF) and act as a barrier to foreign

TABLE 4–1   DEVELOPMENT OF THE PRIMARY VESICLES

PRIMARY VESICLES	SUBDIVISIONS	STRUCTURES THAT ARISE	VENTRICULAR SYSTEM
	Telencephalon	Cerebral hemisphere, corpus callosum, basal ganglia, olfactory tracts	Lateral ventricles and part of third ventricle
Prosencephalon (forebrain) — Wall Cavity	Diencephalon	Thalamus Hypothalamus	Most of third ventricle
Mesencephalon (midbrain)	Mesencephalon	Midbrain	Cerebral aqueducts
Rhombencephalon (hindbrain)	Metencephalon Myelencephalon	Pons Cerebellum	Fourth ventricle
	Spinal cord	Medulla oblongata	Fourth ventricle and part of central canal

substances within the ventricles, preventing them from entering cerebral tissue.

Microglia cells are minute cells that are scattered throughout the CNS and have a phagocytic function. They remove and disintegrate the waste products of neurons.

Schwann cells function similarly to oligodendrocytes, forming the insulating myelin sheaths around axons to facilitate saltatory conduction of impulses in the PNS.

Neurons

Neurons vary from 5 to 100 μm in diameter. As the basic anatomic and functional unit in the nervous system, the neuron has a number of functions: responding to sensory and chemical stimuli, conducting impulses, and releasing specific chemical regulators.

Neurons are classified as unipolar, bipolar, or multipolar. **Unipolar neurons** possess only one process or pole. This process divides close to the cell body. One branch, called the peripheral process, carries impulses from the periphery toward the cell body. The other branch, called the central process, conducts the impulse toward the spinal cord or the brainstem. **Bipolar neurons** are found only in the spinal and vestibular ganglia, the olfactory mucous membrane, and one layer of the retina. The anatomic structure is peculiar to the organ in which it is found. Most neurons in the nervous system are **multipolar.** These neurons consist of a cell body, one long projection (the **axon**), and one or more shorter branches (the **dendrites**).

There are three major components of a neuron: a **cell body,** which constitutes the main part of the neuron; a **single axon,** or **axis cylinder,** which consists of a long projection extending from the cell body; and **several dendrites,** which are thin projections extending from the cell body into the immediate surrounding area. The axon carries impulses **away** from the cell body, whereas the dendrites direct impulses **toward** the cell body.

COMPONENTS OF THE CELL BODY

The main organelles of the neuronal cell body include the nucleus, the cell membrane, and the cytoplasm. There are organelles within each of these structures that are important and are mentioned here briefly.

The **nucleus** is a double-membrane structure that contains chromatin and a prominent nucleolus. **Chromatin** is the thread-like structures in the cell nucleus that consist primarily of **deoxyribonucleic acid (DNA)** and protein. DNA contains genes and the genetic code or information about the cell. The **nucleolus** contains **ribonucleic acid (RNA).** RNA is the "messenger" from the genes of the nucleus; it contains the code for synthesis of specific cellular proteins.

A lipid bilayer is the basic **cell membrane** structure. The cell membrane is a solution of globular proteins dispersed in a fluid phospholipids matrix. The cell membrane creates the parameters of the cell body, enclosing the cytoplasm within its border. The main purpose of the cell membrane is to control the interchange of material between the cell and its environment.

The **cytoplasm** contains smooth and rough endoplasmic reticula, Nissl bodies, Golgi apparatus, mitochondria, lysosomes, neurotubules, and neurofibrils. The **endoplasmic reticulum** of the cytoplasm is a network of tubular membranous structures. There are two types of endoplasmic reticulum, smooth and rough. The smooth endoplasmic reticulum serves as the site for enzyme reactions. **Centrioles** are found in the cytoplasm and take part in cell division. **Nissl bodies** are masses of granular (rough) endoplasmic reticulum with ribosomes, which are the protein-synthesizing machinery of the neuron. The endoplasmic reticulum system connects with the nucleus at that portion of the reticulum called the Golgi apparatus. Substances formed in different parts of the cell are transported throughout the cell by means of this system. The **Golgi apparatus** provides for two interrelated functions: further modification of protein by adding carbohydrates and temporary storage and separation of protein types, depending on their function and destination. It is also responsible for the formation of substances important for the digestion of intracellular material.

Mitochondria are structures that serve as the site for production of most cellular energy. Cell nutrients are oxidized to produce carbon dioxide and water. The energy released is used to produce adenosine triphosphate (ATP). **Lysosomes** isolate the digestive enzymes of a cell from the cytoplasm to prevent cell destruction. They are involved in digestion of phagocytosis products and worn-out organelles.

The elongated axons or dendrites can extend 1 meter or more from the cell body. These fibers require protein and other substances produced in the cell body that must be transported from the cytoplasm by a process called *axoplasmic flow*. **Neurotubules** carry out part of axoplasmic transport. **Neurofibrils** are delicate thread-like structures within

the cytoplasm and the axon hillock that assist in the transport of cellular material.

CELL PROCESSES: AXONS AND DENDRITES

Axons and **dendrites** constitute the cell processes. Dendrites usually extend only a short distance from the cell body and branch profusely. By contrast, an axon can extend for long distances from the cell body before branching near the end of the projection.

Many axons in the PNS are covered by a myelin sheath composed of a white, lipid substance that acts as an insulator for the conduction of impulses. Nerve fibers enclosed in such a sheath are referred to as **myelinated;** those without the myelin sheath are referred to as **unmyelinated** (Fig. 4-1).

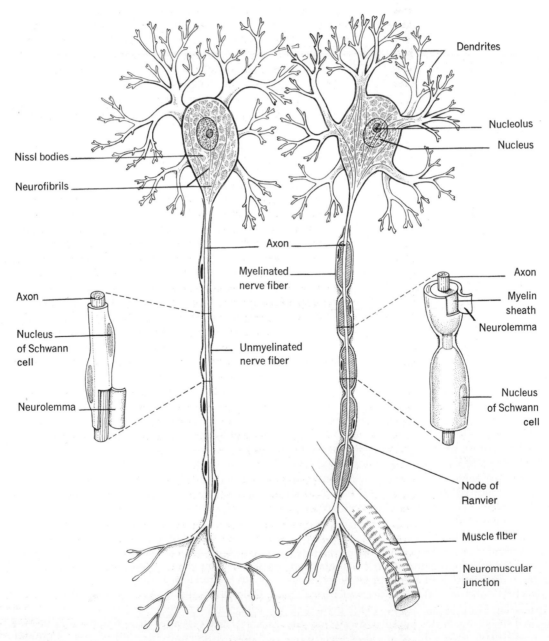

Figure 4-1 • Typical neurons: unmyelinated fiber (*left*); myelinated fiber (*right*). (From Chaffee, E. E., & Lytle, I. M. [1980]. *Basic physiology and anatomy.* Philadelphia: J. B. Lippincott.)

As a rule, larger neuron fibers are myelinated, whereas smaller fibers are unmyelinated.

The **myelin sheath** is formed by Schwann cells that encircle the axons. When several **Schwann cells** are wrapped around an axon, their outer layer (sheath of Schwann) encloses the myelin sheath. This outer layer is called the **neurolemma** and is said to be necessary for the regeneration of axons. The myelin sheath itself is a segmented, discontinuous layer that is interrupted at intervals by the **nodes of Ranvier.** The distance from one node to the next is called an **internode.** Each internode is formed by, and surrounded by, one Schwann cell. At the junction between each of the two successive Schwann cells along the axon, a small noninsulated area remains where ions can easily flow between the extracellular fluid and the axon. It is this area that is known as the node of Ranvier. In the CNS, the oligodendroglial cells provide the myelination of the neurons, similar to the role of the Schwann cells in the PNS. Myelination abnormalities can result in dysfunction in the central nervous system such as multiple sclerosis or peripheral nervous system such as Guillain-Barré syndrome.

PHYSIOLOGY OF NERVE IMPULSES

Resting Membrane Potential of the Neurons

Although a resting neuron is not conducting an impulse, it is considered to be a charged cell. The difference in electrical charge on either side of the membrane is called the **potential difference** and is related to the unequal distribution of potassium and sodium on either side of the membrane. The neuronal cell membrane is electrically polarized to a resting membrane potential of about -80 mV. By convention, the outside side of the membrane is considered to be at 0 mV; therefore, at a resting potential of -80 mV means the inside of the membrane is 80 mV negative to the outside. The resting membrane potential results from the separation of charges across the cell membrane.

The cell membrane is both semipermeable and selectively permeable. The area outside the cell is called the interstitial space; the area inside the cell is called the intracellular space. Sodium ions (Na^+) and chloride ions (Cl^-) are found in much greater concentrations in the interstitial space than in the cell. The potassium ion (K^+) and organic protein material are found in high concentrations within the cell. Diffusion is responsible for the movement of Na^+ and K^+ to the other side of the membrane. If they ever reach equilibrium there will no longer be a resting membrane potential. The maintenance of the resting membrane potential lies with K^+ and Na^+. Two transport proteins are primarily responsible for the resting membrane potential: a K^+ leak channel that permits K^+ to diffuse out of the cell, and the sodium potassium pump (Na^+,K^+-ATPase). The Na^+,K^+-ATPase pumps two K^+ back into the cell at the same time that it pumps three Na^+ out of the cell. Both processes keep the concentration gradient across the cell membrane constant. The concentration of dissolved ions in a solution is a potential source of energy to drive cellular processes.

Action Potential of the Neuron

The fluid and ions in the intracellular space create a highly conductive solution. The large diameter (10 to 80 μm) allows for unrestricted conduction of impulses from one part of the interior of the cell to the other. Various stimuli can change the permeability of the cell membrane to certain ions, resulting in alterations in the membrane potential (Fig. 4-2). The stimuli must be of sufficient magnitude to conduct an impulse and thus create an **action potential,** which is the fundamental unit of signaling in the nervous system.

Many simultaneous discharges at the synaptic junction must occur to create a sufficient effect on the cell membrane. The membrane potential reverses, and the intracellular surface becomes positive (approximately $+20$ to $+40$ mV). When the action potential is realized, there is a sudden reversal of the sodium and potassium relationship across the cell membrane of the axon. This event is called **depolarization.** The neuron receives an influx of sodium and loses potassium to the interstitial space; the time required is only a few milliseconds. With the change in polarity, an impulse is conducted from one neuron to the next at the same amplitude and speed. The cell repolarizes and returns to its resting membrane potential. This sequence of events occurs during the conduction of an impulse in an unmyelinated nerve.

Saltatory Conduction

In myelinated nerves, an action potential hops from one node of Ranvier to the next as a means of rapidly conducting an impulse. This is called **saltatory conduction.** Although ions cannot flow out through the myelin sheath of myelinated nerves, the break in the myelin sheath at the nodes of Ranvier (see Fig. 4-1) provides a perfect route of escape. At this point, the membrane is several times more permeable than many unmyelinated nerves. Impulses are conducted from node to node rather than continuing along the entire span of the axon, as is the case in unmyelinated nerves. Saltatory conduction is advantageous because it increases the velocity of an impulse and conserves energy (because only the nodes depolarize). The velocity of an impulse depends on both the thickness of the myelin and the distance between the internodes. As these two factors increase, the velocity of the impulse also increases.

Synapse

The junction between one neuron and the next at which an impulse is transmitted is called the **synapse.** There are three anatomic structures that are necessary for an impulse to be transmitted at a synapse. These include the presynaptic terminals, the synaptic cleft, and the postsynaptic membrane (Fig. 4-3).

Presynaptic terminals are either excitatory or inhibitory. An excitatory presynaptic terminal secretes an excitatory substance into the synaptic cleft, thereby exciting the effector neuron. The inhibitory presynaptic terminal secretes an inhibitory transmitter that, when secreted into the synaptic cleft, inhibits the effector neuron. The excitatory or inhibitory

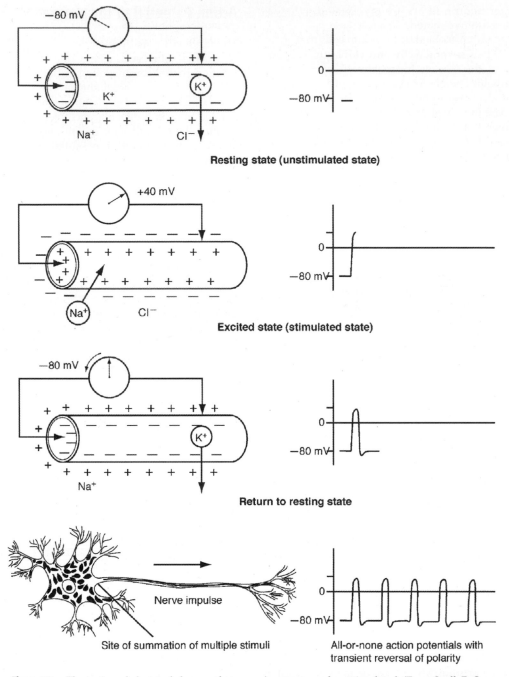

Figure 4-2 • The ionic and electrical changes that occur in a neuron when stimulated. (From Snell, R. S. [1997]. *Clinical neuroanatomy for medical students* [4th ed.]. Philadelphia: Lippincott Williams & Wilkins.)

transmitter secretions arise from the **synaptic vesicle** in the presynaptic terminal of the axon. Mitochondria in the axon supply the ATP to synthesize new transmitter secretions. The **synaptic cleft** is the microscopic space (200 to 300 Å) between the presynaptic terminal and the receptor area of the effector cell. The **postsynaptic membrane** is that part of the effector membrane distal to the presynaptic terminal.

When an action potential spreads over the presynaptic terminal, the membrane depolarizes, emptying some of the contents of the presynaptic vesicles into the synaptic cleft. The released transmitter changes the permeability of the postsynaptic membrane. This results in either excitation or inhibition of the neuron, depending on the type of transmitter substances secreted into the synaptic cleft.

Neurotransmitters

Chemical substances found in the CNS that excite, inhibit, or modify the response of another cerebral cell or cells are called **neurotransmitters.** The presynaptic terminals of one neuron release the chemical that affects particular postsynaptic cells of another neuron. Generally, each neuron releases the same transmitter at all of its separate terminals.

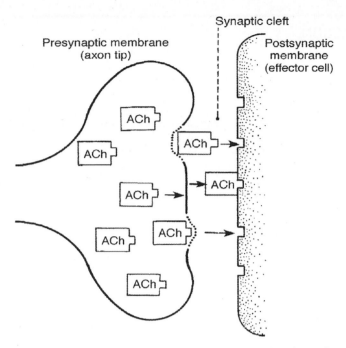

Figure 4-3 • Conduction at synapses. Diagram shows the release of a neurotransmitter (in this case acetylcholine [Ach]) from the presynaptic membrane (axon tip) into the synaptic cleft, where it bonds to the receptor sites of the postsynaptic membrane (effector cell). (From DeMyer, W. [1998]. *Neuroanatomy* [2nd ed.]. Baltimore: Williams & Wilkins.)

Over 100 neurotransmitters have been identified. They include specific **amines** (acetylcholine, serotonin), **catecholamines** (dopamine, epinephrine, and norepinephrine), **amino acids** (γ-amino butyric acid [GABA], glutei acid, lysine, and substance P), and **polypeptides** (endorphins and enkephalins). Table 4-2 summarizes the major neurotransmitters.

Postsynaptic Membrane–Excitation and Inhibition

The postsynaptic membrane (the dendrite cell body region of the effector neuron) initiates its response to stimuli by decremental conduction through the synapse; that is, the impulse becomes progressively weaker during more prolonged periods of excitation. Stimulation of the effector cell at the dendrite cell body can create an action potential. For the action potential to be fired, however, the intensity of an impulse must be sufficient to fire the initial segment of axon (just distal to the axon hillock), where the action potential is initiated. It is said that any factor that increases the potential inside the cell body at any given point also increases the potential throughout the cell body.

Because of differences in the cell membrane and shape of the cell, the intracellular voltage necessary to elicit an action potential will vary at different points on the cell membrane. The most sensitive point is the initial segment of the axon, but the impulse must be of sufficient magnitude to depolarize the axon. **Excitation** is the response of the postsynaptic membrane to the neurotransmitter substance that lowers the membrane potential to form an **excitatory postsynaptic potential** (EPSP). The potential is a small depolarization that conducts itself by decrement. The cell membrane is made more permeable to sodium, potassium, and chloride. Sodium ions rush into the neuron, whereas potassium ions leave the cell through the postsynaptic membrane.

Inhibition acts on a cell so that it is more difficult for it to fire. The inhibitory neurotransmitters increase permeability to only potassium and chloride ions at the synaptic membrane. The membrane potential is raised to form the **inhibitory postsynaptic potential** (IPSP).

Presynaptic Inhibition

Another type of inhibition, **presynaptic inhibition,** results from inhibitory knobs being activated on the presynaptic terminal fibrils and synaptic knobs of an axon. When the inhibitory knobs are activated, they secrete a neurotransmitter substance that partially depolarizes the terminal fibrils and excitatory synaptic knobs. As a result, the velocity of the action potential that occurs at the membrane of the excitatory knob is depressed. This action greatly reduces the quantity of excitatory neurotransmitter released by the knob and suppresses the degree of excitation of the neuron.

FUNCTIONS AND DIVISIONS OF THE NERVOUS SYSTEM

The nervous system controls the motor, sensory, autonomic, cognitive, and behavioral functions of the body. It is divided into a hierarchy with three major functional units:

- Spinal cord level—the lowest functional level; controls automatic motor responses, such as reflexes
- Brainstem and subcortical level—the second functional level; controls blood pressure, respirations, equilibrium, and primitive emotions
- Cortical level—the highest level; responsible for cognition (storage of information, thinking, memory, and abstraction)

The nervous system is also divided into the CNS and the PNS. The CNS is composed of the brain and spinal cord. The PNS includes the 12 pairs of cranial nerves (CNs), the 31 pairs of spinal nerves, and the autonomic nervous system, which subdivides into the sympathetic and parasympathetic nervous systems.

CRANIAL AND SPINAL BONES

The purpose of the skull and vertebral column is to protect the most vulnerable parts of the nervous system—the brain and spinal cord.

Skull

The **skull** is the bony framework of the head; it is composed of the eight bones of the cranium and the 14 bones of the face. Knowledge of the anatomy of both the external and internal

TABLE 4–2   NEUROTRANSMITTERS: SOURCE AND ACTION

NAME	SECRETION SOURCE	ACTION
Amines		

Acetylcholine (ACh)
  First neurotransmitter identified
	Neurons in many areas of brain
	  Large pyramidal cells (motor cortex)
		Usually excitatory
		Inhibitory effect on some of parasympathetic nervous system (e.g., heart by vagus)

Chief transmitter of parasympathetic nervous system	Some cells of basal ganglia
	  Motor neurons that innervate skeletal muscles
	  Preganglionic neurons of autonomic NS
	  Postaganglionic neurons of parasympathetic NS
	  Postganglionic neurons of sympathetic NS	

Serotonin (5-HT) Controls body heat, hunger, behavior, and sleep	Nuclei orginating in the median raphe of brainstem and projecting to many areas (especially the dorsal horns of the spinal cord and hypothalamus)	Inhibitor of pain pathway cord; helps to control mood and sleep
Catecholamines		
Dopamine (DA) Affects control of behavior and fine movement	Neurons on the substantia nigra; many neurons of the substantia nigra send fibers to the basal ganglia that are involved in coordination of skeletal muscle activity	Usually inhibitory

Norepinephrine (NE)
  Chief transmitter of sympathetic nervous system
	Many neurons whose cell bodies are located:
	  In brainstem and hypothalamus (controlling overall activity and mood)
	  Most postganglionic neurons of sympathetic NS
		Usually excitatory, although sometimes inhibitory
		
		Some excitatory and some inhibitory

Amino Acids		
γ-aminobutyric acid (GABA)	Nerve terminals of the spinal cord, cerebellum, basal ganglia, and some cortical areas	Excitatory
Glutamic acid	Presynaptic terminals in many sensory pathways; cerebellum mossy fibers	Excitatory
Glycine	Synapses in spinal cord	Inhibitory
Substance P	Pain fiber terminals in the dorsal horns of the spinal cord; also, the basal ganglia and hypothalamus	Excitatory
Polypeptides		
Enkephalin	Nerve terminals in the spinal cord, brainstem, thalamus, and hypothalamus	Excitatory to systems that inhibit pain; binds to the same receptors in the CNS that bind opiate drugs
Endorphin	Pituitary gland and areas of the brain	Binds to opiate receptors in the brain and pituitary gland; excitatory to systems that inhibit pain

NS = nervous system; CNS = central nervous system.

surfaces of the bones (Figs. 4-4 and 4-5) is helpful in understanding the pathophysiology of craniocerebral trauma.

The **cranium** is defined as that part of the skull that encloses the brain and provides a protective vault for this vital organ. The bones that compose the cranium are the frontal, occipital, sphenoid, and ethmoid, as well as the two parietal and temporal bones.

The **frontal bone** forms the forehead and the front (anterior) part of the top of the skull. The supraorbital arches form the roofs of the two orbits. Frontal sinuses are also located in this bone. The inner table of the frontal bone has a highly irregular bony surface.

The **occipital bone** is the large bone at the back (posterior) of the skull that curves into the base of the skull. The significant markings include the large hole (foramen magnum) in the base of the skull and also the occipital condyles located on either side of the foramen magnum that fit into depressions on the first cervical vertebra.

The **sphenoid bone** is a wedge-shaped bone thought to resemble a bat's wings. The significant bone markings include a body, lesser wings, greater wings, the pterygoid process, the sella turcica (Latin for "Turk's saddle"), and the clivus. The **clivus** is the slanted dorsal surface of the body of the sphenoid bone between the sella turcica and basilar

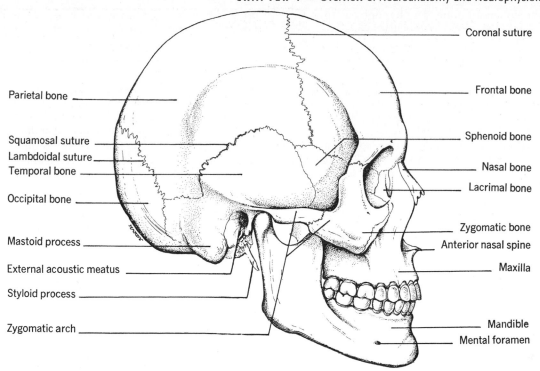

Figure 4-4 • Lateral view of the skull.

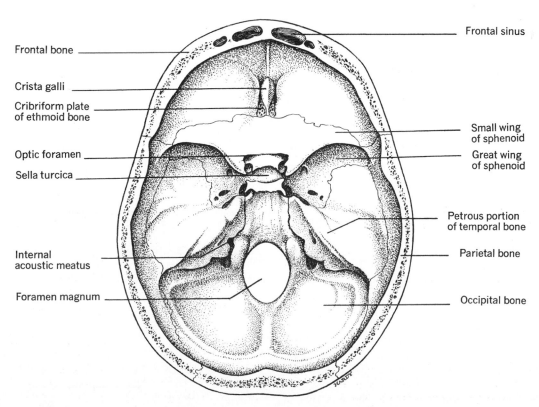

Figure 4-5 • View of the base of the skull from above, showing the internal surfaces of some of the cranial bones.

process of the sphenoid bone. The hypophysis (pituitary gland) is located in the region of the sella turcica.

The **ethmoid bone,** largely hidden between the two orbits, contains both perpendicular and horizontal plates as well as two lateral masses. The horizontal plate, also called the cribriform plate, forms part of the base of the skull through which the olfactory nerves (first CNs) travel. The perpendicular plate forms part of the nasal septum, whereas the lateral masses are part of the ethmoid sinuses.

The **temporal bones** are situated at the sides and base of the skull and consist of three anatomic divisions: the squamous, mastoid, and petrous portions. The temporal bone is highly irregular, both on the internal and external surfaces.

The **squamous portion** is very thin just above the auditory meatus. It contains the zygomatic process externally; internally, there are numerous eminences and depressions to accommodate the contour of the cerebrum. Two well-marked internal grooves are evident for the branches of the middle meningeal artery, a common point of trauma with head injury.

The **mastoid portion** is perforated by many foramina, including a larger foramen, the mastoid foramen, which contains a vein that drains the lateral sinus and a small artery to supply the dura mater. The mastoid process is also contained in this portion of the temporal bone.

The **petrous portion** is so named because it is extremely dense and stone-like in its hardness. There is a pyramidal process that is directed inward and is wedged at the base of the skull between the sphenoid and occipital bones. The internal plate of the petrous portion of the temporal bone is proximal to the branches of the middle meningeal artery.

The **parietal bones,** which fuse on the top of the skull, form the sides of the skull. Externally, they are smooth and convex; internally, the surface is concave with some depressions to accommodate the convolutions of the cerebrum and the grooves for the middle meningeal artery. With these exceptions, the bone has a regular inner surface.

SUTURES OF THE SKULL

The bones of the skull join at various places, known as suture lines. The four major sutures of the skull include the following (see Fig. 4-4):

Sagittal suture: the midline suture formed by the two parietal bones joining on the top of the skull
Coronal suture (frontoparietal): connecting the frontal and parietal bones transversely
Lambdoidal suture (occipitoparietal): connecting the occipital and parietal bones
Basilar suture: created by the junction of the basilar surface of the occipital bone with the posterior surface of the sphenoid bone

SPINE

The spine is a flexible column formed by a series of bones called **vertebrae,** each stacked one on another to support the head and trunk. The vertebral column is made up of 33 vertebrae: 7 cervical vertebrae, 12 thoracic or dorsal vertebrae, 5 lumbar vertebrae, 5 sacral vertebrae (fused into one), and 4 coccygeal vertebrae (fused into one) (Fig. 4-6). Each vertebra consists of two essential parts, an anterior solid segment or **body,** and a posterior segment or **arch.** Two **pedicles** and two **laminae** supporting seven processes (four articular, two transverse, and one spinous) make up the arch (Fig. 4-7).

The cervical vertebrae are smaller than those in any other region of the spine. The first cervical vertebra is called the **atlas,** whereas the second cervical vertebra is known as the **axis.** Each of these two vertebrae has a unique appearance.

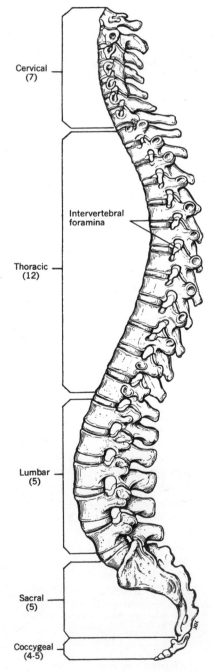

Cervical
(7)

Intervertebral
foramina

Thoracic
(12)

Lumbar
(5)

Sacral
(5)

Coccygeal
(4-5)

Figure 4-6 • Lateral view of the adult vertebral column.

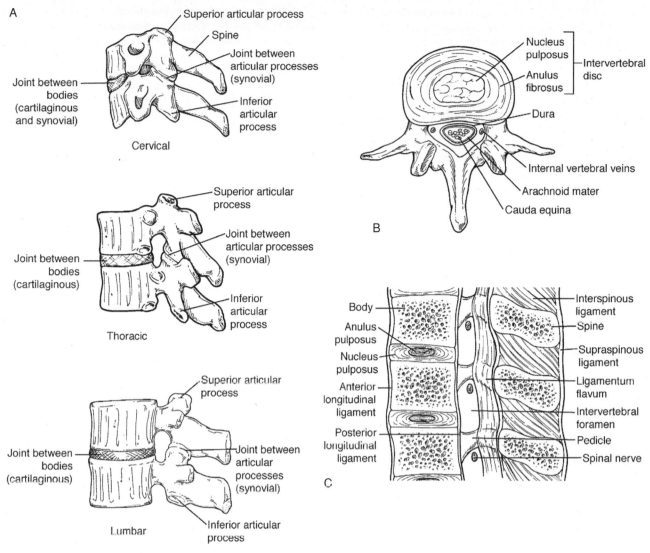

Figure 4-7 • (A) Cervical, thoracic, and lumbar vertebrae. (B) Third lumbar vertebra seen from above, showing the relationship between the intervertebral disc and the cauda equina. (C) Sagittal section through three lumbar vertebrae, showing the ligaments and the intervertebral discs.

The axis has a perpendicular projection called the **odontoid process** on which the atlas sits (Fig. 4-8). The thoracic or dorsal vertebrae are intermediate in size, becoming larger as they descend the vertebral column. The lumbar vertebrae are the largest segments in the spine (see Fig. 4-7).

The vertebral bodies are the largest part of the vertebrae, above and below which flattened surfaces are found for attachment of fibrocartilage. There are apertures for spinal nerves, veins, and arteries. The vertebrae are connected by means of the articular processes and the intervertebral fibrocartilage.

The arch of the vertebrae is composed of two pedicles, two laminae, a spinous process, four articular processes, and two transverse processes. The two **pedicles** are short, thick pieces of bone. The concavity above and below the pedicles creates the intervertebral notches from which the spinal nerves emanate. The two **laminae** are broad plates of bone. They complete the neural arch by fusing in the midline and enclose the spinal foramen, which protects the spinal cord. The upper and lower borders are rough in order to allow for the attachment of the ligamenta subflava. The **spinous process** projects backward from the laminae and serves as the attachment for muscles and ligaments. The four **articular processes** (two on either side) provide stability for the spine. The two **transverse processes** provide stability for the spine and serve as points of attachment for muscles and ligaments.

LIGAMENTS OF THE SPINE

The most important ligaments of the vertebral column are the anterior and posterior longitudinal ligaments and the ligamenta flava (see Fig. 4-7). The **anterior longitudinal ligament** consists of longitudinal fibers firmly attached to the anterior surface of the vertebral bodies and intervertebral discs. The **posterior longitudinal ligament** is attached to the posterior surface of the vertebral bodies within the spinal canal. The **ligamentum flavum** consists of yellow elastic

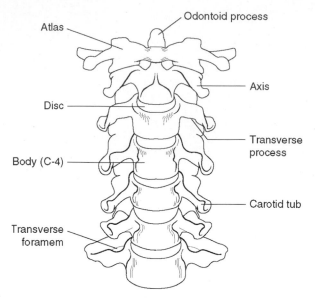

Figure 4-8 • The cervical spine. Note odontoid process of C2 and the atlas, C1, positioned on top of C2.

fibers that connect the laminae of adjacent vertebrae. The attachment pattern is unique in that the attachment is from the lower margin of the anterior surface of the superior lamina to the posterior surface of the upper margin of the inferior lamina.

The **supraspinous ligament** joins the spinous process tips from C7 to the sacrum. The **interspinous ligaments** connect adjacent spinous processes from their tips to their roots. The interspinals fuse with the supraspinals posteriorly and with the ligamentum flavum anteriorly. Such an arrangement controls vertebral movement to prevent excessive flexion. If violent force in any direction occurs, these ligaments can be ruptured, possibly causing injury to the vertebrae and spinal cord (see Chaps. 18 and 19).

INTERVERTEBRAL DISCS

The **intervertebral discs** are fibrocartilaginous disc-shaped structures located between the vertebral bodies from the second cervical vertebra to the sacrum. They vary in size, thickness, and shape at different levels of the spine. The purpose of the intervertebral disc is to cushion movement. The central core, the **nucleus pulposus,** is surrounded by a fibrous capsule called the **annulus fibrosus.** As a result of aging and trauma, discs lose their water content and the tissue is more prone to injury.

MENINGES

Meninges cover both the brain and spinal cord. The layers, from the outermost layer inward, are called the **dura mater,** the **arachnoid,** and the **pia mater** (Fig. 4-9).

The **dura mater** is a double-layer, whitish, inelastic, fibrous membrane that lines the interior of the skull. The outer layer

of the dura is actually the periosteum of the bone. The inner layer is the thick membrane that extends throughout the skull and creates compartments. The dura lines various foramina that exit at the base of the skull. Sheaths for the nerves passing through these foramina are also formed by the dura.

Four folds of dura (Fig. 4-10) are situated within the skull cavity to support and protect the brain. They include the following:

Falx cerebri, a double fold of dura, descends vertically into the longitudinal fissure between the two hemispheres of the brain and partially divides the frontal lobe into a left and right side.

Tentorium cerebelli is a tent-like double fold of dura that covers the upper surface of the cerebellum, supports the occipital lobes, and prevents them from pressing on the cerebellum. The falx cerebri attaches midline to the tentorium. (The tentorium is an important anatomic point to note. The area above the tentorium is termed **supratentorial,** whereas the area below it is called **infratentorial.** The nursing care given differs based on these two classifications, as discussed in Chap. 17.) In addition, the opening in the tentorium from which the brainstem emerges is called the tentorial notch. Herniation through this opening is called uncal herniation.

Falx cerebelli is found between the two lateral lobes of the cerebellum.

Diaphragma sella is a horizontal process that forms a small circular fold, thus creating a roof for the sella turcica.

The spinal dura is a continuation of the inner layer of the cerebral dura. The outer layer of the dura terminates at the foramen magnum, where it is replaced by the periosteal lining of the vertebral canal. The spinal dura encases the spinal roots, spinal ganglia, and spinal nerves. The spinal dural sac terminates at the second or third sacral level.

The second meningeal layer, the **arachnoid membrane,** is an extremely thin, delicate layer that loosely encloses the brain. The subdural space separates the dura mater from the arachnoid layer. Bleeding within this space (subdural hemorrhage) can occur with head injury. The subarachnoid space is not really a clear space because there is much spongy, delicate connective tissue between the arachnoid and pia mater layers. CSF flows in the subarachnoid space. The cisterna magnum is a space between the hemispheres of the cerebellum and the medulla oblongata. The arachnoid layer of the spinal meninges is a continuation of the cerebral arachnoid (see Fig. 4-9). The arachnoid is a delicate, gossamer network of fine, elastic, fibrous tissue; it also contains blood vessels of varying sizes, which may be damaged by lumbar or cisternal puncture, resulting in hemorrhage.

The innermost layer of the meninges is called the **pia mater.** It is a mesh-like, vascular membrane that derives its blood supply from the internal carotid and vertebral arteries. The pia mater covers the entire surface of the brain, dipping down between the convolutions of the surface. Because the pia covers the gray matter, vascularity increases and minute perpendicular vessels extend for some distance into the cerebrum. The pia mater of the spinal cord is thicker, firmer, and less vascular than that of the brain.

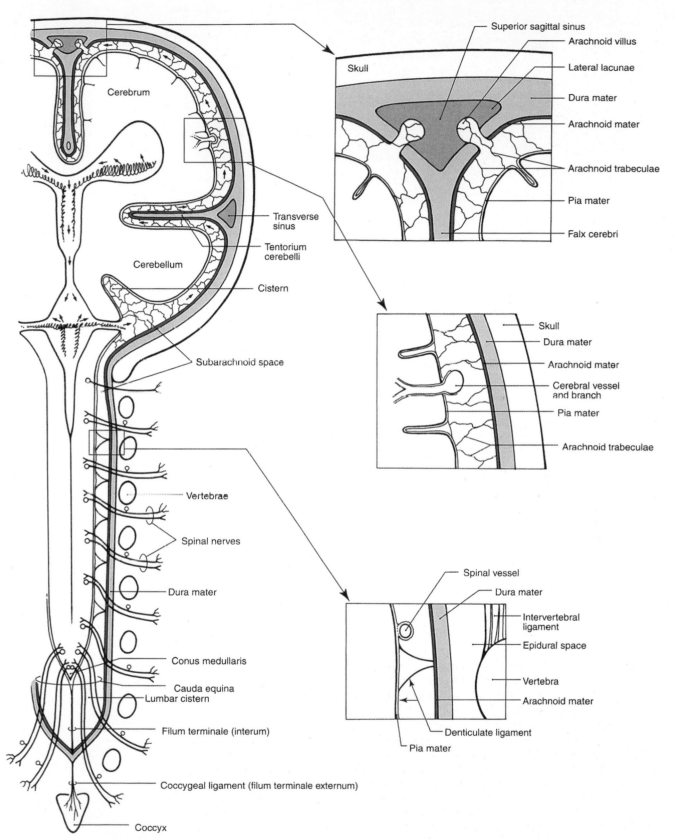

Figure 4-9 • The central nervous system and its associated meninges. The *top right box* shows the superior sagittal sinus and arachnoid villi. Arachnoid villi remove cerebrospinal fluid (CSF) from the ventricles and deposit the CSF into the venous circulation. The *middle right box* shows the layers of tissue from the skull through the three layers of the meninges. The *bottom right box* shows the layers of spinal meninges. (From Haines, D. E. [2000]. *Neuroanatomy: An atlas of structures, sections, and systems* [5th ed.]. Philadelphia: Lippincott Williams & Wilkins.)

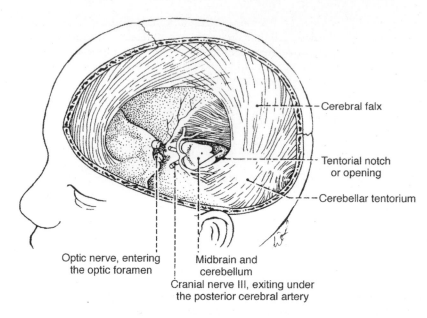

Cerebral falx

Tentorial notch
or opening

Cerebellar tentorium

Optic nerve, entering
the optic foramen

Midbrain and
cerebellum

Cranial nerve III, exiting under
the posterior cerebral artery

Figure 4-10 • Cranial dura mater folds. With the skull and cerebral hemisphere removed, the falx cerebri and the tentorium cerebelli are shown. Note that cranial nerve III (oculomotor nerve) exits under the posterior cerebral artery. With lateral transtentorial herniation, the oculomotor nerve may be caught between the tentorium and posterior cerebral artery, resulting in dilation of the pupil. (From DeMyer, W. [1998]. *Neuroanatomy* [2nd ed.]. Baltimore: Williams & Wilkins.)

Spaces of the Meninges

Three spaces located within the meninges are important to note. The **epidural** or **extradural space** is a potential space located between the skull and outer layer of the dura layer of the brain. In the vertebral column, the epidural space is between the periosteum and the single dural layer. The **subdural space** is between the inner dura mater and arachnoid layer. This is a narrow space and is the site of subdural hemorrhage with certain injuries. The third space is the **subarachnoid space,** which is between the arachnoid and pia mater layers and contains CSF.

CEREBROSPINAL FLUID

Cerebrospinal fluid is normally a clear, colorless, odorless solution that fills the ventricles of the brain and the subarachnoid space of the brain and spinal cord. The purpose of CSF is to act as a shock absorber, cushioning the brain and spinal cord against injury caused by movement, and to provide nutrients to the neural components. The specific gravity of CSF is 1.007 (see Chap. 5 for CSF normal values). CSF differs from other extracellular fluids in the percentage of composition of various factors. It is composed of water, a small amount of protein, oxygen, and carbon dioxide. The electrolytes—sodium, potassium, and chloride and glucose, an important cerebral nutrient—are also present. An occasional lymphocyte may be present. Normally, CSF pressure is in the range of 60 to 180 mm of water pressure in the lateral recumbent position, which is the position assumed for a lumbar puncture. With the patient in the sitting position, a normal lumbar puncture will register 200 to 350 mm of water pressure. Fluctuation in pressure occurs in response to the cardiac cycle and respirations. The amount of CSF in adults is approximately 125 to 150 mL.

FORMATION OF CEREBROSPINAL FLUID

Cerebrospinal fluid, which is produced by active transport and diffusion, is formed from three different sources. The major source of CSF is the secretions from the choroid plexus, a cauliflower-like structure located in portions of the lateral, third, and fourth ventricles (Fig. 4-11). The **choroid plexus** is a collection of blood vessels covered with a thin coating of ependymal cells. CSF is constantly secreted from these surfaces. It is estimated

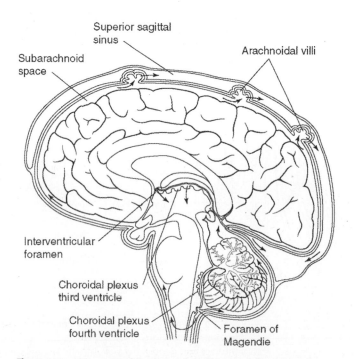

Superior sagittal
sinus

Subarachnoid
space

Arachnoidal villi

Interventricular
foramen

Choroidal plexus
third ventricle

Choroidal plexus
fourth ventricle

Foramen of
Magendie

Figure 4-11 • Diagram of the flow of cerebrospinal fluid from the time of its formation from blood in the choroid plexuses until its return to the blood in the superior sagittal sinus.

that the amount of CSF produced daily by the choroid plexus is about 500 mL, or 25 mL/hr. A lesser proportion of CSF is secreted from the second source, the ependymal cells, which line the ventricles and blood vessels of the meninges. Finally, CSF is also produced by the blood vessels of the brain and spinal cord. The amount produced from this source is small.

Ventricular System

The two **lateral ventricles,** one on either side of the midline, are located in the lower and inner parts of the cerebral hemisphere. Each lateral ventricle consists of a **central cavity** or **body** and three **horns.** The central cavity is located in the lower part of the parietal lobe. The **anterior horn** curves forward and outward into the frontal lobe; the **posterior horn** curves backward and inward into the occipital lobe; and the **middle or lateral horn** descends into the temporal lobe. The curved corpus callosum forms the undersurface of the central cavity and the roof of the anterior, middle, and posterior horns.

The singular **third ventricle** is a midline inner brain–cavity structure. The two optic thalami form the side walls. The floor is formed by the tuber cinereum (infundibulum, pituitary), corpora albicantia, and crus cerebri. The ventricle is bounded by the fornix in the front and pineal body in the back. The singular, diamond-shaped **fourth ventricle** is laterally bounded by the pons and the superior cerebellar peduncles. The roof is formed by the superior cerebellar peduncles and medulla. The floor of the fourth ventricle is continuous with the central spinal canal.

Flow of Cerebrospinal Fluid

Cerebrospinal fluid circulation has been termed the "third circulation." It is a closed system. Fluid formed by choroid plexuses in the two lateral ventricles passes into the third ventricle by way of the two foramina of Monro. The single cerebral aqueduct or aqueduct of Sylvius connects the third and fourth ventricles. CSF flows through the two lateral foramina of Luschka and midline through the foramen of Magendie to the cisternal magnum. At this point, the CSF enters the subarachnoid space. The foramen of Magendie allows CSF to circulate around the cord, whereas the foramen of Luschka directs the CSF around the brain (Fig. 4-12).

Expanded areas of the subarachnoid space are called **cisterns.** CSF may be aspirated from some of these areas for analysis. The major cisterns are the **cisterna magnum,** between the medulla and cerebellar region, and the **lumbar cistern,** between vertebrae L-2 and S-2.

Cerebrospinal Fluid Absorption

Most of the CSF produced daily is reabsorbed into the **arachnoid villi,** which are projections from the subarachnoid space into the venous sinuses of the brain (see Fig. 4-11). CSF drains into the superior sagittal sinus. Arachnoid villi are very permeable and allow CSF, including protein molecules, to exit easily from the subarachnoid space into the venous sinuses. CSF flows in one direction through the arachnoid villi (most of which are located in the subarachnoid space of the cerebrum), which have been compared with pressure-sensitive valves. When CSF pressure is greater than venous pressure, CSF leaves the subarachnoid space. As pressures are equalized, the valves close. Dysfunction of CSF flow is seen in hydrocephalus.

CEREBROVASCULAR CIRCULATION

The blood vessels that supply the nervous system form an extensive capillary bed, particularly in the gray matter of the brain. About **20% of the oxygen** consumed by the body is used for the oxidation of glucose to provide energy. The brain is totally dependent on glucose for its metabolism. A lack of oxygen to the brain for 5 minutes can result in irreversible brain damage.

The brain receives **approximately 750 mL/min of blood, or 15% to 20% of the total resting cardiac output.** These figures remain relatively constant because of various control systems affecting the brain. Blood flow rates to specific areas of the brain correlate directly to the metabolism of the cerebral tissue. The brain is supplied by two pairs of arteries: the **two internal carotid arteries** and the **two vertebral arteries.** Cerebral circulation is also divided into the anterior and the posterior circulation. The **anterior circulation** refers to the common carotids and their distal branches including the internal carotid arteries, the middle cerebral arteries, and the anterior cerebral arteries. The **posterior circulation** refers to the vertebral arteries, the basilar artery, and the posterior arteries.

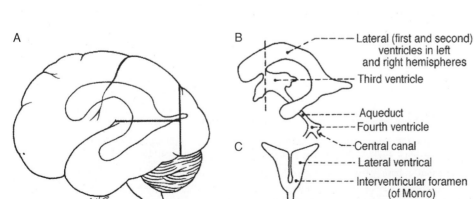

A

B ---- Lateral (first and second)
ventricles in left
and right hemispheres
-- Third ventricle

-- Aqueduct
-Fourth ventricle

C
--Central canal
-- Lateral ventrical
-- Interventricular foramen
(of Monro)
---- Third ventricle

Figure 4-12 • The cerebral ventricles. (*A*) Lateral aspect of the left cerebral hemisphere showing the contour of the lateral ventricles and their relation to the cerebral lobes. (*B*) Lateral outline of the four ventricles. (*C*) Frontal (coronal) section of the lateral and third ventricles at the level of the dotted line (*B*), showing their communicating interventricular foramen. (From DeMyer, W. [1998]. *Neuroanatomy* [2nd ed.]. Baltimore: Williams & Wilkins.)

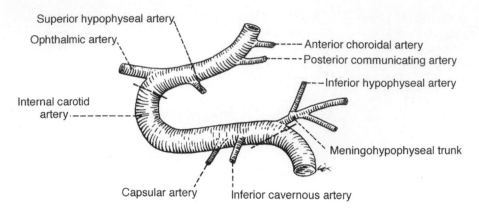

Figure 4-13 • Lateral view of the left carotid artery at the siphon or parasellar region. The *lower interrupted line* is where the carotid artery enters the cavernous sinus, and the *upper interrupted line* is where it exits. (From DeMyer, W. [1998]. *Neuroanatomy* [2nd ed.]. Baltimore: Williams & Wilkins.)

Internal Carotid Arteries

The internal carotid arteries originate from two different vessels: the **left common carotid,** which originates directly from the aorta, and the **right common carotid,** which arises from the **innominate artery** also originating from the aorta. The common carotids branch to form the external and internal carotid arteries. The external carotid artery supplies the face, scalp, and other extracranial structures. The internal carotid artery enters the cranial vault through the foramen lacerum in the floor of the middle cranial fossa. As the internal carotid passes through the bone and dura at the base of the skull and approaches the upper brain, it passes forward through the cavernous sinus just lateral to the pituitary fossa. It curves sharply several times and roughly forms an "S," called the **carotid siphon** (Fig 4-13). Most of the hemispheres, excluding the occipitals, the basal ganglia, and the upper two thirds of the diencephalon, are supplied by the internal carotid arteries (Fig. 4-14).

The first intracranial branch from the internal carotid artery is the ophthalmic artery. The terminal branches of each carotid include the posterior communicating artery, the anterior cerebral artery, and the middle cerebral artery. Table 4-3 summarizes the major branches of the carotid arteries and the areas supplied (also see Fig. 4-14). See also Chapter 25 for further discussion of cerebral vascular territories and stroke.

CHARACTERISTICS OF THE CEREBRAL CIRCULATION

The following lists the outstanding characteristics of cerebral circulation:

Cerebral arteries have thinner walls than arteries of comparable size in other parts of the body. Cerebral arteries have an internal elastic tissue and scanty smooth muscle.

The veins (other than sinuses) have even thinner walls in proportion to their size and lack a muscle layer. The veins and sinuses have **no** valves. The venous return does not retrace the course of corresponding arteries but follows a pattern of its own. The dural sinuses are unique to cerebral circulation.

The distribution of the arteries with rich surfaces (arteries anastomosed by localized "end-artery" distribution of branches penetrating the nervous tissue) is distinctive.

TABLE 4–3   MAJOR INTERNAL CAROTID ARTERIAL BRANCHES AND THE CEREBRAL AREAS THEY INNERVATE

ARTERY	AREA SUPPLIED
Ophthalmic	Orbits and optic nerves
Posterior communicating (Pcom)	Connects the carotid circulation with the vertebrobasilar circulation
Anterior choroidal	Part of choroid plexuses of lateral ventricles; hippocampal formation; portions of globus pallidus; part of internal capsule; part of amygdaloid nucleus; part of caudate nucleus; part of putamen
Anterior cerebral (ACA)	Medial surfaces of frontal and parietal lobes; part of cingulate gyrus and "leg area" of precentral gyrus
Recurrent artery of Heubner	Special branch of ACA, penetrates the anterior perforated substance to supply part of basal ganglia and genu of internal capsule (also called medial striate artery)
Middle cerebral (MCA) (has several branches)	Entire lateral surfaces of the hemisphere except for the occipital pole and the inferolateral surface of the hemisphere (supplied by posterior cerebral artery)
Lenticulostriate (from MCA)	Part of basal ganglia and internal capsule
Anterior communicating (Acom)	Connects the two ACAs

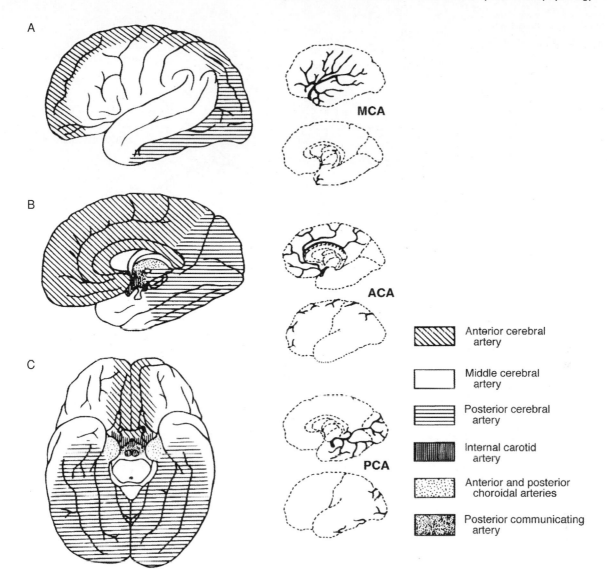

Figure 4-14 • Surface distribution of the anterior, middle, and posterior cerebral arteries. (*A*) Lateral view of the left cerebral hemisphere. (*B*) Medial view of the left cerebral hemisphere. (*C*) Ventral view of the cerebrum. ACA = anterior cerebral artery; MCA = middle cerebral artery; PCA = posterior cerebral artery. (From DeMyer, W. [1998]. *Neuroanatomy* [2nd ed.]. Baltimore: Williams & Wilkins.)

Vertebral Arteries

The **vertebral arteries,** originating from the **subclavian arteries,** enter the skull through the foramen magnum, ventrolateral to the spinal cord. The two vertebral arteries unite at the level of the pons to become the singular **basilar artery** (Fig. 4-15). The basilar artery subdivides into the two posterior cerebral arteries that supply part of the cerebrum (Fig. 4-16).

In general, the vertebral arteries and their branches supply the cerebellum, the brainstem, the spinal cord, the occipital lobes, the medial and inferior surfaces of the temporal lobes, and the posterior diencephalon.

Before they begin to supply blood to the brain, the vertebral arteries give off recurrent branches that anastomose with the anterior and posterior spinal arteries and with a posterior meningeal branch. In its intracranial course, the vertebral arteries give rise to direct bulbar arteries to the medulla, the anterior spinal artery, the **posterior inferior cerebellar artery (PICA),** sometimes the posterior spinal artery, and small branches to the basal meninges. The first branch off the basilar artery is the **anterior inferior cerebellar artery (AICA).** The basilar artery is also the origin of the pontine arteries, the internal auditory arteries, the superior cerebellar arteries, and the posterior cerebral arteries. Table 4-4 summarizes the major branches of the vertebral arteries and the areas supplied.

Circle of Willis

The circle of Willis, which is located at the base of the skull, is divided into anterior (carotid portion) and posterior

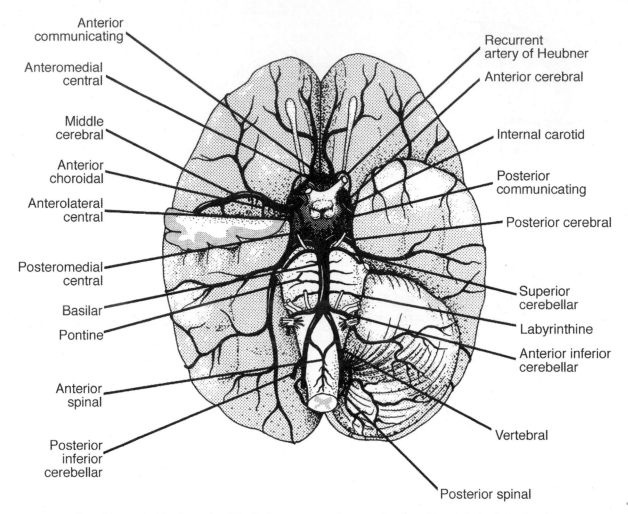

Figure 4-15 • The blood supply of the brain, as seen on the ventral surface. (The right cerebellar hemisphere and the tip of the right temporal lobe have been removed.) (From Barr, M. L., & Kiernan, J. A. [1993]. *The human nervous system* [6th ed.]. Philadelphia: J. B. Lippincott.)

TABLE 4–4   MAJOR VERTEBRAL ARTERIAL BRANCHES AND THE CEREBRAL AREAS THEY INNERVATE

ARTERY	AREA SUPPLIED
Vertebral Branches	
Anterior spinal (only one artery)	Anterior two thirds of spinal cord
Posterior spinals	Posterior one third of spinal cord
Posterior inferior cerebellar (PICA)	Undersurface of the cerebellum; medulla; and choroid plexuses of fourth ventricle
Basilar Artery Branches	
Posterior cerebral (PCA)	Occipital lobes, medial and inferior surfaces of the temporal lobes, midbrain, and choroid plexuses of third and lateral ventricle
Posterior choroidals (from PCA) Medial posterior choroidal Lateral posterior choroidal	 Tectum, choroid plexus of third ventricle, and superior and medial surfaces of the thalamus Penetrating the choroidal fissure and anastomosing with branches of the anterior choroidal arteries
Anterior inferior cerebellar (AICA)	Undersurface of the cerebellum and lateral surface of the pons
Superior cerebellar (SCA)	Upper surface of the cerebellum and midbrain
Pontine	Pons

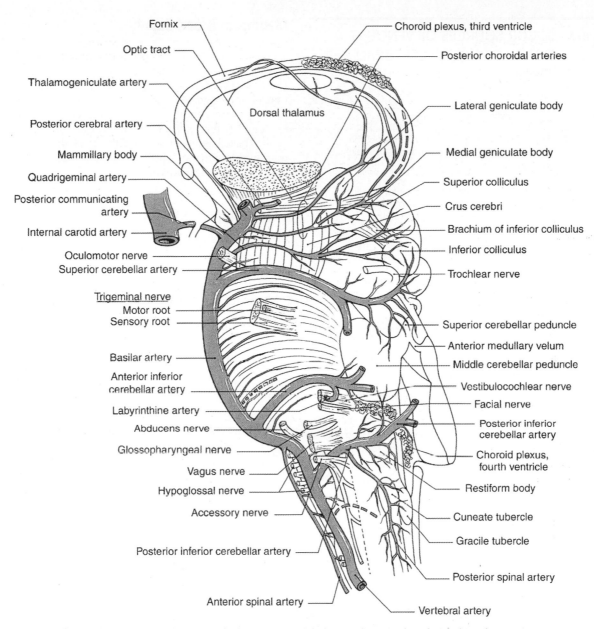

Figure 4-16 • The blood supply to the brainstem and thalamus, showing the relationship of structures and cranial nerves to arteries. (From Haines, D. E. [2000]. *Neuroanatomy: An atlas of structures, sections, and systems* [5th ed.]. Philadelphia: Lippincott Williams & Wilkins.)

(vertebrobasilar portion) circulation (see Fig. 4-15). The composition of each portion includes these elements:

- Middle cerebral arteries, the anterior cerebral arteries, and the anterior communicating artery, which connects the two anterior cerebral arteries
- Two posterior cerebral arteries; two posterior communicating arteries connect the middle cerebral arteries with the posterior cerebral arteries, thus uniting the internal carotid system with the vertebral-basilar system

The circle of Willis encloses a very small area that is little more than 1 inch square, or about the size of a quarter. Functionally, the carotid circulation and the posterior circulation usually remain separate. At one time, the circle of Willis was thought to be a protective mechanism by which blood was shunted to compensate for alterations in cerebral blood flow or pressure. However, collateral circulation through the circle depends on the patency of its components. The vessels of the circle of Willis, particularly the communicating arteries, may be anomalous. Nevertheless, in *favorable instances,* the circle does permit an adequate blood supply to reach all parts of the brain, even after one or more of the four supplying vessels has been ligated.

Venous Drainage

Unlike venous drainage in other parts of the body, which closely follows an arterial pattern, cerebral venous drainage is chiefly managed by vascular channels created by the two

TABLE 4–5 MAJOR SOURCES OF VENOUS DRAINAGE OF THE CEREBRAL CIRCULATION AND THE AREAS DRAINED

VENOUS STRUCTURE	AREA DRAINED
Superior longitudinal (sagittal) sinus	Superior cortical veins of the convexity of the brain; drains CSF
Inferior longitudinal sinus	Medial surface of the brain
Straight sinus	Joins the superior longitudinal sinus; the vein of Galen drains into the straight sinus
Transverse sinus	Area of the ears; collects blood from superior longitudinal and straight sinuses and drains it into the internal jugular vein
Cavernous sinus (contains several cranial nerves and internal carotid artery)	Inferior surface of the brain, including the orbits

CSF = cerebrospinal fluid.

dural layers called **dural sinuses.** There are no valves in dural sinuses. A few dural sinuses deserve mention; these are included in Table 4-5 along with the areas they supply (Fig. 4-17). **Emissary veins** join extracranial veins with the venous sinuses. **Bridging veins** connect the brain and dural sinuses and are often the cause of subdural hemorrhage. Cerebral veins empty into the dural sinuses, which, in turn, empty into the **jugular veins,** which return the blood to the heart.

Meningeal Blood Supply

The meninges are supplied with arterial blood by the anterior, middle, and posterior meningeal arteries. The main route for the arterial supply of the dura mater is through the middle meningeal branches of the external carotid artery. Each vessel ascends through a foramen in the base of the skull and is then situated between the dura mater and the skull. These vessels may be torn as a result of a head injury, thereby causing an epidural hematoma, which requires immediate medical attention.

Blood Supply to the Spinal Cord, Spinal Roots, and Spinal Nerves

The upper cervical cord receives its arterial blood supply from the vertebral arteries through recurrent branches. Below this region, the spinal cord receives its arterial blood supply, in part, from the anterior spinal artery and the two posterior spinal arteries, which arise from the vertebral arteries. The **anterior spinal artery** runs the full length of the cord midventrally, whereas the two **posterior spinal arteries** run full length along each row of the dorsal roots. As these three vessels pass down the cord, they receive feeders from deep cervical, intercostal, lumbar, and sacral arteries. Additional blood supply comes from **radicular arteries** (which supply blood to only one nerve root) and **radiculospinal arteries** (which supply blood to about six spinal cord segments). The large **artery of Adamkiewicz** originates from the aorta and enters the cord at about the second lumbar (L-2) ventral root level (range, T-10 to L-2) and supplies most of the caudal third of the cord.

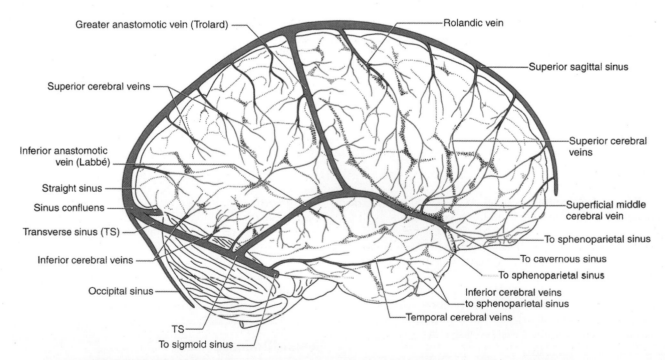

Figure 4-17 • The cranial venous sinuses. Lateral view of the right cerebral hemisphere and part of the venous drainage from the brain. Communications between veins and sinuses or between sinuses are also indicated. (From Haines, D. E. [2000]. *Neuroanatomy: An atlas of structures, sections, and systems* [5th ed.]. Philadelphia: Lippincott Williams & Wilkins.)

The venous system of the spine includes an intradural and extradural system. The intradural veins follow the pattern of the arteries, whereas the extradural intravertebral veins form a plexus extending from the cranium to the pelvis and having many communications along the way with veins of the neck, thorax, and abdomen.

BLOOD–BRAIN BARRIER

For the CNS to function normally, a very stable environment must be maintained within that body system. The so-called blood–brain barrier (BBB) is a descriptive term for the network of endothelial cells (cells that compose the walls of capillaries) and the projections from the astrocytes located in close proximity to the neuron. Astrocytes are large stellate cells with numerous radiating cytoplasmic processes. Extensions of astrocytes called **perivascular feet** surround the brain capillaries.

Capillaries in the brain, unlike those in other areas, do not have pores between adjacent endothelial cells. Therefore, the brain cannot derive molecules from blood plasma by a nonspecific filtering process. Instead, molecules within cerebral capillaries are transported through the endothelial cells by active transport, endocytosis, and exocytosis. This creates a highly selective BBB that guards the entrance into neurons. Before molecules in the blood can enter neurons in the CNS, they pass through both the capillary endothelial cells and the astrocytes. The tight junctions between the endothelial cells and the astrocytes are largely responsible for the BBB. Because of this barrier, most drugs are prevented from affecting the brain and spinal cord. This has implications for selection of drugs that must cross the BBB to treat a number of cerebral conditions.

The movement of substances into the brain depends on particle size, lipid solubility, chemical dissociation, and the protein-binding potential of the drug. In general, drugs that are lipid soluble and undissociated at body pH rapidly enter both the brain and the CSF. When compared with other body organs, the CNS is very slow in its uptake of dyes and both organic and inorganic anions and cations (e.g., sodium, potassium, glutamic acid) from the circulating blood. The barrier is very permeable to water, oxygen, carbon dioxide, other gases, glucose, and lipid-soluble compounds.

BRAIN (ENCEPHALON)

The brain constitutes approximately 2% of body weight. The average weight of the brain of a young male adult is about 1400 g. The brains of older people weigh less, with the average weight being about 1200 g.

The brain is divided into three major areas: the cerebrum, the brainstem, and the cerebellum (Fig. 4-18). The **cerebrum** is composed of the cerebral hemispheres, thalamus, hypothalamus, and basal ganglia. In addition, the olfactory and optic nerves (CNs I and II) are located in the cerebrum. The **brainstem** includes the midbrain, pons, and medulla. The midbrain, which contains the cerebral peduncles and corpus quadrigemina, is a short segment between the hypothalamus and the pons.

Another means of subdividing the brain is by fossae. The **anterior fossa** contains the frontal lobes; the **middle fossa** contains the temporal, parietal, and occipital lobes; and the **posterior fossa** contains the brainstem and cerebellum.

Cerebrum

The cerebrum comprises **two cerebral hemispheres** that are incompletely separated by the great longitudinal fissure. A **fissure,** similar to a **sulcus** only deeper, is a large, predictable

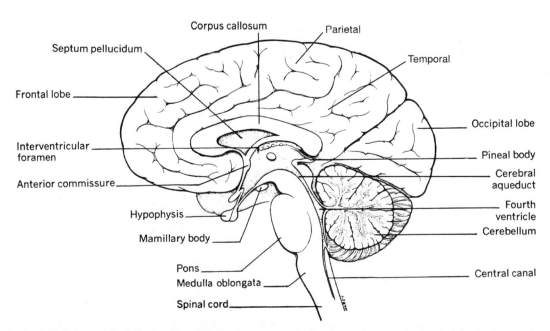

Figure 4-18 • Midsagittal section of the brain. (From Chaffee, E. E., & Lytle, I. M. [1980]. *Basic physiology and anatomy.* Philadelphia: J. B. Lippincott.)

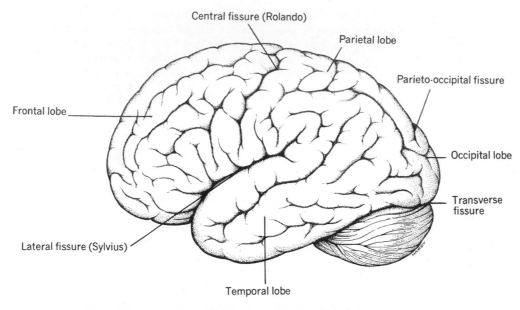

Figure 4-19 • Lateral aspect of the left cerebral and cerebellar hemispheres.

separation in the cerebral hemisphere. The following are some important fissures that are landmarks in studying the gross anatomy of the brain:

- The **great longitudinal fissure** is a midsagittal fissure that separates the cerebral hemispheres into a left and right side. The hemispheres are joined at the bottom of the fissure by the corpus callosum.
- The **lateral fissure of Sylvius** separates the temporal lobe from the frontal and parietal lobes.
- The **central fissure of Rolando** separates the frontal lobe from the parietal lobe.

The last major fissure is the **parieto-occipital fissure,** which separates the occipital lobe from the parietal and temporal lobes (Fig. 4-19).

The surface of the hemispheres consists of numerous "wrinkles," or **gyri** (also called **convolutions**). The gyri fold in on one another, thereby substantially increasing the surface area of the brain. Each hemisphere is covered by a cerebral cortex of gray matter that is 2 to 5 mm thick and contains billions of neurons.

Under the cerebral cortex is **white matter,** which serves as an association and projection pathway. The white matter of the cerebral hemispheres contains nerve fibers and neuroglia of various sizes. Three types of myelinated nerve fibers comprise the center of the hemisphere. They are the transverse fibers, the projection fibers, and the association fibers (Fig. 4-20).

- **Transverse (commissural) fibers** are tracts of fibers that interconnect corresponding parts of the *two* hemispheres. The **corpus callosum** is the largest commissure. It is an arch-shaped structure that crosses the great longitudinal fissure.
- **Projection fibers** connect the cerebral cortex with the lower portions of the brain and spinal cord.
- **Association fibers** connect various areas within the *same* hemisphere.

The cerebral hemispheres are composed of pairs of frontal, parietal, temporal, and occipital lobes. **Brodmann** is credited with mapping the cortical areas of the brain based on slight histologic differences of the cells. Almost 100 different areas of the cerebral cortex have been identified. This method of classification provides a basis for the discussion of functional areas of the brain (Figs. 4-21 and 4-22). The following are some Brodmann areas along with their functional classifications:

- **Area 4**—primary motor cortex or primary motor strip
- **Areas 3, 1, and 2**—primary somatic sensory areas
- **Areas 41 and 42**—primary receptive areas for sound
- **Area 17**—primary receptive area for vision

The primary sensory and motor areas perform highly specialized functions.

Other areas of the brain that do not perform primary functions are called **association areas.** Functions of the association areas are more general but nonetheless important. Functional loss of a sensory association area greatly reduces the ability of the brain to analyze characteristics of sensory experience. It should be mentioned that the cerebral cortex is closely associated, both anatomically and functionally, with the thalamus. Many afferent and efferent pathways connect with specific parts of the thalamus to perform various complex functions.

GENERAL FUNCTIONS OF THE CEREBRAL CORTEX ACCORDING TO LOBES

Frontal Lobe

The major functions of the frontal lobes are to:

- Perform high-level cognitive functions such as reasoning, abstraction, concentration, and executive control
- Provide for storage of information (memory)

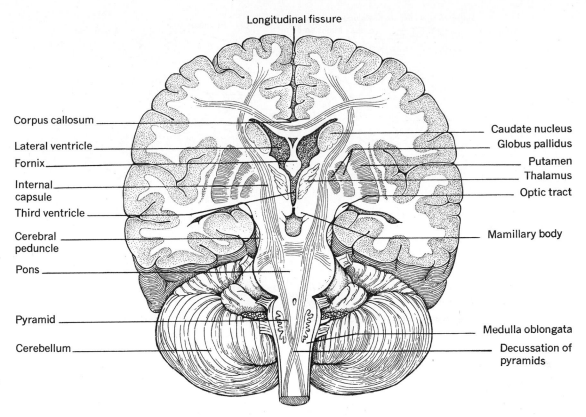

Figure 4-20 • Oblique coronal section through the cerebrum and brainstem. (From Chaffee, E. E., & Lytle, I. M. [1980]. *Basic physiology and anatomy.* Philadelphia: J. B. Lippincott.)

- Control voluntary eye movement
- Influence somatic motor control of activities such as respirations, gastrointestinal activity, and blood pressure
- Motor control of speech in the dominant hemisphere (usually the left hemisphere)

The **motor cortex (area 4),** located anterior to the central fissure, contains giant Betz cells or pyramidal cells that

control voluntary motor function. The various muscles are spatially arranged on the strip so that the feet are located in the area of the longitudinal fissure and the muscles of the face are located at the opposite end of the motor strip. Note the large area allocated to the hand (Fig. 4-23).

Areas **6** and **8** of the cortex are called **motor association areas,** or the premotor cortex. There is a connection between these areas and the oculomotor, trochlear, abducens,

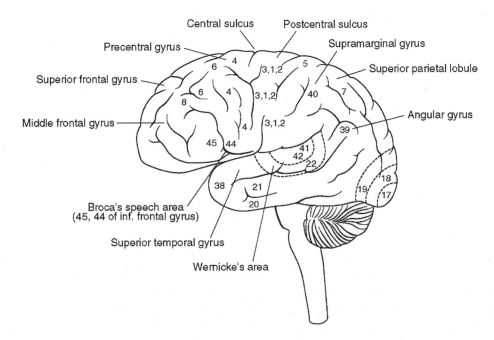

Figure 4-21 • Lateral view of the brain depicting the most significant areas of Brodmann.

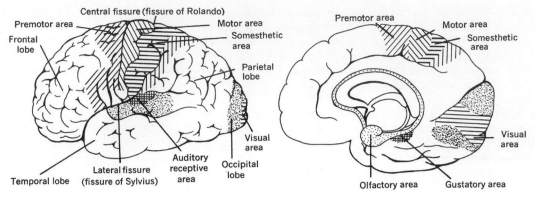

Figure 4-22 • Diagram of the localization of function in the cerebral hemisphere. Various functional areas are shown in relation to the lobes and fissures—lateral view (*left*) and medial view (*right*).

glossopharyngeal, vagus, and spinal accessory CNs. Stimulation of the lateral portion of area 6 results in massive generalized movements, such as the turning of the eyes and head, movement of the trunk, and flexion and extension of the extremities, particularly the hands. Area 8 is concerned with the eye field and coordinates eye movement.

Broca's area (areas 44 and 45), located at the inferior frontal gyrus, is classified as an association area because it is critical for motor control of speech. Damage to this area in the dominant hemisphere results in the inability of the patient to express his or her thoughts (nonfluent aphasia).

Parietal Lobe

Posterior to the central fissure is the **primary sensory cortex (areas 3, 1,** and **2),** which is arranged in the same topographic scheme as the motor strip; that is, the feet are controlled by an area in the longitudinal fissure, and the muscles of the face are controlled by the temporal region. Area 1 receives fibers responsible for cutaneous and deep sensibility sensations. The fibers in area 2 are concerned with deep sensibility, whereas those in area 3 interpret the cutaneous sensations of touch, position, pressure, and vibration.

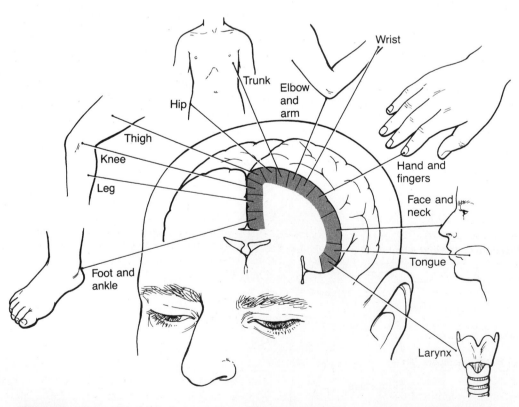

Figure 4-23 • Areas of the brain that control specific areas of the body. Size indicates relative distribution of control. (From Bullock, B. L. [1996]. *Pathophysiology: Adaptations and alterations in function* [4th ed.]. Philadelphia: Lippincott-Raven.)

Input from the thalamus also reaches the primary sensory cortex. The purpose of the primary sensory cortex is to analyze only gross aspects of sensation and send the results of its interpretation to the thalamus and other cortical areas. It is the function of the **sensory association areas (areas 5 and 7)** to analyze the specific characteristics of sensory input.

In the parietal lobes, sensory input is interpreted to define size, shape, weight, texture, and consistency. Sensation is localized, and modalities of touch, pressure, and position are identified. In addition, a person's awareness of the parts of his or her body is a parietal lobe function. The nondominant parietal lobe processes visuospatial information and controls spatial orientation, whereas the dominant lobe is involved in ideomotor praxis.

Temporal Lobe

The **primary auditory receptive areas (areas 41 and 42)** are located in the temporal lobes. The **auditory association area** occupies a part of the superior temporal gyrus **(area 22)** and is also known as **Wernicke's area.** This area is usually largest in the dominant hemisphere. If Wernicke's area is damaged in the patient's dominant hemisphere, words are heard but they are meaningless to the person (fluent aphasia). Thus, affected persons would be able to verbalize but would unknowingly make many errors in content because of a failure to comprehend what has been said by others or by themselves.

A very important area, called the **interpretive area,** is located in the supramarginal and angular gyri of the temporal lobe. This area is at the junction of the lateral fissure where the temporal, parietal, and occipital lobes meet. It provides an integration of the somatic, auditory, and visual association areas and plays an important role in visual, auditory, and olfactory perception; learning; memory; and emotional affect. Types of thoughts that might be experienced are greatly detailed memories of past experiences, conversations, artwork, music, and taste. Memory that requires more than one sensory modality is stored, in part, in the angular gyrus of the temporal lobe. Any destruction of the **dominant temporal lobe** and angular gyrus in an adult will result in great impairment of intellectual ability.

Occipital Lobe

The **primary visual cortex** is **area 17** of the occipital lobe. The **visual association areas** are **18** and **19.** Neurons of the **lateral geniculate bodies** give rise to fibers that form the geniculocalcarine tract (optic radiation) to the cortex of the occipital lobes. The major functions of the occipital lobes are visual perception, some visual reflexes (i.e., visual fixation), and involuntary smooth eye movements (smooth pursuit system).

DOMINANCE OF A CEREBRAL HEMISPHERE

Cerebral dominance is an important consideration. It is generally accepted that most people have one cerebral hemisphere that has become more highly developed than the other. At birth, both hemispheres have an equal capacity for development. As a child develops, the attention of the mind is directed to one specific hemisphere, which develops rapidly in relation to the other side. Left hemispheric dominance is found in 90% of the population; these are right-handed people. Surprisingly, most, but not all, left-handed people also have a dominant left cerebral hemisphere. Many "split brain" studies have been conducted on the left and right hemispheres of the brain. The left side of the brain controls language, whereas the right side is the nonverbal or perceptual hemisphere.

CORPUS CALLOSUM

The **corpus callosum,** as mentioned previously, is a thick area of nerve fibers directed transversely, through which every part of one hemisphere is connected with the corresponding part of the other hemisphere. When the fibers of one hemisphere pass into the opposite hemisphere, they permeate the hemisphere in all directions, terminating in the gray matter of the periphery. As a result of this connective process, the two hemispheres are intricately linked.

BASAL GANGLIA

The **basal ganglia** are the several masses of subcortical nuclei located deep in the cerebral hemispheres. Their anatomic parts include the **lenticular nucleus** (composed of the **globus pallidus** and **putamen**), the **caudate nucleus,** the **amygdaloid body,** and the **claustrum.** The lenticular nucleus and the caudate nuclei are collectively called the **corpus striatum.** The lenticular nuclei and the caudate nucleus are functionally closely related to the thalamus, subthalamus, substantia nigra, and red nucleus. These structures compose the basal ganglia system for motor control of fine body movements, particularly of the hands and lower extremities. Disorders of this area produce Parkinson-like symptoms.

DIENCEPHALON

The **diencephalon,** a major division of the cerebrum, is divided into four regions: the thalamus, hypothalamus, subthalamus, and epithalamus. The thalamus and hypothalamus are the major areas of importance. These four areas are next discussed along with the internal capsule and hypophysis (pituitary gland), which are located in this region.

Thalamus

The **thalamus** consists of a pair of egg-shaped masses of gray matter located in the ventromedial part of the hemispheres that has connections to multiple areas of the brain. The thalamus is divided into anterior medial and lateral groups, and each group includes specific nuclei. The lateral border of the thalamus is the posterior limb of the internal capsule, and the third ventricle lies medially to the thalamus. The thalamus is the last station where impulses are processed before they ascend to the cerebral cortex. All sensory pathways (with the exception of olfactory pathways) have direct afferent and efferent connections with the thalamic nuclei. The thalamus plays a role in conscious pain awareness, in focusing of attention, in the reticular activating system, and in the limbic system.

Epithalamus

The **epithalamus** is the most dorsal portion of the diencephalon. It is composed of the pineal body, which is thought to have a role in growth and development. The pineal body secretes melatonin, which is important in the sleep-wakefulness cycle. The epithalamus is also involved in regulating food and water intake.

Hypothalamus

The **hypothalamus** is located in the basal region of the diencephalon, forming part of the walls of the third ventricle. The optic chiasma, the point at which the two optic tracts cross, is located at the rostral area of the hypothalamic floor. The stalk of the pituitary, **infundibulum,** connects the hypophysis with the hypothalamus. The hypothalamus regulates important physiologically based drives such as appetite, sexual arousal, and thirst. It is the center for the autonomic nervous system, particularly the sympathetic portion. The hypothalamus controls:

Temperature, by monitoring the blood temperature that flows through the hypothalamus and then sending afferent impulses to the sweat glands, peripheral vessels, or muscles (for shivering)

Water metabolism, through the regulation of antidiuretic hormone

Hypophyseal secretions (e.g., growth hormone, follicle-stimulating hormone)

Visceral and somatic activities, by many excitatory-inhibitory functions of the autonomic nervous system (e.g., heart rate, peristalsis, pupillary dilation and constriction)

Visible physical expressions in response to emotions, such as blushing, dry mouth, and clammy hands

Sleep-wakefulness cycle

Circadian rhythms

Subthalamus

The **subthalamus** is located below the thalamus and is closely related to the basal ganglia in function.

▨ INTERNAL CAPSULE

Many nerve fibers coming from various parts of the cerebral cortex converge at the brainstem, forming the corona radiata. As the fibers enter the thalamus-hypothalamus region, they are collectively termed the **internal capsule.** The internal capsule is a **massive bundle of sensory and motor fibers** connecting the various subdivisions of the brain and spinal cord. Although it includes only a small area of tissue, it is a critical anatomic area that controls major sensory and motor function. It is part of the white matter of the cerebrum and contains both radiation and projection fibers. The internal capsule is formed by fibers of the crus cerebri, with additional fibers from the corpus striatum and optic thalamus laterally.

All afferent sensory fibers going to the cortex pass through the internal capsule in the following succession: the brainstem to the thalamus to the internal capsule to the cerebral cortex. All efferent motor fibers leaving the cortex for the brainstem pass through the internal capsule according to the following schemata: cerebral cortex to the internal capsule to the brainstem.

▨ HYPOPHYSIS (PITUITARY GLAND)

The **hypophysis,** also called the **pituitary gland,** is a small gland that is located above the sella turcica at the base of the brain and is connected to the hypothalamus by the **hypophyseal stalk** (also called the **infundibulum**). The hypothalamus controls pituitary secretions. The hypophysis is divided into two lobes, the anterior and the posterior. The anterior lobe secretes six major hormones related to metabolic function of the body: (1) **growth-stimulating hormone** (GSH), (2) **adrenal-stimulating hormone** (adrenocorticotropic hormone [ACTH]), (3) **thyroid-stimulating hormone** (TSH), (4) **prolactin,** (5) **follicle-stimulating hormone** (FSH), and (6) **luteinizing hormone** (LH).

The posterior lobe produces **vasopressin,** also called **antidiuretic hormone** (ADH), and **oxytocin.** ADH controls the rate of water secretion into the urine, thereby controlling the water content of the body. Commonly, abnormal secretion of ADH accompanies intracranial surgery, a pituitary adenoma, or cerebral trauma.

Relationship Between the Hypothalamus and Hypophysis in Neuroendocrine Control

The control center for the autonomic nervous system and the neuroendocrine system is the **hypothalamus.** The following two pathways of hypothalamic connection to the hypophysis enable hypothalamic influence of the endocrine glands: (1) nerve fibers that travel from the supraoptic nuclei and paraventricular nuclei to the posterior lobe of the hypophysis (**hypothalamohypophyseal tract**); and (2) long and short portal blood vessels that connect sinusoids in the median eminence (portion of the hypophysis) and the infundibulum with the capillary plexuses in the anterior lobe of the hypophysis (**hypophyseal portal system**) (Fig. 4-24).

Hypothalamohypophyseal Tract

The precursors of the hormones vasopressin and oxytocin are synthesized in the nerve cells of the **supraoptic** and **paraventricular nuclei.** The precursor material then passes

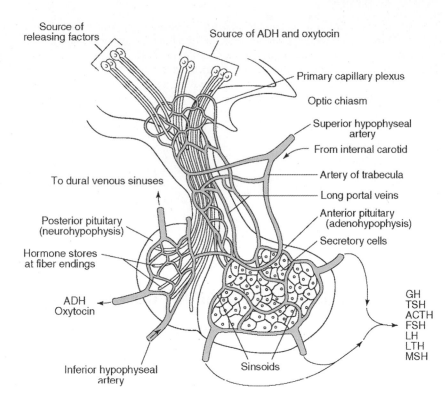

Source of
releasing factors

Source of ADH and oxytocin

Primary capillary plexus

Optic chiasm

Superior hypophyseal
artery

From internal carotid

To dural venous sinuses

Artery of trabecula

Long portal veins

Posterior pituitary
(neurohypophysis)

Anterior pituitary
(adenohypophysis)

Secretory cells

Hormone stores
at fiber endings

ADH
Oxytocin

GH
TSH
ACTH
FSH
LH
LTH
MSH

Inferior hypophyseal
artery

Sinsoids

Figure 4-24 • Diagrammatic and schematic representation of hypophyseal nerve fiber tracts and the portal system. Releasing factors produced by cell bodies in the hypothalamus trickle down axons to the proximal part of the stalk where they enter the primary capillary plexus and are transported via portal vessels to sinusoids in adenohypophysis for control of secretions. Antidiuretic hormone (ADH) and oxytocin, produced by other cell bodies in the hypothalamus, trickle down axons for storage in the neurohypophysis until needed. ACTH = adrenocorticotropic hormone; FSH = follicle-stimulating hormone; GH = growth hormone; LH = leuteinizing hormone; LTH = luteotropic hormone; MSH = melanocyte-stimulating hormone; TSH = thyroid-stimulating hormone.

along the axons and is released at the axon terminals, where it is absorbed into the capillaries of the posterior hypophyseal lobe. **Vasopressin** is produced mainly in the nerve cells of the supraoptic nucleus. The functions of vasopressin are to increase water absorption in the kidney's distal convoluted tubules and to initiate vasoconstriction. The other hormone, **oxytocin,** is produced mainly in the paraventricular nucleus and is responsible for uterine contraction and for stimulating the growth of those cells of the mammary glands responsible for milk production.

Hypophyseal Portal System

The hypophyseal portal system is derived from the superior hypophyseal artery. On entering the median eminence and dividing into capillaries, the capillaries drain into long and short descending vessels that terminate in the anterior lobe of the hypophysis. The release-stimulating hormones and release-inhibiting hormones are delivered to cells of the anterior hypophysis so that the appropriate releasing or inhibiting hormone is synthesized and secreted (e.g., TSH, FSH). Feedback systems from afferent fibers in the hypothalamus, as well as from the target organ, help to regulate the level of the various hormones.

BRAINSTEM (MIDBRAIN, PONS, AND MEDULLA)

The second major subdivision of the brain is the brainstem (Fig. 4-25). Many significant anatomic parts are found in the brainstem and are discussed in relationship to the three major divisions, the midbrain, pons, and medulla.

Midbrain

The **midbrain** is a small, 1.5-cm segment of the upper brainstem lying between the diencephalon and the pons. The midbrain can be divided into the tectum (the roof), the tegmentum (the posterior portion), and the crus cerebri (the cerebral peduncle). The anterior surface extends from the mamillary bodies of the diencephalon to the pons. The **crus cerebri** consists of two rope-like bundles of fibers separated by a deep **interpeduncular fossa.** The rope-like bundles include the corticospinal and corticobulbar tracts centrally and are flanked by corticopontine fibers. Many small penetrating blood vessels emanate in the floor of the interpeduncular fossa. The optic tracts are noted just above the crus cerebri.

The base of the midbrain, also called the **basis pedunculi,** consists of the **cerebral peduncles** (comprising the corticospinal, corticobulbar, and corticopontine tracts) and the substantia nigra. The crus cerebri and tegmentum are collectively called the **cerebral peduncles.** The **substantia nigra** lies between the crus cerebri and peduncles. Because of melanin pigment in the substantia nigra cell bodies, the neurons appear brownish.

On the posterior part of the tectum are four rounded masses: two superior colliculi (optic system) and two inferior colliculi (auditory system). The superior and inferior colliculi are collectively termed the **corpus quadrigemina.** The **superior colliculi** process visual stimuli and also integrate visual and auditory motor reflexes. The **inferior colliculi** are nuclei to relay auditory information.

The **superior cerebellar peduncles** are efferent fibers coming from the dentate nucleus of the cerebellum passing rostrally and near the posterior surface of the midbrain. The crossing of the tracts to the opposite side is called the point of

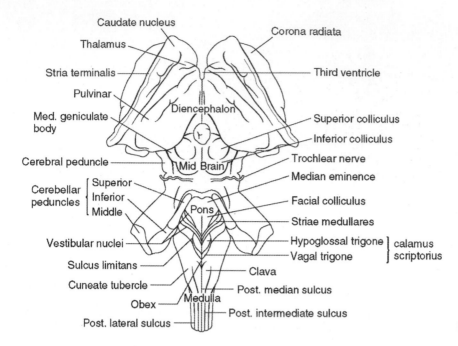

Figure 4-25 • Dorsal view of the brainstem.

cerebellar decussation. The fibers then proceed to the red nuclei and the thalamus.

The **red nuclei** are globular gray masses located at the anterior-central tegmentum. Crossed fibers from the cerebral cortex and superior cerebellar peduncles enter the red nuclei or pass around its edges. The **rubrospinal** and **tectospinal tracts** emanate from this area. They form a relay station for many of the efferent cerebellar tracts. On the lateral surface of the midbrain are the **medial geniculate bodies,** which are the auditory-sensory relay centers. Functionally, the midbrain serves as the pathway for the cerebral hemispheres and the lower brain and as the center for auditory and visual reflexes. CNs III and IV nuclei are located in the midbrain. The midbrain contains the aqueduct of Sylvius.

Pons

The **pons,** about 2.5 cm long, is the bridge between the midbrain and the medulla. The anterior surface of the pons is composed of a band of thick, transverse fibers. The **basal sulcus,** a midline furrow, matches the course of the basilar artery. The anterior area is called the **basis pontis** and is composed of crossing fibers of the middle cerebellar peduncles. The **tegmentum** contains spinothalamic tracts, the lateral lemnisci, the medial longitudinal fasciculi, and part of the reticular formation (regulates consciousness). Several tracts cross through the pons. The inferior, middle, and superior cerebellar peduncles are pathways for the corticospinal tract, and they also connect to the cerebellum. Many other pathways pass through this region connecting higher cerebral regions with the lower levels of the nervous system. The pons contains the fourth ventricle and some control of respiratory function.

Four CNs, V through VIII, have nuclei in the pons. CN V exits laterally from the midpons. At the pontomedullary junction, CN VI exits medially and CNs VII and VIII exit

laterally. About 70% of the neurons of CN VI are motor neurons located in the floor of the fourth ventricle; they innervate the lateral rectus muscle. The remaining 30% of neurons are internuclear neurons, whose axons cross midline, ascend in the **medial longitudinal fasciculus (MLF),** and connect with the medial rectus motor neurons on the opposite side. The abducens is the center for conjugate horizontal gaze. CN VI has the longest intracranial course and is, therefore, more vulnerable to injury and dysfunction.

Medulla

The **medulla oblongata,** also approximately 2.5 cm long, is continuous with the spinal cord and level with the foramen magnum and rootlet of the first cervical nerve; it connects with the pons rostrally. On the posterior surface, the point of division between the pons and medulla is an imaginary transverse line that passes between the caudal margins of the middle cerebellar peduncles. Part of the fourth ventricle is located in the medulla. Anteriorly, the pyramidal (corticospinal) tracts decussate or cross; the pyramidal tracts from the left cross to the right side (and vice versa). The point of decussation forms a ridge on either side of the **median fissure.** In the caudal medulla rostral to the pyramidal decussation, axons from the nucleus gracilis and cuneatus loop anterior-medially around the central gray matter as the **internal arcuate fibers.** These fibers cross the midline to the opposite side and continue as the **medial lemniscus.** Laterally, the **olive** is a prominent oval swelling of convoluted bands that includes the inferior olivary nuclei; they receive fibers from the dentate nucleus of the cerebellum, red nucleus, basal ganglia, and cerebral cortex. Axons from the inferior olivary nuclei form the **olivocerebellar tract** (goes from the inferior cerebellar peduncle to the opposite cerebellar hemisphere). The dorsal spinocerebellar tract is found in a ridge called the **tuberculum cinereum.**

The **MLF** is located in the paramedian area dorsal to the medial lemniscus. The MLF extends rostrally from the cervical cord to the upper midbrain level. It transmits information for the coordination of head and eye movement. In addition to motor and sensory tracts, there are also cardiac, vasomotor, and respiratory centers in the medulla.

CNs IX through XII emanate from the medulla. CNs IX, X, and XI exit the brainstem in the postolivary fissure, whereas CN XII exits from the preolivary fissure.

CEREBELLUM

The **cerebellum,** located in the posterior fossa, is attached to the pons, medulla, and midbrain by the three paired cerebellar peduncles. The organization of the cerebellum allows it to be conceptualized in many ways. The cerebellum consists of three major layers: (1) the cortex, which is the outer gray covering; (2) the white matter, which forms the connecting pathways for efferent and afferent impulses joining the cerebellum with other parts of the CNS; and (3) the four pairs of deep cerebellar nuclei.

The cerebellum can also be divided from side to side and anteriorly to posteriorly. From the anterior to posterior direction, the cerebellum is composed of an **anterior lobe,** a **posterior lobe,** and a **flocculonodular lobe.** Approaching it from side to side, it is divided into midline structures and lateral structures. The midline of the anterior and posterior lobes is called the **vermis,** and the lateral portions are the **cerebellar hemispheres.** The midline of the flocculonodular lobe is the **nodulus;** the lateral portion is the **flocculus.**

The **anterior lobe** uses impulses from the spinocerebellar proprioception to regulate postural reflexes. The **posterior lobe** controls coordination of voluntary muscle activity and muscle tone. The **flocculonodular lobe** is the primary connection with the vestibular apparatus for coordination of location in space and movements. Afferent and efferent nerve fibers are found in the **inferior, middle,** and **superior cerebellar peduncles.** The **cerebellar peduncles** receive direct input from the spinal cord and brainstem and convey it to the deep cerebellar nuclei (**dentate, globose, emboliform,** and **fastigial nuclei**) and cerebellar cortex. The result is both an excitatory and inhibitory influence on the cerebellar nuclei; the excitatory influences predominate. An excitatory effect on the brainstem and thalamic nuclei maintains a tonic discharge to the motor system.

The cerebellum is integrated into many connective efferent and afferent pathways throughout the brain, thus providing muscle synergy throughout the body. All sensory modalities are circuited through the cerebellum, which provides information about muscle activity. Impulses to provide "corrections" are sent after sensory data are evaluated. In other words, there are many feedback loops in which cerebellar function is the center of the circuit receiving and sending impulses to maintain muscle activity. In summary, the cerebellum controls fine movement, coordinates muscle groups (agonist and antagonist muscles), and maintains balance through feedback loops.

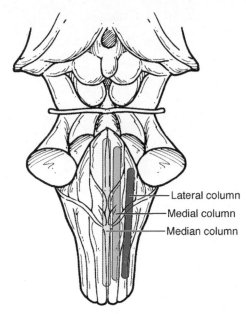

Figure 4-26 • The median, medial, and lateral columns of the reticular formation. (From Snell, R. S. [1997]. *Clinical neuroanatomy for medical students* [4th ed.]. Philadelphia: Lippincott Williams & Wilkins.)

SPECIAL SYSTEMS WITHIN THE BRAIN

Three special systems require further discussion: the reticular formation, the reticular activating system, and the limbic system.

The **reticular formation (RF)** is a net (reticulum) of a continuous network of nerve cells and fibers from the axis of the CNS that extends from the spinal cord; through the medulla, pons, midbrain, subthalamus, hypothalamus, and thalamus; to the cerebrum. The RF is subdivided into lateral, medial, and median columns (Fig. 4-26). The RF receives input from most of the sensory systems and has efferent fibers that descend and influence nerve cells at all levels of the CNS. The exceptionally long dendrites of the neurons of the RF permit input from widely placed ascending and descending pathways. Through its many connections, the RF can control skeletal muscle activity, control somatic and visceral sensation, control the autonomic and endocrine systems, influence biologic clocks, and influence the reticular activating system (control of consciousness).

The **reticular activating system (RAS)** is a diffuse system that extends from the lower brainstem to the cerebral cortex, from which it disperses (Fig. 4-27). The RAS controls the sleep-wakefulness cycle; consciousness; focused attention; and sensory perception that might alter behavior. The brainstem and thalamic portions of the RAS have different functions. Stimulation of the brainstem portion results in activation of the entire brain. Wakefulness is controlled by the brainstem. Stimulation of the thalamic portion relays facilitory impulses, causing a generalized activation of the cerebrum and cognition. Stimulation of selective thalamic areas activates specific areas of the cerebral cortex. This selective stimulation plays a role in directing one's attention during certain mental activities.

The **limbic system** is a group of subcortical nuclei and fiber tracts that form a border around the brainstem. The system

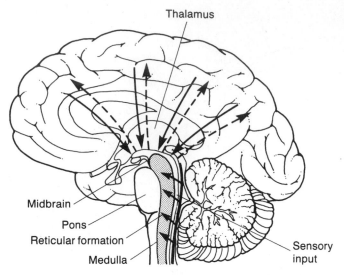

Figure 4-27 • The anatomic components of the reticular activating system related to consciousness.

includes the **hypothalamus,** the **cingulate gyrus,** the **fornix,** the **hippocampus,** the **anterior nucleus** of the **thalamus,** the **uncus,** and the **amygdaloid nucleus** (a part of the basal ganglia). Connections exist with the mamillary bodies, the olfactory tract, and the upper RF of the midbrain (Fig. 4-28). The major connections of the limbic system are called the **circuit of Papez.** The complex function of the system involves basic instinctual and emotional drives, such as fear, sexual drive, hunger, sleep, and short-term memory. These emotional reactions are expressed through endocrine, visceral, somatic, and behavioral reactions through neural pathways that connect with the hypothalamus, brainstem, spinal cord, and hypophysis. Destruction or injury in these areas from trauma or drugs causes symptoms that impact memory and behavior.

SPINAL CORD

The spinal cord is an elongated mass of nerve tissue that occupies the upper two thirds of the vertebral canal and usually measures 42 to 45 cm long and about 1 cm in diameter at its widest point in the adult. The spinal cord extends from the upper borders of the atlas (first cervical vertebra) to the lower border of the first lumbar vertebra (Fig. 4-29). As the cord reaches the lower two levels of the thoracic region, the cord becomes tapered and is called the **conus medullaris.** A nonneural filament called the **filum terminale** joins the dural tube at levels of the second sacral vertebra, where it becomes invested by dura, and continues as the coccygeal ligament to the posterior surface of the coccyx. The three meninges surround the spinal cord for protection.

The Spinal Cord in Cross Section

When viewed in cross section (Fig. 4-30), the spinal cord appears to be a gray *H* or butterfly shape surrounded by white matter. The **gray matter** consists of cell bodies and neuronal projections (axons and dendrites). The **white matter** includes longitudinally running fiber tracts, some of which are myelinated. Each **funiculus** (column) contains ascending and descending tracts. There are two midline sulci, the **anterior median fissure** and the **posterior median sulcus.** The lateral surface contains both **posterolateral** and **anterolateral sulci** that serve to divide the white matter into the anterior, lateral, and posterior funiculi.

Cross sections of the cord at various levels show striking differences in the shape and extent of gray and white matter. The gray matter of the cord contains the **posterior (dorsal)** and **anterior (ventral) horns.** The **anterior horns** are smaller in the thoracic and upper lumbar segments because the muscle mass of the trunk is less than that of the extremities, and these horns are made up largely of cell bodies of neurons that innervate skeletal muscles. In the lumbosacral region, the

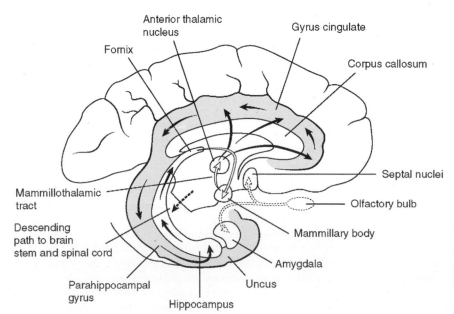

Figure 4-28 • Papez circuit (*arrows*) is depicted in this schematic view of the limbic system. The *solid arrows* represent the hypothetical circulation of impulses during the experiencing of emotions. The *thick dotted arrow* indicates the descending path to the brainstem and spinal cord for the expression of emotions. The olfactory afferent fibers (*lightly dotted arrows*) are also shown.

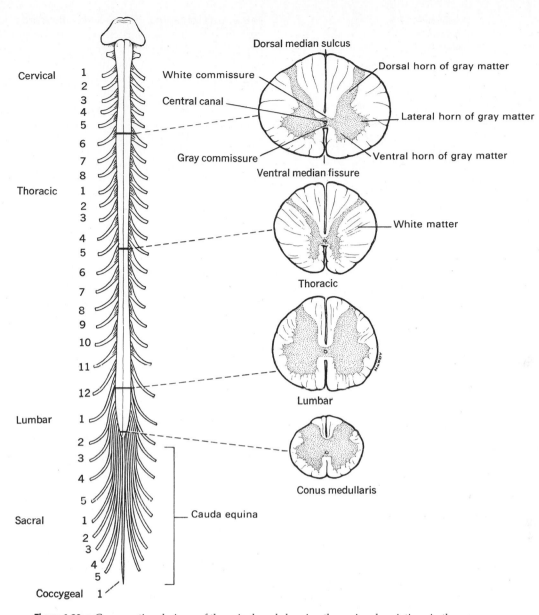

Figure 4-29 • Cross-sectional views of the spinal cord showing the regional variations in the gray matter. (From Chaffee, E. E., & Lytle, I. M. [1980]. *Basic physiology and anatomy.* Philadelphia: J. B. Lippincott.)

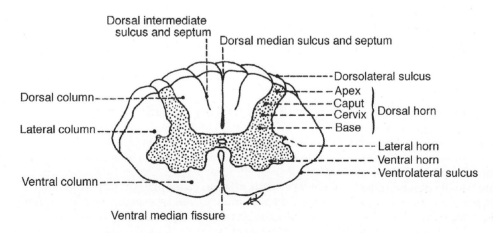

Figure 4-30 • Cross section of the spinal cord. (From DeMyer, W. [1998]. *Neuroanatomy* [2nd ed.]. Baltimore: Williams & Wilkins.)

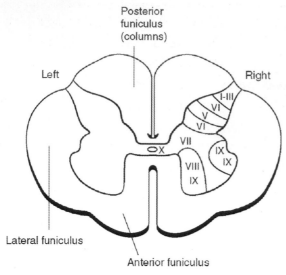

Figure 4-31 • The three funiculi of the spinal cord.

anterior horns are larger than those of the cervical area because of the greater muscle mass in the lower extremities. There is more white matter, compared with gray matter, in the cervical region than in the lumbosacral region. This difference exists because the white matter in the cervical region is made up of connecting fibers that span the entire spinal cord and the brain, whereas the white matter of the lumbosacral cord contains only fibers serving the caudal end of the cord.

On cross section, the gray matter of the spinal cord is divided into sections I through X, called the **laminae of Rexed** (Fig. 4-31). Each lamina extends the length of the cord. Numbering of the laminae begins at the most dorsal point of the posterior horn; lamina IX is located at the most ventral point of the anterior horn. Therefore, the posterior horn contains laminae I through VI. Cells receive and send information about sensory input from the spinal nerve. Lamina VII is located in the intermediate gray zone and extends into the anterior horn. Within this area are the nucleus dorsalis and the intermediolateral gray columns. The anterior horn contains laminae VIII and IX. Lamina VIII contains neurons that send commissural axons to the opposite side of the cord. Lamina IX contains alpha and gamma motor neurons that innervate skeletal muscles. The area surrounding the central canal is the site of lamina X. See also Chapter 27 for discussion of chronic pain implications.

Spinal Nerves

Spinal nerves are part of the PNS. There are 31 pairs of spinal nerves exiting from the spinal cord, including 8 cervical, 12 thoracic, 5 lumbar, 5 sacral, and 1 coccygeal. A typical spinal nerve has a dorsal root by which afferent impulses enter the cord and a ventral root by which efferent impulses leave. Dorsal root fibers are usually absent in the first cervical and the coccygeal roots; therefore, there are no corresponding dermatomes for these segments. The first

pair of cervical spinal nerves leaves the cord above the C-1 vertebra, and spinal nerves of C-2 through C-7 leave by way of the intervertebral foramina, above their corresponding vertebrae. Given that there are seven vertebrae and eight pairs of spinal nerves, the C-8 spinal nerve leaves the cord by way of the intervertebral foramina below the C-7 vertebra. All spinal nerves from T-1 to the caudal end of the cord leave by way of the foramina immediately below the corresponding vertebrae.

In the cervical region, the spinal nerves are almost on a horizontal plane with the corresponding vertebra; however, because the spinal cord is shorter than the vertebral column, the spinal nerves become increasingly oblique as they descend the spinal cord. The lumbar and sacral spinal nerves develop long roots, collectively referred to as the **cauda equina.**

There are two enlargements in the spinal cord to accommodate innervation to the extremities. The cervical (**brachial**) enlargement innervates the upper extremities and extends from the C-5 to the T-1 spinal levels. The lower extremities are innervated by the **lumbosacral** enlargement, which extends from the L-1 to the S-3 levels. See also Chap. 18 for further discussion of segmental spinal levels and sensory areas (homunculus).

DORSAL (SENSORY) ROOTS

The **dorsal roots (posterior roots)** (see Fig. 4-30) convey sensory input (afferent impulses) from specific areas of the body known as **dermatomes** (Fig. 4-32). Dorsal root fibers are usually absent in the first cervical and the coccygeal roots; therefore, there are no corresponding dermatomes for these segments. There is considerable peripheral overlap between one dermatome and another so that no demonstrable sensory deficit will be found unless the sensory component of two or more spinal nerves is interrupted. Interruption of one sensory nerve root may result in paresthesia or pain in that dermatomal area.

Afferent impulses are directed from the dermatomal area through the dorsal root to the dorsal root ganglia, in which the cell bodies of the sensory component are located. The sensory fibers are of two types:

General somatic afferent (GSA) fibers, which carry sensory impulses for pain, temperature, touch, and proprioception from the body wall, tendons, and joints
General visceral afferent (GVA) fibers, which carry sensory impulses from the organs within the body (Fig. 4-33 and Table 4-6)

VENTRAL (MOTOR) ROOTS

The **ventral roots** convey efferent impulses from the spinal cord to the body. The motor fibers are of two types:

General somatic efferent (GSE) fibers, which innervate voluntary striated muscles and have axons originating from the alpha and gamma motor neurons of lamina IX

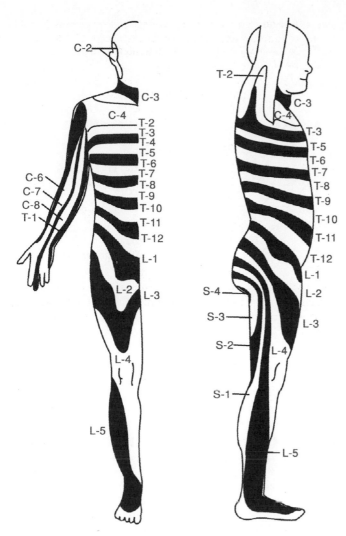

Figure 4-32 • Cutaneous distribution of the spinal nerves (dermatomes). (From Conn, P. M. [1995]. *Neuroscience in medicine.* Philadelphia: J. B. Lippincott.)

TABLE 4–6	SENSORY NERVE ROOTS AND THE AREAS THEY INNERVATE (DERMATOME)
SPINAL NERVES	**DERMATOME**
C-2	Back of head (occiput)
C-3	Neck
C-4	Neck and upper shoulder
C-5	Lateral aspect of shoulder
C-6	Thumb; radial aspect of arm; index finger
C-7	Middle finger; middle palm; back of hand
C-8	Ring and little finger; ulnar forearm
T-1–T-2	Inner aspect of arm and across shoulder blade
T-4	Nipple line
T-7	Lower costal margin
T-10	Umbilical region
T-12–L-1	Inguinal (groin) region
L-2	Anterior thigh and upper buttocks
L-3–L-4	Anterior knee and lower leg
L-5	Outer aspect of lower leg; dorsum of foot; great toe
S-1	Sole of foot and small toes
S-2	Posterior medial thigh and lower leg
S-3	Medial thigh
S-4–S-5	Genitals and saddle area

General visceral efferent (GVE) fibers, which include the preganglionic and postganglionic autonomic fibers that innervate smooth and cardiac muscle and also regulate glandular secretion (see Fig. 4-33)

Impulses to the motor end-plate of voluntary muscle fibers are conveyed by **alpha motor neurons;** impulses to the motor end-plates of intrafusal muscle cells of the neuromuscular spindles are conveyed by **gamma motor neurons.** Both these motor neurons (alpha, gamma) are also called lower motor neurons. Table 4-7 provides a list of myotomes, which are areas of motor innervation to specific muscle groups.

CLASSIFICATION OF NERVE FIBERS

Nerve fibers can be classified by various criteria, including the diameter of the fiber, thickness of the myelin sheath, and speed of conduction of the impulse. Large fibers conduct impulses quickly, and the thicker the myelin sheath, the faster the speed of the impulse conductivity.

Sensory fibers are classified into groups I through IV, depending on their conduction velocities. Group I fibers are the quickest to conduct impulses, whereas group IV fibers have the slowest velocity. Group I is further divided to include I_a fibers (spindle primary afferent or annulospiral endings) and I_b fibers (from Golgi tendon organs). Group II conveys sensation from the myelinated skin and joint receptors (spindle secondary afferent or flower-spray endings). Group III fibers convey sensations of discriminative pain, cold, and some touch. Group IV fibers are unmyelinated and convey nociception and thermal sensation. Another system uses the capital letters A, B, and C to classify both sensory and motor fibers. Type A is either a small, lightly myelinated sensory fiber for touch, pressure, pain, and temperature or alpha or gamma motor neurons of lamina IX. The greatest diameter and velocity are characteristic of type A fibers. Type B fibers have a smaller diameter and are lightly myelinated preganglionic motor fibers. Type C fibers have a small diameter and are unmyelinated. They include motor postganglionic fibers and sensory fibers for pain and temperature.

Plexuses

A **plexus** is a network of interlacing nerves. Sometimes a plexus is formed by the primary branches of the nerves, such

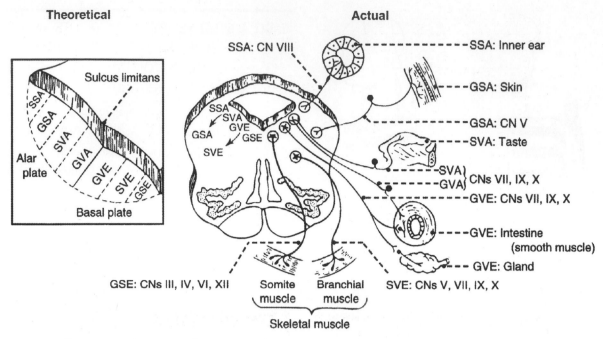

Figure 4-33 • Components of autonomic nervous system in the medulla. CN = cranial nerve; GSA = general somatic afferent; GSE = general somatic efferent; GVA = general visceral afferent; GVE = general visceral efferent; SSA = special somatic afferent; SVA = special visceral afferent; SVE = special visceral efferent. (From DeMyer, W. [1998]. *Neuroanatomy* [2nd ed.]. Baltimore: Williams & Wilkins.)

as the cervical, brachial, lumbar, and sacral plexuses. Other plexuses are formed by the terminal funiculi at the periphery. The following are the major plexuses:

The **cervical plexus** is formed from the ventral branches of the first four cervical nerves of the spine. The resulting

TABLE 4-7   MOTOR NERVE ROOTS (MYOTOMES) AND AREAS THEY INNERVATE

SPINAL NERVES	MUSCLES
C-1–C-4	Neck (flexion, lateral flexion, extension, rotation)
C-3–C-5	Diaphragm (respirations)
C-5–C-6	Shoulder movement and flexion of elbow
C-5–C-7	Forward thrust of shoulder
C-5–C-8	Adduction of arm from front to back
C-6–C-8	Extension of forearm and wrist
C-7, C-8, T-1	Flexion of wrist
T-1–T-12	Control of thoracic, abdominal, and back muscles
L-1–L-3	Flexion of hip
L-2–L-4	Extension of leg; adduction of thigh
L-4, L-5, S-1, S-2	Abduction of thigh; flexion of lower leg
L-4–L-5	Dorsal flexion of foot
L-5, S-1, S-2	Plantar flexion of foot
S-2, S-3, S-4	Perineal area and sphincters

branches innervate the muscles of the neck and shoulders. This plexus also gives rise to the **phrenic nerve,** which supplies the diaphragm.

The **brachial plexus** is composed of the ventral branches of the lower four cervical and first thoracic spinal nerves. Important nerves that emerge from this plexus are the radial and ulnar nerves.

The **lumbar plexus** originates from the ventral branches of the first four lumbar nerves. The femoral nerve arises from this plexus.

The **sacral plexus** arises from the ventral branches of the last two lumbar and first three sacral nerves. The sciatic nerve arises from this plexus.

MOTOR SYSTEM

Movement is the result of complex higher-level structures, descending spinal cord tracts, segmental spinal cord circuits, and muscles. The major higher-level structures involved in movement are the cerebral cortex, basal ganglia, cerebellum, brainstem, spinal cord, and final common pathway (Fig. 4-34). Figure 4-35 shows the motor pathways.

Nearly all voluntary muscle activity originates from the corticospinal tract (motor cortex, in large part from area 4). Other fibers originating in areas 4 and 6 do not initiate voluntary muscle activity, but act as inhibitors or suppressors of the lower motor neurons. Without these controls, lower motor neurons would fire excessively in response to reflex stimuli or discharge spontaneously, resulting in hyperreflexia or spasticity. Other tracts originate in the brainstem and also modify muscle function. The basal ganglia exert an

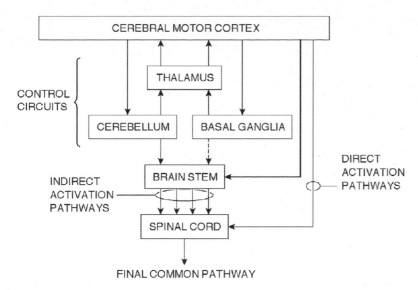

Figure 4-34 • Schematic representation of the motor system. (From Westmoreland, B. F., et al. [1994]. *Medical neurosciences.* Boston: Little, Brown and Company.)

inhibitory effect on lower motor neurons by synapses with the reticular formation. Damage to the basal ganglia results in increased motor tone. The cerebellum's role in movement is indirect through its effect on the vestibular nuclei, red nucleus, and basal ganglia. The tracts affected by these structures include the vestibulospinal, rubrospinal, and reticulospinal tracts. These tracts, in turn, affect the lower motor neurons.

Descending Motor Pathways: Upper Motor Neurons and Lower Motor Neurons

Descending motor pathways are divided into **upper motor neurons (UMNs)** and **lower motor neurons (LMNs). UMNs** are the facilitory and inhibitory descending supraspinal pathways that modify LMNs and are located entirely in the CNS. UMNs include the neurons themselves and their fibers within the corticospinal tract and corticobulbar tracts originating in the cerebral cortex; the rubrospinal and tectospinal tracts originating in the midbrain; and the reticulospinal and vestibulospinal tracts emanating from the pons and medulla. **LMNs** are located in both the CNS and PNS. Voluntary striated muscles are innervated by alpha and gamma neurons and are the **final common pathway** or final linkage between the CNS and voluntary muscles. LMNs are the GSE components of the spinal nerves and of CNs III, IV, VI, and XII and the special visceral efferent components of CNs V, VII, IX, X, and XI.

Voluntary muscle activity is the sum of neural control of the alpha and gamma motor neurons of muscle and motor components of the CN nuclei. Final neural pathways influence the muscle by way of the myoneural junction. The major tract for voluntary movement is the corticospinal tract, which is also known as the pyramidal tract. The tracts cross over to the other side of the spinal cord at the level of the medulla. This explains why voluntary control on the left side of the body (e.g., arm and leg) is by the right side of the brain and vice versa. A summary of the major descending motor tracts is found in Table 4-8.

SENSORY SYSTEM

Sensory receptors, which are located throughout the body, convey afferent impulses for interpretation of stimuli. Sensory input may be integrated into spinal reflexes or it may be relayed to the higher centers of the brain by way of ascending pathways. The impulses are analyzed and can influence unconscious and conscious activities by way of efferent responses. There are various types of receptors that convey specific types of stimuli: **exteroceptors** are stimulated by touch, light pressure, pain, temperature, odor, sound, and light; **proprioceptors** convey a sense of position, movement, and muscle coordination; **interoceptors** provide visceral information concerning pain, cramping, and fullness; and **chemoreceptors** are stimulated by chemicals (e.g., lactic acid).

Pain and Temperature

The pain and temperature pathways are so closely related throughout the body that they are treated collectively as one system. The **anterolateral system** is made up of the **anterior spinothalamic, lateral spinothalamic** (Fig. 4-36), and **spinoreticulothalamic** tracts. These are the major tracts that convey pain and temperature sensation. The afferent impulse enters the cord by way of the **posterolateral tract of Lissauer** and crosses to the opposite side of the spinal cord. Impulses ascend the cord to terminate in the thalamus, with synapsing occurring within the reticular formation of the brainstem.

Proprioception

The posterior funiculus is totally enveloped by two ascending tracts—the **fasciculus gracilis** and **fasciculus cuneatus.** These tracts ascend the cord uncrossed until they reach the area of decussation in the medulla. After the fibers decussate in this area, they proceed initially to the thalamus and then to areas 1 through 3 of the cerebral cortex. These are the major tracts that convey the sensation of **proprioception,** which includes position and movement, vibration, two-point discrimination, deep pressure, and touch.

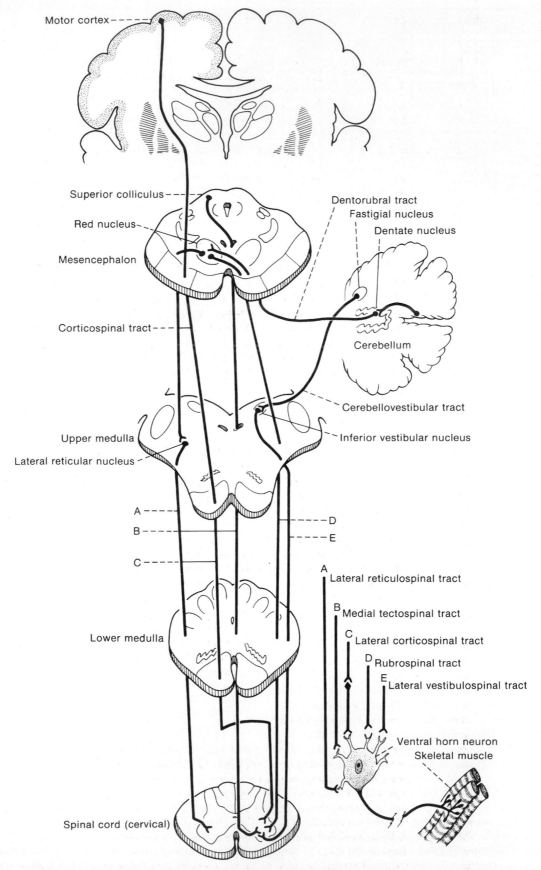

Figure 4-35 • The most important descending motor pathways that act upon the anterior horn cell of the spinal cord (final common pathway). (From Haerer, A. F. [1992]. *DeJong's the neurologic examination* [5th ed.]. Philadelphia: J. B. Lippincott.)

TABLE 4–8   MAJOR SPINAL CORD TRACTS

NAME	ORIGIN	TERMINATION	CROSSED	FUNCTION	DYSFUNCTION
Ascending Tracts					
Fasciculus gracilis	Spinal cord at sacral and lumbar levels	Medulla → thalamus → cerebral cortex (sensory strip)	Yes	Conscious proprioception, fine touch,* and vibration sense from lower body	Lower body Astereognosis Loss of vibration sense Loss of two-point discrimination Loss of proprioception
Fasciculus cuneatus	Spinal cord at thoracic and cervical levels	Medulla → thalamus → cerebral → cortex (sensory strip)	Yes	Conscious proprioception, fine touch,* and vibration sense from upper body	Upper body Astereognosis Loss of vibration sense Loss of two-point discrimination Loss of proprioception
Posterior spinocerebellar	Posterior horn	Cerebellum	No	Conduction of sensory impulses from muscle spindles and tendon organs of the trunk and lower limbs from one side of the body to the same side of cerebellum for the subconscious proprioception necessary for coordinated muscular contractions	Ipsilateral uncoordinated postural movements
Anterior spinocerebellar	Posterior horn	Cerebellum	Some	Conduction of sensory impulses from muscle spindles and tendon organs of the upper and lower limbs from both sides of the body to the cerebellum for the subconscious proprioception necessary for coordinated muscular contractions	Ipsilateral uncoordinated postural movements
Lateral spinothalamic	Posterior horn	Thalamus → cerebral cortex	Yes	Interpretation of pain and temperature	Loss of pain and temperature sensation contralaterally below the level of the lesion
Anterior spinothalamic	Posterior horn	Thalamus → cerebral cortex	Yes	Conduction of sensory impulses for pressure and crude touch† from extremities and trunk	Because one branch of the first neuron immediately synapses with a second, which ascends ipsilaterally for many levels, cord injury rarely results in complete loss of pressure and crude touch sensation
Descending Tracts					
Lateral corticospinal	Motor cortex (area 4) → internal capsule → midbrain → pons → medulla	Anterior horn; all spinal levels in laminae IV through VII and IX	80%-90% cross at the medulla	Controls voluntary muscle activity	Voluntary muscle paresis/paralysis
Anterior corticospinal	Motor cortex (area 4) → internal capsule → midbrain → medulla → anterior funiculus of the cervical and upper thoracic levels	Anterior horn (at each level of cord, axons cross to other side)	Not at medulla; synapse with cells of lamina VIII	Controls voluntary muscle activity	Voluntary muscle paresis/paralysis
Corticobulbar	Areas 4, 6, and 8 of cortex → internal capsule → brainstem	Brainstem; connects with cranial nerves V, VII, IX, X, XI, and XII	Yes	Controls voluntary head movement and facial expression	Because of bilateral innervation, facial expression is usually not affected

(continued)

TABLE 4–8   MAJOR SPINAL CORD TRACTS *(Continued)*

NAME	ORIGIN	TERMINATION	CROSSED	FUNCTION	DYSFUNCTION
Descending Tracts					
Rubrospinal	Midbrain (red nucleus)	Anterior horn	Yes	Facilitates flexor alpha and gamma motor neurons and inhibits extensor motor neurons; also influences muscle tone and posture, particularly of the arms	Altered muscle tone and posture
Reticulospinals Pontine reticulospinal Medullary reticulospinal	Reticular formation (brainstem)	Anterior horn	No	Facilitate extensor motor neurons, particularly of the legs; input to gamma motor neurons	Altered muscle tone and posture
Vestibulospinals	Reticular formation (brainstem)	Anterior horn	No	Convey autonomic information from higher levels to preganglionic autonomic nervous system neurons to influence sweating, pupillary dilatation, and circulation	Altered muscle tone and sweat gland activity
Lateral vestibulospinal			No	Facilitates extensor alpha motor neurons and inhibits flexors	Altered muscle tone and postural equilibrium
Medial vestibulospinal			No	Inhibits fibers to upper cervical alpha motor neurons; influences extraocular movements and visual reflexes	Altered muscle tone and equilibrium in response to head movement

*Fine touch is the ability to identify various objects (e.g., a key) that are placed in the hand with the eyes closed.

†Crude touch refers to light touch, which may be tested with a wisp of cotton placed in the hand with the eyes closed.

Coordination of Muscle Contraction

The anterior and posterior spinocerebellar tracts convey impulses of proprioception for the coordination of locomotion in the lower extremities. The fasciculus cuneatus and spinocerebellar tracts convey similar information from the upper half of the body. A summary of the major ascending sensory tracts is found in Table 4-8.

AUTONOMIC NERVOUS SYSTEM

The **autonomic nervous system** (ANS), part of the PNS, consists of visceral sensory fibers, ascending visceral sensory pathways, visceral reflex arcs, and descending pathways that regulate the activities of the viscera, which includes all smooth (involuntary) muscles, cardiac muscles, and glands (Fig. 4-37). The purpose of the ANS is to maintain a relatively stable internal environment for the body. The three major subdivisions of the ANS are the sympathetic, parasympathetic, and enteric systems.

The **enteric system** is a highly complex neuronal network extending over the full extent of the gastrointestinal tract. It consists of two interconnected plexuses: the myenteric (or Auerbach's) plexus and the submucous (or Meissner's) plexus. It is composed of local sensory neurons, interneurons, and visceral motor neurons in the walls of the alimentary canal. All of these neurons and their processes lie entirely outside the CNS. The enteric system is responsible for the normal coordinated gut motility and secretions that persist even in the total absence of neuronal input between the gut and the CNS.

The **sympathetic system** is activated during stress situations such as fright, fight, or flight phenomena. During these stressful periods, the heart rate and blood pressure increase, and there is vasoconstriction of the peripheral blood vessels.

The **parasympathetic system** stimulates those visceral activities associated with conservation, restoration, and maintenance of a normal functional level. The parasympathetic system decreases heart rate and increases gastrointestinal activity (Table 4-9, page 79).

The sympathetic and parasympathetic systems, which function in an antagonistic relationship, innervate most body organs. These systems are activated primarily by centers located in the spinal cord, brainstem, and hypothalamus. The transmission of impulses from the CNS to the viscera always involves two different neurons. The **preganglionic neuron,** which is the first neuron, has its cell body in the CNS. Its axon terminates in an autonomic ganglion on the **postganglionic neuron.** This postganglionic neuron, which is the second neuron, has its cell body in the ganglion and its axon innervates the end-organ.

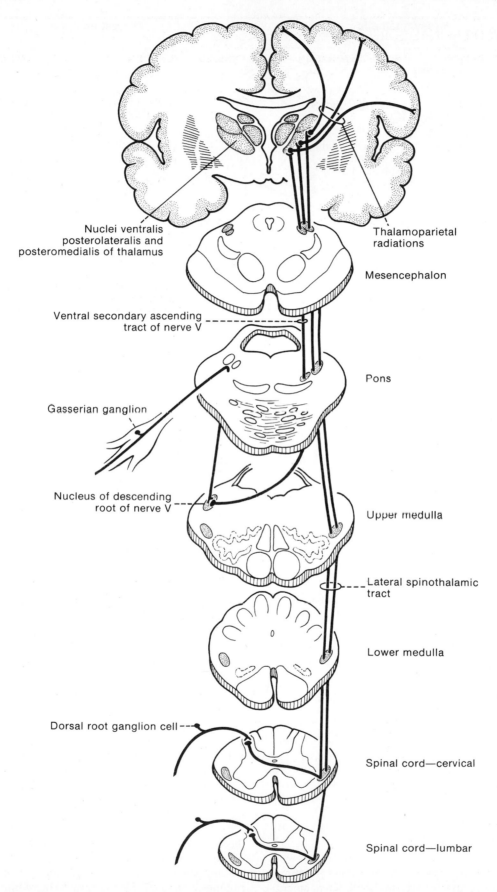

Figure 4-36 • The lateral spinothalamic (sensory) tract. (From Haerer, A. F. [1992]. *DeJong's the neurologic examination* [5th ed.]. Philadelphia: J. B. Lippincott.)

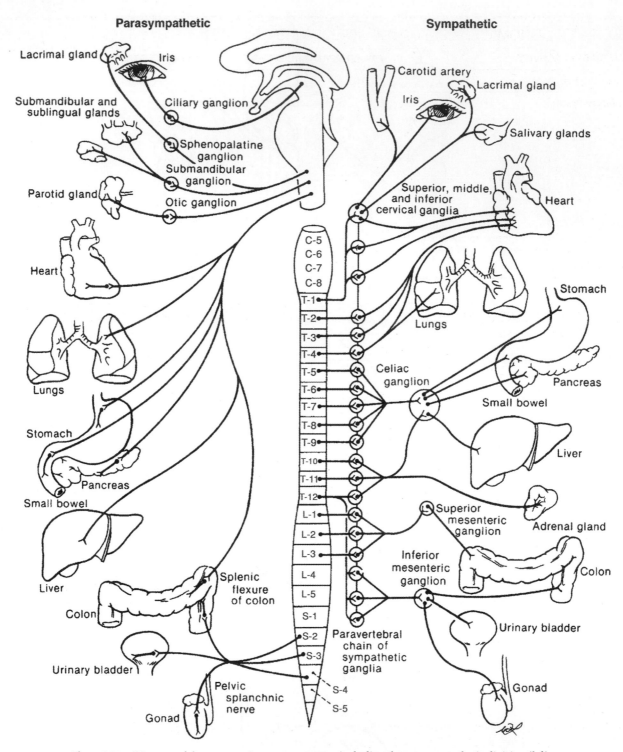

Figure 4-37 • Diagram of the autonomic nervous system, including the parasympathetic division (*left*) arising from cranial nerve (CN) III, CN VII, CN IX, and CN X and from spinal cord segments S-2 through S-4. The sympathetic division (*right*) arises from spinal cord segments T-1 through T-12. (From DeMyer, W. [1998]. *Neuroanatomy* [2nd ed.]. Baltimore: Williams & Wilkins.)

Sympathetic Nervous System

The sympathetic nervous system is also called the **thoracolumbar system** because its preganglionic fibers emerge from cell bodies in the **intermediolateral nucleus of lamina VII.** The sympathetic nervous system extends through the thoracic and upper two lumbar levels (T-1 through L-2). These preganglionic fibers leave the spinal cord with the motor fibers of the ventral roots. After traveling less than 1 cm, the sympathetic fibers pass into the **white rami communicantes**—a branch of the spinal nerve—which, in turn, enters the **sympathetic chain** or trunk, also called the

TABLE 4–9   AUTONOMIC EFFECTS OF THE NERVOUS SYSTEM

STRUCTURE OR ACTIVITY	PARASYMPATHETIC EFFECTS	SYMPATHETIC EFFECTS
Pupil of the Eye	Constricted	Dilated
Circulatory System		
Rate and force of heartbeat	Decreased	Increased

Blood vessels
  In heart muscle
  In skeletal muscle
  In abdominal viscera and the skin
	Constricted
	*
	*
		Dilated
		Dilated
		Constricted

Blood pressure	Decreased	Increased
Respiratory System		
Bronchioles	Constricted	Dilated
Rate of breathing	Decreased	Increased
Digestive System		
Peristaltic movements of digestive tube	Increased	Decreased
Muscular sphincters of digestive tube	Relaxed	Contracted
Secretion of salivary glands	Thin, watery saliva	Thick, viscid saliva
Secretions of stomach, intestine, and pancreas	Increased	*
Conversion of liver glycogen to glucose	*	Increased
Genitourinary System		

Urinary bladder
  Muscular walls
  Sphincters
Muscles of the uterus
	Contracted
	Relaxed
	Relaxed; variable
		Relaxed
		Contracted
		Contracted under some conditions; varies
		  with menstrual cycle and pregnancy

Blood vessels of external genitalia	Dilated	*
Integument		
Secretion of sweat	*	Increased
Pilomotor muscles	*	Contracted (gooseflesh)
Medullae of Adrenal Glands	*	Secretion of epinephrine and norepinephrine

* No direct effect.

(From Chaffee, E. E., & Lytle, I. M. [1980]. *Basic physiology and anatomy* [3rd ed]. Philadelphia: J. B. Lippincott.)

paravertebral ganglia. (The sympathetic chain consists of a chain of ganglia located on either side of the spinal cord that extends from the base of the skull to the coccyx. These ganglia are all interconnected by longitudinal fibers, thus forming a continuous chain.) In the sympathetic chain, the fibers may synapse in three possible places. First, the fibers may synapse immediately with postganglionic fibers located in the chain at the level of entry. Second, the fiber may travel up or down the trunk to synapse in one of the chain ganglia above or below the point of entry. Third, the fiber may pass on to synapse with a postganglionic neuron in an outlying sympathetic ganglia (**prevertebral ganglia** or collateral ganglia).

Some fibers from the postganglionic neuron in the sympathetic chain return to the spinal nerve by way of the **gray rami communicantes** at all levels of the spinal cord.

Each spinal nerve receives a gray ramus, which controls the blood vessels, sweat glands, and piloerector muscles of the hairs.

Sympathetic preganglionic fibers leave the spinal cord to enter the sympathetic chain in only the thoracic and upper lumbar regions; none of the sympathetic preganglionic fibers enters the chain in the cervical, lower lumbar, or sacral regions. Sympathetic innervation to the head is supplied by sympathetic fibers extending from the thoracic chain. In this way, the neck and all structures of the head are innervated. Sympathetic fibers also pass downward from the sympathetic chain into the lower abdomen and legs.

The sympathetic outflow is distributed in the following way: T-1 to T-5 innervate the head, creating three ganglia (superior cervical, middle cervical, and cervicothoracic stellate). Of those sympathetic fibers directed to the head, those from T-1 and T-2 innervate the eye for pupillary dilation; T-2 through T-6 innervate the heart and lungs; and T-6 through L-2 innervate the abdominal viscera through the thoracic and lumbar splanchnic nerves. The thoracic splanchnic nerves carry the preganglionic fibers to the prevertebral ganglia of the abdomen. The celiac, superior mesenteric, and aorticorenal ganglia arise in this area. The lumbar splanchnic nerves terminate in the inferior mesenteric and hypogastric ganglia.

The preganglionic sympathetic nerve fibers pass directly to the adrenal medulla without synapsing. These fibers are cholinergic and end directly on the special cells of the medulla that secrete epinephrine and norepinephrine.

Sympathetic Neurotransmitter

The neurotransmitter released by the postganglionic fibers is **norepinephrine** (noradrenaline). This is why the sympathetic system is termed **adrenergic.** Acetylcholine is secreted at the preganglionic terminal and is quickly deactivated by cholinesterase. There are few exceptions in the postganglionic neurons in the sympathetic nervous system. The piloerector muscles and most sweat glands in the palms of the hands receive cholinergic postganglionic sympathetic neurons.

Parasympathetic Nervous System

The parasympathetic system is also called the **craniosacral system** because its preganglionic fibers emerge either with CNs III, VII, IX, and X or from the second, third, and fourth sacral segments of the spinal cord. The specific parasympathetic innervation to these CNs includes the following:

- Oculomotor (III) supplies the ciliary muscles for accommodation and constrictor sphincter muscles of the pupil.
- Facial (VII) innervates many glands of the head, such as lacrimal, submandibular, sublingual, nasal, oral, and pharyngeal areas.
- Glossopharyngeal (IX) innervates the parotid glands.
- Vagus (X) synapses with terminal ganglia located adjacent to, or within, the various viscera throughout the body.

The sacral portion of the parasympathetic system arises from cell bodies in the intermediate gray matter of sacral segments S-2 through S-4. These fibers pass through the pelvic splanchnic nerve to synapse in the terminal ganglia with the postganglionic neurons, which innervate the descending colon, rectum, bladder, lower ureters, and external genitalia. The parasympathetic system is involved with the mechanisms of bladder and bowel evacuation and, unlike the sympathetic system, is designed to respond to a specific stimulus in a localized area for a short period of time.

Parasympathetic Neurotransmitters

The parasympathetic system secretes **acetylcholine** at the postganglionic neuron. This is why the parasympathetic system is termed **cholinergic.** Acetylcholine is also secreted at the preganglionic synapse and is quickly deactivated by **cholinesterase.**

Spinal Reflexes

A **reflex** is a stereotypical response, mediated by the nervous system, to a particular stimulus of sufficient magnitude. The simplest type of stereotypical neural pathway is called a **reflex arc.** There are five components to a reflex arc, including the following (Fig. 4-38):

Receptor—specific sensory fibers that are sensitive to the stimulus
Sensory (afferent) neuron—relays the impulse through the posterior root to the CNS
Interneuron—an association or connecting neuron located within the CNS
Motor (efferent) neuron—relays the impulse through the anterior root to the effector organ
Effector—a specific organ that responds

Reflexes can be classified by the extent of the regional involvement of the spinal cord. This classification includes **segmental, intersegmental,** and **suprasegmental reflexes.**

A reflex arc which passes through only one anatomic segment is called a **segmental reflex.** A knee-jerk reflex is an example of both a segmental and a simple or monosynaptic reflex. A monosynaptic reflex includes an afferent limb that synapses directly with an efferent limb. Most reflexes, however, are more complex and polysynaptic.

An **intersegmental reflex** involves several spinal segments. A flexor or withdrawal reflex is an example of an intersegmental reflex.

A **suprasegmental reflex** involves interaction between the brain centers that regulate cord activity and the segments of the cord itself. An example of a suprasegmental reflex is extension of the legs in response to movement of the head.

Another classification system useful in clinical practice divides reflexes into stretch, cutaneous, and pathologic reflexes.

Muscle stretch reflexes, also called deep tendon reflexes (DTRs), are elicited by striking a tendon that stretches the neuromuscular spindles of the muscle group. The knee-jerk reflex, a stretch reflex, results in contraction of the quadriceps and extension of the leg in response to tapping the patellar tendon. Other common stretch reflexes involve the biceps, triceps, and ankle.

Cutaneous reflexes, also termed superficial reflexes, are initiated when the skin or mucous membrane is stimulated by light stroking or scratching, resulting in a specific response in a muscle or muscle group. The withdrawal reflex, which is a flexor reflex, is an example of a cutaneous reflex that is a protective reflex. In response to a noxious cutaneous stimulus to the fingers, the hand is flexed and withdrawn. Another cutaneous reflex is contraction of the superficial abdominal muscles in response to light, rapid stroking of the skin on the abdomen.

Pathologic reflexes are those reflexes that should not be present and indicate organic interference with CNS function. The method of eliciting these reflexes usually involves stimulation of the skin in a particular area. Presence of a Babinski sign is a common pathologic reflex.

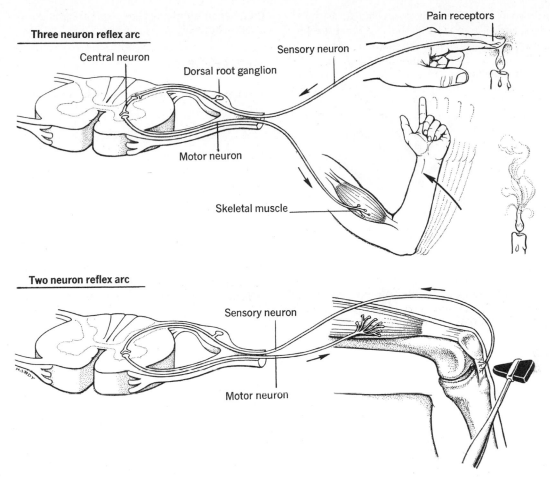

Figure 4-38 • Diagram of a flexor reflex (*top*) and a stretch reflex (*bottom*). (From Chaffee, E. E., & Lytle, I. M. [1980]. *Basic physiology and anatomy.* Philadelphia: J. B. Lippincott.)

Micturition

Micturition, also called voiding or urination, is the process of evacuating urine from the bladder. In the infant and young child, micturition is a simple reflex initiated by distention of the bladder by urine. Between 2 and 3 years of age, the maturation of spinal cord segments, along with the conscious inhibitory ability of the cerebral cortex, results in voluntary control of micturition. The average capacity of the urinary bladder is 700 to 800 mL. Stimulation of the stretch receptors by a volume of 200 to 300 mL of urine will trigger the micturition reflex and a concurrent conscious desire to void.

Two main anatomic parts constitute the smooth muscle urinary bladder: (1) the body, which is the **detrusor muscle;** and (2) the **trigone,** a small, triangular area at the base of the bladder that includes the bladder–ureter junction, the urethra, and the external sphincter (a voluntary skeletal muscle). The external sphincter is located at the opening of the bladder and is normally contracted to prevent dribbling.

Micturition is primarily a parasympathetic function. The micturition reflex is mediated by S-2, S-3, and S-4 spinal segments, from which the preganglionic parasympathetic fibers synapse within the terminal ganglia located in the bladder wall by way of the pelvic splanchnic nerves (Fig. 4-39). Short postganglionic parasympathetic fibers innervate both the detrusor muscle and internal sphincter. Parasympathetic stimulation that is caused by the stretching of the bladder wall results in contraction of the detrusor muscle and relaxation of the internal sphincter. Although there is some sympathetic innervation to the bladder, its role is not certain. Micturition is primarily a parasympathetic function.

The external sphincter is under voluntary control and is mediated by the pudendal nerve. It can be voluntarily contracted, but it relaxes by reflex action when urine is released from the internal sphincter.

Defecation

The act of evacuating the large bowel is called **defecation.** Several physiologic mechanisms are involved in defecation. **Peristalsis** is the wave-like movement of smooth muscles within the wall of the large intestines. There are two important reflexes related to defecation. The gastrocolic and duodenocolic reflexes that result from distention of the stomach and duodenum after eating facilitate peristalsis and mass movement along the gastrointestinal tract toward the rectum.

There are also two defecation reflexes. The first, the **intrinsic defecation reflex,** is triggered by feces entering the rectum. Pressure on the rectal wall sends afferent impulses

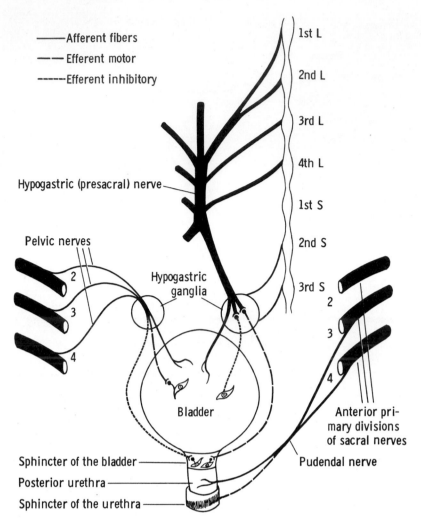

— Afferent fibers
— — Efferent motor
------ Efferent inhibitory

1st L
2nd L
3rd L
4th L
1st S
2nd S
3rd S

Hypogastric (presacral) nerve

Pelvic nerves

Hypogastric ganglia

2
3
4

Bladder

Anterior primary divisions of sacral nerves

Pudendal nerve

Sphincter of the bladder
Posterior urethra
Sphincter of the urethra

Figure 4-39 • Diagrammatic representation of the innervation of the bladder and urethra. (From Chaffee, E. E., & Lytle, I. M. [1980]. *Basic physiology and anatomy*. Philadelphia: J. B. Lippincott.)

through the **mesenteric plexus** to initiate peristaltic waves in the descending colon, sigmoid, and rectum, forcing feces toward the anus. Peristalsis relaxes the internal anal sphincter, and if the external anal sphincter is also relaxed, defecation occurs. The intrinsic defecation reflex is a weak reflex and must occur in combination with another reflex for defecation to occur.

This second reflex, the **parasympathetic defecation reflex,** involves the sacral segments (S-3, S-4, S-5) of the spinal cord. Stimulated afferent fibers in the rectum send signals to the spinal cord, and signals are sent back to the descending colon, sigmoid, rectum, and anus through the parasympathetic nerve fibers in the pelvic nerves. The parasympathetic signals do three things: intensify peristalsis, relax the internal anal sphincter, and augment the intrinsic defecation reflex. A powerful bowel evacuation can occur if the external anal sphincter is relaxed.

Conscious Control of Defecation

During infancy, defecation is a purely reflex action. However, in early childhood voluntary control is learned so that defecation can be postponed until a socially acceptable place to evacuate the bowel is found. Voluntary consciousness now

controls the external anal sphincter. If the sphincter is relaxed, defecation can take place. If contraction of the sphincter prevents defecation, the defecation reflexes soon cease, remaining inactive for several hours until more feces enter the rectum and once again initiate the defecation reflexes. The frequency of defecation among people varies from once per day to two or three times per week.

CRANIAL NERVES

The 12 pairs of CNs are part of the peripheral nervous system. Besides being named, each CN is also identified in Roman numerals. The number is based on the descending order in which the CNs and their nuclei attach to the CNS. CN I connects to the brain in the cerebral hemispheres, whereas CN XII attaches at the lower medulla (Fig. 4-40).

The anatomic locations of connection of the CNs are as follows: I and II are in the cerebral hemispheres; III and IV are in the midbrain; V, VI, VII, and VIII are in the pons; and IX, X, XI, and XII are in the medulla. There are a few exceptions to the schemata: CNs VII and VIII have dual citizenship in both the pons and, to a lesser degree, the medulla. CN V, primarily

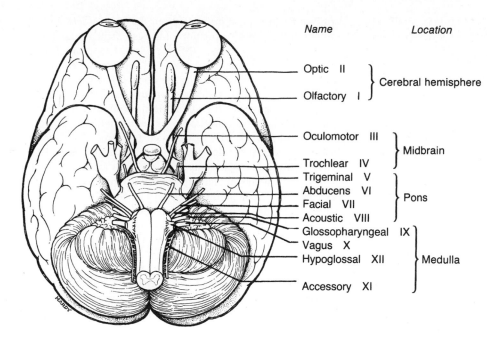

Figure 4-40 • Diagram of the base of the brain showing entrance or exit of the cranial nerves. The eyeballs are shown schematically in relation to the optic nerves. The right column indicates the anatomic location of the connection of each cranial nerve to the central nervous system.

associated with the pons, also has branches in the midbrain and medulla (Fig. 4-41).

As a rule, CNs do not cross in the brain (with the exception of CN IV). There are three sensory CNs (I, II, and VIII), five motor CNs (III, IV, VI, XI, and XII), and four CNs with mixed functions (V, VII, IX, and X).

Classification of nerve fibers is similar to spinal nerves in some cases and dissimilar in other instances. CNs that have functions similar to those of spinal nerves are categorized as **general;** those with specialized functions (olfactory and gustatory) are **special.** The GSA, GVA, GSE, and GVE fibers are similar to spinal nerves of those categories and have already been discussed with spinal nerves. Fibers that are specific to CNs include **special somatic afferent** (SSA), **special visceral afferent** (SVA), and **special visceral efferent** (SVE). SSA fibers convey sensory impulses from the special sense organs in the eye (vision) and ear (hearing and balance). SVA fibers convey impulses from the olfactory and gustatory receptors. SVE fibers innervate striated skeletal muscles from the brachial arches (jaw muscles, facial expression muscles, and muscles of pharynx and larynx).

Olfactory Nerve (Sensory) (CN I)

The olfactory nerve is a pure SVA nerve for the sense of smell. The receptors for smell are located in the superior nasal mucosa of each nostril. The **olfactory** nerve is composed of multiple small fibers from bipolar chemoreceptor cells called olfactory cells. The axons penetrate the skull through the cribriform plate to terminate in the **olfactory bulb.** From the bulb, the **olfactory tract** continues backward to the base of the frontal lobes where the two principal areas—the medial olfactory area and the lateral olfactory area—are located. The **medial olfactory area** is located anteriorly and superiorly to the hypothalamus (septum pellucidum, gyrus subcallosus, paraolfactory area, olfactory trigone, and medial part of the anterior perforated substance). The **lateral olfactory area** is composed of the prepyriform area, the uncus, the lateral part of the anterior perforated substance, and part of the amygdaloid nucleus. Olfaction is unique among the sensory systems, in that impulses in this system project to the cortex without being relayed by thalamic nuclei.

Optic Nerve (Sensory) (CN II)

The **optic nerve,** another pure SSA nerve, arises from the retina of the eyeball and is a part of the visual system. The **fundus** or **optic disc** represents the point where the optic nerve joins the retina and can be visualized by using the

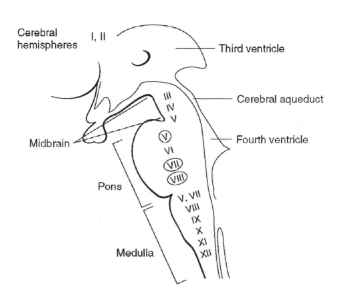

Figure 4-41 • Lateral view of sites of cranial nerves and their nuclei within the cerebral hemispheres and brainstem (midbrain, pons, or medulla).

ophthalmoscope (it is the only CN that can be visualized). The optic disc is a natural blind spot because it does not contain any rods or cones. The **macula** is a 3-mm circular area on the retina, located near the posterior pole of the orbit that is the point of clearest vision. The **scotoma** is an expected blind spot on the retina.

Vision is complex not only because many steps are involved in the process, but also because the visual tracts cut through all the lobes of the cerebral hemispheres. Therefore, visual deficits are common with many intracranial problems.

The **rods and cones** of the retina are the photoreceptors that are stimulated by light, thereby initiating nerve impulses that are conducted to the cerebral cortex (Fig. 4-42). Each **optic nerve** (4.5 to 5.0 cm long) runs posteriorly until it meets the optic nerve from the other side at the **optic chiasma.** The **visual pathways** posterior to the retina include a number of structures. The optic nerves come together at the optic chiasma, above the sella turcica. A partial decussation takes place at the chiasma whereby the nasal half of each optic nerve crosses to the other side and the temporal half of each optic nerve remains uncrossed. The **optic tracts** proceed laterally and posteriorly to terminate in the **lateral geniculate bodies** (a flattened area in the posterolateral surface of the thalamus). Before reaching the lateral geniculate body, a few fibers leave the optic tract to go to the pretectal areas. These fibers become the afferent limb of the light reflex.

The **lateral geniculate body** is the terminal point of the optic tract; the geniculocalcarine tract originates from the cells of the geniculate bodies. The **geniculocalcarine tract** passes through the retrolenticular part of the internal capsule and forms the **optic radiations.** The upper fibers of optic radiations pass posteriorly in the *parietal lobe* and terminate in the superior portion of the calcarine cortex (occipital lobe); the lower fibers (**Meyer's loop**) loop anterolaterally around the temporal horn of the *temporal lobe* and terminate in the inferior calcarine cortex. The **calcarine cortex,** also called the **primary visual cortex,** is organized such that the upper part of the visual field terminates in the inferior calcarine cortex and the lower visual field terminates in the superior cortex. The primary cortex (area 17) is located in the walls of the calcarine fissure and receives primary visual stimuli. The **visual association areas** (areas 18 and 19) are located in the **peristriate cortex** of the temporal and occipital lobes, lateral to the primary cortex. The visual association areas are necessary for visual impressions, recognition of colors and formed objects, and visual memory. In addition, eye movements activated by visual stimuli are controlled by the association areas.

Visual System

When the visual system is considered, it includes not only the optic nerves, visual pathways, and visual cortex, but also eye movement itself. Eye movement is addressed here to complete the discussion of the visual system.

Conjugate gaze and eye movement are complex processes for which the following areas have specific functions:

Brainstem for premotor conjugate gaze and vergence eye movement (**vergence** movements are both eyes moving medially to look at a near object or laterally to look into the distance)

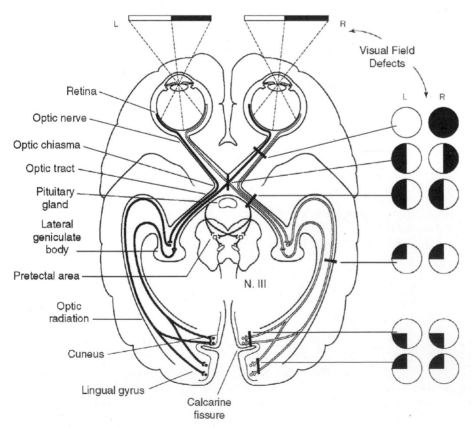

Figure 4-42 • Fields of vision.

Thalamic-midbrain centers for vertical gaze and vergence
Paramedian pontine reticular formation of the pons for horizontal eye movement

Five subsystems have been identified to enable the fovea to find and fixate on a target, stabilize an image on the retina, and maintain binocular focus during head or target movement.

Saccadic system (a **saccade** is a rapid, refixational eye movement): saccades may be voluntary or involuntary
Pursuit system: provides for eyes to track slowly moving targets
Vestibular system (semicircular canals): maintains a stable image on the retina during head movements
Optokinetic system: enables stabilization of images on the retina during sustained head rotation, such as spinning
Vergence eye movement system: allows the eyes to move convergently and divergently to maintain binocular fixation on a target moving toward or away from the subject

The frontal-parietal gaze center (posterior portion of middle frontal gyrus, area 8; and ventral parietal lobe, area 7a) and the occipital gaze center (areas 18 and 19) are important. The **frontal gaze center** is responsible for rapid (saccadic) voluntary control of conjugate gaze to a point of interest. Its fibers pass through the anterior internal capsule to the pons and connect with the lower centers. The **occipital gaze center** controls involuntary slow-tracking eye movement or visual pursuit. The center is responsible for fixing the eyes on an object and maintaining that visual fixation as the object moves through the visual field. Its fibers pass medially to the optic radiations and down through the posterior portion of the internal capsule, connecting with the conjugate eye movement centers in the midbrain and pons.

The MLF extends from the thalamic-midbrain region to the anterior horn cells of the spinal cord; it coordinates the movement pathways of the eye and neck for gaze. The MLF connects and integrates fibers from the following areas of eye movement: brainstem oculomotor, trochlear, and abducens nuclei; fibers from the synapse of cerebellar nuclei and the semicircular canals; and the horizontal gaze center of the pons. Convergence of the eyes is not well understood and seems to be mediated by pontine and medullary structures, but not by the MLF. Divergence is controlled by centers located near the abducens nuclei.

The **paramedian pontine reticular formation (PPRF)** is located in the pons and receives fibers from the superior colliculus, the vestibular nuclei, and other parts of the reticular formation. The PPRF is also known as the lateral gaze center. It sends fibers to the ipsilateral abducens nucleus (lateral movement) and through the MLF to cells of the contralateral oculomotor nucleus that supply the medial rectus muscle, thus coordinating horizontal movement. Therefore, the descending pathways for horizontal conjugate gaze include the PPRF and the MLF. Much less is known about vertical movement. The oculomotor and trochlear nuclei, located in the brainstem, are involved in vertical eye movement: vertical and torsional saccadic innervation arise in the midbrain; the vertical gaze-holding impulses are integrated in the midbrain; and the vestibular and pursuit impulses ascend to the midbrain from the lower brainstem.

Oculomotor Nerve (Motor) (CN III)

The oculomotor nerve innervates four of the six extrinsic muscles responsible for movement of the eye. These muscles are the medial, superior, and inferior recti and the inferior oblique; they are controlled by GSE fibers. The eyes are rotated by these muscles in the following manner: medial recti—inward (medially); superior recti—upward and outward; inferior recti—downward and outward; and inferior oblique—upward and inward (Table 4-10).

TABLE 4–10   CRANIAL NERVE FUNCTION RELATIVE TO EYE MOVEMENT

CRANIAL NERVE	MUSCLE	MOVEMENT OF EYEBALL
Oculomotor (III)*	Medial rectus	Inward or medially on the horizontal plane
	Superior rectus	Upward and outward
	Inferior rectus	Downward and outward
	Inferior oblique	Upward and inward
Trochlear (IV)	Superior oblique	Downward and inward
Abducens (VI)	Lateral rectus	Outward or laterally on the horizontal plane

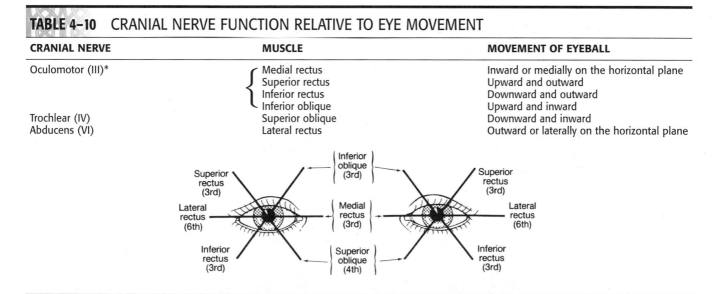

Note that the eye muscles function in pairs: The superior and inferior recti turn the eye upward and downward when the eye is looking outward (temporally); the inferior and superior obliques turn the eye upward and downward when the eye is looking inward; and the medial and lateral recti turn the eye inward (nasally) and outward (temporally) on the horizontal plane.

* The oculomotor nerve also innervates the levator palpebrae oculoris muscle, which elevates the upper eyelid and the muscles that control the iris and ciliary body.

(Figure from Bates, B. [1980]. *A guide to physical examination*. Philadelphia: J. B. Lippincott.)

The oculomotor nerve has two other functions. First, it innervates the levator palpebrae superioris, which is responsible for elevating the upper eyelid (also GSE fibers). Second, it provides motor innervation to the intrinsic smooth muscles of the iris for pupillary constriction and to the muscles within the ciliary body for lens accommodation (both GVE functions).

The eye is innervated by both parasympathetic and sympathetic fibers to control pupillary size. Parasympathetic innervation is responsible for **pupillary constriction.** The parasympathetic preganglionic fibers arise in the **Edinger-Westphal nucleus** (the visceral nucleus of CN III) and then proceed in CN III to the ciliary ganglion. Here, the preganglionic fibers synapse with postganglionic parasympathetic neurons that send fibers through the ciliary nerves into the eyeball. These nerves excite the ciliary muscles and the pupillary sphincter of the iris, resulting in pupillary constriction.

Pupillary dilation is the result of sympathetic innervation of the pupil originating in the intermediolateral horn cells of spinal cord segments C-8 to T-2. Proceeding from here, sympathetic fibers enter the sympathetic chain and pass upward to the superior cervical ganglion, where they synapse with postganglionic neurons. These fibers radiate along the carotid artery and smaller arteries until the eye is reached. Here, the sympathetic fibers excite the radial fibers of the iris and cause pupillary dilation.

Accommodation is the mechanism by which an automatic adjustment or accommodation of the curvature of the lens is made to focus images on the retina for visual acuity. Accommodation results from the contraction or relaxation of the ciliary muscles of the eye. Contraction of the smooth muscle fibers of the ciliary body causes the **suspensory ligaments** to relax and the lens to become thicker. Relaxation of the **ciliary body's** smooth muscle fibers results in tension of the suspensory ligaments and elongation of the lens.

Trochlear Nerve (Motor) (CN IV)

The trochlear nerve, a GSE nerve, supplies the superior oblique muscle. It is responsible for moving the eye downward and inward. The **trochlear nucleus** is located immediately caudal to the oculomotor nucleus at the level of the inferior colliculus in the midbrain. It exits the brainstem dorsally, the only CN to exit from the dorsum (posterior part) of the brainstem. Small bundles of fibers curve around the periaqueductal gray matter and decussate in the superior medullary velum; the trochlear emerges caudal to the inferior colliculus. The superior oblique muscle is supplied by crossed fibers.

Trigeminal Nerve (Mixed) (CN V)

The trigeminal nerve is unique in that its main components are located in the pons with additional components in the midbrain and medulla. The trigeminal nerve has both GSA and SVE components. Pain, temperature, and light touch are conveyed from the entire face and scalp, the paranasal sinuses, and the nasal and oral cavities by the GSA component. The SVE motor component supplies the muscles of mastication, which arise from the brachial arches.

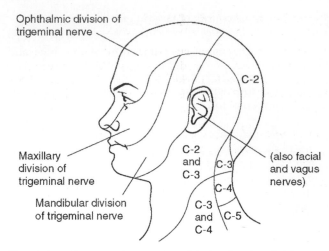

Figure 4-43 • Cutaneous innervation of the head and neck. The boundaries between the territories supplied by the three divisions of the trigeminal nerve do not overlap appreciably, as do the boundaries between spinal dermatomes. (From Barr, M. L., & Kiernan, J. A. [1988]. *The human nervous system* [5th ed.]. Philadelphia: J. B. Lippincott.)

The GSA fibers arise from the cell bodies in the **trigeminal ganglion.** The sensory components of the trigeminal nerve are divided into three sensory branches: **ophthalmic, maxillary,** and **mandibular** (Fig. 4-43). Axons travel centrally from the ganglion to enter the lateral aspect of the pons. Fibers for touch synapse directly on the **main sensory nucleus of V** that is located in the dorsolateral tegmentum of the pons. Pain and temperature fibers follow a different course. They turn caudally and descend via the dorsolateral medulla and upper three or four segments of the cervical spinal cord as the **spinal tract of the trigeminal nerve.** The peripheral path followed by sensory fibers after the trigeminal ganglion is as follows:

1. The **ophthalmic division (V1)** passes through the superior orbital fissure to innervate the upper face.
2. The **maxillary division (V2)** exits the skull via the foramen rotundum to innervate the midface.
3. The **mandibular division (V3),** joined by the motor root, exits the skull via the foramen ovale to innervate the lower face.

The SVE fibers that innervate the muscles of mastication arise from cell bodies in the **motor nucleus of V,** which is located medial to the main sensory nucleus in the pons. The axons follow a ventrolateral path and exit from the lateral surface of the pons.

Abducens Nerve (Motor) (CN VI)

The abducens is a GSE nerve that innervates the lateral rectus muscle and rotates the eye laterally on the horizontal plane. The abducens nerve arises from the **abducens nuclei** located in the floor of the fourth ventricle of the midpons. Axons follow an anterior course through the tegmentum and basis pontis to the pontomedullary junction. The abducens then ascends to the pontine base through the cavernous sinus and exits the cranium through the superior orbital fissure to the lateral rectus muscle. The lateral rectus muscle abducts the eye.

Facial Nerve (Mixed) (CN VII)

The facial nerve has its nucleus primarily in the pons, but it also has connections to the medulla. It has SVE, GVE, and SVA components. The **facial nucleus** is located in the pons and has two branches: SVE fibers (arise in one branch and innervate the muscles of facial expression), and GVE and SVA fibers. The SVE branch is responsible for closing the eye, smiling, whistling, showing the teeth, wrinkling the nose, and grimacing. The parasympathetic GVE fibers originate in the superior salivatory nucleus and control tearing and salivation of the lacrimal, sublingual, and submandibular glands. The sensory fibers originate in the **geniculate ganglion;** these SVA components mediate taste to the anterior two thirds of the tongue and sensation from the skin lining the external auditory meatus.

The SVE innervation of the muscles of facial expression can be divided into the muscles of the lower part of the face and the muscles of the upper part of the face. **Crossed fibers** project from the cerebral cortex to the facial nuclei that supply the contralateral lower part of the face (the area below the eye). **Crossed and uncrossed fibers** project to motor cells that innervate the upper part of the face. Movement of the upper face (e.g., wrinkling the brow) comes from bilateral input from the cortex to the facial nerve nucleus. Because the upper facial muscles receive both crossed and uncrossed fibers, the upper part of the face is spared with central cerebral injury such as in stroke. The upper motor lesion (e.g., stroke) results in a paralysis that is limited to muscles of the contralateral lower face (below the eye). If the facial nerve is injured (Bell's palsy), the entire side of the face (upper and lower face) would be affected. Therefore, the deficits on the affected side would include an "ironed out" forehead, an inability to close the eye, and a flattening of the nasolabial fold.

Vestibulocochlear Nerve (Sensory) (CN VIII)

The vestibulocochlear nerve is divided into two branches: the cochlear, which is concerned with hearing, and the vestibular, which influences balance, maintenance of body position, and orientation in space. Because these branches represent two distinct systems, they are discussed separately.

In the **auditory system,** the **cochlear nerve** has SSA fibers that carry impulses from the cell bodies in the spiral ganglion of the cochlea. Vibrations proceed through the tympanic membrane and activate the three small bones of the middle ear (malleus, incus, and stapes). These vibrations then continue to the cochlea of the inner ear where the basilar membrane with the **organ of Corti** (hair-like mechanoreceptors) sends fibers to the spiral ganglion of the cochlea. The spiral ganglion contains the bipolar cells of the cochlea (dorsal and ventral cochlear nuclei) that connect to the brainstem. The primary auditory receptive areas of the cortex are 41 and 42. From here, the impulses proceed to the auditory association area where recognition of the particular sound takes place.

In the **vestibular system,** the **vestibular nerve** has SSA fibers. The vestibular receptor end-organs in the vestibular system include the three cristae ampullares, one located in each of the semicircular canals, and the maculae of the utricle and saccule. All these structures are sensitive to movement in a particular direction. The vestibular ganglion of the vestibular nerve receives input from the vestibular receptors and the cerebel-lum. The vestibular nuclei have projections into the following areas: spinal cord, by way of the lateral and medial vestibular spinal tracts (inhibitory and facility influence to extensor muscle tone and spinal reflexes); cerebellum; reticular formation; and, through the MLF, the nuclei of CNs III, IV, and VI.

Glossopharyngeal Nerve (Mixed) (CN IX)

The glossopharyngeal nerve is a mixed nerve with SVA, GVE, GSA, GVA, and SVE fibers. The vagus nerve is closely related, both anatomically and physiologically, to the glossopharyngeal nerve. The glossopharyngeal nerve has five branches, all of which penetrate the skull through the jugular foramen. The glossopharyngeal nerve innervates the stylopharyngeus of the pharynx (SVE); taste receptors from the posterior third of the tongue (SVA); parasympathetics of the parotid gland (GVE); sensation from the back of the ear (GSA); and sensation from the pharynx, tongue, eustachian tube, carotid sinus, and carotid body (GVA).

The SVE fibers of the stylopharyngeus muscle originate in the nucleus ambiguus. The GVE fibers carry parasympathetic fibers to the parotid gland and terminate in the otic ganglion. The cell bodies for sensory innervation are located in the inferior and superior petrosal ganglia.

Vagus Nerve (Mixed) (CN X)

The vagus nerve is also a mixed nerve with SVE, GVE, GSA, GVA, and SVE fibers. It branches into several segments. The functions include innervation of the striated muscles from the brachial arches (soft palate, pharynx, and larynx [SVE]); the parasympathetic innervation of the thoracic and abdominal organs (GVE); sensory innervation from the external auditory meatus (GSA); sensory innervation from the pharynx, larynx, and thoracic and abdominal viscera (GVA); and sensory innervation from the taste receptors of the posterior pharynx (SVA).

The SVE fibers (soft palate, pharynx, and larynx) come from the nucleus ambiguus found in the lateral medullary region dorsal to the inferior olive. The GVE components include preganglionic parasympathetic fibers coming from the dorsal motor nucleus to supply the thoracic and abdominal viscera. Preganglionic vagal neurons from the nucleus ambiguus innervate the heart. The preganglionic fibers synapse with the postganglionic neurons in the cardiac, pulmonary, esophageal, or celiac plexuses or within the visceral organs. The cell bodies for sensory innervation are dispersed throughout the body in a number of ganglia.

Spinal Accessory Nerve (Motor) (CN XI)

This spinal accessory nerve is an SVE nerve that innervates the sternocleidomastoid and upper portion of the trapezius muscle, allowing one to shrug the shoulders and rotate the head. The two roots of the spinal accessory nerve originate in the lower medulla and the upper five cervical spinal cord segments. It ascends in the spinal canal and enters the skull through the foramen magnum, where it is joined by the minor accessory component originating in the nucleus ambiguus; the spinal nerve leaves the cranial cavity through the jugular foramen to innervate the sternocleidomastoid and trapezius muscles.

Hypoglossal Nerve (Motor) (CN XII)

The hypoglossal nerve is a GSE nerve that innervates the intrinsic muscles of the tongue to permit normal speech and swallowing. The paramedian area of that caudal medulla in the floor of the fourth ventricle is the location of the hypoglossal nucleus. The fibers exit from the ventral medulla, between the medullary pyramids and the olive. The fibers then pass through the hypoglossal canal in the occipital condyle and innervate the striated muscles of the tongue.

RESOURCES

Professional

Published Material

Aird, T. (2000). Functional anatomy of the basal ganglia. *Journal of Neuroscience Nursing, 32*(5), 250–277.

Bear, M. F., Connors, B. W., & Paradiso, M. A. (2006). *Neuroscience: Exploring the brain* (3rd ed.). Philadelphia: Lippincott Williams & Wilkins.

Conn, P. M. (Ed.). (2003). *Neuroscience in medicine* (2nd ed.). Totowa, NJ: Humana Press.

Jennes, L., Traurig, H. H., & Conn, P. M. (1995). *Atlas of the human brain*. Philadelphia: J. B. Lippincott.

Johnson, L. R. (2003). *Essential medical physiology* (3rd ed., Chaps. 4–6, 9, 48–59). San Diego: Academic Press.

Kandel, E. R., Schwartz, J. H., & Jessell, T. M. (2000). *Principles of neural science* (4th ed.). New York: McGraw-Hill.

Kingsley, R. E. (2000). *Concise text of neuroscience* (2nd ed.). Philadelphia: Lippincott Williams & Wilkins.

Miller, N. R., & Newman, N. J. (2004). *Walsh & Hoyt's clinical neuro-ophthalmology* (6th ed.). Philadelphia: Lippincott Williams & Wilkins.

Minton, M. S., & Hickey, J. V. (1999). A primer of neuroanatomy and neurophysiology. *Nursing Clinics of North America, 34*(3), 555–572.

Nolte, J. (2002). *The human brain: An introduction to its functional anatomy* (5th ed.). St. Louis, MO: Mosby, Inc.

Parent, A. (1996). *Carpenter's human neuroanatomy* (9th ed.). Baltimore: Williams & Wilkins.

Robertson, D., Biaggioni, I., Burnstock, G., & Low, P. A. (Eds.). (2004). *Primer on the autonomic nervous system* (2nd ed.). San Diego: Academic Press.

Snell, R. S. (2005). *Clinical neuroanatomy* (6th ed.). Philadelphia: Lippincott Williams & Wilkins.

CHAPTER
5

Diagnostic Procedures and Laboratory Tests for Neuroscience Patients

Joanne V. Hickey

Diagnostic procedures and laboratory tests for neuroscience patients continue to develop and become more sophisticated and specific as technology is integrated into clinical practice. Development of diagnostic technologies has resulted in a cadre of highly specialized health care professionals skilled in the techniques of testing and the interpretation of the findings that influence treatment decisions. The ongoing expansion of computed tomography (CT) and magnetic resonance imaging (MRI) technologies has relegated some highly utilized diagnostics such as cerebral angiography to a narrowed scope of fewer diagnostic work-ups as noninvasive CT angiography and magnetic resonance angiography replace the traditional invasive angiography. More and more is being learned about the genetic basis of disease. The emerging knowledge of genetics and genomics is becoming important in the diagnosis of subtypes of neurological diseases such as familial Parkinson's disease and familial cerebral aneurysms. The rapid development of genetic testing will influence how patients are diagnosed and treated.

More and more diagnostic procedures are scheduled as outpatient procedures in special hospital areas (e.g., radiology departments, special procedures departments) or in central diagnostic facilities that report results to referring physicians. Outpatient procedures are driven by cost-containment demands, proven safety of outpatient diagnostic procedures, and patient convenience. On the day of the diagnostic procedure, the patient reports to a special hospital area (e.g., 23-hour unit, ambulatory center) or other facility, undergoes the procedure, recovers in a special unit, and is discharged, usually without an overnight stay. In other instances, diagnostics are ordered during hospitalization.

The variations of entry points for diagnostic procedures create special challenges for patient and family education and preparation. Patient education, a key responsibility of the nurse, has been transformed (see the following section). The nurse may not see the patient until arrival for the test, or there may not be a nurse present at all. Nurses should recognize changes in the patient teaching practices and the collaborative responsibility of all health care team members involved in the patient's care. This sensitivity must be incorporated into interactions with patients and families to ensure patient and family understanding and to provide opportunities for questions.

PATIENT AND FAMILY TEACHING

Focus of Patient Teaching

Patients undergoing a diagnostic procedure need a general explanation of the procedure with special emphasis on what to anticipate and their role as participants. For example, patients who are about to undergo a brain CT scan should be told that they must remain very still while the scan is being taken to ensure accuracy and high-quality graphics. Adapt the explanation to the patient's level of understanding and desire for information. If a patient's level of consciousness (LOC) is altered sufficiently to affect attention, comprehension, understanding, memory, and appreciation of causal associations, provide a simple explanation. Repetition and reinforcement of information may be necessary because of cognitive deficits (e.g., memory), anxiety, or fear. Include information about where the procedure will be conducted, who will be there, and where the patient will be taken on completion of the procedure.

The large number of people undergoing diagnostic procedures on an outpatient ambulatory basis presents special challenges for education and preparation. Education may be provided through a direct patient–nurse conference, a telephone call, mailed printed material (e.g., instructions and booklets), videotape or audiocassette, e-mail, or referral to a website. Regardless of educational media used, there is always a need for follow-up to answer questions and clarify information.

OUTPATIENT PROCEDURES

For outpatient procedures, nurses must be knowledgeable about procedures and related protocols and also be sensitive to the anxiety or fear related to the diagnostic process. Patients and families are often aware that the purpose of the procedure is to rule in or rule out certain diagnoses. As a result, they are often anxious and fearful and need emotional support and education.

HOSPITALIZED PATIENTS AND PROCEDURES

For hospitalized patients, the care nurse assumes responsibility for ensuring that the appropriate patient education has been provided. Portions of education may be delegated to other personnel, but the nurse oversees the process and is the person responsible. Depending on the stability of the patient, unit personnel may accompany the patient to the diagnostic procedure. Sometimes it is an absolute necessity for a registered nurse to accompany the patient, such as when frequent suctioning is required or the patient is hemodynamically fragile or needs frequent monitoring. Follow a transport protocol, such as one published by the Society of Critical Care Medicine,[1] to ensure patient safety. For the patient with impaired cognitive function or with a high anxiety level, presence of the nurse may make the difference between success and failure of the diagnostic procedure. It is often necessary for the patient to cooperate, lie quietly, or follow instructions. The familiar nurse is often able to gain the patient's cooperation. Judicious use of sedation before and during the procedure is also useful and sometimes necessary.

At other times, the unit care nurse completes components of preprocedural preparation in the clinical unit. Auxiliary personnel who are solely responsible for patient transport then take the patient to the designated area. After the patient has arrived at the procedure site, technicians and/or the physician are the principal personnel involved. Therefore, it is most important that a proper explanation of the procedure and what to expect be provided to the patient beforehand.

INFORMED CONSENT

Written consent is required for many diagnostic procedures, although there may be some variation among institutions. Adhere to institutional policies and procedure manuals. If a patient has an altered LOC, cognitive deficits, or other impairments that will affect ability to give informed consent, a family member must provide written consent and it must be witnessed. It is usually the physician's responsibility to obtain written consent after explaining the procedure and the risks and answering questions. The nurse may be asked to witness the consent.

X-RAYS OF THE HEAD AND VERTEBRAL COLUMN

Skull/Facial X-Rays

Skull films are ordered infrequently because CT scans and MRI provide much more detailed anatomic information than is available from skull films. If a CT scan is ordered, the need for skull films is eliminated. One of the most frequent reasons for ordering skull films is to determine whether a skull fracture is present. When skull films are ordered, they usually include anteroposterior (AP) and lateral (LA) radiographic views (Fig. 5-1). Other angles may be included in the series to provide information about specific areas such as the orbits or paranasal sinuses. Films provide information

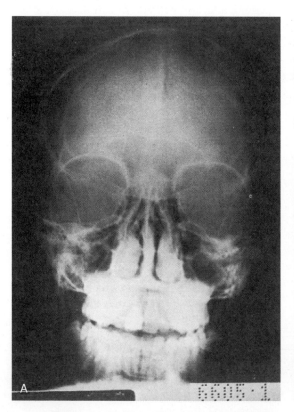 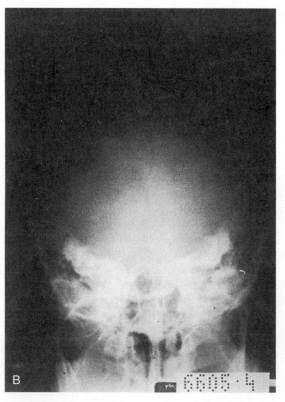

Figure 5-1 • Anterior (*A*) and posterior (*B*) x-ray (radiographic) views of the skull.

about the presence of a skull or facial fracture; unusual calcification or presence of air; the size and shape of skull or facial bones; and bone erosion, particularly of the sella turcica. Skull films are reviewed in an orderly fashion beginning with identification of certain landmarks. For example, the pineal body, normally calcified in the adult, is a midline structure. If it is skewed to one side, it suggests that pressure from a space-occupying lesion is responsible for the midline deviation. Abnormal calcification areas raise suspicion of a calcified component located within a tumor; bone erosion suggests the presence of an intracranial lesion close to bone. Fractures through the base of the skull or paranasal sinuses may produce pneumocephalus or air pockets in the cranial vault or brain.

Patient Preparation and Postprocedural Care

Other than encouraging the patient to lie still for the few moments necessary to take the films, no preparation or postprocedural care is required.

SPINAL X-RAYS

Spinal films are simple radiographs of various regions of the spine: cervical (Fig. 5-2), thoracic, lumbar, or sacral. The most commonly obtained views are the AP and the LA. Because the vertebrae are highly irregular anatomic structures, it is easy to overlook a fracture. This is why both AP and LA films are necessary to rule out a fracture. Indications for spinal films include trauma to the back or vertebral column or back pain with motor or sensory impairment.

In the emergency department, AP and LA films of the cervical region are ordered to rule out cervical fracture. To view the seventh cervical vertebrae, it is often necessary to pull the shoulders downward, especially of muscular men. Viewing of the odontoid process to determine a fracture or instability of C-1 and C-2 vertebrae may require an open-mouth view. Flexion-extension films are used to evaluate the presence of spinal injury. When ordered, the patient must be cooperative and cognitively intact to be able to report pain or onset of neurological symptoms. These films are taken under the direct supervision of the physician. An MRI or CT scan may replace or follow a spinal x-ray for more detailed information.

Abnormalities found on spinal films may include wedging or compression of a vertebra; bone decalcification (osteoporosis); irregular bone calcification (osteophyte/spur); narrowing of the vertebral canal; vertebral fractures and/or dislocations; and spondylosis.

Patient Preparation and Postprocedural Care

There is no preparation or postprocedural care required other than to encourage the patient to lie still for the few moments necessary to take the films.

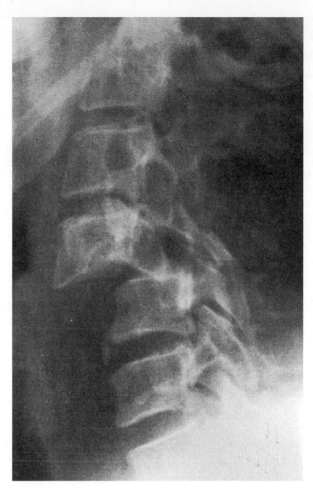

Figure 5-2 • X-ray showing an abnormality of the cervical spine. (From Errico, T. J., Bauer, R. D., & Waugh, T. [1991]. *Spinal trauma.* Philadelphia: J. B. Lippincott.)

ANATOMIC IMAGING TECHNIQUES OF THE BRAIN

The CT scan and MRI are the anatomic imaging cornerstones of the diagnostic work-up for neurological and neurosurgical patients and are readily available technologies (Table 5-1). These technologies have made many previously ordered procedures such as skull and spinal films obsolete.

Computed Tomography

Computed tomography, first introduced in 1972 by Hounsfield, is based on use of conventional ionized radiation that is attenuated as it passes through the skull, cerebrospinal fluid (CSF), cerebral gray and white matter, and blood vessels. More than thirty thousand 2- to 4- mm x-ray beams are directed successively at several horizontal levels in any plane.[2] Detectors measure the degree of attenuation of the exiting radiation. Computers integrate this information and construct the images as cross section images. The thickness of a cross section, which is called a *cut* or *slice*, can vary from 1.5 to 10 mm. Each cut is subdivided into a grid of tiny cubes or volume elements called *voxels*. The degree of

TABLE 5-1 COMPARISON OF INDICATIONS FOR COMPUTED TOMOGRAPHY (CT) AND MAGNETIC RESONANCE IMAGING (MRI)*

CT SCAN	MRI
Detection of acute intracranial blood (e.g., subdural, epidural, intracerebral, or subarachnoid hemorrhage)	Lucunar stroke and small ischemic areas
Initial differentiation of acute ischemic stroke from hemorrhagic stroke	Cerebral trauma after initial screening
Cerebral or cerebellar ischemic infarction in first 12–24 hours; after this, MRI used	MRI used after first 12–24 hours with ischemic infarction
Some tumors when enhancement used	Smaller tumors especially of posterior fossa
Arteriovenous malformation or cerebral aneurysm seen acutely to determine extent of hemorrhage	Dementia (e.g., Alzheimer's disease)
Hydrocephalus	Work-up in epilepsy
Best for detecting abnormal calcification of cranial and vertebral bones	Demyelinating disease (e.g., multiple sclerosis), white matter diseases, and other neurodegenerative conditions
Brain abscess	Spinal cord tumor or trauma Intervertebral disc disease

*Note: The choice between CT and MRI for initial evaluation is not always clear; clinical judgment is imperative in selecting the appropriate test at the appropriate time.

attenuation within each voxel is measured as a numeric value of tissue density and is converted to gray scale values with lower numbers coded as black (i.e. air, CSF) and higher numbers coded as white (i.e., bone). The differing densities of bone, CSF, blood, and gray and white matter are distinguishable in the resulting picture. Films of the various cuts are then arranged sequentially for review.

Clinical Applications

The most recent generation of CT scanners provide extraordinary clarity of the brain, orbits, and spine. Specially, detailed visualization of sulci, caudate and lenticular nuclei, the internal capsule, thalami, optic nerves, the brainstem, the cerebellum, and the spinal cord is provided. One can visualize hemorrhage, cerebral edema, abscess, and tumor as well as the precise size and position of the ventricles and midline structures. A CT without contrast is ordered to rule out bleeding or a hematoma when a cerebral aneurysm is suspected, and to screen for hemorrhage in candidates for thrombolytic therapy with a diagnosis of ischemic stroke. Serial CT scans can be used to follow the resolution of cerebral hemorrhage or edema (Fig. 5-3). Recent advances in CT technology of spiral and helical CT scans have greatly increased the speed of the scanning procedure and have made possible the visualization of cerebral vasculature (i.e.,

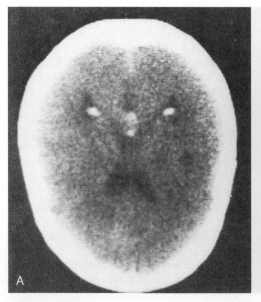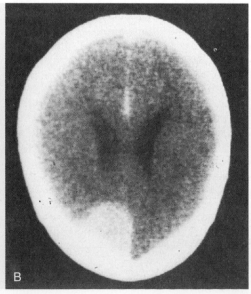

Figure 5-3 • Computed tomography scan of the brain. (*A*) Normal scan. (*B*) Scan showing a large mass in the left frontal lobe.

CT angiography).[2] The newest addition to CT technology is a portable CT scanner. The portability of this equipment allows the scanner to be brought to the emergency room or patient's bedside for scanning and immediate availability of quality images for review. NeuroLogica offers the CereTom, a portable eight-slice scanner.

Procedure

The procedure and equipment are briefly explained to the patient, and reassurance is given that the procedure is painless. No motion will be felt, and a clicking sound from the equipment is to be expected. Even though the technician and radiologist are outside the room, they can see and maintain voice contact with the patient through an intercom system at all times. The patient lies on a movable radiographic table with his or her head carefully positioned and immobilized. The head of the table is inserted into the scanner (Fig. 5-4). A movable circular frame revolves around the head, making clicking sounds while taking numerous scans at different angles.

CT scans are done with or without contrast media. Use of an iodinated radiopaque medium enhances image sharpness and further augments areas of pathology that resulted from breakdown of the blood–brain barrier. If used, contrast medium is administered intravenously. Before administering consider contraindications, which include allergic reaction to shellfish or iodinated dye. CT scanning can begin 10 seconds after infusion of the contrast infusion begins. When contrast

medium is used, a capital "C" will be noted somewhere on the films. The entire CT scanning procedure takes about 10 minutes. Newer-generation scanners have cut the time of scanning.

Advantages and Disadvantages

The advantages of CT scans are many. It is a painless, low-cost, widely available diagnostic tool that requires only minutes to complete, and can be performed on both conscious and unconscious patients. It is useful in rapidly developing neurological conditions when monitoring and life-support equipment is necessary. CT is sensitive to detect acute hemorrhage and calcifications and demonstrates the anatomy of skull and vertebral bones well. CT has drastically reduced the need for more dangerous and expensive diagnostic tests. It is also useful when MRI is contraindicated because of metal aneurysm clips, orthopedic prostheses, foreign objects in the eye, pacemakers, and other metal implants. Finally, the cost of a CT scan varies with the type and complexity of the study; generally it is about half the cost of an MRI.[3]

Some disadvantages are also noted. CT scans include ionizing radiation exposure about equal to that of skull films. By comparison, an MRI does not use radiation. CT scans have decreased sensitivity for detection of many common neurological diseases, lesions adjacent to bone, small soft tissue lesions, posterior fossa (cerebellum and brainstem) lesions, and floor of the middle fossa lesions.[3] Claustrophobia is a *contraindication* for a CT scan. A patient who is unable to tolerate his or her head being in the confined space of a CT scanner is not a candidate for a CT scan.

Patient Preparation and Postprocedural Care

Screen for claustrophobia. All jewelry, eyeglasses, and hair clips or pins are removed from the head and neck. Unless a contrast medium will be administered, there are no dietary restrictions or other screening requirements before the procedure. The need to remain perfectly still is emphasized because movement can cause artifacts that will affect the clarity of the pictures. Agitated or uncooperative patients will require short-acting intravenous sedation such as lorazepam (Ativan) to ensure the necessary quality of the pictures.

Before the contrast medium is administered, a skin test may be done to check for an allergic reaction in high-risk patients. The blood urea nitrogen and creatinine levels are checked for adequate kidney function. Most protocols require the patient to have had nothing by mouth for 4 to 8 hours before the test. Some patients experience flushing or a feeling of warmth, transient headache, a salty taste in the mouth, nausea, or vomiting when the contrast medium is administered; patients should be prepared for these possible reactions.

After the procedure, patients who have received contrast medium should be observed for signs and symptoms of delayed allergic reactions such as hives, skin rash, itching, nausea, headache, or seizures. If symptoms are severe, antihistamines may be ordered. Intravenous hydration or oral fluid intake for hydration to facilitate clearance of contrast medium is very important. Tubular necrosis and acute kidney failure can result from inadequate hydration; older

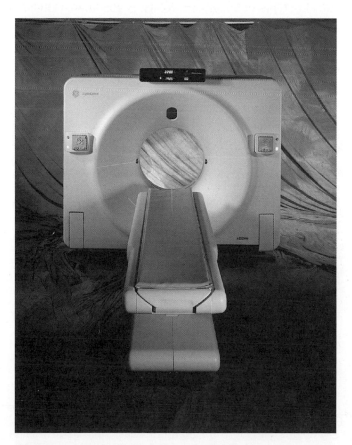

Figure 5-4 • General Electric computed tomography system. (Courtesy of GE Medical Systems, Waukesha, WI.)

patients are at higher risk because of age-related kidney function changes.

Other Uses of Computed Tomography Technology in Diagnostics

CT angiography (CTA) is emerging as an alternative to magnetic resonance angiography (MRA) for imaging extracranial and intracranial blood vessels. The CTA has several advantages over the MRA. It is faster (<32 seconds) than MRA and can be used with intubated patients or those with aneurysmal clips. It offers multiplanar views of the cerebral vasculature and visualization of slow flow or turbulent flow in aneurysms. Finally, it identifies plaque location and characteristics.[4] The limitations include risks associated with iodinated contrast media use and some difficulty in imaging the posterior inferior cerebellar arteries.[5]

Xenon-enhanced computed tomography (XeCT) evaluates cerebral blood flow (CBF). A mixture of oxygen and Xenon is inhaled and the Xenon serves as a contrast medium. The Xenon gas rapidly dissolves in the blood and crosses the lipid-rich blood–brain barrier and enters the brain. The CBF is calculated using the modified Kety-Schmidt equation.[6] After breathing the Xenon and oxygen mixture, the brain is scanned. Upon completion of the scanning, the Xenon is rapidly washed from the cerebral tissue (half-life about 40 seconds).

Adverse reactions include nausea, reversible altered sensorium, or respiratory depression in less than 0.1 cases.[7] Cerebrovascular disorders are the main clinical applications of XeCT, and it has been used to study cerebrovascular physiology. Currently, XeCT is useful to determine viability of cerebral tissue globally and regionally and can be used as part of brain death criteria.

Patient Preparation and Postprocedural Care

There is no special preparation or postprocedural care required other than to monitor for any adverse reaction.

Magnetic Resonance Imaging

The second major diagnostic tool for anatomic imaging of the brain and spinal column is the MRI. It is a noninvasive, painless diagnostic procedure that provides better resolution slice images of anatomic structures of the brain and other soft tissue. The technology uses strong magnetic fields rather than ionized radiation, and thus requires special, copper-lined rooms for shielding from the strong magnetic fields create by the MRI. Current technology uses hydrogen atoms (protons) because hydrogen is the most abundant element in tissue and yields the strongest magnetic signal. The presence of thermal energy causes each proton to spin like a top.[8] New developments are occurring in MRI technology, and new knowledge is being integrated into practice.

In MRI technology, in a strong magnetic field, protons within the tissue align themselves in the longitudinal direction of the magnetic field.[3] A computer-programmed brief (few milliseconds) burst of **radio-frequency** (RF) pulse is applied to the magnetic field, which changes the axis of the alignment of the atoms from the longitudinal to the transverse plane. This effect of rotating the atoms about the axes in a uniform manner is known as **resonance.** When the RF is turned off, the atoms return to their original alignment, an effect known as **relaxation.** The RF energy that was absorbed and then emitted results in an MR signal that is detected by electromagnetic receiver coils and stored. Application of the RF is repeated several times as a **pulse sequence** with the signals being measured and stored after each pulse application. Depending on how quickly these atoms return to their original state, the computer can determine what kind of tissue is represented by the signal returned. It is the *intensity* of the returned signal reported as hypo-, iso-, or hyperintense that correlates to tissue type.[9] Computer programs analyze the stored data and an image constructed from the combined data.

The terms *T1* and *T2* refer to the weighted relaxation time constants for protons; these weights may be altered to highlight certain features of the tissue structure.[10] In a T1-weighted image, the CSF appears very dark, gray matter is lighter, and white matter is bright. The cortical border and cortical–white matter junctions are well defined. In a T2-weighted image, the CSF appears white and there is poor color discrimination between gray and white matter. The T2 image highlights alterations in white matter such as infarction, demyelination, and edema.[2]

Pulse sequences refer to the different imaging techniques generated by manipulating the timing of the RF pulses. The pulse sequence variables that are manipulated to produce different types of images are known as **echo time (TE)** and **repetition time (TR).** The type of image selected depends on the type of tissue under study and the suspected pathology. This ability to manipulate pulse sequence and components enhances the usefulness of MRI. Some of the more common pulse sequences include spin-echo, inversion recovery, gradient echo, and fluid attenuation inversion recovery (FLAIR) sequences. Each type has characteristics that make it useful in special circumstances. For example, the superiority of FLAIR compared with T1-weighted images and T2-weighted images has been shown in many disorders, including stroke, multiple sclerosis, infections, and cerebral hemorrhage.

Gadolinium-diethylenetriamine pentaacetic acid (gadolinium) is the paramagnetic agent used as a contrast medium for MRI studies. It enhances the process of proton relaxation during the T1 sequence of MRI, resulting in sharper definition, and highlights the surrounding regions of lesions where the blood–brain barrier has been disrupted.

Contraindications

In the last few years, new MRI-friendly materials from the manufacturers of neurological and orthopedic equipment have become available. It is imperative to screen patients accurately for the presence of any devices that are contraindications for MRI *before* scheduling the procedure. The *absolute contraindications* for MRI include the following:

- Patients with ferromagnetic devices, such as artificial pacemakers, defibrillators, implanted stimulators of the brain or spinal cord, cochlear implants, prosthetic devices (e.g., metallic hip replacements, orthopedic pins), artificial limbs, respirators, and other metallic equipment

- Patients with older ferromagnetic intracranial aneurysm clips or metal bullet or other metal fragments in the orbits or brain
- Women in the first trimester of pregnancy (gadolinium contraindicated during entire pregnancy)[11]
- Placement of a vascular stent, coil, or filter within the past 6 weeks[11]

The following are *relative contraindications*:

- Agitated, uncooperative patients or patients with uncontrolled movement disorders
- Grossly obese patients who cannot fit into the MRI tube
- Claustrophobic patients who cannot tolerate the closeness of the tube to their faces
- Critically ill patients requiring a ventilator and intravenous (IV) pump (some ventilators are specially designed nonmagnetic; IV pumps are generally magnetic and cannot be used)[11]

Clinical Applications

Because MRIs are not obscured by bone, the technique is excellent in detecting soft-tissue changes that are insensitive to CT scan. These include ischemic and infarcted areas; degenerative diseases (e.g., multiple sclerosis, Alzheimer's disease); cerebral and spinal cord edema; hemorrhage; arteriovenous malformations; small tumors, particularly in the difficult-to-visualize areas of the brainstem, basal skull, and spinal cord; and congenital anomalies. The superb sharpness and precision of detail are superior for diagnosis and location of lesions.

Procedure

The patient is screened for contraindications. After removing all metal objects and credit cards (magnet can desensitize the black strip on the back of a credit card), the patient lies on a padded stretcher that slides into a tunnel-like chamber. The head is placed in a plastic helmet-like structure; the arms are at the side of the body and are held in place with Velcro straps. The head of the table is then rolled several feet into the scanner. The scanner tube has a restricted opening; it has been compared to the opening of a barrel or large pipe (Fig. 5-5). During the scan, noise, caused by the pulsating RF waves, is heard. The patient must be prepared for this and for the requirement to remain absolutely motionless for the scan. Although the patient is alone in the room, voice contact is maintained with the technician through an intercom. If contrast enhancement is desired, gadolinium is administered intravenously. The MRI takes approximately 5 to 50 minutes to complete.

Advantages and Disadvantages

The following are advantages of MRI:

- Provides detailed sagittal (right to left side), axial (top to bottom of the head), and coronal (front to back of the head) images for precise lesion assessment and location

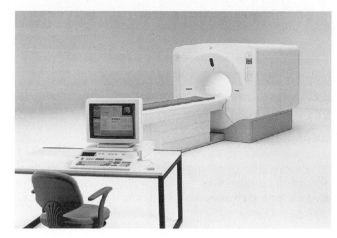

Figure 5-5 • General Electric magnetic resonance system. (Courtesy of GE Medical Systems, Waukesha, WI.)

- Does not use ionizing radiation, thus eliminating radiation exposure risk
- Tissue resolution is far superior with MRI with the exception of bone, which cannot be seen with MRI except for bone marrow
- Provides better differentiation than CT for water, iron, fat, and blood using physical and biochemical characteristics of tissues imaged
- Higher level of gray–white matter contrast obtainable compared with CT
- Can detect soft-tissue changes not seen on radiographs such as small tumors along cranial nerves and other tumors as small as 0.3 mm
- Provides higher-resolution detail of the posterior fossa, skull base, and orbits compared with CT scan

Disadvantages of MRI include its higher cost relative to CT scan and the need to exclude a number of patients who could be adversely affected by the procedure because the strong magnetic field can move or dislodge ferromagnetic material and cause injury to body tissue. The MRI generally takes longer than a CT scan. Also, claustrophobic patients usually have more difficulty tolerating an MRI than with a CT scan because of the length of time for the procedure.

Patient Preparation and Postprocedural Care

Carefully question and screen for the presence of any metal implants or other contraindications. For the patient who is vague about possible contraindications, radiographic screening may be necessary. The patient should be briefed about the procedure and the necessity to remain still for several minutes in very close quarters. Antianxiety medication may be ordered for some patients. All jewelry, eyeglasses, and hair clips or pins and any other metal objects should be removed. Credit cards should not be in the room because the magnetic field will erase the strip on the card. Unless a contrast medium will be administered, there are no dietary restrictions before the procedure.

Several points need attention if contrast medium is to be used. Adequate kidney function is verified through adequate blood urea nitrogen and creatinine levels. Many protocols require nothing by mouth for 4 to 6 hours before the MRI. If contrast media are to be used, skin testing may be done to check for an allergic reaction. There are no special aftercare requirements. When contrast medium is used, adequate hydration is needed.

Newer Magnetic Resonance Imaging Technology

With the rapid evolution of MRI technology, a number of newer noninvasive procedures are being integrated into clinical practice. A few diagnostics will be briefly addressed.

Diffusion-Weighted Imaging and Perfusion-Weighted Imaging

MRI can detect cerebral abnormalities related to ischemia. When MRI uses both diffusion-weighted imaging (DWI) and perfusion-weighted imaging (PWI), it is possible to identify both metabolically impaired and abnormally perfused brain tissue. Both DWI and PWI provide complementary information about tissue changes in neurological events such as stroke. DWI is becoming an important diagnostic tool for detecting the very early stage of ischemic stroke (generally within 2 hours or less of the onset).[2] Other uses include assistance in differentiating between metastatic lesions and abscesses and cytotoxic and vasogenic edema. DWI detects the tiny random movements of water molecules (diffusion) in tissues. This technique allows a map of the average apparent diffusion coefficient (ADC) to be calculated. Shortly after an ischemic stroke, the ADC of the brain tissue is significantly reduced because of cytotoxic edema.[12] Over several days, the rapid initial drop in ADC is followed by a return to close to normal values at approximately 1 week. Subsequently, elevated ADC values are seen at chronic time points. DWI is remarkably sensitive in detecting and localizing acute ischemic brain lesions and allows differentiation of acute regions of ischemia from chronic infarcts. In addition to ischemic stroke, DWI is also used to study lesions and plaque formation in patients with multiple sclerosis.

PWI assesses the perfusion of the microvasculature after rapid injection of a gadolinium contrast agent. Combined DWI and PWI can determine early extent of brain tissue injury and identify the portions of the brain that are not damaged permanently (i.e., the ischemic penumbra). DWI and PWI can guide acute stroke treatment and potentially identify patients who would benefit from thrombolytic therapy and specific stroke investigational treatments. PWI identifies areas lacking blood flow or areas with compromised blood flow that could be considered for reversal before irreversible infarction occurs.

Magnetic Resonance Angiography

MRA is becoming the method of choice for screening the extracranial and intracranial vasculature. Combined with the Doppler ultrasound, MRA is commonly selected for the initial evaluation of carotid bifurcation stenosis to assist in measuring the blood flow rate through vessels and tissue.

Magnetic Resonance Spectroscopy

Magnetic resonance spectroscopy (MRS) is a noninvasive method of studying the biochemistry of living tissue. The technique is based on nuclear magnetic resonance. A region of the brain is selected for analysis and magnetic resonance frequency sequences are applied that detect signals from the electrochemical bonds of various brain tissue. The major chemical bonds used are choline and N-acetyl-aspartate (NAA). Choline is contained primarily in cell membranes of myelin, and NAA is a marker for neuronal function.[2] Choline is elevated in neoplasm and low in stroke. NAA is low in stroke, tumor, multiple sclerosis, epilepsy, and other focal and regional brain abnormalities.[11] MRS has been used in studies of stroke, tumor, multiple sclerosis, and epilepsy patients.

Functional Magnetic Resonance Imaging

Functional magnetic resonance imaging (fMRI) is a way to study brain metabolism and blood flow, and can map functional cortical activity during the performance of cognitive and motor activities in normal patients as well as in patients with neurological and psychiatric disease. This helps scientists better understand areas of cerebral activation during these activities. Applications of fMRI include mapping of brain activation pathways in normal and pathologic states, studying cerebral reorganization, and planning for neurosurgery.

PHYSIOLOGIC IMAGING TECHNIQUES OF THE BRAIN

The major *physiologic neuroimaging* studies are positron emission tomography (PET) and single-photon emission CT (SPECT). These techniques use nuclear medicine technology to evaluate cerebral metabolism and CBF. PET uses positron-emitting radionuclides, and SPECT uses single-photon radioisotopes.

Positron Emission Tomography

PET is not used for routine diagnosis. Used mostly in large medical research centers, the PET measures regional physiologic functions such as glucose uptake and metabolism, oxygen uptake, and CBF patterns. Its elegance of detail demonstrates hypometabolic and hypermetabolic regions of the brain. In neuroscience research, PET is a developing technology providing new understanding about epilepsy, dementia (e.g., Alzheimer's disease), cerebrovascular disease, cerebral trauma, and mental illness. It is used clinically in a limited number of patients for diagnostic purposes (Fig. 5-6).

The technology uses an on-line cyclotron or linear accelerator to create positron-emitting radionuclides. The patient either receives an intravenous injection or inhales a compound that has been labeled with the emission of positron "tag" (i.e., F-fluorodeoxyglucose [FDG]). Once inside the body, the tag concentrates in the area of clinical interest and emits positrons. As the positrons decay, they emit photons that move in diametrically opposite directions and are recorded by detectors

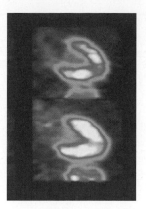

Figure 5-6 • Positron emission tomography scan showing variations in update of isotope.

located on either side of the body. Multiple scanners detect and encode these data into a computerized database that reconstructs cross-sectional images of the tissue.[3]

A major advantage of PET is the clarity of images produced. The major drawbacks of PET are the need for an on-line cyclotron or linear accelerator to manufacture the short-lived isotopes on site. This equipment is very expensive, requiring a highly trained support staff and high-cost physical facility. PET is found only in a few major research centers and is thus not utilized as a routine diagnostic.

Procedure

The patient is placed on a stretcher in the imaging center and prepared for the procedure. An arterial line may be inserted to draw blood samples for measurement of cerebral metabolic rates. No glucose solutions are given. The radiopharmaceutical agent of choice is injected through another venous access. The patient rests quietly in a dimly lit room for about 45 minutes while uptake of the radiopharmaceutical occurs. The head is placed inside the scanner. The scanning portion of the procedure takes about 45 minutes. The patient may be asked to perform cognitive acts such as speaking, mathematical calculations, or reasoning. If blood samples are required, the technician draws them quietly without disturbing the quiet environment created for the study. The entire procedure takes 2 to 3 hours.

Patient Preparation and Postprocedural Care

No caffeine, alcohol, or nicotine should be consumed for 24 hours before the procedure. Maintain NPO status for 6 to 12 hours before the procedure. Glucose solutions should not be used for infusion purposes because they may alter the test results. After completion of the study, force fluids to clear the isotope.

Single-Photon Computed Emission Tomography

SPECT scans are another physiologic imaging study that measures regional CBF and perfusion. The SPECT scan is based on the same principles as PET technology, but the decay of the radioactive "tags" emits only a single photon and a rotating gamma camera (available in many nuclear medicine departments) is used. The radioactive tracers used in SPECT scans are commercially prepared and therefore do not require an on-line cyclotron. The most common tracer used is technetium-99m-hexamethyl-propylamine-oxamine. SPECT tracks the single photons resulting from radioactive decay using the gamma camera, which collects data from multiple angles to reconstruct regional blood flow. It is useful to study cerebral blood flow during hypoperfusion in focal and diffuse cerebral disorders such as dementia, seizures, stroke, and cerebral trauma. It has been useful in confirming brain death.[13]

The major advantage of SPECT is the availability of the technology within many nuclear medicine departments. It detects cerebral perfusion changes and is especially helpful in acute ischemia and monitoring seizure foci. It thus provides excellent perfusion information in stroke, dementia, amnesia, neoplasm, trauma, seizures, brain death, persistent vegetative state, and psychiatric disorders (e.g., schizophrenia and depression). The major disadvantages of SPECT are its cost and technical resolution concerns.

Procedure

The patient lies quietly on a padded stretcher and the isotope is administered. The isotope decays in about 1 hour, so the scan must be conducted within that window of time. The patient must lie quietly during the scan. The entire study takes about 1 to 2 hours.

Patient Preparation and Postprocedural Care

No special preparation is required other than the usual explanation of the procedure to the patient. No special care is required after the procedure.

CEREBROSPINAL FLUID AND SPINAL PROCEDURES

Lumbar Puncture

A lumbar puncture (LP) involves the introduction of a hollow needle with a stylet into the lumbar subarachnoid space of the spinal canal using strict aseptic technique. In the adult, the needle is placed in the interspace between L-3–4 or L-4–5. This location is a safe distance from the end of the spinal cord, which terminates at L-1. Note that the L-3–4 interspace is located at the level of the posterior iliac crests.[14]

The indications for LP can be divided into diagnostic and therapeutic purposes. Diagnostic indications include measurement of CSF pressure; collection of CSF samples for cellular, cytologic, chemical, and bacterial examination; evaluation of spinal dynamics for signs of blockage of CSF flow; and injection of radiopaque media for visualization of parts of the nervous system. Table 5-2 details the characteristics of CSF. Therapeutic purposes include administration of spinal anesthesia; intrathecal injection of antibacterial or chemotherapeutic drugs; and removal of CSF to reduce pressure for

TABLE 5–2   CHARACTERISTICS OF CEREBROSPINAL FLUID (CSF)

PARAMETER	NORMAL VALUE	ABNORMAL FINDINGS
Volume	About 150 mL	↑ with hydrocephalus
Specific gravity	1.007	↑ with RBCs related to subarachnoid hemorrhage or WBCs related to infection
Pressure	100–80 mm H₂O or 8–14 mm Hg	↑ with ↑ intracranial pressure
Color	Crystal clear	Xanthochromia (discoloration) of CSF; usually due to breakdown of RBCs from previous intracranial hemorrhage; appears yellow, orange, or brown. Turbidity (cloudiness): due to ↑ WBCs or ↑ protein from microorganisms in CSF
Total protein count	15–50 mg/dL	Mild ↑ with viral meningitis, subdural hematoma, brain tumor, and multiple sclerosis. Moderate/high ↑ with bacterial or TB meningitis, cerebral hemorrhage, brain and spinal cord tumors, and Guillain-Barré syndrome
White cell count	0–5 cells/mm³	10–200 cells mostly lymphocytes: viral meningitis, multiple sclerosis, CNS tumor, and late neurosyphilis 200–500 cells mostly lymphocytes: TB meningitis, herpes infection of CNS, and meningovascular syphilis >500 cells mostly granulocytes: acute bacterial meningitis
Glucose	40–80 mg/dL (about 2/3 of blood value)	↑ has specific significance; ↓ often seen with all meningitis and subarachnoid hemorrhage

RBC = red blood cell; WBC = white blood cell; TB = tuberculosis; CNS = central nervous system.

conditions such as benign intracranial hypertension (formerly called pseudotumor cerebri).

Contraindications

The contraindications for LP are relative and require careful medical judgment, weighing benefits against risks. First, when clinical evidence (headache and papilledema) indicates a substantial increase in intracranial pressure (ICP), caution is imperative. Performing LP in a patient with high increased ICP may result in brainstem compression, herniation through the foramen magnum, and, ultimately, death. Second, a cutaneous or osseous infection at the proposed puncture site is an absolute contraindication for LP. Third, any patient receiving antiplatelet therapy (e.g., aspirin, ticlopidine [Ticlid], clopidogrel [Plavix]) or anticoagulation therapy (heparin, warfarin [Coumadin]) or who have a low platelet count (<30,000 to 50,000/mm³) or impaired platelet function usually requires reversal of the coagulopathy because of the high risk of hemorrhage at the puncture site and possible spinal cord compression from perispinal or intraspinal bleeding.

Procedure

The LP is usually done at the patient's bedside or in an outpatient facility. The sterile LP set is prepared. The patient is positioned on his or her side along the edge of the bed, arching the back so that the knees are flexed on the chest with the chin touching the knees (Fig. 5-7). This position allows maximal separation of the vertebrae, thereby facilitating insertion of the lumbar needle and reducing potential trauma. The nurse may be called on to assist the patient if this position

cannot be assumed independently. Occasionally, the LP may be performed with the patient seated on the side of the bed. To maximize interspace separation, the patient bends over a pillow that rests on the overbed table.

The lumbar site is aseptically prepared, draped, and locally anesthetized with an intradermal injection of procaine (Novocaine). Strict aseptic technique is essential. The lumbar needle is introduced into the appropriate subarachnoid space, the stylet is removed, and a manometer is affixed to measure and record opening pressure of CSF. A 22-gauge needle is recommended to prevent post-LP puncture headache.[15] The opening pressure is approximately the same as ICP in a patient who is reclining if no CSF obstruction is present. After this measurement has been obtained, the manometer is removed and samples of CSF are collected into sterile test tubes for visual and laboratory examination. The physician may choose to record the exit pressure, for which the manometer would again be necessary. When the procedure is completed, the lumbar needle is removed and a Band-Aid is applied over the puncture site. The tubes of CSF should be sent promptly for laboratory analysis according to physician order.

Traumatic Tap

A traumatic tap occurs when blood from the epidural venous plexus has been introduced into the spinal fluid as a result of insertion of the LP needle. In this instance, the initial sample of CSF contains blood. Such bleeding could be misinterpreted as evidence of subarachnoid hemorrhage. However, in the case of a traumatic tap, CSF clears progressively in successive samples. If there has been hemorrhage into the subarachnoid space from intracranial bleeding, successive samples of CSF will continue to be as discolored

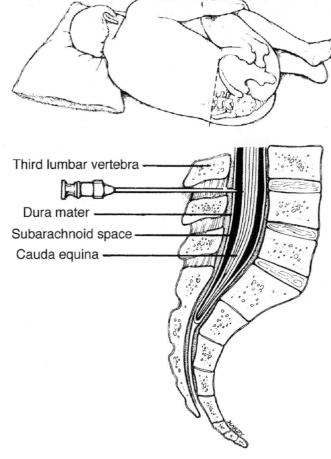

Figure 5-7 • Technique of lumbar puncture. The interspaces between the spines of vertebrae L-3, L-4, and L-5 are just below the line joining the anterosuperior iliac spines. (From Smeltzer, S., & Bare, B. [1996]. *Brunner and Suddarth's textbook of medical-surgical nursing* [8th ed.]. Philadelphia: Lippincott-Raven.)

Third lumbar vertebra

Dura mater

Subarachnoid space

Cauda equina

as the first specimen taken. If the CSF sample with blood is immediately centrifuged, fluid from the traumatic tap would result in a clear column of fluid and red blood cells (RBCs) precipitating to the bottom of the tube. If there was cerebral hemorrhage, the centrifuged sample would result in a column of xanthochromic (discolored) CSF; there would be no precipitated RBCs.

Adverse Effects

Headache occurs in about a third of patients. When headache is severe, vomiting and some neck stiffness may be noted. Analgesics and bedrest are the usual treatment. Headache may be related to low CSF pressure; it is treated with an autologous "blood patch" to prevent leakage of CSF at the puncture site. Finally, bleeding into the spinal meningeal space can result in the development of a hematoma. The patient must be monitored for deterioration of sensory and motor function in the lower legs after an LP. Deterioration in neurological function requires investigation, and if a hematoma is present, rapid surgical removal is necessary to prevent paralysis.

Patient Preparation and Postprocedural Care

In preparing the patient for an LP, the bladder should be emptied immediately before the procedure for patient comfort. Usually, no dietary restriction or preprocedural medication is warranted. The nurse should check the coagulation studies for abnormalities and review the medication sheet for any antiplatelet or anticoagulant drugs that have been ordered.

Care of a patient who has undergone LP includes the following:

- Have the patient lie flat in bed 6 to 8 hours following the procedure, depending on physician preference, hospital protocol, and continued signs of headache.
- Monitor neurological and vital signs frequently; note particularly changes in sensory or motor function of the legs (immediately report changes to the physician).
- Force fluids after completion of the procedure.
- Administer analgesics (for headache) as needed.

Following LP, mild to severe headache may occur, caused by leakage of CSF at the puncture site or by irritation of the spinal roots. Acetaminophen (Tylenol), 650 mg orally (PO) every 4 hours, is used for mild headaches, whereas methylmorphine (codeine phosphate), 30 mg PO, may be ordered for severe headaches. Because headaches are supposedly aggravated by an upright position, the patient is advised to lie flat to relieve headache. An autologous "blood patch" can be used to seal the site of CSF leakage with good results for severe headache. Other possible symptoms that can occur after LP include backache or spasms in the lower back or thighs, transient voiding problems, nuchal rigidity, and a slight rise in temperature. If the LP is done on an outpatient basis, the patient may be discharged 1 to 2 hours after completion. Instruct the patient to lie flat for 6 to 8 hours at home.

Myelography

Myelography is a diagnostic procedure ordered to visualize the lumbar, thoracic, or cervical subarachnoid space or the entire spinal axis, for diagnosis of a spinal cord compression, spinal cord lesion (e.g., tumor, vascular abnormality), vertebral bone displacement, or intervertebral disc herniation. Any partial or complete obstruction that hinders the flow of CSF and contrast medium will be visualized on the films. Ordering of an MRI has significantly decreased the number of myelograms performed; if an MRI is inconclusive, a myelogram may be ordered.

Procedure

The LP is performed and approximately 10 mL of CSF is removed. A water-soluble contrast medium (e.g., Isovue, Amipaque, Iohexol) is injected into the subarachnoid space and the head tipped down on a tilt table to visualize the entire spinal subarachnoid space. Radiographic films of the spinal cord and vertebral column are taken.

A few points need to be made about radiopaque media. In the past, oil-based media were used. Since the introduction of water-soluble contrast media, use of oil-based media has almost completely ceased. After the water-based contrast medium is injected into the CSF, it diffuses upward through the CSF and penetrates into the nerve root sleeves, nerve rootlets, and narrow areas of the subarachnoid space. Upward diffusion occurs regardless of the position of the patient. The head is kept elevated about 30 degrees, and the patient is kept quiet to reduce the rate of upward dispersion of the contrast medium. Upward dispersion is controlled to prevent the contrast medium from entering the cranial vault, which could result in seizures. The head is maintained elevated in postprocedural care, including transfer, to prevent seizures. In addition, confusion, hallucinations, depression, hyperesthesia, chest pain, and arrhythmias can result from the contrast medium.

Patient Preparation and Postprocedural Care

In preparation for the procedure, the patient should be well hydrated. Omit the meal prior to the myelogram. Explain the need to force fluids (3 L) for the first 24 hours after the procedure. After the procedure, the patient is transported back to his or her room or the recovery area with the head of the stretcher elevated 30 degrees at all times. In addition, the following points should be followed (there may be slight variations among institutional practice guidelines):

- Keep the patient on bedrest for 4 to 8 hours with the head of the bed elevated 30 degrees.
- Keep the patient quiet for a few hours after the procedure.
- The patient's head must be elevated (chair or bed) for a total of 12 hours.
- Force fluids to 2400 to 3000 mL per 24 hours.
- Monitor neurological and vital signs.
- Maintain an intake and output record.
- After 4 hours, resume diet as tolerated if there is no nausea or vomiting.
- Do not give any phenothiazine derivatives for 48 hours (increase possibility of seizures).
- Monitor for symptoms such as back pain, spasms, elevated temperature, difficulty voiding, nuchal rigidity, nausea, and vomiting.
- Treat nausea with an antiemetic according to physician's order.
- Treat headache with analgesics as needed.

CEREBROVASCULAR STUDIES

Cerebrovascular studies are broadly classified as noninvasive and invasive. The most common types of studies used in clinical practice are discussed below.

Transcranial Doppler

The transcranial Doppler (TCD) uses the principles of Doppler technology to provide information about the patency, flow velocity, turbulence, and directional flow of blood in basal cerebral arteries. Refinement of the technology over the last decade has greatly increased its use in clinical settings to evaluate cerebrovascular flow. It is inexpensive, noninvasive, safe, and portable, and can be done at the bedside in a short period of time.

Basics of Ultrasonography and Doppler Ultrasound

Ultrasound technology uses the transmission of ultrasonic pulsed-wave frequency through tissue and the reflection of the sound at tissue interfaces. Christian Doppler built on this knowledge and added the concept of "Doppler shift." Doppler shift is the change in the frequency of the pulsed wave resulting from the movement between the source of sound and the detector. The frequency shift detected is that of the red blood cells traveling through the lumen of the vessel. The application of fast Fourier transform (FFT) to analyze change in frequency of the returning signal further adds precision and additional information. The FFT visually displays the spectral waveform, offers information on direction of flow, and provides a means to establish norm values. In 1982, Aaslid and associates determined that it was possible to send an ultrasound beam through a thinning of the skull and analyze the Doppler signal reflected from basal cerebral arteries through the skull. This concept, which became known as TCD, has been recognized as a breakthrough in evaluating intracranial blood flow.

The TCD does not provide an actual image of the vessel or measure of CBF. Rather, it provides information on vessel patency, flow velocity, turbulence, and directional flow about the moving column of blood in a major artery. With vessel stenosis, there is accelerated flow velocity of red blood cells through the stenosis and concurrent disturbance of blood flow and turbulence distal to the stenosis. The higher the numerical value recorded, the narrower the blood vessel. The numerical value provides information about the presence or absence of vasospasm. The newer models of TCD provide colored printouts and descriptive data about the waveforms of the specific blood vessel (Fig. 5-8).

Procedure

A Doppler ultrasonic hand-held probe, which sends low-frequency pulsed sound waves, is placed on the skin over the thinned-skull area of the temporal bone or "window." The sound waves reflect back the velocity of the blood flow. These data are amplified, and graphic recordings of the waveforms common to each vessel, as well as sound recordings of the blood flow, are produced. The test takes 10 to 30 minutes.

Clinical Applications

Because the TCD is noninvasive and does not use radioactive isotopes or radiation, serial evaluations can be done without potential harm to the patient. For example, serial studies may be conducted to monitor changes over time of the evolution or resolution of vasospasm. Current application of TCD includes the following:

- Detection and monitoring of vasospasm with cerebral aneurysms
- Detection of intracranial stenosis and occlusion (e.g., middle cerebral artery, basilar artery disease)

- Evaluation of impact of extracranial stenosis on intracranial blood flow including collateral blood flow
- Identification of feeder arteries of arteriovenous malformations
- Evaluation and monitoring of intracranial blood flow during surgery (e.g., cardiopulmonary bypass)
- Evaluation of vasomotor tone
- Monitor effect of thrombolytic agents on blood vessel in acute stroke
- Adjunct data in diagnosis of brain death

B-Mode Imaging and Duplex Scanning

Principles of ultrasonography are being used in other ways, including B-mode imaging and duplex scanning. **B-mode (brightness-modulated) imaging**, or real-time ultrasonographic angiography, offers visualization of the structural detail of both the vessel walls and atherosclerotic plaques by recording the reflection of ultrasonic waves introduced through a probe. Two-dimensional images of a pulsating blood vessel in longitudinal and transverse sections allow visualization of most of the vessel's circumference. The image is reflected on a display screen in tones of gray. A photograph of the image can be taken to provide a permanent record. The purpose of the procedure is to detect minimal plaque formation and stenosis of carotid vessels. Poor-quality images can result if the patient has a short, thick neck because the carotid bifurcation is high in the neck and difficult to scan. The procedure takes approximately 30 to 45 minutes.

Duplex scanning of the carotids is based on the combination B-mode imaging and pulsed-wave Doppler principles to produce hemodynamic and anatomic information. This dual modality allows evaluation of flow dynamics, the vessel wall, and lumen anywhere along carotid, vertebral, or innominate arteries.[5]

Patient Preparation and Postprocedural Care

Patient preparation is the same for all noninvasive carotid studies. Regardless of the test to be performed, an explanation of what to expect is necessary. For all these tests, the patient will be asked to remain still. Beyond this, there is no other patient preparation.

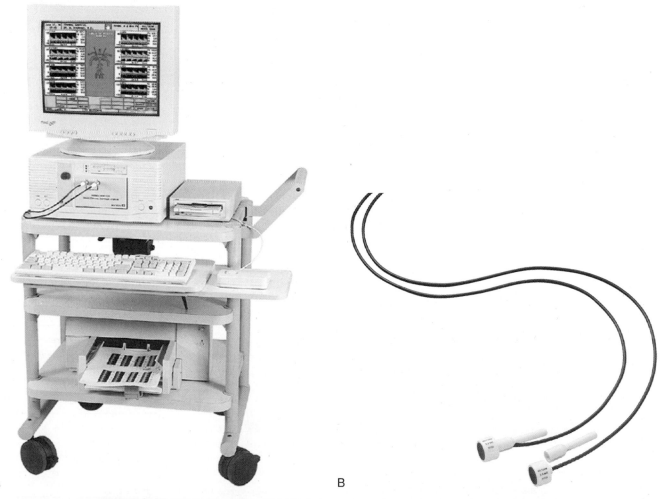

A   B

Figure 5-8 • Transcranial Doppler (TCD). (*A*) Neurovision instrumentation for transcranial Doppler can be wheeled to the bedside for patient evaluation. The monitor displays the data that are stored in the computer; the display can also be printed. (*B*) These are probes that the technician uses to slide over the areas to be evaluated. (*continued*)

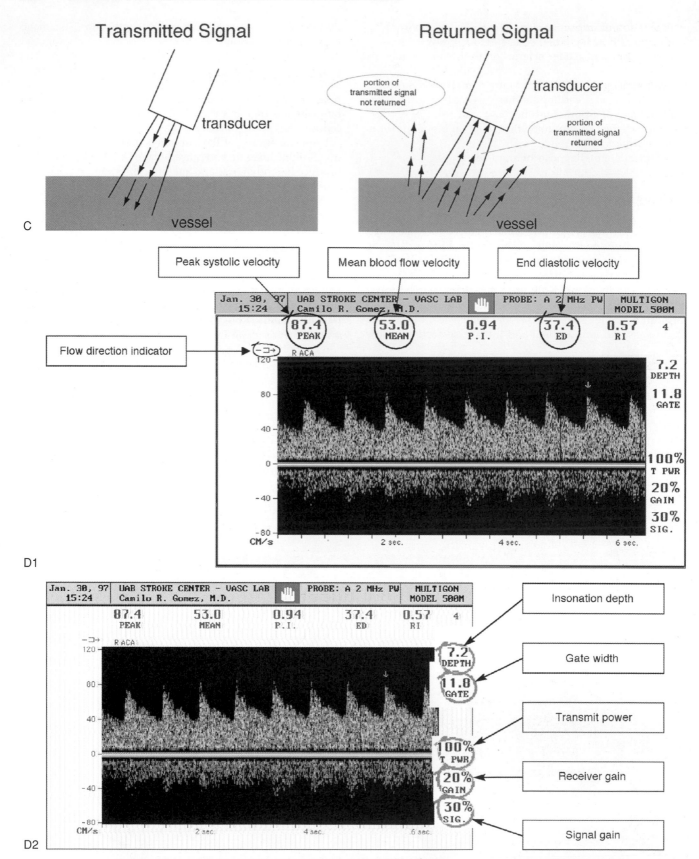

Figure 5-8 • (*Continued*) (*C*) The basic principle of signal transmission and return through the probe. (*D*) The various data elements that are collected and recorded (*D1* and *D2*). (Photos courtesy of Multigon Industries Inc., C. R. Gomez M. D., and Emily Stern.)

Other than cleansing the skin of any gel used as a conductor in Doppler studies, there is no specific aftercare required.

Cerebral Angiography

Cerebral angiography has been the "gold standard" diagnostic procedure for aneurysms, arteriovenous malformations, and other cerebrovascular abnormalities. With the advent of CT, MRI, CTA, and MRA, the previous wide use of cerebral arteriogram is expected to decrease.[2] The lumen of the blood vessels can be visualized to determine patency, narrowing or stenosis, thrombosis, vasospasm, abnormalities such as an aneurysm, and displacement of cerebral vessels. Causes of displacement include space-occupying lesions such as hematomas, cysts, tumors, and abscesses. Cerebral angiography can be performed using local anesthesia or during general anesthesia for a vascular procedure such as an aneurysm clipping to check the position and integrity of the clip.

Procedure

The patient is placed in a supine position on the procedure table. A wide area around the puncture site is shaved. A local anesthetic is usually administered; procaine (Novocaine) is often the drug of choice. The puncture site is aseptically cleansed. A needle is placed in the femoral (the femoral route is the most common) or brachial artery and a cannula is then threaded through the needle and along the aorta and the arterial branches.[2] The contrast medium is injected through a catheter at the origins of the carotid and vertebral arteries and their branches. Radiographic films are then taken at various time intervals after injection for visualization of the intracranial and extracranial blood vessels (Fig. 5-9). When the examination is completed, direct manual pressure is applied to the puncture site for 5 to 10 minutes to prevent bleeding into the subcutaneous space.

Possible complications related to cerebral angiography include allergic reactions to contrast medium, seizures, stroke, thrombosis, symptoms of carotid sinus sensitivity

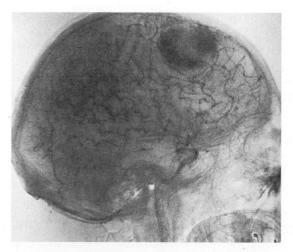

Figure 5-9 • Cerebral arteriogram (angiogram) showing an abnormal, large, space-occupying lesion at one o'clock.

(hypotension, syncope, and bradycardia), aphasia, and visual deficits.

Patient Preparation and Postprocedural Care

After explaining the procedure and the possible risks (e.g., stroke) to the patient, informed consent is obtained. Preoperative medication is usually administered half an hour before the procedure. The choice of drugs used varies from physician to physician and may include any of the following: pentobarbital (Nembutal); atropine sulfate, intramuscularly (IM), to protect against the effect upon the carotid sinus; and diazepam (Valium). Preparation for the examination is similar to that for any operative procedure. Dentures and eyeglasses are removed. Usually nothing by mouth for 6 to 8 hours before the examination is ordered. Baseline vital and neurological signs are recorded. The skin is shaved at the puncture site immediately before the procedure, usually in the procedure suite. The patient is told that, during injection, a burning sensation may be felt for a few (4 to 6) seconds behind the eyes or in the jaw, teeth, tongue, and lips. Even the fillings in the teeth may feel warm. The need to lie still during the procedure is emphasized.

When the angiogram is completed, the patient is returned to his or her room. An Angio-Seal is used at the puncture site so there is no need for a pressure dressing. Nursing responsibilities include the following:

- Maintain the patient on complete bedrest for 4 to 6 hours (according to hospital policy).
- Keep the involved extremity immobilized for 4 to 6 hours to prevent bleeding; in most instances, the upper leg is immobilized for a femoral artery puncture. This means that the patient cannot bend at the hip.
- Observe the puncture site (pressure dressing) frequently for bleeding.
- Monitor vital signs and neurological signs frequently. After the initial period of monitoring every 15 to 30 minutes, check these signs every 1 to 4 hours for a 24-hour period.
- Check pedal pulses in the affected leg if a femoral puncture was performed or radial pulse if the brachial artery was used; also check the color and temperature of the extremity.
- Maintain an accurate intake and output record.
- Force fluids to clear the contrast medium (a toxic response may include acute kidney failure due to contrast medium).
- Apply an ice bag to the puncture site to promote comfort.

Digital Subtraction Angiography

In evaluating the carotid arteries, invasive digital subtraction angiography (DSA) is a refinement of angiographic technique using digital computer enhancement to produce images for visualization of the carotids and other cerebral vessels. The image produced is made more distinct by the elimination of surrounding and interfering anatomic structures. This is accomplished by recording images before and after injection of contrast medium and subtracting the first image from the second.

The purposes of DSA include assistance in the diagnosis of the following conditions:

- Atherosclerotic disease (stenosis, occlusions, large plaques)
- Vascular lesions (arteriovenous malformations, aneurysms, carotid cavernous fistulas)
- Postoperative evaluation of endarterectomy, aneurysm clipping, arteriovenous malformation repair, and anastomosis

Procedure

The antecubital area, usually of the right arm, is cleansed and lidocaine is injected locally so that the antecubital vein (usual approach) or the brachial artery can be incised. A catheter is advanced into the superior vena cava, and contrast medium is injected. Selected vessels are visualized with an image-intensifier video system that displays vessels on a monitor. Images are taken and stored on magnetic tape. The images, which are collected before contrast injection, are received by the computer and are then subtracted from those taken after injection so that the image of the desired area is enhanced. The remaining contrast-enhanced images can be manipulated by the computer to focus on specific problems that might otherwise not be visualized.

On completion of the procedure, which takes from 30 to 45 minutes, the catheter is removed. Pressure is applied to the puncture site for several minutes, and a sterile dressing is applied.

Patient Preparation and Postprocedural Care

Screen patients for any history of allergic reaction to iodine or shellfish. Explain the procedure to the patient. Oral intake is withheld for 2 hours before the procedure. During the procedure, patients are required to hold their breath on command, remain motionless, and lie in the supine position on the x-ray table.

Vital signs and neurological signs are checked and the patient observed for the unlikely occurrence of stroke, allergic reaction, hemorrhage, or hematoma at the injection site. Force fluids to between 2000 and 3000 mL/24 hours to facilitate excretion of the contrast medium. Other possible but rare complications are venous thrombosis and infection.

BIOPSIES

Biopsy of the brain, muscle, nerve, or artery may assist in diagnosis under certain conditions when noninvasive methods such as imaging studies provide inconclusive diagnostic information, when a structure is superficial with easy accessibility, and when the area does not involve a critical area such as the motor strip. **Brain biopsy** may be warranted for diagnosis of brain tumor, infectious disorders such as herpes simplex encephalitis or brain abscess, and certain degenerative diseases such as Creutzfeldt-Jacob disease. **Muscle biopsy** is useful to differentiate underlying weakness of neurogenic or myopathic origin and to diagnose certain inflammatory diseases. Electromyographic findings are not

definitive in ruling in or ruling out myopathies or neuropathies. Therefore, a muscle biopsy is complementary to other studies when there is a question about the accuracy of the diagnosis. On rare occasion, **nerve biopsy** may be done to aid in the diagnosis of infection or inflammatory changes, vasculitis, or neoplasms. Finally, for patients who experience facial pain and nonspecific neurological symptoms, a **temporal artery biopsy** may be considered. A small piece of temporal artery is removed and examined for evidence of temporal arteritis.

Patient Preparation and Postprocedural Care

In preparing the patient, explain the procedure. A surgical permit may need to be signed depending on hospital policy. Medication for sedation may be ordered before the procedure. After the procedure, observe the dressing for bleeding. Vital signs and neurological signs should be monitored.

NERVOUS SYSTEM ELECTRICAL ACTIVITY AND CONDUCTION

Electroencephalography

An electroencephalogram (EEG) is a noninvasive, painless, diagnostic procedure that records the spontaneous electrical activity from the cerebral cortex using 8 to 24 scalp electrodes, amplifies the impulses, and records each tracing from the multiple electrodes on graph paper for interpretation (Fig. 5-10). This cortical activity is the summation of innumerable excitatory and inhibitory synaptic potentials on the cortical neurons that are further influenced by subcortical structures. The EEG records the frequency, amplitude, and characteristics of cerebral waveforms on paper moving at a standard speed of 3 cm/sec. The conventional ink-recorded EEG is gradually being replaced by computer technology. The electrical signal is digitally processed and displayed on a computer screen as a number of channels of recordings representing different cerebral areas for review.

Clinical Application

With the advent of CT and MRI, EEG, formerly a standard diagnostic tool in the neurological work-up, is now generally limited to the evaluation of patients with seizures or those suspected of having seizures. It is, however, the standard diagnostic tool for this patient population. It is also used to evaluate the cerebral effects of many systemic metabolic diseases, to study sleep, and in the operating room to monitor cerebral activity of anesthetized patients.[2]

An abnormal EEG is rarely diagnostic for a particular disease because a variety of conditions can produce similar EEG changes. It provides complementary data to anatomic imaging studies such as CT and MRI. Although pattern changes are nonspecific, some changes are highly suggestive of specific conditions such as particular types of epilepsy, herpes simplex encephalitis, and dementia-related disorders.

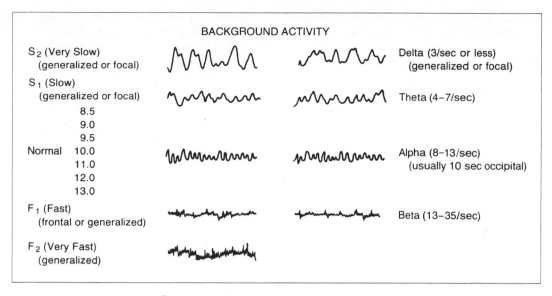

Figure 5-10 • Electroencephalogram classifications.

Abnormal EEGs are also found with brain tumors, abscesses, subdural hematomas, cerebral trauma, cerebrovascular disease, and diffuse degenerative diseases. The EEG is useful in follow-up observation of patients with altered states of consciousness and is an important criterion in the determination of brain death.

For patients who have intractable seizures unresponsive to drug therapy, continuous EEG monitoring and videotaping may be helpful. This provides continuous data about cerebral electrical activity and behavioral changes that can be correlated to determine the type and characteristics of the seizure activity. It often helps in identifying epileptogenic areas in the brain. If this is unsuccessful, electrodes can be inserted surgically into the cerebral cortex. This approach allows for better localization of epileptogenic foci amenable to surgical excision for better control of seizures.

Continuous EEG monitoring is also helpful for detection of seizure activity in patients with subclinical seizures (without physical manifestations). For example, a comatose patient who appears to be improving based on clinical indicators and CT or MRI but who does not awaken may have undiagnosed subclinical seizures that are altering consciousness. Data from the continuous EEG may prompt new treatment to control seizure activity.

Procedure

After a patient has been oriented to the test environment, he or she is made comfortable in an easy chair or on a stretcher. Cooperation is very important to the quality of the test data. A series of small electrodes (8 to 24, although 16 to 21 is most common) are symmetrically affixed to the scalp in standard locations with an adhesive substance. Extra electrodes (e.g., nasopharyngeal and sphenoidal) are available to record activity from the undersurface of the temporal lobes. Routinely, brain waves are recorded at rest, after hyperventilation, with strobe light stimulation, and during drowsiness or sleep. Hyperventilation and strobe light stimulation are stressors and may precipitate abnormal focal or generalized brain wave changes not detectable under normal circumstances. Wave types vary with activity and specific stimulation.

A baseline of spontaneous brain wave activity at rest with the eyes closed is recorded. The patient is then instructed to breathe deeply (20 times/min) for 3 minutes. This hyperventilation may activate characteristic seizure patterns or other abnormalities. Next, strong strobe light stimulation is applied by flashing the strobe light at a frequency of 1 to 20 per second with the eyes open and closed. The occipital EEG leads may show waves corresponding to each flash of light or abnormal discharges.[2] The last recording phase is that of drowsiness or sleep. An EEG takes at least 60 minutes and produces about 150 to 300 pages of recording paper.

A **sleep deprivation** technique is often used to demonstrate suspected abnormalities that are not evident on routine EEG. The patient is kept awake for most of the night before the EEG. Sleep deprivation stresses the brain and, therefore, may evoke abnormal waves not seen in the normal state. An all-night EEG is useful in studying sleep problems.

Patient Preparation and Postprocedural Care

Explain the procedure and expectations for patient involvement during the EEG. Preparation is very important to allay anxiety and ensure patient cooperation. Anxiety can block alpha waves and produce head and neck muscle tension, resulting in recording artifacts.

Because anticonvulsants, stimulants, tranquilizers, and depressants can alter brain wave activity and mask or suppress abnormal brain waves, the physician may withhold selected medications for 24 to 48 hours before the EEG. Coffee, tea, colas, and chocolate are withheld from the regular diet to exclude dietary stimulants. To promote sleep during the EEG, the patient should go to sleep late and arise early. Napping before the test is discouraged. If a sleep deprivation study is required, the patient should be prevented from sleeping the night before the EEG. The patient's hair should be clean and no oils, sprays, or lotions should be used before the test. After the EEG, the hair is washed to remove the electrode-affixing paste. Resume drugs withheld specifically for the EEG.

Classification of Brain Waves

Classification of brain waves is based on the number of cycles per second, which are recorded in hertz (Hz) units. Four common EEG rhythms include:

Delta rhythms (1 to 3 Hz) are not normally present in adults who are awake; they are normally seen in stages 3 and 4 of sleep (slow-wave sleep).

Theta rhythms (4 to 7 Hz) originate from the temporal lobes; there may be a very small amount of delta waves over the temporal regions in normal adults. Theta activity increases slightly in persons over the age of 60 years.

Alpha rhythms (8 to 12 Hz) are most prominent in the occipital and parietal regions. Opening of the eyes, mental effort, anxiety, apprehension, and sudden noise or touch can block alpha waves.

Beta rhythms (>12 Hz) are most prominent in the frontal and central areas. Opening of the eyes, mental activity, anxiety, or apprehension triggers beta waves. They are especially prominent in patients receiving barbiturates and benzodiazepine drugs.

Normal age-related EEG variations are categorized as follows: children and teenagers (younger than 20 years of age); adults (20 to 60 years of age); and older adults (older than 60 years of age). In the older-than-60-years group, EEG patterns are similar to those in the 20- to 60-year group with a few exceptions: alpha waves are slower; beta waves are more prominent; there are more sporadic, generalized slow waves; and intermittent temporal slow waves are evident. Thus, age-related variations must be considered in the interpretation of EEGs.

Common Abnormal Electroencephalographic Abnormalities

Not to be confused with abnormal EEG findings are artifacts. Artifacts are abnormal deflections on the graphic recording that are not caused by cerebral activity but rather by other physiologic activities, such as eye movement, muscle contraction, or heart action.

An EEG is abnormal when it contains lower frequency or higher amplitude than normal. Both delta waves (<4 Hz) and beta waves (>12 Hz) meet these criteria. Spikes or sharp waves are transient high-voltage waveforms that have a pointed peak and a duration of 20 to 70 milliseconds. When spikes occur in epileptic patients or those genetically predisposed to seizures, they are called *epileptiform discharges*. Spikes can be divided into focal, multifocal, and generalized events. For example, the patient with temporal lobe seizures will have characteristically abnormal electrical discharges over one anterior temporal lobe, whereas absence epilepsy is evidenced by widespread, bilateral, synchronous 3-Hz discharges. The normal EEG includes a range of variations that must be differentiated from a true form of epilepsy and abnormal activity related to cerebral lesions (Fig. 5-11).

Slow-wave (defined as 1 to 7 Hz) findings are classified as either focal or diffuse abnormalities. **Focal slow waves** may be related to gray or white matter dysfunction in a localized area that is secondary to a tumor, hemorrhage, or other space-occupying lesion. Focal lesions directly involve either the cerebral cortex or the thalamocortical projection pathways. The finding of a focal abnormality indicates the need for further diagnostic testing, such as a CT scan or MRI. As the lesion enlarges and affects the diencephalon, slow waves can become diffuse. **Diffuse slow waves** are usually seen with toxic (drug toxicity), metabolic (e.g., hepatic), degenerative (e.g., Alzheimer's disease), infectious (e.g., encephalitis), or postictal conditions. Generally, a pattern of diffuse slowing does not point to a specific diagnosis but only provides collaborating diagnostic information. A few forms of dementia, however, do have a characteristic wave pattern.

The electrocerebral silence or "flat" EEG indicates the absence of brain waves and is one finding seen in brain death (others include absence of brainstem function and loss of brainstem reflexes). Brain death is never declared on the basis of a flat EEG only (see Chap. 3 for further discussion).

Abnormal EEGs must be viewed within the context of clinical presentation and circumstances when the EEG was recorded.

Electromyography and Nerve Conduction Velocity Studies

Electromyography (EMG) and nerve conduction velocity studies (NCVSs) are electrophysiologic studies, known collectively as electromyoneurography, which are usually ordered together. An EMG may be ordered for patients thought to have myasthenia gravis, Eaton-Lambert syndrome, or peripheral nerve injury or neuropathies, or when it is unclear whether the primary problem is a myopathy or neuropathy. It can also differentiate among lesions of the anterior horn cell, root, plexus, and specific nerves and muscles.

NCVSs are conducted when nerve damage is suspected because of clinical symptoms of motor weakness or atrophy. They are helpful in the diagnosis of neuropathies (e.g., those induced by diabetes, alcoholism, or nutritional deficiencies and compression of or trauma to the peripheral nerves). Both studies can be used to follow the progression of peripheral nerve disorders and their response to treatment.

Procedures

By inserting small needle electrodes into the muscle, an EMG records muscle activity at rest, during voluntary movement, and with electrical stimulation. Patterns of muscle activity are displayed on an oscilloscope and compared with standardized norms.

NCVSs measure the conduction time and amplitude of electrical stimulation along two or more points of a peripheral nerve using a cathode (negative electrode) and an anode (positive electrode). The recorded response has a simple, biphasic waveform with initial negativity and maximal amplitude. Amplitude, duration, and latency times are measured and compared with standardized norms.

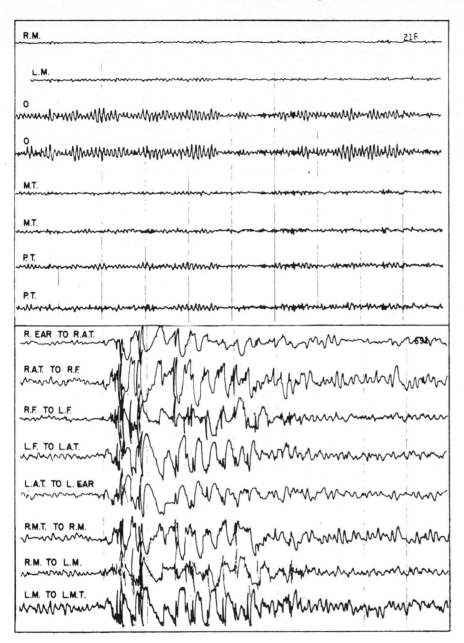

Figure 5-11 • Comparison of a normal electroencephalogram (*top*) with that of an epileptic patient during a tonic–clonic seizure (*bottom*). Note the sharp, spiky waves recorded during the seizure.

Patient Preparation and Postprocedural Care

Explain the procedure to the patient, emphasizing the importance of cooperation. Some discomfort from the needle electrodes and the electrical stimuli is to be expected.

There is no aftercare required except to cleanse the skin of any contact gel.

Evoked Potentials

Evoked potentials (EPs) are a noninvasive means of applying a stimulus to sensory organs or peripheral nerves and recording the minute electrical potentials created. Using a computerized averaging program, the stimulus is repeated several times, allowing a return to the resting state between stimuli. Each evoked response is measured and the data are stored in the computer. After a number of potentials have been stored, the computer then calculates the average curve. The interpretation of EPs is based on the prolongation of the latencies of the waveforms after the stimulus, the interwave latencies, and asymmetries in timing, which are compared to established norms. Value of brainstem auditory evoked responses (BAERs) and somatosensory evoked potentials (SSEPs) is founded on two characteristics. The first is the close relationship between the EP waveforms and specific anatomic structures. This specificity allows localization of conduction defects to within an approximate centimeter for BAERs and a few centimeters for SSEPs. Second, EPs are unaffected by intravenous sedatives, high-dose barbiturates, and general anesthesia. These characteristics provide reliable indicators of physiologic anatomy that are useful in critical care environments.[16]

EPs are part of a battery of tests to diagnosis: lesions of the cerebral cortex, ascending pathways of the spinal cord or thalamus; evaluation of the extent of central nervous system (CNS) injury; diagnosis of neuromuscular disease; and prognostic evaluation of comatose patients.[17] The MRI has mostly replaced EPs for diagnosis of acoustic neuromas and other cerebellopontine angle tumors, subclinical lesions of multiple sclerosis, and brainstem lesions.[11]

EPs are classified into three categories based on the type of stimulus provided and the sensory system stimulated. Each system stimulated produces a characteristic wave formation. The three sensory systems used in EPs are the visual, auditory, and somatosensory pathways.

Visual Evoked Potentials

In visual evoked potentials (VEPs), checkerboard patterns and flashing lights provide stimuli. The retina is stimulated, allowing the pathways to the occipital cortex to be evaluated. Each eye is tested separately. The response is recorded with electrodes over the occipital region. If the patient wears eyeglasses, they should be worn during the procedure. The cooperation of the patient is necessary during testing. VEPs are used in the diagnosis of optic neuropathies such as optic neuritis often related to multiple sclerosis and optic nerve lesions such as tumors.

Brainstem Auditory Evoked Responses

BAERs are primarily used to evaluate brainstem function. The stimuli provided through headphones include a series of clicks that vary in rate, intensity, and duration. Five wave formations, based on the site of origin, are recorded: wave I from the acoustic nerve, wave II from the cochlear nucleus, wave III from the superior olivary complex, wave IV from the lateral lemniscus, and wave V from the inferior colliculus. BAER testing can be conducted on alert or comatose patients. It has been used in diagnosing lesions in multiple sclerosis, acoustic neuroma, coma prognosis, and hearing loss (especially in infants). BAERs are also used intraoperatively to monitor the eighth cranial nerve for surgical injury.

Somatosensory Evoked Responses

Somatosensory evoked responses (SSERs) are used to confirm lesions in the somatic sensory systems. Transcutaneous painless electrical stimuli are applied to the median, peroneal, and tibial peripheral nerves and the EPs recorded. SSERs are helpful in evaluating the possibility of lesions in spinal roots, posterior columns, and brainstem disorders such as Guillain-Barré syndrome; ruptured lumbar and cervical discs; multiple sclerosis; and lumbar and cervical spondylosis.[16]

TESTING OF THE SPECIAL SENSES

Audiometric Studies

Audiometric testing assesses the auditory branch of the eighth cranial nerve for type and cause of hearing loss. Testing is divided into pure-tone audiometry and speech audiometry. The basis for *pure-tone audiometry* is that the louder the sound stimulus (pure or musical tone) necessary before the patient perceives it, the greater the hearing loss. The decibel (dB) is the unit of measure of loudness. *Speech audiometry* is based on the ability of the patient to understand and discriminate between sounds of the spoken word. In testing, a soundproof room and earphones are used to screen out ambient noise. A graphic representation of testing results is interpreted to differentiate between conduction and sensorineural hearing loss. **Conduction loss** results from outer ear or middle ear dysfunction or impairment to both structures. The inner ear is not involved. In such cases, a hearing aid is helpful. **Sensorineural loss** occurs in diseases of the inner ear or nerve pathways. This type of hearing loss is characterized by loss of sensitivity to and discrimination of sounds. Hearing aids are not very effective with this form of hearing loss. Hearing loss in the neuroscience patient is usually related to head injury, meningitis, acoustic neuroma, or drug toxicity.

Caloric Testing

Caloric testing is designed to evaluate the vestibular portion of the eighth cranial nerve and the presence or absence of the oculovestibular reflex. The underlying principle of the procedure is that thermal stimulation of the vestibular apparatus (the balance-sensing mechanism in the inner ear) with cold water will elicit the oculovestibular reflex. The test is *contraindicated* in patients with a ruptured tympanic membrane or cervical injury. Patients with diseases involving the vestibular branch of the eighth cranial nerve (e.g., acoustic neuroma or Ménière's disease) will not have the normal eye movements associated with caloric testing; instead, these movements will be diminished or absent.

Procedure

After tympanic membrane intactness is confirmed and the cervical neck is stable, the patient's head is tilted backward at a 60-degree angle from the horizontal plane to allow maximal stimulation of the lateral semicircular canal, the canal that is most responsible for reflex lateral movement. The external auditory canal is slowly irrigated with 10 mL of ice-cold water. The cold irrigation causes convection currents in the endolymph of the labyrinths, resulting in a change in the baseline firing of the vestibular nerve and slow conjugate deviation of the eyes toward the stimulated ear (see Chap. 6). In the normal waking state with an intact oculovestibular reflex, there is an initial conjugate eye movement (lasting about 30 seconds) toward the side being irrigated with the cold water (slow phase). This is controlled by the brainstem. The lateral gaze is corrected shortly by a rapid component of nystagmus that pulls the eyes back to the midline (fast phase). The rapid component is controlled by the cerebral cortex.

As a patient becomes lethargic, the fast component becomes less pronounced. Deterioration into obtundation and coma results in loss of the fast component because the cerebral cortex is depressed. As the patient slips into a deep coma, the lateral deviation toward the side of irrigation (slow component) may be lost. This indicates that the oculovestibular reflex (a reflex controlled by the brainstem) is absent; this is a poor prognostic indicator.

In the emergency department, the oculovestibular reflex may be tested on an unconscious patient. If there is tonic deviation of the eyes toward the side being irrigated, brainstem function is intact. This is considered a positive prognostic sign. With a brainstem lesion, the caloric reflex is absent. Absence of the reflex is associated with a poor prognosis.

Warm water irrigation produces reversal of endolymphic flow. This results in conjugate eye deviation with the slow phase away from the stimulated ear and normal correction phase toward the irrigated ear. The type of nystagmus is named by the direction of the fast phase. The mnemonic **COWS** (**C**old **O**pposite, **W**arm **S**ame) refers to the **fast phase** of nystagmus. It is also possible to irrigate both ear canals simultaneously with cold water, which results in slow downward deviation; conversely, simultaneous warm water irrigation results in slow upward deviation.

Patient Preparation and Postprocedural Care

In conscious patients, fasting is maintained for at least 8 hours before the procedure. In unconscious patients, this is obviously not a consideration. Caloric testing in normal patients can precipitate nausea, vomiting, or dizziness. Maintain bedrest until nausea, vomiting, vertigo, or dizziness has subsided. A normal diet can be resumed when the patient feels ready.

Genetic Testing

The explosion of knowledge about genetics and the translation of that knowledge into clinical practice are beginning to shape a new health care paradigm. Individual genes responsible for a particular neurological disease have been identified and tests are available for people who wish to be tested. Other neurological diseases, such as stroke, are caused by complex multifactorial genes. Because of the complexity of stroke and other neurological conditions, researchers have not identified the genetic basis for the problem. As more is learned about complex diseases, diagnostic tests will be developed to identify a person at risk before the disease is evident. This change suggests that prevention strategies may be available in the future. Understanding the genetic basis of neurological diseases will also lead to new treatments options. We are at the beginning of a monumental shift in how neurological diseases are diagnosed and treated as the genomics of disease are unraveled.

NEUROPSYCHOLOGICAL EXAMINATION

A neuropsychological examination is a comprehensive assessment of cognition and behavior. A licensed neuropsychologist conducts the examination. The purposes of a neuropsychological examination include the following:

- To ascertain the presence or absence of cognitive deficits
- To determine whether brain dysfunction is localized (focal) or diffuse
- To plan, manage, and evaluate an individualized rehabilitation program
- To determine competency for self-care and decision making
- To document disability for insurance purposes
- To provide information about competency for legal matters and need for a guardian

A number of frameworks are available that address neuropsychological function. One approach is to conceptualize behavior as three functional and integrated systems that include cognition, emotionality, and executive functions.[18] *Cognition* produces the information aspect of behavior; *emotionality* is the feelings and motivation of behavior; and *executive function* is how behavior is expressed. Skill performance is examined in great depth and detail to determine cerebral function. A major benefit of extensive testing is that subtle behavioral changes may be discovered that would not be detected with less refined testing methods or anatomic imaging studies. The comprehensiveness of the examination is reflected in the time required for testing, which is approximately 6 to 10 hours.

Components of a Neuropsychological Evaluation

The examination is tailored to the patient's needs, abilities, and limitations. The specific tests included in the battery of tests vary depending on the patient's age, the nature of the problem, the deficits present, and the specific questions asked by the physician in the referral note. Information about the type of neurological insult, premorbid function and personality, personal and family history, and data from other diagnostic tests is correlated with data from the neuropsychological examination. Components of the examination evaluate the following cognitive functions:

Attention: vigilance (the ability to sustain attention over a period of time, concentration), self-regulation, and screening out of distracting environmental stimuli

Visual perception and visual reasoning: picture completion, picture arrangement, judgment of line orientation, visual search

Memory and learning: short term, immediate, long term; new learning such as remembering word lists; verbal and nonverbal memory (testing includes sentence repetition, serial digit learning, and auditory-verbal learning tests)

Language: understanding of single words and sentences; reading; speaking; and auditory discrimination

General intelligence: verbal and nonverbal; includes information, comprehension, and similarities; naming objects; arithmetic calculations

Constructional ability: drawing to command; drawing to copy; block designs; visual organization of a picture and its parts; right–left orientation; clock setting

Map orientation: being able to read a map

Conceptualization: metaphors and proverbs

Abstraction: verbal and nonverbal abstract reasoning

Perceptual motor speed: ability to plan ahead and shift from one concept to the other

Emotional status: assess for depression, suicidal ideation, anxiety, paranoia, and other abnormal responses

Depression inventory or other inventories of emotional status may be administered in some situations.

COMMON NEUROPSYCHOLOGICAL DEFICITS ASSOCIATED WITH CEREBRAL DYSFUNCTION

Many patients with organic brain dysfunction develop cognitive and behavioral deficits as a result of cerebral trauma, stroke, CNS degenerative disorders (e.g., Alzheimer's disease), and CNS infections (e.g., encephalitis, meningitis). Common deficits include a decreased ability to concentrate, screen irrelevant information, solve problems, sequence complex actions correctly, and learn new tasks. In addition, there may be increased irritability, emotional lability, deficits of memory, logical reasoning, perceptual deficits, and general slowing of all cognitive functions. These cognitive and behavioral deficits cause serious difficulty in activities of daily living and social and vocational readjustment into the family, community, and work setting. Diagnosing the specific deficits and developing a plan for rehabilitation are necessary to help the patient achieve the highest possible level of function and independence.

Because of the focus and time required for neuropsychological evaluation, patient selection is important. The patient must be alert, able to actively participate, and have the physical endurance to complete the examination. The physician should be specific in documenting why neuropsychological evaluation is desired. Timing of testing is critical. There is some natural recovery that occurs over time after cerebral insult. Seeking neuropsychological evaluation too soon after the insult does not allow sufficient time for spontaneous improvement to be captured. In addition, natural recovery can be so rapid that findings on the examination from one day may be outdated on the next day. Often evaluation is postponed for 3 to 6 months after injury to allow for natural recovery. In some instances, a modified version of the evaluation may be requested.

SUMMARY

The major diagnostic procedures commonly used with a neurological patient population have been discussed. Some laboratory studies specific to a condition are included in the pertinent chapter. In caring for patients, the nurse must view the patient holistically and recognize that stabilization and recovery require close monitoring of various laboratory data.

REFERENCES

1. Society of Critical Care Medicine. (1993). Guidelines for the transport of critically ill patients. *Critical Care Medicine, 21*(6), 931–937.
2. Ropper, A. H., & Brown, R. H. (2005). *Adams and Victor's principles of neurology* (8th ed., pp. 11–34). New York: McGraw-Hill.
3. Gilman, S. (1998). Imaging of the brain. *New England Journal of Medicine, 338*(12), 812–819.
4. Griggs, R. C., Jozefowicz, I. A., & Aminoff, M. J. (2004). Approach to patients with neurological disease. In L. Goldman & D. Ausiello (Eds.). *Cecil's textbook of medicine* (8th ed., pp. 2196–2205). St. Louis, MO: Elsevier Health Sciences.
5. DeWalch, D. R., & Proenza, R. M. (2006). Limiting the damage from ischemic stroke. *The Clinical Advisor*, September, 35–42.
6. Wintermark, M., Sisay, M., Barbier, E., Borbely, K., Dillon, W. P., Eastwood, J. D., et al. (2005). Comparative overview of brain perfusion imaging techniques. *Stroke, 36*, e83–e99.
7. Latchaw, R. E., Yonas, H., Pentheny, S. L., & Gur, D. (1987). Adverse reactions to xenon-enhanced CT cerebral blood flow determination. *Radiology, 163*, 251–254.
8. Johnson, L. C., Richards, T. L., Archbold, K. H., & Landis, C. A. (2006). Functional magnetic resonance imaging in nursing research. *Biological Research in Nursing, 8*(1), 43–54.
9. Liebenberg, W. A. (2005). *Neurosurgery explained: A basic and essential introduction* (pp. 123–161). London: Vesuvius Books.
10. Conn, P. M. (1995). *Neuroscience in medicine* (p. 624). Philadelphia: J. B. Lippincott.
11. Greenberg, M. S. (2006). *Handbook of neurosurgery* (6th ed., pp. 126–148). New York: Thieme.
12. Grossman, R. I. (2004). Radiologic imaging procedures. In L. Goldman & D. Ausiello (Eds.). *Cecil's textbook of medicine* (8th ed., pp. 2205–2211). St. Louis, MO: Elsevier Health Sciences.
13. Wijdicks, E. F. M. (1997). *The clinical practice of critical care neurology* (p. 126). Philadelphia: Lippincott-Raven.
14. Boon, J. M., Abraham, P. H., Meiring, J. H., & Welch, T. (2004). Lumbar puncture: Anatomical review of a clinical skill. *Clinical Anatomy, 17*, 544–553.
15. Armon, C., & Evans, R. W. (2005). Addendum to assessment: Prevention of post-lumbar puncture headaches. Report of the therapeutics and technology assessment subcommittee of the American Academy of Neurology. *Neurology, 65*, 510–512.
16. Ropper, A. H., Gress, D. R., Diringer, M. N., Green, D. M., Mayer, S. A., & Bleck, T. P. (2003). *Neurological and neurosurgical intensive care* (4th ed., pp. 129–153). Philadelphia: Lippincott Williams & Wilkins.
17. Shpritz, D. W. (1999). Neurodiagnostic studies. *Nursing Clinics of North America, 34*(3), 593–606.
18. Lezak, M. D. (1995). *Neuropsychological assessment* (3rd ed.). New York: Oxford University Press.

Comprehensive Neurological Examination

Joanne V. Hickey

PURPOSES

The purposes for conducting a neurological physical examination by the physician are to determine whether nervous system dysfunction is present, to diagnose disease of the nervous system, and to localize disease within the nervous system. Although diagnosis of disease is usually the responsibility of the physician, advanced practice nurses also may conduct the neurological examination. It is the *purpose* of the data collection that differentiates medical practice from nursing practice. The nursing purposes are (1) to determine whether nervous system dysfunction is present, (2) to identify functional deficits and how they impact on the individual's ability to function in activities of daily living and other aspects of life, and (3) to determine the human responses to actual or potential health problems precipitated by the dysfunction. The data collected creates a database for planning care that is patient centered. Advanced practice nurses may overlap with physicians in the purposes of the examination based on legal authority to practice in advanced practice roles.

The neurological physical examination is included in this text for several reasons. First, the neurological physical examination provides a comprehensive database of critical information about the patient's neurological function. As part of the patient's record, it is available to nurses and other health care providers to review. Second, a review of these data by nurses may be helpful in identifying areas of special consideration in neurological assessment, as well as special observations to be made and documented. These points should be noted in the patient's individualized care plan. Third, potential multidisciplinary collaborative problems may be suggested by the dysfunction identified. For example, a patient with ataxia, a symptom of cerebellar dysfunction, will usually have problems with balance and coordination and needs supervision when ambulating to prevent falls. The potential for falls and injury must be considered by all providers and noted on the care plan or clinical pathway. Finally, although nurses independently establish an individualized nursing database about the patient's neurological function, collaborative practice and relationships suggest a sharing of information so that each participant understands the database on which other participants provide care. The comprehensive neurological examination recorded on admission provides a baseline for understanding a patient's problems and needs.

THE NEUROLOGICAL EXAMINATION

Circumstances of the Examination

The circumstances surrounding the neurological examination can vary greatly. A patient may be seen in the physician's office, an ambulatory care center, an emergency department, or a hospital setting. The acuteness and urgency of the clinical presentation influences the initial completeness of the examination. The patient's overall condition and level of consciousness (LOC) are key factors that influence a collection of elements of the neurological examination. Many parts of the neurological examination require cooperation and the ability to follow directions. If a person has periods of confusion but can be reoriented, most aspects of the neurological examination can be completed so long as the examiner takes time to reorient and redirect the patient. However, in the case of a comatose patient, data collection is limited to responses to painful stimuli, reflexes, and a few special techniques for assessment. Other parts of the neurological examination will have to be deferred until the patient's condition improves.

Types of Examinations

The major components of a neurological examination are listed in Box 6-1. Neurological examinations may be classified as a screening or an extended examination. A **screening neurological examination** refers to a comprehensive neurological examination for persons who come for a general assessment because of signs and symptoms that may be of neurological origin. A screening examination may suggest the need for further neurological investigation and an extended neurological examination and diagnostics. An **extended neurological examination** is an extension of the screening examination whereby the examiner follows leads from abnormal findings and expands the investigation with additional special tests to determine the presence or absence of dysfunction. A **problem-focused examination** is a subset of an extended examination. It is confined to a particular neurological system or region that is related to specific complaints or signs and symptoms. This chapter focuses on an initial comprehensive neurological *screening examination* (Box 6-2). It also includes components of the extended examination that further explores specific areas of the

---

> **BOX 6–1   Major Components of the Neurological Examination**
>
> - Level of consciousness
> - Mental status examination
> - Cranial nerves
> - Motor system
> - Sensory system
> - Cerebellar system
> - Reflexes
> - Other special tests

nervous system that require more refined techniques for evaluation.

Role of the Nurse During the Examination

The nurse may or may not be present during the neurological examination. If present, the role of the bedside nurse is supportive by providing brief explanations, emotional support, physical support, and assistance, as needed, with the conduct of the examination. Sometimes, the examiner may prefer to examine the patient alone, particularly if the patient is easily distracted by the presence of another person in the room. Additionally, some patients tend to reveal more information to the examiner when the exchange is one to one.

Equipment

The usual equipment necessary to conduct a neurological examination includes the following:

- Ophthalmoscope
- Reflex hammer

> **BOX 6–2   Components of the Comprehensive Neurological Screening Examination**
>
> 1. Level of consciousness
> 2. Mental status and cognitive function examination
> 3. Cranial nerves II to XII
> 4. Motor tone, muscle bulk, and motor strength in major muscle groups; in addition, note any abnormal movements
> 5. Sensory function of pinprick and light touch in medial and lateral aspects of face, extremities, and trunk; vibration and position in thumbs and great toes
> 6. Coordinated or rapid alternation of movements of extremities; finger–nose test; gait; and station
> 7. Reflexes including major superficial (e.g., corneal, gag), deep tendon (e.g., biceps, triceps, brachioradialis, quadriceps, Achilles), and pathologic reflexes (e.g., Babinski's sign)
>
> Note: Abnormal findings or specific symptoms may require an extended evaluation.

- Tuning fork (128-Hz for vibration on bony prominences and 512-Hz for hearing)
- Stethoscope
- Tongue blade
- Pointed/sharp instrument: for instance, picky end of a broken wooden applicator (to test noxious stimuli)
- Wisp of cotton or fluffed cotton swab (to test corneal reflex and light touch sensation)
- Flashlight
- Tape measure
- Snellen or Rosenbaum eye chart

Approach

A comprehensive neurological examination is always preceded by a complete medical history and a general physical examination. The general physical examination will include the chief complaint, present illness, past medical history, family and social history, and review of systems. Typically, abnormal neurological findings in the general physical examination prompt the physician or advanced practice nurse to conduct a comprehensive neurological examination or to refer the patient to a neurologist for a comprehensive evaluation. The person conducting the comprehensive neurological examination will want to review the findings of the history and physical examination.

Generalized neurological signs and symptoms may accompany primary disease in another body system, and may even be the first evidence of such disease. In addition, neurological symptoms of either organic or psychogenic origin may include symptoms referable to other systems as a result of central or autonomic nervous system effects on visceral function. Therefore, all signs and symptoms must be adequately investigated within the context of all body systems before a neurological diagnosis is made.

Chief Complaint and History of Present Illness

After reviewing the patient's medical record or referral information, the chief complaint and history of the present illness are collected. It is advisable to start at the beginning in collecting the complete medical history even though this has already been documented by another practitioner. An explanation to the patient will help in gaining cooperation. For example, one can say, "I know that you have answered some of these questions before. However, I like to start from the beginning and collect this information without being influenced by what is in your chart so I can make an unbiased assessment of you." Often an examiner with neurological expertise will delve into areas not included in a general physical examination. This information may be critical in making a timely and accurate diagnosis. The examiner may wish to speak with a reliable family member or significant other to collect additional information about the past medical history and chronological development of the neurological problem, especially if the patient's cognitive function is altered.

A complete accounting of the present illness, including onset, duration, and sequence of symptoms, must be established in defining the clinical problem. Consider the defining characteristics of signs and symptoms, associated symptoms, and relieving/aggravating factors for each symptom.

Every patient with neurological complaints should be directly questioned about each of the following symptoms[1]:

Loss/change in intellectual abilities, onset of memory problems, difficulty with concentration, personality change, depression, or loss of drive
New onset or change in headache patterns
Seizures and loss of consciousness
Dizziness or vertigo
Loss or blurring of vision (one eye or both) or diplopia
Loss of hearing or tinnitus
Incoordination or gait difficulty
Weakness, involuntary movements
Paresthesias, sensory loss, or pain
Speech difficulties
Dysphagia
Bladder, bowel, or sexual dysfunction
Sleep difficulties (insomnia or increased sleep)

Past Medical History

A chronological past medical history is collected, including surgical procedures. Ask the patient about a history of hypertension, heart disease, stroke, diabetes mellitus, head trauma, alcohol or drug abuse, and exposure to toxins, which may suggest risk factors. A detailed history of all prescribed and over-the-counter medications is imperative because of the high incidence of drug interactions and side effects.

Family and Social History

A family history should be collected, including drawing of a family tree for two to three generations. This information is helpful to suggest risk of diseases seen in families. If a neurogenetic disorder is considered, a three-generation family pedigree is drawn. However, the patient would probably be eventually seen by a practitioner specializing in medical genetics who would collect the history related to the family pedigree. The patient's social history includes use of recreational drugs, alcohol consumption, and cigarette smoking. A history of high-risk sexual behavior should be elicited in light of the many neurological complications associated with acquired immune deficiency syndrome (AIDS).

Reviews of Systems

The review of the major body systems to determine the presence or absence of symptoms is conducted to collect information on all symptoms experienced by the patient that may be related to the current health problem.

CONDUCTING THE NEUROLOGICAL EXAMINATION

The neurological examination is conducted in a systematic, hierarchical, stepwise approach that proceeds from the highest level of function (cerebral cortex) to the lowest (reflexes) and from the general functions to specific functions. It encompasses a review of LOC, mental status/cognitive function, cranial nerves, motor system, sensory system, cerebellar system, reflexes, and special standardized scales of neurological function such as the Mini-Mental Status Examination. By approaching the neurological examination with a conceptual framework in mind, the likelihood of forgetting a part is diminished. The examiner may decide to defer certain parts of the examination. Deciding which parts can be deferred without loss of key data is difficult. The judgment and experience of the examiner will guide these decisions. The examiner must be competent in the appropriate techniques for testing function, know when further investigation is warranted, and be familiar with the expected range of normal, age-based responses. More information about specific findings in the neurological examination is included in Chapter 7. This chapter includes the neurological examinations for both the conscious, cooperative patient and the comatose patient.

The examination begins with an explanation about the examination to gain patient cooperation. The patient profile information is collected on age, gender, race, marital status, and occupation. Establish the patient's hand dominance (i.e., left- or right-handedness). Handedness and cerebral dominance for language are closely aligned. Asking the patient if he or she is left-handed or right-handed is not sufficient because some left-handed people have been taught to write with their right hand. Helpful questions are "What hand do you use for throwing a ball?" or "What eye do you use to focus a camera?"

LEVEL OF CONSCIOUSNESS

A complete discussion of the various components of the LOC is found in Chapter 7. See discussion in the Mental Status Examination section.

MENTAL STATUS EXAMINATION

Many parts of the **mental status examination** are integrated into the history-taking portion of the interview. This provides a natural context for collecting information without creating an artificial test environment that could make the patient uncomfortable or anxious. The basic mental processes are the foundation to proceed to complex functions. Higher-level cognitive functions such as memory and abstraction cannot be reliably tested if basic mental functions such as attentiveness or arousal are absent. In appraising mental status the examiner must determine whether there is any dysfunction present, whether the dysfunction is global or focal, and if global, whether it is an acute confusional state or dementia.

The mental status examination focuses on three general and often overlapping areas: (1) general impression of awareness and mental function, (2) reception and interpretation of sensory stimuli (general cognitive function), and (3) higher-level cognitive function (Box 6-3). An *extended mental status examination* is warranted if abnormalities are found in the screening examination. Referral for neuropsychological testing may be necessary for selected patients.

BOX 6–3   Comprehensive Mental Status Examination

I. General impression of awareness and mental function
   A. Level of alertness
   B. General appearance and behavior
   C. Mood and emotional state
   D. General thinking processes
   E. Content of thought
II. Reception and interpretation of sensory stimuli (general cognitive function)
   A. Orientation
   B. Personal identification
   C. Attention
   D. Comprehension
III. Higher-level cognitive functions
   A. Memory (immediate, short term, long term)
   B. Calculations
   C. General fund of information
   D. Abstract thinking, reasoning, and judgment
   E. Language and speech
   F. Constructional ability
   G. Motor integrative function

General Impression of Patient Awareness and Mental Function

Beginning with the interview and history collection, the following areas are evaluated: level of alertness and awareness; general appearance and behavior; mood and emotional state; and thinking processes along with content of thought.

Level of Alertness

What the examiner must determine before conducting the neurological examination is whether the patient is awake or comatose. If the patient is comatose, *proceed to the neurological examination for the comatose patient found later in this chapter*. If the patient is awake, is attention sufficiently intact so he or she can cooperate and follow instructions to elicit maximum functional ability? If the answer is "yes," you can proceed with the complete neurological examination. If the answer is "no," you will need to limit the neurological examination to what can be collected within the limitations of the LOC and defer other components until the LOC is sufficient to complete the neurological examination. Delirium and dementia can affect the mental status examination. If dementia is suspected, the Mini-Mental Status Examination is a good screening tool.

Appearance and General Behavior

In an ambulatory setting, a patient's attire should be appropriate for the setting and his or her age. A neat and clean appearance reflects good grooming and good personal hygiene habits. An unkempt appearance, conversely, might suggest depression or chronic organic brain disease. **Posture and movement** convey clues about mental state or possible disease process. A slumped posture coupled with slow movements suggests depression or possibly Parkinson's disease, whereas pacing suggests anxiety. **Facial expression** is assessed for appropriateness and variations in expression in relation to topics under discussion. In addition, observe for changes in the characteristics of the skin, features, or hair that are suggestive of other conditions such as hypothyroidism, Cushing's syndrome, or vitamin B_{12} deficiency. Finally, **affect and manner** provide a composite of the openness, approachability, and responsiveness of the patient to the environment and other people.

Mood and Emotional State

Ask the patient about his or her perception of his or her mood. Questions that are helpful include "How are your spirits?" "What makes you angry?" and "What makes you sad?" Reactions to the topic being discussed and to the people around should be noted. Abnormal responses might include hostility, evasiveness, anger, tearfulness, or depression. If depression is suspected, a standardized depression screening scale can be administered to further evaluate the patient. Of special concern is any suggestion related to suicide, which must be taken seriously. A direct inquiry can be made. One can ask "Have you ever thought about killing yourself?" or "Do you ever feel that life is not worth living?" Special observation, supervision, and further evaluation are warranted if suicidal tendencies are suspected. In addition, reports of family or friends can be very helpful in evaluating changes in mood.

Thinking Processes and Content of Thought

The overall characteristics of the thinking processes are evaluated both in response to questions and spontaneous conversation. **Thought processes** refer to the subjective responses to life experiences and how they are verbally expressed. Indicators of intact thought processes are clarity, cohesiveness, relevance, and logical progression and organization of thoughts. Table 6-1 lists disorders of thought processes. **Thought content** refers to themes in expression of ideas. By active listening, reflecting, and exploring the answers provided, the examiner can evaluate the presence of abnormal themes such as compulsive behaviors (i.e., compulsions, obsessions, phobias), anxieties, feelings of unreality, depersonalization, persecution or control by others, delusions, and perceptual deficits (i.e., illusions and hallucinations).

Perception is a person's subjective interpretation of real or perceived stimuli. Illusions and hallucinations are common abnormal perceptual findings. **Illusions** are the misinterpretation of real external stimuli. **Hallucinations** are a subjective sensory perception in the absence of real external stimuli and may be categorized as auditory, visual, olfactory, gustatory, tactile, or somatic. Evidence of illusions or hallucinations may indicate depression, mental illness, or organic disease necessitating further evaluation.

Throughout the interview note the characteristics of speech. **Speech** is the motor activity for the expression of language, and is controlled by the lower cranial nerves and their supranuclear connections. Listen to the **fluency** (i.e., rate, flow, melody of speech, content, use of words) of speech. Note the quality, volume, tone, articulation, inflections, and spontaneity of the speech. Slow monotone speech may be

TABLE 6-1   VARIATIONS/ABNORMALITIES IN THOUGHT PROCESSES

ABNORMALITY	DESCRIPTION OF SPEECH	OBSERVED IN
Circumstantiality	Delay in reaching the point because of unnecessary detail although the content of the descriptions is connected	Obsessive compulsive disorder and many people without mental illness
Derailment	Shift from one subject to another that is unrelated or marginally related without realizing that the subjects are not connected	Schizophrenia, manic episodes, and other psychiatric disorders
Flight of ideas	A continuous flow of accelerated speech with abrupt changes from topic to topic; ideas do not progress to sensible conversation	Manic episodes (common)
Neologisms	Invented or distorted words, or words with new and highly idiosyncratic meanings	Schizophrenia, other psychotic disorders, and aphasia
Incoherence	Largely incomprehensible because of illogic, disconnected, abrupt changes in topic or disordered grammar or word use	Severely disturbed patients with psychosis (e.g., schizophrenia)
Blocking	Sudden interruption in midsentence or before completion of an idea; person attributes this to losing the thought	Normal persons and patients with schizophrenia
Confabulation	Fabrication of facts or events in response to questions to fill in the gaps in an impaired memory	Patients with amnesia
Perseveration	Persistent repetition of words or ideas	Patients with schizophrenia and other psychosis
Echolalia	Repetition of the words and phrases of others	Manic episodes and schizophrenia
Clanging	Words chosen on the basis of sound rather than meaning, as in rhyming and punning speech	Schizophrenia and manic episodes

Adapted from Bickley, L. S. (1999). *Bates' guide to physical examination and history taking* (7th ed., p. 114). Philadelphia: Lippincott Williams & Wilkins.

suggestive of depression, whereas rapid and loud speech is common in manic states. Problems with *articulation* (i.e., clarity and distinctness of the spoken word) are associated with dysarthria. **Dysarthria** is a disorder of articulation in which basic language (i.e., grammar, comprehension, and word choice) is intact. The sounds produced are distorted and often nasal and are usually related to deficits in the throat muscles. An interruption of speech inflections and rhythm (i.e., speech melody) is called **dysprosody**. The resulting speech is monotone and halting.

Reception and Interpretation of Sensory Stimuli

The reception and interpretation of sensory stimuli, including awareness and responsiveness of self, the environment, and the impressions made by the senses, are referred to as *sensorium*. The areas included in the evaluation include **orientation; personal identification; attention and concentration;** and **comprehension**. These functions may be clouded by focal or diffuse cerebral conditions, such as a brain tumor, vascular and degenerative disease, or encephalitis.

Orientation

Orientation is the awareness of **time, place,** and **person** and is evaluated by direct questioning.

Time: the time of day, day of the week, month, season, date, and year, as well as any upcoming holiday or one in the immediate past may be asked. For some patients, however,

a more direct approach, using specific questions (e.g., "What day is it today?") is indicated.
Place: ask the patient to give the present location, such as "I am at Mercy Clinic in Detroit, Michigan"
Person: ability of the patient to give his or her own name

Personal Identification

In the context of evaluation, ask the patient's name, address, and background information such as date and place of birth, history of the illness, and specific dates of significant life events; this will provide insight into awareness of time, place, and person. This information should be corroborated using the medical record or verification by a family member.

Attention and Concentration

Attention is the ability to focus on a particular sensory stimulus while excluding others; **concentration** is sustained attention. In an acute confusional state, attention and concentration are severely impaired. By contrast, both are intact with focal lesions. Attention and concentration are tested in a number of ways, including number series, serial 7s, and spelling backwards.

Number Series. Read a series of digits to the patient and then ask him or her to repeat the numbers. The series should start with a short list, with each digit being enunciated clearly and paced at 1-second intervals. Number series can begin with two digits, then progress to a maximum of six digits (e.g., 7, 2; 9, 5, 2). Avoid consecutive numbers or digits that form easily recognizable combinations, such as the date 1776. If the patient makes an error in repeating the digits, provide a second chance with another series of digits of similar length. Stop after two consecutive failures in a series of any length. In the second part of this test (beginning with the shortest list of digits), the patient is asked to repeat a series in reverse order. Normally, a person should be able to repeat correctly five to seven digits forward and four in reverse order.

Serial 7s. Another common method is to ask the patient to start with 100 and subtract 7s. Normally, one should be able to complete this task with few errors in 90 seconds. In practice, if a patient can accurately complete five subtractions, this is usually sufficient. Patients unable to do serial 7s should be instructed to complete serial 3s in a similar manner.

Spelling Backwards. Say a five-letter word and ask the patient to spell it backward. The word commonly used is W-O-R-L-D.

Comprehension

Evidence of the level of comprehension and perception can be noted throughout the examination. **Comprehension** is the ability to grasp and to understand the meaning of visual, auditory, and other stimuli within the context of the total situation accurately. Comprehension, perception, attention, reasoning, and making decisions are complex processes; they contribute to other mental functions such as memory, judgment, general knowledge, and intelligence.

Higher-Level Cognitive Functions

Higher-level cognitive functions include several higher cognitive and integrative functions. In evaluating responses, consider what someone of comparable cultural and educational background would be expected to know. Testing of these higher-level intellectual abilities includes:

- Memory (immediate, short-term, long-term)
- Calculations
- General fund of information
- Abstract thinking, reasoning, and judgment
- Language and speech
- Constructional ability
- Motor integrative function

Memory

Memory is the ability to register, store, and retrieve information. **Registration**, the ability to receive information through the various senses, is closely related to attention. Without the ability to attend, information will not register. **Storage** is the process whereby selected new information is learned; it is mediated by the limbic structures, including the hippocampi, the mamillary bodies, and the dorsal medial nuclei of the thalami. After the sensory input has been received and registered, that information is held temporarily in short-term memory or working memory. Next, the information is stored in a more permanent form (long-term memory). Stored information is reinforced by repetition or by association with other information already in storage. **Retrieval**, the final step, is the ability to access previously learned information.

Memory can be subdivided into three general categories and includes immediate memory, short-term memory, and long-term memory. **Immediate memory**, also called *primary memory*, is the retrieval of information within seconds or minutes after presentation as in repeating a series of digits. **Short-term memory**, also referred to as *recent memory*, is the ability to remember current, day-to-day events such as the date, the name of the health provider, what was eaten for breakfast, or a recent news event. **Long-term memory**, also referred to as *remote memory*, refers to the recollection of personal and historic facts or events. The clinical significance between short-term memory and long-term memory is that short-term memory requires the *ongoing ability* to learn new information. See Table 6-2 for a comparison of memory types.

In testing immediate memory, give the patient three unrelated words to remember (e.g., lilies, courage, and screwdriver). Ask the patient to repeat each word after you. Then, ask the patient to tell you those three words; this tests immediate memory. Instruct the patient to remember those three words because you will be coming back to them in a few minutes. Go on with the examination. In 3 to 5 minutes, ask the patient to tell you what those three words were. Normally, the patient should be able to remember the three words; this is a test of short-term memory. In testing long-term memory, the following are suggestions for typical personal and historical information:

- Date/place of birth:
  When were you born?
  Where were you born?

TABLE 6–2   COMPARISON OF TYPES OF MEMORY

TYPES OF MEMORY	PRIMARY PURPOSE	ACCESSIBILITY/ CAPACITY	DURATION	ANATOMIC SITE	TESTING METHOD	CLINICAL PRESENTATION
Immediate (primary)	Register new information	• Rapid accessibility • Limited capacity	Seconds to minutes	Reticular activating system (RAS)	Immediately repeat a series of numbers	Lack of any memory
Recent (short term)	Retention and recall of information that has been previously registered	• Slow accessibility • Much larger capacity	Minutes to years	Limbic system	Repeat names of three objects after being distracted for 3–5 min	Inability to recall information previously registered
Remote (long term)	Permanently retain information	• Slower accessibility • Unlimited capacity	Years	Association cortex	Correctly recall important personal events of the past	Cannot recall highly significant past material

Adapted from Tasman, A., & First, M. B. (2004). *DSM-IV-TR mental disorders: Diagnosis, etiology, and treatment* (pp. 276–277). Hoboken, NJ: Wiley.

- School information:
  Where did you go to school?
  When did you attend school?
  Where is your school located?
- Vocational history:
  What do you do for work?
  Where do you work?
  How long have you worked there?
- Family history:
  What are your spouse's and children's names?
  How old are they?
  What was your mother's maiden name?

Memory can be affected by a number of focal and diffuse organic conditions as well as emotional states. **Amnesia** is defined as a defect in memory function and may be an isolated deficit or one component of global cognitive dysfunction. Amnesia is classified into specific categories as follows:

Retrograde amnesia: loss of memory for events that occurred *before* a brain insult
Antegrade or posttraumatic amnesia: loss of memory for events *after* a brain insult
Psychogenic amnesia: loss of memory for an emotionally charged event

Calculations

Serial 7s give some indication of subtraction ability. In addition, simple calculation problems should be asked such as:

How much is a quarter, a dime, and a nickel?
How much is 3×9?
How much is $11 + 7$?

General Fund of Information

To evaluate the patient's general knowledge, consider the patient's cultural and educational background. Ask about current events or general information that you would expect an average adult to know who lives in the area. Examples of questions are:

Who is the president of the United States?
Name the last five presidents from the current president back.
What is the capital of England?

Abstract Thinking, Reasoning, and Judgment

An appraisal of abstract thinking, reasoning, and judgment may begin while taking the history, but a closer evaluation is warranted.

Abstract Thinking. Abstract thinking is the ability to appreciate subtle relationships and meaning in events and between objects. This can be evaluated through the use of proverbs and similarities. Ask the patient what is meant by the following proverbs:

All that glitters is not gold.
Rome wasn't built in a day.

People who live in glass houses should not throw stones.
Rolling stones gather no moss.

A literal, concrete interpretation may indicate organic brain disease, mental illness, mental retardation, or simply limited education.

Similarities. In evaluating ability to recognize similarities, ask the patient to explain how two given objects are alike, such as:

A rose and a carnation
A piano and a violin
Silk and linen

Reasoning. The ability to use intellectual faculties to discover, formulate, or draw a conclusion is called **reasoning**. This can be evaluated by asking the patient to define or differentiate between combinations such as a mistake and a lie, or sadness and hopelessness.

Judgment. The process of forming an opinion or evaluation about something is called **judgment**. It often includes a component of **insight**, the act of seeing the inner nature of things or of seeing intuitively. The examiner can evaluate a patient's judgment and insight by asking questions such as "What seems to be the problem?" or "Why are you here today?" A person might say that he or she is here to be evaluated because of certain signs and symptoms. Conversely, a patient might say that there is nothing wrong, but his or her spouse insisted on the visit. The latter suggests a lack of insight due to denial, being unaware of the relationship of symptoms to illness, or parietal lobe syndrome. To appraise judgment, ask questions such as "How are you going to manage at home after hospitalization?" or "What activity limitations do you need to follow?" The examiner can determine how accurate and reasonable judgments are based on the patient's age and education.

Language and Speech

Language is the basic tool for human communication and often the medium for demonstrating most cognitive functions. Normally, a person can understand the spoken and written word and also express thoughts verbally and in writing. Disturbances of language and speech are divided into three areas:

1. Disorders of central language processing result in *aphasia*.
2. Disorders of motor programming of language symbols result in *apraxia of speech*.
3. Disorders of the motor mechanism of speech result in *dysarthria*.

Language and speech are evaluated throughout the patient–provider interaction. If there are deficits in the language system, it will be difficult, if not impossible, to test cognitive skills such as memory, proverb interpretation, or oral calculations. Word comprehension, repetition, naming, fluency, reading, and writing are all essential elements of the language system and all are tested (Table 6-3).

TABLE 6-3   TESTING OF LANGUAGE AND SPEECH

ELEMENT OF LANGUAGE	THE FOLLOWING ASSIST QUESTIONS IN DETERMINING ABILITY TO UNDERSTAND THE SPOKEN AND WRITTEN WORD AND TO EXPRESS THOUGHTS ORALLY AND IN WRITING
Fluency	Ask the patient to describe his or her work. Avoid questions that can be answered by "yes" or "no." Another approach is to show the patient a picture and ask what is happening in the picture. Listen to the flow of speech.
Word comprehension	Ask the patient to follow a one-step command such as "point to your hair." If this is successfully completed, give a two-step command such as "point to the door, then tap your knee." Then give a three-step command.
Repetition	Ask the patient to repeat simple words such as "cat"; if successful, increase the complexity to a word such as "moratorium." Finally, pose a more challenging phrase, such as repeat "no ifs, ands, or buts."
Naming	Ask the patient to name objects that you introduce. Include 10–20 objects from a variety of categories (colors; clothing and room objects; body parts; parts of an object). For example, point to the watch stem, watch crystal, shin, or coat lapel.
Reading comprehension	Ask the patient to read a few sentences from a newspaper or magazine. Write a message in large print on a paper such as "Close your eyes." Ask the patient to read the sign and follow the request.
Writing	Ask the patient to write a sentence from your dictation. Next, ask the patient to write a sentence about anything of his or her own choosing.

Aphasia is a language disorder due to a dominant hemisphere lesion that produces a defect in the expression or comprehension of any component of spoken language. Aphasia used to be subdivided into nonfluent (expressive) aphasia and fluent (receptive) aphasia, but is now classified on a functional basis. The main types of aphasias include **Broca's aphasia, Wernicke's aphasia,** global aphasia, conduction aphasia, anomic aphasia, transcortical aphasia, and verbal apraxias. See Table 6-4 and Table 6-5 for summarization of aphasias and Figure 6-1 for anatomic locations. Most patients have varying degrees of expressive and receptive language deficits, emphasizing the interrelatedness of cortical function.

Repetition is impaired in Broca's, Wernicke's, conduction, and global aphasias. However, when repetition is preserved in a patient with Broca's aphasia, it indicates transcortical motor aphasia and the lesion is anterior to Broca's area. Preservation of repetition in Wernicke's aphasia is termed transcortical sensory aphasia, and the lesion is posterior to Wernicke's area. Aphasia must be distinguished from other speech production disorders, including speech apraxia, mutism, and dysarthria. **Motor speech (verbal) apraxia** results from a focused lesion in Broca's areas (areas 44 and 45). It is characterized by a partial or complete inability to form the articulatory movements of the lips, tongue, and

TABLE 6-4   TYPES OF APHASIAS WITH ANATOMIC CORRELATIONS

TYPE	DESCRIPTION/CLINICAL CORRELATION	ANATOMIC AREA OR LESION
Broca's aphasia	Unable to convert thoughts into meaningful language Agrammatism (inability to organize words into sentences) Telegraphic speech (use of content words without connecting words) Distorted production of speech sounds Impaired repetition Normal reception of language is intact	Broca's area (frontal lobe areas 44 and 45), underlying white matter, or basal ganglia
Wernicke's aphasia	Fluent speech that is unintelligible because of pronunciation errors and use of jargon Impaired comprehension of verbal and written language, but no focal motor deficit Impaired repetition	Wernicke's area (superior temporal gyrus, area 22)
Conduction aphasia	Impaired repetition	Connections between Broca's and Wernicke's areas
Anomic aphasia	Impaired naming ability with preservation of other language functions	Lesion outside the language areas; possibly lower temporal lobe lesion or of generalized cerebral dysfunction
Transcortical aphasia	Impaired expression or reception of speech, but *repetition is spared*	Arterial border zones
Subcortical aphasia	Fluent, dysarthric speech and hemiparesis	Left caudate nucleus or the left thalamus
Global aphasia	Combined features of Wernicke's aphasia and Broca's aphasia Impaired comprehension and expression of speech Impaired repetition Commonly associated with a dense contralateral hemiplegia	Perisylvian or central regions; commonly seen with left middle cerebral artery infarction

Adapted from Benarroch, E. E., Westmoreland, B. F., Daube, J. R., Reagan, T. J., & Sandok, B. A. (1999). *Medical neurosciences: An approach to anatomy, pathology, and physiology by systems and levels* (4th ed., p. 567). Philadelphia: Lippincott Williams & Wilkins.

TABLE 6–5   CLASSIFICATION OF APHASIA: RELATIVE SEVERITIES

	FLUENCY	AUDITORY COMPREHENSION	REPETITION	NAMING	READING	WRITING
Broca's	−	+	−	−	−	−
Global	−	−	−	−	−	−
Wernicke's	+	−	−	−	−	−
Conduction	+	+	−	+/−	+	+
Anomic	+	+	+	−	+	−
Transcortical, mixed	−	−	+	−	−	−
Transcortical, motor	−	+	+	−	−	−
Transcortical, sensory	+	−	+	−	−	−
Verbal apraxia	−	+	−	−	−	+

+, function is relatively intact.
−, function is abnormal.
+/−, involvement is mild or impairment equivocal.
Modified from Campbell, W. W., & Pridgeon, R. P. (2002). *Practical primer of clinical neurology*. Philadelphia: Lippincott Williams & Wilkins.

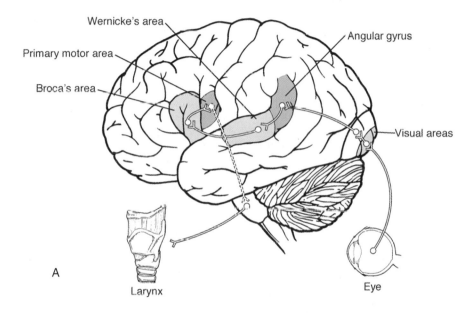

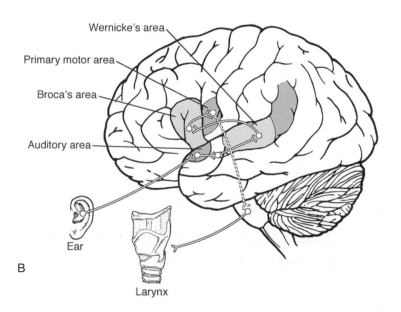

Figure 6-1 • Probable anatomic pathways involved in (*A*) reading a sentence and repeating it out loud and (*B*) hearing a question and answering it. Note that Wernicke's area is connected to Broca's area by a bundle of nerve fibers called the *arcuate fasciculus*.

lower jaw to produce individual sounds that constitute words. The patient knows what he or she wants to say but is unable to execute the motor aspects of speech.[2] **Mutism** is a lack of speech production caused by lesions of the prefrontal areas and cingulate gyrus. **Dysarthria** is the inability to articulate spoken words; it involves the motor component of speech but *not* a deficit with language. Clear speech involves coordinated and modulated activity of muscles supplied by cranial nerves (CNs) V, VII, IX, X, and XII as well as the respiratory muscles. Dysarthria occurs with disorders of the direct and indirect motor pathways, the motor control circuits, and the lower motor neuron system. This is discussed with the section on assessment of the CNs.

Constructional Ability

Construction ability, the ability to reproduce figures or draw a figure on command, can be assessed easily if the patient has motor function in his or her writing hand. This ability can be tested in a number of ways. One option is to draw two five-sided figures that overlap to form a four-sided figure, and then ask the patient to copy it. Another option is to ask the patient to draw a clock with all the numbers and to set the clock at a given time. A variation for this drawing is a daisy with petals equally arranged around the center. Abnormalities of visuospatial function and construct abilities are seen in right, but also in left or bilateral, parietal-occipital lesions. Patients with a nondominant parietal lesion may have a hemi-spatial neglect syndrome resulting in nothing being drawn on one half of the clock or flower (Fig. 6-2 shows sample drawings).

Motor Integrative Function: Apraxia

Performing a skilled act on demand requires integrated functions of several areas of the cerebral cortex. Three steps are necessary to execute a purposeful, skilled act successfully, as detailed in Table 6-6. To perform a skilled motor act, a person must understand what the act entails, remember the steps long enough to complete the act, and possess normal motor strength. If a patient is unable to perform a learned skilled motor act (in response to a verbal command) in the absence of paralysis, comprehension deficit, uncooperative behavior, or other obvious reasons, the term **apraxia** is applied. Ask the patient to pantomime activities for you such as brushing the teeth, combing the hair, blowing out a match, and expressing surprise.

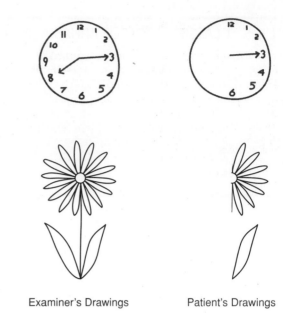

Examiner's Drawings   Patient's Drawings

Figure 6-2 • Examples of impaired performance on a test for copying given to a patient with unilateral neglect.

CLINICAL PEARLS: A decrease in the level of alertness occurs *only* if there is dysfunction of both cerebral hemispheres or the brainstem. There is no one-to-one correlation between a mental status exam task and a single cognitive function; mental tasks are complex and require a number of cerebral areas and cognitive functions. None of the focal deficits in the mental status exam has any *localizing* significance.

CRANIAL NERVE EXAMINATION

The next part of the neurological examination focuses on the central nervous system. There are 12 pairs of CNs. Each CN has a left and a right nerve; each side must therefore be evaluated separately. There may be dysfunction on one side only or on both sides. Findings from each side are compared for symmetry. This chapter is organized to include details of testing, discussion of findings, and abnormal findings. See Chapter 4 for a review of the anatomy and physiology of cranial nerves.

TABLE 6-6   PURPOSEFUL MOTOR ACTS AND APRAXIA

STEPS	ACTIVITY	DEFICITS	APRAXIA TYPE
1	Comprehend concept or idea Remember long enough to accomplish the act	General suppression of cerebral function, rather than a lesion in one specific area	Ideational apraxia
2	Formulate an organized plan to accomplish the task	Lesion at the junction of the frontal, temporal, parietal, and occipital lobes	Ideokinetic or ideomotor apraxia
3	Create a mental image of the action Actually execute the detailed plan	Lesion involving premotor frontal cortex The disability is usually limited to one extremity without weakness or loss of movement	Kinetic apraxia

Olfactory Nerve (Sensory) (CN I)

Testing of the olfactory nerve is often deferred unless the patient reports deficits or there is reason to believe that this function is compromised. If indicated, the sense of smell is tested by obstructing one nostril while testing the other. A piece of cotton that has been saturated with a common, odoriferous, nonirritating substance is placed under the unobstructed nostril. Cinnamon, cloves, coffee, or peppermint are possible odors that patients should be able to identify if CN I is intact.

Abnormalities

Anosmia is an inability to smell. It is an early sign in the diagnosis and localization of frontal lobe tumors. There are several causes of anosmia, some of which are attributable to neuropathologic conditions such as meningiomas of the sphenoid ridge and olfactory groove, gliomas of the frontal lobe, and parasellar lesions with pressure on the olfactory bulbs or tracts. Common non-neurological causes of anosmia include the common cold, sinusitis, or inflammation of the nasal cavity. The typical syndrome with *sphenoidal ridge meningioma* is one of unilateral optic atrophy or papilledema, exophthalmos, and ipsilateral anosmia. A *meningioma of the olfactory groove or cribriform plate area* includes unilateral anosmia progressing to bilateral anosmia, often accompanied by unilateral ipsilateral optic atrophy, and contralateral papilledema.[3]

Optic Nerve (Sensory) (CN II)

The optic nerve is the only CN that can be examined directly. Testing encompasses an evaluation of visual acuity and visual fields and an ophthalmoscopic examination. Each eye is evaluated individually while the other eye is covered.

Visual Acuity

Visual acuity can be evaluated informally by asking the patient to read from printed material, such as a newspaper. A standard Snellen chart is available in office or clinic settings for formal testing. Each eye is checked individually. From a distance of 20 feet, the patient is asked to read the line on the chart with the smallest letters that he or she is able to read. The number beside each line of letters signifies the number of feet at which letters can be read by a person with normal vision. This becomes the denominator in recording vision. Normal vision is 20/20. When vision is defective, the patient may only be able to see the larger letters at 20 feet. For example, persons with 20/40 vision are able to see at 20 feet what those with normal vision can see at 40 feet.

An adaptation of the Snellen chart, the Rosenbaum Pocket Vision Screener, is designed for quick bedside use. The chart is held at a distance of 14 inches from the patient. Normal vision in this instance is 14/14. The ratio is calculated in the same manner as for the Snellen test.

Visual Fields

A **visual field** is the area of vision normally seen with one eye. Each visual field extends 60 degrees on the nasal side, 100 degrees on the temporal side, and 135 degrees vertically (60 degrees superiorly and 75 degrees). Figure 6-3 displays normal visual fields. The **confrontation test** provides a rough estimate of the scope of each visual field. This is a test in which the examiner "confronts" the patient by sitting 2 feet in front of him or her at eye level. The patient is asked to

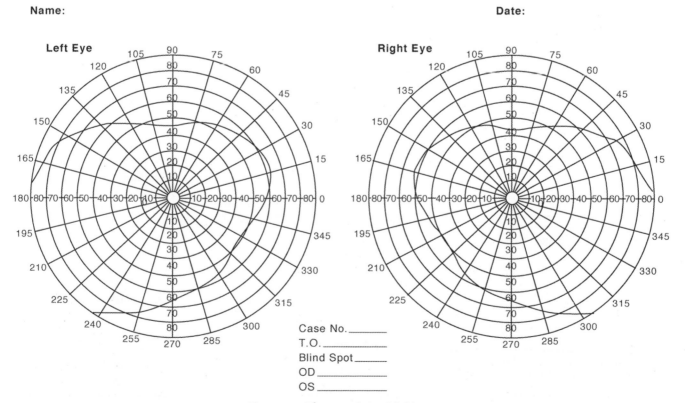

Figure 6-3 • The normal visual fields.

cover one eye lightly and looks at the examiner's eye directly opposite (i.e., the patient's left eye will be looking at the examiner's right eye). The examiner then closes one eye, the one the visual field of which is *not* being currently used, thus isolating the visual field in the other eye and superimposing it on that of the patient's visual field. A pencil or a moving finger is then introduced from the periphery into the patient's field of vision; each quadrant (upper and lower) is checked individually. The patient is asked to indicate when the object is first seen. The examiner uses his or her own visual field as the norm for comparison to the patient's visual field.

The confrontation test is designed to reveal only gross defects of the visual fields. If any defects are found, the visual fields should be plotted by an ophthalmologist using the standard and more sensitive **perimetric test** or a **tangent screen**. Visual field testing can reveal field cuts related to characteristic deficits along the visual pathway (i.e., optic nerve, optic tract, lateral geniculate body, geniculocalcarine tract, or occipital lobe). Chart 6-1 shows specific field cuts; Figure 6-4 shows field cuts in a person with right homonymous hemianopia.

With bilateral occipital or occipitoparietal infarctions, there may be cortical blindness resulting in complete loss of vision often with denial or unawareness of the deficit. Cortical blindness is referred to as **Anton's syndrome**. Because the pupils still react to light, cortical blindness may be difficult to differentiate from hysterical blindness.

CHART **6-1**   Visual Field Defects Produced by Selected Lesions in the Visual Pathways

VISUAL PATHWAYS	VISUAL FIELDS	BLACKENED FIELD INDICATES AREA OF NO VISION

VISUAL PATHWAYS

Left visual field   Right visual field

Temporal — Nasal — Temporal

Left eye   Right eye

Optic nerve — 1
Optic tract — 2   3

Optic radiation — 5   4

VISUAL FIELDS

BLIND RIGHT EYE (RIGHT OPTIC NERVE)

A lesion of the optic nerve and, of course, of the eye itself, produces unilateral blindness.

BITEMPORAL HEMIANOPIA (OPTIC CHIASM)

A lesion at the optic chiasm may involve only those fibers that cross over to the opposite side. Because these fibers originate in the nasal half of each retina, visual loss involves the temporal half of each field.

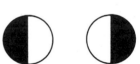

LEFT HOMONYMOUS HEMIANOPIA (RIGHT OPTIC TRACT)

A lesion of the optic tract interrupts fibers originating on the same side of both eyes. Visual loss in the eyes is therefore similar (homonymous) and involves half of each field (hemianopia).

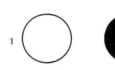

LEFT HOMONYMOUS QUADRANTIC DEFECT (OPTIC RADIATION, PARTIAL)

A partial lesion of the optic radiation may involve only a portion of the nerve fibers, producing, for example, a homonymous quadrantic defect.

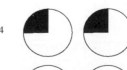
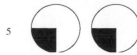

Name:

Date:

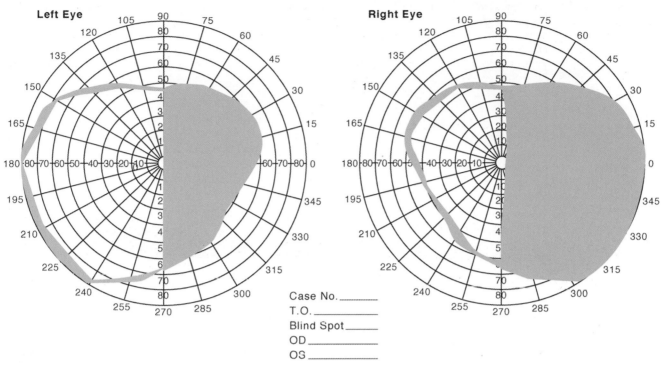

Left Eye

Right Eye

Case No. _____
T.O. _____
Blind Spot _____
OD _____
OS _____

Figure 6-4 • Right homonymous hemianopia in a patient with a neoplasm of the left occipital lobe.

Ophthalmoscopic Examination

The **ophthalmoscopic examination** is conducted with an ophthalmoscope, which contains a special lens that is used to visualize the retina by shining a beam of white light directly into the eye. The room is darkened and the examiner sits directly opposite the subject. To examine the patient's right eye, the examiner holds the ophthalmoscope in the right hand and looks through the instrument with the right eye while the patient focuses on an object straight ahead (Fig. 6-5). Shine the beam of light on the pupil and look for the red reflex—an orange glow reflected from the retina. Move closer toward the pupil, staying focused on the red reflex. The termination of the optic nerve, visible as a prominent, tube-like structure at the back of the eyeball and slightly to the nasal side of center, is called the **optic disc**. Bring the optic disc (fundus) into focus by adjusting the ophthalmoscope lens (Fig. 6-6). The normal disc is round or slightly oval with sharply defined margins. The outer portion of the disc is elevated slightly above the center, or physiologic cup. Another area of the retina is the **macula lutea**, which has the highest density of visual receptors. The center of the macula, called the **fovea**, represents the point of greatest visual acuity.

Four main pairs of blood vessels exit and enter the optic disc; they are followed peripherally in all directions to compare the diameters of the arteries and veins and to determine whether the veins are tortuous. Normally, the **diameter of the veins** is about 30% greater than the diameter of arteries in a ratio varying from 2:3 to 4:5. Retinal venous pulsation is seen in 80% of normal people. The presence of retinal venous

pulsation indicates normal intracranial pressure; the absence may be normal or reflect raised intracranial pressure. As the retina is examined, any abnormalities, such as hemorrhage, swelling, and exudate, should be noted. Table 6-7 summarizes common ophthalmological findings.

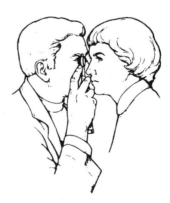

Figure 6-5 • Technique for the proper use of the ophthalmoscope. Turn on the ophthalmoscope light and adjust the output to the small round beam of white light. Use your index finger to adjust the lens for proper focus; begin by adjusting the lens to zero diopters. *Red lens numbers* indicate *minus* diopters (turn the lens control counterclockwise) and are used with a **myopic** (nearsighted) patient. *Black lens numbers* indicate *plus* diopters (turn the lens control clockwise) and are used for a **hyperopic** (farsighted) patient or for one who has undergone surgical lens removal. Instruct the patient to look straight ahead. Hold the ophthalmoscope with your **right** hand and use your **right** eye to look into the patient's **right** eye. Hold the thumb of the opposite hand on the patient's eyebrow above the eye that you are examining.

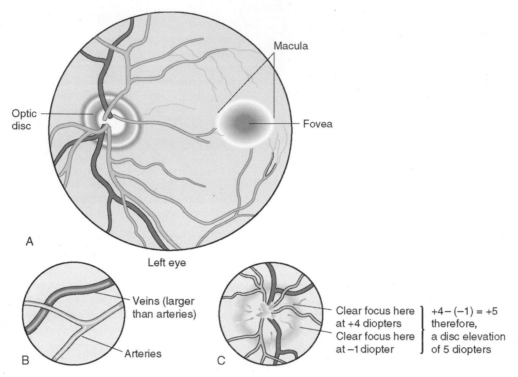

Figure 6-6 • The retina as seen through the ophthalmoscope. The ophthalmoscope is capable of visualizing *only a portion of the retina* at any one time. In examining the retina (*A*) identify the optic disc; ascertain the sharpness of the disc margins; identify the macula and fovea (bright reflection in the center); (*B*) compare the diameters of the veins to the arteries; follow the vessels in each quadrant from the disc to the periphery; and note any exudate, hemorrhagic areas, or abnormalities present. **Measurements within the eye.** Lesions are recorded in relationship to the optic disc as **disc diameters.** For example, in A, the macula is about 2 disc diameters from the disc. (*C*) For an elevated optic disc due to papilledema, note the **differences in diopters** measurement of the two lenses used to focus clearly on the disc and on the uninvolved retina.

Oculomotor (CN III), Trochlear (CN IV), and Abducens (CN VI) Nerves (All Motor)

Cranial nerves III, IV, and VI are tested together because all three supply the extraocular eye muscles (Fig. 6-7). In addition, the oculomotor nerve controls the levator palpebrae superioris muscle, which raises the upper eyelid, and the parasympathetic innervation to the pupil (which causes constriction of the pupil).

Injury to an extraocular muscle compromises the corresponding extraocular movement (EOM). Injury to the oculomotor nerve can result in an inability to focus the eyes medially on the horizontal plane, upward and outward, downward and outward, and upward and inward. The trochlear nerve allows you to look at the tip of your nose. A damaged trochlear nerve results in compromised downward and inward movement of the eye, whereas injury to the abducens nerve causes loss of lateral ocular movement on

TABLE 6–7   COMMON ABNORMAL OPTIC DISC FINDINGS

TYPE	DESCRIPTION	CAUSES
Papilledema (choked disc)	Margins of the disc are distorted and swollen; the disc has a reddish hue because of congestion; patient has normal vision	Increased intracranial pressure; pseudotumor cerebri
Papillitis	Margins of the disc are distorted and swollen; patient has severe visual loss; resembles early papilledema	Vascular, toxic, demyelinating, or inflammatory optic neuritis
Optic atrophy	Paleness (the disc is light pink, white, or gray owing to decreased blood supply); visual acuity is decreased	Primary cause: multiple sclerosis Secondary causes: neuritis or prolonged increased intracranial pressure
Retrobulbar neuritis	Inflammatory lesion of the posterior portion of the optic nerve; no swelling of disc; loss of vision	Hemorrhage, diabetes, or retinitis
Optic neuritis	Inflammation of the disc; associated with loss of vision secondary to a central scotoma	Inflammatory process
Cotton wool patches (seen during fundus examination)	Whitish or grayish oval lesions that look like cotton balls; smaller than disc	Hypertension

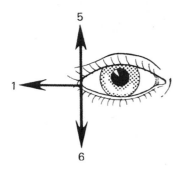
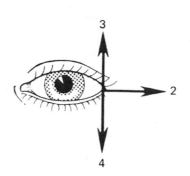

Figure 6-7 • Sequence of eye-testing movements. (*Note:* Numbers indicate the appropriate sequence of movement.)

the horizontal plane. Trochlear nerve dysfunction is rare. The abducens nerve has the longest intracranial course and is frequently involved with neurological disease.

Observations Related to the Eye and Eye Movement

In assessing CNs III, IV, and VI, begin with focused observations on the position of each orbit, upper eyelid, and pupil. Next, examine EOMs for gaze palsy, internuclear ophthalmoplegia, diplopia, and nystagmus. **Gaze** is the act of focusing in a particular direction. It includes coordinated eye and head movements and is the result of complex reflexes of the visual and vestibular systems and the cerebral cortex. Terms related to the eyes are defined in a later section.

Position of Eyes, Eyelids, and Pupils.

The **position of the eyes** is noted by looking at the position of the eyeball from frontal and lateral views, as well as by looking down from above the patient's head. Abnormal protrusion of one or both eyeballs is termed **proptosis** or **exophthalmos**. Abnormal recession of an eyeball within the orbit is termed **enophthalmos**. In assessing the **upper eyelid**, the patient is asked to look straight ahead. The width of the palpebral fissure in each eye is noted and a comparison is made. The **palpebral fissure** is the space between the upper and lower eyelids. One lid may droop compared with the other. The term for a drooping upper eyelid is **ptosis**. Note also edema of the eyelid, if present. Edema can result from trauma to the eye or orbit and may occur in the upper eyelid, the lower eyelid, or both. Next, the position of the eyelids in relation to the pupil and

the iris in each eye is noted and compared. This also helps the examiner to note a slight ptosis.

EOM Evaluation. The six EOM muscles are evaluated next. Ask the patient to follow the examiner's finger or a pencil through the six cardinal directions of gaze in an "H" sequencing (see Fig. 6-7). Observe for full, symmetric movement of both eyes. **Conjugate eye movement** refers to both eyes moving in the same direction, at the same speed, and in constant alignment. By contrast, **dysconjugate gaze** is the lack of alignment between the two visual axes. Table 6-8 summarizes other eye movement abnormalities. Reflex eye movement in the unconscious patient can be tested. The **oculocephalic reflex** (doll's eye response) and the **oculovestibular reflex** (caloric stimulation) are used in the unconscious patient and provide information about the presence or absence of brainstem reflexes. Both are discussed later in this chapter.

Other Ocular Signs. *Diplopia.* The term **diplopia** is used to describe double vision or seeing two separate images of the same object in visual space. With normal vision, the visual images fall on the same point of each retina when the eyes move. By contrast, diplopia results when the visual images fall on each retina at *different* points, rather than on the same points. The lack of parallelism can cause double vision, and it can be confined to focusing in a particular direction. The patient is asked whether or not he or she is seeing double. If the answer is yes, is the double image side by side or one on top of the other? If the images are side by side, the examiner

TABLE 6–8   EYE MOVEMENT ABNORMALITIES WITH POSTERIOR FOSSA LESIONS

ABNORMALITY	DESCRIPTION	CAUSE/LESION
Wall-eyed bilateral internuclear ophthalmoplegia (INO)	Bilateral outward eye deviation that occurs with bilateral INO	Pentine infarction or demyelination
"One-and-a-half" syndrome	Impairment of all horizontal conjugate eye movements, except for abduction of the contralateral eye	Parapontine reticular formation (PPRF)
Ocular bobbing	Episodic, intermittent, usually conjugate, downward, brisk eye movement followed by a return to the resting position by a "bobbing action"	Severe destructive lower pontine lesions, pontine hemorrhage, or infection
Skewed deviation	Misalignment of the eyes observed in the vertical plane that is not due to a lesion of the third or fourth cranial nerve. Vertical diplopia results	Pons, usually on side of the higher eye, but may be in the cerebellum
Parinaud's syndrome	Paralysis of conjugate upward gaze; also includes paresis of convergence, convergence-retraction nystagmus, pupillary hyporeactivity, and light-near dissociation	Midbrain tectal area; often caused by a pinealoma, a vascular lesion, or hydrocephalus

needs to determine whether a dysfunction in CN III (oculo-motor) or VI (abducens) is the cause. Instruct the patient to follow your finger to the left and right on the horizontal plane. Is the diplopia worse when the patient focuses to the left or the right? The deficit is on the side where the diplopia is worse. If the images are one on top of the other, the examiner needs to determine if a dysfunction in CN III or IV (abducens) is the cause. Instruct the patient to follow your finger up and down both on the inward (inner aspect of the eye) and outward (outer aspect of the eye) on the vertical plane. Is the diplopia worse when the patient looks up or down? The deficit is in the direction that diplopia is most severe. Note that trochlear nerve involvement is uncommon. Diplopia is usually preceded by blurring of vision.

Gaze Disorders. If the eyes move conjugately but have limited movement in one direction, it is called **gaze palsy**. The underlying problem is due to a malfunction of either the frontal gaze center, brainstem gaze center, or connecting pathways between the two. If the brainstem gaze center is affected, the neurons of the center cannot be activated by voluntary reflex. This is called **nuclear gaze palsy**. A lesion of the cortical gaze center affects voluntary gaze only and reflexes can activate the brainstem gaze center; this is called **supranuclear gaze palsy**.

Ophthalmoplegia. Ophthalmoplegia is defined as paralysis of the eye muscles (see Table 6-9). For example, **internuclear ophthalmoplegia (INO)** is due to a lesion of the medial longitudinal fasciculus resulting in impairment of adduction in the ipsilateral eye and nystagmus in the contralateral eye on gaze away from the side of involvement. The lesion lies between the nuclei of CN VI and opposite CN III. Convergence is intact, thus ruling out a lesion of CN III. There is no diplopia. The most common cause in the elderly is brainstem infarction and in younger people it is multiple sclerosis. Other causes include trauma and neoplasms. Occasionally

TABLE 6–9   TYPES OF OPHTHALMOPLEGIAS

TYPE OF OPHTHALMOPLEGIA	DESCRIPTION
External	Paralysis of one or more of the extraocular muscles
Internal	Paralysis of one or more intraocular muscles
Nuclear	Paralysis caused by a lesion involving the nuclei of the motor nerves of the eye (cranial nerve III, IV, or VI)
Internuclear	Paralysis caused by injury or a lesion of the medial longitudinal fasciculus located within the brainstem
Supranuclear	Paralysis caused by injury or a lesion to the conjugate eye movement centers located in the frontal, frontal-parietal, and occipital lobes
Parinaud's syndrome or dorsal midbrain syndrome	A type of supranuclear ophthalmoplegia; conjugate upward gaze paralysis; caused by a lesion in the dorsal mid-brain

INO is associated with metabolic disorders such as hepatic encephalopathy, and may also be seen in myasthenia gravis.

Nystagmus. Nystagmus is a common, involuntary drift of the eye with a fast correction in the opposite direction. Nystagmus is described by the direction of the fast component. The movement may be rhythmic to-and-fro oscillation of the eyes that may be horizontal, vertical, rotary, or mixed in direction. The tempo of the movements can be regular, rhythmic, pendular, or jerky, with a noted fast and slow movement component. True nystagmus is a pathologic condition caused by a lesion in the central or peripheral vestibular pathways or their cerebellar connections as well as toxic-metabolic disorders, weakness of gaze, and blindness (Table 6-10).

TABLE 6–10   COMMON TYPES OF NYSTAGMUS

TYPE OF NYSTAGMUS	DESCRIPTION	LOCATION OF LESION	COMMENT
Gaze-evoked nystagmus	With normal eye movement, there may be three or fewer beats at the extremes of eye position; fast phase in direction of gaze	–	Normal finding
Optokinetic nystagmus	Rapid, alternating motion of the eyes normally noted when eyes try to fixate on a moving target; presence indicates physiologic continuity of the optic pathways from the retina to the occipital cortex. Because it is involuntary, a positive response provides reliable verification of intact vision in a patient feigning blindness	–	Normal finding
Retraction nystagmus	Irregular jerks of the eyes backward into the orbit, precipitated by upward gaze	Midbrain tegmentum	–
Convergence nystagmus	Slow, spontaneous, drifting, ocular divergence with a final quick, convergent jerk	Midbrain	–
See-saw nystagmus	Rapid, pendular, dysconjugate see-saw movement accompanied by deficits of visual fields and visual acuity	Proximal optic chiasm	–
Downbeat nystagmus	Irregular jerks precipitated by downward gaze	Lower medulla	–
Vestibular nystagmus	Mixed nystagmus that can be horizontal, rotational, or both, resulting from vestibular disease	Vestibular pathway	–
Toxic nystagmus	Multidirectional gaze-evoked nystagmus; most often drug induced with toxic levels of phenytoin (Dilantin), barbiturates, and bromides; can also result from cerebellar or central vestibular dysfunction	–	Usually due to drug toxicity

Other Findings

Trauma to the peripheral portion of the CN can result in nerve fiber degeneration, followed by unpredictable regeneration. Because of the proximity of other CNs to each other, the regenerating fibers from one nerve can be misdirected to a nearby cranial nerve, forming connections with adjacent nerves. Such an atypical regeneration is called a **misdirection syndrome**. Two are mentioned—the pseudo-Graefe lid sign and Gunn's syndrome. The **pseudo-Graefe syndrome** is an atypical connection between CNs III and IV. Any attempt to look downward is followed by upper eyelid retraction, medial rotation of the eye, and constriction of the pupil. **Gunn's syndrome** involves CNs III and V. As the mouth is opened and the jaw moves to one side, ptosis of the eyelid changes to lid retraction.

Examination of the Pupils

To assess the pupils, the patient should be directed to focus on a distant object located straight ahead. (With a comatose patient, the pupils are examined however they are found.) The pupils are examined for size, shape, and equality. The normal diameter of a pupil is 2 to 6 mm, with an average diameter of 3.5 mm. When the pupils are compared with each other, their diameters should be equal; however, about 12% to 17% of the normal population has discernibly unequal pupil size (**anisocoria**) in the absence of a pathologic condition.

The shape of the pupils is also noted and compared. Normally, the pupils are round; however, in patients who have had cataract surgery, the pupils assume a keyhole shape. An ovoid pupil indicates pupillary dysfunction; it may be seen in early uncal herniation.

Sensitivity to light or **photophobia** may be noted when checking the pupils, or the patient may complain of this problem. The etiology is unclear, but the finding is associated with conditions such as meningitis.

Pupillary Reflexes

A few important reflexes relating to pupillary responses and eye movement can be tested.

Direct Light Reflex. The sensory receptors for the light reflex are the rods and cones of the retina. Afferent impulses follow the normal visual pathway as far as the lateral geniculate bodies. Rather than entering the geniculate body, sensory impulses enter the pretectal area (near the superior colliculus). Connecting neurons synapse in the **Edinger-Westphal nucleus** (oculomotor nucleus) located in the midbrain. From here, the parasympathetic fibers proceed to the ciliary ganglion to the pupilloconstrictor fibers of the iris, causing the pupil to constrict. When the light is withdrawn, the pupil normally dilates because of sympathetic stimulation. A three-neuron chain begins in the posterior hypothalamus. The first neuron descends dorsally in the brainstem and cervical spinal cord to synapse in the **intermediolateral cells** at the C7 to C12 levels. The second neuron leaves the nervous system through the ventral spinal roots and ascends in the sympathetic chain and synapses in the superior cervical ganglion (at level of carotid bifurcation). The third neuron reaches the iris and Müller's muscles by ascending along the internal carotid artery, then traverses the cavernous sinus and the ciliary ganglion as the long ciliary nerves. The post-

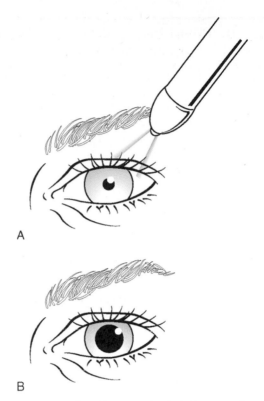

Figure 6-8 • Direct light reflex. (*A*) A bright light is introduced from the temporal area; the pupil normally rapidly constricts when exposed to the light. (*B*) The pupil rapidly dilates when the light is removed.

ganglionic sympathetic fibers synapse with the pupillodilator muscles, resulting in pupillary dilation.

The direct light reflex refers to the constriction and dilation of the pupil when a light is shone into that pupil and withdrawn (Fig. 6-8). Each pupil is tested individually and the results are compared. Response to light is recorded as:

- **Brisk:** very rapid constriction when light is introduced
- **Sluggish:** constriction occurs but more slowly than expected
- **Nonreactive or fixed:** no constriction or dilation is noted

Normally, pupillary constriction is brisk, although age may affect the briskness of reaction. Pupils in younger people tend to be larger and more responsive to light than those in older people. In addition to the constriction of the pupil that occurs with direct light stimulation (direct light response), there is a somewhat weaker constriction of the nonstimulated pupil. This is called the **consensual light reflex**, which occurs as a result of fibers crossing from each side that cross both the optic chiasm and the posterior commissure of the midbrain. See Table 6-11 for pupillary abnormalities.

Near-Point Reaction. In testing the near-point reaction, patients are asked to focus on the examiner's finger, which is positioned 2 to 3 feet directly ahead of them, and to follow it with their eyes as it is rapidly moved closer to their face. Three reflex responses normally occur:

- **Convergence:** the medial recti muscles contract, thus directing both eyes toward the midline. This occurs so that

TABLE 6–11 PUPILLARY ABNORMALITIES CLASSIFIED BY AFFERENT AND EFFERENT PUPILLARY DEFECTS

DEFECTS	DESCRIPTION	CAUSE/COMMENT
Afferent Defects		
Amaurotic pupil (blind eye)	Blindness in one eye results in loss of the sensory limb of the light reflex. If oculomotor nerve (the motor limb) of reflex remains intact, a light directed into the **intact eye** produces normal direct and consensual reactions. In the **blind eye,** you will find • No direct light response • No consensual response • A direct light response in the intact eye • A consensual response in the blind eye (from light shone into the intact eye) • A near pupillary response in both eyes	Disease of the retina or optic nerve
Marcus-Gunn pupil (swinging flashlight sign)	Use a bright light. There is a normal bilateral light response (constriction) when the light is shone into the intact eye, but pupillary dilation occurs when the flashlight is quickly switched to the diseased eye.	Lesions/atrophy of the retina or optic nerve
Argyll-Robertson pupil	Pupils are small and irregularly shaped; they react to accommodation but not to direct light.	Seen with neurosyphilis (tabes dorsalis)
Efferent Defect: Large Pupil		
Adie pupil (tonic pupil)	Unilateral dilated pupil that reacts slowly to light after prolonged stimulation; it accommodates slowly. The pupil also dilates slowly in darkness. Often associated with diminished knee and ankle reflexes Usually women 20 to 30 yr old who are affected Diagnosed by inserting 2.5% methacholine or 0.1% pilocarpine into both eyes; the affected pupil promptly contracts, but the normal pupil does not.	Postganglionic denervation of the parasympathetic pupillary innervation Cause unknown, although noted to occur following a viral infection
Mydriatic pupils (large pupils)	Enlarged pupils that result from use of certain drugs, listed in next column; unilateral large pupil in accidental topical ocular application of anticholinergic agents Large pupil can result from direct trauma	Hallucinogens, antihistamines, glutethiamide, anticholinergics, and dopamine Trauma can damage nerve endings of iris sphincter muscle
Efferent Defect: Small Pupil		
Horner's syndrome	Unilateral, small pupil; both pupils react to direct light and accommodation; with a miotic pupil, there is ptosis of the eyelid, and usually loss of sweating on the affected side.	Lesion of descending sympathetic fibers in ipsilateral brainstem or upper cord, or the ascending sympathetic fibers in neck or head; results in unilateral interruption or complete loss of sympathetic innervation to the pupil
Miotic pupils (small pupils)	Small pupils that result from use of certain drugs, listed in next column Also seen in pontine hemorrhage or pontine infarct Direct orbital injury to the eye with destruction of the sympathetic innervation and interruption of the inhibitory pathways to the oculomotor nuclei (Edinger-Westphal nucleus) Miosis following trauma usually results from intraocular inflammation	Miotic drugs (acetylcholine chloride, carbachol, demecarium bromide, echothiophate iodide, isoflurophate, physostigmine, pilocarpine, and others); and narcotics

the image in each eye will remain focused on the fovea; without this reflex, diplopia would occur.

- **Accommodation:** to sharply focus the image on the fovea, the lenses thicken as a result of tension in the ciliary muscles; the ciliary muscles are innervated by the postganglionic parasympathetic neurons in the ciliary ganglion.
- **Pupillary constriction:** the pupils constrict as an optic adjustment to regulate depth of focus. (This pupillary con-

striction does not depend on light and is regulated separately from the light reflex.)

Trigeminal Nerve (Mixed) (CN V)

The trigeminal nerve is composed of both sensory and motor components. To assess the sensory component, the three sensory vectors of the face are tested (Fig. 6-9). The **ophthalmic**

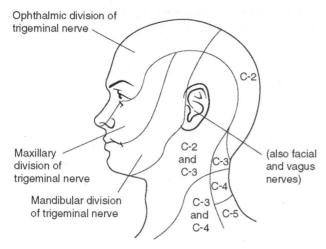

Figure 6-9 • Sensory vectors of the face and neck. Note the three vectors of the trigeminal nerve (CN V): ophthalmic, maxillary, and mandibular divisions.

division innervates the frontal sinuses, the conjunctiva and cornea, the upper lid, the bridge of the nose, the forehead, and the scalp as far as the vertex of the skull. The **maxillary division** innervates the cheek, the maxillary sinus, the lateral aspects of the nose, the upper teeth, the nasal pharynx, the hard palate, and the uvula. The **mandibular division** innervates the chin, the lower jaw, the anterior two thirds of the tongue, the gums and floor of the mouth, and the buccal mucosa of the cheek.

With the patient's eyes closed, ability to appreciate **light touch** is tested by touching the forehead, cheek, and jaw with a wisp of cotton. The patient is instructed to respond every time the skin is touched. **Pain perception** is evaluated with the "picky" (broken) and dull ends of a wooden applicator or by the pinprick method. After demonstrating the difference between sharp and dull, the skin is touched with the sharp end and occasionally with the dull end. The patient is asked to respond "sharp" or "dull." Accuracy of response is noted and a comparison between findings on each side of the face is made.

Next, the motor component (i.e., the muscles of mastication) is evaluated. The strength of the masseter and temporal muscles is evaluated by palpating them when the jaw is clenched and opened. Differences in muscle tone or atrophy should be noted.

Facial Nerve (Mixed) (CN VII)

The facial nerve has both sensory and motor components. The sensory component includes the sense of taste on the anterior two thirds of the tongue. Testing of this function is often deferred. However, if tested, each side of the protruded tongue is tested separately. There are four basic modalities of taste: sweet (tip of tongue), sour (sides of tongue), salty (over most of tongue but concentrated on the sides), and bitter (back of tongue, controlled by CN IX). The patient is asked to identify the taste of sugar placed on the tip of the tongue, after which a sip of water is given. The same procedure is used with sour and salty substances. If bitter is tested on the posterior third of the tongue, it should be recognized that it is innervated by the glossopharyngeal nerve. Sensation to the external ear is also supplied by the facial nerve.

The motor component is tested by observing the symmetry of the face at rest and during deliberate facial movements,

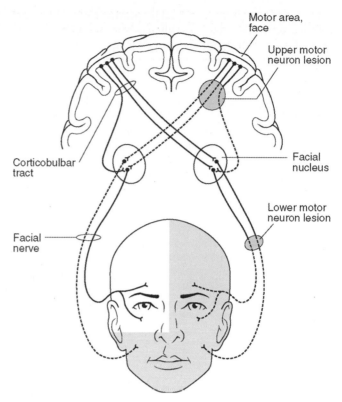

Figure 6-10 • Innervation to the face by the facial nerve.

such as smiling, showing the teeth, whistling, pursing the lips, blowing air into the cheeks, wrinkling the nose and forehead, and raising the eyebrows. Note the nasolabial folds for symmetry. In addition, ask the patient to close the eyes tightly. The examiner should not be able to open the patient's eyes. The facial nerve also controls tearing and salivation.

When weakness is noted, it is important to observe whether the entire side of the face or just the lower face (below the eyes) is affected.

There are two types of facial weakness (Fig. 6-10). If the lower portion of one side of the face is involved, the lesion is said to be caused by a central (involves the central nervous system) problem, an **upper motor neuron lesion** (as seen in association with stroke). This involves the corticobulbar tracts, resulting in contralateral weakness of the *lower face* with normal function of the upper face. Wrinkling of the forehead is left intact because of bilateral innervation of the upper face from the corticobulbar fibers. The lower face, by contrast, has only unilateral contralateral cortical innervation so that retraction of the corner of the mouth to smile is compromised. The second type of facial weakness involves the *total side face* with ipsilateral facial muscle involvement. The lesion is said to be peripheral (involves the peripheral nervous system) or a **lower motor neuron lesion.** Specifically, the condition is called **Bell's palsy.**

In addition to muscle weakness, note any evidence of spasms, atrophy, or tremors of the facial muscles.

Acoustic Nerve (Sensory) (CN VIII)

The acoustic nerve is a pure sensory nerve and is divided into two branches, the **cochlear nerve** for hearing and the **vestibular nerve**, which contributes to equilibrium, coordination, and orientation in space.

Hearing is evaluated in several ways. Much information can be collected in observing the patient. Ability to understand soft and loud tones and low and high pitches is noted. Signs of hearing deficit include inability to hear high or low tones, turning the head toward the speaker when listening, or lip reading. Certain sounds are heard more loudly and at a greater distance. For example, *a*, *e*, and *i* are heard at a greater distance than consonants such as *l*, *m*, and *r* and vowels such as *o* and *u*. "Seventy-six" and "sixty-seven" can be heard at a greater distance than "ninety-nine." To test **hearing**, direct the patient to cover one ear. Standing on the opposite side, 1 to 2 feet away from the ear, whisper a few numbers or a word. An alternative is to rub your fingers together. The patient should be able to hear it. Test the other ear. Hearing should be equal in both ears.

Next, check for **lateralization** and **air** and **bone conduction**. **Weber's test** is used to evaluate lateralization, whereas **Rinne's test** evaluates air and bone conduction. Both tests require the use of a 512-Hz tuning fork (Fig. 6-11). For **Weber's test**, place a lightly vibrating tuning fork firmly vertex of the patient's head

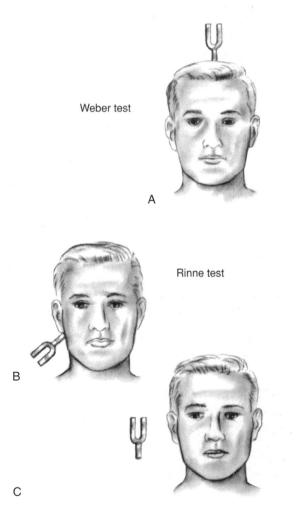

Weber test

A

Rinne test

B

C

Figure 6-11 • Weber test and Rinne test. Note the placement of a vibrating tuning fork (512 Hz) for each test. (*A*) Weber test for lateralization. Place the vibrating fork firmly on the top of the head or on the middle of the forehead. Normally the sound is perceived midline. Rinne test for comparing bone and air conduction: place the base of the vibrating tuning fork on the mastoid process until the patient can no longer hear it (*B*); then, quickly place the fork near the external auditory canal, with one side toward the ear (*C*). Normally, the sound can be heard longer through air than through bone (AC > BC).

or in the middle of the forehead. Inquire whether the patient hears the vibration more on the left side, on the right side, or in the middle. Normally, the sound is heard in the middle or equally in both ears. If one ear is occluded, the vibration is heard better or more loudly in the occluded ear.

In **Rinne's test**, air conduction and bone conduction are compared. Place the base of a lightly vibrating tuning fork firmly on the mastoid process. Ask the patient to inform you when the vibration is no longer heard. Quickly place the vibrating fork near the ear canal with the vibrating portion toward the ear. Ask the patient to inform you when it can no longer be heard. Normally, the sound should be heard longer through air than through bone (AC greater than BC). In evaluating hearing acuity, it is important to differentiate between **conduction loss** and **sensorineural loss**. The findings for unilateral loss for each are as follows:

TYPE OF DEAFNESS	RINNE	WEBER
Conduction deafness	BC > AC	Lateralizes **to** deafer ear
Sensorineural deafness	AC > BC	Lateralizes **away from** deafer ear

Abnormal findings from either test warrant further investigation with more sensitive testing.

In considering the vestibular nerve, certain tests of vestibular function are closely related to the examination of other portions of the nervous system (i.e., motor system and cerebellar testing). However, all patients with a major complaint of vertigo should receive a **Dix-Hallpike positional test**. It consists of seating the patient on the edge of an examining table and moving him or her backward rapidly so that the head is hanging backward while the eyes remain open. If no nystagmus or vertigo develops in 20 seconds, the patient is returned to the sitting position. The head is repositioned to the right, and the downward procedure repeated. If no nystagmus or vertigo develops in 20 seconds, return the patient to the sitting position. Reposition the head to the left and repeat the procedure (Fig. 6-12). Note the onset, duration, and direction of the nystagmus. In benign paroxysmal positional vertigo (BPPV), nystagmus is noted when the head is turned to either side. The nystagmus beats upward and also has a rotatory component so that the top part of the eye beats toward the down ear. The characteristics of the nystagmus are a latency of 2 to 5 seconds and a duration of 5 to 60 seconds, and it is followed by a downbeating nystagmus when the patient is placed upright in the sitting position. Further evaluation is required with persistent vertigo. If the patient complains of vertigo or dizziness, this should be investigated.

CLINICAL PEARLS: The dizziness or vertigo feels like swirling with a vestibular problem, but feels like walking on a boat (side to side) when it is related to cerebellar dysfunction.

Glossopharyngeal (CN IX) and Vagus (CN X) Nerves (Both Mixed)

The glossopharyngeal and vagus nerves are tested together because of their intimate association of function in the pharynx.

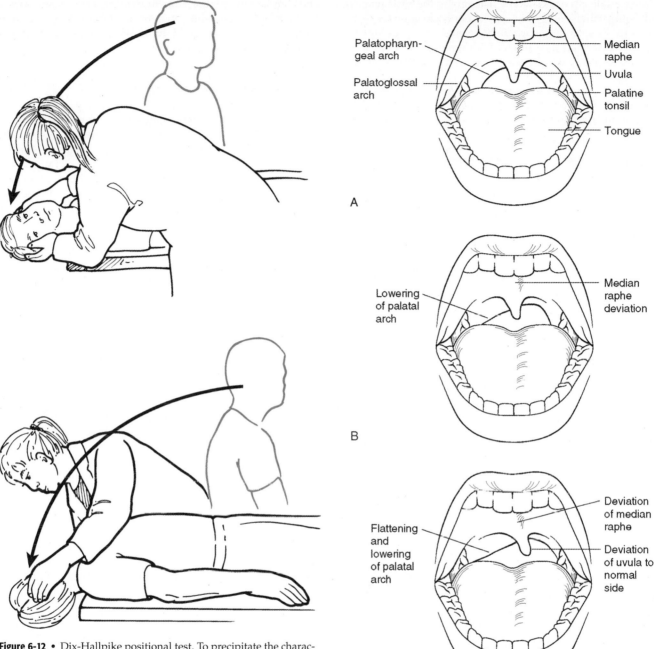

Figure 6-12 • Dix-Hallpike positional test. To precipitate the characteristic nystagmus of benign paroxysmal positional vertigo (BPPV), the patient is rapidly brought into a head position that makes the posterior canal vertical and also brings it through a large angular displacement.

Figure 6-13 • Observing the palate. (A) Normal palate with mouth open and at rest. (B) Right unilateral vagus paralysis with mouth at rest. (C) Right unilateral vagus paralysis when saying "ah."

The glossopharyngeal nerve supplies sensory components to the pharynx, tonsils, soft palate, tympanic membrane, posterior third of the tongue, and secretory fibers of the parotid gland. It also supplies motor fibers to the stylopharyngeal muscle of the pharynx, whose role is to elevate the pharynx. The patient is asked to open the mouth and say "ah." Upward movement of the soft palate and uvula should be noted. The vagus nerve provides parasympathetic fibers to the viscera of the chest and abdomen. Sensory fibers innervate the external ear canal, pharynx, larynx, and viscera of the chest and abdomen. The vagus also provides motor control to the soft palate, larynx, and pharynx.

The soft palate is examined with the patient's mouth open. Normally, when the patient says "ah," the palate elevates and the uvula remains midline. Check to see whether the uvula deviates to one side or the other (Fig. 6-13). The gag reflex is innervated by CNs IX and X. After warning the patient that you are going to check the gag reflex, touch the posterior pharyngeal wall with a tongue blade or applicator first on the left side and next on the right side. A gag response should be stimulated on each side.

Voice quality is evaluated by listening to the patient speak and noting hoarseness; a soft, whispery voice; or no voice. Difficulty in speaking, such as hoarseness or speaking in a whisper, is termed **dysphonia.** Both are due to paralysis of the soft palate **(palatal paralysis)** and can result in nasal-sounding speech. **Dysarthria** refers to defective articulation that may be caused by a motor deficit of the tongue or speech muscles. Slurred speech should be noted, as should difficulty in pronouncing the letters *m, b, p, t,* and *d* and the number *1.*

Spinal Accessory Nerve (Motor) (CN XI)

The accessory nerve, as it is sometimes called, is tested in two segments. First, the trapezius muscle is palpated and its strength evaluated while the patient shrugs the shoulders against resistance provided by the examiner's hands. Second, the patient is asked to turn his or her head to one side and push the chin against the examiner's hand, thereby allowing the sternocleidomastoid muscle to be palpated and its strength evaluated. The same procedure is then repeated on the other side. The symmetry of the trapezius and sternocleidomastoid muscles is noted, along with any muscle wasting or spasm.

Hypoglossal Nerve (Motor) (CN XII)

The patient is asked to open his or her mouth. The tongue is first inspected as it lies on the floor of the oral cavity. Note any atrophy or fasciculation of the tongue. Ask the patient to protrude the tongue. Note asymmetry, atrophy, or deviation from midline. Next, direct the patient to move the tongue from side to side. Note the symmetry of movement. Finally, ask the patient to push the tongue against the inside of each cheek as the examiner palpates externally on the cheek for strength and equality. With a deficit of CN XII, the tongue will deviate toward the weaker side. With unilateral wasting and fasciculation, consider possible unilateral lower motor disease. If the tongue moves in and out when protruded, consider cerebellar disease, essential tremor, or extrapyramidal disease.[4]

▓ MOTOR SYSTEM EXAMINATION

The motor examination comes next and proceeds from the neck, to the upper limbs, to the trunk, and, finally, to the lower extremities. Limb evaluation proceeds from proximal to distal. It is impractical to test all muscles, but major groups are assessed; a more detailed examination can be conducted if deficits are noted in a particular area. The symmetry of each muscle or muscle group is noted. Evaluate muscle size, muscle tone, and muscle strength. Finally, evaluate gait and posture. Throughout the examination, note any involuntary movements.

Muscle Size

Inspect symmetric muscles for both size and contour. When in doubt, a tape measure can be used to measure a muscle and compare it with the same muscle on the opposite side of the body. Measurements must be taken from the same reference point for accuracy. Note muscle wasting, atrophy, or hypertrophy.

Muscle Tone

Muscle tone is the normal state of partial contraction of a muscle and is assessed by passive movement. With the patient relaxed, the joints are put through the normal range of motion (e.g., flexion and extension) by the examiner. The systematic evaluation proceeds from the shoulder, elbow, wrist, and fingers in the upper extremities and from the hip, knee, and ankle in the lower extremities. Findings from the left side and the right side are then compared. Variation in normal muscle tone can result in increased tone referred to as **hypertonia** or decrease in muscle tone referred to as **hypotonia.** Hypotonia manifests itself as hypotonicity or flaccidity, whereas hypertonia manifests itself as spasticity or rigidity.

Hypotonia is defined as decreased tone and may be seen in lower motor neuron lesions, spinal shock, and some cerebellar lesions. **Flaccidity** refers to loss of muscle tone. It is due to a lower motor neuron lesion at any point from the anterior horn cell to the peripheral nerves. The muscle is weak, soft, and floppy. See discussion of lower motor neuron disease.

Spasticity refers to increased motor tone **(hypertonia).** Tone is greater with rapid passive movement, and less pronounced when the rate is slower. In addition, tone is often greater at the extremes of range of motion. Spasticity results from injury to the upper motor neuron of the corticospinal tract at any point from the cortex to the spinal cord.

Rigidity refers to increased tone associated with an extrapyramidal lesion in the basal ganglia. See Table 6-12 for muscle tone variations.

Muscle Strength

Muscle strength is evaluated by asking the patient to move a muscle actively against gravity and then with resistance provided by the examiner. Muscle strength can be rated using a scale of 0 (no muscle contraction detected) to 5 (active movement against full resistance). Muscle strength is recorded together with the maximum grade achievable on the scale (e.g., 4 out of 5 with 5 being the maximum achievable grade). Compare the functional level of each muscle and compare it to the functional level on the opposite side. See Table 6-13 for grading system. (*Note:* Sometimes an examiner will use a plus [+] or a minus [−] in the "4" category to indicate how strong the patient's muscle strength was against the examiner's resistance. A "4+" indicates that a large amount of resistance by the examiner was necessary for the patient's muscle to be finally overcome.)

Note that the pattern of muscle extremity evaluation includes both proximal and distal muscle groups. When considering patterns of dysfunction, differentiating between proximal and distal deficits is important. Symmetric weakness of the **proximal muscles** suggests **myopathy,** a muscle disorder. By contrast, symmetric weakness of **distal muscles** suggests **polyneuropathy,** a peripheral nerve disorder. Note also that weakness on the same side as a lesion or on both sides simulta-

TABLE 6-12 MUSCLE TONE VARIATIONS

MUSCLE TONE VARIATION	DEFINITION	ASSOCIATED WITH
Hypotonicity	Decrease or loss of muscle tone; muscle feels soft and flabby to palpate; there is increased ease with passive movement	Lower motor neuron disease, spinal shock, and some cerebellar lesions
Hypertonicity	Increased muscle tone	Pyramidal and extrapyramidal lesion
• **Rigidity**	Increased tone resistance to passive movement throughout movement; due to steady contraction of flexors and extensors	Extrapyramidal lesions
Cogwheel rigidity	A series of stepwise, ratchet-like, small, regular jerks that are felt on passive movement	Parkinson's disease
Lead-pipe rigidity	Uniform resistance throughout passive movement	Some forms of Parkinson's disease
Paratonia or Gegenhaltem	Resistance increases throughout flexion and extension; becomes less prominent when the patient is distracted	Bilateral frontal lobe lesions often related to stroke
• **Spasticity**	Resistance to passive movement for portions of the movement; due to loss of suprasegmental influence on the tonic contractions of the muscle; usually greatest in the flexors of the upper extremity and the extensors of the lower extremity	Upper motor neuron lesions
Clasp-knife spasticity	Resistance to passive movement with sudden giving away toward the completion of joint flexion or extension	Upper motor neuron paralysis

neously suggests a spinal cord lesion. Weakness on one side, however, suggests a lesion in the brain on the side opposite to the weakness (see Chap. 36 for discussion of neuropathies).

UPPER EXTREMITIES

Table 6-14 summarizes the major muscles, innervating peripheral nerve, and motor action evaluated in the upper extremities. Table 6-15 summarizes the order and method of evaluation of the upper extremity muscles (Fig. 6-14). In evaluating function, make your directions to the patient clear and succinct. Demonstrate movements and cue as necessary.

LOWER EXTREMITIES

In examining the lower extremities, proceed from the hip to the feet. By positioning the hands appropriately, the examiner

TABLE 6-13 GRADING OF MUSCLE STRENGTH

GRADE	STRENGTH
5	Active movement against gravity and full resistance; normal muscle strength
4	Active movement against gravity and some resistance; the examiner can overcome the muscle resistance
3	Active movement against gravity
2	Active movement of the body part when gravity is eliminated
1	A very weak muscle contraction is palpated; only a trace of a contraction is evident, but no active movement of the body part is noted
0	No muscle contraction is detectable

provides resistance to movement. Table 6-16 summarizes the major muscles, innervating peripheral nerve, and motor action evaluated in the lower extremities. Table 6-17 summarizes the order and method of evaluating the lower extremity muscles (Fig. 6-15). Make your directions to the patient clear and succinct. Demonstrate movements as necessary.

Gait and Posture

Gait is evaluated with the motor examination or at the end of the cerebellar examination. **Gait** is the manner of walking, and **posture** is the position or orientation of the body in space. Any patient able to ambulate, even with assistive devices (cane, walker), should be observed walking, preferably without shoes or stockings. The examiner should be prepared to protect the patient from falls and injury. Observe the patient walking back and forth naturally in the room. The points to note include gait (e.g., smooth or staggering); position of feet (e.g., broad based or normal); symmetry of arm and leg movement (do arms swing naturally?); presence of any uncoordinated movements or tremors; height of step (i.e., shuffling, high, normal); and length of step (i.e., short, long, normal). Note how easily the patient can turn around and how many steps are required to turn. Next, have the patient walk heel to toe (called **tandem walking**), walk on the toes only, and walk on the heels only. An alternative is to ask the patient to hop on one foot and then the other. Chart 6-2 and Table 6-18 list the most common gait disturbances seen with neurological conditions.

Involuntary Movements

Any involuntary movements should be noted. In observing for involuntary movement, consideration is given to rate (cycles per second), distribution (proximal muscles, distal muscles), and relationship to movement (increasing or decreasing with movement). Common abnormalities of movement include tremors, choreiform movements, clonus,

TABLE 6-14   SUMMARY OF MAJOR MUSCLES, PERIPHERAL NERVE INNERVATION, AND MUSCLE ACTION OF THE UPPER EXTREMITIES

SPINAL LEVEL	MUSCLE	PERIPHERAL NERVE INNERVATION	ACTION
C-5, C-6, C-7	Serratus anterior	Long thoracic	Movement of shoulder
C-5, C-6	Deltoid and supraspinatus	Suprascapular and axillary	Abduction of shoulder
C-5, C-6	Biceps brachii	Musculocutaneous	Flexion of elbow
C-5, **C-6**	Brachioradialis	Radial	Flexion of elbow
C-7, C-8	Triceps brachii	Radial	Extension of elbow
C-6, C-7	Extensor carpi radialis longus (C-6) and extensor carpi ulnaris (C-7)	Radial	Extension of wrist
C-7, C-8	Flexor carpi radialis (C-7) and flexor carpi ulnaris (C-8)	Medial and ulnar	Flexion of wrist
C-7	Extensor digitorum communis, extensor indicis proprius, and extensor digiti minimi (all C-7)	Radial	Extension of fingers
C-8, T-1	Flexor digitorum superficialis (C-8), flexor digitorum profundus (C-8), and lumbricals (C-8, T-1)	Median and ulnar	Flexion of fingers
T-1	Dorsal interossei (T-1) and abductor digiti quinti (5th finger)	Ulnar	Abduction of fingers
C-8, **T-1**	Palmar interossei	Ulnar	Adduction of fingers
C-8, **T-1**	Opponens pollicis	Median	Opposition of thumb

Bold type indicates primary innervation.

myoclonus, athetosis, tics, spasms, and ballism. Table 6-19 summarizes involuntary movements.

> **CLINICAL PEARLS:**   For motor problems, the examiner collects most of the information from the *physical examination*; for sensory problems, the examiner collects most of the information from the *history*.

SENSORY SYSTEM EXAMINATION

In evaluating the sensory system, the examiner determines the patient's ability to perceive various types of sensations with the **eyes closed**. Each side of the body is compared with the other, as are sensory perceptions at the distal and proximal portions of all extremities. The testing proceeds in an orderly fashion. The body areas commonly evaluated include the face, neck, deltoid regions, forearm, hands (top side), chest, abdomen, thighs, lower legs, and feet (top surface). Compare the left and right sides of the body. The perianal area is assessed only in special circumstances, such as when a sacral injury is suspected. Sensory function is rated according to the following scale:

2: normal
1: present, but diminished (abnormal)
0: absent

A detailed sensory examination is part of the **extended examination** and is undertaken when numbness, pain, trophic changes, or other sensory abnormalities are present. The three main sensory pathways entering the spinal cord are:

- Pain-temperature (anterior and lateral spinothalamic tracts)
- Position and vibration (posterior columns)

- Light touch (involves the anterior and lateral spinothalamic tracts and posterior columns)

Discrimination sensations involve some of the above sensory tracts; it also involves the cerebral cortex, especially the parietal lobe.

The following list shows the sensory modalities with testing methods (Table 6-20). A map of dermatomes (see Chap. 4) should be used to guide the examination or to focus a detailed examination of a particular area. Light touch, pain, and vibration are the modalities tested.

Superficial Sensation

- Light touch: a wisp of cotton is used to lightly touch various areas of the skin.
- Pain: a broken wooden applicator that is "picky" at one end or other "picky" instrument is used to stimulate the skin. A pin-wheel, or a disposable prepacked pin, that can be disposed of safely after use may be used (never use a needle or anything that will break the skin). To prevent transmission of blood-borne diseases, the instrument for testing should never be used on another patient. The skin is touched arbitrarily with the sharp or dull side. The smooth bottom of the applicator is used for a "dull" source of stimuli. (If pain sensation is intact, testing for temperature sensation is usually omitted.)
- Temperature: a tube of hot water and one of cold water are applied in succession to the same areas used in other tests. The patient is asked to identify "hot" or "cold." A cool tuning fork can also be used; it is placed directly on the skin in a particular location and then moved to the same area on the opposite side of the body. The patient is asked if it feels the same on both sides of the body.

TABLE 6–15 SUMMARY OF EVALUATION OF UPPER EXTREMITIES MOTOR FUNCTION

FUNCTION BEING EVALUATED	LETTER IN FIG. 6-14	DIRECTIONS TO PATIENT	EXAMINER AND OBSERVATIONS
Shoulder movement C-5, C-6, C-7	A	"Extend your arms parallel to the floor and push with your palms against the wall" (Fig. A-1). (*Alternately, you can ask the patient to push against your hands.*)	Observe the scapula for increased prominence of the scapular tip (**winging**). Normally, each scapula is close to the thorax. Winging suggests serratus anterior muscle weakness (Fig. A-2).
Adduction of shoulder C-5, C-6	B	"Flex your elbow slightly and move your upper arm away from your body." (*Alternately, ask the patient to position his or her arms like "chicken wings."*)	Try to push the abducted upper arms down against resistance.
Flexion of elbow **C-5,** C-6	C	"Flex your elbow and make a muscle with your palm parallel to the shoulder."	Try to pull the flexed forearm open.
Flexion of elbow C-5, **C-6**	D	"Flex your elbow and make a muscle while your palm is pointed at midline" (midsaggital line).	Try to pull the flexed forearm open.
Extension of elbow C-7, C-8	E	"Push me away with that same arm."	Provide resistance, thus trying to prevent extension.
Pronator drift	F	(*May examine patient when he or she is standing or sitting.*) "Outstretch both arms in front of you parallel to the floor with hands open and palms up." (*The elbows should be fully extended, the wrists extended also.*) "Now close your eyes (*and stay that way for 20 or 30 seconds*)."	Observe for slow pronation of the wrist, slight flexion of the elbow and fingers, and a downward and lateral drift of the hand; called *pronator drift.* Suggests *mild hemiparesis* and may be noted before any significant weakness noted.
Extension of wrist **C-6,** C-7	G	"Extend your wrist and don't let me straighten it."	The examiner attempts to straighten the wrist. If straightened, it suggests wristdrop.
Flexion of wrist **C-7,** C-8	H	"Flex your wrist and don't let me straighten it."	The examiner attempts to straighten the wrist.
Extension of fingers C-7	I	"Put your fingers straight out and don't let me push them down."	Try to push the fingers down.
Flexion of fingers **C-8,** T-1	J	"Flex your fingers and don't let me straighten them."	Try to straighten the fingers.
Abduction of fingers **T-1**	K	"Put your hand on the table and spread your fingers. Try to resist my attempt to bring the fingers together."	Try to push the fingers together.
Adduction of fingers C-8, **T-1**	L	"Put your hand on the table with the fingers slightly spread. Try to resist my attempt to pull your fingers outward."	Try to pull the fingers outward.
Opposition of thumb C-8, T-1	M	(*The thumbnail should be parallel to the palm.*) "Touch the tip of your little finger with your thumb."	Try to pull the thumb away from the little finger with your index finger or thumb.

Bold type indicates primary innervation.

Deep Sensation

- Vibration: a 128-Hz tuning fork is placed on the bony prominence of the big toe and thumb; perception of vibration is a normal finding.
- Deep pressure pain: the Achilles tendon or gastrocnemius muscle belly and forearm muscles are squeezed. The patient should perceive this pressure, and it should feel the same on both sides of the body.
- Proprioception: the thumb and then the large toe are moved up or down. The patient should be able to identify "up" or "down."

Discriminative Sensation (Usually, Not All Modalities Are Tested)

- **Two-point discrimination:** a part of the body is touched simultaneously with sharp objects to determine if one or two pricks can be felt. (Note: the presence of receptors varies in different parts of the body.)
- **Point discrimination:** the patient is asked to name the location at which he or she was touched with the wooden end of an applicator or the examiner's hand.
- **Recognition of shape and form:** the patient is asked to identify common objects placed in his or her hand such as

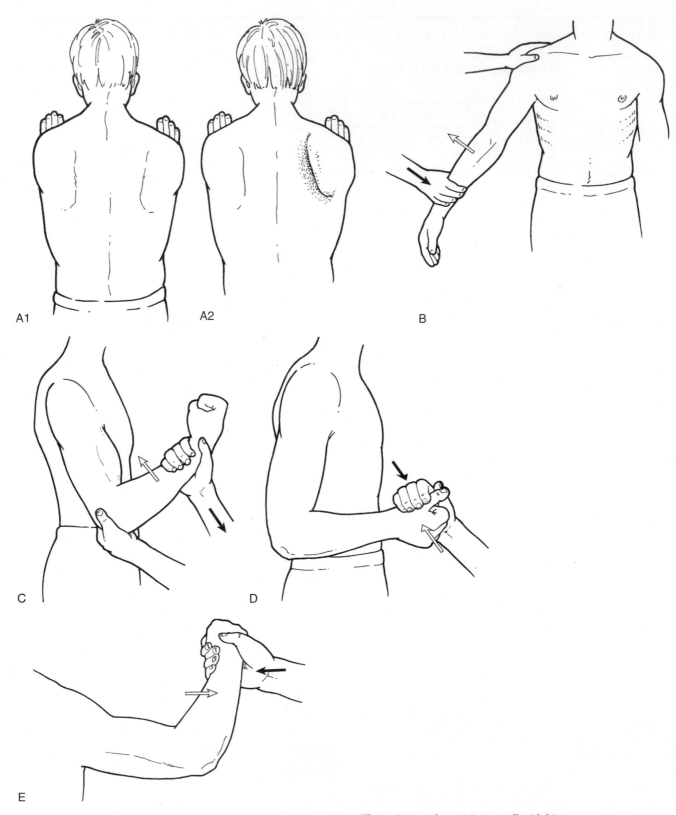

Figure 6-14 • (*A1*) Examination of the serratus anterior. The patient pushes against a wall with his arms extended horizontally in front of him; normally, the medial border of the scapula remains close to the thoracic wall. (*A2*) Winging of scapula. (*B*) Examination of the deltoid. The patient attempts to abduct his arm against resistance; the contracting deltoid can be seen and palpated. (*C*) Examination of the biceps brachii. On attempts to flex the forearm against resistance, the contracting biceps muscle can be seen and palpated. (*D*) Examination of the brachioradialis. On flexion at the semipronated forearm (thumb up) against resistance, the contracting muscle can be seen and palpated. (*E*) Extension of the forearm. On attempts to extend the partially flexed forearm against resistance, contraction of the triceps can be seen and palpated. (*continued*)

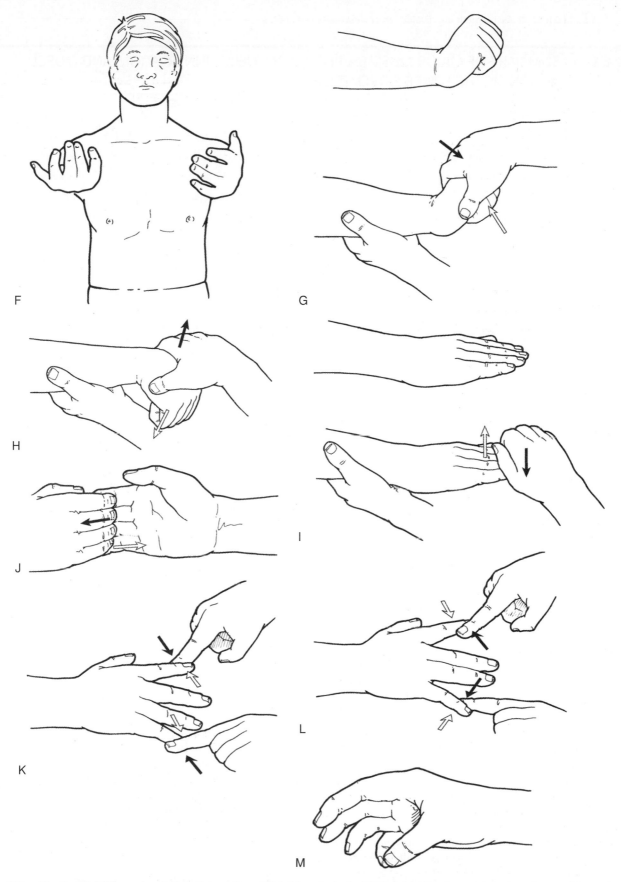

Figure 6-14 • (*Continued*) (*F*) Pronation drift-drift in patient with left hemiparesis. (*G*) Examination of wrist extension. On attempts to extend the hand at the wrist against resistance, the bellies of the extensors carpi radialis longus, carpi ulnaris, and digitorum communis can be seen and palpated. (*H*) Examination of the wrist flexors. (*I*) Examination for finger extension. (*J*) Examination of the flexor digitorum profundus. The patient resists attempts to extend the distal phalanges while the middle phalanges are fixed. (*K*) Examination of the abduction of the fingers. The patient resists the examiner's attempt to bring the fingers together. (*L*) Adduction of the fingers. The patient attempts to adduct the fingers against resistance. (*M*) Opposition of the thumb and little finger.

TABLE 6-16 SUMMARY OF MAJOR MUSCLES, PERIPHERAL NERVE INNERVATION, AND MUSCLE ACTION OF THE LOWER EXTREMITIES

SPINAL LEVEL	MUSCLE(S)	PERIPHERAL NERVE INNERVATION	MUSCLE ACTION
T-12, **L-1, L-2**, L-3	Iliopsoas	Branches from T-12, L-1, L-2, L-3	Hip flexion
L-2, L-3, L-4	Adductor brevis, adductor longus, and adductor magnus	Obturator	Hip adduction
L-4, **L-5**, S-1	Gluteus medius	Superior gluteal	Hip abductors
L-5, S-1, S-2	Gluteus maximus	Inferior gluteal	Hip extension
L-2, L-3, L-4	Quadriceps	Femoral	Knee extension
L-5, **S-1**, S-2	Hamstrings	Sciatic	Knee flexion
L-4, **L-5**	Tibialis anterior, peroneus tertius, extensor digitorum longus, extensor hallucis longus	Deep peroneal	Ankle dorsiflexion
S-1, S-2	Gastrocnemius and soleus	Tibial	Ankle plantarflexion
L-4, L-5	Tibialis posterior	Tibial	Foot inversion
L-5, **S-1**	Peroneus longus and brevis	Superficial peroneal	Foot eversion

Bold type indicates primary innervation.

a key, a pen, or a coin. Inability to recognize objects by touch is called **astereognosis.**

- **Texture discrimination:** the patient is asked to differentiate among various textures (e.g., silk, wool).
- **Graphesthesia:** a letter or number is written on the palm with a dull-pointed object; the patient is then asked to identify the symbol.
- **Extension phenomenon:** touch the patient in the same location on both sides of the body simultaneously; alternate with touching only one side and determine if the patient can tell the difference. If sensation is normal, being touched on the skin on both sides of the body simultaneously should result in both stimuli being perceived.

CEREBELLAR SYSTEM EXAMINATION

The following outlines the most common methods used to evaluate balance and coordination. (Gait, discussed with the motor examination, may be included at the end of the cerebellar examination.) The patient is instructed to do *one* of the following in each category:

Upper Extremities

- The examiner raises his or her index finger to locate it about 2 feet and central-midface from the patient. The patient is given the instruction, "With your left hand, touch my finger, then touch your nose; do this as fast as you can." Be sure that the upper arm is extended and parallel to the floor. This should be evaluated with the patient's eyes open and then closed. Repeat with other arm.
- Instruct the patient to rapidly pronate and supinate the hand in the other palm; repeat with other hand.
- Instruct the patient to rapidly tap his or her index finger on the thumb; then tap all four fingers, one at a time, against the thumb as rapidly as possible. Repeat with other hand.

If the finger-to-nose test is smooth and on the mark, further evaluation of the upper extremities is not necessary. **Dysmetria** is the inability to control accurately the range of movement in muscle action with resultant overshooting of the mark, especially of hand movement. Overshooting is also called **past-point**.

Lower Extremities

- While lying on the back or sitting, the patient is instructed to slide one heel down the shin of the opposite leg, then repeat the procedure on the opposite side.
- While lying on the back or sitting, the patient is instructed to draw the number 8 with the foot in the air; repeat with the other foot.

Balance

Tandem walking is tested (Fig. 6-16). Protect the patient from falls. If the patient sways to one side, it may be an early indicator of cerebellar dysfunction on the side to which he or she sways.

Romberg's test assesses vestibular control of balance in space and is a test of proprioception. Ask the patient to stand erect with feet together, first with eyes open (visual input) and then with eyes closed (without visual input). To protect the patient from injury, stand beside him or her with your arms positioned to provide support should he or she begin to fall. If the patient maintains balance with the eyes open but sways or falls when the eyes are closed, **Romberg's sign** is positive. The patient deviates to the side of the lesion.

REFLEXES

Testing reflexes provides an important indication of the status of the central nervous system in both conscious and

TABLE 6–17   SUMMARY OF LOWER EXTREMITY MOTOR EVALUATION

FUNCTION BEING EVALUATED	LETTER IN FIG. 6-15	DIRECTIONS TO PATIENT	OBSERVED RESPONSE
Hip flexion (iliopsoas) **L-1, L-2,** L-3	A-1 and A-2	(*Position the patient supine.*) "Flex your thigh against the resistance provided" (Fig A-1).	*Alternate method:* have patient sit on the edge of the examining table with legs dangling. Stabilize the pelvis by placing your hand over the iliac crest and the other hand over the distal femoral portion of the knee; apply resistance as the patient attempts to raise knee off the table (Fig. A-2).
Hip adductors **L-2, L-3,** L-4	B	"Lie on your back: extend your legs; now separate them about 6 inches." (*The examiner places both hands firmly between both knees.*) "Try to bring your knees together."	Provide resistance against the inward movement. Determine how much resistance that the patient can overcome.
Hip abductors, gluteus medius and minimus L-4, **L-5,** S-1	C	(*The examiner places both hands on the lateral thighs just above the patient's knees.*) "Spread both legs against my hands."	After the legs are abducted, provide resistance and try to push the legs together. Determine how much resistance that the patient can overcome.
Hip extension (gluteus maximus) **L-5, S-1,** S-2	D	(*One examiner's hand is positioned on the posterior thigh and the other on top; feel for a muscle contraction on the posterior thigh.*) "Push your leg down against the bed."	*Alternate method:* ask the patient to stand from a sitting position without using the arms.
Knee extension (quadriceps) L-2, **L-3, L-4**	E-1 and E-2	(*With the patient prone, the examiner supports the partially flexed knee and places his or her other hand on the top of the lower leg about 4 inches above the ankle and provides resistance against extension*) (Fig. E-1). "Straighten your lower leg."	Stabilize the thigh by placing one hand just above the knee. Place the other hand just above the ankle and provide resistance. Palpate the quadriceps for a contraction with the stabilizing hand. *Alternate method:* sitting on the side of the examining table: direct the patient to extend the knee (Fig. E-2).
Knee flexion (hamstrings) **L-5, S-1,** S-2	F-1 and F-2	(*The examiner grasps the partially flexed knee about 4 inches above the ankle and stabilizes the hip with the other hand; provides resistance against flexion.*) "Flex your knee."	*Alternate methods:* have patient sit on the edge of the examining table with legs dangling. Ask patient to bend the knee and keep it bent while you provide resistance (Fig. F-2) or ask patient to squat in a deep knee bend (should be able to flex both knees symmetrically).
Dorsiflexion of ankle (tibialis anterior) L-4, **L-5**	G	(*The examiner positions the ankle in neutral position and then places the other hand on the top of the foot near the fifth metatarsal.*) "Pull your toes toward your nose."	Anchor the ankle by stabilizing the heel; with your flattened fingers on the top of the foot, provide resistance to dorsiflexion. *Alternative method:* ask patient to walk on heels.
Plantarflexion of ankle (gastrocnemius) **S-1,** S-2	H	(*The examiner positions the ankle in neutral position and then places the other hand on the ball of the foot near the fifth metatarsal.*) "Press down like on the gas pedal."	Anchor the ankle by stabilizing the heel; with your palm on the bottom of the foot, provide resistance to plantarflexion. *Alternative method:* ask the patient to walk on toes.
Foot inversion L-4, L-5	I	(*Position your thumb to dorsiflex and invert the foot.*) "Try to move your foot outward and down."	Try to force the foot into plantarflexion and eversion by pushing against the head and shaft of the first metatarsal; the tendon of the tibialis posterior can be seen and palpated behind the medial malleolus.
Foot eversion S-1	J	(*Secure ankle by stabilizing the heel and place your other hand that forces plantarflexion and eversion. Provide resistance to the eversion by pushing on the fifth metatarsal with the palm.*) "Turn your foot outward."	*Alternative method:* ask patient to walk on the medial borders of feet.

Bold type indicates primary innervation.

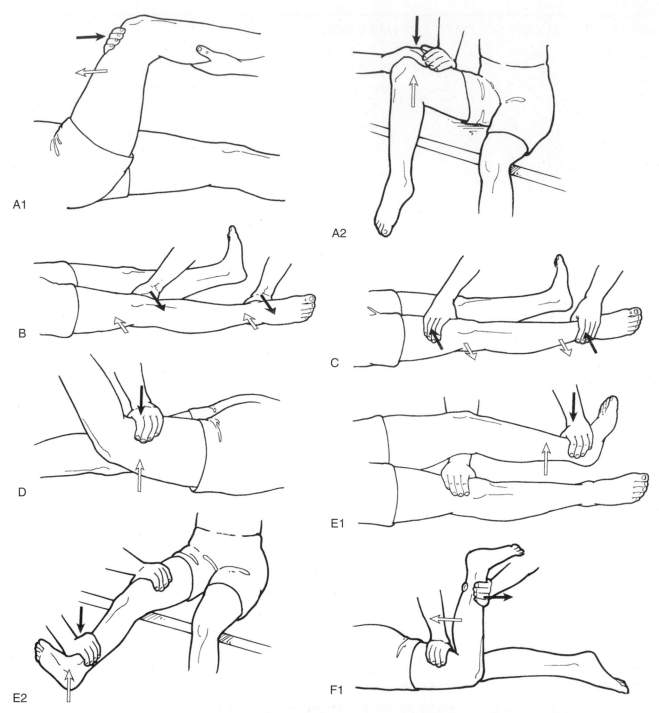

Figure 6-15 • (*A1*) Examination of the flexors of the thigh. The patent attempts to flex the thigh against resistance; the knee is flexed and the leg rests on the examiner's arm. (*A2*) Examination of hip flexion. (*B*) Examination of adduction of the thigh at the hip. The recumbent patient attempts to adduct the extended leg against resistance; contraction of the adductor muscles can be seen and palpated. (*C*) Abduction of the thigh at the hip. The recumbent patient attempts to move the extended leg outward against resistance; contraction of the gluteus medius and tensor fasciae latae can be palpated. (*D*) Examination of the extensors of the thigh at the hip. The patient, lying prone with the leg flexed at the knee, attempts to extend the thigh against resistance; contraction of the gluteus maximus and other extensors can be seen and palpated. (*E1*) Examination of extension of the leg at the knee. The supine patient attempts to extend the leg at the knee against resistance; contraction of the quadriceps femoris can be seen and palpated. (*E2*) Examination of the quadriceps for knee extension. (*F1*) Examination of the hamstring muscle for knee flexion. (*continued*)

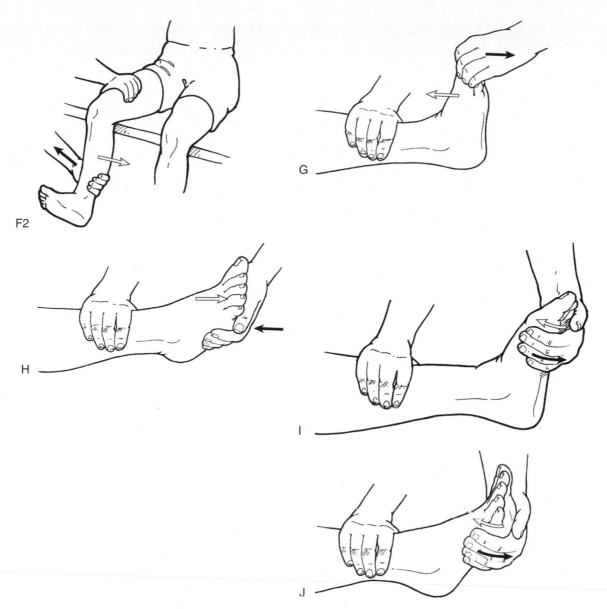

Figure 6-15 • *(Continued)* (*F2*) Muscle test for the quadriceps. (*G*) Examination of dorsiflexion (extension) of the foot. The patient attempts to dorsiflex the foot against resistance; contraction of the tibialis anterior can be seen and palpated. (*H*) Examination of plantarflexion of the foot. The patient attempts to plantar flex the foot at the ankle joint against resistance; contraction of the gastrocnemius and associated muscles can be seen and palpated. (*I*) Examination of inversion of the foot. The patient attempts to raise the inner border of the foot against resistance; the tendon of the tibialis posterior can be seen and palpated just behind the medial malleolus. (*J*) Examination of eversion of the foot. The patient attempts to raise the outer border of the foot against resistance; the tendons of the peronei longus and brevis can be seen and palpated just above and behind the lateral malleolus.

unconscious patients. A stimulus is mediated by a definite pathway through the receptor organ, afferent limb, spinal cord or brainstem, efferent limb, and effector organ. The reflex is modified by the simultaneous activity of other pathways, particularly the corticospinal tract. Alterations in reflexes may be the earliest signs of a pathologic condition. Reflexes are classified into three categories: (1) muscle-stretch reflexes (also known as deep tendon reflexes or

DTRs), (2) superficial or cutaneous reflexes, and (3) pathologic reflexes.

Muscle-Stretch Reflexes

The muscle-stretch reflexes are evaluated first. These reflexes occur in response to a sudden stimulus, such as the percussion

CHART **6-2** Gait Changes Associated With Anatomic Correlations

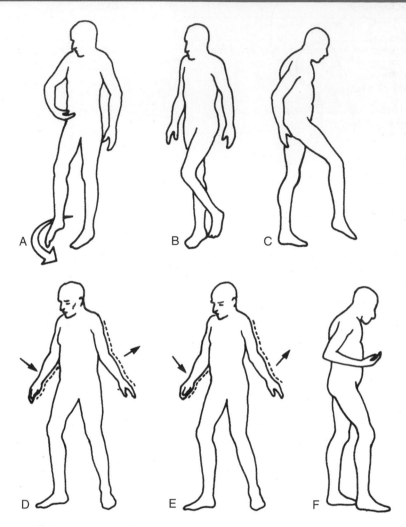

A Spastic hemiparesis is associated with unilateral upper motor neuron disease. One arm is flexed, close to the side, and immobile; the leg is circled stiffly outward and forward (circumducted), often with dragging of the toe.

B Scissors gait is associated with bilateral spastic paresis of the legs. Each leg is advanced slowly and the thighs tend to cross forward on each other at each step. The steps are short. Patients look as if they were walking through water.

C Steppage gait is associated with foot-drop, usually secondary to lower motor neuron disease. The feet are lifted high, with knees flexed, and then brought down with a slap on the floor. Patients look as if they were walking up stairs.

D Sensory ataxia is associated with loss of position sense in the legs. The gait is unsteady and wide-based (the feet are far apart). The feet are lifted high and brought down with a slap. Patients watch the ground to guide their steps. They cannot stand steadily with feet together when the eyes are closed (positive Romberg test).

E Cerebellar ataxia is associated with disease of the cerebellum or associated tracts. The gait is staggering, unsteady, and widely based, with exaggerated difficulty on the turns. The patient cannot stand steadily with feet together, whether eyes are open or closed.

F Parkinsonian gait is associated with the basal ganglia of Parkinson's disease. The posture is stooped, the hips and knees slightly flexed. Steps are short and often shuffling. Arm swings are decreased and the patient turns around stiffly—"all in one piece."

Adapted from Staab, A. S., & Hodges, L. C. (1996). *Essentials of gerontological nursing: Adaptation to the aging process.* Philadelphia: J. B. Lippincott.

hammer that causes the muscle to stretch (Chart 6-3). Although there are many muscle-stretch reflexes, the *major* reflexes included in a screening examination are evaluated. It is important to use the proper technique to elicit a particular reflex. With the muscle relaxed and the joint at midposition, the tendon is tapped directly using a percussion or reflex hammer. Normally, contraction of the muscle occurs with a quick movement of the limb or structure innervated by the muscle. Both sides of the body are tested and the results are compared. The briskness of the response should also be

TABLE 6–18   DESCRIPTION OF GAIT DISTURBANCES

NAME	DESCRIPTION	CAUSES
General Gait Disturbances		
• Steppage gait	Associated with foot drop and flaccidity of the leg. To compensate for foot drop, the patient lifts the upper leg high to clear the foot from floor; as a result, the foot slaps the floor	Can be unilateral when caused by a lesion involving the external popliteal nerve. It is bilateral in cases of peroneal muscle atrophy (as in Charcot-Marie-Tooth disease) or bilateral L-5 and S-l involvement (poliomyelitis or some polyneuropathies)
• Waddling gait	Broad base and lateral jerking movement of the hips and trunk	Weakness of the gluteal, psoas, and truncal muscles
• Hypotonic gait	Hyperextension of the knees, wide-based flail-like movements of the legs accompanied by a high step; the heel touches first, followed by the slap of the foot as the toes touch the floor	Degeneration of the posterior columns (loss of proprioception)
Special Gait Disturbances Classified According to Anatomic Areas		
• Cerebellar gait	Wide-based, staggering, lurching, and uncoordinated gait	Any disease involving the cerebellum (tumor, multiple sclerosis, Friedreich's ataxia)
• Corticospinal gaits		
Hemiplegic	Unilateral; the arm is "semiflexed" with the elbow held close to the waist; fingers are flexed and wrist-drop is noted; the extended, spastic, stiff leg is swung in a semicircle when walking; the foot is inverted, and foot-drop is evident	Stroke
Spastic	Shuffling, with the legs stiff	Bilateral involvement of the corticospinal tract
Scissor	The legs cross, one in front of the other, with each step; the knees are brought inward; and the person often walks on toes because of the swaying motion. Bilateral condition	Severe spasticity of the adductor muscles of the legs
Basal Ganglia Gaits		
• Parkinsonian	Loss of automatic arm swinging is evident while walking; head and body are flexed forward; the arms are semiflexed and adducted; and the legs are rigid and flexed. A slow, shuffling gait is typical. After walking begins, the person may propel forward with increased momentum	Defect in the basal ganglia
• Athetoid	Sudden, worm-like movements of the arms, head, and legs, which make forward progress difficult	Defect in the basal ganglia

noted. The muscle-stretch reflex ranges are graded on a scale from 0 to 4, as follows:

4+: very brisk, hyperactive; muscle undergoes repeated contractions or clonus; often indicative of disease

3+: more brisk than average; may either be normal for that patient or indicative of disease

2+: average or normal

1+: minimal or diminished response

0: no response

Note that all reflexes present are indicated by a plus sign; there are no minuses used in reflex grading of DTRs. Findings can be documented using a stick figure on which the magnitude of the reflex is recorded (Fig. 6-17).

Superficial Reflexes

Superficial reflexes are elicited by light, rapid stroking or scratching (depending on the tissue being tested) of a particular area of the skin, cornea, or mucous membrane. Table 6-21 lists the most common superficial reflexes tested (Fig. 6-18). These reflexes are initiated by cutaneous receptors stimulated by stroking. The grading of superficial reflexes differs from the scale used with muscle-stretch reflexes. Superficial reflexes are graded as either present (+) or absent (0). If they are present but weak, they may be recorded as "weak."

Pathologic Reflexes

There are several reflexes referred to as *primitive reflexes* because they are seen in the early stages of development and subsequently disappear. If they do reappear, they are evidence of disinhibition resulting from dementia. Table 6-22 lists the most common primitive reflexes. Another primitive reflex is a **flexion reflex**, a general term encompassing various polysynaptic reflexes. Also known as the *withdrawal reflex*, it moves the limb away from the source of stimulation, thus resulting in flexion. Because the stimulus is polysynaptic, there is an after-discharge in the interneuronal relays, and the motor response outlasts the stimulus. Activation of the flexor motor neurons in the leg is typically widespread, so that flexor muscles at the *ankle, knee,* and *hip* contract to withdraw the whole limb; this triple contraction is sometimes referred to as a **triple flexion** response.

TABLE 6–19 INVOLUNTARY AND ABNORMAL MOVEMENTS

TYPE	DESCRIPTION	COMMENTS
Tremors	• Involuntary trembling movement of the body or limbs resulting from contraction of opposing muscles; tremors are characterized by rate, distribution, and relationship to movement	• Seen with certain organic diseases; some forms of tremors are psychogenic in origin
• Physiologic	• The occasional tremors seen in healthy people and precipitated by extreme fatigue or stress	
• Essential (familial, senile)	• Tremors occur when muscles are brought into action to support or move an extremity; they may also affect the jaw, lips, and head (head nods from side to side or to and fro) • Absent at rest • Tremor has characteristics similar to those of parkinsonian tremors	• Improvement is usually noted with alcohol ingestion, sedatives, and propranolol
• Toxic	• Tremors are caused by toxic states (e.g., uremia) or ingestion of toxic substances (e.g., drug withdrawal)	
• Cerebellar	• Tremors occur during movement and increase toward the end of the purposeful act	• Caused by cerebellar lesions • May be seen in multiple sclerosis
• Parkinsonian	• These regular, rhythmic tremors are described as "pill-rolling tremors" (alternating flexion-extension of the fingers and adduction-abduction of the thumb) • Observed at rest • Associated with increased muscle tone	• Basal ganglia disorder seen in Parkinson's disease
• Resting tremors	• Tremor occurs when the patient is at rest and is diminished by purposeful activity	
• Intentional tremors	• Tremor is increased or precipitated by purposeful activity	
Choreiform movements	• Characterized by irregular, jerky, uncoordinated movements and abnormal posture • Represent a more generalized condition than tremors • May be evidenced by grimacing and difficulty in chewing, speaking, and swallowing • Increase with purposeful activity, making it difficult to complete the simplest of motor functions	
Clonus/myoclonus	• Sudden, brief, jerking contraction of a muscle or muscle group	
Athetosis	• Involuntary, repetitive, slow gross movements, particularly affecting posture • Arms tend to swing from a widely abducted base	• Movements described as snake-like
Tics	• Involuntary, compulsive, stereotyped movements • Described as "nervous habits" • Repeated at irregular intervals • Often involve the face	• Often psychogenic in origin
Spasms	• Involuntary contraction of large muscle groups (arms, legs, neck)	• Oculogyric spasms, as seen in Parkinson's disease, are an example; these spasms are characterized by a fixed, upward gaze controlled by extraocular muscles
Ballism	• More or less continuous, gross, abrupt contractions of the axial and proximal muscles of the extremities • Violent flail-like movements	• May involve one side of the body (hemiballismus) • Caused by a destructive lesion in or near the contralateral subthalamic nucleus

Normally, the toes show plantarflexion in response to stimuli applied to the sole of the foot. Of the pathologic reflexes, the plantar reflexes are very important. **Babinski's reflex** is the most common plantar reflex assessed (Fig. 6-19). Stimulation of the plantar surface of the foot (from heel to toes along lateral aspect of foot) is followed by dorsiflexion of the toes, especially the great toe, and separation or fanning of the toes. A positive plantar reflex is related to disease of the corticospinal tract at any level from the motor cortex through the descending pathways.

The grading of pathologic reflexes involves noting the presence or absence of the pathologic sign. The presence of a pathologic sign (+) is abnormal, whereas absence of a pathologic sign (−) is normal.

THE NEUROLOGICAL EXAMINATION OF THE COMATOSE PATIENT

Coma is a pathologic state of unconsciousness characterized by the following: an unarousable sleep-like state; the eyes remain closed at all times; no speech or sound is noted; and there is no spontaneous movement of the extremities. If movement of the extremities occurs, it is a reflex response to painful stimuli such as flexor or extensor posturing (see Chap. 7 for discussion of LOC). Coma is a *symptom* of a wide variety of disease entities resulting from a cerebral structural lesion or a metabolic condition. For coma to occur there must be bilateral hemispheric dysfunction, brainstem dysfunction,

TABLE 6-20   SENSORY SYSTEM ASSESSMENT

SENSORY MODALITIES	DESCRIPTION/TECHNIQUE
Primary Sensory Modalities	
Superficial sensations Superficial tactile (light touch) sensation	A wisp of cotton is used as the stimulus. Patients are asked to close their eyes and signify with a word, such as "yes," when they feel a light touch. The examiner lightly touches the skin with the cotton wisp, beginning at the head and working downward. Each side of the body is assessed. Light touch sensation is often preserved when other sensory modalities are compromised in lesions of the spinal cord. This occurs because of an overlap of innervation.
Superficial pain sensation Within a few segments after entering the cord, fibers conveying pain and temperature synapse and cross the midline through the ventral commissure to the opposite lateral spinothalamic tract. This is important to note because there may be dissociation of pain and temperature loss with preservation of the ability to feel light touch.	A pin or other sharp object is used as the stimulus. Care must be taken to prevent injury to the patient. The same systematic procedure is followed as for light touch.
Temperature sensation Note that the tracts conveying pain and temperature both cross to the opposite side of the spinal cord.	Two test tubes, one filled with cold water and the other filled with warm water, are used as stimuli. Alternate: use a cold tuning fork. Following the same procedure as for light touch and pain, the patient is systematically touched and responses are noted.
Deep Sensations	
Sense of motion and position	Passive motion is tested in the upper extremities on the thumb and in the lower extremities on the big toe. The sides of the toe and thumb are lightly grasped by the examiner's index finger and thumb and moved up or down. Note that the thumb and toe should be touched lightly so that the pressure needed to move the appendage is not apparent to the patient. As the examiner moves the thumb and toe, the patient is asked to identify the direction of movement (up or down).
Deep pain	The Achilles tendon, calf, and forearm muscle are squeezed on each side of the body. Note the patient's sensitivity to this stimulus.
Vibration sensation	Using a vibrating tuning fork, place the instrument on the bony prominences (thumb and big toe). The patient is instructed to signal when the vibration is first felt and when it is no longer present. Compare the sensitivity of the two sides; compare proximal and distal portions of the same extremity. If abnormality is detected, more extensive testing is conducted.
Cortical discrimination (complex somatic sensations requiring cerebral cortex interpretation) Two-point discrimination	A small pair of calipers or another sharp instrument is used as the stimulus. Alternate: touch patient simultaneously or singularly.
Note: Body areas vary in sensitivity in discriminating simultaneous stimuli	The patient, with eyes closed, is simultaneously touched with two sharp objects and then asked whether he or she is being touched by one or two objects. This testing procedure continues over the surface of the body.
Point localization	The patient's skin is lightly touched at a particular point while his or her eyes are closed and is asked to identify where he or she was touched. Compare each side of the body for response.
Stereognosis	With the eyes closed, common objects, such as a pencil, comb, or coin, are placed in the patient's hand. The patient is then asked to identify the object.
Texture discrimination	With eyes closed, the patient is asked to differentiate between materials of varying textures. Each side of the body is tested and compared.
Traced-figure identification	The examiner traces a number or letter on the patient's palm, back, or other part of the body with his or her finger or an applicator stick; the patient is asked to identify the figure traced. Each side of the body is tested.
Double simultaneous stimulation (extinction)	Two corresponding body parts are touched simultaneously. The patient is asked to identify the area touched. The examiner notes whether the patient is aware of being touched on both sides.

or both. Sometimes the cause of the coma is obvious (cerebral trauma), and other times it is not (e.g., drug toxicity).

The examiner should think about the underlying cause and pathophysiology. Consciousness has two components, arousal and awareness. Arousal is a state of wakefulness due to activation of the reticular activating system (RAS). The RAS is a diffuse neuronal network located in the cerebral hemispheres and upper portion of the brainstem. Awareness includes self-awareness and cognitive function. Arousal must be intact for awareness to be apparent.

A **supratentorial lesion** (i.e., cerebral hemispheric lesion) that progresses to coma is the result of a *mass effect* of the lesion that expands and affects the bilateral hemisphere and then produces pressure on the rostral brainstem (location of a portion of the RAS). It begins with *asymmetric* signs and symptoms such as a monoplegia or aphasia. As the pathologic

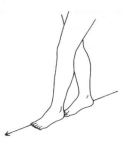

Figure 6-16 • Assessment of cerebellar function. The integrity of the cerebellum can be tested by having the patient walk heel to toe along a line (tandem gait). With cerebellar hemispheric involvement, the patient often falls toward the side of the lesion, and there is ataxia. With midline cerebellar dysfunction, the gait is wide-based and tandem gait walking cannot be performed. (From Weber, J. [1992]. *Nurse's handbook of health assessment* [2nd ed.]. Philadelphia: J. B. Lippincott.)

process proceeds to coma, a rostral-caudal pattern occurs; that is, dysfunction of the hemispheres, then thalamus, then midbrain, then pons, and finally the medulla occurs. An **infratentorial lesion** (i.e., a primary lesion in the brainstem) affects the RAS directly. Coma occurs without the rostral-caudal pattern of dysfunction. Infratentorial lesions are much less common than supratentorial lesions. In **metabolic conditions,** the brain is affected diffusely through the blood-

stream. The progressive rostral-caudal pattern does not occur; instead, *symmetric* deficits are seen.

Components of the Neurological Examination for a Comatose Patient

The neurological examination of a comatose patient is limited because of the patient's inability to participate in the examination actively. However, a good profile of the nervous system can be constructed by observing the patient and collecting focused data. The purpose of the examination is refocused to identify symmetric and asymmetric deficits that will help in determining the underlying problem. The following outlines the areas addressed in the neurological examination:

- Past medical history
- Review of general parameters (e.g., skin, scalp, mouth odor, ears)
- Vital signs, including respiratory pattern
- Level of consciousness
- Pupillary size and response to light
- Eyelids, gaze, and extraocular movement
- Facial symmetry
- Other reflexes (corneal, gag, swallowing reflexes)
- Motor tone and response to pain

CHART 6-3   Evaluation of Muscle-Stretch Reflexes

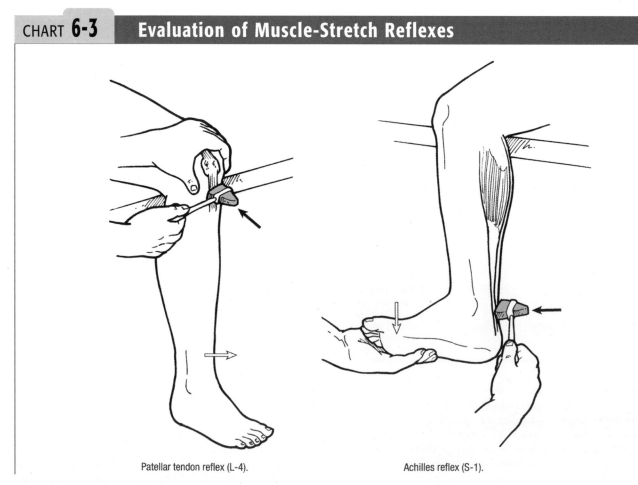

Patellar tendon reflex (L-4).   Achilles reflex (S-1).

(continued)

CHART **6-3**   Evaluation of Muscle-Stretch Reflexes   (Continued)

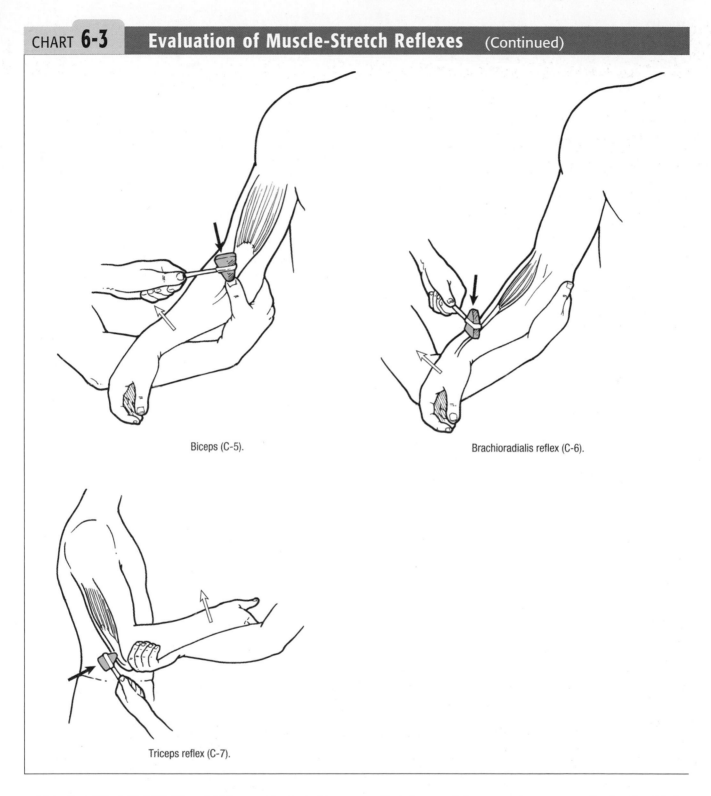

Biceps (C-5).

Brachioradialis reflex (C-6).

Triceps reflex (C-7).

Note that CNs I, II, VIII, XI, and XII cannot be tested in a comatose patient. Only components of the other cranial nerves can be tested in a comatose patient. The past medical history provided by a family member, if present, may be helpful in suggesting the underlying cause of coma in a non-trauma patient. For example, a history of diabetes mellitus or drug or alcohol use could be related to the current problem. Knowledge of the circumstances related to the onset of coma as well as length of coma is important.

Begin by examining general components. Look at the skin for color, evidence of a bleeding disorder, needle marks, or bruises. Check the scalp for possible fracture of boggy areas suggestive of trauma. Note the odor from the mouth and any drainage from the nose or mouth. The ears are examined with an otoscope for evidence of trauma, infection, or drainage. Next, assess the vital signs (see Chap. 7 for a discussion of vital signs).

Now move from the general to the specifics of a neurological function. Take a few minutes to look at the patient lying

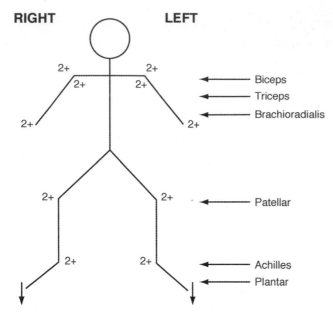

Figure 6-17 • Alternative method of recording the commonly tested muscle-stretch reflexes.

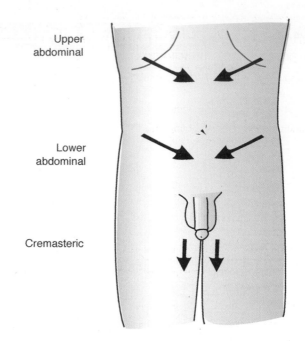

Figure 6-18 • The abdominal and cremasteric reflexes. Test the abdominal reflexes by lightly but briskly stroking each side of the abdomen and below the umbilicus in the direction illustrated. Use a key or a tongue blade to stroke the skin. Note the contraction of the abdominal muscles and the deviation of the umbilicus toward the stimulus. Obesity may mask an abdominal reflex. In this situation, use your finger to retract the patient's umbilicus away from the side to be stimulated. Feel with your retracting finger for the muscular contraction. Not routinely done. If tested the cremasteric reflex is assessed by lightly scratching the inner aspect of the upper thigh. Note the elevation of the testicle on that side. Abdominal and cremasteric reflexes may be absent in both upper and lower motor neuron disorders. (From Bates, B. [1983]. *Guide to physical examination* [3rd ed.]. Philadelphia: J. B. Lippincott.)

in the bed. Note the predominant position of the extremities, position of the head and neck, presence of spontaneous movement, and the position of the eye when the lids are opened.

Level of Consciousness

The *depth* of the coma is important to ascertain. This is done by providing a verbal stimulus (calling the patient's name or clapping your hands loudly over the patient's head) and observing the response. If there is no response, a noxious

TABLE 6–21   MAJOR SUPERFICIAL (CUTANEOUS) REFLEXES

REFLEX	INNERVATION	TEST
Corneal	CNs V, VII	Touch cornea lightly with a wisp of cotton; lids should quickly close.
Gag	CNs IX, X	Stimulate the back of the pharynx with a tongue depressor; a retching or gagging response should be elicited.
Swallowing	CNs IX, X	Stimulate one side of the uvula with a cotton applicator; the uvula should elevate.
Upper abdominals	T-8–T-10	Stroke the outer abdomen toward the umbilicus using a tongue blade; the umbilicus should move up and toward the area being stroked (see Fig. 6–18).
Lower abdominals	T-10–T-12	Stroke the lower abdomen toward the umbilicus using a tongue blade; the umbilicus should move down and toward the area being stroked (see Fig. 6–18).
Cremasteric (male)	L-1–L-2	Lightly stroke the inner aspect of the thigh or lower abdomen; elevation of the ipsilateral testicle should occur (see Fig. 6–18).
Bulbocavernous (male)	S-3–S-4	Apply direct pressure over the bulbocavernous muscle behind the scrotum, or pinch the glans penis; the muscle should contract, raising the scrotum toward the body.
Perianal	S-3, S-4, S-5	Scratch the tissue at the side of the anus with a blunt instrument; there should be a puckering of the anus. Additionally, if a gloved finger is inserted into the rectum, a contraction should be felt.

CN, cranial nerve.

TABLE 6–22 PATHOLOGIC (PRIMITIVE) REFLEXES

REFLEX	DESCRIPTION	ASSOCIATED CONDITIONS
Grasp reflex	Palmar stimulation results in a grasp response.	Most common in association with dementia and diffuse or bifrontal brain impairment
Snout reflex	Puckering of lips in response to gentle percussion in the oral region	As above
Sucking reflex	Sucking movement of the lips in response to light touching, striking, or tapping on the lips, stroking the tongue, or stimulating the palate. Note: may be noticed when the patient is being suctioned or when mouth care is given	As above
Rooting reflex	Stimulation of the lips results in deviating the head toward the stimuli	As above
Palmomental reflex	Ipsilateral contraction of the chin (mentalis and perioral muscles) following a scratching stimulation of the palm (thenar area) of the hand	May be found in unaffected people, but common in dementia
Glabellar reflex (Myerson's sign)	Blinking eyes each time the glabellar area between the eyes is tapped. Normally, the patient blinks only the first few times tapping is initiated.	Seen in Parkinsonism

stimulus is provided by putting pressure on a nail bed of the hand or pinching the muscles of the shoulders.

Pupillary Response

Pupillary size and response to direct light are evaluated. Normally, pupils are 3 to 4 mm in diameter (smaller in the elderly) and are equal in size and reaction to light. See Chapter 7 for a discussion of pupillary responses and size.

Eyelashes, Eyelids, Gaze, and Ocular Movement

Spontaneous blinking, then loss of blink in response to touching of the eyelashes, and finally the loss of the corneal reflex (see page 150) are among the most dependable signs of deepening coma. Observe and stimulate the eyelashes. Raise the eyelids, release them, and observe. In coma, the eyelids close slowly once they are released; in the absence of coma, the lids will close rapidly.

Look at the eyes (with lids held open) for spontaneous movement. **Roving-eye movement** is characterized by spontaneous, slow, and random deviation. It is seen in comatose patients with intact brainstem oculomotor function. Absence of roving-eye movement indicates brainstem dysfunction. Next, look at the eyes for position in the head or a gaze preference. Lesions in the cortex or brainstem above the level of the ocular motor nuclei may impair conjugate movement of the eyes, thus producing one of the following gaze disorders:

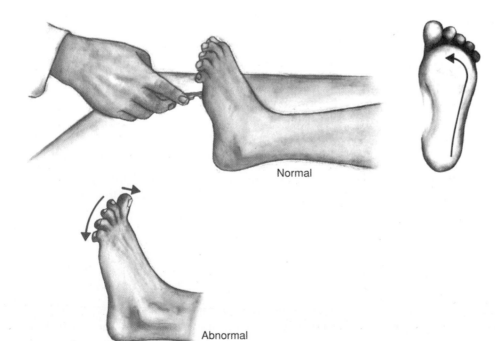

Normal

Abnormal

Figure 6-19 • Babinski reflex. With a blunt object, such as a key, stroke the lateral aspect of the sole from the heel to the ball of the foot, curving medially across the ball. Use the lightest stimulus that will provoke a response. Note any movement of the toes, normally flexion. Dorsiflexion of the great toe, with fanning of the other toes, indicates upper motor neuron disease.

Cranial Nerve Paralysis

- A slight downward deviation of one eye suggests an oculomotor nerve (CN III) palsy, whereas a medial deviation of one eye suggests an abducens (CN VI) palsy.
- When considering abnormalities of eye movement, differentiate between pontine and frontal gaze palsy.

Hemispheric Lesions (Involve Frontal Gaze Center)

- With a large, acute **hemispheric lesion**, both **eyes deviate toward the side of the lesion** and away from the hemiparesis. The palsy is usually temporary and tends to resolve in minutes to hours.
- Seizure discharges involving the frontal gaze centers can result in gaze deviation, so that both **eyes deviate away from** the discharging focus. This may last several days.

Pontine Lesions (Horizontal Gaze Disorders From Lesion at Pontine Gaze Centers)

- **Pontine gaze palsies** are usually bilateral and cause eye **deviation away from the side of the lesion** and toward the hemiplegia; the gaze palsy lasts much longer than frontal gaze palsies.
- Pontine gaze palsies are caused by infarcts, hemorrhages, gliomas, abscesses, Wernicke's encephalopathy, and multiple sclerosis.

Midbrain Lesion (Upward Gaze Disorders)

- Lesions of the dorsal midbrain affect the center for voluntary upward gaze and may therefore produce upward gaze paralysis.
- **Parinaud's syndrome** includes upward gaze paralysis, nystagmus on downward gaze, paralysis of accommodation, midposition pupils, and light-near dissociation.

In the comatose patient, eye movement is tested by stimulating the vestibular system (semicircular canals of the middle ear) by passive head movement or by ice-water irrigation against the tympanic membrane. These tests are usually performed by the physician. Before moving the patient's neck, be sure that there is no possibility of the existence of a cervical fracture or injury. The **oculocephalic reflex (doll's eye movement)** is elicited by briskly turning the head horizontally from side to side or vertically up and down while holding the eyelids open (Fig. 6-20). Moving the head side to side tests CNs III and VI. Moving the head up and down tests only CN III. If the reflex is intact, the eyes move conjugately in the opposite direction to the head movement. (Note that this reflex is not present in the normal, alert person.) If present, the oculocephalic reflex verifies intact brainstem gaze centers, the medial longitudinal fasciculus, and ocular motor nerves. If the reflex is absent, the eyes follow the direction of the head movement. Absence of the reflex indicates severe brainstem dysfunction from the pons to the midbrain level. If the eyes do not move, it is a poor prognostic sign and the patient probably will not regain consciousness.

Oculovestibular or Cold Caloric Testing

If the oculocephalic response is inconclusive, the **oculovestibular reflex (caloric)** can be assessed (Fig. 6-21). This is a more sensitive test of brainstem function. Before testing, the ear is examined to be sure that there is no perforation of the tympanic membrane, an absolute contraindication to proceeding. Additionally, any major wax deposit in the ear should be removed. Raise the patient's head 30 degrees. In the comatose patient, unilateral irrigation with at least 30 to 50 mL of cold water (33°C) over 30 seconds results in slow eye deviation toward the irrigated ear if the brainstem is intact. Wait at least 5 minutes before testing the other side. Using cold irrigant is the most common method of testing the oculovestibular reflex.

There are other ways of assessing vestibular function. Bilateral irrigation with warm water (44°C) can also be used. If the brainstem is intact, the eyes deviate away from the side of the irrigation. Another possibility is simultaneous bilateral irrigation. Bilateral irrigation with cold water causes downward deviation of the eyes; bilateral irrigation with warm water induces upward deviation if the brainstem is intact. The response can be remembered by the mnemonic **COWS** (**C**old **O**pposite **W**arm **S**ame).

The importance of the oculocephalic and oculovestibular reflexes is that their presence or absence provides important information on brainstem function that is useful to determine the depth of coma and to predict patient outcome. Full reflex eye movement in the comatose patient is solid evidence of an intact brainstem from the pons to the midbrain level and excludes a mass lesion in the brainstem. The oculovestibular reflex is used as part of the criteria for determining death.

The following are a few abnormal patterns noted in unilateral cold water oculovestibular testing:

- Lesion of the oculomotor nerve or nucleus (e.g., rostralcaudal herniation): there is no movement toward the side of irrigation on the affected side with unimpaired contralateral abduction.
- Downward deviation of one or both eyes is suggestive of sedative drug intoxication.

Facial Symmetry

Observe for facial symmetry when the patient is at rest and stimulated. Loss of nasolabial fold or weakness of one side of the mouth may be noted with hemiplegia.

Other Reflexes

The corneal and gag reflexes are two other important brainstem reflexes to assess. These cutaneous reflexes are tested by lightly touching the cornea and mucous membrane. A wisp of cotton from an applicator is used to stimulate the cornea. A complete response is a brisk and immediate blinking of the eye. The response may also be diminished or absent. Assess each eye for response. Asymmetry in corneal responses indicates either an acute lesion of the opposite hemisphere or an ipsilateral lesion in the brainstem. Note that wearers of contact lens may have this reflex abolished. Loss of the corneal reflex is due to a lesion affecting CNs V and VII.

In an intubated patient, the gag and swallowing reflex can be tested by tugging gently on the endotracheal tube. If the reflex is intact, the patient will gag or cough. In a nonintubated patient, the gag reflex can be tested by sequentially

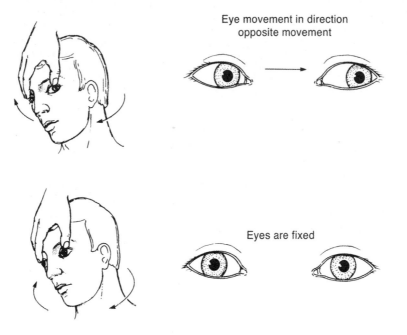

Assessment Technique for the Oculocephalic Reflex

1. Briskly rotate the head from side to side, or
2. Briskly flex and extend the neck.

Eye movement in direction opposite movement

Eyes are fixed

Findings

• When the head is rotated, the eyes should move in the direction opposite to the head movement *(top)*. (If the head is rotated to the left, the eyes appear to move to the right.) Alternative method: When the neck is flexed, the eyes appear to look upward; when the neck is extended, the eyes look downward.
• When the doll's eye reflex is absent, the eyes do not move in the sockets and thus follow the direction of passive rotation. Loss of the oculocephalic reflex in the comatose patient indicates a lesion at the pontine–midbrain level of the brainstem.

Figure 6-20 • Oculocephalic reflex. Eye movement in the unconscious patient can be assessed by the physician by means of the oculocephalic response (doll's eye phenomenon). In the presence or suspicion of a cervical fracture or dislocation, this test is contraindicated. (*Note:* If the presence of the oculocephalic reflex is questioned or the conduction of the test is contraindicated, the oculovestibular reflex is tested. In many hospital emergency departments, the oculovestibular reflex is tested more often than the oculocephalic reflex unless there are contraindications.)

stimulating *each side* of the posterior pharynx with a tongue blade or a cotton-tipped applicator. An immediate gag response is noted if the reflex is intact. Abnormal findings include a diminished or absent gag reflex and indicate a lesion involving CNs IX and X.

Deep tendon reflexes and the plantar response (Babinski's sign) are included. See previous sections of this chapter for discussion and Figure 6-19.

Motor Tone and Response to Pain

In the comatose patient, the examiner relies on observing predominant posture, muscle tone, and response to painful stimuli. Note any abnormal posturing (decorticate or decerebrate) as the patient lies in bed (see Chap. 7 for discussion). To assess muscle tone, grasp each forearm a few inches above the wrist and raise the arm to a vertical position. The hand is flexed at almost a right angle in a comatose patient. Lower the arm to

12 to 18 inches from the bed and release the arm. A flaccid arm drops rapidly and flails in a comatose patient, compared with a slow descent in a noncomatose patient. To assess the legs, flex both legs so that both heels rest on the bed. Release the legs at the knees. In acute hemiplegia, the flaccid leg drops rapidly and externally rotates at the hip, and the leg extends. A normal leg slowly extends to its original position.

Next, a painful, central stimulus is provided by pinching the trapezius or pectoralis major muscles of the neck or by applying firm pressure to the supraorbital area. Pressure on the nail beds may also be used, but because it is peripheral stimulation, some suggest that it may not be as reliable as central stimulation. Possible responses to painful stimuli are:

• Purposeful: localization/push the painful stimuli away
• Nonpurposeful: movement of the stimulated area, but no attempt to push the stimuli away
• No response: no reaction to painful stimuli

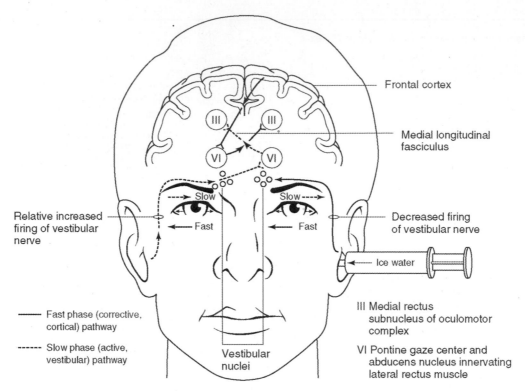

Figure 6-21 • Physiology of the oculovestibular reflex (cold calorics). Infusion of ice water into the ear of a comatose patient will elicit the oculovestibular reflex if both the cerebral hemisphere and brainstem are intact. With an intact brainstem, a signal passes through pathways from the medulla to the midbrain, generating a slow movement of the eyes to the side of the ice-water infusion. This is followed by a rapid corrective movement of the eyes, generated by an intact ipsilateral side of the cerebral hemisphere. The ice-water infusion test can be repeated in the other ear of the comatose patient to test the integrity of the other side of the brainstem.

In considering depth of coma on a continuum for prognostic purposes and change over time, a purposeful response suggests moderate severity, a promising response. Abnormal posturing may also be noted. Decortication is associated with a direct lesion of the thalamus or a large hemispheric mass that compresses the thalamus. Decerebration suggests midbrain dysfunction, which is an upper brainstem structure, and is thus considered more ominous than decortication. Finally, flaccid paralysis is seen in the final stages of cerebral demise.

Posturing may follow several patterns. Bilateral symmetric posturing is seen in both structural and metabolic disorders. Asymmetric posturing suggests a disorder in the contralateral cerebral hemisphere or brainstem.

Reflexes

Deep tendon reflexes, some cutaneous reflexes, and some pathologic reflexes can be tested. The cutaneous reflexes evaluated include the corneal and gag reflexes (see earlier discussion). The patient is also examined for presence of Babinski's reflex (see Fig. 6-19). Table 6-21 provides the most common primitive reflexes, especially the grasping, sucking, and rooting reflexes. Note also triple flexion in the section on pathologic reflexes found earlier in this chapter.

SUMMARY

The neurological physical examination is the foundation for diagnosis of neurological problems and results in a comprehensive assessment of neurological function through an organized and systematic approach. Regardless of whether the patient is fully alert and interactive or comatose, the examiner must be competent in implementing the appropriate technique for testing each function and be confident about findings. Knowledge of neurological anatomy, physiology, pathophysiology, and patterns of signs and symptoms helps to localize dysfunction and is the foundation for diagnostic reasoning skills. Based on the findings of the neurological examination, the examiner determines the need for additional diagnostic investigations that lead to a working diagnosis and a comprehensive treatment plan.

REFERENCES

1. Campbell, W. W. (2005). *DeJong's the neurological examination* (6th ed., pp. 19–36). Philadelphia: Lippincott Williams & Wilkins.
2. Strub, R. L., & Black, F. W. (2000). *The mental status: Examination in neurology* (4th ed., p. 47). Philadelphia: F. A. Davis.
3. Campbell, W. W. (2005). *DeJong's the neurological examination* (6th ed., pp. 114–115). Philadelphia: Lippincott Williams & Wilkins.
4. Fuller, G. (2000). *Neurological examination made easy* (2nd ed., p. 98). New York: Churchill Livingstone.

RESOURCES

Books

Bickley, L. A., & Szilagyi, P. G. (2005). *Bates' guide to physical examination and history taking* (9th ed.). Philadelphia: Lippincott Williams & Wilkins.

Blumenfeld, H. *Neuroanatomy through clinical cases.* Sunderland, MA: Sinauer Associates, Inc.

Brazis, P. W., Masdeu, J. C., Biller, J., & Brazis, P. (2001). *Localization in clinical neurology* (4th ed.). Boston: Little Brown & Co.

Campbell, W. W. (2005). *DeJong's the neurologic examination* (6th ed.). Philadelphia: Lippincott Williams & Wilkins.

DeMyer, W. E. (2004). *Techniques of the neurological examination* (5th ed.). New York: McGraw Hill.

Fuller, G. (2000). *Neurologic examination made easy* (2nd ed.). New York: Churchill Livingstone.

Goetz, C. G. (2003). *Textbook of clinical neurology* (3rd ed.). Philadelphia: W. B. Saunders.

The Guarantors of Brain. (2000). *Aids to the examination of the peripheral nervous system* (4th ed.). Philadelphia: W. B. Saunders.

Hoppenfeld, S. (1976). *Physical examination of the spine and extremities.* Norwalk, CT: Appleton & Lange.

Hoppenfeld, S. (1977). *Orthopaedic neurology: A diagnostic guide to neurologic levels.* Philadelphia: J. B. Lippincott.

LeBlond, R. L., DeGowin, R. L., & Brown, D. D. (2004). *DeGowin's diagnostic examination* (8th ed.). New York: McGraw-Hill.

Lezak, M. D. (2004). *Neuropsychological assessment* (4th ed.). New York: Oxford University Press.

Members of the Mayo Clinic Department of Neurology. (1998). *Mayo clinic examinations in neurology* (7th ed.). St. Louis, MO: Mosby.

Miller, N. R., Newman, N. J, Biousse, V., & Kerrison, J. B. (2004). *Walsh & Hoyt's clinical neuro-ophthalmology—the essentials* (6th ed.). Philadelphia: Lippincott Williams & Wilkins.

Patton, J. P. (1998). *Neurological differential diagnosis* (2nd ed.). New York: Springer.

Ropper, A. H., & Brown, R. H. (2005). *Adams and Victor's principles of neurology* (8th ed.). New York: McGraw Hill.

Strub, R. L., & Black, F. W. (2000). *The mental status examination in neurology* (4th ed.). Philadelphia: F. A. Davis Co.

Tasman, A., & First, M. B. (2004). *DSM-IV-TR mental disorders: Diagnosis, etiology, and treatment.* Hoboken, NJ: Wiley.

Young, G. B., Ropper, A. H., & Bolton, C. F. (1997). *Coma and impaired consciousness: A clinical perspective.* New York: McGraw Hill.

Journal Articles

Bronstein, A. M. (2003). Vestibular reflexes and positional manoeuvres. *Journal of Neurology, Neurosurgery, & Psychiatry, 74,* 289–293.

Dick, J. P. R. (2003). The deep tendon and the abdominal reflexes. *Journal of Neurology, Neurosurgery, & Psychiatry, 74,* 150–153.

Larner, A. J. (2003). False localizing signs. *Journal of Neurology, Neurosurgery, & Psychiatry, 74,* 415–418.

Schott, J. M., & Rossor, M. N. (2003). The grasp and other primitive reflexes. *Journal of Neurology, Neurosurgery, & Psychiatry, 74,* 558–560.

Electronic Resources

Gelb, D. (2004). The detailed neurological examination. UpToDate.

Oommen, H. J. (2005). Neurological history and physical examination. http://www.emedicine.com/neuro/index.shtml.

Neurological Assessment

Joanne V. Hickey

The purposes of this chapter are (1) to provide an overview for establishing and updating a database for a hospitalized neuroscience patient, and (2) to provide a framework for understanding the purpose, organization, and interpretation of data from the systematic neurological assessment conducted at the bedside. Some content that appears in Chapter 6 has also been included in this chapter for the convenience of the reader.

ESTABLISHING A NURSING DATABASE

On admission of a patient, the nurse begins to collect a comprehensive database by completing a nursing admission history and general admission assessment before conducting a neurological assessment. Most nursing departments have adopted a specific format for this purpose as part of their documentation system. The data may be entered in a written format or typed into a computerized documentation system. Regardless of how the data are entered or stored, the database is the foundation for ongoing assessment, planning, implementation, and evaluation of care and outcomes. The database is key to maintain continuity of care across levels of care through discharge and follow-up.

One section of the database includes demographics, route and circumstances of admission, vital signs, weight, and other general information (e.g., eyeglasses, hearing aid). The largest section includes a comprehensive systematic assessment often based on body systems or functional patterns. The circumstances of admission affect data collection. Ideally, the nurse has an opportunity to interview the patient and family on admission. The interview is not only a mechanism for gathering data and dispensing information, but also an opportunity to establish rapport with the patient and family.

Throughout the interview, the nurse should be alert for any misconceptions or misunderstandings held by the patient or family. Information should be corrected and clarified as necessary and appropriate referrals made. Identify high-risk patients and families who have problems that will affect recovery negatively, such as drug abuse or family dysfunction. Early identification can result in timely interventions and referrals.

For a patient with altered consciousness or cognitive deficits, enlist a family member to help you learn about the patient's personality and behavior before the current illness.

This baseline information is useful for future comparison throughout the course of hospitalization. In the event of an emergency admission, some data gathering will be postponed until the patient is stabilized or family can be reached. As soon as possible, the nurse should interview the patient and family to develop a plan of care. If care maps are used, the appropriate care map should be reviewed and modified as necessary.

The neurological assessment is the core nursing database for identifying nursing diagnoses and collaborative problems and for planning care. The accuracy of these assessment data and the nurse's critical thinking skills form the foundation of neuroscience nursing practice.

The taxonomy of nursing diagnoses may be a helpful framework to use when analyzing data from neurological assessment. However, there are many collaborative problems that require an interdisciplinary collaborative approach. For example, *increased intracranial pressure* (ICP) is a problem that requires collaboration of the entire health care team. A patient with increased ICP will require supportive and restorative care, along with definitive treatment for the underlying cause. Nurses participate as collaborative team members with physicians, physical therapists, occupational therapists, speech therapists, physiatrists, nutritionists, and social workers to address the comprehensive patient needs. Care includes various supportive, preventive, maintenance, and restorative strategies. Examples of collaborative problems include safety measures to prevent falls and injury, prevention of the complications of immobility, adaptation of activities of daily living (ADLs), maintenance of a patent airway, maintenance of adequate blood pressure, and nutritional-hydration support.

OVERVIEW OF NEUROLOGICAL ASSESSMENT

Purposes

The purposes of the care nurse's neurological assessment are different, in some respects, from those conducted by the physician, the advanced practice nurse, and other health care professionals. The care nurse's purposes are to:

- Establish a neurological database
- Identify the presence of nervous system dysfunction
- Determine the effects of nervous system dysfunction on ADLs and independent function

- Detect life-threatening situations
- Compare current data to previous assessment data to determine trends and need for change in interventions
- Provide a database on which nursing diagnoses and collaborative problems will be based

A baseline assessment of neurological signs is made to determine deviations and trends in clinical status. A comparison is made between current assessment data and previously collected data to determine whether neurological signs are stable, deteriorating, or improving. Changes in neurological signs may develop rapidly in a few minutes, or subtly over a period of hours, days, weeks, or even months. There are various sources from which information about the neurological status can be derived, including the nursing admission history and comprehensive assessment, nurses' notes, neurological assessment sheets, and intershift nurses' reports. Other parts of the medical record are also a rich source of data (e.g., comprehensive neurological examination) and should be reviewed.

Nursing management of the neurological patient is based on highly developed nursing assessment and clinical reasoning skills. The nurse must know which parameters to assess, the proper technique for assessment, the appropriate method of documentation, and how to interpret the data to decide what action, if any, should be taken.

In analyzing data from the neurological assessment, the following questions should be asked:

- What do I see?
- What does it mean?
- How does it relate to previous assessments?
- How am I going to proceed?

The third question, "How does it relate to previous assessments?" is critical because data are compared with the previous baseline assessments as well as trends of multiple data points over time to denote change. The assessment can reveal no change, subtle change, or dramatic change from previous findings. Generally, a change of any kind is important to note because it usually reflects an intracranial change.

A change in any of the data included in the neurological assessment must be considered in conjunction with changes in other areas evaluated in the assessment. For instance, a rapidly developing hematoma or cerebral edema will affect multiple assessment data, such as the level of consciousness (LOC) and motor function. If, however, the pupil appears to be dilated and fixed (a new finding from the previous assessment) and the patient continues to be well oriented and maintains motor function, then the pupillary signs should be rechecked and other possible explanations explored.

Critical thinking skills are inherent in the assessment process, both to detect subtle and substantive changes in the neurological assessment data and overall clinical condition, and to incorporate this information within the context of the overall patient profile. Well-developed critical thinking skills are the foundation for all patient management decision making.

Components of the Neurological Assessment

The components included in a neurological assessment depend on the patient's state of consciousness and coopera-tiveness as well as clinical stability. A comprehensive baseline must be established. A **neurological assessment** is focused on selected critical components that are sensitive to change and that provide an overview of the patient's overall condition. The nurse must decide what other components, if any, should be added to best monitor the patient's condition. An assessment in the intensive care unit for an unconscious patient is quite different from the assessment in an intermediate care unit for a patient who is recovering from a stroke. This neurological assessment at a minimum includes:

- LOC (orientation and cognition)
- Pupillary signs
- Motor strength of extremities (e.g., arms, hand grasps, pronator drift, legs, feet)

FREQUENCY OF ASSESSMENT AND DOCUMENTATION

The frequency and extent of the neurological assessment will depend on the stability of the patient and the underlying condition. For a stable patient who is doing well, an assessment may be ordered by the physician every 4 to 8 hours. However, a patient who is very unstable may warrant assessment every 5 to 15 minutes to monitor changes and the need for or response to an intervention. The nurse should use independent clinical judgment to determine the need to assess the patient more frequently or to expand the assessment to include more parameters. A physician order is not required to assess the patient more frequently than what might be included on the physician order sheet or unit standard because assessment is within the nurse's scope of practice.

Most facilities use a standardized neurological assessment form or computerized assessment template to document neurological data. It may be necessary to add a narrative description to expand on the data recorded or to add other pertinent information to the data set. Most forms or computer documentation systems allow for these important additional entries.

CONCEPT OF CONSCIOUSNESS

Consciousness is a state of general awareness of oneself and the environment and includes the ability to be oriented to time, place, and person. It results from a diffuse yet organized neuronal system located in the brainstem, diencephalon, and cerebral hemispheres.

Consciousness is multifaceted and divided into two components:

- **Alertness** or **wakefulness:** the appearance of wakefulness; reflects activity of the reticular activating system
- **Awareness** or **cognition:** content of cognitive mental functions; reflects cerebral cortex activity

Awareness or cognition is largely a cerebral cortical function, whereas alertness requires both the cerebral hemispheres and the brainstem. Consciousness can be viewed as analogous

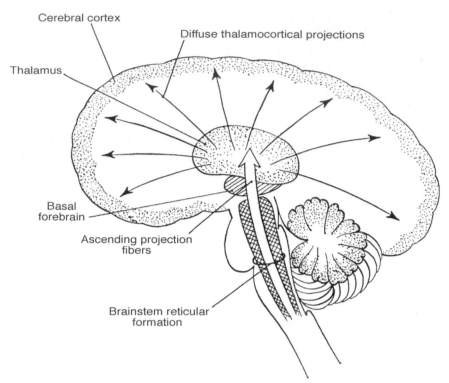

Figure 7-1 • Lateral view of the brain showing the components of the consciousness system.

to a double helix. The difficulties inherent in assessing altered consciousness and underlying pathologic states, then, can be compared to the difficulty of trying to separate the strands of a double helix into distinct entities. As a result, consciousness terminology and concepts tend to be somewhat vague. For example, the level of alertness is described by terms such as *clouding of consciousness, drowsiness, obtundation, stupor,* or *coma,* and is assessed by evaluating the content of consciousness, especially as represented by the quality of the patient's perception of self and the environment. Because consciousness cannot be measured directly, it is estimated by observing behavioral indicators in response to stimuli. *Consciousness is the most sensitive indicator of neurological change*; as such, a change in the LOC is usually the first sign to be noted in neurological signs when the brain is compromised. This is true because the brain is sensitive to slight hypoxia or change in adequate blood supply. Consciousness is a dynamic state that is subject to change; it can occur rapidly (within minutes) or very slowly, over a period of hours, days, or weeks. When an assessment is conducted, the patient's alertness and behavior merely provide an estimate of consciousness *at a given point in time.*

> **CLINICAL PEARLS:** Consciousness is the earliest and most sensitive indicator of neurological change, and is usually the first sign to be noted in neurological signs when the brain is compromised.

Anatomic and Physiologic Basis of Consciousness

A centrally positioned neuronal system located in the brainstem, diencephalon, and cerebral hemispheres (i.e., from brainstem to cerebral cortex) controls consciousness. This system includes portions of the brainstem reticular formation; neurochemically defined nuclear groups of the brainstem; thalamic nuclei; basal forebrain (portions of the ventral and medial cerebral hemispheres); ascending projections to the thalamus and cerebral cortex; and widespread areas of the cerebral cortex (Fig. 7-1).

The **reticular formation** (RF) is a complex network of nuclei and nerve fibers in the central portion of the brainstem, extending from the pyramidal decussation in the medulla to the basal forebrain area and thalamus. The term *reticular* means forming a network. The long radiating dendrites and axons have numerous collaterals that project for long distances centrally with many interconnections and afferent input from various sensory and motor sources.[1] The **reticular activating system** (RAS) is a part of the RF. The multiple ascending pathways, channeled through the RF, receive synaptic input from multiple sensory pathways and send sensory impulses to the thalamus and then to all parts of the cerebral cortex. These impulses, sent to different parts of the cerebral cortex, cause a sleeping person to awaken. Ongoing impulses keep a person alert and awake.

Alterations in Consciousness

Degree of Dysfunction

Alteration of LOC can vary in severity from slight to severe. An altered LOC indicates brain dysfunction or brain failure. The longer the duration and the more severe the dysfunction, the poorer the prognosis is for a complete recovery. LOC can change rapidly, as in association with an epidural hematoma, or very slowly over a period of weeks, as noted with a chronic subdural hematoma.

Major Causes

Alterations in the LOC may occur because of:

- Direct destruction of the anatomic structures of consciousness by a disease process (structural)
- Toxic effects of endogenous or exogenous substances on the structures (metabolic)
- Alterations in the energy substrates necessary for function of the anatomic structures involved in consciousness (e.g., seizures, cerebral edema)

Specifically, use the mnemonics "A-E-I-O-U" and "TIPSS" to recall the major causes of altered consciousness. **A-E-I-O-U** stands for **a**lcohol, **e**pilepsy, **i**nsulin, **o**pium, and **u**remia, whereas **TIPSS** stands for **t**umor, **i**njury, **p**sychiatric, **s**troke, and **s**epsis. A psychiatric cause should be considered only after all other possibilities have been ruled out.[2]

Coma

Various states of altered LOC are discussed in this chapter. However, a few points should be made about coma. Coma is the result of (1) bilateral, diffuse cerebral hemispheric dysfunction; (2) involvement of the brainstem (midbrain and pons, which includes the RAS); or (3) both. A focal hemispheric lesion (e.g., small brain tumor) will not result in coma; only diffuse hemispheric conditions (e.g., diffuse cerebral edema) result in coma. Coma is not a disease itself, but reflects some underlying disease processes involving either (1) primary problems with the central nervous system (CNS) or (2) metabolic or systemic conditions. The following is a summary of the major causes of altered consciousness.[3]

CLINICAL PEARLS: Coma is the result of bilateral, diffuse cerebral hemispheric dysfunction, involvement of the brainstem (midbrain and pons, which includes the RAS), or both.

Supratentorial Lesions. A lesion must affect the cerebral hemispheres **directly and widely** to cause diffuse bilateral cerebral hemispheric dysfunction and subsequent coma. Common lesions and associated secondary cerebral edema that can have diffuse effects on the brain include subcortical destructive lesions such as a thalamic lesion, hemorrhagic lesions (intracerebral, epidural, subdural hematomas), infarctions, tumors, abscesses, and cerebral injuries.

Subtentorial (Infratentorial) Lesions. Subtentorial lesions **directly compress or destroy** the neurons of the RAS that lie in the central gray matter of the diencephalon, midbrain, and upper pons. Common compression lesions and associated secondary cerebral edema include basilar artery aneurysms, cerebellar or brainstem hemorrhage, abscess, tumor, or infarction. Common destructive lesions include pontine hemorrhage and brainstem infarction.

Metabolic Disorders. Altered consciousness may also be attributable to metabolic causes and systemic disease, such as deprivation of oxygen and other key metabolic requirements (hypoxia, ischemia hypoglycemia, or vitamin deficiency). It may also be caused by disease of organs excluding the brain, such as the following:

- Nonendocrine organs
  - Kidney (uremic coma)
  - Liver (hepatic coma)
  - Lungs (carbon dioxide narcosis)
- Hypofunction or hyperfunction of endocrine organs
  - Thyroid (myxedema and thyrotoxicosis)
  - Parathyroid (hypoparathyroidism and hyperparathyroidism)
  - Adrenals (Addison's disease, Cushing's disease, pheochromocytoma)
  - Pancreas (diabetes mellitus and hypoglycemia)
- Electrolyte and acid-base imbalance
- Pharmacologic agents
  - Sedatives: barbiturates and nonbarbiturates, hypnotics, tranquilizers, ethanol, opiates, and bromides
  - Acidic toxins: paraldehyde, methyl alcohol, ethylene glycol, and ammonium chloride
  - Psychotropic drugs: amphetamines, lithium, tricyclic antidepressants, and others
  - Other drugs such as steroids, cimetidine, salicylates, and anticonvulsants

The most common metabolic causes of altered LOC seen in a hospitalized population are hypoxia, hypoglycemia, and sedative drug overdose. It is routine practice in most emergency departments to draw blood for glucose levels and toxicology screening, as necessary.

In assessing a comatose patient, the nurse should be aware that several problems outside the CNS can cause a decreased LOC. A comparison of the changes that accompany coma caused by metabolic disorders and those occurring with nervous system structural lesions is summarized in Table 7-1.

TABLE 7–1   COMPARISON OF COMA CAUSED BY METABOLIC AND CENTRAL NERVOUS SYSTEM STRUCTURAL LESIONS

OBSERVATION	METABOLIC COMA	CNS STRUCTURAL COMA
Motor system deficits	Diffuse abnormal motor signs (tremors, myoclonus, and, especially, asterixis); symmetric	Focal abnormal signs that are unilateral; asymmetric
Motor abnormalities	Coma precedes motor abnormalities	Coma follows motor abnormalities
Pupils	Bilaterally reactive	Unilaterally nonreactive, or later, bilaterally nonreactive
Progression of neurological deterioration	Partial dysfunction affects many levels of the CNS while other functions are retained	Orderly rostral-caudal deterioration with supratentorial lesions
Electroencephalogram	Diffusely but not locally slow	May show slowed activity, but will also show abnormal focal areas

CNS, central nervous system

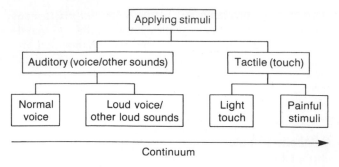

Figure 7-2 • Assessment of consciousness: Applying stimulation.

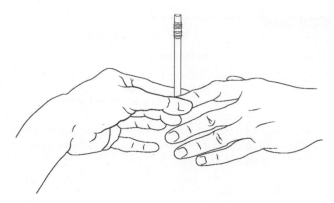

Figure 7-3 • Applying pressure to the fingernails is one kind of stimulus used in assessing the patient's level of consciousness.

Level of Consciousness Assessment

The LOC is assessed by applying stimuli and observing the response. The technique used depends on the type of stimuli applied. Auditory and tactile stimuli are the two used to assess consciousness and are considered on a continuum (Fig. 7-2).

Auditory Stimuli. Sound is the stimulus that is applied first. A normal speaking voice is used initially. If the patient responds, then the nurse can talk to him or her and ask questions to assess orientation and response to questions (discussed in the next section). If the patient does not respond to a normal voice volume, a louder voice or a loud noise, such as that produced by clapping the hands, is used. If a response is elicited, the nurse can then assess orientation by asking questions.

Tactile Stimuli. If there is no response to auditory stimulation, tactile stimulation is attempted. The patient's arm is gently shaken while calling his or her name. If no response is elicited by this means, painful (or noxious) stimuli are applied.

The most common method of applying painful stimuli is to apply firm pressure to the nail beds (fingernails) or web spaces between the fingers or toes and then observe the motor response (Fig. 7-3). However, this provides a peripheral stimulus; the response elicited *could* be a reflex response. A central stimulus, such as firmly grasping the trapezius or pectoralis major muscle, is another method of providing painful stimuli. The response elicited by a central stimulus is more reliable in comatose patients. Some practitioners suggest using the "sternal rub" (vertically rubbing the tissue along the sternum). However, the soft tissue above the sternum bruises easily in most people. Applying supraorbital pressure is another form of stimulus; it is not recommended if a facial fracture is possible. Motor response to painful stimuli is classified according to the following categories:

Purposeful: withdraws from the painful stimuli and crosses midline; may push the examiner's hand away (seen in light coma)

Nonpurposeful: the stimulated area moves slightly, without any attempt to withdraw from the source of pain; painful stimuli to the pectoralis or trapezius may result in a contraction of a muscle or muscles, such as the quadriceps or biceps, but the arm does not cross midline

Unresponsive: patient shows no signs of reacting to painful stimuli (seen in deep coma)

▨IDENTIFYING THE LEVELS OF CONSCIOUSNESS

There is no internationally accepted taxonomy of definitions with which to label LOC, nor is there agreement on the definitive manifestations of the various stages of consciousness. Therefore, no precise terminology exists for conveying information about a patient from one clinician to another. This creates confusion in accurately assessing patients. As a result, the Glasgow Coma Scale is used universally to decrease the subjectivity and confusion associated with assessing LOC in acute situations.

Consciousness can be viewed as a crude continuum, anchored by full consciousness at one end and deep coma on the opposite end (Fig. 7-4). Despite the problems with precise terminology, there are several commonly used terms to describe gradations of consciousness (Table 7-2).

Confusion exists in describing the comatose state because of variations in the definition of coma and the inability to measure consciousness directly. Most texts classify depth of coma by correlating motor responsiveness (purposeful, nonpurposeful, and unresponsive) with painful stimuli with LOC. Clinicians attest that there are gradations of coma, based on motor responsiveness to painful stimuli, which are helpful in evaluating a patient's neurological condition in the clinical setting.

For the purposes of this discussion, **coma** is defined as a sustained pathologic state of unconsciousness and unrespon-

Full consciousness	Confusion	Lethargy	Obtundation	Stupor	Coma		
					Light coma	Coma	Deep coma

Figure 7-4 • Continuum of consciousness. Arousal/wakefulness includes a wide range of levels that can be conceptualized as a crude continuum with "full consciousness" as the anchor on one end and "deep coma" as the anchor on the other end.

TABLE 7–2   LEVELS OF CONSCIOUSNESS

TERMS	DEFINITIONS	COMMENT
Full consciousness	Awake, alert, and oriented to time, place, and person; comprehends the spoken and written word and is able to express ideas verbally or in writing	Demonstrates reliable and responsible behavior
Confusion	Disoriented in time, place, or person; initially becomes disoriented to time, then to place, and, finally, to person; shortened attention span; memory difficulty is common; becomes bewildered easily; has difficulty following commands; exhibits alterations in perception of stimuli; may have hallucinations; may be agitated, restless, irritable, and increasingly confused at night	High risk for falls and injury Requires frequent observation and supervision
Lethargy	Oriented to time, place, and person; very slow and sluggish in speech, mental processes, and motor activities; responds appropriately to painful stimuli	High risk for falls and injury Pull up side rails Needs frequent observation and supervision
Obtundation	Arousable with stimulation; responds verbally with a word or two; can follow simple commands appropriately when stimulated (e.g., when asked to stick out tongue); otherwise appears very drowsy; responds appropriately to painful stimuli	High risk for injury Unable to assume any responsibility for self; needs complete care
Stupor	Lies quietly with minimal spontaneous movement; generally unresponsive except to vigorous and repeated stimuli; incomprehensible sounds and/or eye opening may be noted; responds appropriately to painful stimuli	High risk for injury Unable to assume any responsibility for self; needs complete care
Coma	Appears to be in a sleep-like state with eyes closed; does not respond appropriately to bodily or environmental stimuli; does not make any verbal sounds; differentiation of coma level is based on motor response to painful stimuli	High risk for injury and aspiration Needs standard of care appropriate for comatose, completely dependent patient Priority of care is maintaining patent airway

siveness that includes three gradations: light coma (sometimes called semicoma), coma, and deep coma. The critical element that differentiates depth of coma is the response to painful stimuli:

Light coma (semicoma): unarousable; no spontaneous movement noted; withdraws *purposefully* to painful stimuli; usually, the brainstem reflexes, such as the gag, corneal, and pupillary reflexes, are intact.

Coma: unarousable; withdraws *nonpurposefully* to painful stimuli; brainstem reflexes may or may not be intact; decorticate or decerebrate posturing may be present.

Deep coma: unarousable; *unresponsive* to painful stimuli; brainstem reflexes are generally absent; decerebrate posturing or flaccidity is usually present.

THE GLASGOW COMA SCALE

The **Glasgow Coma Scale** (GCS), developed in Glasgow, Scotland, in 1974, is widely used in the United States and internationally for assessment of comatose patients. The scale was developed to standardize observations for the objective and accurate assessment of LOC. The GCS is especially useful for monitoring changes during the first few days after acute injury or in unstable comatose patients.

The scale is divided into three subscales: eye opening, best verbal response, and best motor response (Fig. 7-5). Each subscale has a variety of categories. The information collected can be plotted on a graph to provide a visual record of deterioration, improvement, or stabilization. In interpreting

the GCS, the numeric values of each subscale are added for a total score. The range of possible scores is 3 to 15. A score of 15 indicates a fully alert, oriented person, whereas a score of 3, the lowest possible score, indicatives deep coma. Patients with a score of 8 or below are usually unconscious. Unconscious patients require a high standard of nursing care appropriate for an unconscious patient. These patients usually need to be in an intensive care setting.

CHANGES IN LEVEL OF CONSCIOUSNESS

Changes in the LOC are, to some extent, predictable in that a patient who has been in a coma and now is arousable with repeated stimulation is described as displaying improvement in LOC. Clinicians frequently say "The patient appears to be lighter." What they are actually implying is that the LOC appears to have improved since the last examination or the overall trend is one of improvement. The crude continuum of LOC aids the clinician in assessing changes in the patient's condition. It is possible, and indeed probable, that all the levels of consciousness are not observable in a particular patient as he or she recovers from injury.

A few final points about the LOC should be kept in mind:

1. A patient with a brain injury who is evaluated during the posttraumatic period may arrive at an extended plateau of consciousness in the recovery process. For example, a patient can be comatose for a period of time and then become restless and agitated. This state may persist for days before it is followed by full consciousness. The pattern

Scoring of Eye Opening

- 4 Opens eyes spontaneously when the nurse approaches
- 3 Opens eyes in response to speech (normal or shout)
- 2 Opens eyes only to painful stimuli (*e.g.*, squeezing of nail beds)
- 1 Does not open eyes to painful stimuli

Scoring of Best Motor Response

- 6 Can obey a simple command, such as "Lift your left hand off the bed"
- 5 Localizes to painful stimuli and attempts to remove source
- 4 Purposeless movement in response to pain
- 3 Flexes elbows and wrists while extending lower legs to pain
- 2 Extends upper and lower extremities to pain
- 1 No motor response to pain on any limb

Scoring of Best Verbal Response

- 5 Oriented to time, place, and person
- 4 Converses, although confused
- 3 Speaks only in words or phrases that make little or no sense
- 2 Responds with incomprehensible sounds (*e.g.*, groans)
- 1 No verbal response

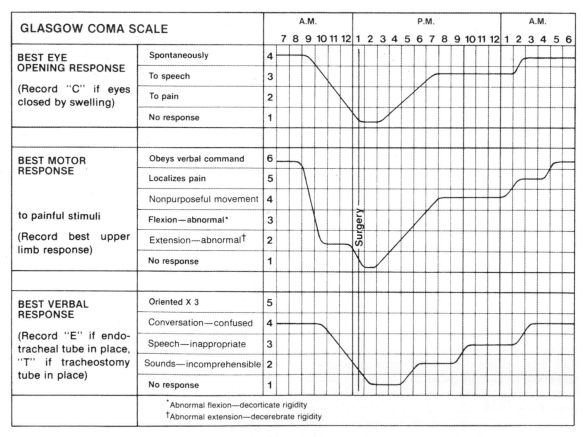

Figure 7-5 • Glasgow Coma Scale.

of recovery is based on the type, extent, and site of the injury and secondary injuries.

2. If the patient is sedated with very ultra-short-acting drugs such as propofol, turn off the drug about 10 minutes before assessing the patient so that the drug's effect will not cloud assessment of LOC.

3. It is important to record the time of observation of postoperative patients who have undergone intracranial surgery. It makes a great difference whether there is a 1-hour or 4-hour interval between observations that indicate how rapidly the neurological status of the patient might be changing following surgery.

| CHART **7-1** | **Special States of Altered Consciousness** |

VEGETATIVE AND PERSISTENT VEGETATIVE STATE

According to the American Academy of Neurology current published practice parameters, the **vegetative state** is a clinical condition of complete unawareness of the self and the environment accompanied by sleep-wake cycles with either complete or partial preservation of hypothalamic and brainstem autonomic functions. The criteria include the following:

- No evidence of awareness of self or environment and an inability to interact with others
- No evidence of sustained, reproducible, purposeful, or voluntary behavioral responses to visual, auditory, tactile, or noxious stimuli
- No evidence of language comprehension or expression
- Intermittent wakefulness manifested by the presence of sleep-wake cycles
- Sufficiently preserved hypothalamic and brainstem autonomic functions to permit survival with medical and nursing care
- Bowel and bladder incontinence
- Variably preserved cranial nerve (pupillary, oculocephalic, corneal, vestibular-ocular, gag) and spinal reflexes

The **persistent vegetative state (PVS)** is defined as a vegetative state present at 1 month after acute traumatic or nontraumatic brain injury, and present for at least 1 month in degenerative/metabolic disorders or developmental malformations.

Discussion about the definition and clinical course of PVS has been a topic of intense interest in the last few years and has raised many ethical questions about quality of life. In 1989, the American Academy of Neurology published guidelines on the vegetative state. The Multi-Society Task Force on PVS has built on their work.

Further, PVS is defined as a vegetative state present 1 month after acute traumatic or nontraumatic brain injury or lasting for at least 1 month in patients with degenerative or metabolic disorders or developmental malformations.

Recovery of consciousness is unlikely or rare for both adults and children in the following situations:

- Posttraumatic PVS after 12 months
- Nontraumatic PVS after 3 months
- Degenerative metabolic disorders or congenital malformations after several months

The life expectancy of all PVS patients is substantially reduced; survival ranges from 2 to 5 years; survival beyond 10 years is very unusual.

PVS presents special ethical, moral, and legal issues that are discussed in Chapter 4.

LOCKED-IN SYNDROME

The term **locked-in syndrome** refers to a state in which full consciousness and cognition are intact but severe paralysis of the voluntary motor system makes movement and communications impossible. Usual cause is the interruption of the descending corticobulbar and corticospinal tracts at or below the pons; however, breathing is left intact. The locked-in syndrome can also be associated with peripheral motor neuron disease or paralysis produced with neuromuscular blocking drugs. Patients with this version of the locked-in syndrome can usually establish simple communications through eye blinking and vertical eye movement. The locked-in syndrome may be seen in certain cerebrovascular diseases with ventral pontine infarction and such conditions as myasthenia gravis and poliomyelitis. The diagnosis is established by clinical examination.

* American Academy of Neurology. (1989). Position of the American Academy of Neurology on certain aspects of the care and management of the persistent vegetative state patient. *Neurology, 39,* 125–126.
† Multi-Society Task Force on PVS. (1994). Medical aspects of the persistent vegetative state (Part 2). *New England Journal of Medicine, 330*(22), 1572–1579.
‡ Multi-Society Task Force on PVS, p. 1573.
§ Plum & Posner, 1980 (see ref. 4); American Academy of Neurology, 1989.

4. Recovery from an altered LOC is influenced by age, type of injury, and premorbid health status. Younger patients (especially those under 20 years) have a much better prognosis for recovery than do older patients.
5. As a rule, the longer the coma, the worse the outcome. Absence of corneal, gag, pupillary, or oculocephalic/ oculovestibular reflexes initially or during the course of illness indicates a poor outcome. Decortication, decerebration, or flaccidity of the motor system also denotes a poor prognosis.

Special States of Altered Consciousness

According to the classic text by Plum and Posner, nearly all comatose patients begin to awaken from their comatose state within 2 to 4 weeks after injury, regardless of the severity of brain damage, if they survive at all.[4] After a sleep-wakefulness cycle has been re-established, the patient is no longer comatose, even though there is no apparent awareness of or interaction with the environment. A few special states of altered

consciousness are seen in the clinical setting and discussed in the literature. These special states include persistent vegetative state and locked-in syndrome and are included in Chart 7-1. See Chart 7-2 for nursing management of the patient with an altered LOC. Interdisciplinary collaborative efforts are usually required to manage a comatose patient.

Cognition

Assessment

Consciousness has been conceptualized as having two components: alertness and cognition. Alertness (wakefulness) has already been discussed in the previous section. **Awareness or cognition** represents the sum of cognitive and affective function and is controlled by the cerebral cortex. As part of the assessment of LOC, the nurse assesses orientation to time, place, and person. However, this provides limited information about the patient's overall cognitive function. Therefore, in the awake patient, the nurse conducts a cognitive

CHART **7-2**	**Nursing Management of the Patient With an Altered Level of Consciousness**

The following are some basic management points for a patient with altered level of consciousness (LOC):

1. **Maintaining a patient airway is a top priority.** The patient should not be left lying on his or her back because of the increased possibility of aspiration. Position to facilitate drainage of oral secretions.

2. A change in the LOC is the **most sensitive indicator of neurological change** and, therefore, the first neurological sign that changes with altered neurological status. The LOC should be assessed periodically (as often as every 5 to 10 minutes in the acute, unstable patient and every 4 hours in the stable patient). Regardless of all the technological advances in health care, the observations of the nurse who knows the patient are still the most sensitive "sensors" of neurological changes. The nurse who is well acquainted with the personality and behavior pattern of the patient can best evaluate whether behavior changes are caused by pain, fatigue, or neurological deterioration. The nurse has the responsibility of advising the physician of changes in the LOC.

3. When the LOC has deteriorated, the nurse should talk to the patient in a calm, normal, reassuring voice, explaining in simple terms what is being done and orienting him or her to the environment. If the patient normally wears glasses or a hearing aid, they should be worn.

4. When talking to the patient, the nurse should try to screen out external environmental stimuli that might increase confusion. Also, a group of people entering the room and talking to the patient can be both overwhelming and confusing. In essence, it creates a sensory overload for fragile, recovering neurological circuits and can result in confusion and misinterpretation of stimuli.

5. After patients begin to awaken and verbalize, they often recognize a void of time for which they cannot account. This can be very frightening. The nurse should fill the gaps of time by briefly recounting what has happened during the lapse. Also, when the patient begins to make incorrect statements, the nurse should matter-of-factly correct any misconceptions.

6. The nurse is responsible for **protecting the patient from injury.** As the LOC deteriorates, the nurse must assume total responsibility for the patient's safety. The methods employed depend on the availability of staff (usually fewer staff on evenings and nights), the patient's degree of agitation and impulsive behavior, the location of his or her room in relationship to the nurses' station, and the use of supportive equipment (ventilator, CVP and IV lines, ICP monitoring catheter, and others). Regardless of the circumstances, the standard of care for this patient requires much more nursing time and intervention than that required for an alert, oriented patient. The nurse should observe the patient frequently; talk in a calm manner; maintain the bed in low position, unless contraindicated; maintain all siderails in up position; and use restraints as necessary to protect the patient from injury, according to hospital policy.

7. Nighttime and darkness often lead the patient to misinterpretation of environmental and other stimuli. A night light and periodic visits by the nurse can help to control confusion, fear, and hallucinations.

8. The family and other visitors need instruction about how to visit a patient with altered LOC or cognitive functions. The specific guidelines will depend on the particular patient. The nurse should be available to intervene if problems occur during the visit, as well as to evaluate the effects of the visit on the patient and the visitors. If the patient is upset, the possible reasons for the reaction should be explored. Family members may need support after the visit to express their concerns and fears.

CVP, central venous pressure; ICP, intracranial pressure; IV, intravenous.

---

assessment, or mental status examination, to determine the effect of neurological disease on the patient's ability to function in day-to-day living.

There are several areas to address in cognitive assessment (see Chap. 6). The following list includes the major areas covered in a mental status assessment:

- Orientation to time, place, and person
- Attention and vigilance (the ability to sustain attention over a period of time) as well as the ability to focus and concentrate on a task, which requires self-regulation and screening out of distracting environmental stimuli
- Memory (immediate, short term, long term)
- General fund of information (e.g., name the presidents starting with current president and going back from the present)
- Language and speech demonstrating an understanding of the written and spoken word, as well as the ability to use language appropriately (e.g., identifying any difficulty with word finding or misuse of words) (see Chap. 6, Table 6-4)
- Calculation

- Abstract thinking, reasoning, problem solving, insight, and judgment
- Special integrative function (skilled motor acts for apraxias, and motor-sensory integration for agnosias)
- Construction ability (ability to draw or copy on command; helpful to identify neglect syndrome)

Assessment of Cognitive Function at the Bedside

In clinical practice, the question is raised about how much of the mental status examination should be conducted and how frequently should particular parameters be assessed. The answer is, "it depends." It depends on the type of clinical setting, the patient's level of consciousness and ability to cooperate, and the purposes of the assessment. In the acute care setting, especially in the intensive care environment, the LOC is usually so depressed that assessing higher-level function is impossible. As the patient begins to regain consciousness, an abbreviated bedside assessment will help the clinician to determine progress. For example, asking the patient to show you two fingers is a simple command that requires understanding of the spoken word and the motor ability to respond to the command. The following is a sample of questions that can be asked at the bedside to assess cognitive and motor function:

- What is the name of this place?
- What is the date?
- Show me two fingers.
- Stick out your tongue.
- Look toward me.
- Wiggle your thumb or toes.
- How much is a quarter, a dime, and a nickel?

Some cognitive functions are assessed within the context of providing care and observing the patient during ADLs. Deficits may be obvious because of their impact on ADLs. Higher-level deficits may be subtle because the patient may appear to be functional, having devised ways to compensate for deficits. Standardized instruments such as the Mini-Mental Status Examination[5] may also be used to assess cognitive function. The Rancho Los Amigos Scale (see Chap. 11), an eight-level scale developed originally to follow recovery in brain trauma patients, is also used in rehabilitative settings for determining behavioral patterns and related interventions for other neurological patients.[6] The general collaborative problem of **cognitive deficits** may be made. It will require interdisciplinary collaboration to define the particular deficits present and to develop and implement a collaborative plan of care.

RECOVERY AND REHABILITATION

Some improvement in cognitive function is often evident during the course of acute hospitalization due to the natural recovery of the brain. Most natural recovery occurs in the first 3 to 6 months after injury; recovery can still occur after this time, but at a much slower rate. Many patients will have persistent cognitive deficits that will require rehabilitation. In most hospitals, the occupational therapist can perform a short (approximately 30 minutes) cognitive assessment screening to determine areas affected by cognitive deficits. If necessary, a neuropsychologist can conduct a detailed cognitive assessment (several hours) to pinpoint deficits and develop a treatment program. Often, a consultation with the neuropsychologist is postponed to allow for natural recovery. Specific patient management will depend on the overall assessment. Some patients will require only short-term cognitive rehabilitation, whereas others will require long-term treatment. Patients with dementia will have persistent cognition deficits that become worse over time.

CRANIAL NERVE ASSESSMENT

Occasionally, the nurse may be required to conduct a comprehensive cranial nerve (CN) assessment at the time of admission to establish a baseline (see Chap. 6) and at key critical points such as postoperatively. In the real world of clinical practice, however, cranial assessment is often abbreviated. There are two reasons for this. First, the patient may be unable to cooperate and follow specific commands (e.g., smile, stick out the tongue) or to report subjective changes in neurological function (e.g., double vision). The inability to cooperate or to participate is often the result of altered consciousness (e.g., coma) or cognitive-perceptual deficits. Second, after a comprehensive assessment, it is often appropriate to tailor the assessment to the patient's specific condition.

Such tailoring implies an understanding of the pathophysiology of the specific condition and the need to monitor specific functions that are at high risk for dysfunction. For example, a patient who is admitted with a diagnosis of an acoustic neuroma (a tumor involving the eighth CN) requires assessment of CN VIII function to determine hearing loss and vertigo. Assessment of function would also be required for CN V (sensory loss to the face), CN VII (deficits in motor function of the face), and CNs IX and X (loss of gag reflex or difficulty speaking). The reason for assessment of these cranial nerves is their anatomic proximity in the posterior fossa to CN VIII. As the tumor grows, it may impinge on a number of adjacent cranial nerves, causing dysfunction. Because consciousness is usually not affected by an acoustic neuroma, the patient is able to cooperate with the assessment.

Table 7-3 summarizes the components of cranial nerve assessment as conducted in actual clinical practice (see also Chap. 6). Pupillary signs are of particular importance and can be assessed in all patients regardless of LOC or ability to cooperate. Other CNs can be tested at the bedside only in conscious, responsive patients. Still other cranial nerves can be tested in both conscious and unresponsive patients, using alternative techniques. The following sections describe these practical bedside techniques.

ASSESSMENT OF VISUAL FIELDS (OPTIC NERVE)

The visual field can be easily and quickly assessed for a conscious, cooperative patient at the bedside. This is done by asking the patient to focus on your nose and then introducing a varying number of fingers with both hands simultaneously into the bilateral upper quadrants; repeat in the bilateral lower quadrants (see Chap. 6, Chart 6-1). You can quickly ascertain whether the patient has full visual fields or gaps in the visual fields. If a deficit is noted, further assessment may be necessary.

ASSESSMENT OF PUPILS (OCULOMOTOR NERVE)

Examination of the pupils is an extremely important part of patient assessment that can be carried out in either a conscious or unconscious patient. The general points to note when assessing the pupils include their size, shape, and reaction to light. Accommodation is **not** evaluated in every

TABLE 7–3   SUMMARY OF CRANIAL NERVE ASSESSMENT AT THE BEDSIDE

CRANIAL NERVE	ASSESSMENT	COMMENTS
I Olfactory	**Sense of smell** Usually deferred	Deficits noted in only a few cases, usually with lesion in the parasellar area
II Optic	**Vision** Monitor while working with patient; observe for difficulty with ADLs Ask patient to identify how many fingers are being held up or to read menu or newspaper Use Rosenbaum Pocket Vision Screener to assess vision in each eye Monitor for visual field cuts by checking upper and lower quadrants while patient focuses on your nose	Common deficits; deficits can cause blindness in one eye, bitemporal hemianopsia, or homonymous hemianopsia
III Oculomotor	**Pupil constriction; elevation of upper eyelid** Assess size, shape, and direct light reaction of pupils	Changes are common with a number of progressing neurological problems
III Oculomotor, IV Trochlear, and VI Abducens	**Extraocular movement** Tested together in conscious, cooperative patient; ask patient to follow a pencil tip through the six cardinal eye movements	Deficits are common; inability to move the eyes in one or more directions is called strabismus
V Trigeminal	**Sensation to face; mastication muscles** Often deferred If assessed, patient must be cooperative and able to accurately report facial sensation from stimulation **Afferent limb of corneal reflex**	Deficits found in trigeminal neuralgia and sometimes with acoustic neuroma Corneal reflex assessed in trigeminal neuralgia; can assess reflex in unconscious patient
VII Facial	**Muscles for facial expression; efferent limb of corneal reflex** Ask cooperative patient to smile, show teeth, puff cheeks, wrinkle brow; observe for symmetry of face In comatose patient, tickle each nasal passage, one at a time, by inserting a cotton-tipped applicator; observe for facial movement	Total unilateral facial weakness called Bell's palsy Unilateral from below the eye and down, seen in stroke Note the difference between central and peripheral facial involvement
VIII Acoustic	**Hearing and balance** Usually deferred May note deficit while working with patient	Deficits with acoustic neuroma, cerebellar pontine angle tumors, Ménière's disease
IX Glossopharyngeal and X Vagus	**Palate, pharynx, vocal cords, and gag reflex;** tested together because of overlap In conscious patient, have patient open mouth and say "ah"; assess gag reflex Unconscious patient: assess gag reflex	Deficits common in posterior fossa lesions Gag reflex is a brainstem reflex and has prognostic value in unconscious patient
XI Spinal accessory	**Shrug shoulders and move head side to side** Usually deferred	Deficits common in posterior fossa lesions
XII Hypoglossal	**Movement of tongue** In conscious patient, ask him or her to stick out the tongue	Deficits common in posterior fossa lesions

Note: This table summarizes **assessment at the bedside**. Although a baseline assessment of all cranial nerves is recommended, this may not always be possible. In addition, although frequent assessment of particular cranial nerves is critical in certain conditions, it may be safely deferred in other conditions. ADLs, activities of daily living.

assessment. The findings in one pupil are always compared with the findings in the other pupil, and differences between the two are noted. Data are documented in the neurological database.

Size

Normally, the pupils are equal in size, measuring about 2 to 6 mm in diameter with an average diameter of 3.5 mm. Two methods are used to record pupillary size: the millimeter scale (most common) and descriptive terms. If the millimeter scale is used, the examiner, using a diagrammatic gauge, estimates the size of each pupil by comparing the gauge with the patient's pupils (Fig. 7-6). The examiner then records a numeric value ranging from 2 to 9 mm to signify the size of each pupil. If descriptive terms are used to evaluate the size

of the pupils, the following terms are used: pinpoint, small, midposition, large, and dilated (Chart 7-3).

Shape

Shape is assessed simply by looking at the contour of the pupils. Normally, both pupils are round. Abnormal pupillary shapes are described as ovoid, keyhole, or irregular (Chart 7-4).

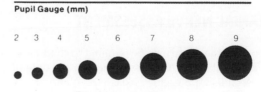

Pupil Gauge (mm)

2   3   4   5   6   7   8   9

Figure 7-6 • Pupil gauge.

CHART 7-3   Nursing Assessment of Pupillary Size

In assessing pupillary size using either descriptive terms or a gauge, each pupil is assessed individually and then the findings for each pupil are compared. This is very important because pupils are normally equal (see note on anisocoria).

DESCRIPTIVE TERM	DEFINITION	FINDINGS
Pinpoint 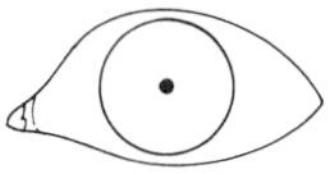	The pupil is so small that it is barely visible or appears as small as a pinpoint.	Seen with opiate overdose, pontine hemorrhage, and ischemia
Small 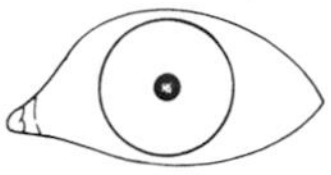	The pupil appears smaller than average but larger than pinpoint.	Seen normally if the person is in a brightly lit place; also seen with miotic ophthalmic drops, opiates, pontine hemorrhage, Horner's syndrome, bilateral diencephalic lesions, and metabolic coma
Midposition 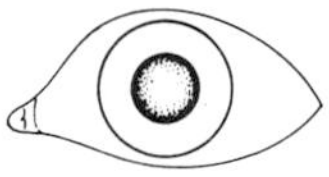	When the pupil and iris are observed, about half of their diameter is iris and half is pupil.	Seen normally; if pupils are midposition and nonreactive, midbrain damage is the cause
Large 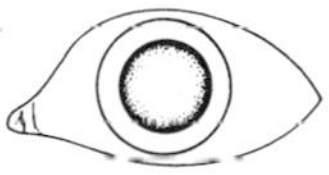	The pupils are larger than average, but there is still an appreciable amount of iris visible.	Seen normally if room is dark; may be seen with some drugs, such as amphetamines; glutethimide (Doriden) overdose; mydriatics; cycloplegic agents; and some orbital injuries
Dilated 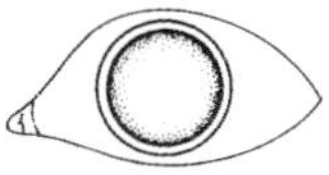	When the pupil and iris are observed, one is struck by the largeness of the pupil with only the slightest ring of iris, which is barely visible.	Abnormal finding; bilateral, fixed, and dilated pupils are seen in the terminal stage of severe anoxia–ischemia or at death.

Note: **Anisocoria** is the term used to describe inequality in size between the pupils. About 17% of the population has slight anisocoria without any related pathologic process. It is, therefore, important to make a baseline assessment of pupillary size and compare subsequent assessments with the baseline. If pupillary inequality is a new finding, it should be reported. If the patient is admitted with slight pupillary inequality and no other abnormalities are detected on the neurological assessment, the pupil inequality may not be significant.

CHART 7-4   Nursing Assessment of Pupillary Shape

DESCRIPTIVE TERM	DEFINITION	FINDINGS
Round 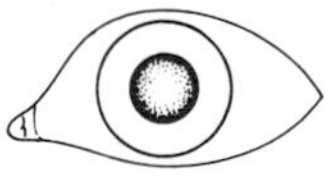	Like a circle	Normal findings
Ovoid 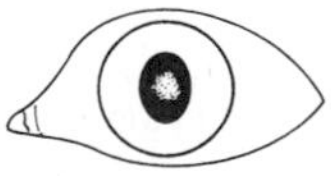	Slightly oval; "ovoid"	Almost always indicates intracranial hypertension and represents an intermediate phase between a normal pupil (round) and a fully dilated fixed pupil; an early sign of transtentorial herniation
Keyhole 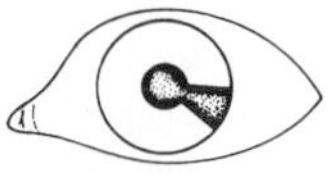	Like a keyhole	Seen in patients who have had an iridectomy (excision of part of the iris). An iridectomy is often part of cataract surgery, a common procedure in the elderly population. (The reaction to light is very slight.)
Irregular 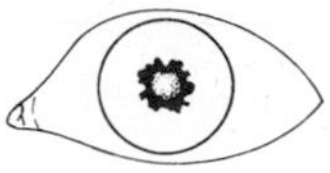	Jagged	Seen in Argyll-Robertson pupils and with traumatic orbital injuries

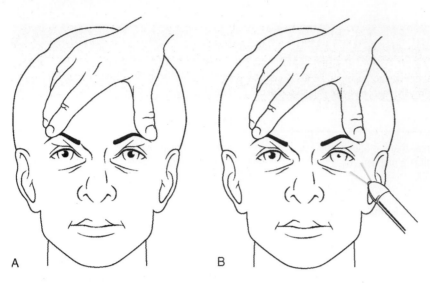

Figure 7-7 • Evaluating pupillary reactions by checking pupil size (*A*) and reaction to light (*B*).

Reaction to Light

When light is shone into the eye, the pupil should immediately constrict. Withdrawal of the light should produce an immediate and brisk dilation of the pupil. This is called the **direct light reflex** (Fig. 7-7). Introducing the light into one pupil should cause similar constriction to occur simultaneously in the other pupil. When the light is withdrawn from one eye, the opposite pupil should dilate simultaneously. This response is called the **consensual light reaction.**

Pupillary reaction to light is recorded using descriptive terms or symbols (Chart 7-5). The descriptive terms that are used include brisk, sluggish, and nonreactive or fixed. Plus and minus signs are recorded if a symbol recording system is used. (Common abnormal pupillary responses and findings are found in Chart 7-6. Refer also to Chap. 6 for more information on pupillary assessment.)

CHART 7-5   Nursing Assessment of Pupillary Light Responses

DESCRIPTIVE TERM	SYMBOL	FINDINGS
Brisk	++	Normal finding
Sluggish	+	Found in conditions that cause some compression of the oculomotor nerve (cranial nerve III); seen in early transtentorial herniation, cerebral edema, and Adie's pupil
Nonreactive or fixed	−	Found in conditions that include compression of the oculomotor nerve; seen with transtentorial herniation syndromes and in severe hypoxia and ischemia (terminal stage just before death)
Swollen closed	c	One or both eyes are tightly closed because of severe periorbital edema; the pupillary light reflex may be difficult to assess.

One other response—the Hippus phenomenon—is included; this does not usually appear on assessment sheets but may be observed in the clinical area and, therefore, needs to be recorded.

Hippus phenomenon	None	With uniform illumination of the pupil, dilation and contraction are noted. This may be considered normal if pupils are observed under high magnification. The Hippus phenomenon is also observed in patients who are beginning to experience pressure on the third cranial nerve. This is often associated with early transtentorial herniation.

Note: On some pupillary assessment sheets, other symbols are used in place of descriptive terms.

| CHART **7-6** | **Common Abnormal Pupillary Responses** (*Note:* Compare findings with previous assessment data, document, and report new findings to the physician.) |

OCULOMOTOR NERVE COMPRESSION

Observation

One pupil (R) is larger than the other (L), which is of normal size. The dilated pupil (R) does not react to light, although the other pupil (L) reacts normally. Ptosis may be seen in the dilated pupil.

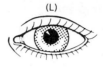

Ptosis

Interpretation

A dilated, nonreactive (fixed) pupil indicates that the control for pupillary constriction is not functioning. The parasympathetic fibers of the oculomotor nerve control pupillary constriction. The most common cause of interruption of this function is compression of the oculomotor nerve, usually against the tentorium or posterior cerebral artery.

Compression of the oculomotor nerve is caused most often by cerebral edema and uncal herniation on the same side of the brain as the dilated pupil.

Action

Compare with data from previous assessments. If the dilated pupil is a new finding, it should immediately be reported to the physician because the process of rostralcaudal downward pressure must be treated without delay. In this situation changes in LOC, motor function, sensory function, and possibly vital signs would be expected.

BILATERAL DIENCEPHALIC DAMAGE

Observation

On examination, the pupils appear small but equal in size, and both react to direct light, contracting when light is introduced and dilating when light is withdrawn.

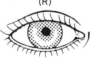

Interpretation

The sympathetic pathway that begins in the hypothalamus is affected. Because both pupils are equal in size and respond equally to light, the damage is bilateral. Therefore, it can be assumed that there is bilateral injury in the diencephalon (thalamus and hypothalamus).

Because metabolic coma can also result in bilaterally small pupils that react to light, this diagnostic possibility must be ruled out.

Action

Compare findings with previous assessments to determine change. Consider metabolic coma by reviewing blood chemistry findings and other data. For example, diabetic acidosis may result in a metabolic coma because of a high blood glucose level.

HORNER'S SYNDROME

Observation

One pupil (L) is smaller than the other (R), although both pupils react to light. The eyelid on the same side as the smaller pupil (L) droops (ptosis). Inability to sweat (anhidrosis) on the same side of the face as the ptosis is common. The symptoms of a small reactive pupil, ptosis, and anhidrosis combine to form Horner's syndrome.

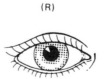

Interpretation

There is an interruption of the ipsilateral sympathetic innervation to the pupil that can be caused by hypothalamic damage, a lesion of the lateral medulla or the ventrolateral cervical spinal cord, and, sometimes, occlusion of the internal carotid artery.

Action

If this is a new finding, it should be reported.

(continued)

CHART 7-6   **Common Abnormal Pupillary Responses** (*Note:* Compare findings with previous assessment data, document, and report new findings to the physician.)   (Continued)

MIDBRAIN DAMAGE

Observation

Both pupils are at midposition and nonreactive to light.

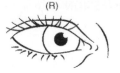
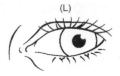

Interpretation

With midposition, nonreactive pupils, neither sympathetic nor parasympathetic innervation is functional. This finding is often associated with midbrain infarction or transtentorial herniation.

Action

Compare findings with previous assessment data. Consider also changes in other components of the assessment. The pupils should be evaluated in conjunction with other neurologic assessments. Report new findings to the physician.

PONTINE DAMAGE

Observation

Very small (pinpoint), nonreactive pupils are seen.

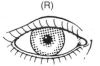
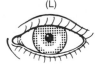

Interpretation

This finding indicates focal damage of the pons often due to hemorrhage or ischemia. *Bilateral* pinpoint pupils may occur from opiate drug overdose, so this possibility should be ruled out.

Action

Compare findings with previous assessment data. Report findings to the physician immediately. Other changes in neurological status, such as a decreased LOC and respiratory abnormalities, would be expected.

BILATERAL DILATED UNREACTIVE PUPILS

Observation

Both pupils are dilated and nonreactive (fixed).

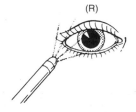
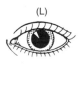

Interpretation

This finding is characteristic of the terminal stages of severe anoxia and death.

Action

Emergency action (code) is necessary to attempt to resuscitate the patient, although the possibility of reversal is low. Oxygen therapy at high concentrations and a patent airway must be ensured to provide oxygen for the ischemic cerebral cells. Other signs and symptoms of neurological deterioration will be present.

ASSESSMENT OF EXTRAOCULAR MOVEMENT (OCULOMOTOR, TROCHLEAR, AND ABDUCENS NERVES)

Extraocular movement and the position of the eyeballs are assessed. In the normal healthy person, one would expect the following:

- The eyes move conjugately in the orbital sockets.
- The eyes blink periodically.
- No nystagmus or abnormal eye movement is noted.
- The eyeball neither protrudes nor is sunken in the orbits.
- The upper eyelid does not droop and the palpebral fissures are equal bilaterally.

Some of the data are collected simply through focused observation of the patient for 10 to 15 seconds. Other components require a cooperative patient.

ASSESSMENT OF THE CONSCIOUS, COOPERATIVE PATIENT

The Eyeballs

The position of the eyeballs within the eye sockets is assessed by observing the eyes frontally, in profile, and from above the patient's head. If no abnormality is noted, most clinicians will not comment about position in the documentation.

- Abnormal protrusion of one or both eyeballs is termed **proptosis or exophthalmos.**
- Abnormal recession of one or both eyelids is termed **enophthalmos.**

Eyelids

The patient is asked to look straight ahead; observations of each eye are then made and compared. The width of each palpebral fissure is observed. The palpebral fissure is the space between the upper and lower eyelid. Next, the position of the eyelid in relation to the pupil and iris is evaluated. Normally, the lid slightly covers the outer margin of the iris. A narrowed palpebral fissure usually indicates a droopy eyelid, also known as **ptosis.** Ptosis is seen in Horner's syndrome and conditions that affect the oculomotor nerve, such as transtentorial herniation syndromes and myasthenia gravis with ocular involvement.

Note the presence of edema of the eyelids. Edema can result from trauma to the orbital area and may occur in the upper eyelid, the lower eyelid, or both.

Movement of the Eyes

Extraocular movement is assessed in conscious patients by asking them to follow a pencil or the examiner's finger through the six cardinal directions of gaze in an "H" sequencing (Fig. 7-8; also see Chap. 6, Fig. 6-7). Inability to move either eye in any direction should be noted. When both eyes move in the same direction, at the same speed, and maintain a constant alignment, the gaze is termed **conjugate gaze.** A lack of parallelism between the two visual axes or movement in opposite directions is called **dysconjugate gaze.** If the dysfunction is limited to a specific movement or movements, an ophthalmoplegia is present. **Ophthalmoplegia** is defined as paralysis of one or more eye muscles (see Chap. 6, Table 6-9 for a summary of ophthalmoplegias).

The patient is asked whether double vision **(diplopia)** is present. If the answer is yes, is the double image side by side or one on top of the other? This will help determine if the problem is CN III (oculomotor) or CN VI (abducens) on the horizontal plane or CN III or CN IV (trochlear) on the vertical plane. See Chapter 6 for further discussion.

Abnormal Movements

The patient is asked to focus straight ahead and then to follow the examiner's finger (see Fig. 7-8). Any abnormal eye

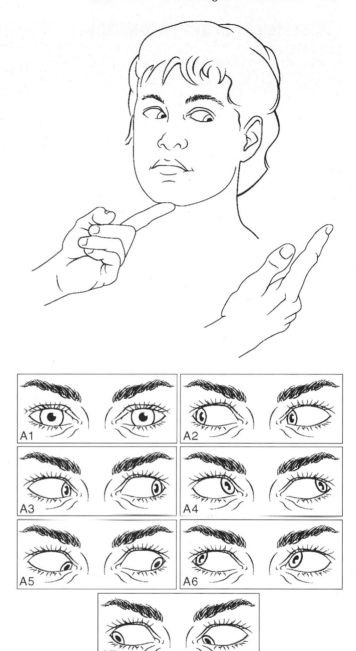

Figure 7-8 • Extraocular movements.

movements should be noted. **Nystagmus** is defined as involuntary movement of an eye, which may be horizontal, vertical, rotary, or mixed in direction. The tempo of the movements can be regular, rhythmic, pendular, or jerky, with the movement having a fast and slow component. Nystagmus can result from several problems. If present, the nurse should document the characteristics of the movement and include any information about related characteristics (e.g., focusing the eye in a certain direction). Specific types of nystagmus are found in Chapter 6, Table 6-10. Periodic blinking is normal and expected. The nurse should assess blinking by observing the patient. In association with some conditions, such as Parkinson's disease, blinking is decreased.

ASSESSMENT OF THE UNCONSCIOUS PATIENT

General Observations

The unconscious (comatose) patient appears to be in a sleep-like state, with or without the eyes closed. If the eyes are closed, the eyelids can gently be raised to inspect the position and movement of the eyes. The eyes may assume a prolonged stare without any discernible movement, or they may move slowly from side to side. Absence of any movement suggests that the eye movement center in the brainstem is not functioning. This is a poor prognostic sign. Conversely, slow movement from side to side indicates an intact brainstem. See Chapter 6 for assessment of the unconscious patient.

Eyelids

After the eyes are inspected, the eyelids are released. In coma, the lids slowly cover the eyes.

Eye Movement

Because the patient is unconscious and therefore unable to follow commands, voluntary eye movement cannot be assessed. Although not routinely done by the nurse, the physician may wish to evaluate the eye movement brainstem centers to determine if they are intact. For this evaluation, the **oculocephalic reflex (doll's eye response)** (see Fig. 6-20) or **oculovestibular reflex (cold caloric)** can be assessed, provided there are no contraindications (see Fig. 6-21). (If the eyes do not move, the brainstem is not functioning, a poor prognostic sign.) The physician may choose to evaluate these reflexes in some patients to determine brainstem function for prognostic purposes or as part of brain death criteria.

Frequency of Assessing Eye Movement

Ocular movement function does not change as rapidly as other components of the neurological assessment. The nurse should assess eye movements once during a shift and more often if the patient is unstable.

Assessment of Facial Movement (Facial Nerve)

If the examiner wishes to assess the facial nerve in the conscious, cooperative patient, the patient is asked to smile and show his or her teeth while the examiner observes for symmetric bilateral facial movements. In the unconscious patient, the easiest and quickest way to assess the facial nerve is to stimulate one nostril and then the other with a cotton-tipped applicator. The patient should respond to the stimulation with a facial contraction. The examiner can determine whether there is symmetric bilateral facial movement.

Selected Reflexes

The corneal, gag, and swallowing reflexes, all brainstem reflexes, can be assessed in both the conscious and unconscious patient. These brainstem reflexes are helpful in determining the intactness of the brainstem. In the conscious patient or unconscious patient, touch each cornea with a wisp of cotton and observe for a blinking action. Another way to check the corneal reflex in an unconscious patient is to drop a small amount of sterile water or saline (from a plastic ampule) onto the cornea. If the reflex is intact, the eye will blink. Recall that the corneal reflex is mediated by CNs V and VII.

To assess the gag and swallowing reflexes in the conscious patient, ask the patient to stick out his or her tongue so that a cotton-tipped applicator can be used to touch the posterior pharynx on each side. For an unconscious patient, gentle tugging on an endotracheal tube will cause gagging if the reflex is intact. Alternatively, a cotton-tipped applicator can be used to stimulate each side of the posterior pharynx. In both cases, there should be an immediate retraction of the pharynx or gagging if the reflex is intact. Recall that the gag and swallowing reflexes are mediated by cranial nerves IX and X. Checking these reflexes provides data about intactness of brainstem function.

ASSESSMENT OF MOTOR FUNCTION

The assessment of motor function is conducted in an orderly fashion, beginning with the upper limbs and proceeding to the neck and trunk and, finally, to the lower extremities. Limb evaluation proceeds from proximal to distal.

The purposes of the neurological assessment are a little different from those of the neurological physical examination, which includes a detailed examination of the motor system. The neurological assessment provides a baseline from which to denote change. A sampling of a few key muscles or muscle groups provides a good indicator of function and change. In the neurological assessment, the motor assessment usually focuses on the arms and legs.

Noting motor function helps the nurse to consider the patient's functional level, the effect on independence in ADLs, and the need for adaptation of activities or assistive devices.

The technique used to evaluate motor function depends on the patient's LOC. In the conscious and alert patient, the assessment can be conducted by observing responses to directions such as "Squeeze my hands." The aphasic or apraxic patient may have difficulty following directions and may need cueing.

In an unconscious patient or one who is unable to participate, the nurse must rely on special testing techniques and observations for data. The basic approach to assessment of motor function is detailed in Chart 7-7. A few additional points will help to guide the assessment process. In assessing motor function, the following should be considered: (1) muscle size, (2) muscle tone, (3) muscle strength, (4) presence of involuntary movement, and (5) posture and gait, if appropriate for the patient's condition. When one muscle or muscle group is assessed, it is always compared with the same muscle or group on the opposite side of the body for symmetry.

Muscle Size and Tone

The muscle or muscle group is observed for size. It is also palpated at rest and then during passive movement for tone.

CHART 7-7   Nursing Assessment of Motor Function at the Bedside

CONSCIOUS PATIENT WHO IS ABLE TO FOLLOW SIMPLE COMMANDS

A sampling of the strength of key muscles in the extremities will provide an overview of motor function. Other muscle groups of interest can be added (see Chap. 6 and Fig. 6-10 for more information).

Upper Extremities

A. Deltoids
B. Biceps
C. Triceps
D. Hand grasps
E. Pronator drift

Lower Extremities

F. Hamstrings
G. Quadriceps
H. Dorsiflexion
I. Plantarflexion

UNCONSCIOUS PATIENT

Unconscious patients can exhibit abnormal muscle tone or motor responses that appear as stereotyped postures and are initiated by noxious stimuli (see decortication and decerebration).

Upper Extremities: Unconscious Patient

- First observe for spontaneous movement with patient lying in bed.
- Apply a noxious stimulus. *Note:* **Apply a noxious stimulus centrally rather than peripherally. An example of a central stimulus is pinching the pectoralis major muscle. A peripheral stimulus, such as pressing on the nail bed, may result in a reflex response and confuse findings.**

- Observe for withdrawal of the arm on the stimulated side. A purposeful response is present if the arm crossed the midline to noxious stimulus.

Sometimes added to the assessment:
- With the patient lying on his or her back, position the forearms perpendicular to the bed, holding the patient's arms upright by the hands or wrists.
- The movement of both arms is then observed as the extremities are released simultaneously.
- A paralyzed or paretic arm will fall more quickly than an intact arm. The weaker arm may strike the patient's face as it falls.

Lower Extremities: Unconscious Patient

- Observe for spontaneous movements.
- Apply noxious stimuli; observe for motor response.

Sometimes added to the assessment for paralysis or paresis, although often impractical because of abnormal posturing and increased tone:
- Position flat on the back with the knees flexed so both feet are flat on the bed.
- The knees are simultaneously released and the movement of the legs is observed.
- The paralyzed or paretic leg will fall to an extended position with the hip outwardly rotated. The normal leg will maintain the flexed position for a few moments and then gradually assume its previous position.

Common abnormalities in muscle tone include spasticity, rigidity, and flaccidity.

Spasticity refers to increased resistance to passive movement, often more pronounced at the extremes of range of motion and often followed by a sudden or gradual release of resistance. Spasticity is caused by injury to the corticospinal system. **Rigidity** is a state of increased resistance. **Flaccidity (hypotonia)** refers to decreased muscle tone. The muscle is weak, soft, and flabby and fatigues easily. See Table 6-13 for variations in muscle tone.

Decortication and decerebration, special states of muscle tone seen in some unconscious patients, require more detailed explanation (see next section).

Muscle Tone in the Unconscious Patient

In the unconscious patient, observe the patient lying in the bed for position and abnormal movement. Muscle tone can be assessed by guiding the extremities through passive range of motion. Rigidity, flaccidity, and spasticity can be noted by these simple maneuvers.

Unconscious patients can exhibit abnormal muscle tone or stereotyped postures initiated by noxious stimuli. The particular posture assumed varies according to the anatomic level of injury and motor tract interruption. This response results from rostral-caudal (head-to-toe) deterioration, which can occur when a hemispheric lesion extends into the midbrain or when a midbrain or upper pons lesion is present.

Decortication and Decerebration. The abnormal postures that may be noted are called *decortication* and *decerebration*, and each can be correlated to structural cerebral dysfunction (e.g., hemisphere or upper brainstem). **Decortication** is characterized by adduction of the arm at the shoulder with flexion at the elbow and pronation and flexion at the wrist; the legs extend at the hips and knee. This posture implies a structural lesion of the cerebral hemisphere or diencephalon (*above* the midbrain); the decortication is contralateral to the hemispheric lesion (Fig. 7-9). **Decerebration** includes extension, adduction, and internal rotation (hyperpronation) of the arm; there is flexion of the wrist and fingers; the legs are extended and the feet are plantarflexed. Decerebration is

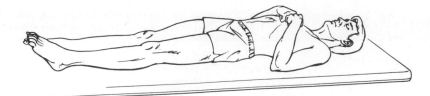

A *Flexor or decorticate posturing response*

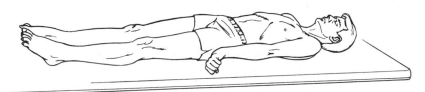

B *Extensor or decerebrate posturing*

Figure 7-9 • Abnormal rigidity. (*A*) Decorticate rigidity. In decorticate rigidity, the upper arms are held tightly to the sides, with elbows, wrists, and fingers flexed. The legs are extended and internally rotated. The feet are plantarflexed. This posture implies a destructive lesion of the corticospinal tracts within or very near the cerebral hemispheres. (*B*) Decerebrate rigidity. In decerebrate rigidity, the jaws are clenched and the neck extended. The arms are adducted and stiffly extended at the elbows, with forearms pronated, wrists, and fingers flexed. The legs are stiffly extended at the knees, with the feet plantarflexed. Decerebration is caused by a lesion in the diencephalon, midbrain, or pons, although severe metabolic disorders, such as hypoxia or hypoglycemia, may also produce it. (From Fuller, J., & Schaller-Ayers, J. [1994]. *Health assessment: A nursing approach* [2nd ed.]. Philadelphia: J. B. Lippincott.)

caused by a structural lesion of the upper brainstem, although severe metabolic disorders may also be the cause. The decerebration is contralateral to the upper brainstem lesion. Decortication and decerebration are the result of rostral-caudal deterioration. **Rostral-caudal deterioration** describes the progressive deterioration in cerebral and brainstem function that occurs with the expansion of a supratentorial lesion, thus producing pressure on the brainstem and a pattern of progressive neurological dysfunction (see Chap. 13). Early recognition and reversal of the process are imperative if permanent severe brainstem damage or death is to be prevented.

Intermittent Decortication and Decerebration. If there is a difference in an ischemic response or structural dysfunction between the deep cerebral hemispheric structures and upper brainstem, variations in adequate blood supply to these regions may cause intermittent decortication or decerebration. Clinically, the patient can change from bilateral decerebration to bilateral decortication (or vice versa), from unilateral decerebration to unilateral decortication, or with decortication on one side and decerebration on the other. Both decerebration and decortication are poor prognostic signs, although decerebration is a more ominous sign than decortication.

ASSESSMENT OF MUSCLE STRENGTH

In the **conscious, cooperative patient**, muscle strength is assessed by active and active resistive movements. What muscle should be assessed as part of the abbreviated neurological assessment at the bedside? Depending on the patient's condition, pronator drift and hand grasps must be tested at the very least. For the lower extremities, depending

on the patient's condition, asking the patient to move each leg and wiggle his or her toes and feet provides minimal data on function. A more extensive examination of both upper and lower extremities is found in Tables 6-15 and 6-17. See Table 7-4 for grading motor strength and Chart 7-7 for a summary of motor function assessment at the bedside. See Chapter 6 for assessment of the unconscious patient.

In the **unconscious patient**, muscle strength is surmised through observing the patient lying in bed and by applying noxious stimuli and noting response. The following responses are possible in response to painful stimuli:

Purposeful: localization/pushes the painful stimuli away
Nonpurposeful: movement of the stimulated area, but no attempt to push the stimuli away
Unresponsive: patient shows no signs of reacting to painful stimuli (seen in deep coma)

TABLE 7–4   GRADING OF MUSCLE STRENGTH

GRADE	STRENGTH
5	Active movement against gravity and full resistance; normal muscle strength
4	Active movement against gravity and some resistance; the examiner can overcome the muscle resistance
3	Active movement against gravity
2	Active movement of the body part when gravity is eliminated
1	A very weak muscle contraction is palpated; only a trace of a contraction is evident, but no active movement of the body part is noted
0	No muscle contraction is detectable

Upper Extremities

The unconscious patient is first observed for spontaneous movement as he or she lies in the bed. A noxious stimulus is then applied to elicit a motor response. *Note:* Apply a noxious stimulus centrally rather than peripherally. An example of a central stimulus is squeezing the pectoralis major muscle. A peripheral stimulus, such as pressing on the nail bed, may result in a reflex response. Observe for withdrawal of the arm on the stimulated side. A purposeful response will be evident if the arm crosses the midline as the arm attempts to withdraw from the noxious stimulus. To assess each arm for paresis, place the patient in a neutral supine position. Position the forearms perpendicular to the bed, holding the patient's arms upright by the hands or wrists. The movement of both arms is then observed as the extremities are released simultaneously. A paralyzed or paretic arm will fall more quickly than an intact arm. The weaker arm may strike the patient's face as it falls.

Lower Extremities

Observe for spontaneous movements. Apply a noxious stimulus to observe for any movement. Although often impractical, the legs can be assessed for paralysis or paresis. The patient is positioned flat on the back with the knees flexed so both feet are flat on the bed. The knees are simultaneously released and the movement of the legs is observed. The paralyzed or paretic leg will fall to an extended position with the hip outwardly rotated. The normal leg will maintain the flexed position for a few moments and then gradually assume its previous position.

INVOLUNTARY MOVEMENT, POSTURE, AND GAIT

The presence of involuntary movements, such as tremors, choreiform movements, myoclonus, athetosis, tics, spasms, or ballism, is noted (see Table 6-19). **Posture** is the position or orientation of the body in space; **gait** is the manner of progression in walking. First, the patient's position while he or she is lying in bed is observed. Next, if weight bearing and ambulation are possible, observe the patient's posture while he or she is standing still. The patient is then observed while walking and the following characteristics are noted: erect, stooped, or leaning toward one side; position of the arms in relationship to the body; and quality and amount of movement in the lower extremities. A description of common gait abnormalities appears in Table 6-18 and Chart 6-2.

SENSORY ASSESSMENT

The sensory assessment is usually deferred unless the patient has spinal cord disease (secondary to trauma, neoplasm, infectious processes, or stenosis), intervertebral disc disease, Guillain-Barré syndrome, or other conditions that affect the spinal cord or spinal nerves. The decision to include a sensory assessment is left to the judgment of the clinician. A sensory assess-

ment is conducted in the patient who is conscious, cooperative, and able to respond appropriately. If a sensory assessment is conducted, the sensory modalities that can be assessed include:

- Superficial sensation
- Light touch (cotton-tipped applicator)
- Pain (pin-prick)
- Deep sensation
- Proprioception (the big toe and thumb are moved in various positions)

Pain and **light touch** are the most frequently assessed modalities. The technique for assessment follows these basic principles:

- With the patient's eyes closed, begin either at the face or feet and systematically assess and compare findings on both sides of the body. If you are assessing a patient with spinal cord or spinal nerve deficits, starting at the feet and working upward is helpful to determine the highest level of intact sensory function.
- Ask the patient to tell you when the sensory stimulation is felt.
- Record the highest level of function on each side of the body (there may be unilateral sensory functional loss).

Table 4-6 includes a list of dermatome levels. Table 6-20 discusses sensory assessment in greater detail. Chart 18-4 includes the sensory assessment for spinal cord injury.

FREQUENCY AND DOCUMENTATION OF SENSORY DATA

The frequency of assessment depends on the patient's acuity and stability. Patients with acute spinal cord trauma, acute transverse myelitis, or acute Guillain-Barré syndrome should be assessed for the highest level of function every 1 to 4 hours. In a patient whose condition is stable, assessment once a shift is probably frequent enough to keep the nurse aware of functional level. Documentation of findings can be done in several ways. If a special Spinal Cord Assessment Sheet or dermatome territory map is used, data are entered using a check-mark format. Data may also be recorded in a narrative format, using dermatome landmarks to monitor function (e.g., highest sensory level is one finger above the umbilicus).

ASSESSMENT OF CEREBELLAR FUNCTION

To assess cerebellar function at the bedside, a sample of upper extremity and lower extremity function is acceptable. See Chapter 6 for more details about assessment. For upper extremities assessment, ask the patient to touch your finger and then his or her nose, and to continue doing this movement as fast as possible. Assess first with eyes open, then with eyes closed. Note the smoothness of the movement and accuracy of touching the target. An alternative method is to ask the patient to rapidly pronate and supinate the hand onto the palm of the other hand several times.

For the lower extremities, ask the patient to run the heel of one foot down the shin of the other leg. Ataxia and dysmetria are abnormal findings. If the patient is ambulatory, the Romberg test can be used. However, be prepared to support the patient if he or she begins to sway or fall. In addition, observe the patient for any involuntary movements that may be associated with cerebellar dysfunction. Cerebellar function cannot be tested in the unconscious patient. Data that suggest cerebellar dysfunction may be noted by nystagmus (see Table 6-10).

VITAL SIGNS AND CLINICAL IMPLICATIONS

Vital sign data are collected from all patients, but in patients with neurological problems there can be special considerations, particularly with increased ICP or brainstem pathophysiology. The relationship between vital signs and neurological function is based on neuroanatomy and changes in hemodynamics. The brain requires a constant, large volume of oxygen-rich blood to support adequate cerebral perfusion pressure (CPP). Without adequate CPP, cerebral ischemia develops, which affects cerebral metabolism, and neurological dysfunction occurs.

The following are homeostatic mechanisms important to understanding cerebral hemodynamics.

CNS Ischemic Response

When cerebral blood flow to the brainstem vasomotor center is compromised sufficiently to cause ischemia, the chemosensitive cells within the vasomotor center respond directly by sending efferent commands that strongly stimulate both the vagal and sympathetic nerves. Blood flow to all other tissue, including the kidney, is reduced in favor of maintaining the required flow to the brain and heart. There is a significant rise in arterial pressure. The cerebral ischemic response is interesting in that simultaneous stimulation of both the vagus and the sympathetic nerves results in an increase in myocardial contractility along with slowing of the heart rate because the vagus nerve has the stronger influence on the sinoatrial node. Therefore, the cerebral ischemic response is characterized by profound bradycardia.[7]

Cushing's Response (Reflex)

A special type of CNS ischemic response that results from increased ICP is called *Cushing's reflex* (also called Cushing's response). When cerebrospinal fluid (CSF) pressure approaches the pressure found within the intracranial cerebral arteries, the cerebral arteries become compressed and begin to collapse, compromising cerebral blood flow. To compensate, Cushing's reflex is activated, causing the arterial pressure to rise. When the arterial pressure has risen to a higher level than the CSF pressure, cerebral arterial flow is re-established and the ischemia is relieved. Thus, the arterial pressure is established and maintained at a new, higher level to provide adequate blood flow. Cushing's reflex is a compensatory response that helps protect the brain from loss of adequate blood flow.

Clinically, the nurse should realize that changes in vital signs are *late* findings in rostral-caudal deterioration. Therefore, do not wait for changes in vital signs before intervening, because it may be too late to prevent irreversible neurological damage or even death. In the discussion that follows, it is evident that the assessment of vital signs should be both quantitative and qualitative. The numeric value of each vital sign is important, but the characteristic descriptive pattern and rhythm provide diagnostic indicators of intracranial pathophysiology and neurological progression.

Anatomy and Physiology Related to Vital Signs

The vital sign "centers" are located within the brainstem. Complex networks of neurons in the brainstem reticular formation participate in the regulation of cardiovascular, respiratory, and other visceral functions. Rather than being discrete anatomic centers for a particular function, neurons for autonomic functions are intermingled and functionally related and have reciprocal connections. Observation of a physiologic response, such as inspiration, is seen when a particular area of the RF is stimulated. The RF receives visceral sensory input polysynaptically through collaterals from ascending spinal cord sensory pathways, through descending fibers from the hypothalamus, and from the limbic system through the dorsal longitudinal fasciculus, medial forebrain bundle, and mamillotegmental tracts.

Heart Rate and Blood Pressure

Control of heart rate and blood pressure are also mediated by circuits at multiple levels within the nervous system. Inputs to the caudal nucleus solitarius, also known as the cardiorespiratory nucleus, and the circuits in the medullary RF are primarily responsible for heart rate and blood pressure. The ventrolateral medulla contains a group of **vasomotor neurons** that control blood pressure.

The nucleus solitarius receives input from baroreceptors in the carotid body and aortic arch via cranial nerves IX and X. Control of heart rate and blood pressure is then mediated by circuits, many which project directly from the nucleus solitarius to parasympathetic and sympathetic preganglionic neurons in the brainstem and spinal cord. Presympathetic neurons in the rostral ventrolateral medulla project to sympathetic neurons in the spinal cord intermediolateral cell column and are critical for maintaining normal arterial blood pressure, mediating sympathetic reflexes, and serving as relay stations for sympathetic pathways.[8] Other neurons in the ventrolateral medulla, the cardiovagal neurons, control heart rate. Finally, portions of the medullary RF coordinate various respiratory and cardiovascular reflexes.

Respirations

Respiration involves a multiple-level network of control systems. Selected neurons within the RF control visceral motor neurons and respiratory motor neurons (Fig. 7-10). The numerous inputs to respiratory circuits include chemoreceptors from blood oxygen level and pH. Many of the projections to the respiratory circuits come from the cardiorespiratory

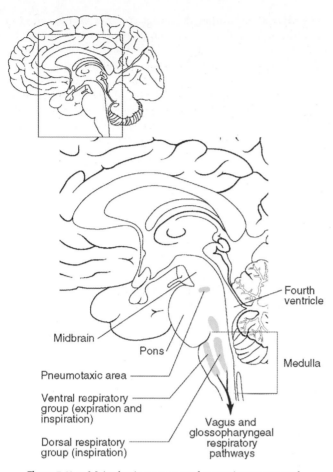

Figure 7-10 • Major brainstem areas for respiratory control.

portion of the nucleus solitarius (located in the medulla). In addition, there are inputs from stretch receptors located in the lungs. Other nuclei in the medulla participate in respiratory rhythms; some are active during inspiration, while others are active during expiration. Ultimately, these nuclei project to spinal cord lower motor neurons in cervical spinal segments C-3 to C-5 to excite efferent neurons of the phrenic nerve that contract the diaphragm during inspiration, or to lower motor neurons at thoracic levels controlling thoracic inspiratory and expiratory muscles.[8] Respiratory neurons found in the parabrachial area (pons) are called pontine dorsal or the **pneumotaxic center**, whereas the nucleus solitarius (medulla) and ventrolateral medulla neurons together are called the **ventral respiratory groups**. These excitatory neurons sustain vasomotor tone and respirations. The several respiratory groups include **inspiratory neurons** that project to the spinal phrenic motor neurons and **expiratory neurons** that project to the intercostal respiratory motor neurons. Interneurons located proximal to the ventral respiratory groups are key for the generation of respiratory rhythm.

The **ventral respiratory groups** have a role in controlling inspiration and expiration. The **pneumotaxic center** transmits impulses of varying magnitude for inspirations. The primary function of the center is to limit inspiration; however, by limiting respirations, it exerts a secondary effect on the rate of breathing. Strong pneumotaxic signals can increase the rate of breathing (e.g., 30 to 40 per minute), whereas weak signals will reduce the rate to only a few

breaths per minute. The Hering-Breuer reflex also has an effect on turning off respirations.

The **Hering-Breuer reflex** is a protective reflex that prevents excessive lung expansion. Stretch receptors located in the bronchi and bronchioles throughout the lungs transmit signals through the vagus nerve to the dorsal respiratory group when the lungs are overinflated and expiration is initiated. This reflex has a function similar to that of the pneumotaxic center in that it limits the duration of inspiration through a feedback loop that "turns off" inspiratory effort and reduces the time of inspiration so that the respiratory rate is increased.

Body Temperature

Control of body temperature is complex. No single center within the nervous system controls body temperature. On the contrary, thermoregulation is a process that involves a continuum of neural structures from the hypothalamus and limbic system through the lower brainstem and reticular formation to the spinal cord and sympathetic ganglia.[9] The preoptic region, located in and near the rostral hypothalamus, appears to have a primary role in thermoregulation. The preoptic region includes the medial and lateral aspects of the peroptic area, the anterior hypothalamus, and septum.[10]

In living cells, heat is derived from biochemical reactions. At the mitochondrial level, energy derived from the catabolism of metabolites, such as glucose, is utilized in oxidative phosphorylation to convert adenosine diphosphate to adenosine triphosphate. Heat generated by deep-lying vital organs is distributed throughout the body via the circulatory system. The nervous system monitors the temperature of various body parts and the rate of heat loss from body surfaces (e.g., conduction, convection, radiation, and evaporation).[11] Regulation of heat is accomplished by an integrated response of the sweat glands, peripheral vessels, and skeletal muscles for shivering. Through these structures, the body can conserve or divest itself of body heat. In a warm environment or in the presence of an elevated core temperature, cutaneous blood flow increases so that heat is transported from the core to be dissipated at the skin surface. Conversely, in a cold environment or in the presence of a decreased core temperature, cutaneous blood is diverted to the body core.

Other Functions

Coughing, hiccuping, sneezing, yawning, shivering, gagging, and vomiting are heavily dependent on circuits in the pontomedullary RF. Lesions of the brainstem can interfere with these functions or cause abnormalities in their presentation.[8]

Assessment of Vital Signs

Respirations

The respiratory patterns may be helpful in localizing levels of brainstem involvement, but metabolic abnormalities may affect the respiratory centers and result in patterns resembling those due to neurological disease. Therefore, a thorough review of the metabolic status of the patient must be included to accurately interpret respiratory changes. Abnormal respiratory patterns generally suggest brainstem dysfunction and progression of pathophysiology, a prognostic indicator of poor outcome. See Table 7-5 for a discussion of abnormal respiratory patterns and anatomic site of dysfunction.[12] Clinically, it is not always possible to observe abnormal respiratory patterns because the patient may be intubated and connected to a ventilator that is set for a particular mode, rate, and rhythm, thus overriding an inadequate respiratory pattern. In some cases, respiratory changes may not be seen until just before death.

Note the rate, rhythm, and characteristics of the inspiratory and expiratory phases of respirations. In addition to neurological causes of respiratory changes, a number of other etiologies should also be considered, such as acidosis, alkalosis, electrolyte imbalance, congestive heart failure, anxiety, and various respiratory complications (e.g., atelectasis, pneumonia, pulmonary edema). Drugs, particularly narcotic analgesics, sedatives, and anesthetics, may have a depressant effect on the respiratory system. Morphine sulfate depresses the respiratory rate in addition to causing constriction of the pupils. Because it causes respiratory depression and masks the neurological signs of pupillary response, use of morphine sulfate is limited in neurological patients. Small doses of morphine sulfate may be ordered to decrease rapid respirations as long as ongoing monitoring and respiratory support are available via a pulse oximeter or other monitoring device.

Changes in respirations can be due to many neurological and non-neurological causes. The nurse must consider the complete data set when assessing respiratory function and planning interventions. Metabolic, cardiac, and respiratory conditions can trigger changes in respiratory function. Trauma to the cervical spine may produce respiratory distress; if the injury is above the phrenic segment (C-3 to C-5), total arrest will occur.

The role of the nurse in relation to respiratory function includes (1) periodically assessing and documenting the rate, rhythm, and characteristics of respirations; (2) implementing interventions to maintain a patent airway and promote respiratory function; (3) assessing for secondary conditions that may cause changes in respiratory pattern or rate; (4) assessing for respiratory complications or insufficiency; and (5) notifying the physician if respiratory problems occur.

Pulse and Heart Rate

The rate, rhythm, and quality of the pulse and heart rate should be assessed, documented, and compared with previous data. Common changes that may occur in rate and rhythm are tachycardia, bradycardia, and cardiac arrhythmias. A bounding or thready pulse is a common change in pulse quality, and often accompanies rising ICP. A thready pulse is seen in the terminal stages of neurological demise, or with hemorrhage. **Tachycardia** in a neurological patient can indicate that a patient is hypoxic, experiencing terminal stages of high ICP, or bleeding internally in the abdominal, thoracic, or pelvic cavity. **Bradycardia** can occur in the later stages of progressive increased ICP as part of Cushing's response. The blood is pumped to the edematous brain against great pressure and resistance so that the pulse is decreased to a rate of 40 to 60 per minute and bounding. Additionally, **hypotension and bradycardia** may be secondary to cervical spinal cord injury with interruption of descending sympathetic pathways.

Cardiac arrhythmias are rather common in neurological conditions. Arrhythmias are seen more often in patients who have blood in the CSF (e.g., subarachnoid hemorrhage, severe head injury), have undergone posterior fossa surgery, or have increased ICP. If there is evidence of abnormalities in cardiac rate or rhythm, a rhythm strip should be obtained immediately to document and identify the problem. Treatment should be instituted as necessary. Continuous cardiac monitoring is important in unstable, acute patients.

Blood Pressure

In assessing blood pressure, the nurse monitors for hypotension, hypertension, and pulse pressure. A comparison is made with previous assessment data.

Hypertension in the neurological patient may be associated with sympathetic stimulation resulting from massive hypothalamic discharge or a rising ICP. An elevated systolic blood pressure, widening pulse pressure, and bradycardia are seen in the advanced stages of increased ICP and are known as **Cushing's reflex**.

Hypotension is rarely attributable to cerebral injury. When it is seen with severe neurological injury, it occurs as a terminal event and is accompanied by tachycardia. Inadequate cerebral perfusion denies cerebral tissue of an adequate oxygen supply, and the regulatory mechanisms no longer function. In this stage of decompensation, deterioration is rapid and death results. The suspicion of occult internal hemorrhage (thoracic, abdominal, pelvic, or long bone) should be raised when **hypotension and tachycardia** are seen together. **Hypotension and bradycardia** may be seen in patients with cervical spinal injury as a result of interruption in the descending sympathetic pathways.

Temperature

The temperature and the route by which it was taken should be recorded on the clinical flow sheet. If a continuous temperature-monitoring device is being used, this should also be noted on the flow sheet. If the temperature is elevated and the patient has been placed on a hypothermia blanket, the temperature should be monitored frequently (e.g., every 30 minutes) until it drops to an acceptable level. Shivering increases ICP and must be avoided.

Hypothermia is seen in certain conditions such as spinal shock when autonomic innervation is lost; metabolic or toxic coma of any origin; drug overdose, especially in barbiturate overdose; and destructive brainstem or hypothalamic lesions. Specific treatment depends on the cause. A variety of interventions can be implemented to maintain normal body temperature such as application of warm blankets and/or a warming blanket and adjustment of the thermostat for a comfortable room temperature.

Hyperthermia is much more common than hypothermia. Fever is a complex, coordinated autonomic, neuroendocrine, and behavioral response that is adaptive and is often part of the acute-phase reaction to an immune challenge.[13] Fever can originate from infectious and noninfectious conditions. It is important that this determination is made to save needless diagnostics and inappropriate antimicrobial therapy. Regardless of the cause, the clinical presentation of fever is stereotypical and largely independent

TABLE 7–5 RESPIRATORY PATTERNS ASSOCIATED WITH LESIONS AT VARYING LEVELS OF THE BRAIN

The following abnormal respiratory patterns are seen in conditions that affect the respiratory centers of the brainstem directly and indirectly. *Primary brainstem injury* occurs as a result of direct injury, ischemia, infarction, or a tumor located in the brainstem respiratory centers. *Secondary brainstem injury* can occur as a result of ischemia secondary to impending herniation from a supratentorial lesion (e.g., cerebral edema, space-occupying lesion) or, rarely, an infratentorial lesion; or CNS depression from metabolic conditions or drug overdose. However, increased ICP with impending herniation is the major cause of abnormal respiratory patterns.

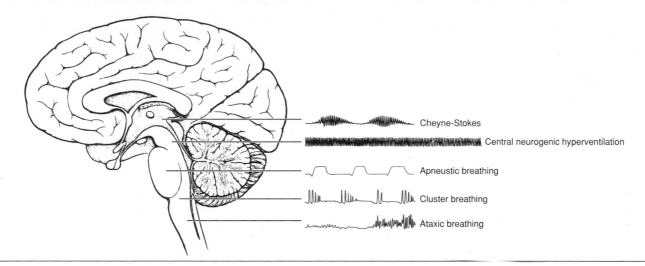

PATTERN AND LOCATION	DESCRIPTION
Cheyne-Stokes Respirations	

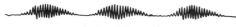

├─One Minute─┤

Lesion: may be associated with bilateral widespread cortical lesions but most often associated with bilateral thalamic dysfunction; may also result from bilateral damage anywhere along the descending pathway between the forebrain and upper pons; can also be associated with metabolic abnormalities as seen in uremia and heart failure patients	• Rhythmic waxing and waning pattern • Brief periods of hyperpnea alternating with short period of apnea • Pattern due to two factors: (1) increased sensitivity to carbon dioxide resulting in change in depth and rate, and (2) decreased stimulation from respiratory centers resulting in apnea

Central Neurogenic Hyperventilation

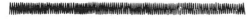

├─One Minute─┤

Lesion: midbrain and upper pons

• Prolonged and rapid hyperpnea from 40–70 breaths per minute
• Rare, and must be differentiated from reactive hyperventilation related to metabolic abnormalities
• May lead to respiratory alkalosis

Apneustic Breathing

├─One Minute─┤

• A prolonged inspiratory gasp with a pause at full inspiration in which the breath is held and then released

Lesion: lower pons

Cluster Breathing

├─One Minute─┤

• Clusters of periodic respirations that are irregular in frequency and amplitude, with varying periods of apnea between clusters of breaths

Lesion: lower pons or upper medulla

Ataxic Breathing

├─One Minute─┤

• Completely irregular, unpredictable pattern in which inspiratory gasps of varying amplitude and length are interspersed with periods of apnea

Location: medulla

CNS, central nervous system; ICP, intracranial pressure.

of the causative agent. Fever may be associated with any of the following conditions.

Infectious Origins.

Various organisms such as *Staphylococcus aureus, Escherichia coli, Pseudomonas aeruginosa,* and others cause infections. Infections can result from open head wounds (meningitis), contaminated postoperative wounds or shunts, nosocomial pneumonia, and intravenous lines and tubes (central and peripheral lines, urinary catheters [urosepsis], ventriculostomies). Nonneurological causes of infection must be considered in the differential diagnosis such as septicemia, gram-negative sepsis, endocarditis, community-acquired pneumonia, ventilator-associated pneumonia (VAP), septic pulmonary emboli, antibiotic-associated diarrhea/colitis, and intraabdominal or pelvic infection resulting from perforation, trauma, or surgery. Treatment is based on the selection of a sensitive antimicrobial drug. In addition, strict aseptic dressing technique and line- and tube-change protocols can significantly reduce infections. The relationship of good mouth care to VAP is well established by a number of studies, thus establishing an imperative for mouth care protocols as a preventive strategy.

Noninfectious Origins

- **Non-neurological,** noninfectious, common causes of fever include acute myocardial infarction, acute pulmonary embolism/infarction, acute pancreatitis, gastrointestinal hemorrhage, phlebitis, hematomas, attacks of acute gout, fevers related to malignancies, and drug hypersensitivity reactions.
- **Drug-induced fever** is caused by an immune response to a drug. Common causative drugs include anticonvulsants such as phenytoin (Dilantin) and carbamazepine (Tegretol); analgesics; phenothiazines; anticholinergic drugs; and antibiotics. The diagnosis is established by withdrawal of the drug and subsequent rechallenge. Cultures of blood, urine, and sputum are negative, and the patient looks better clinically than the temperature would suggest.
- **Posterior fossa syndrome** mimics meningitis with a number of symptoms that include stiff neck. However, unlike meningitis, CSF cultures are negative. Posterior fossa syndrome is seen in patients who have had posterior fossa surgery or blood in the CSF and is often related to subarachnoid hemorrhage.
- **Neuroleptic malignant syndrome (NMS)** is an adverse reaction to antipsychotic agents such as butyrophenones, phenothiazines, and thioxanthenes. The most common cause of NMS is haloperidol. The etiology is believed to be the result of CNS dopamine receptor blockade, or withdrawal of exogenous dopaminergic agonists.[14] Signs and symptoms usually occur within several days of initiation of treatment and include "lead pipe" muscular rigidity, altered mental status, autonomic dysfunction (e.g., diaphoresis, labile blood pressure, dysrhythmias), and a high fever of up to 41.5°C (107°F). The dosage and serum concentration of the drugs are usually within normal therapeutic ranges. Discontinuing of the drug and supporting therapy are the components of a treatment plan.

- **Malignant hyperthermia** (MH) is a rare, pharmacogenetic problem of skeletal muscles characterized by hypermetabolism that occurs on exposure to a triggering agent or agents. Anesthetic agents, particularly inhalation anesthetics, and succinylcholine and halothane are most commonly associated with MH. Since it is related to anesthetics, it occurs in the perioperative period, although it can reoccur within the first 24 to 48 hours after an initial event. Tachycardia is the most common first sign occurring within the first hour of induction of anesthesia. Other signs and symptoms include increased carbon dioxide production, skin cyanosis with mottling, and marked hyperthermia up to 45°C (113°F). In addition, hypotension, dysrhythmias, rhabdomyolysis, electrolyte abnormalities, and disseminated intravascular coagulation can occur.[14] Management includes immediate discontinuation of the offending agent and supportive care (e.g., airway management, cardiac support) and cooling interventions. Dantrolene is the specific drug used to treat MH.

Central Fever.

Central fever is a much debated concept and is defined as a fever caused by a central neurogenic etiology seen with space-occupying lesions, trauma or a lesion that involves the hypothalamus or base of the brain, or traction of the hypothalamus or brainstem. High fever—up to 41.5°C—is the cardinal finding, and perspiration is absent. This is a diagnosis of exclusion and is made only after all other causes of fever have been ruled out.

Effects of Steroids on Temperature.

The neurological patient may be treated with large doses of steroids, often dexamethasone (Decadron). Steroids are anti-inflammatory agents that mask the classic clinical signs of infections, such as an elevated temperature and white blood count.[15] Therefore, monitor the patient for signs of infection such as cloudy or foul-smelling urine; yellowish, foul-smelling sputum; or adventitious breath sounds. Cultures and blood counts should be monitored for evidence of infection.

Management of Elevated Body Temperature.

How aggressively should an elevated temperature be treated? Most clinicians who manage neurological patients will treat an elevated temperature when it reaches a certain level (38° or 39°C) because of the effect on the brain. An elevated temperature increases overall body metabolism and cell metabolism of all systems, including the brain, which, in turn, produces an increase in carbon dioxide and lactic acid by-products of cell metabolism. Carbon dioxide, a potent cerebral vasodilator, will cause an increase in ICP in a patient who may already have high ICP. If the oxygen supply to cerebral tissue is insufficient, cerebral ischemia develops. Usual treatment is acetaminophen and possibly a cooling blanket for high temperatures. Reviews of the evidence-based practices followed by nurses to reduce fever found no scientific basis for many practices.[16] The conclusions from randomized controlled trials are that elevated body temperature independently contributes to increased length of stay, higher mortality rates, and poorer patient outcomes in neurological intensive are units.[17] Therefore, aggressive treatment of an elevated body temperature to prevent neurological deterioration is critical. Evidence-based practice guidelines are available for evaluating new fever in critically ill adult patients.[18] Mild therapeutic hypothermia is being used to improve neurological outcomes from stroke and traumatic brain injuries. This will be discussed in later chapters. Guidelines have been published by the Society of Critical Care Medicine[18]; although they were published in 1998, they are still current and comprehensive.

The cause of the elevated temperature must be investigated carefully. The nurse should listen to the patient's chest for adventitious breath sounds. The urine and the sputum should be considered for possible culture. Finally, all dressings and drainage, if present, should be assessed.

SUMMARY

The neurological assessment is the foundational database for the nurse to use in identifying nursing diagnoses and collaborative interdisciplinary problems, planning care, implementing interventions, and evaluating outcomes. It is essential that the nurse develop the skills and knowledge to conduct this assessment competently and engage in the clinical reasoning for patient management and positive patient outcomes.

REFERENCES

1. Blumenfeld, H. (2002). *Neuroanatomy through clinical cases* (pp. 588–592). Sunderland, MA: Sinauer Associates, Inc.
2. Masferrer, R. (2000). Advanced neurological assessments: Clinical and radiographic correlations. 8th International Nurse Practitioner Conference, San Diego, California, September 28, 2000.
3. Rubino, F. A. (2002). Approach to the comatose patient. In J. Biller (Ed.). *Practical neurology* (2nd ed., pp. 54–65). Philadelphia: Lippincott Williams & Wilkins.
4. Plum, F., & Posner, J. (1980). *The diagnosis of stupor and coma* (3rd ed., pp. 178–180). Philadelphia: F. A. Davis.
5. Folstein, M. F., Folstein, S. E., & McHugh, P. R. (1975). Minimental state: A practical method for grading the cognitive state of patients for the clinician. *Journal of Psychiatric Research, 12*, 189–198.
6. Retrieved June 25, 2008, from http://www.waiting.com/levelsofcoma.html Rancho Los Amigos Scale/The levels of Coma.
7. Johnson, K. R. (Ed.). (1998). *Essential medical physiology* (2nd ed., pp. 212–213). Philadelphia: Lippincott-Raven.
8. Blumenfeld, H. (2002). *Neuroanatomy through clinical cases* (pp. 605–606). Sunderland, MA: Sinauer Associates, Inc.
9. Mackowiak, P. A., & Boulant, J. A. (1996). Fever's glass ceiling. *Clinical Infectious Diseases, 22*, 525–536.
10. Mackowiak, P. A. (1998). Concepts of fever. *Archives of Internal Medicine, 158*, 1870–1881.
11. Boulant, J. A. (1980). Hypothalamic control of thermoregulation: Neurophysiological basis. In P. J. Morgane & J. Pankepp (Eds.). *Handbook of the hypothalamus* (vol. 3, part A, pp. 1–82). New York: Marcel Dekker Inc.
12. Berger, J. R. (2004). Clinical approach to stupor and coma. In W. G. Bradley, R. B. Daroff, G. M. Fenichel, & J. Jankovic (Eds.). *Neurology in clinical practice: Principles of diagnosis and management* (4th ed., pp. 50–58). Philadelphia: Butterworth Heinemann.
13. Saper, C. B., & Breder, C. D. (1994). The neurological basis of fever. *New England Journal of Medicine, 330*(26), 1880–1886.
14. Mechem, C. C. Severe hyperthermia: Heat stroke; neuroleptic malignant syndrome; and malignant hyperthermia. Retrieved October 19, 2005, from http://www.uptodateonline.com/application/topic/topicOutline.asp?file=cc_medi/13742
15. Rhen, T., & Cidlowski, J. A. (2005). Antiinflammatory action of glucocorticoids — New mechanism for old drugs. *New England Journal of Medicine, 353*(16), 711–723.
16. Henker, R. (1999). Evidence-based practice: Fever-related interventions. *American Journal of Critical Care, 8*(1), 481–487.
17. Diringer, M. N., Reaven, N. L., Funk, S. E., & Uman, G. C. (2004). Elevated body temperature independently contributes to increased length of stay in neurologic intensive care unit patients. *Critical Care Medicine, 32*(7), 1489–1495.
18. O'Grady, N. P., Barie, P. S., Bartlett, J., Bleck, T., Garvey, G., Jacobi, J., et al. (1998). Practice parameters for evaluating new fever in critically ill adult patients. *Critical Care Medicine, 26*(2), 392–408.

RESOURCES

Books and Chapters

Berger, J. R. (2004). Clinical approach to stupor and coma. In W. G. Bradley, R. B. Daroff, G. M. Fenichel, & J. Jankovic (Eds.). *Neurology in clinical practice: Principles of diagnosis and management* (4th ed., pp. 43–64). Philadelphia: Butterworth Heinemann.

Bickley, L. A., & Szilagyi, P. G. (2005). *Bates' guide to physical examination and history taking* (9th ed.). Philadelphia: Lippincott Williams & Wilkins.

Blumenfeld, H. (2002). *Neuroanatomy through clinical cases*. Sunderland, MA: Sinauer Associates, Inc.

Brazis, P. W., Masdeu, J. C., Biller, J., & Brazis, P. (2001). *Localization in clinical neurology* (4th ed.). Boston: Little Brown & Co.

Campbell, W. W. (2005). *DeJong's the neurological examination* (6th ed.). Philadelphia: Lippincott Williams & Wilkins.

DeMyer, W. E. (2004). *Techniques of the neurological examination* (5th ed.). New York: McGraw Hill.

Fuller, G. (2000). *Neurologic examination made easy* (2nd ed.). New York: Churchill Livingstone.

Goetz, C. G. (2003). *Textbook of clinical neurology* (3rd ed.). Philadelphia: W. B. Saunders.

The Guarantors of Brain. (2000). *Aids to the examination of the peripheral nervous system* (4th ed.). Philadelphia: W. B. Saunders.

Hoppenfeld, S. (1976). *Physical examination of the spine and extremities*. Norwalk, CT: Appleton & Lange.

Hoppenfeld, S. (1977). *Orthopaedic neurology: A diagnostic guide to neurologic levels*. Philadelphia: J. B. Lippincott.

Jennett, B. (2002). *The vegetative state: Medical facts, ethical and legal dilemmas*. Cambridge, UK: Cambridge University Press.

LeBlond, R. L., DeGowin, R. L., & Brown, D. D. (2004). *DeGovin's diagnostic examination* (8th ed.). New York: McGraw-Hill.

Lezak, M. D. (2004). *Neuropsychological assessment* (4th ed.). New York: Oxford University Press.

Members of the Mayo Clinic Department of Neurology. (1998). *Mayo clinic examinations in neurology* (7th ed.). St. Louis: Mosby.

Miller, N. R., Newman, N. J, Biousse, V., & Kerrison, J. B. (2004). *Walsh & Hoyt's clinical neuro-ophthalmology—the essentials* (6th ed.). Philadelphia: Lippincott Williams & Wilkins.

Strub, R. L., & Black, F. W. (2000). *The mental status examination in neurology* (4th ed.). Philadelphia: F. A. Davis Co.

Tasman, A., & First, M. B. (2004). *DSM-IV-TR mental disorders: Diagnosis, etiology, and treatment*. Hoboken, NJ: Wiley.

Young, G. B., Ropper, A. H., & Bolton, C. F. (Eds.). (1998). *Coma and impaired consciousness: A clinical perspective*. New York: McGraw Hill.

Journal Articles

Bronstein, A. M. (2003). Vestibular reflexes and positional maneuvers. *Journal of Neurology, Neurosurgery, & Psychiatry, 74,* 289–293.

Lower, J. (2002). Facing neuro assessment fearlessly. *Nursing, 32*(2), 58–65.

Meeker, M., Du, R., Bacchetti, P., Privitera, C.N., Larson, M. D., Holland, M. C., et al. (2005). Pupil examination: Validity and clinical utility of an automated pupillometer. *Journal of Neuroscience Nursing, 37*(1), 34–40.

Neatherlin, J. S. (1999). Foundation for practice: Neuroassessment for neuroscience nurses. *Nursing Clinics of North America, 34*(3), 573–592.

Saper, C. B., & Breder, C. D. (1994). The neurological basis of fever. *New England Journal of Medicine, 330*(26), 1880–1886.

Electronic Resources

Gelb, D. (2004). The detailed neurological examination. UpToDate. www.uptodate.com

Oommen, H. J. (2005). Neurological history and physical examination. http://www.emedicine.com/neuro/topic632.htm

General Considerations in Neuroscience Nursing

CHAPTER

8

Nutritional Support for Neuroscience Patients

Joanne V. Hickey and Theresa Dildy

Recognition of the critical role of nutrition in health and disease is reflected in standards of nutritional assessment and therapeutics based on a large body of scientific evidence and knowledge. The clinical dietitian is the recognized clinical expert prepared in nutritional therapeutics who is a member of the interdisciplinary team. For nurses who provide holistic comprehensive care for neuroscience patients, meeting nutritional needs of the patient is a critical component in the recovery process that requires an appropriate knowledge base and collaboration with a clinical dietitian. Injury, physiologic dysfunction, and stress often change the basic requirements and utilization of nutrients for energy, cellular function, and repair of injured tissue. Additionally, a patient with a neurological condition may have neurological deficits, such as an altered level of consciousness or paresis/paralysis of the muscles for arm movement or swallowing, which further complicates ingestion of nutrients. Consideration of these multiple and complex factors, plus the effect of an illness on both the neurological and other systems, requires the expertise and collaborative efforts of the interdisciplinary team. This chapter briefly addresses nutritional requirements and nutritional therapeutics as applied to a neuroscience patient population. The reader is referred to other standard texts, periodicals, and websites for more detailed information.

BASIC NUTRITIONAL REQUIREMENTS

Recommended dietary reference intakes (DRIs), updated in 2004, are the recognized guidelines for nutritional sufficiency.[1] The DRIs are based on scientific evidence and are approved by the National Academy of Sciences and Institute of Medicine, Food and Nutrition Board. The DRIs outline target intake levels of essential nutrients for healthy people. Nutrient requirements include macronutrients (energy, protein, lipids) and micronutrients (vitamins, minerals). It is important to keep in mind that the nutritional need can differ greatly in *patients who are ill*, especially if a malabsorption syndrome is present. Recommended daily allowances (RDAs) cited apply only to oral intake unless otherwise noted; there are some variations for parenteral routes of administration.

Essential Nutrient Requirements in Health and Illness

The essential nutrient requirements of adults in health and illness vary. These requirements will be briefly addressed from the perspective of energy, carbohydrate, fat, protein, fluid, electrolyte, vitamin, and trace elements based on recommendations of A.S.P.E.N.[2] The Institute of Medicine defines *estimated energy requirement* (EER) for healthy adults as the dietary energy intake predicted to maintain energy balance in a healthy adult of a defined age, gender, weight, height, and level of physical activity consistent with good health.[3]

In calculating EER age, physical activity, height, and intensity of activity are included. Energy requirements can also be measured with indirect calorimetry that results in the resting energy expended (REE). This indirect method of estimating REE requires special equipment that measures the ratio of carbon dioxide expired to the amount of oxygen inspired. The values collected are used in a mathematical equation to determine nutritional needs. Other options to estimate REE in the hospitalized patient are the Harris-Benedict equations, and more recently, the Ireton-Jones equations.[4] The advantage of the Ireton-Jones calculations is that it is normed to sick populations so that the stress of illness has already been calculated into the equation. The Harris-Benedict equations must be adapted to sick patients. A few basic rules are useful for calculating energy requirements as outlined in the A.S.P.E.N guidelines.[2] Energy requirements are based on kilocalories per kilogram of body weight with a range of 20 to 35 total kcal/kg body weight/day. Energy comes from carbohydrates and fats. Carbohydrates should be provided at a rate not to exceed 7 g/kg/day, while fat should not exceed a rate of 2.5 g/kg/day. For critically ill patients fat intake is limit to 1 g/kg/day.

Carbohydrates are defined as starches and sugars that are used by the body for energy. When metabolized, 1 g of carbohydrate yields 4 calories. Carbohydrates are classified as monosaccharides, disaccharides, or polysaccharides. For carbohydrates to be used by the body, they must be broken down into glucose (a monosaccharide), the simplest form of sugar. Glucose is oxidized to release energy and is the source of energy for cerebral cell metabolism. Glucose may also be stored as a reserve in the liver (and in muscle tissue to a lesser degree) in the form of glycogen through a process called **glycogenesis.** Hydrolysis of glycogen to glucose is called **glycolysis** (the anabolic enzymatic conversion of glucose to lactate or pyruvate, resulting in energy stored in the form of adenosine triphosphate [ATP], such as occurs in muscles). In addition, excess glucose can be converted into fat and stored in the body as adipose tissue.

Fats occurring as organic substances in the body are called **lipids** and include triglycerides (fats and oils), phospholipids (e.g., lecithin), and sterols (e.g., cholesterol).[5] The major function of fats is energy production, although they are also important for the manufacture of other fat-related compounds, such as cholesterol, triglycerides, phospholipids, and lecithin. The major sources of fat in the normal diet are butter, margarine, oil, bacon, meat, fats, egg yolks, nuts, and legumes. When 1 g of fat is oxidized, 9 calories are generated.

Fatty acids are the basic units of structure in lipids; they can be divided into essential fatty acids and nonessential fatty acids. An **essential fatty acid** is one that cannot be manufactured in the body. There are two essential fatty acids that are polyunsaturated; they are linoleic acid (omega-6 fatty acid) and α-linolenic acid (omega-3 fatty acid). Essential fatty acids play a role in maintaining skin and growth in children. As part of phospholipids, essential fatty acids are a component of cell membranes and are precursors of *eiconsanoids*, a group of hormone-like substances involved in inflammation and blood clotting. Prostaglandins, thromboxanes, and leukotrienes are types of eiconsanoids related to essential fatty acids.[5] Although the body cannot make essential fatty acids, it does store them so that deficiencies are rare under normal conditions. Under normal circumstances, **nonessential fatty acids** do not cause specific deficiency disorders if not ingested in sufficient amounts because they can be manufactured in the body.

All food contains a mixture of saturated, monounsaturated, and polyunsaturated fatty acids. The saturation characteristic is important because it influences the fat's physical traits and its impact on health. Discussion about the role of omega-3 and omega-6 fatty acids in health is of interest. Omega-3 polyunsaturated oils are found in fish such as salmon, herring, trout, mackerel, and swordfish and also in some plant oils such as canola oil, flaxseeds, walnuts, and hazelnuts, whereas omega-6 polyunsaturated oils are found in plant oils such as sunflower, corn, soybean, and cottonseed oils. Both omega-6 and omega-3 fatty acids have immune-modulating properties and both have an effect on inflammation, blood clotting, and lipid levels. However, these are often opposing functions; therefore, it is important that both omega-6 and omega-3 fatty acids are present in the diet in a balanced ratio.

Protein is a class of energy-yielding nutrients composed of carbon, hydrogen, and oxygen plus nitrogen, which is unique to protein. When metabolized, 1 g of protein yields 4 calories. The building blocks of protein are amino acids, the primary function of which is to build and repair body tissue. Almost all nitrogen ingested comes from protein, and most of the nitrogen lost from the body is in the form of nitrogenous end-products found in the urine as urea, creatinine, uric acid, and ammonium salts. A small amount of nitrogen loss occurs through the stool and skin. **Nitrogen balance** is defined as when protein synthesis and protein breakdown occur at the same rate. **Positive nitrogen balance** is present when protein synthesis exceeds protein breakdown, whereas **negative nitrogen balance** occurs when protein breakdown exceeds protein synthesis. In the clinical setting, nitrogen balance is determined by calculating protein intake and urine urea nitrogen (UUN) excretion for the same 24-hour period and comparing findings.

Proteins are composed of amino acids. There are 20 common amino acids that are classified as either essential or nonessential. **Essential amino acids** are necessary for normal growth and development and cannot be manufactured by the body. **Nonessential amino acids** are defined as amino acids that are not necessary for normal growth and development and can be manufactured by the body. Protein can also be classified as either complete or incomplete. A **complete protein** is one that contains all essential amino acids in sufficient quantity and appropriate proportions to supply the body's needs. Proteins of animal origin, such as milk, meat, cheese, and eggs, are examples of complete proteins. An **incomplete protein** is defined as one that is deficient in one or more essential amino acids. Incomplete proteins are of plant origin and include grains, legumes, and nuts.

The RDA of protein for healthy adults is 0.8 g/kg regardless of gender or age.[3] For a patient who is in a catabolic state, the requirement is higher, ranging from 1.2 to 2.0 g/kg/day.[7] In addition, adequate kilocalories must be provided with the protein to ensure proper protein utilization. Note that patients with certain diseases, such as renal failure and end-stage liver disease, may require a protein-restricted diet.

Fluid, electrolytes, vitamins, and trace elements are all essential to health. The typical *fluid* requirement for adults is 20 to 40 mL/kg per day or 1 to 1.5 mL/kcal of energy expended.[6] In the clinical setting, there are great variations dependent on disease (e.g., heart failure, ascites), which may require fluid restriction, and hypermetabolic states (e.g., perspiration, diarrhea), which may require an increased fluid intake. Fluid supplement is individualized based on intake and output measurements and clinical condition. Relying on the thirst mechanism to trigger drinking is unreliable, especially in elderly persons, because there tends to be impairment of thirst, which leads to underhydration. When adequate fluid intake cannot be achieved by the oral route, the enteral or parenteral routes are alternative options that will be discussed later in the chapter. See Chapter 9 for further discussion of fluid imbalance. The major *electrolytes* in the body are sodium, potassium, chloride, calcium, magnesium, and phosphorus. Electrolytes are involved in metabolic activities and are essential to the normal cellular function. Electrolyte imbalances are common in disease states and require careful physical and laboratory monitoring and correction as part of therapeutic intervention.

Certain **vitamins** cannot be stored in the body, so that deficiencies can develop if an adequate diet is not consumed daily. Other vitamins can be stored in the body so that deficiencies are not apparent for weeks to months of inadequate vitamin intake. Vitamins are classified as either water soluble or fat soluble. **Water-soluble vitamins** are vitamin C and the B-complex vitamins (i.e., thiamine, riboflavin, niacin [nicotinic acid], pyridoxine, pantothenic acid, biotin, folic acid, and cobalamin). The **fat-soluble vitamins** are vitamins A, D, E, and K. Vitamins are needed for recovery and maintenance of cellular and system functions. Although there are recommendations for vitamin and trace mineral requirements for a healthy person on an oral diet, the recommendations can be extrapolated with caution for patients who are ill.[2]

In summary, this brief review provides a backdrop to consider the nutritional requirements and the impact of neurological conditions and nutritional modifications needed for recovery and maintenance.

METABOLIC CHANGES AND CHARACTERISTICS OF ACUTE STRESS

Profound metabolic changes result in response to acute illness such as neurotrauma, sepsis, and major surgery. Patients have increased energy and nutrient needs and require nutritional support. Because of the complexity of the stress response to injury and subsequent changes in nutrient metabolism, the nutrition prescription and implementation are challenging.[7]

After acute episodic events such as neurotrauma, sepsis, and major surgery, a *shock phase* occurs lasting about 24 to 48 hours and is characterized by hypoxia, acidosis, and hypoglycemia, which result in hypovolemia, hypotension, and tissue hypoxia. The sympathetic nervous system (SNS) and the hypothalamic-pituitary-adrenal axis (HPAA) are stimulated and precipitate a number of complex humoral responses. The focus in the shock phase is physiologic stabilization as evidenced by hemodynamic stability and restoration of oxygen delivery and cellular perfusion. The metabolic response follows the physiologic stabilization and has two components, an *acute-phase response* and the *adaptive response*. The *acute-phase response* is a hypermetabolism catabolic state, which peaks 3 to 6 days after initial insult and then gradually subsides to an adaptive phase in 2 to 3 weeks.[7,8] The HPAA and SNS are further activated by the hypermetabolic state triggering the release of cortisol, glucagon, insulin, growth hormone, and catecholamines.[9] Concurrently, the immune system is activated through proinflammatory mediators such as prostaglandins and cytokines (interleukin [IL]-1 to -16 and tumor necrosis factor-α [TNF-α]).[10] If the patient is well stabilized, he or she transitions into the adaptive phase. The *adaptive phase* is characterized by anabolism and recovery. However, the transition to the adaptive phase may be delayed by a second insult, such as sepsis or surgery, that could lead to accelerated catabolism and loss of lean body mass; chronic dysfunction of carbohydrate, protein, and fat utilization; profound weight loss; negative nitrogen balance; lactic acidosis; recurring hyperglycemia; malnutrition; and stress starvation.[7,10,11]

Approximately 50% of hospitalized patients exhibit either hypoalbuminemic malnutrition or marasmic-type malnutrition. *Hypoalbuminemic (protein) malnutrition*, the most common in hospitalized patients, is diagnosed by laboratory findings of reduced serum albumin, transferrin, prealbumin, or retinol-binding protein levels, with albumin being the most commonly used diagnostic. *Marasmic malnutrition* is characterized by loss of 20% or more of usual body weight over the

preceding 3 to 6 months or less than 90% of ideal body weight.[9] Malnutrition is associated with increased mortality, nosocomial infections, sepsis, pressure ulcers, and pneumonia. Therefore, attention to nutritional needs is critical for achieving best outcomes.

NUTRITIONAL ASSESSMENT

The nutrition care process is a series of steps that includes nutrition screening, nutrition assessment, and nutrition support.[12] All patients should have a nutrition screening by a registered nurse to determine presence of nutritional risk. The Joint Commission (JC) notes that "a nutritional screening, when warranted by the patients' needs or condition, is completed within no more than 24 hours of inpatient admission."[13] The nutrition screen is usually part of the admission history and assessment conducted by the nurse within 24 hours of admission. An example of a simple screening tool with established validity and reliability is found in Figure 8-1.[14] Patients identified as "at nutritional risk" usually have altered nutritional intake, malabsorption, or altered metabolism problems and require a more comprehensive nutrition assessment.[15,16] Identification of a patient at risk usually triggers the need for an in-depth assessment by a registered dietitian (RD). A nutritional assessment is a systematic process of collecting, verifying, and interpreting data to make decisions about the nature and cause of nutrition-related problems. The data set collected depends on the practice setting and patient acuity, but usually includes a thorough history, physical examination, and laboratory studies.[2,12] The RD assumes responsibility for conducting the nutritional assessment, estimating nutritional requirements, and recommending a nutritional support plan. The nurse implements the nutritional plan, provides education for the patient and family, and monitors both response to therapy and complications. Implementation includes safe administration of nutrients by the oral, enteral, or, on occasion, parenteral route.

The prevalence of malnutrition in hospitalized patients is reported at a rate of 30% to 55%.[17] Therefore, malnutrition has an impact on patient outcomes and must be carefully addressed. Malnutrition is a common comorbidity that places patients at risk for complications such as pressure ulcers, pneumonia, and other infections; delayed wound healing; failure to wean from a ventilator; and difficulty refeeding. In addition, documented increased length of stay, higher costs, and increased mortality make nutritional support an important therapeutic intervention for improved outcomes.[18] Nutritional assessment is the cornerstone for addressing nutritional needs.

Components of the Nutritional Assessment

History

The history includes acute and chronic diseases, medications (including supplements), diagnostic procedures, surgeries, and other therapies (e.g., immunosuppressants).[19] It includes a review of systems to collect information about recent weight change, anorexia, nausea, vomiting, diarrhea,

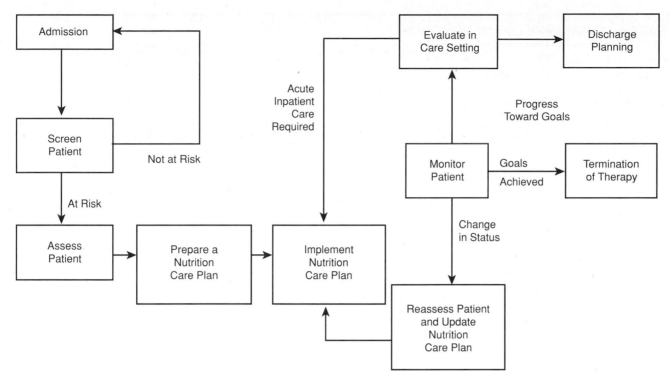

Figure 8-1 • Adult nutrition and screening and assessment algorithm. (Reprinted from A.S.P.E.N. Board of Directors and Task Force on Standards for Specialized Nutrition Support for Hospitalized Adult Patients. Russell, M. K., Andrews, M. R., Brewer, C. K., Rogers, J. Z., & Seidner, S. L. [2002]. Standards for specialized nutrition support: Adult hospitalized patients. *Nutrition in Clinical Practice*, 17, 384–391, with permission from the American Society for Parenteral and Enteral Nutrition.)

and other positive findings. Determine whether there has been unexplained weight loss or weight gain. An involuntary weight loss of 10% or more in 1 year is significant. Reference data for body weight is available from the National Health and Nutrition Examination Surveys (NHANES).[20] Information on recent dietary changes and what constitutes normal daily dietary intake is noted. This information can be collected from the medical record, a family member, or the patient.

Physical Examination

Physical inspection includes a *comprehensive assessment* with attention to special components such as skin (turgor, dryness, edema, bruising, scaling, dermatitis, seborrhea); mucous membranes (dryness, color, bruising, bleeding, especially gums); tongue (swelling, papillary atrophy); eyes (pale or dry conjunctiva, sunken eyeballs); dry, dull-looking hair or hair loss; and muscles (atrophy, wasting). Note the patient's weight and how it compares with usual weight. This is more useful than actual weight because many critically ill patients retain fluid, so that their current weight may not correlate with current nutritional status.[21]

Anthropometric measurements such as skinfold thickness and midarm muscle circumference are not useful in critically ill patients because of frequent clinical conditions such as fluid retention and edema. Anthropometric measurements are more useful in less severely ill patients. When used, triceps or subscapular skinfold thickness (SFT) estimate body

fat, and midarm muscle circumference estimates lean body muscle (protein stores). These data are not helpful in patients who are obese or edematous.[22]

Laboratory Studies

Blood and Urine Studies. A few blood and urine laboratory tests are used to indirectly estimate nutritional status. However, caution needs to be exercised because these studies are greatly affected by organ function (especially liver and renal), infection, inflammation, administration of intravenous fluids, medications such as steroids, and the acute stress response. Serum hepatic transport proteins are considered markers for malnutrition. Albumin, transferrin, and prealbumin, all synthesized in the liver, are used to assess for malnutrition.[2] These proteins are referred to as negative acute-phase proteins because they decrease in serum concentration at least 25% due to decreased hepatic synthesis in response to chronic or acute inflammation. By comparison, proteins that increase in concentration at least 25% associated with inflammation and increased hepatic synthesis are called positive acute-phase proteins (C-reactive proteins).[23] Serum *albumin* is a good marker of malnutrition in patients who are not in a stressed state because it is a measure of visceral protein stores.[9] It has a long half-life of approximately 21 days and thus is a poor marker of the effects of short-term feeding in hospitalized patients. *Transferrin* has a half-life of 8 to 10 days and is helpful to monitor response to nutritional support. Prealbumin (half-life, 2 to 3 days) can be useful for monitoring rapid changes

TABLE 8-1   MARKERS OF MALNUTRITION

	NORMAL	MILD DEPLETION	MODERATE DEPLETION	SEVERE DEPLETION
Albumin	3.5–5.0 mg/dL	2.8–3.4 mg/dL	2.1–2.7 mg/dL	<2.1 mg/dL
Transferrin	212–360 mg/dL	150–211 mg/dL	100–149 mg/dL	<100 mg/dL
Prealbumin	18–45 mg/dL	15–17 mg/dL	11–14 mg/dL	<10 mg/dL

Note: These ranges are unreliable in acute renal or hepatic failure. Serum albumin is unreliable after fluid resuscitation or acute stress response. Values may differ slightly by laboratory.

in nutritional status. Table 8-1 compares markers of malnutrition.[24] Note that these values are unreliable in acute renal or liver failure.

Nitrogen represents the end-product of protein metabolism. Nitrogen balance studies, such as 24-hour *UUN* collection, compare adequacy of protein intake in relation to protein need with a goal of nitrogen balance (zero).

Nitrogen balance = g protein intake/6.25 − urinary nitrogen (mostly urea) + fecal losses + obligatory losses (usually 2 to 4 g; corrects for obligatory and insensible protein losses through the skin, lungs, and stool)

The study may be unreliable in patients with severe nitrogen retention conditions (renal or hepatic failure) or if protein intake is incomplete or urine samples for the collection period have been spilled or inadvertently discarded.

The Immune System. Malnutrition is closely correlated with alternations in immune response as measured by total lymphocyte count (TLC) and delayed hypersensitivity reaction (DHR) skin-test antigens.[25] The TLC is calculated by multiplying the white blood cell count by the percentage of lymphocytes.[26] Infections and immunosuppressant drugs alter the TLC and thus are not helpful in patients with advanced age, immunodeficiency syndromes, radiotherapy, hypoalbuminemia, metabolic stress, infection, cancer, or chronic illness.[2] The second test mentioned is DHR; in malnutrition, the reaction is delayed or fails to react to several skin-test antigens. The DHR may not be helpful in the critically ill because of a decreased cellular immunity response (a decrease in the synthesis of antibodies and the antibody response). C-reactive protein (CRP) is the most commonly identified indicator of inflammation and an elevated CRP is a marker of ongoing acute stress response.

ESTIMATING NUTRIENT REQUIREMENTS

Estimating the actual nutrient requirements of a patient is important because there are serious adverse effects from both overfeeding and underfeeding. *Overfeeding* with high glucose infusions can lead to hyperglycemia, hypokalemia, edema, a fatty liver degeneration, and an increased risk of nosocomial infections.[27] Overfeeding also increases carbon dioxide production (V_{CO2}), which in turn may lead to difficulty weaning from a ventilator because the minute ventilation cannot be increased. The RD is the member of the interdisciplinary team who will estimate nutrient requirements. As

previously mentioned, there are both direct (Harris-Benedict equations and Ireton-Jones equations) and indirect (indirect colorimetry) methods available to the RD to calculate nutritional requirements of a patient. The nurse will implement the prescribed nutrition support ordered for the patient.

PROVIDING NUTRIENTS

A nutritional plan of care for the neuroscience patient should provide adequate nutrients using the safest and most physiologically normal route of delivery. For many patients the oral route remains a viable option for nutrient delivery. But for others with end-stage neurological disease or a severe acute neurological insult, nutritional support with enteral and/or parenteral nutrition may be required to meet the nutrient needs of the patient. If nutritional support is required, a series of questions need to be answered.

- What route (enteral or parenteral) of administration should be used?
- If enteral feeding is used, where should the tube be placed?
- When should the feeding begin?
- What feeding should be given?
- What are the energy and protein requirements for this patient?

Patients Needing Nutritional Support

The following patients will need nutritional support: those expected to receive nothing by mouth for more than 7 to 10 days, those with hypermetabolic states (sepsis, multitrauma), or those with pre-existing undernourishment (loss of 10% or more of usual body weight). In neuroscience populations, comatose, multitrauma, and septic patients are candidates for nutritional support, as well as those with severe dysphagia.

Providing Adequate Energy and Protein Requirement

Using the formulas previously discussed, the *basal caloric requirement* for most hospitalized patients is about 2100 kcal if the patients do not exceed 200 lb. Even with correction factors for fever and sepsis, patients' total energy requirements are usually less than 3000 kcal/day. Previous published reports of significantly increased kcal/day have not been substantiated by more recent studies or studies focused on head-injured patients.[28] In addition, protein catabolism is high after head injury according to many studies. Reports state that higher levels of protein (2.2 g/kg/day) were needed to reverse a negative nitrogen balance in this population. A general rule of thumb for *caloric requirements* for seriously ill patients is *25 to 35 kcal/kg/day of ideal body weight* and *1.5 g/kg/day for protein* (up to 2.5 g/kg/day is recommended for the sickest patients). These are *initial goals,* which can then be increased, as necessary, based on laboratory data (e.g., prealbumin, UUN balance) and changing clinical condition (e.g., increased fever). Recommendations vary about the allocation of calories from carbohydrate, protein, and lipid sources, but generally about 20% protein, 30% lipid, and 50% carbohydrate is recommended.[21] If hepatic or renal disease is present, special formulas are available.

There is growing evidence supporting permissive underfeeding during periods of stress (sepsis, trauma, serious illness).[29] The natural anorexia associated with stress may be advantageous by blunting cytokine responses, oxidant production, organ injury, and hypermetabolism. Prospective and retrospective patient trials have demonstrated the benefits of moderate, short-term underfeeding including lower infection rates, fewer days on the ventilator, and fewer days in the intensive care unit. Guidelines for permissive underfeeding are:

- Begin feeding early (within 24 hours of admission, if hemodynamically stable).
- Strive to provide 33% to 66% of calculated needs.
- Maintain this level of moderate underfeeding for 3 to 5 days.
- As the patient improves, advance feeding to the 100% of calculated requirements over the next 3 to 5 days, as tolerated.

Route of Administration

Enteral feeding, rather than parenteral nutrition, is clearly the preferred route for administering nutritional support. There are good reasons for preferring enteral nutrition over parenteral nutrition. First, nutrients to the intestinal lumen protect the integrity of the gastrointestinal (GI) tract. They preserve optimal gut function, maintain the gut barrier from translocation of microorganisms, and support gut-associated immune system IgA secretion. Second, enteral nutrition is safer, more convenient, and less expensive than parenteral nutrition. Beginning feeding at as low a rate as 10 mL/hr at a continuous rate will maintain the integrity of the endothelial lining of the GI tract and decrease the incidence of sepsis.

The use of the enteral route for feeding is evaluated based on the availability of the GI tract and the adequacy of intestinal function. Conditions to consider when assessing the adequacy of the enteral route include length of intestines (e.g., short from previous surgical procedure), adequate gastric and small bowel motility, and conditions that are potential exclusions for enteral feeding. These conditions include severe diarrhea, bowel disease (e.g., Crohn's disease, inflammatory colon disease), acute GI bleeding, obstructive small bowel or colon lesions, paralytic ileus, acute inflammation of the pancreas or biliary tract, and dependence on high doses and/or multiple pressors to maintain hemodynamic stability.

Most neurological patients will not require parenteral nutrition (PN). For those patients who need nutritional support but who do not have a usable GI tract for enteral feeding (see discussion above), PN is useful. PN is a method of administering a highly concentrated hypertonic solution of essential macro- and micronutrients intravenously to provide the nutritional needs of the patient over an extended period. Total PN is employed when the GI tract is completely unusable. Partial PN is useful when enteral feeding alone does not meet nutrient requirements. Neuroscience patients who are good candidates for PN include multitrauma patients with GI injuries that interfere with digestion and absorption of nutrients.

Feeding Tubes and Site of Placement

When there is an intact intestinal tract, three possibilities exist for delivering food to the alimentary tract. First, oral feeding is always the preferred method of nutritional support. However, in many hospitalized neurological patients this is not possible for a number of reasons, including coma, high risk for aspiration, and multitrauma. In that case, temporary oral-gastric or nasogastric tubes into the stomach or nasoduodenal tube into the duodenum are available. Because a feeding tube is an extraordinary method of providing nutrition, there are ethical considerations that must be weighed. See Chapter 4 for a discussion of artificial feeding.

The feeding tube is inserted through the nose and into the stomach or upper small bowel. The type and the size of feeding tube chosen vary; each has certain advantages and disadvantages. Larger-bore, rigid feeding tubes can cause erosion of the nasal passages, esophagus, and stomach, but the larger bore of the tube ensures better delivery of the feeding without occlusion. Smaller, more pliable tubes are less likely to erode tissue but are more likely to become occluded. Most continuous infusion enteral feeding is performed through small-bore tubes designed for nasogastric or nasoduodenal placement. The size of these small-bore tubes ranges from about 6- to 12-Fr gauge. *For neuroscience patients with a basal skull fracture, facial fractures, or leakage of cerebrospinal fluid, insertion of a tube nasally is contraindicated.*

There continues to be controversy about the merits of tube placement in the stomach or duodenum. A critical review of the evidence suggests that bypassing the stomach does increase tolerance to feedings, but it does not reduce the risk of aspiration or pneumonia.[30] Further, enteral feeding should not be delayed to establish small-bowel access. Most patients are able to tolerate some gastric feeding early in the course of illness. Small-bowel placement is reserved for those who cannot tolerate gastric feeding, although some physicians prefer the small-bowel site routinely.

Many serious problems can develop from prolonged nasogastric intubation. Possible problems include erosion and/or necrosis of the nares or nasal septum, sinusitis, peptic esophagitis from gastric reflux along the tube, and gastric erosion or ulcers. The need for prolonged tube feeding (i.e., 6 weeks or longer) is an indication for a simple surgical procedure whereby a gastrostomy or jejunostomy tube is sutured into position on the abdominal wall. After the tube is inserted, it is usually left to gravity drainage for the first 24 hours. When bowel sounds have returned, a feeding is begun and advanced as tolerated. The insertion site is treated like any other surgical wound with daily stoma dressing care according to hospital protocol and monitoring of the incision for signs or symptoms of infection. Another enteral tube placement option for long-term feeding is percutaneous endoscopic gastrostomy (PEG). It involves the placement of a 16- to 18-gauge latex or silicone catheter through the abdominal wall directly into the stomach using an endoscopic approach. This approach does not require anesthesia and has a low complication rate. The tube can be used for feeding within 24 to 48 hours of placement.

Beginning Feedings

Current research-based evidence supports starting enteral feeding as soon as possible following admission to the intensive care unit.[30] Early nutritional support within 12 to 48 hours blunts the hypercatabolic state and sepsis related to serious illness. A common finding in patients with such critical illness is decreased motility of the GI tract that lasts about 5 to 7 days or longer if the patient remains critically ill. Motility and nutrient absorption of the small bowel usually are functional even after severe trauma. Bowel sounds are a poor index of small bowel motility.

After insertion of a nasogastric or nasoduodenal tube, feedings are not begun until an x-ray film of the abdomen confirms appropriate tube placement. Feeding should be started at 25 to 30 mL/hr and increased by 10 to 25 mL/hr every 1 to 4 hours as tolerated until the caloric goal is achieved. Tolerance is evaluated by measurement of gastric residuals (<200 mL) and presence of abdominal distention, vomiting, or diarrhea. If the gastric residual is greater than 200 mL, the feeding is held for 2 hours and then resumed. Feeding can be increased at a slower rate (e.g., 10 mL every 6 to 12 hours), but this is often not necessary and delays achievement of the caloric intake goal. The goal rate should be achieved by the third day of therapy, if not earlier. Feedings can be administered intermittently a few times a day (running over an hour or two) or continuously with a food pump.

Selection of Feeding Formula

There are a number of available enteral nutrition products. These products are classified as standard, high protein, very high protein, disease specific, with fiber, elemental, and volume restricted. Most formulas are complete formulas; that is, they provide recommended daily requirements of micronutrients (vitamins and minerals) in addition to the macronutrients of carbohydrate, protein, and fat. Some patients may need additional vitamin or mineral supplements beyond what is provided in the formula for deficiencies (e.g., for patients with a history of alcoholism, thiamine, and folate). In some cases thiamine is supplemented to avoid metabolic acidosis.[31] Most enteral formulas, with the exception of elemental formulas, are isotonic at full strength. Dilution of a feeding does not generally enhance tolerance and may delay achievement of caloric intake goals. Feeding formulas, therefore, should *not* be diluted.

In recent years, interest has been increased in the immunomodulating properties of various nutrients such as branch-chained amino acid, nucleotides, arginine, glutamine, and omega-3 fatty acids.[32] There are a variety of commercial immune-enhancing formulas available on the market. According to the recommendations of the U.S. Summit on Immune-Enhancing Enteral Therapy held in 2000, immune-enhancing formulas may be beneficial for several patient populations including patients with severe brain injury and ventilator-dependent nonseptic medical and surgical patients at risk for infection. However, in two studies on patients with severe sepsis, there may have been an increased mortality rate when fed an immune-enhancing diet.[33] Therefore, use of immune-enhancing diets in patients with severe sepsis requires further study.

PROBLEMS ASSOCIATED WITH TUBE FEEDINGS

Overview of Problems

Infectious and metabolic complications frequently occur in critically ill patients on nutritional support. The most common metabolic complication is undernutrition.[32] The associated major problems are underfeeding and overfeeding. *Underfeeding* is related to starvation, depletion of protein stores, delayed wound healing, high risk for skin breakdown, high risk for nosocomial infections, respiratory muscle weakness and ventilator dependency, and increased mortality and morbidity. The causes of underfeeding are multifactorial, and delay in initiating feeding is common. Diarrhea, vomiting, GI tract dysfunction, and electrolyte imbalance are but a few of the problems that can interfere with adequate nutritional support in the patient receiving enteral feeding. *Overfeeding* is related to complications such as hyperglycemia, azotemia, hypertonic dehydration, electrolyte imbalance (especially potassium, magnesium, phosphorous), edema, metabolic acidosis, hypercapnia (related to failure to wean from a ventilator), hyperlipidemia, hepatic steatosis (fatty degeneration), refeeding syndrome, and an increased risk of nosocomial infections. The most common cause of overfeeding is overestimating daily caloric needs for the patient. These potential problems and considerations are presented in Table 8-2.

Medications

An important consideration in patients receiving enteral nutrition is that of medications. The size and location of the feeding tube, as well as the specific drug, must be considered.

Tube

The diameter of the tube is important. The smaller the diameter of the tube, the more likely it is to become clogged. Thick liquids such as antacids should not be administered through a tube smaller than 10-Fr. gauge.[34] Determining the location of the tube (stomach, duodenum, jejunum) affects drug metabolism. First, drugs administered beyond the pyloric valve are absorbed more rapidly. Additionally, some drugs, such as antacids and sucralfate, should not be delivered beyond the pylorus. Other drugs with enteric coatings or

TABLE 8–2   POTENTIAL PROBLEMS WITH ENTERAL TUBE FEEDINGS

PROBLEM	POSSIBLE CAUSES	CONSIDERATIONS
Diarrhea	Multifactorial and common in the acute care setting Drugs (e.g., antibiotics; liquid medications containing sorbital [elixirs]) Visceral protein depletion (alters oncotic gradient) Stress-associated GI dysfunction (e.g., malabsorption) Infections (*Clostridium difficile*), other infectious disease causes, bacterial overgrowth Impaction GI tract problems: inflammatory bowel, disease, pancreatic insufficiency, short gut syndrome These causes are more common than the tube feeding itself or its administration	Attempt to identify underlying cause Rule out *C. difficile* (stool culture) and other infections (stool smear for ova, parasites) It is rarely necessary to stop enteral feeding
Vomiting	Feeding too soon after intubation or suctioning Too rapid a rate of infusion Underlying GI problems	Allow patient a rest period before beginning feeding Run infusion slowly Explore possibilities
Gastric distention	Decreases lower esophageal sphincter pressure and predisposes to reflux and high risk for aspiration	Observe for distention Monitor gastric residuals; hold if >200 mL for 2 hr Keep head of bed at 30-degree angle
Dehydration	Rapid infusion of hyperosmolar carbohydrates that cause hyperglycemia → osmotic diuresis → dehydration Excessive protein and electrolytes (have an osmotic effect); no other source of fluid given (no IVs, no free water)	Observe for signs and symptoms of dehydration Monitor glucose and acetone levels every 4–6 hr May need regular insulin on sliding scale Adjust/change formula Administer slowly Administer free water Monitor electrolytes
Aspiration	Feeding tube not in stomach/jejunum Vomiting (see under Vomiting for description) *Note:* Aspiration can cause pneumonia or acute respiratory distress syndrome; every precaution should be taken to prevent aspiration.	Check position of tube *before* beginning feeding Elevate head of bed at 30 to 45 degrees Have suction equipment handy
Hyperglycemia	Often seen with dehydration Overnutrition Hyperosmolar condition Precipitates glycosuria that, if untreated, will result in osmotic diuresis and hyperosmolar nonketotic coma Impairs immune response and increases infection rate	Monitor glucose 4–6 hr May need regular insulin on sliding scale Adjust/change formula Administer slowly Administer free water
Electrolyte imbalance	Potassium (K), phosphorous, magnesium are most common Patients with renal, hepatic, or cardiac disease are especially prone to such problems These may decline when nutritional support is beginning due to protein synthesis	Monitor electrolyte blood levels Adjust or change formula to a restrictive formula as necessary (e.g., low-K formula) Supplement electrolytes as needed
Other disease-related intolerances	Renal or hepatic disease (some patients may not tolerate even normal levels of amino acids; only 20% of cases need to limit protein) Electrolyte imbalances may increase with renal failure	Change feeding to a disease-specific program Monitor renal and liver blood studies
Migrating feeding tube	Can become dislodged during care, pulling by patient, or from effect of tube on GI tract Can cause aspiration or peritonitis	Check position of tube periodically
Refeeding syndrome	Seen when severely malnourished patient begins enteral or parenteral nutrition With refeeding, phosphate, potassium, and magnesium move from the extracellular to the intracellular space causing hypophosphatemia and hypomagnesemia	Monitor serum phosphate, potassium, and magnesium If low, replace as necessary
Catheter occlusion	More likely with small-bore catheter especially when used to administer medications	Flush tube frequently Do not administer medications through small-bore tube

slow-release drugs (e.g., verapamil hydrochloride [Calan SR] or diltiazem [Cardizem]) should not be crushed, because this may increase the rate of absorption for the slow-release drugs or expose drugs to breakdown in the stomach and cause gastric irritation.

Drug Administration Guidelines

A number of guidelines to provide effective drug administration are outlined by Alpers et al.[35]:

- Use liquid preparation of a drug, if available.
- Crushing or dissolving of tablets is discouraged. If absolutely necessary, dissolve in at least 10 to 15 mL of water.
- Hard gelatinous capsules should be opened and dissolved in at least 10 to 15 mL of water.
- Drugs irritating to the GI tract should be dissolved in large amounts of water before administration.
- Do not add drugs to the enteral feeding.
- Stop the feeding before administering the medications.
- Flush the feeding tube with water to remove residual formula *before* administering the drug.
- Flush the feeding tube with 10 to 30 mL of water *after* administering the drug.
- For patients on an intermittent gastric feeding schedule, adjust the timing of medication to the feeding schedule according to the need for drug delivery on a full or empty stomach.

Drugs With Special Administration Requirements With Enteral Feedings

A few drugs commonly administered to neuroscience patients need special mention.

Impaired absorption of phenytoin (Dilantin) with concomitant administration of enteral feedings is well documented in the literature.[36,37] There is debate over the mode of interaction but proposed reasons include that calcium caseinate protein sources may impair phenytoin absorption, phenytoin may bind to the enteral tube, and there is a reduced gastrointestinal transit time with enteral feedings versus oral feedings. The A.S.P.E.N. Nutrition Support Practice Manual provided the following strategies to maintain therapeutic phenytoin levels and provide adequate protection from seizures[38,39]:

- Hold the tube feeding for 2 hours before and 2 hours after administering the phenytoin dose; adjust the tube-feeding schedule to accommodate the targeted total 24-hour requirement.
- Dilute the phenytoin in water (30 to 60 mL) before administration; the water enhances dissolution and improves absorption.
- Monitor drug blood levels frequently when changing from an established therapeutic parenteral dose to a suspension form administered via the feeding tube.
- Phenytoin toxicity can occur as the patient transitions from tube feeding to oral feedings; monitor the phenytoin levels closely until stable.

- Consider the use of intravenous phenytoin or fosphenytoin in difficult situations.

Carbamazepine suspension (Tegretol) is another commonly prescribed anticonvulsant drug. Dilute the suspension to prevent adherence of the drug to the wall of the feeding tube. Flush well after administration.

Monitoring Patients Receiving Enteral Feedings

The following outline suggests laboratory studies helpful in monitoring patients receiving enteral feedings so that abnormalities and deficiencies can be identified and treated appropriately.

- **Electrolytes:** sodium, potassium, chloride, and bicarbonate (baseline and twice per week)
- **Other chemistries:** glucose (baseline until stable, and then three times weekly; patients with diabetes will need it more frequently)
- **Renal function:** creatinine levels and blood urea nitrogen (BUN) (baseline and twice per week)
- **Liver function:** as needed based on patient profile
- **Other laboratory data:** calcium, phosphorus, magnesium, albumin, prealbumin (baseline and once per week); triglycerides, cholesterol (baseline and as indicated); hematocrit (baseline and twice per week); prothrombin time (as needed)

Depending on the patient's underlying problems, other laboratory studies may be indicated.

THE NURSE'S ROLE: MEETING THE NUTRITIONAL NEEDS OF PATIENTS

The importance of nutrition in recovery from neurological illness is well established. The nurse works collaboratively with the clinical dietitian and other members of the health care team to meet the nutritional needs of the patients regardless of neurological deficits or acuity of illness. Along the continuum, many hospitalized neuroscience patients require enteral nutritional support. Others may need assistance with re-establishing oral nutrition within the limitations imposed by neurological illness. The nurse begins with conducting a nutritional assessment to establish a baseline and plan of care. The nurse's plan of care is designed to complement the overall nutritional goals for the patient. When nutritional therapeutics are ordered, the nurse implements the protocol and monitors the patient's response to therapy providing information to the health care team.

Based on a nutritional assessment, various collaborative problems and nursing diagnoses can be made. Because of the complexity of neurological illness that impacts on the nutritional goal, several potential collaborative problems must be kept in mind; they include starvation, paralytic ileus, hypoglycemia, hyperglycemia, negative nitrogen balance, electrolyte imbalance, sepsis, and aspiration pneumonia. Other problems may be added, such as renal or hepatic failure based on complications that may occur as a result of neurological insult. The following patient problems/nursing diagnoses are often identified for the patient with problems related to nutritional need:

- Nutrition, Altered, More Than Body Requirements
- Nutrition, Altered, Less Than Body Requirements
- Fluid Volume, Deficit or Risk of
- Fluid Volume Excess
- Swallowing, Impaired
- Aspiration, Risk for

Ongoing Nursing Assessment

The nurse can monitor the patient's nutritional status with the following:

- Once stabilized, weigh the patient twice per week, on designated days, and note trends in weight (stable, losing, gaining).
- Observe skin turgor, tongue, mucous membranes, muscle tone, and muscle bulk daily for evidence of dehydration.
- Record and monitor intake and output and daily balance.
- Maintain a calorie count with the help of the clinical dietitian.
- Monitor tolerance to oral or enteral feeding; use as basis for progress of feeding to caloric goal.
- Monitor appropriate laboratory data (electrolytes, glucose, prealbumin, creatinine, BUN).

Administering Enteral Feedings

Enteral feedings may be administered in one of two ways: continuously with the use of a food pump or intermittently with the use of a gavage bag. The continuous method is recommended for postpyloric feeding, whereas either method can be used for feedings going into the stomach. Most commercial formulas in *open systems* (i.e., bags that are manually filled) are designed to hang for up to 4 hours without refrigeration after being spiked with connecting tubing. Most commercial formulas in *closed systems* (i.e., aseptic 1-L bottles) are designed to hang for 24 hours without refrigeration after they are spiked with the administration tubing, although some formulas are manufactured to hang longer. The nurse should follow hospital policy regarding length of time that it is left hanging.

A few comments about aspiration for residual are warranted. Before initiating a feeding into the stomach (e.g., nasogastric or gastrostomy tube), it is recommended that the tube be aspirated to determine whether retained formula is present. The expectation is that if the GI tract is working properly, there will be minimal or no formula present from the last feeding. Most centers use residual volumes as a guide to monitoring tolerance and subsequent feedings, but there is variation about the cut-off amount to hold a feeding. The range is from 100 mL to 200 mL, although there are few

data on which to base any recommendation. One report noted that no patients were intolerant to feeding even when residuals were greater than 300 mL.[40] In most centers, intermittent feeding is held for 2 hours if the amount of residual exceeds the cut-off point set by that facility or by that physician, generally between 100 mL and 200 mL. After the 2-hour delay, the residual is rechecked before administering the next feeding.

Special nursing protocols are followed for safe administration of the feeding to prevent complications (e.g., aspiration, pneumonia). In addition, the previous section offers suggestion for ongoing monitoring. While the feeding is in progress, monitor the patient frequently to detect complications and to assess efficacy of the nutritional support. Because of anatomic considerations, there are some differences in administering enteral feedings into the stomach compared with feeding delivered below the level of the pylorus. These commonalties and differences are included in Table 8-3. The following are a few other nursing responsibilities in managing a patient receiving enteral feeding:

- Check the position of the tube to be sure it has not migrated.
- If the patient has a tracheostomy tube in place, *deflate* the cuff; keep it *deflated* for 1 hour after completion of the feeding. The purpose of this action is to prevent aspiration.
- Intermittent feedings should be administered over a period of 30 to 60 minutes, depending on the amount of the feeding.
- Record the amount and type of feeding on the intake and output record.
- Observe the patient for signs and symptoms of abdominal distention, regurgitation, aspiration, nausea/vomiting, diarrhea, or intolerance to the feeding.

In the past, blue food coloring added into the feeding was used as a means of assessing pulmonary aspiration of enteral formula in intubated patients based on questionable evidence of sensitivity, specificity, and safety of this method. A Food and Drug Administration Public Health Advisory issued in 2003 reported blue discoloration, refractory hypertension, metabolic acidosis, and death in some patients receiving tube feedings containing FD&C Blue No. 1 dye.[41] Case reports reveal that critically ill patients, especially those with increased intestinal permeability, are at risk for these complications. Other disadvantages of adding blue dye to enteral feedings include contamination of the formula and the potential to induce an allergic response.

Oral Feeding

Oral feeding is always the first choice for nutritional intake. If enteral feeding is used, the goal is to return the patient to oral feeding as soon as possible. When the patient appears ready to progress to oral feedings, a swallowing study is usually conducted by the speech therapist to assess for dysphagia or silent aspiration. A dysphagia diet and/or the need for thickened liquids are common recommendations

TABLE 8-3   COMPARISON OF MANAGEMENT OF A PATIENT RECEIVING ENTERAL FEEDING BY NASOGASTRIC OR GASTROSTOMY TUBE VERSUS NASODUODENAL OR JEJUNOSTOMY TUBE

FOCUS	NASOGASTRIC TUBE OR GASTROSTOMY TUBE FEEDING	NASODUODENAL TUBE OR JEJUNOSTOMY TUBE FEEDING
Site of feeding infusion	Stomach	Small intestines (duodenum or jejunum, both postpyloric valve structures)
Type of formula selected	Appropriate for particular patient	Same
Intermittent/gavage or continuous feeding	Some controversy; either method acceptable, although more support for intermittent method	Continuous Intermittent/gavage *not recommended* because of somatic response of the small bowel to feeding
Initiation of feeding	Follow physician orders A typical order for intermittent method is: Begin with 100–150 mL/q4h of formula and add water	Follow physician orders A typical order is: Slow constant infusion rate of isotonic or slightly hypotonic formula at 25–50 mL/hr
Advancing infusion rate (based on patient tolerance)	Follow physician orders A typical order for intermittent method is: Advance 50 mL every one or two feedings up to a maximum of about 400 mL q4h	Follow physician orders A typical order is: If after 8–24 hr rate is tolerated, increase infusion rate by 25–50 mL/hr, until goal is reached Usually tolerated well
Achieving caloric goal (hourly rate set to achieve total calculated daily caloric requirement)	Goal is to achieve calculated daily total caloric requirements within ≤3 d or less Usually achieved with good team collaboration and communications	Goal is the same Usually goal achieved in <3 d
Temperature of material being fed	Follow manufacturer's instructions Most commercially prepared formulas can hang without refrigeration (see previous description) as follows: Open system can hang for up to 4 hr Closed system can hang for up to 24–48 hr	Same
Elevation of head of bed	At least 30 degrees before beginning feeding, and leave elevated for at least 2 hr after completion of feeding; designed to decrease aspiration risk	30 degrees while feeding
Flushing of feeding tube	Use at least 30 mL of warm water every feeding and as needed to ensure patency	Use at least 30 mL of water q4h and as needed to maintain patency
Aspiration for residual	Before each intermittent feeding; if residual exceeds the cut-off point, hold feeding for 2 hr and then recheck before administering another feeding	Do not aspirate tube that is placed beyond the pyloric valve

(see Chap. 11 for a discussion of dysphagia). Before beginning to feed the patient by the oral route, the nurse should:

- Assess the gag reflex. Do not initiate oral feedings if the gag reflex is not intact, because of the risk of aspiration.
- Observe for the presence of any facial weakness. Paresis or paralysis may be confined to only one side of the face. Deficits can cause difficulty in chewing and "pocketing" of food.
- Auscultate the abdomen for the presence of bowel sounds.
- Sit the patient up, if possible, thus decreasing the risk of aspiration.
- In the tracheostomized patient, the cuff should be *deflated* before beginning to offer oral intake. There is an increased risk of delayed aspiration if food becomes lodged above an inflated cuff, which may, upon deflation, fall into the trachea.

After the preliminary assessment has been conducted and necessary precautions initiated to prevent aspiration, oral nutrition can be begin.

Self-Feeding

Assess the patient's ability for self-feeding. Cognitive, motor, and coordination deficits may interfere with this activity. Several problems that interfere with eating may be identified. These problems and appropriate nursing actions are described in Table 8-4. Although it can be time consuming to supervise a patient, it is an important component in the rehabilitation process and achievement of independence. Every effort should be made to assist the patient in achieving this goal.

TABLE 8-4 POTENTIAL PROBLEMS ASSOCIATED WITH ORAL FEEDINGS

PROBLEM	DESCRIPTION	NURSING ACTIONS
Distractibility/short attention span	Patients become interested in the activity around them and stop eating; patients forget what to do with their food once it is on their eating utensils	Screen patient from the distraction. Take excess dishes off the meal tray. Redirect patient's attention to eating; cue as necessary. Screen patient from excessive environmental stimuli. Break activity of eating into steps and direct the patient in the steps of eating (e.g., pick up the potatoes with your spoon; lift the spoon to your mouth; open your mouth).
Disorientation	Not always aware of time, place, person May think that the food belongs to someone else or that it is poisoned	Provide reality orientation and assist patients in feeding themselves. Give many verbal cues for eating. Correct any misconceptions. Reassure the patient in a calm voice. Be sure the patient is wearing eyeglasses if needed.
Visual deficits Diplopia	Double vision	Apply an eye patch to one eye or cover one lens if double vision is present.
Hemianopia	Loss of vision in half of the visual field	If patient eats food from only one side of the dish, turn the dish; remind the patient to turn his or her head to scan the dish.
Dimness of vision	Visual images may be dim or fuzzy	Provision of a good light may help alleviate dimness.
Motor deficits (plegia or paresis) Muscles of chewing or of the face or tongue Arm or hand	May involve deficits of cranial nerves V, VII, or XII Associated with hemiparesis or hemiplegia; monoplegia of one extremity may be present	Encourage patient to chew food on the unaffected side. Have the patient try to eat with other hand. Use built-up eating utensils. Use special equipment, such as a guard around the plate to prevent food from spilling off the dish. Consult the occupational therapist for suggestions. Prepare the patient's tray (e.g., cut up meat, pour milk).

REFERENCES

1. Dietary Reference Intakes: Recommended Intakes of Individuals. Retrieved September 4, 2006, from www.nal.usad.gov

2. A.S.P.E.N. Board of Directors and the Clinical Guidelines Taskforce. (2002). Guidelines for the use of parenteral and enteral nutrition in adults and pediatric patients. *Journal of Parenteral Enteral Nutrition, 26,* (1 Suppl.), 1SA–138 SA.

3. Institute of Medicine. (2002). *Dietary reference intakes for energy, carbohydrate, fiber, fat, fatty acids, cholesterol, protein, and amino acids (macronutrients).* Washington, DC: National Academy Press.

4. Ireton-Jones, C., & Jones, J. D. (2002). Improved equations for predicting energy expenditure in patients: The Ireton-Jones equations. *Nutritional in Clinical Practice, 17,* 29–31.

5. Dudek, S. G. (2007). *Nutrition essentials for nursing practice* (5th ed.). Philadelphia: Lippincott Williams & Wilkins.

6. Institute of Medicine. (2004). *Dietary reference intakes for water, potassium, sodium, chloride, and sulfate.* Washington, DC: National Academy Press.

7. Cartwright, M. M. (2004). The metabolic response to stress: A case of complex nutrition support management. *Critical Care Nursing Clinics of North America, 16,* 467–487.

8. Kinney, J. M. (1987). Nutrition in the intensive care patient. *Critical Care Clinics, 3*(1), 1–10.

9. Tayek, J. A. (2003). Nutrition and malnutrition in the critically ill patient. In F. S. Bongard & D. Y. Sue (Eds.). *Current critical care diagnosis & treatment* (2nd ed., electronic book).

10. Kim, P. K., & Deustschaman, C. S. (2000). Inflammatory responses and mediators. *Surgical Clinics of North America, 80*(3), 885–894.

11. Baracos, V. E. Overview on metabolic adaptation to stress. In L. Cynhober & F. A. Moore (Eds.). *Nutrition and critical care* (Nestle Nutrition Workshop Series Clinical and Performance Program, vol. 8., pp. 1–13). Vevey, Switzerland: Netc Ltd.

12. Lacey, K., & Pritchett, E. (2003). Nutrition care process and model: ADA adopts road map to quality care and outcomes management. *Journal of American Dietetic Association, 103,* 1061–1072.

13. The Joint Commission. (2006). CAMH refresher core, January, 2006. Standard PC.2.120. Retrieved September 16, 2006, from www.jointcommission.org

14. Kovacevich, D. S., Boney, A. R., Braunschweig, C. L., Perez, A., & Stevens, M. (1997). Nutrition risk classification: A reproducible and valid tool for nurses. *Nutrition in Clinical Practice, 12*(1), 20–25.

15. American Dietetic Association. (1994). ADA's definition for nutrition screening and assessment. *Journal of American Dietetic Association, 94,* 838–839.

16. Shronts, E. P., & Cerra, F. B. (1990). The rational use of applied nutrition in the surgical setting. In M. Paparella (Ed.). *Otolaryngology.* Philadelphia: W. B. Saunders.

17. Trujillo, E. B., Robinson, M. K., & Jacobs, D. O. (1999). Nutritional assessment in the critically ill. *Critical Care Nurse, 19*(1), 67–78.

18. Harrington, L. (2004). Nutrition in critically ill adults: Key processes and outcomes. *Critical Care Nursing Clinics of North America, 16,* 459–465.

19. A.S.P.E.N. Board of Directors. (2002). Standards for specialized nutrition support—adult hospitalized patients. *Nutrition in Clinical Practice, 17*(6), 384–391.

20. U.S. Department of Health and Human Services, Centers for Disease Control and Prevention, National Center for Health Statistics. National Health and Nutrition Examination Survey. Retrieved September 16, 2006, from http://www.cdc.gov/nchs/about/major/nhanes/survey

21. Roberts, P. R. (1999). Nutrition in the intensive care unit. In D. J. Dries & R. K. Albert (Eds.). *ACCP/SCCM combined critical care course: Multidisciplinary board review* (pp. 425–436). Anaheim, CA: Society of Critical Care Medicine and the American College of Chest Physicians.

22. Alpers, D. H., Stenson, W. F., & Bier, D. M. (1995). *Manual of nutritional therapeutics* (3rd ed., pp. 73–114). Boston: Little, Brown.

23. Gabay, C., & Kishner, I. (1999). Acute-phase proteins and other systemic responses to inflammation. *New England Journal of Medicine, 340,* 448–454.

24. Ghanbari, C. (1999). Protocols for nutrition of neuro intensive care unit patients: A guide for residents. *The Internet Journal of Emergency and Intensive Care Medicine, 3*(1).

25. Nompleggi, D. J. The basic principles of nutritional support in the intensive care unit. In R. S. Irwin & J. M. Rippe (Eds.). *Manual of intensive care medicine* (4th ed., pp. 465–467). Philadelphia: Lippincott Williams & Wilkins.

26. Langkamp-Henken, B., & Wood, S. M. (2003). Evaluating immunocompetence. In L. E. Matarese & M. M. Gottschlich (Eds.). *Contemporary nutrition support practice* (pp. 63–76). Philadelphia: W. B. Saunders.

27. Pomposelli, J. J., Baxter, J. K., & Babineau, T. J. (1998). Early postoperative glucose control predicts nosocomial infection rate in diabetic patients. *Journal of Parenteral and Enteral Nutrition, 22,* 77–81.

28. Twyman, D. (1997). Nutritional management of the critically ill neurologic patient. *Critical Care Clinics, 23*(1), 39–49.

29. Zaloga, G. (2005). Permissive underfeeding of critically ill patients. In *Current Topics in Clinical Nutrition.* Minneapolis, MN: Nestle Nutrition.

30. Heyland, D. K. (1998). Nutritional support in the critically ill patient: A critical review of the evidence. *Critical Care Clinics, 14*(3), 423–440.

31. Byers, P. M., & Jeejeebhoy, K. N. (1997). Enteral and parenteral nutrition. In J. M. Civetta, R. W. Taylor, & R. R. Kirby (Eds.). *Critical care* (3rd ed., pp. 457–473). Philadelphia: Lippincott-Raven.

32. Daly, J. M., Lieberman, M. D., Goldfine, J., Shou, J., Weintraub, F., Rosata, E. P., et al. (1992). Enteral nutrition with supplemental argentine, RNA, and omega-3 fatty acids in patients after operation: Immunologic, metabolic, and clinical outcome. *Surgery, 112*(1), 56–67.

33. Kudsk, K. A., Moore, F., Martindale, R. T., et al. (2001). Consensus recommendations from the U.S. Summit on Immune-Enhancing Enteral Therapy. *Journal of Parenteral Enteral Nutrition, 25,* (Suppl.), S61–62.

34. Phelps, S. J., Brown, R. O., Helms, R. A., Christensen, M. L., Kudsk, K., & Cochran, E. B. (1991). Toxicities of parenteral nutrition in the critically ill patient. *Critical Care Clinics, 7*(3), 725–752.

35. Alpers, D. H., Stenson, W. F., & Bier, D. M. (1995). *Manual of nutritional therapeutics* (3rd ed., pp. 316–317). Boston: Little, Brown.

36. Bauer, L. A. (1982). Interference of oral phenytoin absorption by continuous nasogastric feedings. *Neurology, 32,* 570–572.

37. Fleisher, D., Sheth, N., & Kou, J. H. (1990). Phenytoin interaction with enteral feedings administered through nasogastric tubes. *Journal of Parenteral and Enteral Nutrition, 14,* 513–516.

38. Rodman, D. P., Stevenson, T. L., & Ray, T. R. (1995). Phenytoin malabsorption after jejunostomy tube delivery. *Pharmacotherapy, 15*(6), 801–805.

39. Merritt, R. (2005). *The A.S.P.E.N. Nutrition Support Practice Manual* (2nd ed.). Silver Spring, MD: American Society for Parenteral and Enteral Nutrition.

40. McClave, S. A., Snider, H. L., Lower, C. C., McLaughlin, A. J., Greene, L. M., McCombs, R. J., et al. (1992). Use of residual volume as a marker for enteral feeding intolerance: Prospective blinded comparison with physical examination and radiographic findings. *Journal of Parenteral and Enteral Nutrition, 16*(2), 99–105.

41. FDA Public Health Advisory. (2003). *Reports of Blue Discoloration and Death in Patients Receiving Enteral Feedings Tinted with the Dye, FD&C Blue no.1.* Rockville, MD: U.S. Food and Drug Administration.

Fluid and Metabolic Disorders in Neuroscience Patients

Joanne V. Hickey

Several interrelated, complex physiologic mechanisms control fluid, electrolyte, and metabolic balance. One can relate metabolic and electrolyte derangements, which are common in neuroscience patients, to non-neurological problems, neurological problems, or a complication of therapeutics. When assessing the patient's fluid and metabolic status, the nurse should be attuned to the various signs and symptoms of imbalance. As part of the assessment, the nurse reviews blood chemistry values and correlates them with the clinical presentation. This chapter addresses major electrolyte and metabolic imbalances, diabetes insipidus (DI), syndrome of inappropriate secretion of antidiuretic hormone (SIADH), cerebral salt wasting, and hyperosmolar nonketotic dehydration syndrome (HONK). All are common in hospitalized neuroscience patients.

Osmolarity is a measure of the osmoles of solute *per liter* of solution, whereas **osmolality** is a measure of the osmoles of solute *per kilogram* of solvent. Serum osmolarity is a sensitive measure of hydration status and is useful in monitoring hydration, dehydration, and rehydration. The normal range of plasma osmolarity is 282 to 295 mOsm/L, although it can vary slightly from laboratory to laboratory. Water comprises 50% to 60% of the total body weight. The body maintains a near-constant body fluid osmolality primarily by regulating water balance within a narrow range rather than by regulating solute balance.[1] The following formula is useful to *estimate* serum osmolality (mOsm/L).

$$\text{Calculated serum osmolarity} = 2\,(\text{Na}) + \frac{\text{BUN}}{2.8} + \frac{\text{Glucose}}{18}$$

(Na is sodium and BUN is blood urea nitrogen; *18* and *2.8* are derived from the conversion of mg/dL to mOsm/L)

Comparable results can usually be derived by simply doubling the serum sodium.[2]

HYPOTHALAMIC-NEUROHYPOPHYSEAL SYSTEM

The hypothalamic-neurohypophyseal system controls both the intake and the renal excretion of water. The hypothalamus-

neurohypophysis includes the anatomic structures that control water osmolality. The production, storage, and secretion of **arginine vasopressin**, also called **antidiuretic hormone (ADH),** affect the reabsorption of water by acting on the collecting tubules of the kidney. Within the hypothalamus are two pairs of nuclei cell groupings called the **supraoptic nuclei** and **paraventricular nuclei,** so named for their anatomic locations (Fig. 9-1). The perikarya of the magnocellular neurons in the supraoptic and paraventricular nuclei synthesize most antidiuretic hormone (ADH). ADH then bonds loosely with a carrier protein called **neurophysin.** From the supraoptic and paraventricular nuclei, the combined ADH and neurophysin are transported down the **pituitary stalk** or **infundibulum** through terminal nerve fibers and terminal nerve endings. Here ADH is stored in large secretory granules in the nerve endings of the posterior pituitary gland (also called the **neurohypophysis).**

ADH is very potent, and even minute amounts (as little as 2 mcg) have an appreciable effect on water balance. The half-life of ADH is 15 to 20 minutes, with metabolic degradation occurring in the liver and kidney. Even minute changes in volume, concentration, and composition of body fluids respond quickly to ADH. The immediate release and rapid breakdown of ADH account for this quick response. Electrical impulses generated by the supraoptic and paraventricular nuclei control secretion of ADH. Impulses traveling down the nerve fibers and nerve ending tracts cause ADH to be released from the nerve endings. Because of the loose bonding of neurophysin to ADH, the neurophysin immediately separates from ADH. The adjacent capillaries and the circulation then absorb the ADH.

The kidney is the target organ of ADH. With ADH present, the collecting ducts and tubules become very permeable to water so that fluid is reabsorbed and conserved within the body. Conversely, without ADH present, the renal collecting ducts and tubules are almost totally impermeable to water so that fluid is not reabsorbed; therefore, it is excreted in the urine. ADH has two primary actions on the kidneys. First, ADH stimulates sodium chloride NaCl reabsorption by the thick ascending limb of Henle's loop. Second, it increases the permeability of the distal convoluted tubule and collecting ducts to water and urea. These two processes concentrate urine and result in the preservation of water. As the body does not excrete reabsorbed water, there is a diminished rise in plasma osmolality

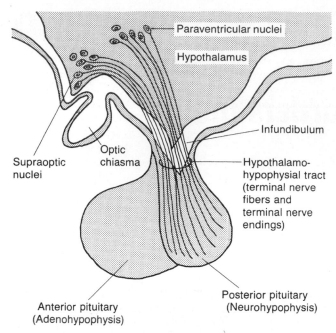

Figure 9-1 • Within the hypothalamus are the supraoptic nuclei and paraventricular nuclei, which produce antidiuretic hormone (ADH). This hormone combines with neurophysin and travels down the terminal nerve fibers and terminal nerve endings to be stored in large secretory granules in the nerve endings of the posterior pituitary gland (neurohypophysis). (The lateral hypothalamic area, where the thirst center is located, is not shown.) (From De Graaff, K. M., & Fox, S. I. [1988]. *Concepts of human anatomy and physiology* [2nd ed.]. Dubuque, IA: Wm. C. Brown.)

and a better maintenance of both blood volume and total body water volume. Reabsorption of water completes the feedback loop and tends to decrease the secretion of ADH.[3]

Regulation of ADH Secretion

Osmoregulation and baroregulation control the secretion of ADH by providing negative feedback loops to control secretion of ADH. **Osmoreceptors** are specialized cells that sense changes in serum osmolality. Located in the hypothalamus near the cells that produce ADH, osmoreceptors respond to changes in concentration of **extracellular fluid** (ECF). Concentrated ECF stimulates the supraoptic nuclei to send impulses to release ADH, which will cause reabsorption of water in the kidney. Conversely, dilute ECF around the hypothalamic osmoreceptors inhibits the generation of impulses for the release of ADH. Hypertonic NaCl or sucrose does stimulate ADH release, but hypertonic urea and glucose do not. Because the osmolality of plasma is determined by the concentration of a number of different solutes, including urea and glucose, the total plasma osmolality alone is not always clearly related to the ADH level.[3] The ability of osmotic particles to cross the osmoreceptor membrane may account for these differences. Changes in osmolality as small as 1% are sufficient to alter ADH secretion significantly.[4]

The **ventromedian nucleus**, also known as the **thirst center**, is within the lateral hypothalamus. The osmoreceptors that stimulate the supraoptic and paraventricular nuclei also stimulate the thirst center. The thirst center, in turn, stimulates the

cerebral cortex, signaling the need to drink fluids. So long as the person is able to respond to this impulse, fluid and electrolyte balance can be maintained. However, motor deficits, dysphagia, or a decreased level of consciousness may interfere with the person's ability to respond appropriately to the thirst stimuli.

Baroreceptors, located in the chest, left atrium, aortic arch, and carotid sinuses, are specialized cells that sense changes in blood volume and blood pressure. Impulses from the baroreceptors travel via the vagus and glossopharyngeal nerves to the supraoptic and paraventricular nuclei. A decreased blood volume of 5% to 10% stimulates the secretion of ADH. An increased ADH level has important vasopressor, as well as antidiuretic, effects. A decrease in the mean arterial blood pressure of 5% or more can also result in an increased secretion of ADH. This action may mediate the rise in ADH secretion during sleep. Under ordinary circumstances, changes in osmolality of body fluids play the most important role in regulating ADH secretion. In situations of severe volume depletion, stimulation of ADH secretion via baroreceptors occurs despite significant hypo-osmolality.

Certain conditions stimulate secretion of ADH, thereby conserving water in the body. They include the upright position, hyperthermia, hypotension, hypovolemia (especially caused by severe blood loss), pain, severe stress, anxiety, nausea, emesis, hypoxia, and trauma. Drugs that increase ADH release include acetaminophen (Tylenol), amitriptyline, anesthetic agents, angiotensin II agents, barbiturates, β-adrenergic agents, bromocriptine, chlorpromazine (Thorazine), chlorothiazide, cholinergic drugs, clofibrate (Atromid-S), cyclophosphamide, haloperidol, histamines, monoamine oxidase inhibitors, meperidine hydrochloride, metoclopramide, morphine, nicotine, phenothiazines, prostaglandin E_2, and vincristine sulfate.[1,3] Other conditions inhibit release of ADH. They include the recumbent position, hypothermia, hypertension, hypo-osmolality, increased blood volume, and sleep. Drugs that decrease ADH secretion include ethanol, α-adrenergic agents, anticholinergic agents, demeclocycline, glucocorticosteroids (e.g., dexamethasone), lithium carbonate, narcotic antagonists, phenytoin, tolazamide, and vinblastine.[1,3] Finally, chlorpropamide, carbamazepine, nonsteroidal anti-inflammatory drugs (NSAIDs), and tolbutamide enhance the effect of ADH.

HYPONATREMIA

Hyponatremia, defined as serum sodium level of less than 135 mEq/L, is one of the most common electrolyte disorders seen in neuroscience patients. The manifestations depend not only on the sodium level, but also on the rapidity of development of hyponatremia. Patients with *acute hyponatremia* (i.e., develops rapidly in <24 to 36 hours) may be symptomatic with mild hyponatremia, whereas patients with chronic hyponatremia (i.e., develops slowly and is present for >36 to 48 hours) may be asymptomatic. The signs and symptoms are nonspecific and related to the effects on the central nervous system (CNS). Patients with a serum sodium between 125 and 130 mEq/L with an acute onset may complain of headache, nausea, myalgia, and generalized malaise.[5] In the range of 115 to 120 mEq/L, mental status changes from lethargy, confusion, disorientation, and agita-

TABLE 9-1   CLINICAL SIGNS AND SYMPTOMS OF ACUTE HYPONATREMIA

SYSTEM	SIGNS AND SYMPTOMS
	(Note: Although significant symptoms do not generally occur until serum sodium is 125 mEq/L, individual thresholds vary widely.)
Neurological (hyponatremic encephalopathy)	Headache Disorientation, confusion, irritability, apathy, lethargy, obtundation Neurological deficits Seizures Weakness Cerebral edema Herniation syndromes Respiratory arrest
Gastrointestinal	Nausea and vomiting Anorexia
Muscular	Cramps Muscle weakness Rhabdomyolysis

tion followed by seizures, coma, and death are noted (see Table 9-1). Cerebral edema may occur, especially with rapid decline of serum sodium.[6]

CLINICAL PEARLS: Symptoms of hyponatremia or hypernatremia are noted primarily in the central nervous system.

Assessment should include not only the neurological system, but also hydration-volume status. Tachycardia, orthostatic hypotension, dry mucous membranes, decreased skin turgor, and sunken eyes are indicators of hypovolemia. The initial laboratory work-up for a patient with hyponatremia includes serum electrolytes, renal function, plasma and urine osmolality, and urine sodium concentration (see Table 9-2).

Hyponatremia is more than a low sodium level. To understand the underlying pathophysiology and basis for treatment, patients should be classified according to a two-tier schemata. First, all hyponatremic patients are categorized into iso-osmolar, hyperosmolar states and hypo-osmolar states based on plasma osmolality.[7] Hypo-osmolality is a state of excess body water, whereas hyperosmolality is a state of depletion of body water. Second, if the hyponatremia is classified as hypo-osmolar hyponatremia, then it is further classified into hypovolemic, euvolemic, or hypervolemic hypo-osmolar hyponatremia.

The first classification is based on plasma osmolality. *Iso-osmolar hyponatremia* (275 to 290 mOsm/kg) is seen with hyperlipidemia and hyperproteinemia (e.g., multiple myeloma). Treatment is directed at the underlying cause of hyperlipidemia or hyperproteinemia. *Hyperosmolar hyponatremia* (>290 mOsm/kg) is commonly seen with hyperglycemia and mannitol administration. This solute replaces sodium as the osmotically active particle in the blood. By stimulating water movement into the extracellular space, hyperglycemia lowers serum sodium (by 1.6 mEq/100 mg/dL glucose), causing hyponatremia with hyperosmolality.[9] This is also true when mannitol is administered. Other molecules

TABLE 9-2   LABORATORY STUDIES TO MONITOR FLUID IMBALANCE

TEST/NORMAL VALUES	DESCRIPTION	ALTERED LEVELS
Serum sodium 135–145 mEq/L	Sodium accounts for most of the total serum osmolality Serum sodium concentration essentially controlled by the water balance in an individual	Sodium ↑ seen in total body water deprivation Sodium ↓ seen with water overload or water intoxication
Urine sodium 30–70 mEq/L	Helpful in evaluating volume status assuming normal renal, adrenal cortical, and thyroid function	In volume overload, urinary sodium excretion and concentration ↑ —in volume overload >70 mEq/L In volume depletion, urinary sodium excretion and concentration ↓ —in volume depleted <25 mEq/L
Plasma osmolality (Osm) 280–295 mOsm/L	Can approximate plasma Osm by doubling the serum sodium concentration More accurate method, see formula on page 195	
Urine Osm 100–800 mOsm/L*	Useful to assess renal function and evaluate abnormalities of water balance Urine Osm may be hypertonic or hypotonic compared to serum Osm	Inability to dilute or concentrate urine can be seen in renal dysfunction or various other causes and in disorders of antidiuretic hormone (ADH) secretion or function
Urine specific gravity 1.010–1.030	An approximate measure of urine Osm if glucose or other chemicals are absent (i.e., they alter specific gravity)	1.001–1.005 in diabetes insipidus (DI)
Vasopressin level	Direct measure of ADH Expensive test available in selected laboratories; requires special handling	↑ seen in nephrogenic DI and in states of inappropriate ADH excess ↓ seen in central DI and states of water intoxication
Water deprivation test	Useful for making a differential diagnosis in states of polyuria Both excess water intake and central ADH deficiency are associated with a low level of ADH; this test distinguishes between the two	Lack of response to exogenous ADH after several hours of water deprivation is diagnostic for nephrogenic DI

*On random testing.

that are small and that are highly permeable to the cell membrane (e.g., ethanol, urea) do not generally cause hyponatremia. However, high levels of urea, as seen in renal failure, may result in hyponatremia because of impaired water excretion. Treatment is directed to the underlying cause such as hyperglycemia.

The most common type of hyponatremia seen in clinical practice is *hypo-osmolar hyponatremia* (<275 mOsm/kg), which can be further subdivided into three categories based on the clinical assessment of *total body volume*. These subcategories are hypervolemic hyponatremia, euvolemic hyponatremia, and hypovolemic hyponatremia.

Hypervolemic hyponatremia (free water gain > sodium gain) is seen in congestive heart failure, cirrhosis, nephrotic syndromes, and renal failure. Patients appear edematous and hyponatremic with a low urine sodium level (<20 mEq/L) and a high urine osmolality (>300 mOsm/kg; or >500 mOsm/kg in renal failure).[8] The increase in free water with an increase in ECF and extracellular volume (ECV) results in a low circulating volume. Low volume stimulates thirst, ADH, and aldosterone secretion. Treatment is directed at fluid restriction and diuresis.

Euvolemic hyponatremia (free water gain and minimal sodium loss) is seen most often in patients with SIADH, discussed later in this chapter. Patients with SIADH have a high urine osmolality (>100 mOsm kg), a high urine sodium (>20 mEq/L), hypo-osmolar hyponatremia, euvolemia, and normal adrenal, thyroid, cardiac, hepatic, and renal function.[7] Other causes of euvolemic hyponatremia include hypothyroidism, adrenal insufficiency, and salt-wasting syndromes. Patients with gastrointestinal (GI) loss of fluid and electrolytes may also present with a urine osmolality greater than 100 mOsm/kg and a urine sodium of less than 20 mEq/L. Treatment varies within the euvolemic category. Patients with SIADH are usually treated with fluid restriction, whereas those with GI loss receive isotonic fluid.

With *hypovolemic hyponatremia* (sodium loss > free water loss), sodium depletion exceeds total body water volume depletion. Hypovolemia triggers thirst and ADH secretion, which leads to water gain and further enhances the hypo-osmolar state. The causes of hypovolemic-hyponatremia are classified into nonrenal sodium loss and renal sodium loss. Nonrenal losses of water and sodium are due to GI losses such as vomiting, diarrhea, and fistula drainage, as well as burns.

In this case, a low urine sodium level (<20 mEq/L) is noted because the kidneys are able to reabsorb sodium so that urine osmolality is more than 300 mOsm/kg. By comparison, renal sodium loss results from diuretics, polycystic kidney disease, renal failure, and mineralocorticoid deficiency (e.g., hypoaldosterone). Urine sodium is more than 20 mEq/L and urine osmolality is less than 300 mOsm/kg.[9] Concurrently, hypokalemia may be present, especially with GI fluid loss or use of diuretics. Treatment is directed at identifying the underlying cause and administering isotonic saline to correct the moderate-to-severe hyponatremia.

Hypovolemic and euvolemic patients may have common characteristics. Urine osmolality and urine sodium concentration help to differentiate. If the urine osmolality is less than 100 mOsm/kg, these patients are euvolemic because they demonstrate maximally dilute urine. The causes are psychogenic polydipsia, resent osmostat, and beer potomania (related to chronic alcoholism). By comparison, when urine osmolality is greater than 100 mOsm/kg and the urine is less than 20 mEq/L, these patients are hypovolemic from extrarenal sodium and water loss such as from the GI tract or skin. If the urine osmolality is greater than 100 mOsm/kg and the urine sodium is greater than 20 mEq/L, these patients may be hypovolemic from renal water loss or euvolemic from SIADH, hypothyroidism, or adrenal insufficiency.[7] Isotonic intravenous fluids are used to treat beer potomania.

Treatment Principles

Treatment of hyponatremia is based on volume status. Hypovolemic patients have decreased whole body sodium and free water loss and require oral or intravenous sodium administration. Isotonic saline is used for concurrent salt and water replacement. Once a euvolemic state has been reached, the intravenous fluid is changed to 0.45% saline to avoid correcting the serum sodium too quickly.[7] By comparison, euvolemic and hypervolemic patients are treated with free water restriction of 800 to 1000 mL/24 hours. Concurrent loop diuretics are useful to promote free water excretion.

Treatment of hyponatremia must be carefully managed and corrected slowly. *Correcting severe hyponatremia too rapidly should be avoided because it can cause cerebral pontine myelinolysis (CPM).* CPM, also known as *osmotic demyelination syndrome (ODS),* can cause pontine and extrapontine myelinolysis, a rare brain demyelinating disorder responsible for severe neurological morbidity and mortality.[10,11] It occurs when water moves too rapidly out of the brain cells during administration of relatively hypertonic saline solution too rapidly.[12] Clinically, after a few days of improvement, symptoms of deteriorating mental status and neurological status, including pseudobulbar palsy and spastic quadriparesis, develop with a poor prognosis. Therefore, in all cases of hyponatremia, *care must be taken to prevent too rapid a correction of hyponatremia.* The therapeutic approach to managing a symptomatic chronic hyponatremic patient follows a controlled gradual raising of serum sodium levels. The serum sodium level should not be increased by more than 0.5 to 1 mEq/L/hr and no more than 12 mEq/L in a 24-hour period.[13,14]

CLINICAL PEARLS: In chronic hyponatremia or hypernatremia, neurological symptoms are much less pronounced because the brain has adapted over time.

HYPERNATREMIA

Hypernatremia is defined as a serum sodium level that exceeds 145 mEq/L. It is characterized by a deficit of total body water in relation to total body sodium and can result from either net water loss or, less frequently, hypertonic sodium gain. Regardless of cause, the primary problem is inadequate water intake. Hypernatremia in neuro-intensive care unit (NICU) patients is most often due to normal saline intravenous solutions containing 154 mEq/L of sodium adding to the sodium load.[15,16] In hypernatremia, intracellular water shifts into the hypertonic extracellular compartment resulting in cellular dehydration and neurological symptoms. As noted with hyponatremia, the symptoms of hypernatremia arise in the central nervous system and the symptoms present depend on the acuteness of development of hypernatremia. Patients with mild hypernatremia may be asymptomatic or experience anorexia, nausea, or vomiting. With advancement of hypernatremia symptoms may include altered mental status, agitation, irritability, lethargy, delirium, weakness, seizures, and coma. Assessment should include not only the neurological system, but also hydration-volume status. Common laboratory tests are found in Table 9-2.

Hypernatremia can be classified according to the clinical volume status of the patient (hypovolemic, euvolemic, and hypervolemic). *Hypovolemic hypernatremia* (free water loss > sodium loss) is caused by either extrarenal or renal loss. Extrarenal losses that result in mild hypernatremia (serum sodium <160 mEq/L) include excessive sweating, diarrhea, and nasogastric suctioning. With extrarenal fluid loss, the urinary sodium is low (<10 mEq/L) and urine osmolality is approximately greater than 700 mOsm/kg. Renal loss is associated with osmotic diuretics use without adequate volume replacement or severe glucosuria in diabetics. In these cases urinary sodium is elevated (>20 mEq/L) and urine is isotonic or hypotonic (<700 mOsm/kg). Regardless of the cause, patients with hypovolemic hypernatremia have severe volume loss with clinical manifestations of tachycardia, poor skin turgor, dry mucous membranes, and orthostatic hypotension. Treatment includes isotonic saline fluid to hemodynamically stabilize the patient and then changed to 0.45 saline to prevent fluid overload.

Patients with *euvolemic hypernatremia* (free water loss) have water loss without hypovolemia as a result of water loss from the intracellular space related to extrarenal and renal causes. Extrarenal causes of free water loss include insensible losses from the skin and respiratory system (e.g., mechanical ventilation) without adequate fluid replacement. The urine becomes concentrated (>700 mOsm/kg) due to stimulation of ADH. By comparison, renal loss of free water results in hypotonic urine (<700 mOsm/kg or >200 mOsm/kg) as a result of central or nephrogenic DI. Patients with DI have a lower urine than plasma osmolality. DI will be discussed later in this chapter. In general, hypovolemic hypernatremia patients require pure water replacement with hypotonic saline or free water replacement.

Hypervolemic hypernatremia (sodium gain) is most frequently seen due to overcorrection of hyponatremia with hypertonic saline or administration of hypertonic enteral feedings. Treatment includes loop diuretics and free water replacement.

CLINICAL PEARLS: Correction of hyponatremia or hypernatremia more rapidly than 0.5 to 1.0 mEq/L/hr can result in ODS or cerebral edema, respectively. The maximum change in serum sodium concentration should be about 10 mEq/L over a 24-hour time period.

OTHER COMMON ELECTROLYTE IMBALANCES

In addition to hyponatremia and hypernatremia, potassium, calcium, magnesium, and phosphorus are other important electrolytes in acute care settings that have been associated with high morbidity and mortality. Relatively small changes in plasma concentrations of potassium, calcium, and magne-

sium can have significant effects on neuromuscular excitability and cardiac rhythm. Balance of these three cations is maintained largely by regulation of their excretion in the urine.[17,18] Table 9-3 outlines common electrolyte imbalances, causes, related conditions, and signs and symptoms.

Potassium (3.5 to 5.0 mEq/L) is the major intracellular ion. An important determinant of the plasma concentration is the balance between the uptake and loss of potassium across the cellular membrane. Potassium cellular uptake is increased by alkalosis, β-adrenergic agonists, insulin, and aldosterone; it is lost from the cell by acidosis.[17] Potassium is important in cellular metabolism for protein and glycogen synthesis, and in maintaining cellular membrane potential.

Calcium (8.5 to 10.5 mg/dL or 4.2 to 5.2 mEq/L) is important for blood coagulation, skeletal and cardiac muscle contractility, and several membrane and cellular functions. About one half of the total calcium and magnesium is found as free ions in the plasma. The free form is physiologically active and is controlled by parathyroid hormone and vitamin D. Parathyroid hormone (PTH) stimulates the release of calcium from bone and its reabsorption in the kidney and gut. Inhibition of PTH is controlled by hypercalcemia and hypermagnesemia. When calcium and magnesium levels fall, they usually fall together because both are bound to albumin. Calcium and magnesium are important in neuromuscular conduction and activation.

Magnesium (1.7 to 2.4 mg/dL or 1.4 to 2.0 mEq/L) is the most common intracellular cation after potassium and the fourth most abundant cation in the body overall. It is regulated by renal excretion. Diuresis, acidosis, phosphate depletion, extracellular fluid expansion, and hypercalcemia result in excessive loss of magnesium.[15] Magnesium is a metabolic cofactor in over 300 enzymatic reactions, including energy use and protein and nucleic acid synthesis. It is necessary in cellular phosphated transfer reactions (sodium-potassium-adenosine triphosphatase [Na-K-ATPase] pump, calcium-adenosine triphosphate [ATP] pump, proton pump) and participates in the regulation of vascular smooth muscle tone, cellular second messenger systems, and signal transduction.[19] Deficiency of magnesium has been associated with failure to wean from a ventilator. Low serum levels of calcium and magnesium increase the risk of muscle twitching and seizures.[15]

Phosphorus (2.0 to 4.5 mg/dL or 2.3 to 4.3 mg/dL or 1.5 to 2.8 mEq/L) is a form of a phosphate ion. It is a key component of DNA and RNA and is essential for intracellular storage and conversion of energy (ATP, creatine phosphate), carbohydrate metabolism, regulatory compounds, and dissociation of oxygen. Low phosphorus and magnesium levels are related to failure to wean from a ventilator.

Correction of Electrolyte Imbalances

A complex interrelatedness exists among electrolytes with overlapping functions and effects. This "big picture" needs to be kept in mind when imbalances are corrected. Several principles guide correction of imbalance and include:

- Estimate the degree of deficit or excess based on laboratory data and clinical signs and symptoms; several formulas are useful to calculate actual deviations.

TABLE 9-3   OTHER COMMON SERUM ELECTROLYTE IMBALANCES

ELECTROLYTE IMBALANCE	CAUSES/RELATED CONDITIONS	SIGNS AND SYMPTOMS
Hypokalemia (<3.5 mEq/L)	GI loss (diarrhea, fistula, cathartics) Shift into cell from insulin therapy Renal losses related to hypoaldosteronism Urinary diuresis Magnesium depletion	ECG changes or cardiac arrhythmias: U waves, prolonged QT interval, depressed ST segment, low, flat T waves
Hyperkalemia (>5.0 mEq/L)	Cellular shift because of drugs and cell lysis Decreased renal excretion due to decreased tubular secretion Tubulointerstitial nephritis	Mild symptoms if the potassium level is 5–7 mEq/L; severe if the level is >7.0 mEq/L. Symptoms include the following: • *Cardiac:* ECG changes/cardiac arrhythmias (tall peaked T waves, widening QRS complex, shortening of the QT interval); ventricular fibrillations leading to cardiac arrest; bradycardia and hypotension • *Neuromuscular:* weakness, hyporeflexia • *Other:* paresthesia, respiratory paralysis
Hypocalcemia (<4.2 mEq/L)	Most commonly resulting from small-bowel resection or inflammation (e.g., Crohn's disease) Liver or renal disease may also cause vitamin D deficiency	Tingling of fingertips Perioral paresthesia Tetany Abdominal cramps Muscle cramps Carpopedal spasms Seizures Prolonged QT interval
Hypercalcemia (>5.2 mEq/L)	Increased GI absorption Vitamin D intoxication Increased bone absorption related to hyperparathyroidism, osteolytic metastases, multiple myeloma, immobilization Increased renal absorption related to hyperparathyroidism or thiazide diuretics	Anorexia, constipation, and abdominal pain Progressive weakness, lethargy, obtundation, and possible coma Deep bone pain Flank pain from renal calculi Muscle hypotonicity Dehydration
Hypomagnesemia (<1.4 mEq/L)	GI magnesium wasting (malabsorption states, diarrhea, short bowel) Renal magnesium wasting (primary tubular disorders) problems Common in ICU patients Common with long-term diuretic therapy	*Neuromuscular:* hyperexcitability with hyperreflexia *Cardiac:* potentially lethal cardiac conduction disturbances (e.g., PVCs, ventricular fibrillations or tachycardia; torsades de pointes; electrocardiographic changes Deficiency of magnesium associated with failure to wean from a ventilator
Hypermagnesemia (>2.0 mEq/L)	Occurs primarily in patients with renal insufficiency or in those receiving excessive magnesium therapy IV or oral (antacids, laxatives)	Symptoms related to level of elevation and include: • *Cardiovascular:* hypotension progressing to prolonged QRS and PR intervals and finally to heart block • *Neuromuscular:* hyporeflexia, muscle paralysis, respiratory weakness • *Other:* nausea, vomiting, and skin warmth
Hypophosphatemia (<1.5 mEq/L)	Phosphate-binding therapy for renal failure (e.g., antacids, sucralfate, calcium carbonate) Other disease states including hyperparathyroidism, paralytic syndromes, alcoholism, diabetic ketoacidosis, hyperglycemia, hyperosmolar states	*Muscular:* muscle weakness and myalgia *Respiratory:* respiratory failure, ventilation dependency, or respiratory muscle fatigue *Renal:* acute tubular necrosis *Neurological:* paresthesia, weakness, numbness, seizures, and altered mental status
Hyperphosphatemia (>2.8 mEq/L)	Acute and chronic renal failure Hypoparathyroidism Diabetic or alcoholic ketoacidosis	When high phosphorus levels are maintained for an extended time, phosphate deposits may develop in the body

GI, gastrointestinal; ECG, electrocardiographic; ICU, intensive care unit; PVC, premature ventricular contraction.

- Determine underlying cause and correct if possible.
- Consider speed of replacement (most often, slow replacement is advocated).
- Consider what other related electrolytes need to be managed for successful correction.
- Individualize therapy (consider whether acute or chronic problem; choice of drugs).
- Calculate the dosage and timeline for correction.
- Monitor the response and other related electrolytes.

Although management and correction of electrolyte imbalances are collaborative problems, the effects of specific imbalances require nursing assessment and monitoring of specific parameters such as vital signs, continuous electrocardiographic waveforms, and neurological signs. The nurse must be aware of the specific electrolyte imbalance, overall plan for correction, and adverse signs and symptoms to provide comprehensive assessment and monitoring of patients for safe correction of imbalances.

SYNDROME OF INAPPROPRIATE SECRETION OF ANTIDIURETIC HORMONE

SIADH is the single most common cause of hyponatremia in hospitalized and, particularly, postoperative patients. Causes of SIADH can be grouped into four categories of CNS disorders, malignancy, pulmonary disorders, and pharmacologic agents. Almost any CNS disorder, including cerebral trauma, infections (meningitis, encephalitis, abscesses), tumors, cerebrovascular disease, aneurysmal subarachnoid hemorrhage, and Guillain-Barré syndrome, can cause SIADH. Malignancy, especially bronchogenic carcinoma (oat cell carcinoma), is well recognized as a cause of SIADH. In addition, pneumonia, especially that caused by *Legionella pneumophila*, tuberculosis, and advanced chronic obstructive pulmonary disease, is implicated. Finally, a number of drugs are associated with an increased secretion of ADH such as oral hypoglycemics, general anesthetics, chemotherapeutic agents, sedatives, tricyclic antidepressants, selective serotonin uptake inhibitors, NSAIDs, opiates, and carbamazepine. The elderly and patients receiving positive pressure breathing ventilation are more prone to SIADH.

The symptoms of SIADH include confusion, lethargy, nausea/vomiting, coma, seizures, and possible fluid overload. The diagnostic criteria for SIADH include[20]:

- Exclusion of renal, adrenal, or other endocrine disease (hypothyroidism or hypoadrenalism)
- Hypo-osmolar hyponatremia (usually <275 mOsm/L) of serum
- Concentrated urine (>100 mOsm/kg) relative to serum
- High urine sodium (>25 mEq/L)
- High ratio of urine to serum osmolality
- Decreased urinary output (400 to 500 mL/24 hours)
- Possible generalized weight gain (more than 5% of body weight)

In SIADH, there is persistent production of ADH or an ADH-like peptide despite body fluid hypotonicity and an expanded effective circulating volume so that the negative feedback mechanisms that normally control the release of ADH fail. As a result, there is excessive retention of water by the kidneys, hyponatremia, and euvolemic or slight expansion of ECF that may cause an increase in body weight by 5% to 10%. The volume expansion results in reduced rates of proximal tubular sodium absorption and consequent natriuresis.

Treatment

The treatment of SIADH depends on its severity and the underlying cause of the problem. The underlying cause should be identified and managed. Usually, SIADH is self-limited in neurological patients. The principles of treatment include the following:

- Restriction of free water (<1000 mL/24 hours). This may be the definitive treatment.
- Slow, judicious replacement of sodium with saline or hypertonic solution (3%) of sodium chloride administered slowly. Correction usually occurs over 3 to 6 days. See discussion of hyponatremia correction for rationale.

- Furosemide (Lasix) 40 mg daily for diuresis
- In some instances, demeclocycline hydrochloride, 150 to 300 mg every 6 hours, to suppress ADH activity

> **CLINICAL VIGNETTE:** A 60-year-old man is admitted with a subarachnoid hemorrhage secondary to a cerebral aneurysmal bleed. His serum sodium on admission is 135 mEq/L and is 120 mEq/L 3 days later. He is also very confused and sometimes stuporous. Based on hemodynamic data, hypervolemia is present. SIADH is diagnosed and he is treated with fluid restriction of 900 mL/d; loop diuretics are added. The nurse must monitor intake and output and also assess neurological signs for deterioration in level of consciousness.

Nursing Management

Assessment

The patient with SIADH should undergo periodic assessment of the following:

- Intake and output (not fluid retention)
- Daily weight for gain, if possible
- Urine and serum osmolalities
- Urine and serum sodium
- Urine specific gravity
- Blood urea nitrogen
- Neurological assessment (lethargy, confusion, muscle weakness and cramping, headache, seizures, coma)

Collaborative Problems and Interventions

The major collaborative problem with SIADH is fluid and electrolyte imbalance. The nurse must monitor the laboratory values for serum and urine sodium and osmolalities. Intake and output must be carefully recorded and monitored. If an intravenous infusion is ordered, it should be administered slowly. Most patients with SIADH are placed on fluid restriction. The reason for this restriction should be explained to the patient and family. A strict intake and output record is maintained to conform to prescribed fluid restriction. Frequent mouth care is provided for comfort, because fluid restriction can cause dry mouth.

Because weight gain is common with SIADH, the patient is weighed daily and recorded. The accumulation of fluid also predisposes the bedridden patient to pressure ulcers. Frequent skin care, turning, and repositioning should be included in the plan of care. The hyponatremia associated with SIADH can lead to neurological changes in the sensorium, muscle cramping, headache, seizures, and even coma. The nurse must be aware of the signs and symptoms of sodium depletion and must notify the physician of any such changes so that definitive action can be taken before serious deficits develop.

DIABETES INSIPIDUS

Diabetes insipidus is a condition of decreased secretion of ADH. DI can be classified into central neurogenic DI and nephrogenic DI. *Central neurogenic DI* is due to compression, traction, or destruction of the posterior pituitary gland by tumors or trauma, resulting in a deficiency of vasopressin also known as ADH. Central neurogenic DI can be subdivided into the following four types: (1) classical severe DI, in which there is failure to synthesize or release ADH; (2) defective osmoreceptor DI, in which very high osmolality fails to trigger secretion of ADH, although the hormone is released in response to hypovolemia; (3) reset osmoreceptor DI, in which secretion of ADH is not triggered until the plasma osmolality is higher than the usual threshold; and (4) partial DI, in which ADH is released at the usual threshold, but the amount of hormone secreted is decreased.[21]

Nephrogenic DI is uncommon and can be acquired through drug toxicity (lithium, demeclocycline, amphotericin B, gentamicin, glyburide, or furosemide). It can be differentiated from neurogenic DI by a lack of response to the administration of ADH.[22] Physiologically, nephrogenic DI arises from end-organ resistance to vasopressin, either from a receptor defect or from medications and other agents that interfere with the aquaporin-2 (AQP_2) transport of water.

Central neurogenic DI (CDI) may be neurogenic or idiopathic. Neurogenic causes include primary brain tumor (30%), head trauma (17%), neurosurgery (9%), metastatic carcinoma (8%), intracranial hemorrhage (6%), and granulomatous disease (5%).[23] The presence of CDI is common in brain death, especially with hemodynamic and respiratory support during an organ donation protocol. Idiopathic DI occurs in 25% of cases. CDI due to trauma or neurosurgical injury is characterized by polyuria that is often triphasic: an initial period of intense polyuria lasting for hours to several days; followed by a period of normal urinary output; and finally the recurrence of transient or permanent polyuria.

Most DI is transient and resolves spontaneously within a few days or a few weeks. Patients may or may not require treatment, depending on the severity of the condition, their ability to balance intake and output, or adequate treatment and fluid replacement. A condition of permanent DI develops only if 80% to 90% or more of the ADH-producing nuclei are destroyed. In this situation, life-long treatment with replacement hormonal therapy is necessary. The diagnostic criteria for DI include:

- Polyuria (urine volumes ranging from 4 to 10 L daily with hourly output exceeding 200 mL)
- Dilute urine (<200 mOsm/L)
- Low urine specific gravity (1.001 to 1.005)
- Hypernatremia
- Normal to high serum osmolality
- Hypovolemia
- Extreme thirst (polydipsia) if the patient is conscious and the thirst center is intact

The diagnosis of DI is based on a history and the clinical finding of polyuria coupled with low urinary specific gravity levels and high serum osmolality. Although rarely done, a water dehydration test may be ordered to determine which type of DI is present when the cause is unclear. If necessary, a magnetic resonance imaging scan is helpful in visualizing the pituitary.

The following summarizes the pathophysiology of DI. Secretion of ADH, also called arginine vasopressin (AVP),

from the posterior pituitary gland is regulated by the paraventricular and supraoptic nuclei (see Fig. 9-1). ADH acts on the target site of the cortical collecting duct of the kidneys. AVP binds to a vasopressin-2 receptor at the basal lateral membrane of the cortical collecting duct. The vasopressin-2 receptor acts with G protein and adenylate cyclase to produce cyclic adenosine monophosphate (AMP). Protein kinase A subsequently is stimulated and acts to promote AQP_2 to recycle vesicles. In the presence of AVP, the exocytic inclusion of AQP_2 protein at the surface of the cortical tubular cells allows water to enter the cell. In the absence of AVP, AQP_2 protein is retrieved by endocytic retrieval mechanisms and returned to the recycling vesicle.

Treatment

The treatment of DI initially includes the replacement of fluids if the patient is unable to take an adequate amount of fluid orally. Administration of ADH as desmopressin (DDAVP) is used, preferably by the intranasal route at a dosage of 5 to 20 mcg daily. Rhinitis and sinusitis may interfere with intranasal absorption of this drug. An oral form of desmopressin is also available, but at a dose 20 times higher than that used for the intranasal route. The increased dosage is necessary because of bioavailability; the recommended starting dose is 0.05 mg twice a day. Aqueous desmopressin can be used IV for acute DI and for brain-death organ protocol. The dosage is 0.5 to 2.0 mcg every 3 hours.[24] Drug therapy recommendations are summarized in Table 9-4. For patients with mild DI, drugs known to stimulate production of ADH or to enhance the kidney's response to ADH may be ordered (see Table 9-4). If the DI is a permanent condition, the patient will require education and ongoing medical management.

Nursing Management

Assessment

The nurse caring for a neurosurgical patient should be aware of the possible development of DI and should monitor the patient accordingly. The following should be assessed:

- Urinary output every 1 to 2 hours
- Urinary specific gravity every 1 to 2 hours
- Intake and output balance for 24-hour time frame
- Serum osmolality and electrolytes
- Signs and symptoms of dehydration
- Daily weight, if possible

When assessing the fractional urinary output for a patient with an altered level of consciousness, an indwelling catheter is usually in place to measure urinary output on a specific time schedule. The amount of urinary output in just 1 hour can be extraordinary. If the urinary output is 200 mL/hr or more for 2 consecutive hours, this should be reported to the physician because large outputs can quickly lead to dehydration. In most instances, neurosurgical patients and those subject to increased intracranial pressure are maintained in a euvolemic state to control intracranial pressure. The nurse will notice very pale (i.e., straw colored) and dilute urine

TABLE 9-4   DRUGS USED IN THE TREATMENT OF DIABETES INSIPIDUS (DI)

NAME	USUAL ADULT DOSE	FREQUENCY	COMMENTS
Desmopressin acetate (DDAVP)	5–40 mcg intranasally in 1–3 divided doses	Daily; adjustment of morning and evening doses separately for adequate diurnal rhythm of water turnover	Causes minimal nasoconstriction; used for severe permanent, or transient complete, central DI
Lypressin nasal spray	Spray intranasally three to four times a day	4–6 h	Nasal mucosa must be intact; useful for mild DI; patient may develop nasal congestion, which will interfere with absorption
Aqueous vasopressin	0.5–2.0 mcg IV	3 h	Short duration; used for patients who have acute DI who have more than 300 mL/hr for 2 consecutive hours
Desmopressin	Starting doses of 0.05 mg orally with subsequent dose adjustment to achieve optimal water balance	In 2 or 3 divided doses	Adjust individual dosage in increments of 0.1–1.2 mg daily divided into 2 or 3 doses. Optimal dosage range is 0.1–0.8 mg daily in divided doses
In milder forms of DI, (in which antidiuretic hormone [ADH] is secreted in small amounts), the following drugs may be used to enhance the secretion of ADH or to increase the response of the kidney to ADH:			
Chloropropamide (Diabinase)	250–750 mg/d PO	Daily	Stimulates release of ADH from the posterior pituitary and enhances its action of small amounts of ADH on renal tubules to augment urine concentrating ability; hypoglycemia in patients taking >500 mg limits its usefulness
Clofibrate (Atromid-S)	500 mg orally four times daily	Four times a day	Useful to curtail polyuria in patients with partial central DI by stimulating release of ADH from the hypothalamus
Carbamazepine (Tegretol)	400–600 mg/d	Daily	Same as for clofibrate; in addition, carbamazepine may increase the sensitivity of the kidney to ADH
Hydrochlorothiazide (Hydrodiuril)	50–100 mg/d (or b.i.d.) PO	Daily or in 2 divided doses	Used in both central and nephrogenic DI

(From Johnson, P. H. [Ed.]. [1998]. *Nurse practitioner's drug handbook* [2nd ed. pp. 307–308]. Springhouse, PA: Springhouse.)

with a specific gravity of 1.005 or less along with large urinary outputs. These two concurrent findings are usual signs of DI in the acute care setting. Other findings include a rising serum osmolality, hypernatremia, extreme thirst (if conscious), and dehydration.

The major collaborative problems associated with DI are electrolyte imbalance, dehydration, and hypovolemia that can lead to altered cerebral tissue perfusion (R/T hypovolemia, dehydration). A major nursing responsibility is managing fluid replacement. The oral route is used if the patient is conscious and able to swallow adequate amounts of fluid. If this is not possible, an IV route is used. The rate of infusion is monitored frequently and the amount of intake compared with the amount of output. In the patient who has triphasic DI, care should be taken to prevent water intoxication during the period of normal urine output. For a patient receiving vasopressin replacement therapy by the intranasal route, monitor for evidence of rhinitis or sinusitis, conditions that would decrease the absorption of the drug. For the patient with permanent DI, a patient teaching plan is developed and implemented. The following information should be included in the teaching plan: (1) explanation of DI; (2) suggestions for adjusting the daily schedule to accommodate the care needs associated with DI; (3) review of the individualized drug protocol (frequency, side effects, overdose); (4) plan for follow-up care; and (5) recommendation to wear a medical alert bracelet.

CLINICAL VIGNETTE: A 35-year-old woman is admitted to the neurotrauma unit following a motor vehicle accident. A computed tomography scan of the brain reveals a basilar skull fracture. Three hours after admission her urinary output increased to 200 mL, 240 mL, 300 mL, and 240 mL for 4 consecutive hours for a total output of 3 L/8-hour shift and was very light in color. This pattern continues. Laboratory data at admission and 24 hours later are as follows: serum sodium is 140 and 155 mEq/L, blood urea nitrogen 14 and 30 mg/dL, and glucose 80 and 85 mg/dL, respectively. She had developed central diabetes insipidus. She received fluid replacement and the problem self-corrected after 2 days.

CEREBRAL SALT WASTING

Cerebral salt wasting (CSW) is a condition characterized by renal loss of sodium leading to true hyponatremia, decreased vascular volume, and decreased extracellular fluid, and increased urine sodium that results from intracranial disease.[25]

TABLE 9-5   COMPARISON OF SIADH, CEREBRAL SALT WASTING, AND DIABETES INSIPIDUS

	SIADH	CEREBRAL SALT WASTING	DIABETES INSIPIDUS
Serum sodium	Hyponatremia	Hyponatremia	Hypernatremia
Vascular volume	WNL or increased	Decreased	Decreased
Extracellular fluid	Increased	Decreased	Decreased
Urine sodium	WNL or increased	Increased	WNL
Urine osmolality	Increased	WNL or increased	Increased

SIADH, syndrome of inappropriate secretion of antidiuretic hormone; WNL, within normal limits.

The underlying cause of why the kidneys fail to reabsorb sodium is unclear. Table 9-5 presents a comparison of SIADH, cerebral salt wasting, and diabetes insipidus. Greenberg[20] recommends caution in patients with subarachnoid hemorrhage (SAH) resulting from cerebral aneurysms. These patients may have CSW with hyponatremia, which may mimic SIADH; however, hypovolemia usually accompanies CSW rather than hypervolemia common in SIADH.[26] In this case, the usual practice of fluid restriction used for SIADH could exacerbate vasospasm and induce cerebral ischemia in the SAH patient. Treatment for CSW is volume and salt replacement with 0.9% normal saline of hypertonic NaCl solution. Replacement of salt follows the rule of gradual correction to prevent CPM as outlined for hyponatremia correction. See collaborative problems for fluid replacement management.

HYPEROSMOLAR NONKETOTIC HYPERGLYCEMIA

Hyperosmolar nonketotic dehydration syndrome is a serious metabolic complication seen in some neurological patients caused by an insulin deficiency that may be precipitated by serious illness. The syndrome can develop slowly and is usually seen in older patients (50 to 70 years of age) with a history of non-insulin-dependent diabetes mellitus. However, some patients without a history of diabetes mellitus have developed HONK. A common criteria used to define HONK is hyperglycemia exceeding 800 mg/dL, associated with an abnormal sensorium and the absence of ketoacidosis.[23] Hyperglycemia can exceed 1000 mg/dL and can occasionally reach 2000 mg/dL.

Some conditions appear to place patients at risk for the development of HONK. The most common associated conditions seen in neurological patients are infections (especially those caused by gram-negative organisms, such as certain pneumonias and acute pyelonephritis), enteritis, acute trauma, severe physiologic stress, hyperalimentation, and drugs known to interfere with diabetic control (e.g., thiazide diuretics, mannitol, steroids, and phenytoin). Most patients who develop HONK have concurrent renal or cardiovascular disease.

Clinically, the patient develops polyuria, which leads to dehydration, marked hypovolemia, high serum osmolality (about 350 mOsm/L), and elevation of serum blood urea nitrogen. Hyponatremia is present. The serum ketone level is negative, and the acetone breath and Kussmaul respiration seen in diabetic coma are usually not present. The skin and mucous membranes are dry, with decreased skin turgor. Neurologically, the level of consciousness deteriorates from confusion to stupor and, finally, to coma. Other neurological findings may include seizures, hemisensory deficits, and visual field cuts.

Treatment of HONK is directed at administration of insulin and replacement of fluids along with electrolyte replacement, as needed. Because of the profound dehydration, vigorous fluid replacement is necessary. According to Kruse,[23] it is important to initiate fluid resuscitation before administering insulin because the hypovolemia can lead to circulatory collapse. Hypovolemic shock can occur because insulin drives the glucose intracellular, decreasing plasma osmolality and causing an osmotic shift of water from the intravascular compartment to the intracellular compartment. Recommended intravenous fluid is normal saline.

The major collaborative problems with HONK are dehydration and hyperglycemia. The major nursing diagnosis related to the care of the patient with HONK is **fluid volume deficit.** The nurse must monitor vital signs, neurological signs, and hemodynamics and provide supportive care to these seriously ill patients. The blood glucose should be monitored every 1 to 2 hours during IV insulin infusion, and electrolytes every 4 to 6 hours until the blood glucose falls below 250 mg/dL. As correction of the hyperglycemia occurs, the hyponatremia can convert to hypernatremia. This is due to the deficit of free water common in HONK. Therefore, close monitoring of the electrolytes is necessary so that the intravenous fluid can be changed accordingly.

SUMMARY

In summary, fluid replacement and management of electrolytes and metabolic disorders with neuroscience patient populations requires knowledgeable nurses who understand the principles of treatment and complications common in the clinical setting.

REFERENCES

1. Reeves, W. B., & Andreoli, T. E. (1999). The antidiuretic hormone: Physiology and pathophysiology. In A. F. Krisht & G. T. Tindall (Eds.). *Pituitary disorders: Comprehensive management* (pp. 79–98). Philadelphia: Lippincott Williams & Wilkins.
2. Janicic, N., & Verbalis, J. G. (2003). Evaluation and management of hypo-osmolality in hospitalized patients. *Endocrinology and Metabolism Clinics of North America, 32,* 459–481.
3. Kettyle, W. M., & Arky, R. A. (1998). *Endocrine pathophysiology* (pp. 55–57). Philadelphia: Lippincott-Raven.
4. Berne, R. M., & Levy, M. N. (1993). *Physiology* (3rd ed., pp. 759–767). St. Louis, MO: Mosby.
5. Ellis, S. J. (1995). Severe hyponatremia: Complications and treatment. *QJM, 88,* 905–909.
6. Verbalis, J. G. (1998). Adaptation to acute and chronic hyponatremia: Implications for symptomatology, diagnosis, and therapy. *Seminars in Nephrology, 18*(1), 3–19.

7. Lin, M., Liu, S. J., & Lim, I. T. (2005). Disorders of water imbalance. *Medical Clinics of North America, 23,* 749–770.

8. Muther, R. S. (1999). Electrolyte disorders: Disorders of serum sodium, calcium, magnesium, and potassium. In S. Kawada (Ed.). *ACCP-SCCM combined critical care course: Multidisciplinary board review* (pp. 233–255). Anaheim, CA: Society of Critical Care Medicine and American College of Chest Physicians.

9. Civetta, J. M., Taylor, R. W., & Kirby, R. R. (1997). *Critical care* (3rd ed., pp. 413–441). Philadelphia: Lippincott-Raven.

10. Wright, D. G., Laureno, R., & Victor, M. (1979). Pontine and extrapontine myelinolysis. *Brain, 102,* 361–385.

11. Laureno, R. (1983). Central pontine myelinolysis following rapid correction of hyponatremia. *Annals of Neurology, 13,* 232–242.

12. Sterns, R. H., Riggs, J. E., & Schochet, S. S. (1986). Osmotic demyelination syndrome following correction of hyponatremia. *New England Journal of Medicine, 314,* 1535–1542.

13. Faber, M. D., Kupin, W. L., Heilig, C. W., & Narins, R. G. (1994). Common fluid-electrolyte and acid-base problems in the intensive care unit: Selected issues. *Seminars in Nephrology, 14*(1), 8–22.

14. Muther, R. S. (1999). Electrolyte disorders: Disorders of serum sodium, calcium, magnesium, and potassium. In D. J. Dries & R. K. Albert (Eds.). *ACCP/SCCM combined critical care course: Multidisciplinary board review* (pp. 233–255). Anaheim, CA: Society of Critical Care Medicine and the American College of Chest Physicians.

15. Ropper, A. H., Gress, D. R., Diringer, M. N., Green, D. M., Mayer, S. M., & Bleck, T. P. (2004). *Neurological and neurosurgical intensive care* (4th ed., pp. 105–112). Philadelphia: Lippincott Williams & Wilkins.

16. Snyder, N. A., Feigal, D. W., & Arieff, A. I. (1987). Hypernatremia in elderly patients: A heterogeneous, morbid, and iatrogenic entity. *Annals of Internal Medicine, 107*(3), 309–319.

17. Schafer, J. A. (1998). Renal regulation of potassium, calcium, and magnesium. In L. R. Johnson (Ed.). *Essential medical physiology* (2nd ed., pp. 395–402). Philadelphia: Lippincott-Raven.

18. Riggs, J. E. (2002). Neurological manifestations of electrolyte disturbance. *Neurological Clinics, 20*(1), 227–239.

19. Salem, M., Munoz, R., & Chernow, B. (1991). Hypomagnesemia in critical illness: A common and clinically important problem. *Critical Care Clinics, 7*(1), 225–252.

20. Greenberg, M. S. (2006). *Handbook of neurosurgery* (6th ed., pp. 13–14). New York: Thieme Medical Publishers.

21. Arvanitis, M. L., & Pasquale, J. L. (2005). External causes of metabolic disorders. *Emergency Medical Clinics of North America, 23,* 827–841.

22. Wijdicks, E. F. M. (1997). *The clinical practice of critical care neurology* (pp. 363–376). Philadelphia: Lippincott-Raven.

23. Saborio, P., Tipton, G. A., & Chan, J. C. M. (2000). Diabetes insipidus. *Pediatrics in Review, 21*(4), 122–129.

24. Wijdicks, E. F. M. (1997). *The clinical practice of critical care neurology* (pp. 363–376). Philadelphia: Lippincott-Raven.

25. Harrigan, M. R. (1996). Cerebral salt wasting syndrome: A review. *Neurosurgery, 38*(1), 152–160.

26. Dooling, E., & Winkelman, C. (2004). Hyponatremia in the patient with subarachnoid hemorrhage. *Journal of Neuroscience Nursing, 36*(3), 130–135.

Behavioral and Psychological Responses to Neurological Illness

Joanne V. Hickey

The purpose of this chapter is to address common behavioral and psychosocial aspects of neuroscience nursing practice and to present interventions as they relate to neurological illness. What is unique about behavioral and psychological responses to neurological disease and illness is the overlay of neurological deficits that influence cognitive processes and control of behavior in light of acute and chronic illness. The cognitive, perceptual, and structural deficits have a profound influence on behavior and psychological responses not found in diseases and illnesses that do not affect the neurological system. The neuroscience nurse is left with interventions designed for patients who are cognitively intact and who have not sustained injury to neurological structures that influence behavioral and psychological responses. As a result, the neuroscience nurse must adapt interventions based on intact neurological function and cognitive ability as they exist in the patient at the time of interaction.

Although often used interchangeably, it is important to distinguish between the terms *disease* and *illness*. *Disease* is a condition based on a pathophysiologic perspective that addresses signs, symptoms, and alteration in structure and function. By contrast, *illness* is the human experience of symptoms and suffering, and refers to how the disease is perceived, lived with, and responded to by the patient and his or her family.[1] Illness is a unique personal experience that is felt within the context of an individual's life. Neurological disease has far-reaching effects, not only on the neurophysiology, but also on the cognitive and affective, personality, and individual characteristics that give a person uniqueness, individuality, and identity. These compounded deficits and devastating losses create stresses for the patient and family that tax coping and adaptive skills. Because many neurological conditions can alter a person's cognitive abilities, patients may lack awareness and insight of change, implications, and impact on their life.

In caring for neurological patients and their families, the nurse must understand and be able to support the patient and family through both the dynamic acute and chronic phases of illness. Family members and significant others are better able to accept physiologic changes in their loved ones than behavioral, cognitive, or personality changes. Changes in a patient's behavior affect group dynamics and interpersonal relationships as well. The normal patterns of family interactions are altered, and family structure changes accordingly. Changes in patterns of interaction and family structure also alter usual methods of decision making and problem solving and the use of effective coping mechanisms. These factors contribute additional stresses to the already stressful experience of neurological illness.

STRESS AND THE STRESS RESPONSE

Stress is defined as "the nonspecific response of the body to any type of increased demands upon it."[2] New models based on psychoneuroimmunology examining the interactions among behavior and neural, endocrine, and immune systems elucidate the complex interactions and their impact on health and illness.[3] The coordinated interaction and integration of physiologic and psychological responses to stress are well documented and included in stress adaptation models. The stress response involves the sympathetic nervous system via direct and indirect mechanisms and has far-reaching effects. What is new is the increased understanding of the detrimental effect of long-term stress on hormonal and neurotransmitters and the immune system in relation to both physiologic and psychological responses.

Selye is credited with the introduction of the term *general adaptation syndrome* into the literature.[2] This syndrome comprises the nonspecific reactions of the hypothalamic-pituitary-adrenocortical system to any type of stress. The general endocrine changes associated with the response are enlargement of the adrenal cortex, shrinkage of the thymus gland, and ulceration of the stomach (stress ulcers).[2] These responses are mediated by the pituitary-adrenocortical axis of the neuroendocrine system and cause a multisystemic response. Much interest and numerous research studies have been devoted to understanding the neuroendocrine influence during stress.

When considering the general adaptation syndrome, three phases can be identified: the alarm reaction, in which the sympathetic system is activated and subsequently activates the neuroendocrine system; resistance to stress, a period of adaptation to the stress; and exhaustion from stress, a time when the coping mechanisms are insufficient or ineffective for continuing to deal with the stress. The degree to which the general adaptation syndrome is implemented and the amount of time during which it is operational depend on the intensity and type of stress experienced. Selye suggested that continued intense stimulation from stress would deplete the organism's ability to respond to stress at all, or to respond effectively.

The concept of stress as a psychological phenomenon has evolved from the work of various theorists. The conceptualization of stress has taken on many diverse models. The critical components that contribute to the understanding of stress have been identified as follows: the stimulus (stressor) must be viewed as a threat by the individual; the stimulus, regardless of whether it is positive or negative, must be viewed as being significant or relevant to the individual's welfare; and the organism's capacity for adaptation must have been exceeded. These critical components address the type and intensity of a stimulus, the individual's perception of the stimulus, and the duration of the stimulus that depletes the capacity to cope.

What kinds of stimuli activate the stress response in the neurological patient? Any intense physical or psychological stimuli, such as forced immobilization, trauma, pain, fear, threat of loss, lack of control, or anxiety, can cause a multisystemic stress response. There are degrees of intensity of stimuli that cause a proportional stress response. For example, one would expect a much less intense stress response in a patient who has been admitted for an elective cranioplasty for cosmetic purposes long after an injury occurred than in a patient who has been admitted for a craniotomy for removal of a brain tumor of unidentified histological origin.

HUMAN ADAPTATION AND COPING

Adaptation is the process of change undertaken by an organism in response to a change in the internal or external environment for the purpose of maintaining equilibrium. Physiologic adaptation supports physiologic survival and homeostasis within the organism, whereas psychological adaptation is directed toward maintaining psychological homeostasis. Adaptation may be positive or negative in that the process either supports or is detrimental to the well-being of that individual. Behaviors that are detrimental to the person are termed *maladaptive behaviors*, whereas those that support well-being are called *adaptive behaviors*. The conceptualization of adaptation is central to the practice of nursing because much of the nurse's focus is directed at supporting healthy adaptation.

Coping refers to an individual's response to stressors in the internal or external environment. Coping is viewed as the individual's attempt to remove stress and restore physical and emotional equilibrium. *Coping mechanisms* are the strategies, skills, or processes used to adapt to stresses and are categorized as effective or ineffective coping mechanisms based on their outcome. The choice of coping mechanisms and the manner in which they are applied affect recovery and the promotion of health.

NEUROLOGICAL CONDITIONS AND THEIR PSYCHOLOGICAL EFFECTS

In the case of neurological illness, the psychological stressors and stress response can be particularly taxing in terms of the person's ability to cope and adapt to the illness. Common concerns and losses precipitated by neurological illness may include the threat to survival and the impact of neurological deficits on independence and quality of life.

When assessing the patient's ability to cope and adapt to the emotional and behavioral responses necessitated by the impact of neurological illness, the nurse seeks both verbal and nonverbal feedback from the patient to validate perceptions, clarify information, and ascertain whether the patient understands the information provided. For the patient with neurological conditions, these interactions may be severely compromised or impossible (e.g., those who are comatose or aphasic) and create additional stress.

GENERAL PRINCIPLES: EMOTIONAL AND PSYCHOLOGICAL RESPONSES TO NEUROLOGICAL CONDITIONS

Certain emotional and psychological responses can be expected in most patients, such as fear and anxiety about impeding surgery. However, there are also individual concerns paramount to the patient. Identifying specific concerns and fears provides an opportunity to acknowledge and address the concerns to alleviate some stress through information and discussion. For example, the shaving of the hair from part of the head may be the biggest fear for a patient. Much can be done to dispel some of the underlying concerns and fears, thus modifying the emotional and behavioral response of the patient.

Initial and Ongoing Assessment

In assessing the psychological responses, data are collected from a number of sources and contexts and are tempered by limitations by the patient's level of consciousness and neurological deficits. Data sources can change over the course of an illness due to recovery or further loss of neurological function. Observe the patient's behavior when alone and while interacting with others (family members, significant others, staff, other patients); note facial expressions, body language, tone of voice, and reactions to particular individuals and situations. Listen to what the patient says and how it is said (e.g., how things are described, use of analogies). Collect information from the patient and family on the patient's personality before onset of illness. Determine also previous emotional/behavioral responses to stress, adjustment patterns and coping mechanisms (e.g., jogging, withdrawal), and support systems. Consult with other health providers about their observations of the patient's behavior.

Assessment is an ongoing process involving data collection, analysis, and identification of patient problems and interventions. Part of assessment is measurement through the use of instruments to determine the nature and degree of particular psychological/emotional responses such as anxiety and depression. It is beyond the scope of this chapter to discuss all available instruments. However, measurement of the degree of dysfunction can help the nurse determine the need for specific interventions and consultation by other

| CHART **10-1** | **Patient Problems and Nursing Diagnoses Related to Emotional and Psychological Responses of Patients and Families to Neurological Conditions** |

The following patient problems and nursing diagnoses are often identified for the patient or family with an altered emotional or psychological response to neurological conditions:

PATIENT PROBLEMS/NURSING DIAGNOSES

- Fear
- Personal Identity Disturbance
- Anxiety
- Hopelessness

- Powerlessness
- Body Image Disturbance
- Altered Role Performance
- Impaired Social Interaction
- Altered Family Processes
- Impaired Verbal Communication
- Ineffective Individual Coping
- Impaired Adjustment
- Ineffective Family Coping: Compromised

health professionals. Measurement at key points over time assists in monitoring change in condition and need for reformulation of interventions.

The catastrophic and disabling nature of most neurological conditions precipitates many emotional and behavioral responses in patients and their families. Common patient problems and nursing diagnoses are listed in Chart 10-1. The nurse is a collaborative member of the team caring for the patient. Interdisciplinary team communications and patient-centered conferences are useful to determine problems and interventions and evaluate outcomes. Other team members include the physician, case manager, social worker, nutritionist, and chaplain. In some special cases a neuropsychologist may be consulted. Case management is a reality of health care delivery, and most patients with complex and long-term neurological problems are assigned a case manager. One of the considerations in managing a patient is the impact of behavior on safety and availability of needed services in care settings within the context of third-party reimbursement. The case manager is critical in finding the best resources available for the patient.

Nursing Interventions

General nursing interventions to help the patient deal with the many emotional and behavioral responses to the stress of neurological illness include the following:

- Provide an open, nonjudgmental, and supportive environment.
- Accept the patient's perceptions and behavior.
- Correct any inaccurate factual information matter-of-factly.
- Develop alternate ways of communication if communication deficits exist.
- Encourage the patient to express feelings in whatever way possible.
- Help the patient use positive adaptive coping mechanisms.
- Include the patient in problem solving and decision making to the degree possible.

- Provide information through patient education adapted to the needs of the patient; provide reinforcement as necessary.
- Help the patient set realistic goals.
- Make referrals to other health care professionals when appropriate.

COMMON EMOTIONAL AND PSYCHOLOGICAL RESPONSES TO THE STRESS ASSOCIATED WITH NEUROLOGICAL CONDITIONS

The general management principles of assessment and nursing intervention discussed in the previous section can be applied to the management of the common emotional and psychological responses seen in many patients with acute or chronic neurological disease. The emotional and psychological responses discussed include anxiety, frustration, anger, hostility, fear, denial, depression, stigma, loss, grief and bereavement, altered body image, sensory deprivation, sensory overload, sleep deprivation, intensive care unit (ICU) psychosis, and family responses. Although these common responses are discussed as separate entities, several responses can occur concurrently and there is overlap in interventions.

Anxiety

Anxiety is a feeling of uneasiness, apprehension, or dread that is associated with an unrecognized, subjective source of anticipated danger. It results from the real or perceived conflicts and frustrations of living. For patients who are unable to speak because of neurological disability or a tracheostomy, their ability to express feelings of frustration, anger, and hostility is negated. This causes anxiety for the patient and perhaps for the nurse. Anxiety is often classified as mild, moderate, or severe to convey the notion that the feeling can range from the mild awareness of fear or anticipatory danger to outright panic. Physiologic alterations in the autonomic system, such as an elevated pulse rate and blood pressure, perspiration, tightness in the stomach, or diarrhea, may accompany this mood state. An anxious patient demonstrates various recognizable behaviors associated with the degree of anxiety including irritability, uneasiness, apprehension, demanding or unreasonable behavior, and often verbal abusiveness. Such a patient is often described as "very difficult."

Approach

Because anxiety is associated with an unrecognized, subjective source of anticipated danger, time should be spent trying to discover the underlying basis. Often, several concerns are responsible for anxiety, some of which cannot be identified on the conscious level. For the patient who cannot communicate, the nurse must try to anticipate potential sources of anxiety and provide information. Alternative methods of communication should be developed, and the nurse must read body language. Recognizing potential sources of anxiety is a major focus of care. To alleviate anxiety, the nurse explains what is going to be done before beginning and then keeps the patient apprised while care is administered. Care is also explained to the "unresponsive" or "unconscious" patient because there is no way to determine whether sensory stimuli are getting through to the brain and being processed. The caregiver must assume that some verbal stimuli will penetrate the barriers of neurological illness, thus providing information and comfort to the patient.

For patients who are able to follow directions and cooperate, relaxation therapy may reduce anxiety. This is a systematic approach to tightening and relaxing muscle groups to relieve muscle tension. Another relaxation technique is the use of imagery. Patients are encouraged to select an image that is particularly relaxing and pleasing. They are taught to close their eyes, relax, and focus on experiencing all the pleasing sensations of being in this chosen setting. Any type of relaxation technique takes time to learn and must be practiced to achieve optimal results. Appropriate patient selection is necessary for this therapy.

Frustration, Anger, and Hostility

Frustration is the feeling that occurs when a course of action or activity cannot be carried out or brought to a desirable conclusion. Irritability, anxiety, and verbal outbursts often accompany frustration. **Anger** is an intense feeling of displeasure and antagonism in response to mounting frustration, conflict, or anxiety. It connotes strong feelings in response to the actual prevention or threat of prevention of achievement or maintenance of a desired goal or state. Anger that is turned inward is called **depression**. The behavioral manifestations of anger may include aggressive or destructive acts, verbal attacks, silence, or depression. **Hostility** is usually seen in association with anger. It is a feeling of antagonism directed toward another and is associated with a wish to hurt, humiliate, or discredit that person. Hostility is generally thought to be the result of frustrated or unfulfilled needs or wishes.

Approach

Allow patients to express feelings in a safe, nonjudgmental environment. Help the patient identify the basis of frustra-

tion or anger. If the source can be identified, it may be possible to alleviate or reframe the problem. Unrealistic goals may be noted, followed by a transition to more realistic goals. Angry patients need the same kind of help and support provided for the anxious patient. If an angry patient is apt to lose self-control and cause injury to self, others, or property, he or she must be controlled. Use a quiet environment, drug therapy, other forms of therapy directed at preventing self-harm, and referrals.

Fear

Fear is a feeling of extreme apprehension or dread associated with a potential or real threat to the well-being, quality of life, and survival of the individual. It may be associated with the unknown, mutilation, loss of control, pain, disability, or other factors. Behavioral manifestations of fear include excitability, irrational behavior, and irrational and inaccurate beliefs about the feared object. Physiologic signs and symptoms of the activated sympathetic nervous system (fight-or-flight response) include pallor, tachycardia, pupillary dilation, dry mouth, and cold, clammy hands.

Approach

Identify the basis of the fear, exploring concerns with the patient. Correct any misinformation. Ongoing verification of the patient's understanding and perceptions as well as clarification and amplification of information is an ongoing and necessary aspect of support.

Denial

Denial is a defense mechanism, sometimes called a temporary protective mechanism, whereby the person refuses to acknowledge the existence or significance of known facts. The known fact is too painful or overwhelming for the person to accept, so its existence is denied. The degree of denial can vary and is likely to be carried out in fantasy or refusal to discuss the facts so that reality is temporarily blocked. Denial can be an effective, temporary method of dealing with a stress-producing situation until the person is able to cope effectively. Sustained denial, however, becomes a negative and ineffective mechanism, in that the person is not willing to incorporate the new information for problem solving and realistic planning.

Approach

The nurse helps the patient to cope and adapt. An enormous amount of stress is associated with this realization. Patients gradually begin to acknowledge some of the more obvious aspects of their illness. Questions are answered honestly and as completely as possible based on the known facts so that patients can gradually face the realities of their illness. Depression and grieving are characteristic of this period. Once the painful information is incorporated into reality, the patient is able to make realistic decisions based on an altered and realistic appraisal.

Depression

Depression is a feeling of sadness and self-depreciation accompanied by difficulty in thinking and conducting usual activities and responsibilities, a lowered energy level, and self-preoccupation. Depression is also described as anger turned inward. The depressed person may be unable to express feelings and instead internalizes them. There are varying degrees of depression, although the characteristic behaviors associated with depression are a sad, expressionless face; flat affect; listlessness; lack of interest in others or the environment; possible crying spells; and a sense of hopelessness. Depressed persons often see no possible resolution to their situation and may contemplate suicide. Allusions to suicide may be made either directly or indirectly and should be taken seriously with special suicide prevention interventions.

Approach

The person who is severely depressed may need psychiatric consultation and help. Drug therapy may be helpful in treating temporary depression. However, the reasons for the depression must be sought, identified, and addressed. Suicide precautions may need to be instituted. Conduct of a suicide assessment on all patients is imperative. Various assessment instruments are available. All health care agencies must have a method of screening for suicidal potential and a policy and procedure to follow when it is identified. Check for the policy and procedure in your practice site.

Stigma

When a person feels devalued or unable to meet minimum societal norms, this is termed **stigma.** The feeling of stigmatization can result from physical or emotional deficits, behavioral abnormalities, or violation of societal laws or codes. The stigmatized person demonstrates characteristic behaviors of feelings of shame, alienation, or being devalued; a decreased feeling of self-esteem or social worth; isolation from normal relationships; rejection of attempts by others to reach out to him or her; suspicion; paranoid behavior; loneliness; hostility; and anger.

Approach

Dealing with patients who feel stigmatized is difficult. The feelings are usually based on deep-seated beliefs and values. The patient needs assistance in exploring his or her feelings for better understanding. The nurse presents reality and corrects any erroneous information that the patient expresses. Support and build the patient's self-esteem. Referrals may be necessary.

Loss, Grief, and Bereavement

Loss, grief, and bereavement are addressed together because they are part of an overlapping response. **Loss** is a state in which a person experiences deprivation or the complete lack of something valued that was previously present and available to him or her. The person who has sustained a significant loss will demonstrate behaviors consistent with grieving and bereavement. The loss of any valued object or function is followed by three stages that lead to healthy resolution: (1) shock and disbelief, (2) development of an awareness (recognition) of the loss, and (3) restitution (reconciliation).[4]

The *shock phase* immediately follows the loss. The patient is stunned and in a state of disbelief. Although intellectualization of the loss is possible, it is not accepted emotionally. Disbelief is overwhelming and verbalization that this cannot be true is common. During the *recognition phase*, the realization that the loss is real begins to occur. Characteristic behaviors include anger, self-blame, depression, and asking, "why me?" The patient is often preoccupied with the loss and what it means personally. The loss is internalized. In the *restitution phase*, there is realistic acceptance of what has happened and gradual interest in others and the environment. A patient begins to revise and accept a realistic self-concept and future and is able to make decisions based on the changes related to loss.

Loss can be sudden or gradual, predictable or unexpected, and temporary or permanent depending on the disease trajectory and how it affects the particular patient. Significant losses include loss of possessions; spouse, family members, or significant others; body parts; physiologic, psychological, or cognitive functions; and life. Certain physiologic functions, such as continence of the bladder and bowel and sexual function, are highly valued. Loss of these functions may be viewed as major, even catastrophic, losses by the person and society and have a great impact on quality of life. The individual's response to the loss depends on the value placed on the loss, societal and cultural values related to the loss, and support available to assist the individual in dealing with the loss.

Cultural values influence an individual's response to loss and adaptation. If the culture places a high value on the lost function, then the impact on the individual's status in the culture is significant. Cultural support in dealing with loss varies. All societies, regardless of whether they are primitive or highly sophisticated, have customs and rituals related to death. However, no such customs exist when there is loss of body function. The loss of body function (disability) may render the person socially unacceptable because of discomfort of others or cultural taboos. For example, the person who has dysphagia may not be a welcome guest at the dinner table. Even if other people are able to accept the patient's difficulty in managing food, the patient may feel humiliated by uncontrolled drooling or liquids and food falling from the mouth.

Approach

During the shock phase, accept the patient's behavior. Denial may be a temporary protective coping mechanism; allow the patient to deny the loss if he or she must. Listen in an accepting, nonjudgmental manner, and refrain from telling the patient that you understand how he or she feels unless you have experienced the same loss. Explore the significance of the loss to the patient within the context of self-concept, lifestyle, and quality of life. An analysis of the meaning of the loss from the patient's and family's perspective is the basis for creating an individualized plan for information, support, and referrals. During the recognition phase, accept the patient's anger. Allow for opportunities for the expression of feelings and to correct any misinformation. Explain the patient's responses to the family. Be supportive of the family. Referrals to other professionals and services are helpful (e.g., referral to the social worker). As the period of restitution emerges, encourage the patient to express his or her views and to plan realistically. Help the patient collect needed information. Be supportive, and help the patient adapt and integrate any alterations (e.g., self-image) into a revised self-concept. Support independent and self-responsibility to the degree possible.

Support groups, both within health care organizations and the community, are available for some patients with particular health problems, such as brain injury or multiple sclerosis. The particular services offered vary, but usually include practical information on how to live with the particular disease and illness, psychological and emotional support, a forum for discussion of mutual problems, and identification and acquisition of resources to assist the patient and family.

Change in Body Image

A concept basic to one's sense of identity, security, self-esteem, and self-concept is body image. **Body image** is defined as the conscious and unconscious perceptions that one has about his or her body as a separate and distinct entity. It is a developmental and social creation that is subject to very slow change in adult life. Illness, disability, and loss of function force a change in body image. If the change can be integrated realistically within the patient's self-concept without altering self-esteem, then the adaptation and adjustment are positive.

Behavioral manifestations associated with a change in body image include those that accompany loss, grief, and bereavement. The change is viewed as a threat or significant loss, and the patient passes through the characteristic stages of shock, recognition, and reconciliation.

Approach

If the nurse views the patient's change in body image within the framework of loss, grief, and bereavement, the nursing intervention will follow a similar approach. Accept the patient's perception of self. Recognize that changing body image is a slow process. Support patients as they begin to recognize the impact of illness on their concept of body image. Help patients to accept and adapt to the change with positive reinforcement.

Sensory Deprivation

Sensory deprivation is defined as a lack of or decreased sensory input from the external or internal environment. There is a lack of or decreased perception of multisensory input of various intensities and meanings to the person. The behavioral manifestations of sensory deprivation vary, depending on the degree of deprivation. They may include abnormalities in feeling states, disorientation, impairment of the ability to think, distortion of perception, and illusions and hallucinations. The patient with neurological disease may experience many neurological deficits that contribute to sensory deprivation, such as an altered level of consciousness, paresis or paralysis, numbness, paresthesias, visual deficits, hearing loss, taste or smell deficits, and cognitive or emotional deficits. Brain injury, spinal cord injury, stroke, multiple sclerosis, and many other neurological conditions contribute to sensory deprivation.

Therapeutic protocols, such as instituting aneurysm precautions, may also cause sensory deprivation.

Approach

The nurse must be sensitive to the high risk of neurological patients for sensory deprivation and recognize the development and presence of the problem. Provide multisensory stimuli to high-risk patients as a compensatory preventive intervention. Sensory input can be provided by talking to the patient; playing the radio, television, or tapes of recorded favorites; providing reality orientation and touch; and positioning to optimize impact. Reality orientation is a process of actively making patients aware of their environment (e.g., describing ongoing activities, weather, date, time, place, people, objects). Sensory deprivation, rather than physiologic deficits of the reticular activating system, may be the cause of a patient's disorientation.

Sensory Overload and Sleep Deprivation

Sudden, excessive, sustained, multisensory experiences that are perceived as confusing, bothersome, meaningless, and extremely stressful to the patient are defined collectively as **sensory overload.** The behavioral manifestations of sensory overload are confusion, disorientation, irritability, restlessness, agitation, panic, and hallucinations. Neurological patients may experience sensory overload from equipment and technology (e.g., ventilator, cardiac monitor), conditions that intensify sensory input (meningitis, encephalitis), or the constant environmental stimuli of unit noise, lights, activity, and nursing care. Intensive care units (ICUs) are particularly high in environmental stimuli, equipment sounds, activity, and care intensity. The deleterious response of patients to sensory overload in ICUs is referred to as ICU psychosis.

Because of constant unit noise and stimuli related to care, sleep deprivation is a common problem in neurological patients. **Sleep deprivation** is defined as a lack of adequate sleep or dream time in relation to earlier or usual sleep patterns. Persons with sleep deprivation experience behavioral, psychological, and physiologic alterations. Behavioral manifestations are similar to those seen in psychosis (alterations in perceptions, cognition, orientation, mood, affect). Patients admitted to ICUs, requiring constant care and monitoring, receiving certain medication, and experiencing extreme stress are prime candidates for sleep deprivation. The strange environment and constant activity of the hospital predispose patients to this common phenomenon. Because of injuries to the brain and their need for attention, neurological patients often experience sleep deprivation.

Approach

Identify the various sensory levels and sources of input in the patient's environment. Every effort should be made to control and moderate the intensity of stimuli. In patients with meningitis or encephalitis, minimize tactile stimuli and all other environmental stimuli.

In assessing for sleep deprivation, consider the complex multidimensional factors related to sleep interruption. Review the patient's 24-hour sleep-wakefulness cycle to determine how much sleep time is actually provided. Plan the nursing care to provide for uninterrupted sleep time. Drug therapy can also have an effect on the quality of sleep and dream time. Certain drugs may alter the depth of sleep and the sleep pattern. Recognize the various factors that influence the patient's ability to sleep and control the environment as much as possible to facilitate sleep. Many units now follow a late evening–nighttime protocol to facilitate sleep by controlling environmental stimuli such as noise and light.

Intensive Care Unit Psychosis

Admission to the alien environment of the ICU is stressful for the patient and family for many reasons. The ICU environment is characterized by strange noises, smells, and bright lights, and the open floor plan characteristic of most ICUs offers little privacy. The pervasive atmosphere is one of urgency, danger, and death being held in abeyance by technology and heroic measures of the staff. Ironically, the patient and family can feel profound isolation within this charged environment. Fear, anxiety, depression, and delirium are common responses to the situation, and the patient or family may panic. Sleep deprivation or an altered sleep-wakefulness cycle contributes to disorientation and misinterpretation of reality. Patients may exhibit agitation, hallucinations, delusions, and psychosis. This phenomenon is called **ICU psychosis**. The changes in behavior can be difficult to interpret. When neurological patients exhibit a change in behavior, one often attributes the change to a neurological cause. *However, psychological responses and drug side effects and interactions must also be carefully considered as possible etiologies.*

Approach

Institute strategies to provide emotional support, reassurance, and information to the conscious patient, and plan activities to allow for periods of uninterrupted sleep. Control environmental stimuli and noise. Provide for the safety needs of agitated patients. In an unconscious patient, provide for "soft stimuli," such as light touch, soft voices, and family visits whereby family members talk quietly to the patient about pleasant topics.

The Family and Significant Others

Neurological illness has serious consequences, not only for the patient, but also for family members and significant others. The family structure, relationships, and coping strategies for dealing with stress and crisis become important considerations for the nurse. Family members will react to illness individually across the entire gamut of responses, including anxiety, anger, depression, denial, grieving, and fear. Neurological illness often takes the form of a chronic condition with permanent or progressive disabilities that compel the patient to depend on family or significant others to meet basic needs. The stresses incurred by neurological illness are significant and require the support and assistance of health professionals for the family to make a realistic adjustment. The ability of the family to accept and adapt will directly influence the emotional well-being of every member of the family unit, including the patient. See Chart 10-1 for patient problems and nursing diagnoses related to the family.

Approach

The role of the nurse in supporting the family includes:

- Assess to determine understanding and perception of the patient's illness.
- Assess the family's style of interactions and support systems.
- Keep the family informed; be prepared to repeat and reinforce information.
- Encourage the family members to express their feelings; correct misinformation, and provide accurate information as necessary.
- Make referrals as necessary.
- Include the family in the care of the patient; provide coaching and education.
- Promote normality.
- Support the family's decision about patient care or plans for posthospital care.
- Be prepared to repeat information.

SUMMARY

In summary, this chapter has addressed common behavioral and psychological responses of patients with neurological disease and illness. The impact of neurological disease on functions that influence intake and processing of cognitive and perceptual information adds to the complexity of supporting patients with cognitive interventions designed for patients with intact neurological function. The nurse can manage some of these common problems, but also can engage the social worker, case manager, and other health professionals as necessary.

REFERENCES

1. Larsen, P. D. (2006). Chronicity. In I. M. Lubkin & P. D. Larsen (Eds.). *Chronic illness: Impact and interventions* (6th ed., p. 4). Boston, MA: Jones and Bartlett Publishers.
2. Selye, H. (1956). *The stress of life.* New York: McGraw-Hill.
3. DeKeyer, F. (2003). Psychneuroimmunology in critically ill patients. *AACN Clinical Issues, 14*(1), 25–32.
4. Engel, G. L. (1964). Grief and grieving. *American Journal of Nursing, 64*, 93.

Rehabilitation of Neuroscience Patients

Joanne V. Hickey

This chapter provides basic information about the principles and concepts of rehabilitation as they apply to neuroscience patient populations. Rehabilitation nursing is a specialty area of nursing practice with a published scope and standards of practice. However, rehabilitation principles and concepts are fundamental components of nursing practice and transcend all practice areas. Understanding of the comprehensive rehabilitation process by neuroscience nurses will facilitate a seamless continuum of care for patients.

FRAMEWORK FOR DISABILITY

The restoration to health or improvement of function is the main focus of rehabilitation. Most definitions of rehabilitation are based on the *International Classification of Functioning, Disability and Health* (ICF) published by the World Health Organization (WHO).[1] The ICF provides a comprehensive description of how people live with their health conditions through a classification of health and health-related domains that describe body functions and structures, activities, and participation. It provides a way to measure the impact disability has on health and how to optimize the ability to remain engaged and functional. The ICF consists of two parts, each of which is divided into two components:

- Functioning and disability
  - Body functions and body structures
  - Activities and participation
- Contextual factors
  - Environmental factors
  - Personal factors

Body functions include the physiology of body systems (includes psychological function), whereas *body structures* include the anatomic parts of the body such as organs, limbs, and their components. *Activity* is defined as the execution of a task or action by an individual; *participation* is involvement in life situations. *Environmental factors* are the physical, social, and attitudinal environment in which an individual lives and conducts his or her life; *personal factors* are the internal influences on functioning and disability unique to the person. This conceptualization of rehabilitation is holistic and recognizes the influence of environmental and personal factors on rehabilitation outcomes.

Disease and health conditions are comparable regardless of cause. This view places mental disorders and physical illness on equal footing in that both can affect the ability to function optimally. **Disease** refers to intrinsic pathology that may or may not be evident clinically. **Impairment** is an abnormality of a psychological, physiologic, or anatomic structure and function; it represents disturbance on the *organ* level. **Disability** is the consequences of impairment as it relates to individual functional performance and activity; it represents disturbance on the *person* level.

CONCEPTS OF REHABILITATION

Rehabilitation is a dynamic process through which a person is assisted to achieve optimal physical, emotional, psychological, social, and vocational potential and to maintain dignity, self-respect, and a quality of life that is as self-fulfilling and satisfying as possible. The major goals of rehabilitation are optimizing function; promoting independence, satisfaction, and quality of life; and preserving self-esteem. To be effective, rehabilitation is a philosophy of care and an integral part of health care delivery.

Rehabilitation is a continuum of functional restoration. In some situations, complete functional restoration is possible, as in the situation of a patient who sustains a mild cerebral concussion. In this instance, complete recovery is the rule. However, when complete recovery of function is not possible and permanent disability is likely, the patient needs help to accept, adjust to, and compensate for the existing deficit and to establish an optimal level of function. An example is a paraplegic patient who has sustained a severed spinal cord injury resulting in permanent paralysis. Present medical therapies cannot restore the severed cord to its premorbid condition, although this may be a future possibility. However, a comprehensive rehabilitation program helps the person live a useful, relatively independent life from a wheelchair.

Another aspect of rehabilitation addresses chronic health problems and degenerative diseases, such as multiple sclerosis. Although currently no cure exists for multiple sclerosis, a rehabilitation program can improve quality of life through health promotion, symptom management, prevention of complications, and patient education to promote optimal independence for the longest possible time. As the disease progresses, rehabilitation offers alternate ways of conducting activities of daily living (ADLs) with adaptive devices and alternate methods of performing skilled acts.

▨ A PHILOSOPHY OF REHABILITATION

A **philosophy** is a set of broad statements about fundamental beliefs and values. The philosophy of rehabilitation offers a framework to shape the overall rehabilitation process; it often includes the following premises:

1. *A person with a disability has intrinsic value that transcends the disability; each person is a unique holistic being who has the right and the responsibility to make informed personal choices regarding health and lifestyle.* Restoring an individual's capacity to the highest level possible assists the person to resume roles such as homemaking, parenting, and gainful employment, thus offering many social, emotional, psychological, and financial returns to society.
2. *Rehabilitation is an integral component of all care administered by all health care providers.* Rehabilitation begins the moment a person seeks health care so that prevention is incorporated into the rehabilitation process. A major goal in educating all health care providers is to prepare them to "think rehab" from the moment of initial contact with the patient.
3. *Comprehensive rehabilitation requires the active participation and collaboration of all health care providers through ongoing communication and management.* Scheduled team conferences, informal discussion, written plans of care, and progress notes provide a means of communication. Multidisciplinary collaboration and management mean that all health team members collaborate to achieve specific, identified, mutual goals.
4. *Rehabilitation requires the active participation of the patient to achieve optimal rehabilitative potential.* The patient must be motivated and actively involved in the rehabilitation process to achieve optimal outcomes.
5. *Rehabilitation actively involves the patient's family or significant others; they are the patient's potential support systems and assist with the transition back to the home and community.* Family members should be reached at their individual levels of understanding, taking into consideration their educational, socioeconomic, and cultural backgrounds to understand the rehabilitative goals and methods selected to meet these goals. The nurse usually interprets this information for the family, helping them to understand how they can best participate. In addition, the family is a rich source of information about the patient's personality and lifestyle that will be helpful in the transition back to the community.
6. *An individual patient and family evaluation is the basis to determine their ability to contribute to the rehabilitation process.* All families cannot contribute in the same way or to the same degree. Because each family and patient present different problems, individual evaluation is necessary.
7. *The patient experiences illness and disability within the context of his or her previous adjustment patterns.* The strengths and weaknesses of the patient's personality are essentially the same during illness. Team members must recognize the social and cultural influences that affect the patient's adjustment patterns and acceptance of care.
8. *Rehabilitation takes place within the context of the patient's whole life: the sociocultural aspects of life, his or her job or vocation, family, home, place in the community, religion, and relationship to self.* When illness strikes, family life is abruptly interrupted and altered. Illness affects not only the patient, but also the family. Therefore, rehabilitation includes the needs of the family.
9. *Rehabilitation is a dynamic process with progress, plateaus, and setbacks.* Only through ongoing assessment and problem solving is achievement of patient goals possible.
10. *Transitions in care include plans for continued rehabilitation services.* Options include acute or subacute inpatient rehabilitation, community re-entry, outpatient rehabilitation, or home health therapies. The patient and family are presented with various care alternatives and helped to evaluate the implications of each choice, including cost and health insurance issues. The patient and family actively participate in the decision-making process of discharge planning to the degree that they are able and willing to participate for a relatively smooth transition and adjustment.

Terminology of Rehabilitation

The following terms are used consistently in rehabilitative health care:

- **Rehabilitative potential:** dormant power for rehabilitation within a person that exists as a possibility that can eventually become actualized
- **Short-term goals:** goals to be achieved in the immediate future (usually set for 1 week); discrete units or steps involved in the learning of a skill that must be achieved before more complex skilled acts can be accomplished; the steps through which long-term goals are achieved
- **Long-term goals:** goals projected for completion in the distant future; can be considered the ultimate objectives of a rehabilitation program
- **Optimal goals:** optimal rehabilitation goals that may be expected barring significant setbacks or complications
- **Realistic goals:** goals that reflect a realistic appraisal of the person and achievable outcome
- **Acute disability:** a disability that has a finite duration and is completely resolved in a short period of time; reversible; temporary
- **Chronic disability:** an ongoing disability that limits the person in some way; permanent; irreversible
- **Interdisciplinary practice model:** health professionals working collaboratively together to achieve measurable functional outcomes for people with disabilities
- **Multidisciplinary team rounds:** activity in which the health professionals round together to assess and monitor progress, functional level, problems, and concerns on some scheduled daily or weekly basis; it provides data for further discussion at team meetings or patient care conferences
- **Family meetings:** planned meetings with one or more health care professionals and family members to discuss patient progress, needs, and planning; recognizes the

importance of the family in the rehabilitation of the patient, and helps to maintain open communication

Framework for Rehabilitation Decisions

Initial decisions related to rehabilitation are based primarily on information gathered during a screening examination. The goal is to determine the best match between the patient needs and available resources. In this complex health care environment, utilization of health care and cost are scrutinized. A key initial decision is whether the person can benefit from rehabilitation. Figure 11-1 summarizes the process of rehabilitation decision making. This information and figure are taken from the Agency for Health Care Policy and

Research (AHCPR) clinical practice guidelines, *Post-Stroke Rehabilitation* (1995), but they are applicable to all initial and subsequent transitional rehabilitation decisions.[2]

Multidisciplinary Team and Outcomes

Depending on patient needs, several health care disciplines may participate in a multidisciplinary collaborative model of practice to provide a comprehensive rehabilitation program. The central focus of care is the patient and family, and each multidisciplinary team member works with the patient and family to achieve optimal outcomes. Although all patients will not require the services of every discipline, they are available for consultation as necessary.

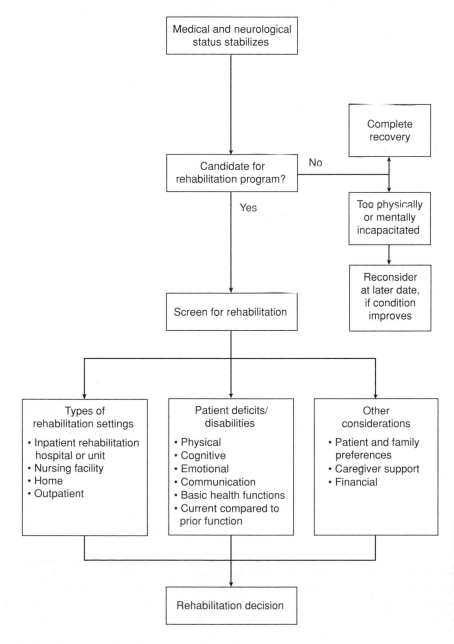

Figure 11-1 • Framework for rehabilitation decisions. (Gresham, G. E., Duncan, P. W., Stason, W. B., et al. [1995]. *Post-stroke rehabilitation.* Clinical practice guideline, No. 16. Rockville, MD: U.S. Department of Health and Human Services. Public Health Service, Agency for Health Care Policy and Research. AHCPR Publication No. 95-0662. May.)

The rehabilitation process begins with a comprehensive functional assessment. The functional independence measure (FIM) is the most widely used standardized instrument to measure severity of disability based on a functional assessment. The FIM assesses self-care, sphincter control, transfers, locomotion, communication, and social cognition. In addition, each health care team member can further assess the patient using other instruments specific to the particular discipline.

After a database has been compiled, a comprehensive rehabilitation plan is developed with identified functional outcome measures. Team conferences are one example of a formal communication mode. Informal communications between and among team members are ongoing. These interactions reinforce interdisciplinary collaboration among team members by promoting continuity of care and moving the plan forward. Because of the complexity of care and the numbers of people involved, it is easy for communications to break down. Therefore, planned, formal, patient-centered conferences are essential for the vitality of the process. Patient outcomes are measured using the FIM, Barthel Index, and other specific instruments.

ASSESSMENT OF ACTIVITIES OF DAILY LIVING

ADLs are a number of self-care and mobility activities. A number of instruments are available to measure independence in ADLs. Independence can be measured by the degree of ability a patient has for successful functioning at home, at work, and in social situations.

The ADLs focus on different aspects of function:

- **Personal ADLs:** bathing, toileting, grooming, eating, oral hygiene, dressing, ambulating (on various surfaces), and communicating. The ability to perform these activities vastly contributes to independent self-care.
- **Instrumental ADLs:** using the telephone, shopping, using transportation to get around in the community, and walking distances outside the home. Independence in these activities is a key marker for independence in basic activities outside the home.
- **Occupational and role activities:** roles in the home, such as homemaking, parenting, and spousal roles, and jobs outside the home. The skills necessary to assume any role or job are identified; the occupational therapist, family counselor, or vocational counselor can assist in assessing critical skills.

Helping the patient relearn ADLs begins with an assessment of the skills that remain intact, those that are lost, and those that can be used with help. The major barriers to relearning ADL skills in the neurological patient are deficits affecting perception, motor activity, communication, vision, and cognitive functions.

The teaching plan is based on the individual patient needs and the principles of learning and teaching. For example, an occupational therapist (OT) helps in making suggestions for teaching the patient ADLs such as self-feeding. If the patient is being seen by the OT, the nurse coordinates nursing activities with those of the OT so that the patient is given the same instructions; this prevents confusion and frustration.

CHART 11-1   Principles of Learning and Teaching

Patient and family education are important components of the rehabilitation process. Effective teaching rests on an understanding of the principles of learning and teaching as applied to the clinical setting.

The following basic principles can serve as a guide in teaching the patient:

- The objectives of the teaching session should be defined clearly; it is wise to write down objectives to identify the expected knowledge and skills outcomes.
- The skills involved in the activity are limited to small, critical units to facilitate learning.
- People learn best when they perceive a need or value in the learning.
- Readiness to learn is important if patients are to benefit from the material presented; sufficient physical and mental function is necessary to learn successfully.
- To enhance participation and concentration, the patient is rested and comfortable before the teaching session begins.
- The nurse demonstrates the skill and then invites the patient to perform the skill under supervision; if the skill is not performed correctly, demonstrate again. Provide sufficient supervision and opportunity for repetition to master the skill.
- The more senses involved in learning, the higher the probability that learning occurs. (For example, the nurse can demonstrate and describe the activity; gestures may also be used.)
- Reinforcement of learning follows throughout with consistency by all staff members working with the patient. Such reinforcement is based on a written teaching plan.
- Consider the patient's age, neurological deficits, educational background, fluency, and intelligence when individualizing a teaching plan that is appropriate for his or her needs.
- Provide positive verbal feedback for accomplishments.
- Motivate the patient to participate actively in the learning process.
- Encourage the patient and family to ask questions.

Each activity that must be relearned is analyzed to identify the critical components involved in the overall task. Use of adaptive devices may be necessary to compensate for neurological deficits and to allow the patient to perform ADLs independently. Simple remedies may provide great self-care benefits. For example, a spoon with a bulky stem may allow the patient with hand contractures to grasp the spoon and feed himself or herself, an unachievable act with a regular spoon. Chart 11-1 details the principles of learning and teaching. The information in Chart 11-2 applies specifically to patients with cerebral injury.

PRINCIPLES OF REHABILITATION NURSING

Principles of rehabilitation are an integral component of independent nursing practice and include the major elements of **prevention, maintenance,** and **restoration.** Many nursing protocols and procedures contain elements of all three components. Preventive measures include special skin

Teaching the Patient With Cerebral Injury

Patients with cerebral injury present special problems in learning because of certain cognitive deficits, such as easy distractibility, short attention span, inability to think abstractly, memory deficits, poor judgment, and inability to transfer learning from one situation to another. An assessment to identify deficits and to develop an individualized teaching plan that reflects modifications designed to compensate for deficits is necessary. A few principles should be remembered when teaching such a patient:

- Be realistic in your expectations.
- Assume a calm and positive attitude toward the patient's ability to learn.
- Develop a written teaching plan for use by all nursing staff; be consistent.
- Plan short teaching sessions with specific goals.
- Choose a time when the patient is not tired.
- Use simple, specific instructions.
- Proceed systematically, in a step-by-step fashion.
- Motivate the patient.
- Facilitate learning by repetition and reinforcement.
- For the patient who is easily distracted, structure the environment to minimize distractions.
- Praise any accomplishment.
- Incorporate behavior modification principles.
- Tailor teaching methods to the patient's functional level (e.g., may need visual aids and demonstration rather than explanation).

slow process requiring ongoing perseverance and effort. The long-lasting reward is that a human being has been helped to achieve maximal potential.

Rehabilitation is a collaborative interdisciplinary process involving health care professionals working together to achieve mutual goals. As the member of the rehabilitation team who spends the most time with the patient on a daily basis, the nurse supports continuity of care through coordination. The nurse coordinates and manipulates the patient's daily schedule so that optimal benefit will be derived from therapy. For example, the patient needs a high energy level for the strenuous activity of mat work or ambulation in physical therapy. Scheduling these activities when the patient is fatigued is counterproductive to the goals of physical therapy. The nurse also assesses and addresses the patient's physical, emotional, and psychological responses to various therapeutic regimens.

The family often approaches the nurse with questions and concerns about the overall plan of care. In some instances, information and clarification are provided. In other instances, referral of questions to other team members for a one-on-one basis or initiation of a family–team meeting is most appropriate. Keeping the lines of communication open is a tedious and difficult job that is compounded by the large number of people involved in the patient's care. The nurse often becomes the clearinghouse for information, concerns, and confrontations.

Patient and family education is key to optimal recovery. Community resources are available through various agencies such as the American Stroke Association. Stroke rehabilitation information can be accessed by telephone or website. The patient and family need to be aware of these resources; they may need assistance in making contact.

Nursing Management of Patients With Impaired Physical Mobility

Assessment

The nurse assesses mobility by conducting a motor function examination and reviewing the data from the FIM. Independence is closely correlated to a person's ability to move individual body parts or the body as a whole. Loss of mobility imposes severe constraints on the individual's freedom and independence.

Nursing management depends on identifying patient and collaborative problems. The following are possible patient problems and nursing diagnoses:

- Impaired Physical Mobility
- Risk for Injury (from falls)
- Risk for Altered Skin Integrity
- Fatigue
- Activity Intolerance
- Depression

The following are possible collaborative problems, although many more preventive focused problems can be cited:

- Pathologic fractures
- Joint dislocation
- Falls

care, proper positioning and realignment, frequent turning, and range-of-motion exercises. The maintenance of intact skills and functions is supported by such activities as getting the patient out of bed to a chair and encouraging the patient to be as independent as possible in ADLs. Instituting exercise programs designed to increase range of motion, teaching ADLs to a patient with a paralyzed limb, and helping a patient to relearn names of common objects are examples of restorative nursing activities. This framework can be kept in mind when planning and administering nursing care to address particular deficits.

A fundamental concept of rehabilitation is to do *with* the patient and not do *for* or *to* the patient. According to the American Nurses Association and the Association of Rehabilitation Nurses, the goal of rehabilitation nursing is to assist people who have disability and chronic illness to attain maximum functional ability, maintain optimal health, and adapt to an altered lifestyle.[3] Rehabilitation nurses assist patients to identify goals that are realistic and attainable and consider the patient's continuing accountability for optimal wellness. After a skill has been mastered, it is expected to be maintained, and also to become a building block for the next functional level. A patient is assisted to do any part of a task even if it is not the complete task. For example, the nurse may soap and squeeze a wash cloth, and the patient may be able to wash one side of the face with this assistance. This begins the cycle to develop the complete skill in the future. Unlike other aspects of nursing, rehabilitation is often a very

The major patient problem of **Impaired Physical Mobility** is exemplified by a patient with limited physical movement including bed mobility, transfers, and ambulating. When considering altered mobility, interventions directed at preventing edema of the extremities, skin breakdown, contractures, subluxation, deconditioning of muscles, pneumonia, and deep vein thrombosis are common collaborative problems in which the nurse plays an important role.

Patients with concurrent cerebral injury and impaired physical mobility may not have sufficient cognitive ability to comprehend fully the extent and implications of their disability or the relationship of prescribed treatment to the maintenance, prevention, and restoration of functional loss. They will need direct supervision. They are at high risk for injury due to falls.

Fatigue and **Activity Intolerance** are related to bed rest deconditioning. Endurance for activity must be developed. As a rule, one day for every day in bed is necessary to build endurance; in elderly patients, it is longer. The nurse deals with these patient problems to help the patient achieve an optimal level of independence.

Interventions

As a member of the multidisciplinary team, the nurse works collaboratively with other team members to assist the patient to regain function. The philosophy of rehabilitation nursing is an integral part of care. The specifics of care depend on the patient's functional deficits and needs as well as expected outcomes.

THE BASIS OF MOVEMENT AND TREATMENT OF MOVEMENT DISORDERS

Normal movement patterns originate in genetically programmed configurations of neurons. Maturation of the central nervous system follows a predetermined pattern of elaboration and refinement of movement. Reflex and voluntary control proceeds in cephalic to caudal and proximal to distal directions. For example, voluntary head movement is learned before voluntary trunk movement. Most motor systems are modifiable within limits, thus providing the basis for developing acquired motor skills.

The maturation and concurrent development of movement and posture follow a deliberate pattern for learning skilled acts. Mobility develops from synchronized coactivated flexor and extensor muscles that provide the stabilizing forces for posture. Hand and finger control develops from visually directed grasping and releasing of objects. Understanding the underlying physiology and pathophysiology of movement patterns is the basis of treatment.

Neurophysiological and Developmental Treatment Approaches

There are at least five recognized rehabilitation treatment approaches for people with motor control deficits related to cerebral injury: the Root approach; the Bobath neurodevelopmental approach; the Brunnstrom approach; proprioceptive

neuromuscular facilitation; and Carr and Shepard motor relearning. Because the Bobath neurodevelopmental approach is used by many nurses, it is discussed here in greater detail.

Bobath Neurodevelopmental Treatment Approach

The Bobath approach is used primarily for patients with hemiplegia caused by stroke, brain injury, and cerebral palsy. The major goal is normalization of muscle tone, posture, movement, and function. Underlying premises include the following[3–5]:

- The sensation of movement is learned and not the movement itself.
- Every skilled activity takes place against a backdrop of basic patterns of postural control, righting, equilibrium, and other protective reactions.
- When cerebral injury occurs, abnormal patterns of posture and movement develop that interfere with the performance of ADLs.
- Abnormal patterns develop because sensation is diverted into the abnormal patterns; this diversion must be stopped to reinstitute control over the motor output in developmental sequence.
- Eliciting the basic patterns of postural control, righting, and equilibrium is necessary, thus providing the normal stimuli while inhibiting abnormal patterns.
- People are allowed to feel, and thus relearn, normal movement patterns and postures.

Nurses can incorporate major principles of treatment into positioning, turning, transferring, and ADLs. These principles include the following[3]:

- Reintegration of function of the two sides of the body is emphasized during movement, ADLs, and bed or chair positioning so that bilateral segmental movement will occur.
- Proximal to distal positioning is recommended (tone in the limbs can be reduced from proximal points, such as the head, shoulder, or pelvic girdle).
- Weight bearing is provided on the affected side to normalize tone. This includes its role in sitting, lying, or rising.
- Tasks should begin from a symmetric midline position with equal weight bearing on the affected and unaffected sides.
- Movement toward the affected side is encouraged.
- Straightening of the trunk and neck is encouraged to promote symmetry and normalization of tone and posture.
- Hemiplegic patients should be positioned in opposition to the spastic patterns of flexion and adduction in the upper extremity and extension in the lower extremity.

Positioning

Positioning the patient in proper body alignment is necessary to prevent development of musculoskeletal deformities, such as contracture and ankylosis; pressure ulcers; and decreased vascular supply, thrombosis, and edema. Positioning of the neuroscience patient may be complicated by nuchal rigidity, spasticity, abnormal posturing (e.g., decerebration), presence of a cast, position restriction secondary to surgery, and lacerations or abrasions associated with multiple

TABLE 11-1   PATTERNS OF MUSCLE RECOVERY IN HEMIPLEGIA

STAGE	NAME	ONSET	DESCRIPTION
I	Flaccidity	From the time of injury to 2 or 3 d after	No tendon reflexes or resistance to passive movement
II	Spasticity (late onset of spasticity indicates a poorer prognosis)	2 d–5 wk	Hyperactive tendon reflexes and exaggerated response to minimal stimuli
III	Synergy (flexion, then extension)	2–3 wk	Simultaneous flexion of muscle groups in response to flexion of a single muscle (e.g., an attempt to flex the elbow results in contraction of the fingers, elbow, and shoulder)
IV	Near normal, possible weakness or slight incoordination may still be present (late return of tendon reflexes indicates a poor prognosis)	1 wk–6 mo	Control of voluntary movement; recovery occurs predictably from the proximal muscles of the extremity to the distal muscles (i.e., voluntary movement of the hand and foot is last to recover and tends to be weaker)

trauma. These specific problems encountered in positioning change as the muscles undergo the various phases of recovery (Table 11-1).

A few basic principles are guides for positioning the patient in bed[6]:

- The unconscious patient should be repositioned every few (e.g., 2 hours) hours around the clock. As consciousness is regained, independent movement in bed and participation in self-care activities are encouraged to maintain muscle strength and tone. Proper positioning should be taught to the patient if he or she has the cognitive ability to participate.
- If spasticity is present, frequent repositioning is necessary. Splinting and casting to inhibit tone may be ordered and applied by a physical therapist.
- Any restrictions of position are posted conspicuously at the head of the patient's bed and included in the nursing care plan (paper or electronic site).
- A sufficient number of pillows are available to maintain body alignment.
- Trochanter rolls and other positioning devices are useful.
- If an arm is weak or paralyzed, it is positioned to approximate the joint space in the glenoid cavity. The affected arm is not pulled. A pillow or small wedge in the axillary region helps prevent adduction of the shoulder.
- Special resting hand splints may be ordered to prevent contracture; remove periodically to assess the skin for pressure ulcers.
- Edema of the extremities, particularly of the hands, is controlled by positioning and elevating the hand higher than the elbow.
- An elastic glove may be ordered to control hand edema.
- Prevention of foot-drop is critical. Foot positioning devices, such as high-top sneakers or special splints, may be ordered.
- Heels are kept off the bed to prevent pressure ulcers from developing. A pillow placed crosswise to elevate the lower legs or heel guards may be applied. (In many instances, the patient will already be wearing elastic stockings and air boots.)

Side-Lying Position

An unconscious patient, or one with a diminished or absent swallowing or gag reflex, is not positioned supine because of the possible aspiration of secretions or occlusion of the airway by the tongue. Therefore, positioning in the true supine position is reserved only for the conscious patient. The side-lying position with the head of the bed elevated 10 to 30 degrees facilitates drainage of secretions from the mouth. The head should be placed in a neutral position. A soft collar or towel roll is useful to maintain the neutral position and prevent hyperflexion, which can partially obstruct the airway and impede venous drainage from the brain. Proper body alignment is maintained through the use of pillows and positioners. With a patient on long-term bed rest, a modified position halfway between the supine and side-lying position may be necessary to relieve pressure on body surfaces. This patient can be positioned in good body alignment with the head turned slightly to facilitate drainage of oral secretions and to maintain a patent airway.

Exercise Programs

Voluntary muscles will lose tone and strength if they are not used. Patients with neurological deficits involving paresis and paralysis and those confined to prolonged bed rest are subject to these deleterious muscle effects of immobility (Table 11-2). Because the flexor and adductor muscles are stronger than the extensors and abductors, contractures of the flexor and adductor muscles will develop quickly if preventive measures are not instituted. An exercise program is followed aggressively to maintain muscle tone and function, prevent additional disability, and aid in the restoration of motor function.

Range-of-motion (ROM) exercises include the full range of movement that each joint of the body can *normally* perform. A patient who cannot carry out independent ROM exercises is assisted in these activities by the nurse. After radiographic studies rule out fractures and the presence of other medical problems or medical treatments or contraindications are verified, ROM exercises begin. Exercises can be classified into the following categories:

- **Passive:** ROM is provided to a body joint by another person or outside force.
- **Active:** voluntary ROM to a body joint is independently executed by the individual.
- **Active assistive:** ROM to a body joint is accomplished by the patient with the assistance of another person.

TABLE 11–2	**EFFECTS OF IMMOBILIZATION ON THE MUSCULOSKELETAL SYSTEM**	
STRUCTURE	**INITIAL CHANGES**	**ADVANCED CHANGES**
Bones	• Skeletal malalignment • Decreased bone mineral density	• Skeletal deformities • Generalized osteoporosis • Fractures
Joints	• Joint stiffness • Changes in periarticular and cartilaginous joint structure • Fibrotic changes of ligaments and tendons • Shortening or stretching of ligaments • Decreased range of motion	• Ankylosis • Contractures • Osteoarthritis
Muscles	• Decreased muscle mass • Decreased muscle strength* • Muscle shortening	• Muscle atrophy

*Decreased muscle strength by 2%–5% per day or 10%–15% per week (Hamilton, L., & Lyon, P. S. [1995]. A nursing driven program to preserve and restore functional ability in hospitalized elderly patients. *Journal of Nursing Administration, 25*[4], 30–37.)

Decline in muscle mass and strength linked to falls, functional decline, increased frailty, and immobility (Gillis, A., & MacDonald, B. [2005]. Prevent deconditioning in the hospitalized elderly. *Canadian Nurse, 101*[6], 16–20.)

- **Active resistive:** ROM is voluntarily provided to a body joint against resistance.
- **Isometric or muscle setting:** exercises are accomplished by alternately tightening and relaxing the muscle without joint movement.

The exercise program prescribed depends on the stage of illness and the particular disabilities. In the acute stages of illness, a physical therapist (PT) comes to the bedside once or twice daily to administer specific exercises. If only ROM exercises are prescribed, nurses will be the care provider administering these exercises. After the patient's condition improves, he or she is taken to the physical medicine department where equipment is available for a more sophisticated, aggressive rehabilitation program. The nurse can reinforce and integrate the skills gained into other aspects of care. In addition, the patient's family is taught how to carry out the prescribed exercises.

Passive Range-of-Motion Exercises

When passive ROM exercises are administered, two factors are considered: the joint being exercised and the placement of the caregiver's hands when administering the exercise properly. One hand is placed above the joint to provide support against gravity and any unwanted movement. The other hand gently moves the joint through its normal ROM.

Passive ROM exercises are usually administered at least four times daily and may be incorporated, in part, with other procedures, such as bathing or repositioning.

- Choose a time when the patient is rested, comfortable, and pain free to gain cooperation.
- Explain the procedure, even if the patient is apparently unconscious.

- Position in proper body alignment, and drape, as necessary, to avoid undue exposure. Drawing the curtains offers privacy and excludes environmental stimuli in the instance of an easily distracted patient.
- Provide a comfortable room temperature to prevent chilling, shivering, and unwanted muscle contractions.
- Maintain good posture to ensure efficient body movement; face the patient to observe facial reaction to the exercises.
- Movements are slow, smooth, and rhythmical.
- Move the body part to the point of resistance and stop.
- Move the body part to the point of pain and stop.
- If the patient becomes excessively fatigued, discontinue the exercises.

Although the PT may move a body part beyond the point of pain or resistance for selected patients, this is not within the scope of nursing practice and is avoided unless specifically prescribed. As the patient's condition improves, self-care is encouraged for as many activities as possible. Because return of motor function is a slow process, the patient is encouraged to carry out the exercises and be reminded of the need to continue with these activities as part of the rehabilitation program.

Other Exercises

Specific exercises, such as lifting hand weights, may be ordered to strengthen a weakened arm. Encourage the patient to engage in these activities. Be sure that the necessary equipment is present. Adapt activities to provide movement for specific muscle groups. For example, providing a ball of yarn for a female patient who enjoys knitting can improve motor function of a weakened hand while providing sensory stimulation.

Balancing and Sitting Activities

After the patient's condition has stabilized and ROM exercises have begun, the next skills to acquire are balancing and sitting. Deconditioning develops rapidly. Patients who have been confined to bed for a long time will progress slowly. The head of the bed is raised gradually over a period of days to overcome orthostatic hypotension. Monitor the physiologic response by assessing the blood pressure, pulse, and skin color and asking the patient whether he or she is experiencing dizziness or lightheadedness. Record baseline signs and symptoms. After the head of the bed is raised the prescribed number of degrees, again assess for a drop in blood pressure; a thready, rapid pulse; paleness; diaphoresis; dizziness; or lightheadedness. If these signs quickly reverse, no action is necessary. Sustained symptoms require lowering the head of the bed slightly until symptoms subside. Although many neurological patients are placed at a 30-degree angle while confined to bed, they will still need a period of adaption to tolerate the vertical position. For those maintained in a flat position or at a 10-degree angle, the adjustment will take longer.

For paraplegic or quadriplegic patients, orthostatic hypotension can be a stubborn problem to manage, because extensive vasomotor paralysis results in a subsequent drop in blood pressure when the vertical position is assumed.

Wearing an abdominal binder or thigh-high elastic stockings and elevating the leg rests of the wheelchair help to combat hypotension. These patients, particularly quadriplegics, may require a special PT program in which a tilt table is used to raise the patient gradually over several days.

Balancing. Balancing, the ability to sit or stand erect, is achieved through consciously using both sides of the body, focusing on the symmetric midline point, and using support devices that help to steady the center of gravity. Use of a back or neck brace for a spinal cord injury patient can make the difference between success and failure. The hemiplegic patient is placed in the sitting position and instructed to support himself or herself with the unaffected arm and hand. The hand is placed flat on the bed slightly behind or at the side as a means of support. Because there is a tendency to slouch to the affected side, the patient is reminded to sit straight and erect, focused on a balanced midline. Some conscious patients who have difficulty balancing while sitting in bed do well when they are helped to sit at the side of the bed or in a chair with their feet flat on the floor.

In unconscious patients, the same process for overcoming orthostatic hypotension is used; however, information regarding the adjustment of these patients is derived from objective signs. Ability to balance is not possible until the level of consciousness improves; however, the patient can be propped to the required position. Conditioning reflexes can be maintained by simply sitting in a chair for 1 to 2 hours.[7]

After balance in the sitting position has been mastered, the patient is ready to begin balancing in the standing position at the bedside.

Sitting. Both conscious and unconscious patients can sit in a chair, although the unconscious patient is not positioned in the sitting position on the side of the bed for obvious safety concerns. The conscious patient may sit on the side of the bed, using the overbed table and pillows for support. The chair selected should provide firm support and have a high back and arms, especially if the patient has motor weakness or paralysis. For the weak, debilitated patient who cannot hold up the head or neck, a high-back chair that extends to the top of the head is most effective. Some patients have a neck brace; apply it for sitting.

A lapboard, pillows, and the overbed table, rolled down to a comfortable height, are helpful for providing added support while positioning a patient in a chair. Pillows or rolls support the arms in the desired position. The feet are positioned flat on the floor. The pressure on the bottom of the feet assists in stretching the heel cord. Foot-drop may develop if stretching of the heel cord is not provided. The head is positioned carefully so that the airway or tracheostomy (if present) is not obstructed. Any equipment that is in place, such as a urinary catheter or feeding tube, is checked to ensure patency and freedom from traction.

If the patient has some intact motor function, necessary equipment is placed nearby, possibly on an overbed table that has been lowered and placed in front of the patient's chair. The call bell is accessible to the patient. Observe the patient to monitor tolerance of the activity. Don't allow the patient to become overtired. It is best to plan a schedule that allows for periods of bed rest and out-of-bed activity based on an individual patient's tolerance and fatigue.

Mobility: Transfer and Ambulation

When considering a patient's mobility, the type(s) of transfer used reflect(s) a continuum from complete dependency to complete independence. For a completely dependent patient two options are possible:

- Two-person lift: physical transfer by at least two nursing staff members; no active patient participation
- Mechanical lift: transfer using a lifting device that is operated by nursing staff members; no active patient participation

After the patient is able to balance and sit, he or she is ready for transfer activities:

- The patient, with assistance from one or more nursing staff members, stands and pivots on the unaffected leg; moderate patient participation is required. A transfer belt is worn around the patient's waist to allow the nurse to grasp it to support the patient. Inspect the transfer belt to be sure it is not worn or defective.
- With the assistance of a slide board, the patient is able to transfer from the bed to the chair with or without assistance.
- Independent transfer is the patient's ability to transfer without assistance.

The degree of assistance necessary for transfer and ambulating is classified as follows:

- Dependent: maximal, moderate, or minimal
- Contact guard: provision of verbal cues and minimal physical support during the activity, such as holding the arm or waist during ambulation
- Supervision: provision of verbal cues only, as necessary

Transfer Activities

Keep in mind a few basic principles for assisting patients:

- As a rule, transfer toward the unaffected side.
- Patients should wear properly fitted, flat shoes rather than slippers, because most slippers offer little support or traction on the floor.
- If a paretic arm is in need of support, support it by gently holding the forearm. Never tug on the paretic arm by pulling on the upper arm or shoulder.
- If balance is unsteady, stand on the affected side, ready to grasp the belt around the patient's waist (can grasp the top of pants or pajama bottoms, but this is not as secure).
- If the patient's knees buckle and additional assistance is required, stand in front of the patient and push with your knee against the patient's unaffected knee to lock the knee in position and prevent buckling. This action enables the patient to bear some of his or her own body weight.
- A walker or four-point cane may be used for support.
- The patient learns to stand erect before ambulation training can begin. If difficulty is encountered in raising the affected foot, a special shoe with a foot brace may be helpful.
- Other transfer activities that may need to be learned, depending on the permanence of the disability, include transferring from the wheelchair to the toilet, bathtub, or automobile.

Transfer Activity: From Lying in Bed to a Sitting Position

Hemiplegic Patients. For the hemiplegic patient who wants to assume a sitting position from a back lying position in bed (Fig. 11-2), these steps are followed:

- Move toward or roll onto the side of the bed on which you intend to sit.
- Slip the unaffected leg under the affected leg at an angle so that the unaffected leg becomes a transfer cradle for the affected limb.
- Place the affected arm on the abdomen or lap.
- Push off the mattress with the unaffected elbow, raising your upper body, while turning your hips toward the side of the bed on which you intend to sit.
- Swing the unaffected leg (on which the affected leg rests) over the side of the bed, and use the unaffected hand to push up.
- Once in the sitting position, lean on the unaffected hand to maintain an erect position.

Paraplegic or Incomplete Quadriplegic Patients. Most transfer activities for quadriplegic and some incomplete quadriplegic patients require direct assistance from facility personnel. A trapeze over the bed and a sliding board can be used to assist paraplegic patients and some quadriparetic patients.

Transfer Activity: From Sitting on the Side of the Bed to a Back-Lying Position

Returning to the back-lying position from a sitting position on the side of the bed involves the following steps (Fig. 11-3):

- Sit slightly above the center on the side of the bed so that you will be in the proper position on the mattress once the back-lying position is assumed.
- Place the affected arm on your lap.
- Slip the unaffected foot under the affected ankle.
- Place the unaffected hand on the edge of the mattress next to the unaffected hip.

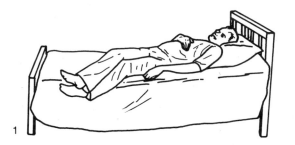

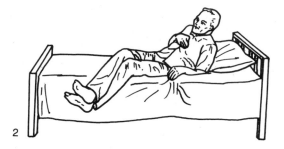

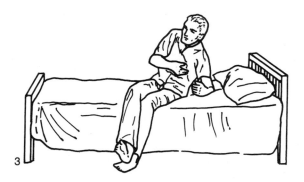

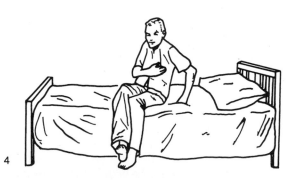

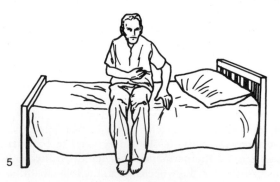

Figure 11-2 • Getting up and sitting on side of the bed. *Clockwise:* (1) Use strong hand to place weak arm across abdomen. Slide strong foot under weak ankle; move both legs to side of the bed on strong side and over side. (2) Grasp edge of mattress as illustrated and push with elbow and forearm against the bed. (3) Come to a half-sitting position, supporting body weight on strong forearm. (4) Move hand to the rear, pushing up to a full sitting position. (5) Move around until sitting securely on side of bed; uncross legs. (*Up and Around.* Reprinted with permission of the American Heart Association.)

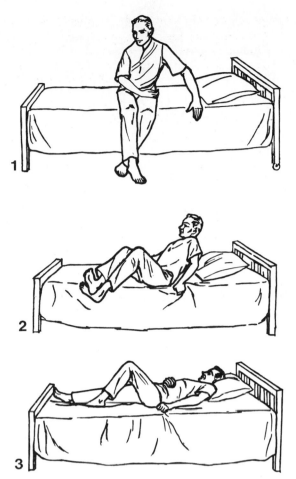

Figure 11-3 • Moving from a sitting position on edge of bed to a back-lying position. (*1*) Place weak arm across the lap. Slide strong foot under weak ankle. (*2*) With strong hand, grasp edge of mattress near the hips and press against bed, lowering body to the bed as the elbow bends. At the same time, swing legs onto bed. (Note: Patient should be seated in the proper spot so that head will be on pillow after lying down.) (*3*) Uncross legs. Bend the strong hip and knee and push against bed with heel to move body up or down in bed to proper position. (*Up and Around*. Reprinted with permission of the American Heart Association)

- Press the hand into the mattress, lowering your body onto the bed while the elbow bends.
- Simultaneously swing the unaffected leg onto the bed as your body is lowered.
- Uncross the ankle and bend the unaffected knee; push up or pull down on the bed, as necessary, with the bending and pulling action of the knee to position yourself comfortably.

Transfer Activity: From a Sitting Position on the Bed to a Chair

Transferring from the bed into a chair requires planning. If a chair is used, it should provide firm support and have arms. In the case of a wheelchair, the wheels of the chair are locked with the footrests up.

Hemiplegic Patients. Hemiplegic patients may complete this type of transfer by following these steps (Fig. 11-4):

- Free any catheter or other tubes that are secured to the bed.
- Place the chair at a slight angle as close as possible to the bed on the unaffected side.
- With feet close together, lean forward slightly, put the unaffected hand on the mattress edge, and push off to a standing position, bearing weight on the unaffected side.
- Once balance has been maintained and is steady enough for momentary release of support, move the strong hand to the farthest armrest of the chair.
- Keep the body weight well forward; pivot on the unaffected foot, and slowly lower to a sitting position.

Paraplegic or Incomplete Quadriplegic Patients. The paraplegic or quadriplegic patient will need a dependent transfer with slide board, which provides less strain on the back than a lift into the chair; the aid of two or three people may be needed, depending on the patient's height and weight. Some paraplegic patients can learn to transfer themselves from the bed to a chair with the use of a slide board.

Transfer Activity: From Chair to Bed

When transferring from a chair to a sitting position on the bed, the following technique is used (Fig. 11-5):

- The chair is at a slight angle, as close to the bed as possible; the patient's unaffected side is closest to the bed.
- Place feet firmly on the floor close to the chair, with the unaffected heel slightly in back of the affected heel and directly under the edge of the seat.
- Move forward in the chair, placing the unaffected hand on the front portion of the arm of the chair.
- Lean forward over the unaffected leg; push off to a standing position so that the feet are slightly apart with most of the weight being borne by the unaffected leg.
- After regaining balance with the support of the armrest, lean slightly forward, reach for the edge of the mattress with the unaffected hand, and pivot on the unaffected foot, slowly lowering to a sitting position.

Ambulation

Hemiplegic Patients. Before hemiplegic patients can ambulate, they must first learn to stand and balance in an upright position. Standing exercises can begin at the bedside and proceed to the parallel bars in the physical medicine department. Standing helps to reinforce a positive body image and feeling of wholeness and also improves overall physical fitness.

Once standing has been mastered, an evaluation is conducted to determine whether any special bracing or support equipment is necessary. If the patient is developing foot-drop or has a tendency to drag the foot, a short plastic leg brace or a brace with a spring is helpful. These types of braces are designed to prevent extreme plantarflexion. If the patient is weak, a crutch, four-point cane, or walker may be necessary (Fig. 11-6). A sling may be applied to the affected arm for balance while walking. The sling is adjusted to approximate the glenoid (shoulder) joint space. Do not pull the affected arm.

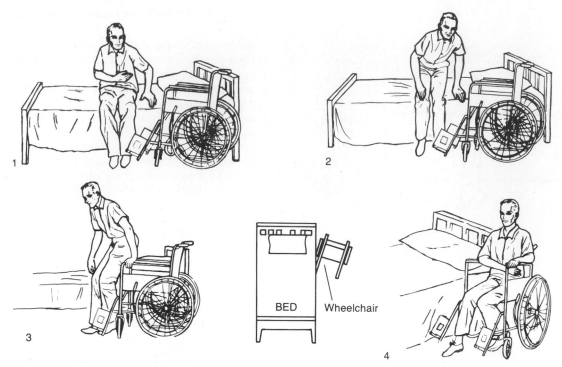

Figure 11-4 • Transfer from bed to wheelchair. *Clockwise:* (1) Place wheelchair at 45-degree angle to bed on patient's stronger side; lock brakes and raise footrest; move to the edge of bed. (2) Push down on bed with stronger arm; push off bed and stand, keeping weight on the stronger leg. (3) Move stronger arm and leg to opposite side of wheelchair. (4) Lean forward and sit down while holding on to wheelchair arm. (*Up and Around.* Reprinted with permission of the American Heart Association.)

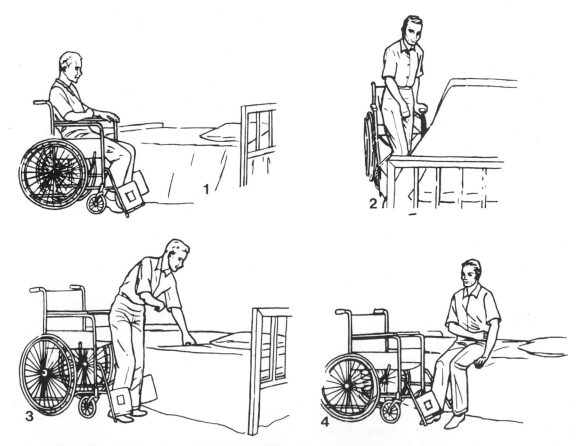

Figure 11-5 • Transfer from wheelchair to bed. *Clockwise:* (1) Place wheelchair at 45-degree angle to the bed on the patient's stronger side; lock brakes and raise footrest; move to edge of chair. (2) Grasp chair arm with stronger arm and push off the chair to a standing position bearing weight on stronger leg. (3) Move strong hand to edge of bed for support. (4) Lean forward, pivot on stronger foot, and slowly sit down. (*Up and Around.* Reprinted with permission of the American Heart Association).

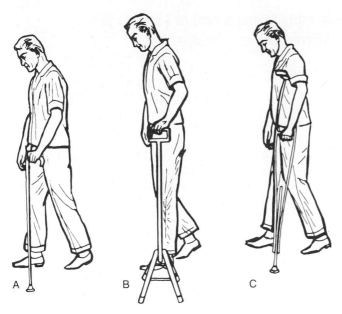

Figure 11-6 • Assistive devices, such as a cane (*A*), a wide-base cane (*B*), or crutches (*C*), may be necessary for ambulation. (*Up and Around.* Reprinted with permission of the American Heart Association.)

Ambulation or gait training often begins at the parallel bars, where the patient learns to bend a knee and then extend it again. This exercise is alternated from one knee to the other. If the affected knee continues to be weak and tends to buckle, a longer leg brace can be designed to compensate for this disability.

When helping the patient to ambulate, the nurse walks on the patient's affected side. Added support is given by grasping the patient's belt or the top of the patient's pants or by applying a safety belt. The patient may feel more secure walking near the wall with the unaffected side nearest the wall. A handrail in the corridor or room is another source of support and security. In the physical medicine department, climbing and descending stairs are taught.

For the patient who is unable to master ambulation, wheelchair mobility may be achieved using the unaffected hand to propel the wheelchair on a level surface. This provides a degree of independence. An electric (i.e., battery-operated) wheelchair is another alternative for providing mobility.

It is impossible to state the exact intervals at which balancing, sitting, standing, and walking are introduced and mastered. Age, severity of illness, other neurological deficits, chronic conditions, endurance, and complications are all factors. Attitude and motivation are important factors in the rehabilitation process. Frequent assessment allows systematic evaluation of the patient's needs so that rehabilitation can progress steadily toward the greatest level of independence.

Paraplegic or Incomplete Quadriplegic Patients. The physiologic and psychological benefits of ambulation need to be considered. Research has contributed greatly to ambulation options for spinal injured people. Some paraplegic and a few quadriparetic patients can walk with the help of braces and canes. For others, ambulation is possible using functional electrical stimulation and a walker.

For a person who needs a wheelchair, the many different types available need to be matched to the needs of the particular patient. Battery-operated wheelchairs that are activated by a breath sensor located near the mouth of the quadriplegic patient provide a degree of independence. Even a quadriplegic patient with an injury at C-5 can use this type of wheelchair. Incomplete quadriplegics with a C-2 to C-5 injury can use chin, eye, or tongue control systems. The paraplegic patient does well in a standard wheelchair or an electric wheelchair operated by hand controls. Wheelchair users can have different chairs for different activities, such as a sports wheelchair for quad rugby, basketball, and others. There is increased awareness of the need to monitor shoulder function in wheelchair users, because shoulder problems increase with age.

Computer-operated equipment programmed to execute many mundane activities, such as closing draperies or turning out lights, has afforded a greater degree of independence to the disabled person. Computer technology for adaptive living is developing rapidly. As the technology improves, the cost decreases, making the equipment more accessible for the patient.

MANAGEMENT OF THE SKIN

The neuroscience patient is at high risk for the development of pressure ulcers because of motor, sensory, and vasomotor deficits related to neurological disease and immobility. According to the AHCPR clinical practice guideline, *Pressure Ulcers in Adults: Prediction and Prevention* (1992),[8] a **pressure ulcer** is any lesion caused by unrelieved pressure resulting in damage of underlying tissue. Many evidence-based practice protocols and guidelines related to pressure ulcers are found at www.guidline.gov.

Nursing Management of the Patient With Altered Skin Integrity

Assessment and Intervention

Pressure ulcers usually develop over bony prominences and are graded or staged to classify the degree of tissue damage observed. **Impaired Skin Integrity** related to immobility or the effects of pressure, friction, shearing, or maceration is the recognized patient problem. The AHCPR *Pressure Ulcers Guideline* (1992)[8] is the foundation on which the standard of practice for prediction, prevention, and early treatment of pressure ulcers rests. This publication set the standard of evidence-based practice. Numerous research-based publications are available to address pressure ulcer prevention and management standards. Health care facilities have identified the guidelines and protocols that they follow to address this problem. Occurrence of pressure ulcers is a common quality indicator used by many benchmarking initiatives.

SENSORY-PERCEPTUAL DEFICITS

Perception is a complex intellectual process of recognizing, interpreting, and integrating sensory stimuli into meaningful information from the internal and external environments. Whereas the left side of the brain is dominant for language, the right side of the brain is dominant for perception of two- and three-dimensional shapes, faces, color, spatial positions, and orientation in space. The parietal lobe is particularly important in perception. Perceptual deficits are often seen in patients with cerebral trauma and stroke and may take many forms, including deficits in perception of self, body image, illness, spatial relationships, agnosia, and apraxia.

Nursing Management of Patients With Perceptual Deficits

Assessment

The major perceptual deficits are summarized in Table 11-3. Several patient problems and nursing diagnoses are applicable; the following are common patient problems that require input from a variety of health team members:

- Sensory/Perceptual Alterations
- Body Image Disturbance
- Impaired Environmental Interpretation Syndrome
- Impaired Memory
- Self-Esteem Disturbance
- Risk for Injury
- Confusion
- Personal Identity Disturbance
- Neglect Syndrome
- Cognitive Deficits

Interventions

Nursing interventions are directed at helping the patient to compensate for any deficits. Patients with perceptual deficits are often impulsive and lack awareness of their deficits. This behavior also places a patient at higher risk for injury.

▨ COMMUNICATION DEFICITS

Aphasia is the loss of ability to use language and to communicate thoughts verbally or in writing.[9] It results from injury to the cortex of the left hemisphere in the posterior frontal or anterior temporal lobes. Aphasia can be subdivided into nonfluent and fluent aphasia. The nursing diagnosis for a patient with aphasia is **Impaired Verbal Communication**. Chart 11-3 summarizes aphasia and the nursing guidelines for working with affected patients. See Chapters 4 and 7 for further discussion of aphasia.

Generally, the greatest degree of spontaneous functional return occurs in the first 3 to 6 months following injury, although substantial deficits may persist. Additional improvement can occur for 2 or 3 more years. Each patient must be viewed as an individual in the rehabilitative process. Age, area of injury, presence of other health problems, and motivation are a few factors having a direct bearing on recovery.

Nursing Management of Patients With Altered Communication

Assessment

The nurse will need to assess the patient's communication system to determine which skills are intact or deficient. Assess the following abilities:

- Speaking in response to an open-ended question, such as "tell me about your hobbies"
- Using vocabulary, grammar, and syntax correctly; note spontaneity, hesitancy in pronunciation, and speed of speech
- Responding appropriately to verbal instructions that are one to three steps in complexity
- Responding appropriately to written instructions that are one to three steps in complexity
- Expressing ideas in writing; writing a response to such requests as "write your name" or "describe this room"

Note difficulty in expressing thoughts verbally, finding the correct word (word finding), forming words or sentences, following written instructions, and expressing ideas in writing. Other abnormal findings include slurring of speech. As a result of stroke, some patients may be unable to speak the primary language and may revert to a language spoken in the past. Several factors associated with neurological illness can mask an accurate assessment of communication skills, such as altered level of consciousness, decreased visual acuity, hearing loss, dysarthria, cognitive deficits (decreased attention or concentration), short-term memory deficits, visual field cuts (hemianopsia), absence of prescription eyeglasses, absence of hearing aid normally worn, and unfamiliarity with the language.

A short attention span or inability to concentrate influences the ability to follow verbal or nonverbal cues. Because concentration and attention seem to vary from day to day or even minute to minute, there can be vacillation in the patient's ability to communicate at any time.

The following are possible patient problems and nursing diagnoses:

- Sensory/Perceptual Alterations
- Impaired Verbal Communication
- Impaired Memory
- Collaborative Problems include cognitive deficits, aphasia, and neglect syndrome

Interventions

To work effectively with the patient, the nurse should assume a calm, reassuring, and supportive manner that conveys acceptance of the patient's behavior. Spending time and assuming an unhurried approach reinforce this message. Guidelines for working with the aphasic patient are included in Chart 11-3. Deficits in the ability to communicate are devastating and frustrating to the patient, and may result in fear and depression.

TABLE 11–3 SUMMARY OF MAJOR PERCEPTUAL DEFICITS AND NURSING MANAGEMENT

DEFICIT	ASSESSMENT	INTERVENTION
Perception of Illness		
• Denial of hemiplegia or other motor or sensory deficits • *Anosognosia*—inability to recognize, denial of, or unawareness of a loss of or defect in physical function	• Fails to use the involved side of the body without being reminded to do so • Shows a lack of concern about the disability and fails to understand how paralysis and other deficits will affect lifestyle • Lacks awareness or denies outright the presence of paralysis or other deficits on the involved side • May deny all sensory input on the affected side	• Accept the patient's perception of self, and provide for the safety and cleanliness of the area. • Provide tactile stimuli to the affected side by touching or stroking the affected side by itself, rather than stimulating both sides simultaneously. • Teach the patient to position the affected extremity carefully and to check its position by looking at it; if the patient completely ignores the area, use positioning to improve his or her perception (e.g., position the patient facing the affected side so that the area is in view).
Body Image		

• *Body image*—concept one has of the sum of one's body parts in relationship to the whole
  • Nursing diagnosis: Body Image Disturbance
• *Unilateral neglect*—a condition in which the patient ignores the hemiplegic side
  • Nursing diagnosis: Unilateral Neglect
	• If asked to draw a clock, will not draw the side of the clock on same side as that on which neglect is present	• Encourage the patient to handle the affected side.
		* Teach visual scanning of the environment to overcome one-sided neglect.
		* Approach the patient from the unaffected side until ready to learn compensatory scanning techniques.
		* Place the food tray toward the unaffected side.
		* Use verbal cues to guide the patient toward the affected side.
		* Provide a mirror, if possible.
		* Position the call light and other equipment on the patient's unaffected side.

Spatial Relationships		

• *Hemianopia*—loss of vision in half of the visual field
  • Nursing diagnosis: Sensory/Perceptual Alterations
 	
• Defects in:
  • Localized objects in space
  • Estimating size
  • Judging distances
  • Remembering arrangement of objects in the environment
  • Finding way to places or back to room
  • Telling time
  • Right-left discrimination
	• Neglects input from the affected side
	
	• Has difficulty walking through a doorway
	• Exhibits impaired recall of the placement of objects in a familiar environment, such as the locations of windows and doors in the room
	• Has difficulty learning the way around the hospital unit (such as how to go from the hospital room to the kitchen and back)
	• Experiences difficulty reading and computing figures because of an inability to move eyes from left to right on a page or to line up numbers accurately to compute figures
	• Is unable to identify left or right
		• See last six interventions listed above (with asterisks).
		• *Note* visual changes commonly present that change about every 6 mo. No ophthalmological check-up is necessary until 6 mo have transpired.
		• Provide verbal cues.
		• Do not allow the patient to wander around the unit alone.
		• Use descriptive terms to identify areas, rather than "left" or "right" directions (e.g., "Lift the unaffected leg" but not "good/bad").
		• Use a mirror to help patients adjust position if they have difficulty maintaining their position.

Agnosia		

• Inability to recognize familiar environmental objects through the senses
  • Visual agnosia: inability to recognize familiar objects by sight (Nursing diagnosis: Sensory/Perceptual Alterations)
  • Auditory agnosia: inability to recognize familiar objects through sound (Nursing diagnosis: Sensory/Perceptual Alterations)
  • Tactile agnosia (astereognosis): inability to recognize familiar objects through the sense of touch (Nursing diagnosis: Sensory/Perceptual Alterations)
	• Ask patient to identify common objects by sight
	• Observe the patient's response to common sounds, such as a ringing telephone
	• With the patient's eye closed, place a common object in his or her hand, and ask the patient to identify the object
		• Use other, intact senses to identify environmental stimuli (e.g., if the patient has visual agnosia, have him or her use voices and sounds to identify familiar objects).
		• Use the drill method of teaching to help the patient relearn objects that cannot be identified.
		• Protect the patient from injury.
		• Interpret the patient's behavior for the family.

Apraxia		

• Inability to carry out a learned, voluntary act in the absence of paralysis
  • Constructional apraxia (Nursing diagnosis: Self-Care Deficit)
  • Dressing apraxia (Nursing diagnosis: Dressing Self-Care Deficit)
	• May exhibit clumsiness or an inability to carry out ADLs correctly; may be unable to sequence components of a skilled act
	• May have difficulty completing the task of drawing a clock and placing the hands at a given time
	• May have difficulty dressing self (e.g., may put both arms in the same sleeve)
		• Encourage patient to participate in ADLs.
		• Correct any misuse of equipment or incorrect actions; guide the patient's hand, if necessary.
		• Reteach any forgotten skills.
		• Protect the patient from injury.
		• Interpret the patient's behavior for the family.

ADLs, activities of daily living.

CHART 11-3 Communication Deficits: Descriptions and Nursing Guidelines

NONFLUENT APHASIA (BROCA'S APHASIA)

- The patient will have difficulty expressing thoughts verbally or in writing.
- The degree of difficulty can range from mild word finding difficulty to limitation of expression to "yes" and "no."
- The ability to understand the written and spoken word remains intact.
- The site of injury is Broca's area (in the frontal lobe close to the area of the motor cortex that controls the movement of the lips, jaw, tongue, soft palate, and vocal cords).
- Broca's area contains the memory for motor patterns of speech.

FLUENT APHASIA (WERNICKE'S APHASIA)

- Wernicke's area (in the temporal lobe flanked by Heschl's gyrus on one side and the angular gyrus on the other) is the site of injury.
- Heschl's gyrus is the primary receptor area for auditory and visual fields.
- Wernicke's area provides the connective pathways that bridge the primary auditory cortex and the angular gyrus.
- The patient hears the sounds of speech, but the parts of the brain that give meaning to the sounds of speech are not activated, so that comprehension of speech is impaired.
- Because the control of the musculature for speech is not impaired, the patient can speak but makes many errors when using words.
- Because patients are unaware of their imperfect messages, they may talk at great length.
- The patient's ability to express words in writing may also be compromised.

GLOBAL APHASIA

- Global aphasia results from a massive stroke or lesion involving Broca's and Wernicke's areas of the brain.
- Global aphasia is a combination of expressive and receptive aphasia whereby the patient is left with little, if any, intact communication system.
- Affected patients can neither understand what they hear or read nor convey their thoughts in speech or writing.
- Prognosis is poor.

MILD NONFLUENT APHASIA

- Stimulate conversation and ask open-ended questions.
- Allow patients time to search for the words to express themselves.
- Disregard choice of incorrect words.
- Be supportive and accepting of the patient's behavior as he or she deals with the frustration of finding the right words of expression.
- Assure patients that their speech will gradually improve with time.

SEVERE NONFLUENT APHASIA

- Accept self-expression by whatever means possible (e.g., pantomime, pointing).
- Do not pressure the patient into self-expression.
- Be supportive of patients, and accept their behavior if they show frustration (by crying or some other means) because of difficulty encountered in expressing themselves.
- Provide a loose-leaf notebook with pictures of common objects so that the patient can point to the picture when unable to say the word.
- Tell the patient that speech skills can be relearned, given time.
- Anticipate the patient's needs.

MILD FLUENT APHASIA

- Stand close to patients (within their line of vision) so that they can also observe lip movements as an added cue to communication.
- Speak slowly and distinctly, using simple sentences and a common vocabulary.
- Use simple gestures as an added cue in speaking.
- Repeat or rephrase any instructions if they are not understood.
- Speak in a normal speaking voice.

SEVERE FLUENT APHASIA

- Use whatever vocabulary the patient can still understand.
- Use very simple sentences or phrases that express only the critical essence of a thought.
- Divide any tasks into small units, working with the individual units to accomplish the task.
- Use pantomime, pointing, touch, and so forth to express ideas.
- Anticipate the patient's needs.

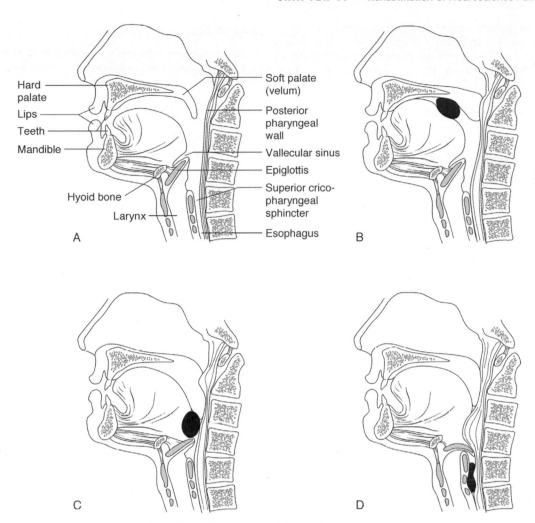

Figure 11-7 • Components of the swallowing process.

SWALLOWING DEFICITS

Swallowing is a complex process of ingesting solid or liquid food while protecting the airway (Fig. 11-7). There are four phases of swallowing:

- **Oral preparatory phase:** food is taken into the mouth and chewed, forming a bolus.
- **Oral phase:** the bolus of food is centered and moved to the posterior oropharynx.
- **Pharyngeal phase:** the swallowing reflex carries the bolus through the pharynx.
- **Esophageal phase:** peristalsis carries the bolus to the stomach.

Several cranial nerves are involved in functions related to swallowing (Table 11-4).

Regardless of whether the food is liquid or solid, protection of the airway is imperative to prevent the most serious of complications—aspiration. Aspiration is serious because it causes a chemical pneumonia. When thinking about aspiration, a picture of someone coughing vigorously comes to mind. This is the case if the gag and cough reflexes are intact. However, there is much discussion about "silent aspiration." A person with diminished or absent gag and cough reflexes can aspirate material without the usual evidence of coughing. In a conscious patient, a moist, wet voice may be noted. Usual

TABLE 11-4   CRANIAL NERVES INVOLVED IN SWALLOWING

CRANIAL NERVE (NUMBER)	MOTOR INNERVATION	SENSORY INNERVATION
Trigeminal (V)	Mandibular muscles for chewing and mastication	Two sensory areas of face (maxillary, mandibular)
Facial (VII)	Facial expression, including movement of lips; submandibular and sublingual salivary glands	Taste to anterior two thirds of tongue
Glossopharyngeal (IX)	Stylopharyngeus muscle to pull up pharynx	Pharynx, tongue, and taste receptors of posterior one third of tongue
Vagus (X)	Muscles of soft palate, pharynx, and larynx	Pharynx and larynx
Spinal accessory (XI)	Sternocleidomastoid and trapezius to hold head up and rotate head	None
Hypoglossal (XII)	Intrinsic muscle of tongue to move tongue	None

symptoms of aspiration are absent. Silent aspiration may first be evident by an elevated temperature or adventitious lung sounds followed by a diagnosis of pneumonia by chest film.

With neurological disease, there can be deficits in the mechanisms controlling swallowing, and aspiration can result. The patient problems associated with swallowing deficits are **Impaired Swallowing** and **Risk for Aspiration**. Aspiration can lead to aspiration pneumonia.

Nursing Management of the Patient With Impaired Swallowing

Assessment

Swallowing is a complex process (see Fig. 11-7 for normal swallowing). The defining characteristics for impaired swallowing are also related to the specific phases of swallowing listed previously (Table 11-5).

Before offering any food or drink orally, the gag and swallowing reflexes are assessed. The gag reflex on each side should be assessed, because an asymmetric response is possible. The examiner can assess the swallowing reflex by placing his or her index finger on the top of the larynx and asking the patient to swallow. If the reflex is intact, the larynx will elevate (the epiglottis closes over the trachea), displacing the examiner's finger. If the gag or swallowing reflex is not intact, *nothing should be given orally* because the patient cannot protect the airway and will aspirate. Diagnostic tests may be ordered to identify the specific etiology of the dysphasia. Common diagnostic tests include the bedside swallow examination, modified barium swallow with video fluoroscopy, and video endoscopy. A review of the video film will help to identify the specific portion of the sequence of swallowing that is problematic.[10]

TABLE 11–5   PHASES OF SWALLOWING

PHASES OF SWALLOWING	CHARACTERISTIC OBSERVATIONS; ALSO OBSERVE FOR EVIDENCE OF ASPIRATION
Oral phase	Drooling or loss of food particles on affected side or chin Pocketing of food Excessive chewing Facial asymmetry or weakness Tongue weakness or limitation of movement Inability to close lips tightly or move lips Weakness or absence of gag reflex Weakness or absence of swallowing reflex Nasal drainage due to nasal regurgitation Loss of internal or external sensation of the oral cavity or face
Pharyngeal phase	Noted delayed or absence of swallowing Coughing while drinking fluids or eating liquids (e.g., soup) History of aspiration pneumonia Wet, gurgling, moist, or nasal voice, particularly during eating Frequent clearing of throat Complaints of burning (from drugs or other irritating material sticking and irritating tissue) or something sticking in back of throat
Esophageal phase	Burping or substernal distress due to esophageal reflux Coughing or wheezing

Interventions

Supervise the patient during mealtime and snack time. There are some general interventions to facilitate swallowing. Specific suggestions, based on specific patient needs, may also be made. Consider these general points:

- Feed or eat in the upright, sitting position at a 90-degree angle; avoid slumping.
- Tilt the head forward and tuck the chin in to prevent food from moving into the posterior oropharynx before it has been chewed; if the patient is unable to maintain head position, the nurse can support the head with the palm of the hand against the forehead.
- Encourage taking small bites and thorough chewing.
- For patients with hemiplegia or hemiparesis, place food on the unaffected side.
- The nurse notes consistency of food that is troublesome. (Some people have more difficulty with solid foods, and others will have more difficulty with liquids.)
- If "pocketing" of food is a problem, have the patient sweep the mouth with his or her finger after each bite to clear the food.
- The speech therapist can be helpful by suggesting an adaptive cup and special techniques to ensure swallowing.
- Discuss with the physician any persistent problems. If oral feeding is contraindicated, a feeding tube or gastrostomy tube can be considered (see Chap. 8).
- If cognitive deficits are present, the patient may have poor impulse control and may stuff the mouth hurriedly with food. If this occurs, the basis of the swallowing problem may be behavioral rather than neurological, and nursing interventions should be directed at managing the behavior and controlling distractions from the focus of eating. This patient requires mealtime supervision and verbal and nonverbal cues.

BLADDER DYSFUNCTION AND RETRAINING

Normal Bladder Function

Bladder control is an integrated function of the brainstem, spinal, and cerebral levels[11] (see Chap. 4).

- **Brainstem pontine level:** the true micturition centers are located in the dorsal pons. During micturition, the medial pontine region is activated, and the lateral pontine region is inhibited. This activity produces coordinated bladder contraction and sphincter relaxation, resulting in bladder emptying. Disruption in the central nervous system *above* the sacral reflex center usually causes a hyperreflexic bladder and is classified as an upper motor neuron (UMN) injury.
- **Spinal level:** the *sacral reflex control center* of the bladder is located in spinal segments S-2 to S-4. The parasympathetic innervation of the pelvic nerve is responsible for bladder emptying, whereas the sympathetic (hypogastric nerve) and somatic (pudendal nerve) innervations promote retention of urine. Micturition involves a supraspinal-spinopontospinal reflex triggered by stimulation of tension receptors, which result in coordination of the contracted detrusor muscle and relaxation of the sphincter. Interruption

of the descending suprasegmental pathways results in micturition through segmental spinospinal sacral reflexes that are triggered by perineal or nociceptive stimulation. The sphincter contractions are not well coordinated. Disruption at the sacral reflex center or in the peripheral nervous system causes an areflexic bladder, which is classified as a lower motor neuron (LMN) injury.

- **Cerebral level:** the micturition centers are controlled by input from the hypothalamus and the medial frontal cortex. Cortical input is responsible for voluntary control of the initiation and cessation of micturition. Lesions of the medial frontal lobes or hypothalamus can interrupt these pathways, resulting in involuntary micturition sometimes called **uninhibited bladder.**

Summary of Effects of Neurological Lesions on Micturition

People with neurological disease or injury may be unable to maintain normal urinary elimination patterns because of dysfunction at the brainstem, spinal, or cerebral levels. Any disruption of the sensory or motor pathways in the central or peripheral nervous systems that have input to the bladder will cause a disruption in urinary elimination patterns.

Types of Bladder Dysfunction: Alterations in Urinary Elimination Patterns

There are many conceptual frameworks regarding altered urinary elimination, including UMN and LMN injury and a classification of neurogenic bladder types. A **neurogenic bladder** is defined as any bladder disturbance that is attributable to motor or sensory pathways in the central or peripheral nervous systems that have input to the bladder. See Table 11-6 for a list of neurogenic bladder types. From a nursing perspective, nurses focus on assisting people to improve function through a functional health pattern framework; this is the approach taken in this chapter.

Alterations in urinary elimination patterns can be classified generally into urinary incontinence (UI) and urinary retention. Each of these two major classifications can be further subdivided into categories based on cause, characteristics, and pathophysiology to treat the problem effectively. It is important to accurately categorize the type of altered urinary elimination pattern present. The following sections discuss UI and urinary retention with emphasis on altered function in neurological patients.

Classification of Urinary Incontinence. Urinary incontinence can be associated with various problems, such as a diminished level of consciousness; cerebral injury, especially to the frontal lobe; or spinal cord injury. The Clinical Practice Guidelines for *Urinary Incontinence in Adults,* published in 1992, has been the definitive resource for health professionals in the management of adult UI in ambulatory and nonambulatory patients in outpatient, inpatient, home care, and long-term care settings.[12] Four major categories identified include urge incontinence, stress incontinence, overflow incontinence, and other types of functional incontinence. **Urge incontinence** is the involuntary loss of urine associated with an abrupt and strong desire to void (urgency). **Stress incon-**tinence is the involuntary loss of urine during coughing, sneezing, laughing, or other physical activities that increase abdominal pressure. **Overflow incontinence** is the involuntary loss of urine associated with overdistension of the bladder. **Functional incontinence** is urine loss caused by factors outside the lower urinary tract; this category includes UI not classifiable into the three categories listed previously. Table 11-7 lists descriptions, related findings, and patient populations associated with each type of UI.

Causes of Urinary Incontinence. The nurse considers the many common causes of transient UI when assessing for risk factors and related contributing factors for UI. Common causes of UI include altered states of consciousness (e.g., confusion, coma); urinary tract infections; atrophic urethritis or vaginitis; depression; excessive urine production related to excess intake; diuresis from drug therapy or endocrine conditions (e.g., hydrochlorothiazide or diabetes mellitus); restricted mobility related to bed rest; Parkinson's disease; restriction of bed rest; deconditioning (e.g., orthostatic hypotension, weakness, fatigue); and fecal impaction. In addition, various drugs may contribute to UI secondarily by clouding the sensorium or by directly affecting the organs of micturition. They include sedative hypnotics; diuretics that may overwhelm bladder capacity and lead to polyuria, frequency, and urgency; anticholinergics with related urinary retention and associated urinary frequency and overflow UI; α-adrenergic agents (e.g., sphincter tone in the proximal urethra can be decreased with α antagonists and increased with α agonists); and calcium channel blockers (e.g., can reduce smooth muscle contractility of the bladder, resulting in urinary retention and overflow UI).

Urinary Retention. Urinary retention is often associated with spinal cord–injured patients. In the acute phase of spinal cord injury, the abrupt interruption of the spinal innervation is lost, which results in spinal shock and an areflexic bladder. The bladder becomes distended, causing overflow UI (Table 11-6 and Table 11-7). The bladder gradually converts to a hypersensitive bladder as the spinal shock diminishes over days or weeks. If the spasticity and hypersensitivity of the bladder are severe, any slight stimulus, such as a minimal amount of urine in the bladder (20 to 50 mL) or stroking of the abdomen, thigh, or genitals, will cause the bladder to empty by reflex.

Nursing Management of Patients With Altered Urinary Elimination Patterns

Assessment

The nurse assesses the patient to determine the altered urinary elimination pattern present (Chart 11-4, page 234). The parameters considered in the assessment include confirming the voiding pattern by monitoring the pattern and characteristics over 24 hours, intake and output record, recent urinalysis and culture, and functional level. Factors that may be contributing to or resulting from the altered elimination pattern must be identified, as should the areas in need of further evaluation before therapeutic interventions are begun. The pathophysiology is considered in relation to normal function. The nurse discusses with the physician and other team members the need for further evaluation and the best

TABLE 11-6   CLASSIFICATION OF NEUROGENIC BLADDER TYPES[*†]

NEUROGENIC BLADDER TYPES	ANATOMIC LEVEL OF DISRUPTION	CHARACTERISTICS AND DESCRIPTION	ASSOCIATED CLINICAL PROBLEM	MANAGEMENT
Uninhibited neurogenic	Lesion in the frontal brain or pontine micturition centers	• Cortical control of initiation and inhibition to suppress voiding urge diminished • Reduced bladder capacity with little or no residual urine • Urgency, frequency, nocturia, urge incontinence	Stroke, traumatic brain injury, multiple sclerosis (MS), and brain tumor	• Timed voiding • Condom-type catheter for male, and "padding" of bed with absorbent pads for female
Reflex neurogenic	Spinal cord lesion above T-12–L-1	• Upper motor neuron (UMN) lesion with disruption of sensory and motor innervation *above* segments S-2–S-4 • Control lost from higher brain centers, resulting in uninhibited, involuntary detrusor contractions and uncontrolled voiding; spinal reflex arc takes over • Inability of distal sphincter to relax in coordination with detrusor contraction; results in ↑ bladder pressure with emptying and large amounts of residual urine	Lower spinal cord lesion or patient with blood supply interruption to cord secondary to trauma, tumor, vascular lesion, or MS	• Reflex triggering techniques • Intermittent catheterization • Drugs
Autonomous or areflexic neurogenic	Spinal cord lesion *at or below* T-12–L-1	• Disruption of sensory and motor innervation of sacral spinal reflex arc (S-2–S-4), a lower motor neuron (LMN) injury • ↓ sensation of bladder fullness, weak or absent detrusor contractions, and ↑ bladder capacity with high residual urine.[†] • Loss of voluntary voiding except with straining; overflow incontinence is common	Spina bifida, meningocele, or herniated intervertebral disc with LMN injury	• Intermittent catheterization • Straining using Valsalva's maneuver • Credé's method
Motor paralytic neurogenic	Anterior horn cells of S-2–S-4 ventral roots	• Partial or complete motor loss of bladder function with intact sensation • Difficulty with starting stream[*] • ↑ bladder capacity; high residual urine; overflow incontinence common	Herniated intervertebral disc, spinal trauma, spinal tumor, and poliomyelitis	• Intermittent catheterization • Straining using Valsalva's maneuver • Credé's method
Sensory paralytic neurogenic	Dorsal roots of sacral reflex center (S-2–S-4) or in sensory pathways to cerebral cortex	• ↓ or absent sensation of pain or fullness in bladder • Infrequent voiding with large output; ↑ bladder capacity with overflow incontinence common	Diabetic neuropathy, tabes dorsalis, syringomyelia, and MS	• Timed voiding • Intermittent catheterization

[*]Ouslander, J. G. (2004). Urinary incontinence. In L. Goldman & D. Ausiello (Eds.). *Cecil textbook of medicine* (22nd ed., pp. 111–114). Philadelphia. Saunders.
[†]Hoeman, S. P. (2002). *Rehabilitation nursing: Process, application, and outcome* (3rd ed.), (pp. 427–432). St. Louis, MO: C.V. Mosby.

approach to the management of the urinary elimination pattern (Chart 11-5, page 235).

Nursing management will depend on the patient problems and related nursing diagnoses, which include:

• Altered Urinary Elimination
• Stress Incontinence
• Reflex Incontinence
• Urinary Retention
• Risk for Altered Skin Integrity
• Urge Incontinence
• Functional Incontinence
• Total Incontinence
• Risk for Urinary Tract Infection

Possible collaborative problems include acute urinary retention; renal insufficiency/renal failure; and renal calculi.

Interventions

Follow the evidence-based protocols as endorsed by the health care practice committee. Various methods of managing altered urinary elimination patterns are discussed in the next section and are all based on evidence-based practice protocols. Within a collaborative interdisciplinary model of practice, input regarding management of urinary function is provided by team members. However, the nurse is primarily responsible for managing the complex multifactorial problem of an altered urinary elimination pattern, integrating

TABLE 11–7 TYPES, DESCRIPTIONS, RELATED FINDINGS, AND PATIENT POPULATIONS ASSOCIATED WITH URINARY INCONTINENCE*

TYPES	DIAGNOSIS/DESCRIPTION	RELATED FINDINGS	PATIENTS AFFECTED AND COMMENTS
Urge	• Diagnosed by urodynamics • Usually associated with urodynamic findings of involuntary detrusor contractions • Urodynamic finding of detrusor hyperactivity with impaired bladder contractility (DHIC) • DHIC can mimic other types of urinary incontinence (UI) and result in wrong treatment.	• If associated with neurological disorder, termed detrusor hyperreflexia • If no neurological disorder, called detrusor instability • Patients with DHIC have involuntary detrusor contractions, yet must strain to empty bladder either completely or incompletely; in addition to urge UI with ↑ postvoid residual volumes, patients with DHIC may also have obstruction, stress UI, or overflow UI.	• Stroke; in suprasacral spinal cord lesions or multiple sclerosis, detrusor hyperreflexia often accompanied by external sphincter dyssynergia; can cause urinary retention, vesicoureteric reflux, and renal damage • Frail elderly often have DHIC.
Stress	Diagnosed by observed urine loss with an ↑ in abdominal pressure, absence of detrusor contraction, or an overdistended bladder	Two possible causes: • Hypermobility or significant displacement of urethra and bladder neck during exertion • Intrinsic urethral sphincter deficiency (ISD); may be related to congenital sphincter weakness	• Patients with myelomeningocele, post-trauma, radiation, or sacral cord lesions; in women may be associated with many surgeries for incontinence • May leak continuously or leak with minimal exertion
Overflow	• Many presentations: constant dribbling, urge UI, or stress UI symptoms	• May be due to (1) an underactive or acontractile detrusor; or (2) a bladder outlet or urethral obstruction, resulting in overdistention and overflow; and (3) weak detrusor from idiopathic causes	• Underactive detrusor related to certain drugs, fecal impaction, diabetic neuropathy, or low spinal cord injury • Outlet obstruction common in men with prostatic hypertrophy, pelvic prolapse in women, and suprasacral spinal cord–injured and multiple sclerosis patients, detrusor external sphincter dyssynergia
Other types of functional UI	• A diagnosis of exclusion • Caused by factors outside the urinary tract, such as chronic impairments of physical or cognitive functioning • May be caused by ↓ bladder compliance	• May be improved or cured by improving functional level, treating other medical conditions, discontinuing certain drugs, adjusting hydration status, or reducing environmental barriers • May have a combined urge UI and stress UI, which is called **mixed UI** • Severe urgency associated with bladder hypersensitivity without detrusor overactivity called **sensory urgency**	• Immobilized and cognitively impaired may also have other types and causes of UI. • Patients with ↓ bladder compliance resulting from inflammatory bladder conditions (chemical or interstitial cystitis) and some patients with myelomeningocele often have **sensory urgency**.

*U.S. Department of Health and Human Services, Agency for Health Care Policy and Research. (1992). *Urinary incontinence in adults*, No. 92-0038. Washington, DC: Author.

Ouslander, J. G. (2004). Urinary incontinence. In L. Goldman & D. Ausiello (Eds.). *Cecil textbook of medicine* (22nd ed., pp. 111–114). Philadelphia: Saunders.

all the components of the treatment plan, and preventing complications, such as urinary tract infection and skin breakdown.

To prevent urinary tract infection, remove the indwelling catheter as soon as possible and use alternate methods of emptying and stimulating the bladder on a regular schedule. Follow all the research-based guidelines for maintaining aseptic technique related to catheters, catheterization, and skin care. Maintain an intake and output record, and review it periodically. Fluid intake is an important factor to adjust when trying to establish continence and regular emptying of the bladder. UI is a risk factor for skin break-

down. Provide for meticulous skin care, and keep the patient dry.

Treatment Options for Management of Altered Urinary Elimination Patterns

The three major categories of treatment outlined for UI are behavioral, pharmacologic, and surgical.[13,14] This can be used as a framework for nursing management and is summarized in Table 11-8. "Acute urinary retention" is a collaborative problem to be addressed with the physician. Management

CHART 11-4   Nursing Assessment for Altered Patterns of Urinary Elimination

CHARACTERISTICS OF VOIDING PATTERN

- Frequency of voiding and time during day and night
- Amount of voiding each time
- Evidence of dribbling (frequency, amount)
- Urgency
- Ability to delay voiding until in appropriate place
- Awareness of full bladder
- Distended bladder
- Sensation of incomplete bladder emptying
- Difficulty starting stream
- Dysuria
- Foul-smelling urine
- Residual urine >150 mL

RELATED FACTORS

Neurological disease or injury
- Cognitive deficits
- Sensory deficits with vision or hearing
- Altered sensorium or consciousness (confusion, coma)
- Neuropathies
- Comorbidity
- Urinary tract infection
- Vaginitis or atrophic urethritis
- Drug therapy that influences urinary output or bladder function
- Depression
- Large amounts of oral or intravenous intake; evaluation of intake and output record
- Environmental barriers to getting to bathroom
- Restricted mobility
- Stool impaction

of acute urinary retention is always directed at using some method of evacuating the bladder to prevent reflux and infection. Chronic urinary retention is usually treated with intermittent catheterization.

Whenever possible, the patient should be involved in selecting treatment options from established methods. As a rule, the least invasive and least dangerous procedure should be the first choice.[15] According to the AHCPR guidelines for UI in adults, behavioral techniques are low-risk interventions that decrease the frequency of UI in most individuals when provided by knowledgeable health care professionals. All behavioral techniques involve educating the patient and providing positive reinforcement for effort and progress.[12] Behavioral techniques include bladder training (retraining), habit training (timed voiding), prompted voiding, and pelvic muscle exercises. These are discussed later in this chapter. Additional techniques that may be used in conjunction with behavioral methods are biofeedback, vaginal cone retention, and electrical stimulation. There are also many drugs that can be used to treat urinary elimination problems. For those interested in the additional techniques and drug therapy, other references should be consulted.

After the particular type of altered urinary elimination pattern has been identified, treatment options are considered.

Behavioral Techniques

The following behavioral techniques have been effective and are recommended by AHCPR in the adult patient with incontinence.[12]

Bladder Training. Bladder training, also called bladder retraining, includes several variations. The time at which a bladder training program is initiated is critical to the success or failure of the program. Patients must be conscious, alert, and oriented. A bedpan, bedside commode, or access to the bathroom is necessary. The patient should be stable and preferably free from urinary tract infection.

Bladder training includes the three primary components of education, scheduled voiding, and positive reinforcement. The patient needs to be educated to understand the physiology, pathophysiology, technique, and desired outcome. The method of education depends on the patient with consideration for any cognitive or perceptual deficits that may interfere with learning.

A bladder retraining program assists the patient to learn to resist or inhibit the sensation of urgency, postpone voiding, and urinate according to a timetable rather than the urge to void. The strategies of a bladder retraining program vary and may include adjusting the fluid loads and postponing voiding so that progressively larger volumes of urine distend the bladder and longer intervals between voiding are achieved.[15] Motivating the patient is an important component of bladder training. The initial goal interval may be 2 to 3 hours, although it is not followed during sleep. Bladder retraining may continue for several months, during which time setting realistic goals, reinforcing patient education, and overall health monitoring and supervision are necessary.

Habit Training. Timed voiding is scheduled toileting on a planned basis with the goal of keeping the person dry by asking him or her to void at regular intervals. Unlike bladder training, there is no systematic effort to motivate the patient to delay voiding and resist the urge. An attempt is made to match the timed voiding with the person's usual voiding schedule. The time interval may be from 2 to 4 hours.

Prompted Voiding. Prompted voiding is a technique used primarily with dependent or cognitively impaired people. Prompted voiding is directed at teaching the incontinent person awareness of his or her incontinence so that toileting assistance is requested either independently or after being prompted by a caregiver. There are three major elements to prompted voiding:

- **Monitoring:** the person is checked by caregivers on a regular basis and asked to report verbally whether he or she is wet or dry.

CHART 11-5 · Diagnostic and Evaluative Procedures for Patients with Urinary Elimination Problems

PATIENT DATA

- Medical history including list of all prescribed and over-the-counter medications
- Physical examination–abdominal, genital, pelvic, rectal, neurological

ADDITIONAL TESTS RELATED TO VOIDING

- Postvoid residual ultrasound and measurement of residual volume
- Provocation stress test
- Data related to urinary elimination–voiding diary, voiding pattern, amount, time of day, related activities, type and amount of fluid intake

LABORATORY TESTS

- Urinalysis
- Blood urea nitrogen, creatinine, protein, complete blood count
- Urine culture

SPECIALIZED TESTS

- Urodynamic tests
- Endoscopic tests including video endoscopy
- Ultrasound
- Imaging tests
  - Upper tract
  - Lower tract with and without voiding

- **Prompting:** the person is asked (prompted) to try to use the bathroom to void.
- **Praising:** the person is praised for maintaining continence and attempting to use the toilet.

Pelvic Muscle Exercises. Pelvic muscle exercises, also called Kegel exercises, comprise a behavioral technique that requires repetitive active exercise of the pubococcygeus muscle to improve urethral resistance and urinary control by strengthening the periurethral and pelvic muscles in women. The woman must gain awareness of her pelvic muscles and be taught the correct exercise method of "drawing in" the perivaginal muscles and anal sphincter as if to control urination or defecation without contracting abdominal, buttock, or inner thigh muscles.[16] Muscles are contracted to a count of 10 and then relaxed to a count of 10. About 50 to 100 of these exercises must be done daily to be effective. It takes about 4 to 6 weeks to notice improvement.

Bladder-Triggering Techniques

A few bladder-triggering techniques facilitate bladder emptying. They include suprapubic stimulation, Valsalva's maneuver, and Credé's maneuver. **Suprapubic stimulation** activates the sacral-lumbar dermatomes by manually tapping the suprapubic area, pulling pubic hairs, or stroking the medial thighs. This is used for patients with UMN lesions.

Valsalva's maneuver is straining against a closed epiglottis while contracting the abdominal muscles and bearing down on the bladder. The straining is sustained or the breath held until the urine flow ceases. This maneuver is used for patients with LMN lesions. **Credé's maneuver** is placing the hands flat just below the umbilical area and pressing firmly down and inward toward the pelvic arch. The purpose of this maneuver is to express urine from the bladder. It may be repeated as many times as necessary to express all of the urine in the bladder. This method is used only with LMN lesions (sacral reflex arc is not intact). Generally, Credé's maneuver is not used in patients with UMN bladder disorders because it triggers sphincter closure and can cause reflux.

Catheters and Catheterizations

In the acute phase of spinal cord injury or other acute conditions, an indwelling catheter for continuous urinary drainage may be necessary. However, it should be removed as soon as possible and an intermittent catheterization schedule established.

TABLE 11-8 · MANAGEMENT OF ALTERED URINARY ELIMINATION PATTERNS

URINARY PATTERNS	PATIENT TYPES	TREATMENT
Urge urinary incontinence	Strokes	Timed voiding; bladder training and prompt every 2 h
Reflex urinary incontinence	Spinal cord injuries with upper motor neuron (UMN) and lower motor neuron lesions	Anticholinergic drugs and intermittent catheterization Condom catheter for men and "padding" for women
Overflow urinary incontinence	Spinal cord injuries with UMN lesion	Intermittent catheterization
Functional urinary incontinence	Various types of patients with functional deficits	Assistance for toileting and timed voiding • May use condom-type catheter for men and "padding" for women
Urinary retention	Spinal cord injuries; some stroke patients	• Intermittent catheterization for life with a goal of 400 mL per catheterization (no voiding on own) • Trigger voiding philosophy for some practitioners

Intermittent Catheterization.
Intermittent catheterization means that the patient is straight catheterized at regular intervals of 2 to 4 hours or more to empty the bladder at regular intervals. Bladder-triggering techniques should be incorporated as a means of emptying the bladder before straight catheterization. After the patient begins to void by reflex, the interval between catheterizations can be extended using the postvoid residual urine amount as a guide. Indications for stopping intermittent catheterization include an adequate amount of urine voided, residual urine volume of 100 to 150 mL or less, or a genitourinary tract free of pathologic changes or infection.

Self-Catheterization.
If intermittent catheterization is needed on a long-term basis or in the home setting, many patients can be taught intermittent catheterization using a "clean technique" rather than the "sterile technique" used in care facilities. This is referred to as self-catheterization. With the clean technique, the patient starts with a clean catheter rather than sterilized equipment. Warm tap water and soap are used to wash the perineal area. Hands must be meticulously washed with soap and water, but sterile gloves are not worn. If the patient is not able to self-catheterize, use of an external condom type catheter connected to a leg bag may be used by male patients. This method can also be used for continuous drainage during sleep.

Indwelling Suprapubic Catheter.
The placement of indwelling suprapubic urinary catheters is often used for quadriplegics. The rationale for placement is the excessive burden of intermittent catheterization for both the patient and his or her caregiver. With all of the other care essentials to complete, the suprapubic catheter is attractive. With intermittent catheterization, the patient may be incontinent between catheterizations, which necessitates changing wet linen. Another attractive feature of an indwelling suprapubic catheter is that it frees the patient from trying to pace fluid intake with the timing of intermittent catheterization.

Padding.
Padding is the placement of absorbent pads in the bed or chair to absorb the urine related to incontinence. Use of padding is preferred to maintaining an indwelling catheter long term for patients who do not respond well to behavioral techniques or are not candidates for behavioral or other techniques.

BOWEL ELIMINATION AND DYSFUNCTION

Normal Function

The act of bowel evacuation is called **defecation.** The anus, the terminal end of the large bowel, is controlled by two sphincters: the involuntary proximal anal sphincter (smooth muscle) and the voluntary distal anal sphincter (striated muscle). Defecation is a coordinated reflex involving sacral segments S-3, S-4, and S-5, which is initiated by stimulated stretch receptors located in the anus that initiate peristaltic waves. These waves propel fecal matter toward the anus and open the proximal sphincter. If the distal sphincter is also open, bowel evacuation will occur.

The sacral reflex for bowel evacuation is weak and is aided by parasympathetic responses (peristalsis caused by ingestion of food and increased pressure within the lower bowel, which opens the proximal sphincter). Additionally, contraction of the abdominal wall aids bowel evacuation by increasing pressure on the bowel. See Chapter 4 for further discussion of defecation.

Types of Altered Bowel Function Patterns

Various neurological conditions and treatment protocols can cause alterations in bowel elimination patterns (constipation, diarrhea, or incontinence). Several risk factors have been identified for these abnormal patterns:

- **Constipation:** fluid restriction, prolonged immobility, nothing by mouth status as a result of swallowing deficits or unconsciousness, decreased bulk in diet, drugs known to decrease peristalsis (e.g., codeine), spinal nerve compression, paralytic ileus, lack of sensation, lack of privacy, interruption of usual bowel routine, and failure to respond to defecation stimuli
- **Diarrhea:** intolerance to tube feeding, antibiotic therapy, and fecal impaction
- **Incontinence:** altered consciousness, cognitive deficits (e.g., social disinhibition, lack of impulse control, inability to recognize and respond to defecation impulses), impaired communication, and neurogenic bowel without sensation or control (related to spinal cord injury above T-11 or involving sacral reflex arc S-2 to S-4)

Nursing Management of Patients With Altered Bowel Elimination Pattern

Assessment

The nurse assesses the patient to identify the functional bowel elimination problem present. Parameters to be considered include bowel elimination pattern (frequency, characteristics of stool, presence of discomfort), presence of bowel sounds and abdominal distention, previous elimination pattern, and presence of risk factors (see previous list). Nursing management depends on the nursing diagnosis. The following are possible patient problems and nursing diagnoses:

- Diarrhea
- Colonic Constipation
- Bowel Incontinence

Possible collaborative problems include:

- Paralytic ileus/small-bowel obstruction
- Gastrointestinal bleeding

Interventions

Nursing management for altered bowel elimination patterns depends on the particular problem identified. However, the goal is for the patient to eliminate a soft, formed stool every 1 to 3 days. An individualized bowel program is developed for each patient following established standards of care and is included in the patient's care plan. See www.guideline.gov for the latest guidelines on constipation. Chart 11-6 provides a sample bowel program. Daily documentation should be included in the record.

CHART 11-6   Sample Bowel Program to Establish Normal Elimination

There are a number of bowel elimination guidelines available (see www.guideline.gov). The following protocol includes the basic components of a bowel program, although there may be slight variations in protocols of various health facilities. Once a normal bowel elimination pattern has been established, an individualized protocol should be followed.

- Make sure the lower bowel is empty; an enema may be necessary before beginning the training program.
- Establish a time of day for a bowel movement based on the patient's previous pattern; adhere to this designated time of day rigidly.
- Encourage a diet high in roughage (whole-grain bread and cereal, fresh fruits, and vegetables); in addition, offer prune juice.
- Unless contraindicated by a fluid restriction, increase fluid intake to 2000 to 2500 mL/d.
- Insert a suppository on the first day. If it does not work, you may wait until the next day.
- On the following day, repeat the insertion of the suppository. If it is effective, continue with the protocol every other day, but daily use may be necessary for some patients.
- If at all possible, the patient should be seated on the commode or taken into the bathroom to defecate.
- Administer medications and collaborate with patient and health team members to adjust regimen individualized to the patient.

If the patient is constipated, the following points may need to be considered:

- Determine which risk factors can be controlled or altered.
- Increase fluid intake if not contraindicated.
- Administer any drugs ordered by the physician as part of the bowel program:
  - Bulk-forming agent (e.g., Metamucil, 15 mL daily)
  - Stool softeners (e.g., docusate sodium, 100 mg three times daily)
  - Mild laxatives (e.g., Milk of Magnesia, 30 mL daily)
  - Suppositories (glycerin or Dulcolax as needed)
- Enemas may be ordered.

The nurse should keep in mind the following guidelines when instituting any bowel program:

- Start with an empty lower bowel and then individualize a bowel program to meet needs.
- Get the patient onto the commode if at all possible.
- Try to establish an evacuation pattern at the same time of day that mimics the patient's preadmission pattern.

In addition to the treatment plan outlined, digital stimulation of the rectum can be used in patients with spinal cord injuries to stimulate defecation. Initiation of Valsalva's maneuver or a push-up on the commode may also aid defecation. (Both hands are placed on the commode seat, and the patient raises himself or herself slightly off the seat.) Autonomic hyperreflexia may be triggered by impaction in patients with high spinal cord injuries (see Chap. 18).

COGNITIVE REHABILITATION

Cognitive deficits are one of the most disabling categories of deficits resulting from brain injury because they have an impact on every aspect of life. Deficits in higher-level cognitive functions can be overlooked without careful assessment of the patient. If they are overlooked, the patient is often set up for failure and will not achieve the highest level of independence and quality of life possible.

Nursing Management of Patients With Cognitive Deficits

Assessment

The patient's cognitive function can be assessed by observing the patient's behavior, interactions, and function in the care setting or by using various assessment techniques and instruments to evaluate cognitive function.

The nurse should observe the patient's reaction to stimuli, ability to perform ADLs, memory, way of dealing with minor stresses, problem-solving abilities, and judgment. The nurse should also identify cognitive deficits that impact on patient safety and implement interventions to protect the patient from injury. Various instruments may be used to assess specific cognitive functions, such as memory, attention span, affect and general behavior, sequencing skills, problem solving, insight, judgment, and abstract thinking. The choice of instruments depends on the cognitive level of the patient. In many facilities, a short (half-hour) cognitive screening assessment may be conducted by the occupational therapy department. The information derived from this evaluation is helpful to the nurse in planning care if cognitive deficits can be identified. Many physicians prefer this approach rather than a lengthy full neuropsychological assessment in the acute care setting because some recovery is expected during the early weeks after cerebral insult. If problems persist, a complete neuropsychological assessment can be ordered 3 to 6 months after injury. Based on this comprehensive assessment, the neuropsychologist can then prescribe a treatment plan.

Interventions

Nurses can provide simple interventions for many cognitive problems in the acute care setting (see Chap. 6). With knowledge of the patient's cognitive deficits, the nurse can identify realistic goals and expectations for the patient. An important role for the nurse is to explain the patient's behavior to the family and be supportive of their concerns. Family members should be told what kind of behavior to expect and how to interact with the patient.

The patient with severe cognitive deficits will require ongoing treatment following discharge to a rehabilitation facility or to the patient's home. If a home discharge is planned, referrals for follow-up care should be arranged.

THE HOME-BASED VENTILATOR-DEPENDENT PATIENT

As higher technology becomes possible in the home, more patients are being managed at home on ventilators. These patients need 24-hour care that is provided by professional and family caregivers. Much planning, coordinating, and family teaching are needed to even consider home-care options. For example, the family must be competent in providing manual resuscitation using an Ambu bag, tracheostomy care, and operating of a home ventilator. In addition, provisions must be made for back-up power with a generator if electrical supply is interrupted. See Chapter 18 for further discussion of the care of the spinal cord–injured patient.

DISCHARGE PLANNING

Some patients will require long-term rehabilitation, which will necessitate the use of community resources or admission to a rehabilitation center or extended care facility. The nurse should evaluate the patient's level of independence in terms of ADLs to assess how much help the patient will need. This information, along with evaluations by other health care team members, will provide a database for designing a comprehensive rehabilitation plan.

Family members must also be assessed to determine their ability to participate in the rehabilitation program. Some families are willing and able to care for the patient at home with the help of various community agencies. Other families do not want to care for the patient or are unable to do so because of other family responsibilities. **Caregiver stress** needs to be considered. The decision of how and where to provide for the long-term rehabilitative needs of the patient must be a collaborative one that includes input from the physician, nurse, other health care team members, family, and patient, if possible.

Regardless of whether the patient is going home to be cared for by family or to an extended care facility, the nurse will need to compile a summary assessment of the patient's needs and abilities in performing ADLs. Referral forms must be completed and sent to appropriate resources. (See Chap. 2 for information about discharge planning.)

REHABILITATION LEGISLATION AND ENTITLEMENT PROGRAMS

The value of rehabilitation for the individual and society is well appreciated and has been supported through many legislative programs. Information about entitlement programs and rehabilitation can be obtained from a variety of sources, such as the following:

- The social worker
- Local and state health departments through their departments of social service, rehabilitation, or vocational rehabilitation
- Special focus groups, such as the Multiple Sclerosis Society and National Head Injury Foundation

REFERENCES

1. World Health Organization. (2001). *International classification of functioning, disability, and health: ICF.* Geneva: Author.
2. U.S. Department of Health and Human Services, Agency for Health Care Policy and Research. (1995). *Post-stroke rehabilitation* (No. 95-0662). Washington, DC: Author.
3. McCourt, A. E. (Ed.). (1993). *The specialty practice of rehabilitation nursing: A core curriculum* (3rd ed., p. 32). Skokie, IL: The Rehabilitation Nursing Foundation.
4. Borgman-Gainer, M. F. (1996). Independent function: Movement and mobility. In S. P. Hoeman (Ed.). *Rehabilitation nursing: Process and application* (2nd ed., pp. 232–233). St. Louis: C. V. Mosby.
5. Bobath, B. (1990). *Adult hemiplegia: Evaluation and treatment* (3rd ed.). Oxford, UK: Butterworth-Heinemann.
6. Gillis, A., & MacDonald, B. (2005). Prevent deconditioning in the hospitalized elderly. *Canadian Nurses, 101*(6), 16–20.
7. Brummel-Smith, K. (2003). Rehabilitation. In C. K. Cassel (Ed.). *Geriatric medicine: An evidence based approach* (4th ed.). New York: Springer-Verlag. Available on-line as e-book.
8. U. S. Department of Health and Human Services, Agency for Health Care Policy and Research. (1992). *Pressure ulcers in adults: Prediction and prevention* (No. 92-0047). Washington, DC: Author.
9. Saver, J. L. (2002). Approach to the patient with aphasia. In J. Biller (Ed.). *Practical neurology* (2nd ed., pp. 27–39). Philadelphia: Lippincott William & Wilkins.
10. Logemann, J. A. (2002). Approach to the patient with dysphagia. In J. Biller (Ed.). *Practical neurology* (2nd ed., pp. 227–235). Philadelphia: Lippincott William & Wilkins.
11. Benarroch, E. E., Westmoreland, B. F., Daube, J. R., Reagan, T. J., & Sandok, B. A. (1999). *Medical neurosciences: An approach to anatomy, pathology, and physiology by systems and levels* (pp. 272–285). Philadelphia: Lippincott Williams & Wilkins.
12. U.S. Department of Health and Human Services, Agency for Health Care Policy and Research. (1992). *Urinary incontinence in adults* (No. 92-0038). Washington, DC: Author.
13. Borgman-Gainer, M. F. (2002). Independent function: Movement and mobility. In S. P. Hoeman (Ed.). *Rehabilitation nursing: Process, application, & outcomes* (3rd ed., pp. 232–233). St. Louis, MO: C. V. Mosby.
14. Young, C. C., & Bradley, W. E. (1997). The diagnosis and treatment of urinary bladder dysfunction. In: P. A. Low (Ed.). *Clinical autonomic disorders, evaluation and management* (2nd ed.). Philadelphia: Lippincott-Raven.
15. Garg, B. G. (2002). Approach to the patient with bladder, bowel, or sexual dysfunction and other autonomic disorders. In J. Biller (Ed.). *Practical neurology* (2nd ed., pp. 366–376). Philadelphia: Lippincott William & Wilkins.
16. Rose, M. A., Baigis-Smith, J., Smith, D., & Newman, D. (1990). Behavioral management of urinary incontinence in homebound older adults. *Home Healthcare Nurse, 8*(5), 10–15.

RESOURCES

Alexander, T. T., Hiduke, R. J., & Stevens, K. A. (Eds.). (1999). *Rehabilitation nursing procedures manual* (2nd ed.). New York: McGraw-Hill.
Association of Rehabilitation Nurses. (2006). *Evidence based rehabilitation nursing: Common challenges and interventions.* Skokie, IL: Author.
Hoeman, S. P. (2002). *Rehabilitation nursing: Process, application, and outcomes* (3rd ed.). St. Louis, MO: Mosby.
National Guideline Clearinghouse. www.guideline.gov
O'Sullivan, S. B., & Schmitz, T. J. (2007). *Physical rehabilitation* (5th ed.). Philadelphia: F. A. Davis Co.
Sarkodie-Gyan, T. (2006). *Neurorehabilitation devices.* New York: McGraw-Hill.

Pharmacologic Management of Neuroscience Patients

Timothy F. Lassiter and Amy I. Henkel

OVERVIEW

Role of the Pharmacist in Patient Management

Historically, the profession of pharmacy has been devoted exclusively to dispensing a high-quality drug product. With advances in technology, pharmacists have been safely able to devote less time to drug distribution services while assuming new roles in multidisciplinary patient management. Pharmacists today undergo extensive training, enabling them to contribute to the care of the patient on a number of fronts.[1] At the same time, as medical science has advanced, pharmacologic management of patients has become increasingly complex. Pharmacists are drug therapy experts whose primary responsibility is preventing and solving drug-related problems and providing drug information to all health care providers and patients. These circumstances have empowered pharmacists to become proactively involved in patient care as part of the multidisciplinary health care team. Pharmacists also develop and implement drug therapy monitoring plans, such as scheduling and reviewing serum drug concentrations, to achieve therapeutic endpoints and avoid toxicity.[1,2]

Impact of Pharmacotherapy on the Nervous System

Pharmacotherapy has a tremendous impact on the assessment and care of the neuroscience patient. For example, many drugs commonly prescribed in the acute care setting can alter the level of consciousness (LOC). This is an obvious desired endpoint for narcotic analgesics, benzodiazepines, and other sedatives. However, many other drugs can also alter the LOC, either as a side effect (clonidine, H_2 receptor antagonists) or as a symptom of toxicity (relative overdose of imipenem in a patient with renal failure). Toxicity is of particular concern in the elderly and any patient in the intensive care unit (ICU). In both cases, patients may be more sensitive to the pharmacologic effects or toxicities of a medication.

This sensitivity is frequently compounded by an impaired ability to eliminate the offending agent because of renal or hepatic insufficiency. Despite the risks involved, properly managed adjuvant pharmacotherapy can indeed save lives. Selection of drug products with a favorable neurological profile increases the potential for a good outcome in the neuroscience patient.

Therapeutic Decision Making

Determining optimal pharmacologic management of the neuroscience patient depends on numerous factors. Ultimately, a risk–benefit assessment must be made for each therapeutic decision. Occasionally, this process results in a drug being prescribed that carries with it a high risk of producing a deleterious effect, but it is also potentially life saving. This is frequently the case when amphotericin B or an aminoglycoside is prescribed. Another example is a patient given sedatives and neuromuscular blockers for ventilator compliance at the expense of a reliable neurological examination.

After a careful risk–benefit assessment has been made, a comparable therapy can be selected over another based on relative cost. Such decisions become more difficult when a more expensive drug can potentially shorten a hospitalization or avoid an expensive adverse effect. Studies that comprehensively examine costs from a pharmacoeconomic perspective are being conducted more routinely in today's health care environment.

COMMONLY USED DRUGS ALONG THE CONTINUUM OF CARE

Discussion of drug therapy in this chapter focuses on practical information necessary to manage the neuroscience patient. Tables are included for a quick reference. Drugs are addressed by body systems. For those who want more detailed information, pharmacology texts should be consulted.

TABLE 12-1   VASOCONSTRICTOR AGENTS

DRUG	DOSE	ADVERSE EFFECTS	COMMENTS
Dopamine	4–8 mcg/kg/min	Tachycardia compared with equipotent dose of dobutamine; skin necrosis with extravasation	Inotropic dose; may begin to see vasoconstrictor effects
	8–20 mcg/kg/min	Tachycardia, hypertension; skin necrosis with extravasation	Prolonged high doses produce organ hypoperfusion and renal dysfunction
Phenylephrine	0.5–5 mcg/kg/min	Reflex bradycardia; skin necrosis with extravasation	May be drug of choice for spinal shock; may be useful when other vasoconstrictors cause excessive tachycardia
Norepinephrine	2 mcg/min, titrate to effect, titrate to effect (typically <30 mcg/min)	Tachycardia; skin necrosis with extravasation	Useful for patients not responding to dopamine; organ hypoperfusion and renal dysfunction with prolonged high doses
Epinephrine	2–10 mcg/min 10–20 mcg/min	Tachycardia Tachycardia	Primarily inotropic effect Vasoconstricting dose; preserves coronary and cerebral flow

Hemodynamic Support and Associated Drugs

In addition to proper fluid management, neuroscience patients in the ICU often require therapy with vasoconstrictors, vasodilators, or inotropes. Proper monitoring is essential and typically includes frequent measurement of mean arterial pressure, heart rate, central venous pressure, urine output, and cardiac output as determined by a pulmonary artery catheter. The goal is to meet the oxygen requirements of the body. More definite therapeutic endpoints, such as specifically targeted oxygen delivery values or a minimum acceptable blood pressure, are controversial. Therapy must be individualized for each patient. Hemodynamic regimens often involve multiple drugs, making physical and chemical compatibility an issue with respect to concomitant fluids and intravenous (IV) access. The pharmacist can help solve these complex problems. Never assume compatibility when appropriate data are lacking.

In the neuroscience patient, recent research has focused on cerebral oxygen delivery and consumption optimization, rather than cerebral perfusion pressure, as a therapeutic endpoint for hemodynamic manipulation. This is particularly useful when vasodilators and other antihypertensives are prescribed because of the complex interrelationships between vascular tone and cerebral perfusion in the setting of an acute neurological insult (see Chapter 16).

Vasoconstrictors

Vasoconstrictors are helpful when hypotension is the result of a loss of vascular tone. This is commonly due to either sepsis or spinal shock. They are relatively contraindicated in untreated hypovolemic or cardiogenic shock. A high-dose requirement of vasoconstrictors for a prolonged period is an ominous sign because these drugs preserve blood pressure at the expense of organ perfusion. Extended periods of vital organ hypoperfusion contribute to multiple organ dysfunction syndrome, which carries with it a high mortality rate.

Dopamine is notable in that its pharmacologic effects are dose dependent. At moderate doses, inotropic (increased cardiac contractility) and chronotropic (increased heart rate) effects predominate. At high doses, it is a potent vasoconstrictor, effectively overriding any selective vasodilatation activity. The use of low-dose dopamine as a renal protective therapy has been widely disproved and fallen out of favor.[3] **Phenylephrine** is a potent vasoconstrictor devoid of direct inotropic or chronotropic activity. Some clinicians consider it the drug of choice for spinal shock, and it is being used more frequently for septic shock. Reflex bradycardia develops occasionally with its use. **Norepinephrine** is a potent vasoconstrictor with concomitant inotropic and chronotropic activity. **Epinephrine** acts as a positive inotropic or chronotropic agent at low doses and a vasoconstrictor with higher infusion rates (Table 12-1).

Regardless of the dose prescribed, great care must be taken to avoid extravasation of these vasoactive substances. This complication can produce extensive skin necrosis due to intense local vasoconstriction. Local instillation of phentolamine is indicated when this occurs.

Inotropic Agents

The inotropic agents are useful when cardiac contractility needs to be increased to optimize cardiac output. Careful titration is necessary because these agents can increase heart rate. Excessive tachycardia can be deleterious due to decreased cardiac output resulting from shortened filling time and diminished stroke volume, or from prolonged excessive myocardial oxygen demand in the setting of ischemic heart disease. The inotropic agents can also cause vasodilatation, which is usually tolerated poorly in this setting (Table 12-2).

Dobutamine is the most frequently prescribed positive inotropic agent. It is usually well tolerated and infrequently causes tachycardia. **Amrinone** and **milrinone** are newer agents that have inotropic activity without direct chronotropic activity. Their ability to raise cardiac output is in part due to their vasodilator activity, so blood pressure must be monitored closely. Amrinone is associated with a high incidence of thrombocytopenia. **Milrinone** is similar to

TABLE 12-2   INOTROPIC AGENTS

DRUG	DOSE	ADVERSE EFFECTS	COMMENTS
Dobutamine	2.5 mcg/kg/min, titrate up to 20 mcg/kg/min	Hypotension, ischemia, tachycardia	Wean slowly (1 mcg/kg/min/h), useful for low cardiac output unresponsive to fluids
Dopamine			See Table 12-1
Epinephrine			Vasoconstrictor
Norepinephrine			Agents, for details
Amrinone	0.75 mg/kg 1 over 3 min, then 5 mcg/kg/min, titrate up to 15 mcg/kg/min	Hypotension, ischemia, thrombocytopenia, tachycardia	Primarily a vasodilator, typically used with dobutamine
Milrinone	50 mcg/kg over 10 min × 1, then 0.375–0.75 mcg/kg/min	Hypotension, ischemia, tachycardia	More potent than amrinone
Isoproterenol	2–10 mcg/min	Tachycardia, hypotension, ischemia	Excessive tachycardia limits use to severe bradycardia only

amrinone but is a much more potent inotropic agent. Milrinone may provide an advantage in right-sided heart failure due to specific effects on the pulmonary vasculature. It is also the most expensive drug in its class. Patients with severely impaired cardiac contractility are sometimes prescribed both milrinone and dobutamine. **Isoproterenol** is used infrequently as an inotropic agent because of its strong concomitant chronotropic activity. It is useful, however, for treating symptomatic bradycardia unresponsive to atropine.

Vasodilators

Vasodilators are routinely prescribed for the neuroscience patient. They can be used in patients with impaired cardiac output to decrease the workload of the heart (afterload) and improve cardiac performance. More typically, they are used to control blood pressure in hypertensive patients with neurological sequelae. Blood pressure goals must be individualized to prevent further damage related to elevated pressures without also worsening cerebral ischemia. As mentioned previously, the most common side effects are hypotension and tachycardia (Table 12-3).

The calcium channel blockers are frequently used agents in this class. **Nicardipine** is available in IV form and is a smooth-acting vasodilator when given as a continuous infusion. **Nifedipine** given orally has been used extensively to treat hypertension in neuroscience patients. It is more potent than nicardipine. Careful monitoring of vital signs and neurological status is required because nifedipine has rarely been associated with worsened ischemic stroke when administered sublingually. **Nimodipine**, although an effective antihypertensive, is only indicated for prevention of cerebral vasospasm. In addition to having antihypertensive properties, calcium channel blockers may help interrupt the development of secondary brain injury after trauma. **Verapamil** and **diltiazem** are effective when given as an IV bolus or infusion for supraventricular arrhythmias. They also lower blood pressure but are not routinely used for acute hypertensive situations. Verapamil and diltiazem are often prescribed chronically to treat hypertension. Sustained-release oral dosage forms are available. They should not be crushed and given through any kind of enteral tube, because this will place the patient at risk for hypotension from the relative overdose. Similarly, immediate-release calcium channel blockers given once daily are likely to be ineffective unless they have a long half-life like amlodipine.

Nitroglycerin is a vasodilator but is often ineffective in managing severe hypertension. **Sodium nitroprusside** is a potent arterial and venous vasodilator that has been used for many years for hypertensive urgencies and emergencies. It should be avoided in patients with acute neurological injury because it tends to override any remaining vascular protection and expose the brain to excessively high pressures. High doses given for a prolonged period can lead to thiocyanate toxicity, particularly if the risk of renal failure is high. Unexplained acidosis is usually the first sign. Concomitant administration of **sodium thiosulfate** has been advocated to prevent thiocyanate toxicity. **Fenoldopam** is a new dopamine receptor agonist that may be an alternative to nitroprusside. It provides effective blood pressure lowering with additional effects on the kidney. Fenoldopam's ability to increase renal blood flow and promote naturesis has been held by some clinicians as a renal sparing therapy.

Beta blockers (**metoprolol, atenolol,** others) are also useful antihypertensives. **Esmolol** is an ultra-short-acting beta blocker that can be given as escalating IV boluses or by a continuous infusion. It is also effective for supraventricular tachycardia. In addition to slowing heart rate, **labetalol** also has peripheral vasodilating effects. Many consider it to be the drug of choice for acutely managing hypertension in the neuroscience population because of its safety record and because it does not cause as much tachycardia as other potent vasodilators. All beta blockers have negative inotropic effects that can limit their use in patients with congestive heart failure. They can also worsen glucose control in patients with diabetes, worsen pulmonary function in asthmatics, and (rarely) cause hyperkalemia. The angiotensin-converting enzyme inhibitor **enalaprilat** is available for IV use in the acute care setting. The relative efficacy of this drug fluctuates depending on the volume status of the patient. Hypovolemic patients tend to have an exaggerated response, whereas fluid-overloaded patients tend to respond poorly. Enalaprilat also can cause hyperkalemia.

TABLE 12-3 VASODILATORS

DRUG	DOSE	ADVERSE EFFECTS	COMMENTS
Calcium Channel Blockers			
Nicardipine	5 mg/hr IV, titrate q15min up to 15 mg/hr *Onset:* 1–5 min	Hypotension, tachycardia	Fluid load can be substantial, typical concentration = 0.1–0.2 mg/mL
Nifedipine	PO: 10–30 mg q6–8h Max daily dose, 180 mg *Onset:* 5–15 min	Hypotension, tachycardia, headache, flushing	SL route has been associated with worsened ischemic stroke
Nimodipine	60 mg PO q4h × 21 d	Hypotension, tachycardia	Only for treatment of vasospasm after aneurysmal subarachnoid hemorrhage, 30 mg q2h has been used in hypotensive patients
Verapamil	PO: 80 mg q8h up to 480 mg/d	Heart block, worsened congestive heart failure, constipation	IV useful for supraventricular arrhythmias, not for acutely elevated BP
Diltiazem	PO: 30 mg q6h up to 360 mg/d IV: 0.25 mg/kg bolus, may repeat × 1 with 0.35 mg/kg. *Infusion range:* 5–15 mg/hr	Similar to those of verapamil, but less pronounced	See verapamil. IV form for supraventricular tachycardia or atrial fibrillation only
Nitroglycerin	20–300 mcg/min *Onset:* 1–2 min	Hypotension, headache, methemaglobinemia	Tachyphylaxis can occur, oral and topical forms available: provide "nitrate free" interval daily to lessen tachyphylaxis
Sodium nitroprusside	0.5–10 mcg/kg/min *Onset:* seconds	Hypotension, cyanide toxicity, especially with concurrent renal failure	Avoid in setting of increased intracranial pressure; some advocate concurrent sodium thiosulfate to minimize risk of cyanide toxicity
Fenoldopam	0.1–1 mcg/kg/min *Onset:* 10 min	Hypotension, headache, nausea, blurred vision	Promotes naturesis and increased renal blood flow, renal protective effect
Beta Blockers			
Labetolol	IV: 10–20 mg over 2 min, may increase to 40–80 mg and repeat q10min up to total of 300 mg—see comments *Onset:* 5 min	Bradycardia, bronchospasm, worsened glucose control in association with diabetes, worsened congestive heart failure	May be the drug of choice for many neuroscience patients; may use continuous infusion starting at 0.5–2 mg/min
Metoprolol	IV: 5 mg q5min up to 15 mg PO: 25 mg q12h up to 100 mg q6h	See labetolol, cardiac selective up to 200 mg/d	IV maintenance doses up to 20 mg q6h have been tolerated, but expensive
Esmolol	500 mcg/kg × 1, then 25–50 mcg/kg/min up to 400 mcg/kg/min *Onset:* 1–3 min	See labetolol	Also useful for supraventricular tachycardia, very short acting
Enalaprilat	0.625–5 mg over 5 min q6h *Onset:* 15 min PO: 2.5–40 mg/d	Hypotension, hyperkalemia rash, cough, laryngeal edema	Intensity of response depends on fluid status of patient; IV form at least twice as potent as oral

Anticonvulsants

Anticonvulsants are a mainstay of therapy for patients with seizure disorders. These agents are effective for control of seizures from various etiologies. Most patients with seizure disorders can be managed with pharmacotherapy alone. More than 20 different drugs are used to control convulsive episodes, but most patients are effectively managed with four to five agents used alone or in combination. A review of commonly used anticonvulsants is presented in Table 12-4. A more complete discussion of selected agents and nursing implications follows.

Phenytoin (Dilantin)

Phenytoin is a member of the hydantoin class of anticonvulsants. It blocks synaptic posttetanic potentiation and subsequent propagation of electrical discharge in the motor cortex. The drug blocks sodium transport and thereby stabilizes membrane sensitivity to hyperexcitable states. Phenytoin is

TABLE 12-4   ANTICONVULSANT AGENTS

DRUG	COMMON DOSES	THERAPEUTIC SERUM LEVEL	ADVERSE EFFECTS	COMMENTS
Barbiturates				
Phenobarbital	3–5 mg/kg/d	15–40 mg/L	Sedation, rash, ataxia, hyperactivity, respiratory depression, hypotension (IV)	Induces hepatic metabolism—may increase elimination of drugs
Primidone (Mysoline)	10–25 mg/kg/d	5–20 mg/L	Sedation, ataxia, nausea, dizziness, rash (similar to phenobarbital)	Active metabolites: PEMA and phenobarbital
Hydantoins				
Phenytoin (Dilantin)	4–8 mg/kg/d	10–20 mg/L	Nystagmus, rash, sedation, fever, gingival hyperplasia, ataxia, hypotension and bradycardia, pain on injection (IV)	IV administration: limit 50 mg/min as direct push into running IV line. Enzyme inducer
Fosphenytoin (Cerebyx)	4–8 mg PE/kg/d	10–20 mg/L	Pruritus, significantly less cardiotoxicity; otherwise similar to phenytoin	150 mg PE/min maximum IV administration
Other Agents				
Carbamazepine (Tegretol, Carbatrol)	10–35 mg/kg/d	4–12 mg/L	Dizziness, ataxia, nystagmus, rash, diplopia, aplastic anemia	Induces own metabolism and metabolism of other drugs
Valproic acid (Depakene, Depakote, Depacon)	15–60 mg/kg/d	50–100 mg/L	Nausea, vomiting, diarrhea, drowsiness, liver toxicity	Hepatic enzyme inhibitor. IV should be divided every 6 hr
Clonazepam	2–20 mg/d	20–80 ng/mL	Drowsiness, ataxia	Tolerance to anticonvulsant effect may occur
Felbamate (Felbatol)	15–45 mg/kg/d	Not established	Nausea, vomiting, diarrhea, anxiety, insomnia, headache, hypophosphatemia, rash	Risk of fatal aplastic anemia, liver failure; use recommended only if benefits exceed risks
Gabapentin (Neurontin)	900–4800 mg/d	Not established	Drowsiness, ataxia, dizziness, fatigue	No known interactions with other anticonvulsants; beneficial in pain management
Lamotrigine (Lamictal)	100–500 mg/d	Not established	Dizziness, diplopia, headache, ataxia, nausea, severe skin rash	Slow dosage titration required; approved for monotherapy
Topiramate (Topamax)	200–900 mg/d	Not established	Drowsiness, dizziness, fatigue, parasthesias, impaired cognition	Dosage titration over 8 wk
Tiagabine (Gabitril)	32–56 mg/d	Not established	Dizziness, somnolence, asthenia, tremor, anxiety, confusion	Rare incidence of serious rash
Oxcarbazepine (Trileptal)	300–1800 mg/d	Not established	Headache, drowsiness, fatigue, dizziness, hyponatremia	Lacks hematologic toxicity seen with carbamazepine
Zonisamide (Zonegran)	100–400 mg/d	Not established	Impaired memory, drowsiness, ataxia, nystagmus, diplopia, nephrolithiasis	Long plasma half-life of 50–68 hr
Levetiracetam (Keppra)	1000–3000 mg/d	Not established	Asthenia, headache, pain, dizziness, somnolence	No titration required; therapy initiated at therapeutic dose
Pregabalin (Lyrica)	75–300 mg/d	Not established	Diplopia, somnolence, ataxia, arthralgias, thrombocytopenia	C-V controlled substance, also for neuropathic pain
Refractory Status Epilepticus				
Midazolam (Versed)	0.1–0.2 mg/kg bolus; maintenance IV at 0.04–2 mg/kg/hr	Not established	Hypotension, respiratory depression	Tachyphylaxis may develop rapidly, requiring frequent dose titrations
Propofol	1–2 mg/kg bolus; maintenance IV at 2–10 mg/kg/hr	Not established	Hypotension, respiratory depression	Cardiac depressant effects at high doses
Pentobarbital	10–20 mg/kg bolus; maintenance IV at 1–5 mg/kg/hr	Not established	Hypotension, respiratory depression, cardiac depressant	Typically requires fluid and/or pressor support

used for management of tonic-clonic and psychomotor seizures. It may be used alone or in combination with other drugs. When used in combination, it is often possible to reduce the adverse effects of the respective agents and achieve a synergistic effect on controlling seizures. Phenytoin is also used prophylactically in neurosurgical patients to prevent seizures in the postoperative period.

Serum Concentration Monitoring. The accepted therapeutic range for phenytoin is 10 to 20 mg/L. At concentrations above this, side effects such as nystagmus, ataxia, and altered cognition are more apparent. The half-life of phenytoin varies considerably among patients and increases with dosage and plasma level. Steady state levels are normally reached in 7 to 14 days but may take up to 28 days in some patients. Except when patients are loaded with phenytoin, obtaining levels more frequently than every 3 to 4 days is rarely necessary.

Phenytoin is highly protein bound, with about 90% of drug in serum bound to albumin. Only the unbound (free) drug is available to exert a pharmacologic effect. Serum phenytoin levels are normally reported as total drug concentrations. Thus, the free concentration is approximately 10% of the total phenytoin concentration, or 1 to 2 mg/L. In patients with hypoalbuminemia, total serum phenytoin levels may appear low when the active free phenytoin component may actually be normal or high. In such patients, measurement of free levels is a better indicator of clinical response. When free phenytoin concentrations are not readily available, total phenytoin levels may be estimated by the following equation:

$$\text{Adjusted phenytoin level} = \text{measured phenytoin} / [(\text{serum albumin}) (0.2) + 0.1]$$

Drug interactions with agents that displace phenytoin from albumin (e.g., valproic acid) will also increase the free concentration and lead to enhanced therapeutic effect or toxicity.

Administration. Phenytoin is available as an IV preparation, chewable tablets, oral suspension, and extended-release capsules. The IV and capsule formulations contain phenytoin sodium, whereas the chewable tablets and suspension contain phenytoin acid. Phenytoin sodium contains 92% phenytoin. In some patients, changing formulations may result in altered serum concentrations due to the different percentages of phenytoin. The extended-release capsule formulation is the only oral form approved for once daily dosing, though daily doses exceeding 400 mg are usually divided.

Administration of phenytoin can present problems for patients receiving enteral feedings. The suspension tends to settle out in the bottle, making it difficult to deliver a specific dose consistently. Vigorous shaking is required to resuspend the drug. When administered concurrently with tube feedings, phenytoin may bind with the feeds, reducing absorption of the drug. Although theoretically possible with all oral forms, this is most frequently reported with the suspension formulation. If serum levels begin declining in patients previously maintained on a fixed dosing regimen, administration may need to be staggered with feedings to allow time for complete absorption. Chewable tablets may be crushed and put down feeding tubes, and the capsules may be emptied and instilled through the tube. The extended phenytoin sodium contained in the capsule formulation retains its delayed release properties even when removed from the capsule shell if administered without crushing.

Parenteral formulations of phenytoin are insoluble in water and contain solvents (propylene glycol and alcohol) to produce a solution. These solvents contribute to the problems associated with parenteral administration. Manufacturers recommend direct push into a running IV line at no more than 50 mg/min. Rates exceeding this lead to cardiac toxicity and hypotension. When administering large loading doses, however, this can be inconvenient. Dilution in various fluids can cause precipitation of the drug. Although not recommended by manufacturers, various researchers have studied administration of phenytoin in 0.45% and 0.9% sodium chloride or lactated Ringer's solution with good results. Most studies mixed the drug in 100 to 500 mL of fluid and used an in-line filter to prevent transmission of microcrystals to the patient. This technique may offer an alternative to IV push when large doses of phenytoin are given. Intramuscular administration is not advisable because absorption is highly erratic, and the extreme alkaline pH of the injection causes tissue damage.

Drug Interactions. Phenytoin is subject to interactions with many other drugs. As mentioned previously, any agents that displace phenytoin from binding sites will potentiate its effect. Warfarin, tricyclic antidepressants, and aspirin are examples of agents that cause displacement interactions. Because phenytoin is metabolized in the liver, drugs inhibiting (e.g., fluconazole, valproic acid) or inducing (e.g., phenobarbital, carbamazepine) hepatic metabolism may alter serum phenytoin concentrations (pharmacokinetic interaction). Additionally, phenytoin can alter effects of other anticonvulsants by unpredictable complex mechanisms. Phenytoin may increase or decrease the action of phenobarbital and valproic acid and decrease the effect of carbamazepine (pharmacodynamic interaction). Patients should be carefully monitored when adding or discontinuing any medications to their regimen when taking phenytoin. Drug–food interactions may also be clinically relevant. Long-term phenytoin administration can lower folic acid levels in patients, whereas folate replacement therapy may decrease its anticonvulsant effects.

Side Effects and Toxicities. With increasing plasma levels, common side effects include nystagmus, drowsiness, ataxia, fatigue, and cognitive impairment. Gastrointestinal (GI) symptoms of nausea, vomiting, or diarrhea are seen frequently. Administering phenytoin with meals can reduce the occurrence of these effects. Some patients may develop a drug-induced fever while on phenytoin. Patients may develop an erythematous morbilliform rash requiring discontinuation of the drug. Gingival hyperplasia is a frequent side effect with long-term phenytoin use. Patients should be counseled on the importance of good oral hygiene to minimize this problem. Rare complications include hepatotoxicity and blood dyscrasias, including thrombocytopenia.

Fosphenytoin (Cerebyx)

Due to the adverse effects associated with parenteral phenytoin, fosphenytoin was developed. It is a water-soluble phosphate ester of phenytoin, which is converted to phenytoin in the blood stream by plasma esterases. Because of molecular weight differences, fosphenytoin is dosed in "phenytoin equivalents," or PEs. Thus, 100 mg PE of fosphenytoin delivers 100 mg of phenytoin. Because it lacks the propylene glycol solvent, fosphenytoin is better tolerated from a cardiovascular standpoint. The maximum rate of administration for fosphenytoin is 150 mg PE/min, compared with 50 mg/min for parenteral phenytoin. Due to the time needed for conversion, faster administration does not equate to faster onset of pharmacologic effect. The formulation has a less basic pH of 9 (compared with pH 12 for phenytoin), so tissue damage and pain from injection are reduced. As a result, fosphenytoin may be given intramuscularly if necessary. As phenytoin is the active component of fosphenytoin, other side effects noted previously with phenytoin are also observed. Pruritus has also been observed in patients receiving fosphenytoin; this is attributed to the phosphate component of the formulation. Although ease of administration and reduced side effects are significant benefits, fosphenytoin is considerably more expensive than phenytoin. Therefore, some health care centers restrict the use of fosphenytoin to patients without central venous access who cannot tolerate enteral phenytoin.

Valproic Acid (Depakene, Depakote, Depacon)

Valproic acid is a carboxylic acid compound that exerts its anticonvulsant activity through increasing brain levels of gamma-aminobutyric acid. There may also be some effect on potassium channels and direct membrane-stabilizing effects. The drug is usually used for treatment of absence seizures or in combination with other agents for control of various convulsive disorders. The enteric-coated formulation, divalproex sodium (Depakote), is metabolized to valproic acid in the gut. An IV formulation, valproate sodium (Depacon), is also available. Dosing is the same for all three products. However, the manufacturer currently recommends that Depacon be dosed no less frequently than 6-hour intervals unless trough serum levels are monitored.

A new extended-release form of divalproex sodium (Depakote ER) is indicated for both seizure control and migraine headache prophylaxis. The tablet is formulated to be administered as a single daily dose, but some epileptologists opt to dose twice daily when used for seizures. Also, there is potential for confusion between the two Depakote formulations, so extra scrutiny is required to ensure that the proper dosage form for the patient is selected.

Serum Concentration Monitoring. The accepted therapeutic range for valproate is 50 to 100 mg/L. However, some studies have shown that higher levels may be necessary for effective seizure control. Most toxicities associated with valproic acid do not seem to be correlated with serum concentration as much as with total dose administered. Steady state plasma levels are normally achieved in 2 to 4 days.

Drug Interactions. Valproic acid is a potent inhibitor of hepatic microsomal enzymes. As such, drugs that are metabolized in the liver are eliminated more slowly from the body. Phenobarbital clearance is decreased considerably when combined with valproic acid. Valproate is greater than 90% bound to plasma proteins, creating the potential for displacement interactions. These effects may occur simultaneously, leading to unpredictable results when valproic acid is combined with other anticonvulsants. Combinations with phenytoin or carbamazepine are representative of this phenomenon, leading to increased toxicities or loss of seizure control when adding or removing agents from a patient's regimen.

Side Effects and Toxicities. Gastrointestinal complaints are the most frequently reported problem with valproic acid therapy; they include nausea, vomiting, indigestion, diarrhea, and anorexia. These can be reduced by administering the dose with food or by changing to an enteric-coated formulation. Central nervous system (CNS) symptoms of drowsiness, ataxia, and tremor are also reported. Hepatotoxicity may occur, usually within the first 6 months of therapy. This has been most commonly reported in children younger than 2 years on multiple anticonvulsants. Minor elevations in liver function test results are often seen and appear to be dose related. Some physicians recommend L-carnitine treatment to protect against hepatotoxicity, but this has not been clearly proved effective. Valproic acid also affects platelet aggregation and may cause thrombocytopenia and other blood dyscrasias. Reduction in dose usually results in an increase in the platelet count.

Carbamazepine (Tegretol)

Carbamazepine is an iminostilbene derivative chemically related to the tricyclic antidepressants. It is believed to reduce polysynaptic responses and block posttetanic potentiation. The drug is useful in the treatment of tonic-clonic, mixed, and psychomotor seizures.

Serum Concentration Monitoring. Serum levels from 4 to 12 mg/L are considered therapeutic for carbamazepine. Steady state levels are initially reached in 3 to 5 days. Carbamazepine, however, has the unique property of inducing its own metabolism (autoinduction). The initial drug half-life of carbamazepine ranges from 25 to 65 hours, but decreases to 12 to 17 hours with long-term dosing. This effect is seen in the first few days of therapy and is normally complete in 3 to 4 weeks. Thus, patients stabilized on a given dose early in the course of therapy may experience decreased levels and loss of seizure control with time. Frequent monitoring and dosage adjustments are necessary in the first few months of treatment to optimize drug therapy.

Drug Interactions. In addition to inducing its own metabolism, carbamazepine can induce the metabolism of other drugs. Interactions have been documented with valproic acid, warfarin, and ethosuximide, resulting in decreased blood levels of these agents. Carbamazepine is 76% bound to plasma proteins; thus, displacement interactions are less a problem than with other anticonvulsants. Other drugs induce (phenobarbital, phenytoin, primidone) or inhibit (valproic acid, cimetidine, erythromycin) the metabolism of carbamazepine and require careful monitoring with concomitant use.

Side Effects and Toxicities. The most common side effects of carbamazepine therapy are drowsiness, dizziness, headache, diplopia, nausea, and vomiting. These may be minimized by slow titration of dose and tend to decrease with time. Serious bone marrow toxicities have been reported, including aplastic anemia, agranulocytosis, and thrombocytopenia; fortunately, these are rare. Leukopenia is the most common blood abnormality seen in about 10% of patients but is usually transient. Skin rashes may occur, ranging from a mildly eczematous form to a Stevens-Johnson syndrome. Carbamazepine may also induce a hyponatremic hypo-osmolar condition similar to the syndrome of inappropriate antidiuretic hormone (SIADH).

Phenobarbital

Phenobarbital is a barbiturate that exerts its anticonvulsant effect by depression of postsynaptic excitatory discharge. Therapeutic levels are between 15 and 40 mg/L. The half-life is extremely long (100 hours); thus, steady state levels will not be reached for 3 to 4 weeks after initiating therapy. However, this does allow for convenient once daily dosing in most patients.

Drug Interactions. Phenobarbital is a potent inducer of hepatic microsomal enzymes. Thus, it may reduce blood concentrations of any drug cleared by the liver, including phenytoin, carbamazepine, and valproic acid. Phenobarbital metabolism may be inhibited by valproic acid or ethanol.

Side Effects and Toxicities. The primary side effects of phenobarbital are sedation, fatigue, and depression. Tolerance to these doses develops with long-term use. In children and the elderly, the drug may produce opposite effects, causing insomnia and hyperactivity. Hypotension can occur with IV administration. Intramuscular injections are painful and can produce tissue necrosis. Respiratory depression can be profound after IV injections, especially when combined with benzodiazepines.

Newer anticonvulsants have been marketed for the management of seizure disorders.

Other Agents

Other anticonvulsants include **felbamate (Felbatol), gabapentin (Neurontin), lamotrigine (Lamictal), tiagabine (Gabitril), topiramate (Topamax), oxcarbazepine (Trileptal), levetiracetam (Keppra), zonisamide (Zonegran), and pregabalin (Lyrica).** These agents are indicated for adjunct use in various convulsive disorders. Lamotrigine, topiramate, and oxcarbazepine have demonstrated efficacy as monotherapy in recent trials and are approved for use as single agents for various seizure types. Some patients have developed severe, life-threatening rashes requiring hospitalization while taking lamotrigine, especially when combined with valproic acid. Patients presenting with a rash while on lamotrigine should normally have therapy discontinued.

Gabapentin and the newer agent levetiracetam are unique among the anticonvulsants because they have not been found to interfere with the metabolism of other seizure medications. This is a desirable property when adding these agents to complex medication regimens. Felbamate has been noted to cause aplastic anemia and liver failure in some patients. Given this, the Food and Drug Administration warned that patients should be withdrawn from felbamate treatment when possible. Current recommendations state that felbamate should only be used in patients refractory to other agents. When the risk of uncontrolled seizures outweighs the potential risk of hematologic or hepatic problems, physicians are encouraged to obtain informed consent and should perform frequent monitoring for associated symptoms.

Oxcarbazepine is an analogue of carbamazepine that appears to lack the hematologic toxicities seen with carbamazepine. Other adverse effects, however, are comparable between the two agents. It also does not appear susceptible to autoinduction as with carbamazepine. In contrast to the classic anticonvulsants, four of the newly available agents have significant elimination via the kidney. Dosage reductions are required for patients with renal impairment managed on gabapentin, topiramate, oxcarbazepine, pregabalin, or levetiracetam.

Long-Term Management of Anticonvulsants

Patients with epilepsy or other secondary seizure disorders often require long-term therapy with anticonvulsants to keep symptoms under control. Maintaining adherence to their medication regimen is crucial, because the most frequent cause of seizures in this population is abrupt withdrawal from anticonvulsants. Patients will need to be counseled on the importance of maintaining dosing schedules, potential side effects and their management, and the possibility for other drugs to interact with their antiepileptic medications. Frequent blood level monitoring may be necessary, especially when titrating doses of newly added agents. Establishing a relationship with a community pharmacist is essential to ensure safe management of this disease. Pharmacists can help patients understand the side effects they encounter and provide close monitoring for drug interactions with prescription and nonprescription medications.

Sedation and Neuromuscular Blockade

The decision to give neuroscience patients sedatives is complex. On one hand, untreated agitation can contribute to ventilator noncompliance, self-extubation, and decannulation; can induce or worsen hypertension; and can elevate intracranial pressure (ICP). However, agitation can also be an important symptom of hypoxemia, evolving sepsis, worsening neurological injury, or pain. Potentially reversible causes of agitation must be identified and treated before giving sedatives because the patient's neurological assessment will be compromised once therapy is started.

After the decision to implement sedation has been made, careful monitoring is important. Aspiration precautions should be instituted when appropriate. Respiratory depression and hypotension are common side effects of sedative regimens, so excessive sedation should be avoided. Prolonged sedation from overzealous administration of these drugs can delay extubation and complicate brain-death protocols. Sedation can also mislead clinicians into suspecting acute neurological deterioration and prompt otherwise unnecessary computed tomography scans. For these reasons it is preferable to titrate sedative administration according to a sedation scale, such as the Ramsay, rather than giving an arbitrary amount. Newer technologies, such as the bispectral index or BIS monitor, may also improve ability to monitor level of sedation. Continuous infusions of sedatives are probably more likely to result in excessive sedation than intermittent administration. Either way, the patient must be allowed to recover at regular intervals to allow neurological assessment. Recent research has focused on developing shorter-acting sedatives to minimize these concerns and make them easier to use. Specific

TABLE 12-5   SEDATION AND NEUROMUSCULAR BLOCKADE

DRUG	DOSE*	ADVERSE EFFECTS	COMMENTS
Benzodiazepines			
Diazepam	0.1–0.2 mg/kg q1–2h *Onset:* 1–3 min	Excessive sedation, respiratory depression, hypotension	Commonly used for initial control of seizures, active metabolite, vein irritant, considerably higher doses may be necessary in patients tolerant to benzodiazepines (see text)
Lorazepam	0.04 mg/kg q2–4h *Onset:* 5–15 min	See diazepam	See diazepam, inactive metabolites, predictable response in critically ill
Midazolam	0.025–0.035 mg/kg q1–2h *Onset:* 1–3 min *Infusion:* 0.05–5 mcg/kg/min	See diazepam, prolonged sedation, especially with continuous infusions	Unpredictable elimination in critically ill patients
Propofol	*Bolus:* 1–2 mg/kg *Infusion:* 5–50 mcg/kg/min	Cardiovascular depression, infection risk with long hang times, hypotension	No withdrawal syndrome, quick recovery, expensive, does not directly lower intracranial pressure
Haloperidol	*Initial:* 2–10 mg; may double q30min until symptoms improve *Onset:* 3–5 min *Maintenance:* 5–40 mg q4h	Extrapyramidal side effects; lowers seizure threshold; hypotension (uncommon)	Works particularly well for delirium, up to 100-mg doses and continuous infusions have been tolerated well
Pentobarbital	3–5 mg/kg over 30 min, then 1 mg/kg/hr *Onset:* <1 min	Cardiac depression	Serum concentration of 30–50 mcg/mL may produce coma with low risk of cardiac side effects; must have level <10 mcg/mL to determine brain death
Dexmedetomidine	0.2–0.7 mcg/kg/hr (may load with 1 mcg/kg over 10 min)	Hypotension, bradycardia	Sedation with arousability maintained, no depression of respiratory drive
Neuromuscular Blockers			
Pancuronium	0.01–0.015 mg/kg q1–2h	Tachycardia	Active metabolite; accumulates in renal failure, "train of four" monitoring with nerve stimulator best for monitoring efficacy
Vecuronium	0.01–0.015 mg/kg; repeat q1h or start 1 mcg/kg/min infusion	Prolonged paralysis increasingly reported	Partially active metabolite may accumulate in renal failure, expensive, use "train of four" monitoring
Cisatracurium	0.1 mg/kg, then 1–3 mcg/kg/min	Minimal histamine release	Does not accumulate in renal or hepatic failure, expensive, monitor "train of four"

*Sedative doses provided are for parenteral management of acute agitation only. Considerably higher doses are occasionally required with long-term use (see text). Chronic oral dosing (where appropriate) will differ and is highly patient specific.

details regarding the use of individual sedatives and neuromuscular blockers can be found in Table 12-5.

Benzodiazepines

Benzodiazepines remain the mainstay for sedation of the neuroscience patient. They can be given as an intermittent IV bolus or a continuous infusion. Benzodiazepines are relatively insoluble in water. This can be an important consideration when fluid limitation is necessary and dose requirements are high. This situation commonly occurs in neuroscience patients with benzodiazepine tolerance for whatever reason (tachyphylaxis) or a history of significant ethanol abuse (accelerated metabolism). The pharmacist should be consulted before dilution when concentrated continuous infusions are required.

Diazepam is the oldest injectable benzodiazepine. It is still frequently used for initial control of seizures. **Lorazepam** has also been available for several years and is particularly use-

ful in patients with hepatic dysfunction because its elimination tends to be preserved under these conditions compared with actions of other benzodiazepines. **Midazolam** is the newest parenteral benzodiazepine, and some clinicians consider it the drug of choice due to its short half-life. However, more recent data have shown that the duration of sedation of all injectable benzodiazepines is roughly equal. In fact, numerous case reports describe long recovery times (i.e., days) after midazolam infusions are stopped in critically ill patients. Midazolam has also been used as a high-dose continuous infusion to control refractory status epilepticus.

Flumazenil is a specific benzodiazepine antagonist that can quickly reverse excessive sedation from these drugs. However, using flumazenil this way is specifically discouraged because it can cause severe withdrawal symptoms and seizures in benzodiazepine-tolerant patients. Patients who receive flumazenil should be monitored closely because it is very short acting. Resedation after it wears off is common.

Other Sedatives

Propofol is a very short-acting sedative that is being used in some ICUs. It is particularly useful when the anticipated duration of sedation is short, because recovery is rapid. Patients with long-term sedation requirements should receive a different agent because the short sedation duration is no longer advantageous. It is the most expensive sedative in routine use. Attempts at using propofol to lower ICP have been disappointing. Individual propofol preparations should not hang for longer than 12 hours because it is provided as a lipid emulsion and is therefore an excellent medium for microbial growth. It is also a significant source of calories that needs to be considered when feeding regimens are titrated. Propofol has also been associated with cardiac toxicity and pancreatic injury; patients should be monitored for symptoms of organ dysfunction with prolonged use.

Dexmedetomidine (Precedex) is a centrally acting alpha agonist with unique sedative properties. It induces sedation, mimicking natural sleep, while allowing the patient to remain easily arousable with no effect on respiratory function. Hypotension may be an issue in patients receiving the drug. **Haloperidol** is a useful sedative and is particularly effective for patients experiencing delirium. Low doses tend to be prescribed, often with disappointing results; however, a properly titrated dose can be safe and effective. Extremely high doses of haloperidol and continuous infusions have been used safely. Conversely, higher doses can cause akesthesias, which may be confused with agitation and lead to adverse effects from continued administration. Close monitoring is key to successful haloperidol use. Haloperidol can lower seizure threshold and is usually not used in patients with known epilepsy. It can also cause hypotension if administered too quickly. The barbiturate **pentobarbital** is usually reserved for inducing pharmacologic coma in the setting of status epilepticus or elevated ICP unresponsive to other treatment. High doses can suppress cardiac function. Serum pentobarbital concentrations can be monitored, but the correlation with efficacy or toxicity is poor. Low concentrations (<10 mcg/mL) need to be documented before declaring brain death in patients who have received high doses of pentobarbital.

Long-Term Management of Sedatives

Long-term sedative use should be reserved for patients in whom agitation secondary to a residual neurological deficit places them or others at risk for harm. Sedatives should be carefully withdrawn at intervals to make sure they are still indicated because excessive or unnecessary sedation can mask or impede neurological recovery. Fall precautions should be observed, even in patients taking these drugs chronically. Aspiration is also a long-term risk. Sudden discontinuation of long-term benzodiazepine therapy can precipitate a withdrawal reaction. Depending on the benzodiazepine, the onset can be delayed for as long as 7 days after cessation of therapy. Extreme agitation with hyperdynamic vital signs is a routine symptom. Seizures are not uncommon. The shorter-acting benzodiazepines alprazolam and lorazepam may have a higher risk of seizure with sudden withdrawal.

Neuromuscular Blockade

Occasionally, a patient may be so combative that neuromuscular blockade (NMB) is warranted. Other indications include short-term paralysis for a bedside procedure or elevated ICP unresponsive to other treatments. NMB is also used to decrease the work of breathing in patients with acute respiratory distress syndrome and increase ventilator compliance, particularly when nonphysiologic modes, such as inverted inspiratory:expiratory ratio, are used. **Pancuronium, vecuronium**, and **cisatracurium** are the most frequently prescribed neuromuscular blockers. Specific details are listed in Table 12-5.

Careful monitoring is important when continuous NMB is prescribed. All neuromuscular blockers are associated with tachyphylaxis. Therefore, as the patient becomes "tolerant" to a drug, higher doses are required. Patients requiring amounts that greatly exceed maximum recommended doses will usually respond to a different agent. Doses should be titrated so that one or two twitches are maintained when a "train of four" is assessed by a nerve stimulator. Failure to monitor carefully increases the risk of excessively prolonged NMB after the drug is stopped. Complete blockade lasting several days after drug discontinuation has been reported, particularly with vecuronium, resulting in abnormal neuromuscular weakness lasting several weeks after initial recovery. In addition, excessive doses waste health care dollars because NMB regimens are very expensive. Patients receiving neuromuscular blockers to improve respiratory status may achieve ventilator compliance goals while technically "subtherapeutic" from a train-of-four perspective. Using this as a therapeutic endpoint is appropriate and should limit episodes of prolonged NMB and reduce drug wastage.

NMB should be stopped regularly to allow a full neurological evaluation, because many signs and symptoms of acute deterioration are masked while the patient is paralyzed. Furthermore, the patient must be adequately sedated (and when appropriate, receive adequate analgesia) at all times while the blockade is in effect. These drugs do *not* have sedative or analgesic properties. Hyperdynamic vital signs may be the only clue that sedation or analgesia is ineffective.

▓ ANTIBIOTICS

Indications

Many neuroscience patients require antibiotic therapy at some point during their hospitalization. Antibiotics are often prescribed as prophylaxis in conjunction with neurosurgical procedures. The initial dose should be infused as close to the time of initial incision as possible (within 2 hours is optimal) for maximal efficacy. Therefore, they are best given in preoperative holding, as opposed to "on call to the operating room (OR)," to avoid ineffective prophylaxis due to unanticipated delays. The value of postoperative doses is controversial.

Occasionally, patients may have an unrelated pre-existing infection, such as a urinary tract infection or community-acquired pneumonia, that requires treatment. In contrast, meningitis and ventricular shunt infections are examples of established CNS infections that require hospitalization for aggressive therapy with antibiotics.

Some patients are admitted with an evolving infection resulting from prehospital events. For example, aspiration of gastric contents during an episode of status epilepticus can lead to bacterial pneumonia in addition to a chemical pneumonitis. Presumptive antibiotics are often prescribed under these circumstances. Trauma victims may present with an open skull fracture or other systemic injuries, such as penetrating abdominal trauma, that require presumptive antibiotics for proper management.

Despite strict adherence to aseptic technique and optimal overall management, neuroscience patients are at high risk for developing nosocomial infections. Neurological impairment increases the risk of pneumonia, as a result of continued aspiration, atelectasis, or prolonged mechanical ventilation. Indwelling devices, such as external ventricular drains, all methods of vascular access, and bladder catheters, are associated with infectious complications. Corticosteroid therapy and inadequate nutritional support also increase risk of nosocomial infection in the neuroscience patient.

General Principles

Proper selection of antibiotics depends on numerous factors. These include the presumed site of infection, local antibiotic sensitivity trends, and patient-specific considerations. For example, pre-existing conditions such as drug allergies, a seizure disorder, or renal dysfunction may preclude use of one antibiotic over another in applicable patients. The selection of an antibiotic regimen for meningitis must take into account the penetration of that drug across the blood–brain barrier.

After a given therapy is selected, the patient is monitored for response and adverse effects. Response is usually determined based on trends in core body temperature, white blood cell count and differential, and results of culture and sensitivity testing. Other tests specific to the infectious source, such as chest radiographs in patients with pneumonia, are also important when grading response. Generally, at least 72 hours are required to gauge the clinical response to a new regimen of antibiotics. Neuroscience patients can be particularly difficult to assess in this capacity. For example, depending on the primary neurological insult, certain patients may remain febrile due to a centrally mediated "resetting" of their core temperature, despite proper treatment of their infection. Corticosteroids can confuse the clinician either by masking an ongoing fever resulting from their antipyretic action or by triggering a sustained leukocytosis. Neuroscience patients may become "colonized" with nosocomial bacteria during a long hospitalization. This results in consistently positive cultures, despite the absence of a clinical infection. Thus, the whole patient must be assessed when determining response to antibiotic therapy.

Compared with other classes of pharmaceuticals, antibiotics (with important exceptions shown in Table 12-6) are remarkably safe to administer. In general, few adverse reactions are related to IV administration. Drug incompatibilities, as always, should be checked before coadministering an antibiotic with another IV fluid or drug infusion. Most IV antibiotics can be given in reasonable volumes of 0.9% normal saline (NS). See Table 12-6 and later discussion of specific antibiotics for details. Known allergies to antibiotics are common because they are so widely prescribed. Therefore, it is necessary to screen each patient for drug allergies before giving the first dose of any antibiotic. The assistance of a pharmacist can be invaluable in assessing the risk of cross-sensitivity in patients with allergies to certain antibiotics requiring treatment for infection.

All antibiotics can disrupt the normal bacterial flora resulting from their antimicrobial action. Often, this does not cause a detectable problem or may elicit only mild diarrhea. Unfortunately, this can also lead to superinfection by allowing other endogenous microorganisms resistant to the antibiotics to multiply unchecked. One possible outcome, pseudomembranous colitis, is characterized by high-output diarrhea (which is occasionally bloody) and can be life threatening. The diagnosis is usually confirmed by the detection of *Clostridium difficile* toxin in a stool sample. Treatment consists of discontinuing the offending antibiotic(s) whenever possible and starting enterally administered antibiotics, such as metronidazole, to treat the *C. difficile* infection. Antidiarrheals and antimotility agents are contraindicated until the cause of the diarrhea has been identified. Another common example of superinfection is a serious nosocomial infection caused by "selected" multiple-drug-resistant microorganisms that typically develops after a lengthy regimen of broad-spectrum antibiotics. The selection of resistant microorganisms (e.g., *Pseudomonas*) through the prolonged use and misuse of antibiotics ultimately affects the ecology of the entire health care facility. The recent emergence of vancomycin-resistant *Enterococcus* (VRE) as a serious nosocomial pathogen is an example. This unfortunate development has an impact on the neuroscience patient in particular, because the propagation of this new pathogen seems to be related to excessive use of vancomycin, which has been commonly prescribed as prophylaxis in neurosurgical patients. The Centers for Disease Control and Prevention (CDC) guidelines discourage the routine use of vancomycin for prophylaxis. Newer antibiotics that are effective against VRE have been developed, but antimicrobial resistance is still a problem.

Specific Antimicrobials

The following is a discussion of specific classes of antibiotics, with special emphasis on nursing implications and application to the neuroscience patient. Specific details regarding dose ranges, clinical use, and adverse effects are listed in Table 12-6.

Beta-Lactam Antibiotics

These antibiotics are the most frequently prescribed class of antimicrobials. This category includes various *penicillins* and *cephalosporins, beta-lactamase inhibitor combinations, monobactams,* and *carbapenems*. They are effective for a wide variety of clinical infections and prophylaxis. Of particular note in the neuroscience patient are the third-generation cephalosporins, which unlike most antibiotics penetrate the blood–brain barrier well. **Ceftazidime** and **ceftriaxone** in particular are useful for gram-negative meningitis and have largely replaced intrathecal instillation of aminoglycosides. Most beta-lactams are eliminated by the kidneys. When high doses of these antibiotics are given to patients with renal failure, subsequent accumulation of the drug can cause neurological side effects, including generalized seizures. Incidence of this adverse drug reaction is probably highest with the carbapenem antibiotic imipenem. A pharmacist can assist with questions regarding the proper dosing of these drugs in patients with renal insufficiency.

A common dilemma encountered in patients prescribed beta-lactam antibiotics is cross-sensitivity. When a beta-lactam

TABLE 12–6   ANTIBIOTICS*

DRUG	DOSE†	ADVERSE EFFECTS‡	COMMENTS‡
Beta-Lactams			
		Adverse effects common to all beta-lactams and related antibiotics include phlebitis, nausea, diarrhea, pseudomembranous colitis, hypersensitivity reactions (see text), rare disturbances in blood counts	All beta-lactams can cause neurotoxicity, including seizures, with prolonged excessive doses
Penicillins			
Penicillin G Ampicillin	5–30 mu/d 4–12 g/d	See above	Particularly useful for *Streptococcus* infections, including *Enterococcus*; weak activity against *Staphylococcus aureus*

Antistaphylococcal penicillins
  Nafcillin
  Methicillin
  Oxacillin
	
	4–12 g/d
	4–12 g/d
	4–12 g/d
		Interstitial nephritis not rare, especially with methicillin, see above	Little activity against anything but *S. aureus* and certain *Streptococcus* strains resistant to methicillin resistant to all 3

Extended spectrum
  Piperacillin
  Ticarcillin
  Mezlocillin
	
	8–18 g/d
	4–24 g/d
	6–18 g/d
		See above, ticarcillin in particular inhibits platelet function	Useful for hospital-acquired gram-negative bacteria; can inactivate aminoglycosides in serum samples, resulting in falsely low values

Cephalosporins			
		See above general adverse effect statement for beta-lactams	Most cephalosporins can falsely elevate creatinine levels
First generation Cefazolin	 2–6 g/d	See above	Most often used for surgical prophylaxis

Second generation
  Cefuroxime
  Cefamandole
	
	2.25–4.5 g/d
	2–12 g/d
		See above
		Hypoprothrombinemia
			Cefuroxime particularly useful for community-acquired pneumonia

Cephamycins
  Cefoxitin
  Cefotetan
	
	3–8 g/d
	2–4 g/d
		See above, can cause hypoprothrombinemia	Expanded spectrum against enterics and anaerobes; good for intra-abdominal infection

Third generation
  Ceftriaxone
  Ceftazidime
  Ceftizoxime
  Cefoperazone
  Cefotaxime
	
	1–4 g/d
	1.5–6 g/d
	2–12 g/d
	2–4 g/d
	2–12 g/d
		See above	All are useful for hospital-acquired pneumonia; ceftazidime and ceftriaxone in particular effective for meningitis

Cefepime	2–4 g/d	See above	Better gram-positive coverage than third-generation agents; use 6 g/d in neutropenia
Beta-Lactamase Inhibitor Combinations			
Ampicillin/sulbactam Ticarcillin/clavulanate Piperacillin/tazobactam Amoxicillin/clavulanate	6–12 g/d 12.4–18.6 g/d 13.5 g/d 1.5–1.75 g/d PO	See above	See information on individual drugs; all have expanded spectrum against enterics, *S. aureus,* and anaerobes
Aztreonam	3–8 g/d	See above	Similar spectrum as ceftazidime, does not cross-react in penicillin-allergic patients
Imipenem/cilastatin	1.5–4 g/d	See above; highest incidence of neurological toxicity, including seizures	Very broad spectrum, usually reserved for patients with known resistant bacteria
Meropenem	1.5–3 g/d	See imipenem—lower risk of seizures	Up to 6 g/d used in meningitis

Aminoglycosides
  Gentamicin
  Tobramycin
  Amikacin
	
	3–5 mg/kg/d
	3–5 mg/kg/d
	15 mg/kg/d
		Nephrotoxicity, possible ototoxicity
		Neuromuscular blockade
			Serum concentration monitoring required to ensure efficacy, minimize toxicity (see text), therapeutic amikacin: peak-25–35; trough, 5–10 mcg/mL

TABLE 12-6 ANTIBIOTICS (Continued)

DRUG	DOSE†	ADVERSE EFFECTS‡	COMMENTS‡

Vancomycin	IV: 2 g/d
	PO: 125 mg q6h
	Intrathecal: 5–10
	  mg q48–72 h
		Red man's syndrome, possible
		  nephrotoxicity, possible ototoxicity
			Role of concentration monitoring
			  controversial: peak-20–40 mcg/mL;
			  trough at least 5 mcg/mL typical
			  therapeutic goals if measured, oral form
			  only useful against Clostridium difficile

Antifungals
  Amphotericin B
	0.25–1.0 mg/
	  kg/d
		Nephrotoxicity, electrolyte depletion
		  fever, chills, hypotension,
		  anaphylaxis
			Drug of choice for the most serious
			  systemic fungal infections, infuse over
			  4–8 hr, not compatible in saline,
			  250–500 mL dilution required

Liposomal amphotericin B	5 mg/kg/d	See above; may be milder than
		  regular amphotericin B
			Several products; not interchangeable;
			  extremely expensive

Fluconazole	100–800 mg/d	Rash, elevated liver function tests	Excellent enteral absorption, limited
			  antifungal spectrum, drug interactions
			  (see text)

Chloramphenicol	50 mg/kg/d	Aplastic anemia, grey syndrome, fever	Excellent penetration across blood–brain barrier

Fluoroquinolones
  Ciprofloxacin
  Moxifloxacin
  Levofloxacin
  Gatifloxacin
	400–1200 mg/d
	400 mg/d
	250–750 mg/d
	200–400 mg/d
		Headache, restlessness, agitation	Significant drug interactions (see text); do
			  not give with antacids, iron, calcium, or
			  sucralfate

Acyclovir	15–30 mg/kg/d	Crystalluria, tremors, seizures	Effective for viral meningitis, infuse over at least 1 hr

Trimethoprim/sulfame-
  thoxazole
	8–20 mg/kg/d
	  (trimethoprim)
		Allergic reactions common, nausea
		  renal failure
			Requires dilution in high volumes of
			  dextrose, interacts with warfarin (see text)

Clindamycin	900–2700 mg/d	Highest risk of pseudomembranous
		  colitis, neuromuscular blockade
		  (rare)
			Effective against anaerobes and S. aureus,
			  useful for aspiration pneumonia and
			  intra-abdominal infection

Metronidazole	1–2 g/d	Diarrhea, metallic taste, disulfiram
		  reaction
			Active against gram-negative anaerobes
			  only; useful in intra-abdominal infections,
			  oral form is drug of choice for treatment
			  of C. difficile

Linezolid	600 mg PO/IV
	  q12h
		Anemia, neutropenia, nausea,
		  diarrhea thrombocytopenia
			IV and oral forms equally effective, active
			  against vancomycin-resistant
			  Enterococcus (VRE) and methicillin-
			  resistant S. aureus (MRSA) very
			  expensive

Daptomycin	4 mg/kg/d	Myopathy, gastrointestinal distress	Active against MRSA and VRE, not indicated for pulmonary infections

*Antimicrobials listed restricted to those most frequently encountered in neuroscience patients.

†All dosing information refers to intravenous administration except where indicated.

‡Adverse effects and comments listed for groups of antimicrobials apply to all antimicrobials in group unless otherwise specified.

is ordered for a patient with a history of hypersensitivity to a similar antibiotic, the allergy must first be characterized. A history of a severe reaction, such as anaphylaxis, to any beta-lactam precludes the use of any related antibiotic, with the possible exception of the monobactam aztreonam. Patients with a history of less severe reactions to a penicillin, such as a rash or hives, should probably not receive another penicillin but will probably tolerate a cephalosporin without incident. Careful monitoring is required, however. The reported incidence of cross-sensitivity of penicillin-allergic patients to a cephalosporin is probably about 5%. Cross-sensitivity with imipenem is about 10%. Aztreonam does not cross-react in penicillin-allergic patients. Because cephalosporin allergies are relatively uncommon, the incidence of cross-sensitivity with other beta-lactam antibiotics is unknown. Chemically distinct antibiotics should probably be used. It is worth not-

ing that allergic-type adverse drug reactions can occur at any time during a course of antibiotics.

Aminoglycosides

The aminoglycosides are powerful antibiotics that are commonly prescribed for nosocomial pneumonia, intra-abdominal infections, and urinary tract infections. They need to be dosed carefully to maximize efficacy and minimize toxicity. Critically ill neuroscience patients often fail to attain therapeutic peak concentrations with typical doses. Furthermore, impaired renal function can lead to excessive aminoglycoside accumulation and cause nephrotoxicity. Therefore, peak and trough serum concentration monitoring is necessary to ensure that the dose selected is safe and effective. These serum samples are usually obtained when the patient has reached a steady state, typically after three to four consecutive, properly timed doses. The recommended time these drug concentrations ("levels") are measured relative to the dose infused varies somewhat. Whatever the strategy, accurate documentation of *actual* infusion times and serum sampling times is critical to allow proper interpretation of aminoglycoside concentrations and prevent inappropriate adjustments. Pharmacists can be of great assistance when questions regarding serum drug concentration sampling arise. Peak concentrations of **gentamicin** or **tobramycin** need to be 6 to 12 mcg/mL to treat most infections adequately, whereas trough concentrations should be less than 2 mcg/mL to reduce the risk of kidney damage.

Recently, an alternative dosing strategy for the aminoglycosides called single daily dosing (SDD) has gained acceptance in many institutions. With SDD, patients with normal renal function receive their entire daily dose as a single 5 to 7 mg/kg infusion. This dosing strategy may increase efficacy and reduce toxicity. Therapeutic peaks for SDD are 12 to 20 mcg/mL, which needs to be considered if an aminoglycoside concentration is reported by the laboratory as toxic. Previously, peaks this high were thought to cause ototoxicity, but this is probably not true. Trough concentrations with SDD are usually undetectable. Therefore, instead of measuring a trough, the second serum level is usually obtained 8 hours after the peak is drawn. Alternatively, the regimen may be evaluated by a single drug concentration measured 6 to 14 hours after an SDD of an aminoglycoside. This number can vary widely and must be compared with a dosing nomogram for proper evaluation. Aminoglycosides should be avoided in patients with myasthenia gravis because they have been shown (rarely) to potentiate neuromuscular junction blockade.

Vancomycin

Vancomycin is a chemically distinct antibiotic that is prescribed for many infections, such as catheter-related sepsis, pneumonia, and meningitis caused by gram-positive bacteria (*Staphylococci, Streptococci*). It is particularly useful in patients with documented allergies to beta-lactam antibiotics. Vancomycin is the drug of choice for the treatment of documented infections with methicillin-resistant *Staphylococcus aureus* (MRSA). Empiric vancomycin prescribing in patients at low risk for MRSA is discouraged by the CDC because of the emergence of *vancomycin-resistant microorganisms*.

An unusual acute flushing or erythematous reaction involving the upper torso and neck, dubbed "red man syndrome," has been associated with the rapid infusion of vancomycin. It resolves spontaneously by slowing down the infusion rate. Hypotension has also been associated with brisk vancomycin administration. To minimize infusion-related adverse effects, each gram of vancomycin should be given over at least 1 hour. Long-standing concerns about the association of excessive vancomycin accumulation with adverse effects, such as ototoxicity and nephrotoxicity, have not been supported in well-designed studies.

Patient-specific vancomycin regimens are calculated based on weight and kidney function. In addition, empiric vancomycin regimens are occasionally monitored with serum drug concentrations (see the section Aminoglycosides). This practice has recently been challenged because the relationship between vancomycin concentrations and efficacy or adverse effects is unclear. The need for vancomycin serum concentration monitoring is less controversial in patients with meningitis, in whom high serum concentrations are needed owing to poor penetration of the drug through the blood–brain barrier. In severe cases of meningitis when aggressive vancomycin therapy is indicated, the drug may be given intrathecally to overcome this problem. Patients receiving strictly prophylactic regimens certainly do not benefit from vancomycin concentration monitoring.

Antifungal Therapy

Antifungals are occasionally prescribed in neuroscience patients, usually for meningitis or urinary tract infections. **Amphotericin B** has been the drug of choice for most serious systemic fungal infections. It is associated with numerous side effects, including hypotension, fever, nephrotoxicity, hypomagnesemia, and hypokalemia. These adverse drug reactions occur to a greater or lesser extent in virtually every patient who receives amphotericin B. Close monitoring is essential. *Potassium supplementation* requirements in excess of 200 mEq/d are not uncommon. Each dose of amphotericin B should be infused over at least 4 hours in an attempt to minimize these side effects, although it can be given faster in otherwise stable outpatients. Some clinicians advocate giving a 1-mg test dose before the first dose because anaphylaxis has been reported rarely, though this practice is increasingly uncommon. There is some evidence that sodium chloride repletion (500 mL of 0.45% to 0.9% NaCl before and/or after the dose) may decrease the risk of nephrotoxicity. Recently, several liposomal amphotericin B products have been marketed. Emerging evidence suggests that the incidence of adverse effects may be lower with these agents. Many centers have developed guidelines regarding their use because of their high cost. The liposomal products all differ and cannot be interchanged. Patients with fungal urinary tract infections may benefit from local treatment with amphotericin B (**not** liposomal), using either intermittent instillations or a continuous bladder irrigation. No systemic absorption occurs, thus avoiding the many side effects mentioned previously.

Fluconazole is an azole antifungal that is usually well tolerated, but resistance has been reported with selected types of isolates. Its excellent blood–brain barrier penetration makes it particularly useful for cryptococcal meningitis in patients with the acquired immunodeficiency syndrome. Oral absorption is almost complete. Fluconazole interacts with several drugs, including warfarin, phenytoin, and cyclosporin. Reducing the dose of these drugs is usually required to prevent toxicity. Newer antifungal agents such as **itraconazole, voriconazole, and caspofungin** have been added to the armamentarium for invasive fungal infections.

Other Antimicrobials

Information about specific antimicrobials not discussed previously is listed in Table 12-6. Specific issues regarding these antimicrobials in neuroscience patients are discussed next.

Chloramphenicol is a broad-spectrum antibiotic that for years was the drug of choice for meningitis. This is due to its excellent penetration into the CNS. Serious hematologic toxicities and the availability of equally effective alternatives limit its use today.

The *fluoroquinolones* (**ciprofloxacin**, others) are useful for many nosocomial and community-acquired infections. Patients with concomitant renal failure require reduced doses to avoid neurological toxicity (see Beta-Lactams). Some fluoroquinolones can interact with several drugs, including warfarin and theophylline. Patients receiving these drugs have an increased risk of toxicity resulting from amplification of their pharmacologic effect when the fluoroquinolone is added. Doses of antacids, oral calcium or magnesium supplements, iron, or sucralfate should not be given within 2 hours of an enterally administered dose of a fluoroquinolone, because absorption of the antibiotic will be impaired. Several new fluoroquinolones have been marketed, with the more recent ones possessing greater activity against gram-positive organisms.

Acyclovir is an antiviral drug that is indicated for patients with serious viral meningitis. IV doses should be infused over at least 1 hour accompanied by adequate fluid intake, to avoid kidney damage from crystallization in the nephrons.

Trimethoprim-sulfamethoxazole is routinely prescribed for urinary tract infections. Occasionally, larger IV doses are prescribed for serious systemic infections with resistant microorganisms, such as *Stenotrophomonas maltophilia, Burkholderia cepacia,* or *Pneumocystis carinii.* Large volumes of IV fluid are required for proper administration. Check with a pharmacist before dilution when fluid restriction or isotonic fluids are important. A history of sulfa allergy, which is common, should always be ruled out before giving trimethoprim-sulfamethoxazole. Dermatologic allergic reactions can be severe (Stevens-Johnson syndrome). Concomitant trimethoprim-sulfamethoxazole can also interact with warfarin and increase the risk of bleeding complications.

Metronidazole and **clindamycin** are two antibiotics with strong activity against anaerobic bacteria. Clindamycin is particularly useful for treating aspiration pneumonia because it also has activity against *S. aureus.* Diarrhea and, uncommonly, pseudomembranous colitis (see previous discussion) are associated with clindamycin. Metronidazole, in addition to being commonly used for intra-abdominal infections, is the drug of choice for pseudomembranous colitis (see previous discussion). The beta-lactamase inhibitor combinations (see Table 12-6) also have excellent antianaerobic activity, thus negating the need for concomitant metronidazole or clindamycin.

Long-Term Management of Antimicrobials

Neuroscience patients usually finish antibiotic therapy for serious infections while still hospitalized. However, home-based IV antimicrobials may rarely be encountered in patients finishing long regimens for difficult-to-treat infections such as fungal meningitis. Proper education of the patient and family is crucial for the safety and efficacy of these comparatively complicated therapies.

Unfortunately, patients with incomplete neurological recovery requiring long-term care are still at an increased risk of developing new infections (see Indications). Prophylactic antibiotics have been prescribed under these circumstances. However, this is generally discouraged because prophylactic antibiotics have not been shown to decrease reliably the risk of clinically significant infections. In addition, when infections occur, they tend to be more difficult to treat because of selection of resistant organisms (see General Principles). Furthermore, avoidable drug interactions, adverse drug effects, and increased health care expenditures are associated with these unnecessary antibiotics. When antibiotics become necessary, proper education of the patient and other caregivers is important, because noncompliance contributes directly to therapeutic failure. Having all prescriptions filled at the same pharmacy can decrease the risk of undetected drug interactions.

STEROIDS

Steroids have several potential indications in the neuroscience patient. However, they can also cause significant side effects. Steroids can have either mineralocorticoid activity or glucocorticoid activity, or both. The mineralocorticoid effect causes sodium and water retention, along with potassium wasting. The anti-inflammatory effect of steroids results from glucocorticoid activity, which causes most of the therapeutic and adverse effects of these drugs. The following discussion is limited to systemic applications of these drugs in neuroscience patients.

Dexamethasone

Dexamethasone is a potent steroid that has nearly exclusive glucocorticoid activity. This is advantageous in patients who require limited fluid intake to prevent edema or minimize swelling. It is usually prescribed for patients with vasogenic edema secondary to tumor. Currently available glucocorticoids are ineffective for the cytotoxic edema that commonly accompanies acute head injury. Dexamethasone has also been used to minimize inflammation after spinal cord surgery.

Other Steroids

Methylprednisolone has mineralocorticoid and glucocorticoid activity. Extremely high doses given for 24 to 48 hours have been shown to improve recovery after spinal cord injury if started within 8 hours of the initial insult.[4,5] However, recent reviews of this research have called to question the magnitude of benefit for this indication.[6] It has also been used for certain neuromuscular disorders (e.g., multiple sclerosis) but can aggravate others (e.g., myasthenia gravis). Fluid and sodium retention limits the usefulness of methylprednisolone in many neuroscience patients.

Hydrocortisone also possesses mineralocorticoid and glucocorticoid activity and closely resembles the cortisol normally produced by the body. It is routinely used in "stress doses" (200 to 400 mg/d) after trauma or major surgery in patients who take long-term steroid therapy. **Corticotropin** or its synthetic form, **cosyntropin**, triggers cortisol secretion from the adrenal glands. Intermittent therapy has helped some patients with multiple sclerosis. It can also be used as a one-time dose to assess adrenal function.

Fludrocortisone is a pure mineralocorticoid. It is used to reverse the temporary sodium wasting that can occur in neuroscience patients. The drug may also be required chronically after pituitary resection. It usually takes 2 to 3 days to assess the maximum effect of fludrocortisone. In patients with diabetes insipidus, desmopressin or vasopressin are preferred treatments due to their rapid onset of action.

Adverse Effects

Most serious adverse effects of steroids result from glucocorticoid activity. Steroids lower glucose tolerance, leading to hyperglycemia and its complications. White blood cell counts rise, but the result is immunosuppression because the cells do not function properly, predisposing the patient to infection. Steroids further confuse the evaluation for infection because they are also antipyretics. They also can prevent or delay wound healing, contribute to muscle atrophy, and cause osteoporosis. Although profound steroid deficiency can make a patient unresponsive to vasopressors, quick IV administration of large doses can cause cardiovascular collapse. An unusual side effect sometimes seen after rapidly infused doses of dexamethasone is anorectal burning. Glucocorticoids can increase potential for GI bleeding. Acid suppressant drugs like H_2 antagonists or proton pump inhibitors are routinely prescribed concomitantly, but have not been conclusively proved effective in preventing this complication. Steroids are appetite stimulants. They can also induce a profound psychological dependence and other neuropsychological changes. Excessive sodium and fluid retention and hypokalemia are common when agents with mineralocorticoid activity are administered. This can be particularly deleterious in patients with underlying heart disease or hypertension.

Long-Term Management of Steroids

Although many neuroscience patients who receive steroids acutely tolerate them fairly well, the incidence of significant adverse effects rises with long-term therapy. Therefore, the risk–benefit ratio needs to be carefully weighed before patients are committed to long-term steroid therapy. After the decision has been made, the minimally effective dose should be used. Drug-free holidays or intermittent ("pulse") therapy should be considered when feasible. However, patients receiving long-term steroid therapy should be instructed never to stop taking it unless instructed to do so by the health care provider. Eventually, the body stops making its own cortisol when high doses of steroids are given for prolonged periods. Abrupt withdrawal can lead to cardiovascular collapse and other complications due to the sudden acute deficiency of this vital hormone. A slow tapering of the dose can minimize these complications. Patients should also be instructed to watch for and report signs of infection (fever, thrush) or GI bleeding (melena, sharp abdominal pain).

▨ DIURETICS

Diuretics are used in neuroscience patients either as part of the hemodynamic management in general or to lower ICP.

The osmotic diuretic **mannitol** is preferred for managing intracranial hypertension because it relieves intracellular edema in addition to prompting a diuresis. Patients with preexisting congestive heart failure should be monitored carefully, because the osmotic load of the drug may shift enough fluid into the intravascular space to cause vascular congestion and pulmonary edema. Serum osmolality should be monitored, especially in patients with renal failure, because the mannitol will accumulate. The drug is ineffective when the serum osmolality exceeds 320 mOsm/kg H_2O. Mannitol is also used to prompt diuresis in an attempt to minimize renal complications after angiography.

Loop diuretics decrease chloride and water reabsorption in the nephron. Therefore, a loop diuretic, such as **furosemide**, may assist in the fluid management of patients with elevated ICP. However, unlike mannitol, it does nothing to reverse intracellular edema directly. Furosemide is also a vasodilator and can lower blood pressure and relieve pulmonary congestion prior to the onset of diuresis. For this reason, IV doses should be given no faster than 10 mg/min. Patients with acute renal failure may receive very large doses in an effort to maintain an adequate urine output. Continuous infusions of furosemide have also been used in this setting. Other, more expensive diuretics, such as bumetanide or torsemide, have been tried, but they provide no advantage over furosemide when given in equipotent doses.

Hypokalemia and hypomagnesemia occur in virtually 100% of patients who receive a loop diuretic. Monitoring serum values and supplementing when necessary are important to minimize the cardiac sequelae associated with these deficiencies. Some clinicians feel that high doses of loop diuretics may be nephrotoxic, but the effects probably result from excessive diuresis and kidney hypoperfusion from hypovolemia. IV doses need to be doubled when switching to enteral therapy, because absorption is only about 50%. Likewise, patients maintained on oral therapy need to have their dose reduced by 50% when converted to a parenteral regimen unless a more vigorous diuresis is desired.

▨ GASTROINTESTINAL AGENTS
Stress Ulcer Prophylaxis

Neuroscience patients in the ICU are at high risk for developing what is called stress-related mucosal damage (SRMD). SRMD can result in hemodynamically significant and occasionally life-threatening upper GI hemorrhage. In addition to being "stressed" as are other critically ill populations, neuroscience patients tend to secrete abnormally large amounts of stomach acid. This risk is further compounded when corticosteroids are concomitantly prescribed. Thus, pharmacologic prophylaxis is routinely prescribed. Whether adequately tolerated upper GI feedings provide acceptable protection against SRMD is controversial. Agents prescribed strictly for SRMD prophylaxis are not typically required as part of the long-term management of neuroscience patients because the risk is only temporary. Due to the costs of administering these drugs, patients should be periodically evaluated for risk of SRMD and have prophylaxis discontinued when appropriate.

TABLE 12-7   STRESS-ULCER PROPHYLAXIS

DRUG	DOSE	ADVERSE EFFECTS	COMMENTS
H$_2$ antagonists			
Ranitidine	IV: 50 mg q8h Infusion: 6.25 mg/h PO: 150 mg q12h	Altered mental status, elevated liver enzymes, thrombocytopenia	Continuous infusions can be titrated based on gastric pH—see text
Cimetidine	IV: 300 mg q8h Infusion: 37.5 mg/h PO: 300 mg q6h	See above	See above, interacts with phenytoin, warfarin, theophylline
Famotidine	IV: 20 mg q12h Infusion: 1.67 mg/h PO: 20 mg q12h	See above	See above, continuous infusion not as well studied as ranitidine and cimetidine
Sucralfate	1 g PO/NG q6h	Constipation, hypophosphatemia	Does not affect gastric pH, do not give through any tube that empties anywhere but the stomach; drug interactions
Omeprazole	PO: 20–40 mg daily	Diarrhea, abdominal pain, drug interations increasingly reported	Not well studied for stress ulcer prophylaxis; do not crush capsule contents for administration by tube
Pantoprazole	PO: 40–80 mg daily IV: 40 mg 1–2x daily	Diarrhea, abdominal pain, phlebitis (IV)	Do not crush tablet for tube use, IV may be given as continuous infusion for gastrointestinal bleeds

Histamine Type 2 Antagonists

Histamine type 2 antagonists (H$_2$ blockers) are effective in preventing SRMD. They act by decreasing stomach acid production. Attempts have been made to correlate a specific targeted gastric aspirate pH with efficacy, but there is no consensus about what that target value should be. A gastric pH that is consistently 3 or lower may need higher doses of H$_2$ antagonists. A continuous infusion that can be titrated according to gastric pH may be indicated, yet tolerance or diminished effect can be seen with long-term infusions. H$_2$ antagonists can also be given enterally in patients with functional GI tracts. Refer to Table 12-7 for specific details.

H$_2$ antagonists are usually well tolerated. They have been associated with acute mental status changes (delirium, sedation), particularly in elderly patients in the ICU. There is also a potential for drug interactions involving these agents. In the neuroscience patient, **cimetidine** can decrease clearance of phenytoin, resulting in potentially toxic phenytoin concentrations. This is particularly significant when cimetidine is started or stopped in a patient already stabilized on a phenytoin regimen. **Ranitidine, nizatidine,** and **famotidine** do not appreciably interact with phenytoin. H$_2$ antagonists may also predispose patients to nosocomial pneumonia. The stomach is usually sterile because it is strongly acidic under normal circumstances. Acid suppression allows bacterial overgrowth, which is then available for aspiration and subsequent infection. However, studies to date comparing acid-reducing SRMD prophylaxis regimens with cytoprotective regimens (see following discussion) have not consistently shown a difference in infectious complications.

Sucralfate

Sucralfate has been extensively studied for SRMD prophylaxis. Many studies have shown it to be as effective as H$_2$ antagonists for preventing SRMD. Sucralfate acts by covering the stomach with a protective coating and stimulating secretion of gastric protective factors. It is not systemically absorbed; therefore, it is ineffective if given through an enteral access tube that empties anywhere but in the stomach. Likewise, suspensions or slurries should not be administered orally, because most of the dose will coat the upper pharynx and esophagus. Because gastric pH is unaffected, it may cause fewer infectious complications. Sucralfate should not be given at the same time as a fluoroquinolone, because absorption of the antibiotic will be impaired. Separating the administration of these drugs by 2 hours will minimize this effect.

Proton Pump Inhibitors

The proton pump inhibitors (PPIs) are strong inhibitors of gastric acid secretion. Examples of drugs in this group include **omeprazole, lansoprazole,** and **pantoprazole.** While their efficacy in treatment of peptic ulcer disease is well established, there are limited trials looking at their use in SRMD. In spite of this, PPIs have proven to raise gastric pH and are often used for SRMD prophylaxis. The only intravenous PPI available is pantoprazole, and its cost somewhat restricts its widespread use for this indication. Oral PPIs are all subject to degradation by stomach acid; thus, all solid dosage forms are enteric coated and should not be crushed. Suspension formulations of PPIs, whether compounded by pharmacy or purchased commercially, are buffered to protect the drug and may be given via feeding tubes.

Other GI Agents

Neurological and neurosurgical patients often experience problems related to the GI tract. Many situations contribute to hypoactive bowel function, including surgery, paralysis, inability to ambulate, and medications such as sedatives and narcotic analgesics. In patients receiving enteral feeds, delayed gastric emptying can lead to increased residuals and possible aspiration. The drugs commonly used for treating these conditions are GI prokinetics and stool softeners or laxatives. *GI prokinetics* stimulate the stomach and intestinal tract to improve gastric emptying and shorten intestinal transit time. The two agents currently used in clinical practice are metoclopramide and erythromycin. Another drug, cisapride (Propulsid), was withdrawn from distribution due to significant drug interactions with certain medications, which potentiated cardiac arrhythmias.

Metoclopramide (Reglan)

Metoclopramide was first introduced to treat diabetic gastroparesis but is often used in various hypoactive GI conditions. It is also used for gastroesophageal reflux disease and as an antiemetic for cancer chemotherapy. Metoclopramide sensitizes GI receptors to acetylcholine. It primarily affects the upper GI tract, with little effect on colon or gall bladder motility. Doses range from 10 to 20 mg given four times daily, 30 minutes before meals or every 6 hours in patients on continuous feeds. Available formulations include tablets, oral liquid, and injection.

Side effects from metoclopramide are related to its dopaminergic actions. The drug antagonizes central and peripheral dopamine receptors. Extrapyramidal and Parkinson-like symptoms may occur in 1% to 9% of patients, but in doses of 20 mg or less the incidence of these side effects is lower. CNS complaints occur in 12% to 24% of patients and consist of drowsiness, restlessness, fatigue, akathisia, and dizziness. GI symptoms reported include nausea and diarrhea. In patients requiring neurological assessments, metoclopramide's CNS actions may affect examination findings.

Erythromycin

Erythromycin is a macrolide antibiotic that has the additional property of stimulating the GI tract. The drug works by stimulating motilin receptors throughout the gut, resulting in increased upper and lower motility. Erythromycin has been studied in diabetics for gastroparesis, as well as in hospitalized patients with decreased bowel function. It has demonstrated efficacy in both groups. Doses are typically smaller than that used for infection, in the range of 125 to 250 mg three to four times daily.

Stool Softeners and Laxatives

These agents are used to promote passage of feces in patients with decreased bowel function. The many available products can be grouped in five primary classes. Bulk-forming laxatives (e.g., psyllium, Metamucil) add fiber to facilitate normal passage of intestinal contents. However, if not given with sufficient fluid, bulk laxatives can have a constipating effect. In fact, these are sometimes given in minimal volume to treat diarrhea. Lubricants (e.g., mineral oil) coat the stool in the intestinal tract to facilitate passage through the colon. Stool softeners (e.g., docusate, Colace) are surfactants that increase the wetting efficiency of intestinal fluid, thus softening fecal mass. Saline laxatives (e.g., milk of magnesia, sodium phosphate) draw water into the bowel through an osmotic process. Finally, stimulant laxatives (e.g., bisacodyl) directly irritate the intestinal wall to promote peristalsis. Overuse of stimulant laxatives can lead to cathartic colon, in which the luminal wall loses tone and functions poorly. Any agent that increases intestinal transit and emptying has the potential to reduce absorption of medications from the gut.

ANTICOAGULANTS AND ANTIPLATELET AGENTS

Drugs that affect coagulation are often encountered in neurological and neurosurgical patients. These may be used to treat primary disease, such as ischemic stroke, or for prophylaxis of embolic complications in immobilized patients. The major anticoagulants used are heparin and warfarin. Antiplatelet agents include dipyridamole, aspirin, ticlopidine, and clopidogrel (Table 12-8).

Heparin

Heparin is used for the treatment and prevention of venous thromboembolism. It acts by combining with antithrombin III, which inhibits the intrinsic clotting cascade (activated factors XII, XI, IX, X, and thrombin). Thus, by inhibiting coagulation, heparin stops formation and growth of thrombi and allows endogenous thrombolytics to eliminate the clot.

Dosing

Traditionally, heparin was dosed by giving a 5000-unit bolus intravenously, followed by a 1000 unit/hr continuous infusion. The rate of infusion is titrated to achieve an activated partial thromboplastin time (aPTT) of 1.5 to 2.5 times control. This normally equates to 50 to 90 seconds in most patients. Recent studies have shown reduced bleeding complications by using a weight-based dosing formula. Patients receive a bolus of 50 to 100 unit/kg, followed by an infusion of 15 to 25 unit/kg/hr. The half-life of heparin ranges from 30 to 150 minutes. Accordingly, serum aPTT measurements should be made 4 to 6 hours after initiation of therapy or any dosage changes. Some institutions are using serum heparin levels or factor X activity levels to guide therapy instead of the aPTT. This is especially useful when other agents such as low-molecular-weight heparin are used in therapeutic doses. For prophylaxis, heparin may also be administered subcutaneously. Common regimens call for 5000 units given every 8 to 12 hours.

Side Effects

The primary complication of heparin therapy is bleeding. The risk of bleeding is greater when the aPTT is above two times the control value. Given its short half-life, reduction or cessation of the infusion will rapidly reverse the effects. Heparin is a combination of different-size polymers, of which only a small portion is believed to cause its anticoagulant effect. Heparin may be reversed by administration of protamine sulfate. A dose of 1 mg of protamine will neutralize approximately 100 units of heparin.

TABLE 12-8 ANTICOAGULANT AND ANTIPLATELET AGENTS

DRUG	DOSE	ADVERSE EFFECTS	COMMENTS
Warfarin (Coumadin)	2–10 mg/d	Bleeding, skin necrosis	INR 2.0–3.0 for most indications; INR 2.5–3.5 for prosthetic valve replacement
Heparin	50–100 U/kg bolus, followed by 15–25 U/kg/hr infusion	Bleeding, thrombocytopenia	APTT 1.5–2.0 × control or 40–80 sec
Enoxaparin (Lovenox)	*Prophylaxis:* 30 mg SQ bid or 40 mg SQ qd *Treatment:* 1 mg/kg SQ q12h or 1.5 mg/kg SQ q24h	Bleeding, pain on injection, thrombocytopenia	Routine laboratory monitoring usually not necessary. Periodic complete blood counts recommended
Aspirin	50–1500 mg/d	GI upset, bleeding	Typical doses range from 81–325 mg/d
Ticlopidine (Ticlid)	250 mg bid	GI upset, bleeding, neutropenia	Routine complete blood counts recommended
Clopidogrel (Plavix)	75 mg qd	GI upset, bleeding	Rare incidence of thrombotic thrombocytopenic purpura
Aspirin/dipyridamole extended release (Aggrenox)	25 mg aspirin/200 mg dipyridamole bid	GI upset, headache	Capsules should be swallowed intact

INR, international normalized ratio; aPTT, activated partial thromboplastin time; GI, gastrointestinal.

Thrombocytopenia is also a complication of heparin therapy. Two primary effects on platelets are seen. One type presents as a slight fall in the platelet count soon after initiation of therapy. This effect is usually transient, with platelet counts tending to stabilize or return to baseline with continued therapy. The second type (autoimmune-mediated heparin-induced thrombocytopenia or HIT) is normally seen after 3 to 5 days of heparin therapy and is characterized by a continual decline in the platelet count. This form of thrombocytopenia is serious and requires cessation of heparin therapy if counts do not stabilize. Measurement of heparin-induced antibodies may be helpful in establishing the diagnosis. Low-molecular-weight heparin (see next section) may be used when this occurs, although it can also rarely cause HIT. Newer agents, the direct thrombin inhibitors, are typically used in current practice for HIT patients requiring anticoagulation. These drugs have no cross-reactivity with the heparin antibodies. Examples of this class include **lepirudin, argatroban, bivalirudin** and **fondaparinux.**

Low-Molecular-Weight Heparin

Low-molecular-weight heparin (LMWH) provides effective anticoagulation while reducing bleeding complications. One such product, **enoxaparin** (Lovenox), is indicated for both prophylaxis and treatment of thromboembolism. Prophylaxis regimens are either 30 mg subcutaneously twice daily or 40 mg subcutaneously once daily. For treatment of active thromboembolic disease, the recommended dose is 1 mg/kg per dose subcutaneously every 12 hours or 1.5 mg/kg per dose daily. The remaining products, **dalteparin** (Fragmin), **tinzaparin** (Innohep), and **ardeparin** (Normiflo), are dosed in anti-factor Xa units. Doses between LMWHs are not interchangeable and must be individualized for each patient. Although the incidence is lower, adverse effects seen with unfractionated heparin are also possible with the low-molecular-weight products.

Warfarin (Coumadin)

Warfarin (Coumadin) is an anticoagulant that prevents synthesis of vitamin K–dependent clotting factors in the liver (factors II, VII, IX, and X). It is used to treat or prevent complications from venous thrombosis, atrial fibrillation with embolization, or pulmonary embolism. Although the anticoagulant effect occurs within 24 hours of initial treatment, the antithrombotic effect is not present for 4 to 7 days. Because warfarin inhibits the *synthesis* of clotting factors, those in circulation are not affected. For this reason, patients are typically maintained on heparin and warfarin for 3 to 5 days to allow for the full antithrombotic effect of warfarin to occur.

Dosing and Therapeutic Monitoring

Normal dosing ranges for warfarin are 2 to 10 mg/d. Doses are titrated to achieve a prothrombin time (PT) of 1.3 to 1.5 times control for deep venous thrombosis or 1.5 to 2.0 times control for prophylaxis in patients with prosthetic heart valves. The World Health Organization now advocates the use of the international normalized ratio (INR) for monitoring warfarin therapy. This method eliminates the variability seen between controls when using the PT. The target INR for most thrombotic conditions is 2.0 to 3.0; for prosthetic heart valves, the desired INR is 2.5 to 3.5. Patients who are ready for discharge prior to full warfarin anticoagulation are commonly "bridged" with an LMWH product as outpatients until the desired PT is achieved.

Side Effects and Drug Interactions

Bleeding is the major concern with warfarin therapy. Warfarin overdoses may be treated by administration of vitamin K, but this will adversely affect continuation of warfarin therapy owing to the synthesis of new clotting factors. Mild bleeding may often be resolved by holding one or more doses. Severe bleeding that is life threatening should be treated with IV fresh frozen plasma. A rare complication of warfarin involves skin necrosis. This occurs within the first 10 days and is due to a hypercoagulable state induced prior to achieving the full antithrombotic effect of the drug. Overlapping heparin administration for the first 5 days of warfarin use helps to minimize this complication. Warfarin is more than 98% bound to albumin, presenting a major bleeding risk from interactions with other highly bound drugs. Because warfarin is eliminated by the liver, enzyme inhibitors can also lead to increased anticoagulant effects.

Antiplatelet Drugs

These drugs prevent platelet aggregation and subsequently reduce formation of arterial thrombi, which could lead to stroke or myocardial infarction. **Aspirin** is the most frequently prescribed antiplatelet agent. It irreversibly acetylates platelet cyclooxygenase, affecting function for the lifespan of the platelet (5 to 7 days). Several studies have shown benefits in neurological conditions, including symptomatic relief of transient ischemic attacks and reduction in incidence of stroke. Doses from these trials ranged from 30 mg/d to 1.5 g/d. Most patients, however, are maintained on doses of 81 to 325 mg/d. In myocardial infarction trials, benefits were also seen with doses in this range. Side effects from these doses are minimal and primarily consist of GI complaints.

Ticlopidine (Ticlid) is another irreversible inhibitor of platelet aggregation and is indicated for patients with cerebral ischemic symptoms or for poststroke patients. It blocks the adenosine diphosphate pathway and has no effect on cyclooxygenase. The recommended dose is 250 mg twice daily, taken with food. Because aspirin and ticlopidine act on platelets through different mechanisms, there may be some beneficial effects to using both together. However, this combination potentiates the effects of aspirin and may lead to toxicities. Ticlopidine is associated with severe neutropenia; thus, routine blood counts are necessary to monitor for this complication. Given this finding, it is rarely prescribed in current practice. Other ticlopidine side effects include diarrhea, rash, and minor bleeding.

Clopidogrel (Plavix) is an analogue of ticlopidine, which was designed to avoid the blood dyscrasias seen with ticlopidine. Benefits have been shown in both neurology and cardiology populations. The standard dose is 75 mg taken once daily, but higher doses may be used during cardiac catheterization procedures. Side effects consist primarily of GI disturbances and rash. Owing to its more favorable safety profile, clopidogrel has largely replaced ticlopidine in clinical practice. Although no problems were observed during clinical trials, cases of thrombotic thrombocytopenic purpura with clopidogrel have been reported.[7]

Aspirin and extended-release dipyridamole (Aggrenox) is the most recent antiplatelet agent introduced for prevention of ischemic stroke. The product consists of 25 mg aspirin plus 200 mg of sustained-release dipyridamole per capsule, given twice daily. Side effects reported are attributable to the individual components and may include gastrointestinal distress, headache, and dizziness.

Long-Term Management of Anticoagulants

Patients with thromboembolic disease often require long-term anticoagulation to prevent further complications. Some conditions in which this may be indicated include deep vein thrombosis, pulmonary embolism, and embolic stroke. The patient must understand the nature of the disease and the need for strict compliance with the medication regimen. Patients should be counseled to watch for any signs or symptoms of bleeding. They should also understand the need for frequent PT monitoring. Dietary counseling is also necessary, because foods rich in vitamin K can blunt the effect of warfarin. Those taking warfarin should be able to identify such foods and maintain consistency in their diet. Patients should be educated about the potential for drug interactions with warfarin. The pharmacist can play a vital role in monitoring the patient's medication regimen for potential problems and offering advice on over-the-counter drugs that may adversely interact with warfarin.

VOLUME EXPANDERS AND INTRAVENOUS FLUIDS

In patients with cerebral ischemic injury from stroke or vasospasm, one cornerstone of treatment involves hypervolemic or hemodilution therapy. This is accomplished by administration of IV fluids (**crystalloids**) or plasma volume expanders (**colloids**). The goal is to increase systemic blood pressure to a level adequate to maintain cerebral perfusion. There is considerable debate among practitioners as to whether colloids or crystalloids are better, so a brief discussion of their respective use follows.

Crystalloids

Crystalloids consist of solutions containing sodium chloride as their osmotic component. When fluids such as 5% dextrose and water (D5W) are infused, the dextrose is rapidly metabolized, leaving free water. This will rapidly equilibrate with extravascular tissues and fluid compartments and can contribute to fluid overload and edema. For this reason, isotonic fluids (0.9% sodium chloride, NS) are preferable for hypervolemic therapy. Because the solution is osmotically consistent with body fluids, the solution remains in the vasculature longer. NS will ultimately equilibrate with other body compartments, so the effect is short lived and requires continuous infusion of large volumes to maintain desired pressures. Alternatively, some clinicians choose to use hypertonic saline solutions (1.8% or 3% sodium chloride) for hypervolemic therapy. These solutions draw fluid from other compartments into the intravascular space, allowing for longer effects on blood pressure with lower administered volumes. Caution should be used when infusing hypertonic solutions through peripheral veins due to the potential for irritation and hemolysis. Using central venous catheters for administration avoids this problem. Frequent electrolyte monitoring is also necessary to avoid hypernatremic complications.

Colloids

Colloid solutions contain osmotically active protein or starch molecules that increase plasma oncotic pressure. As with hypertonic solutions, colloids draw fluid from extravascular spaces and provide more sustained hemodynamic effects. Colloid solutions are normally isotonic, minimizing the potential for hemolysis. The effects from colloid administration usually persist for hours, allowing for intermittent dosing and reduction in total fluid given to the patient relative to crystalloids. **Albumin** is the major contributor to plasma oncotic pressure in the body. Commercially, it is available as a 5% or 25% solution. The 5% solution is isotonic and used when the patient is hypovolemic or when fluid status is not an issue. More concentrated 25% solutions are hypertonic, which is beneficial in fluid-restricted patients or those with cerebral edema. **Plasma protein fraction (Plasmanate, PPF)** comes as a 5% solution of plasma proteins, of which 83% to 90% is albumin. Adverse effects from albumin and PPF are rare and usually arise from hypersensitivity reactions to the proteins. Reactions are more common with PPF than albumin and more prevalent when PPF is infused at greater than 10 mL/min. **Hetastarch** (Hespan, Hextend) is a synthetic colloid used to expand plasma volume. It produces hemodynamic effects much longer than albumin and PPF, ranging from 3 to 12 hours. Recommended doses should not exceed 1500 mL/d; some patients have tolerated larger doses. The large starch molecule in hetastarch adversely affects coagulation and may precipitate bleeding in various patient populations. Case reports of bleeding and neurological deterioration have been noted in neurosurgical patients treated with hetastarch.[8,9] In fact, the manufacturer warns against using it in patients with subarachnoid hemorrhage or in any neurosurgical patient in whom the possibility of intracranial bleeding exists.[10]

ELECTROLYTE MANAGEMENT

Patients hospitalized with neurological conditions often experience electrolyte abnormalities, especially in the ICU. Surgery, fluid balance, medications, and the patient's own pathophysiology may contribute to imbalances in electrolytes. Without correction, such imbalances may worsen the patient's clinical condition. A discussion of important electrolyte disturbances and treatment follows.

Sodium

This is the main extracellular cation in the body. Sodium performs two principal roles: regulating osmotic pressure and water balance between intracellular and extracellular compartments and maintaining acid-base balance. The normal serum level is 135 to 145 mEq/L. Hypernatremia normally results from some form of dehydration and is treated by fluid replenishment. Hyponatremia may result from several causes, which include fluid overload, cerebral salt-wasting syndrome, SIADH, and medications, such as diuretics. Treatment may include fluid restriction for SIADH or sodium replacement. Replacement may be accomplished with hypertonic saline (1.8% or 3% sodium chloride) or by increasing dietary salt intake. Dietary sodium replacements may be added to enteral feeds or taken by mouth in the form of salt tablets. Fludrocortisone (Florinef) is a mineralocorticoid that produces significant sodium retention and increases urinary potassium excretion. It is useful in patients who remain hyponatremic despite aggressive sodium repletion. Doses range from 0.1 to 0.2 mg twice daily.

Potassium

This is the primary intracellular cation and is important in the regulation of acid-base balance, balance of intracellular volume, and maintenance of electrical conduction in cardiac and skeletal muscle. The normal serum range is 3.5 to 5.0 mEq/L.

Hypokalemia is normally due to net body losses (e.g., nasogastric suctioning, vomiting, diarrhea, and diuretics) or redistribution into cells (e.g., alkalosis). Symptoms include confusion, muscle weakness, diminished reflexes, arrhythmias, hypotension, and electrocardiographic (ECG) changes. Treatment consists of potassium replacement through the oral or parenteral route. Many available oral products may be used interchangeably according to patient acceptance. Enteric-coated potassium tablets should be avoided owing to lesions resulting from dose dumping in the intestines. IV potassium replacement must be done carefully to avoid hyperkalemia secondary to a lag in redistribution into cells. Potassium may be administered safely at a rate of 10 mEq/hr in most patients. Rates of 20 to 40 mEq/hr have been used but should be accompanied by close ECG and serum potassium monitoring, which may not be possible in a non-ICU setting. Peripheral infusions of more than 10 mEq/100 mL are associated with burning during administration. Thus, central venous lines or larger veins should be used whenever possible.

Hyperkalemia usually results from excessive potassium repletion, shifts out of cells as with acidosis, and renal failure. Patients experience irritability, nausea, muscle weakness, and ECG changes. Acute therapy for hyperkalemia includes calcium chloride, which is cardioprotective, and sodium bicarbonate or glucose plus insulin, to shift potassium intracellularly. Follow-up or long-term treatment requires exchange resins such as sodium polystyrene sulfonate (Kayexalate), to increase potassium elimination. Severe hyperkalemia may require hemodialysis.

Calcium

The role of calcium in the body is complex and involves various mechanisms, including coagulation, propagation of nerve impulses, insulin release, and cardiac contractility. The accepted normal serum (total) calcium concentration is 8.5 to 10.5 mg/dL. Most laboratories measure total calcium concentrations, but the free or ionized fraction is the active component. Thus, physiologic changes can alter ionized calcium levels and make the total level seem abnormally low or high. Acidosis can raise free levels, whereas alkalosis increases calcium binding to albumin. This can cause a clinically relevant hypocalcemia while total calcium levels appear normal.

Hypoalbuminemia can also result in lowered calcium levels. Total serum calcium values will decrease 0.8 mg/dL for each 1.0 g/dL deviation of albumin below 4.0 g/dL. When the patient's clinical condition complicates interpretation of total serum levels, ionized calcium concentrations may be necessary.

Hypercalcemia most commonly results from malignancy or hyperparathyroidism. Symptoms include nausea, vomiting, bone pain, renal stones, muscle weakness, coma, and cardiac arrhythmias. Treatment modalities include loop diuretics, calcitonin, gallium nitrate, plicamycin, pamidronate, and oral phosphorus supplementation.

Hypocalcemia may result from a number of causes, including poor nutritional status, low serum albumin levels, pancreatitis, vitamin D deficiency, and hypoparathyroidism. Symptoms consist of tetany, abdominal and skeletal muscle cramping, convulsions, irritability, confusion, and cardiac changes. Correction of symptomatic hypocalcemia requires IV replacement. Calcium chloride or calcium gluconate injections are the most common agents used. Most patients receive 1 to 2 g as a single dose repeated as needed based on findings of measurement of blood chemistries. Administration of a 10% solution (1 g/10 mL) at a rate of 1 mL/min is considered safe in most patients. The dose may also be added to maintenance IV fluids. Calcium chloride contains more elemental calcium per gram (13.5 mEq) than calcium gluconate (4.5 mEq).

Magnesium

This is the second major intracellular cation and plays a role in nerve conduction, muscular contractility, and activation of multiple enzyme systems. Normal serum values range from 1.6 to 2.4 mEq/L. Hypermagnesemia almost always results from renal insufficiency and is treated by dialysis or aggressive diuresis. Hypomagnesemia is characterized by paresthesias, muscle weakness, tremor, hyperreflexia, nystagmus, ataxia, seizures, and cardiac arrhythmias. Causes include inadequate intake, reduced GI absorption, primary renal diseases, and iatrogenic renal wasting secondary to medications (e.g., amphotericin, diuretics). Magnesium replacement may be accomplished orally or IV; however, oral magnesium absorption is variable, and large doses can induce diarrhea. Examples of oral regimens include milk of magnesia 5 mL or magnesium oxide 400 mg four times daily. Parenteral magnesium sulfate in doses of 1 to 4 g is commonly used to replenish magnesium stores. Solutions more concentrated than 2 g/100 mL are associated with pain during infusion. A 10% solution may be administered as a bolus at a rate of 1.5 mL/min. As with potassium, a low serum magnesium concentration may indicate a large intracellular deficiency that may require assertive doses over several days to replenish. Follow-up serum measurements are often needed after a "normal" serum level is achieved to ensure intracellular stores are replaced.

Phosphorus

Primarily an intracellular anion, phosphorus is involved in bone formation and is the energy source of adenosine triphosphate to drive numerous physiologic processes. The accepted range for serum phosphorus is 2.5 to 5.0 mg/dL. Hyperphosphatemia is normally a condition accompanying renal failure.

Treatments involve administration of phosphate binders, such as aluminum hydroxide or calcium acetate. Hypophosphatemia occurs most commonly from insufficient nutritional intake, acid-base disturbances, or phosphate-binding drugs (e.g., antacids, sucralfate, calcium salts). Symptoms include malaise, paresthesias, weakness (including respiratory arrest with severe deficiency), confusion, seizures, and coma. Phosphate salts can be given by the oral or parenteral route. Oral intake for moderately low phosphorus levels should start at 50 to 60 mmol/d in three to four divided doses. Doses for IV administration range from 0.08 to 0.25 mmol/kg of lean body weight, depending on the degree of hypophosphatemia and whether the patient is symptomatic. Infusions should be run slowly over 4 to 6 hours to avoid adverse consequences of intravenous phosphate administration.

PHARMACOLOGIC TREATMENT OF MULTIPLE SCLEROSIS

Multiple sclerosis (MS) is an inflammatory autoimmune disorder characterized by the destruction of the myelin sheath around CNS neurons, forming the characteristic plaques and lesions that are seen on magnetic resonance imaging (MRI). Curative measures are still unavailable, and treatment goals focus on improving quality of life and treating complications of the disease for patients diagnosed with MS.

Disease-Modifying Therapies

One of the main focuses of MS treatment is disease modification. This category of therapy focuses on slowing the progression of lesions seen on MRI and reducing the frequency and severity of clinical exacerbations known as acute attacks. Disease-modifying medications currently available for relapsing forms of MS include interferon preparations and glatiramer acetate. The National MS Society recommends the initiation of disease-modifying therapy as soon as possible following a definite diagnosis of MS with active disease.

Interferon Therapy

In 1993, the U.S. Food and Drug Administration (FDA) approved interferon beta-1b (Betaseron), a synthetic analogue of recombinant interferon beta, which was the first agent shown to halt and even reverse disease progression. There are now three interferon preparations available for the treatment of MS: interferon beta-1b (Betaseron), interferon beta-1a (Avonex), and interferon beta-1a (Rebif). The exact mechanism of action is not entirely clear, but the effects of interferons in MS are thought to be due to their ability to enhance immune cell activities. The most common side effects experienced with interferon therapy are flu-like symptoms (chills, fever, malaise, sweating, and myalgia), which can be alleviated by premedication with acetaminophen or ibuprofen and usually lessen after a few months of treatment. It is very important to instruct patients on self-injection techniques, such as rotating injection sites, to help minimize injection-site reactions. Patients should also be cautioned about the possible development of depression and suicidal ideations as side effects of interferon therapy. Because depression is common in MS patients, clinicians should closely monitor patients who develop depression while on these medications because there may be an increased risk of suicide. Patients should be counseled to consult their prescriber immediately if they feel depressed or have any thoughts of suicide. Also, patients should be advised to avoid the use of interferon therapy during pregnancy due to an increased risk of abortion. One limitation of interferon therapy is that some patients develop neutralizing antibodies that can deactivate interferons, and there is debate over how to best manage these patients' medications. Monitoring parameters should include complete blood count with differential and liver function tests at baseline and every 6 months while on interferons to detect potential blood dyscrasias or elevated hepatic enzymes that can occur.

Interferon beta-1b (Betaseron) is dosed as a 0.25-mg (8 million units) subcutaneous (SQ) injection given every other day. It is packaged in vials containing powder for injection that do not require refrigeration. Once reconstituted, the final solution should be used immediately after preparation or kept in a refrigerator and used within 3 hours of reconstitution. The dose is administered by withdrawing 1 mL of the reconstituted solution into a syringe and injecting the mixture subcutaneously into the arms, abdomen, hips, or thighs. Interferon beta-1b contains mannitol and human albumin and is contraindicated in patients with mannitol or albumin hypersensitivity.

Interferon beta-1a (Avonex) is dosed as a 30-mcg (6 million units) intramuscular (IM) injection given once weekly. It is packaged in prefilled syringes and powder for injection that should be stored in a refrigerator. The prefilled syringes should be used within 12 hours once removed from the refrigerator. Once the powder for injection has been reconstituted into solution, the product should be used as soon as possible but may be kept in a refrigerator for up to 6 hours.

When **interferon beta-1a (Rebif)** was approved for MS in 2002, it was the first time the FDA lifted market exclusivity of another product after approving interferon beta-1a (Avonex) for MS in 1996. The approval was based on clinical data demonstrating improved efficacy of Rebif over Avonex in preventing relapses and reducing disease burden seen on MRI over a 24-week period. Interferon beta-1a (Rebif) is given as a three-times-a-week SQ injection with each dose given at least 48 hours apart. The dose is started at 8.8 mcg SQ three times a week and titrated up over 4 weeks to a goal dose of 44 mcg SQ three times a week. Rebif is available in prefilled syringes that should be stored in a refrigerator. Dose administration can be rotated between available injection sites that include the arms, abdomen, hips, and thighs. Because both the Avonex and Rebif formulations of interferon beta-1a contain human albumin and are produced through recombinant DNA technology with Chinese hamster ovarian cells, patients with albumin and hamster protein hypersensitivity should avoid these medications.

Glatiramer Acetate

Glatiramer acetate (Copaxone) is the final agent available for disease modification in MS. It is a mixture of random polymers of the amino acids L-alanine, L-glutamic acid, L-lysine, and L-tyrosine that is antigenically similar to the myelin protein found in the myelin sheath of nerves. The drug's mechanism of action is unknown, but it is thought to suppress T lymphocytes specific for myelin antigen. Glatiramer acetate is given as a 20-mcg SQ injection daily. Most patients experience only mild side effects, with the most common being transient chest tightness, pain, vasodilation, and dyspnea occurring several minutes after injection and lasting less than 20 minutes. The medication is available as vials containing 20 mg glatiramer and 40 mg mannitol that should be stored in a refrigerator and requires reconstitution prior to injection. The reconstituted product contains no preservative and should be used immediately. Glatiramer acetate is contraindicated in patients with mannitol hypersensitivity.

Treatment of Acute Attacks

When MS patients have deterioration in neurologic status that produces function disability, the mainstay of therapy is high-dose use of the corticosteroid methylprednisolone for 3 to 5 days. IV **methylprednisolone (Solu-Medrol)** is administered in divided doses of 500 to 1000 mg/d and may be followed by an oral prednisone taper. While corticosteroid use will not slow disease progression and its mechanism of action in MS is unknown, it is thought to decrease swelling in demyelinating areas to improve patient recovery.

Other Treatment Options

If patients experience progression of MS while on disease-modifying medications, immunosuppressive therapy is an option. **Mitoxantrone (Novantrone)** is a chemotherapeutic agent approved for reducing neurologic disability and/or the frequency of clinical relapses in patients with secondary progressive, progressive relapsing, or worsening relapsing-remitting MS. Mitoxantrone is dosed at 12 mg/m² IV every 3 months and must be diluted in at least 50 mL of NS, D5W, or D5NS prior to administration. The infusion should be given over 5 to 15 minutes into a free-flowing IV infusion of NS, D5W, or D5NS with care to avoid extravasation, because the drug can cause irritation to extravascular tissue even though it has not been proven to be a vesicant. There is a cumulative lifetime dose of 140 mg/m² in patients with MS. Prior to the use of mitoxantrone, an evaluation of left ventricular ejection fraction (LVEF) by echocardiography or multiple gated acquisition (MUGA) scan is recommended, and the drug should not be used in patients with an LVEF less than 50% or a clinically significant reduction in LVEF. Patients should also be monitored for complete blood count with differential prior to each dose of mitoxantrone because myelosuppression occurs in less than 10% of patients, and use should be avoided in MS patients with an absolute neutrophil count less than 1500 cells/mm². Liver function tests should be performed prior to each dose, because mitoxantrone can cause a transient elevation of liver enzymes. Mitoxantrone is classified as pregnancy category D, and its use should be avoided in pregnancy because there is positive evidence of human fetal risk. The drug has moderate emetogenic potential, and a dose of ondansetron 16 mg by mouth (PO) or 8 mg IV plus dexam-

TABLE 12-9   PHARMACOLOGIC TREATMENT OPTIONS FOR PRIMARY MULTIPLE SCLEROSIS SYMPTOMS

SYMPTOM	DRUG AND DOSE	ADVERSE EFFECTS
Spasticity	Baclofen (Lioresal) 5–20 mg tid up to 80 mg/d; continuous intrathecal pump if cannot tolerate or unresponsive to oral therapy	Drowsiness, vertigo, ataxia, weakness
	Tizanidine 4 mg qhs increased to bid or tid frequency up to 36 mg/d	Dry mouth, elevation of liver enzymes, daytime drowsiness
	Diazepam (Valium) 0.5–10 mg 2–4 times/d	Drowsiness, fatigue
	Dantrolene (Dantrium) 25 mg daily up to 100 mg bid–qid	Increased muscle weakness, drowsiness, diarrhea
Urinary (urgency, incontinence, frequency, nocturia)	Oxybutynin (Ditropan) 2.5–5 mg bid or tid up to 5 mg qid; extended-release product 5 mg daily up to 30 mg daily	Dry mouth, constipation, drowsiness
	Tolterodine (Detrol) 1–2 mg bid; extended-release product 2–4 mg daily	Dry mouth
	Tamsulosin (Flomax) 0.4–0.8 mg daily	Headache, dizziness
Fatigue	Amantadine (Symmetrel) 100–200 mg bid	Hypotension, depression, irritability
	Modafinil (Provigil) 100–200 mg daily up to 400 mg/d	Headache, nausea
Sensory (burning, itching, neuralgia)	Carbamazepine (Tegretol) 100 mg bid–tid up to 1200 mg/d	Dizziness, hyponatremia, nausea, ataxia
	Gabapentin (Neurontin) 100 mg tid up to 4800 mg/d	Somnolence, dizziness, ataxia, fatigue
	Amitriptyline (Elavil) 25 mg qhs up to 100 mg/d	Dry mouth, sedation, hypotension
Tremors	Propranolol (Inderal) 20 mg bid up to 320 mg/d	Bradycardia, bronchospasm
	Primidone (Mysoline) 125 mg qhs up to 2000 mg/d in divided doses 3–4 times/d	Drowsiness, ataxia, nausea
	Clonazepam (Klonopin) 0.25 mg bid up to 2 mg/d	Drowsiness, ataxia
Depression	Sertraline (Zoloft) 25 mg daily up to 200 mg/d	Insomnia, dizziness, headache
	Citalopram (Celexa) 20 mg daily up to 60 mg/d	Somnolence, insomnia, nausea
Sexual	Sildenafil (Viagra) 50 mg given 30 min–4 hr before sexual activity; avoid with concurrent use of nitroglycerin	Headache, flushing

ethasone 20 mg PO or IV can be given 30 minutes prior to mitoxantrone as premedication to alleviate nausea and vomiting. Other side effects that commonly occur include headache, alopecia, GI bleeding, diarrhea, abdominal pain, mucositis, stomatitis, upper respiratory tract infection, urinary tract infection, and blue-green discoloration of the urine and sclera.

A number of other agents have been investigated in the treatment of MS. Some of the agents studied include **cyclophosphamide, cyclosporine, azathioprine, natalizumab, alemtuzumab, rituximab, and intravenous immune globulin (IVIg),** but data are limited and further studies are needed.

Symptomatic Management

The main symptoms of MS that may be treated with pharmacologic agents include spasticity, urinary symptoms, fatigue, sensory symptoms (burning, itching, neuralgia), depression, sexual dysfunction, and tremors. Patients experiencing these symptoms can often benefit from nonpharmacologic therapies such as physical therapy and exercise in addition to or as an alternative to medications. Pharmacologic treatment for MS involves initiation of medications at the lowest effective doses and careful titration to effect while

balancing drug side effects. Table 12-9 lists pharmacologic treatment options for primary MS symptoms.

PHARMACOLOGIC TREATMENT OF MYASTHENIA GRAVIS

Muscle weakness and fatigability are the hallmark symptoms of myasthenia gravis (MG), a chronic autoimmune neuromuscular disease in which there is a deficit of acetylcholine receptors at the neuromuscular junctions. Treatment focuses on enhancing neuromuscular transmission with anticholinesterase agents, immunosuppression, thymectomy, and plasmapheresis or IVIg therapy. This section will highlight the pharmacologic treatments with an emphasis on nursing implications of these medications.

Anticholinesterase Drugs

Anticholinesterase agents not only are the first-line treatment for MG symptoms, but are also used in diagnosing the disease. **Edrophonium (Tensilon)** testing is used diagnostically because of the drug's rapid onset within 30 seconds of administration and short duration of action, lasting only 5 minutes. An important note is that atropine must be available for the treatment of possible cholinergic reactions. The test is performed by drawing up 10 mg of edrophonium into a syringe and administering a 2-mg IV test dose over 15 to 30 seconds. If no excessive muscarinic side effects (excessive sweating/salivation, lacrimation, diarrhea, bradycardia, incontinence of stool and urine, pupils <2 mm) are seen, the remaining 8 mg can be given 45 seconds later. If muscle strength improves in an objectively weak muscle, the test is considered positive. Once MG has been diagnosed, the anti-cholinesterase drug **pyridostigmine (Mestinon)** is the first-line medication used to inhibit the destruction of acetyl-choline by acetylcholinesterase and increase impulse transmission at the neuromuscular junctions. Pyridostig-mine has a highly individualized dosing range and is available in liquid syrup, tablets, sustained-release tablets, and IV injection. The drug works quickly within 15 to 30 minutes of administration, with peak effects seen at about 2 hours, and effects last for 3 to 4 hours or longer. The typical dose of the regular release product is 30 to 120 mg PO every 4 to 6 hours. Timing of doses should be individualized; for example, patients who have trouble chewing food may benefit from taking a dose 30 minutes before a meal. If the patient has weakness at night or in the early morning, the sustained-release formulation can be used at bedtime but cannot be crushed. In the setting of myasthenic crisis, in which there is acute weakening and respiratory support is often required, pyridostigmine therapy is usually not effective and may be held until the patient is stabilized. Pyridostigmine has a number of side effects that can be dose limiting, with the most bothersome being gastrointestinal (nausea, abdominal cramps, flatulence, diarrhea, vomiting). Other common side effects include muscle twitching and cramping, blurred vision, urinary urgency, bradycardia, and increased sweating and salivation. Patients can take pyridostigmine with food to reduce some of the gastrointestinal side effects. While anti-cholinesterase therapy benefits most MG patients, symptomatic improvement is usually incomplete and often declines within months, making other forms of therapy necessary.

Immunosuppression

When weakness is not controlled by pyridostigmine, immunosuppressive therapy is indicated, unless there is a contraindication to steroid use. Steroids are commonly used for symptom improvement and disease remission, and the drug of choice is prednisone (Deltasone). Low-dose **prednisone** is started at 15 to 20 mg PO daily and increased by 5 mg every 2 to 3 days until there is a satisfactory response up to 50 to 60 mg/d. Patients usually respond in 2 to 4 weeks and maximal benefit is seen in 6 to 12 months. Therapy can be modified to every-other-day dosing after about 3 months of treatment to minimize steroid side effects, and most patients require at least a small dose of chronic steroid therapy. Initiation of higher-dose steroids can cause a transient steroid-induced weakness that occurs 5 to 10 days after the onset of therapy and lasts 5 to 6 days. Therefore, high-dose steroid therapy is usually reserved for hospitalized patients who are receiving plasmapheresis or IVIg for myasthenic crisis and then titrated to the lowest effective maintenance dose.

If there is an incomplete response to steroid therapy or a contraindication to steroid use, other immunosuppressive agents that can be used include azathioprine (Imuran), cyclosporine (Neoral, Gengraf), and mycophenolate mofetil (CellCept). It is recommended that nurses use special handling precautions such as a mask and gloves when administering these medications to avoid the immunosuppressive effects.

Azathioprine is a derivative of the chemotherapeutic agent 6-mercaptopurine and antagonizes purine metabolism. Azathioprine may not only be useful for patients with an inadequate response to steroid therapy or a contraindication to steroid use (such as uncontrolled diabetes), but it can also be added to steroid therapy so a lower steroid dose can be used. Most patients tolerate azathioprine well, with flu-like symptoms such as fever, chills, and malaise being the most bothersome side effects. Other side effects include nausea, vomiting, diarrhea, thrombocytopenia, leukopenia, anemia, and hepatotoxicity. Azathioprine is started at a dose of 50 mg PO daily for 1 week, and if tolerated, is increased to a target dose of 2 to 3 mg/kg total body weight. One disadvantage of azathioprine is that its therapeutic effects begin slowly and can take 3 to 4 months for a response to occur and up to a year for the full benefits to be achieved. Monitoring parameters should include complete blood count and liver function tests so that bone marrow suppression and liver enzyme elevations can be detected. Azathioprine is contraindicated in pregnancy, and contraception is recommended during therapy.

Cyclosporine inhibits the production and release of interleukin-2 to exert its immunosuppressive effects against MG. While cyclosporine has similar efficacy to azathioprine in MG, it works more quickly, with its effects beginning within 1 to 2 months of therapy initiation. The dose is typically titrated to 5 mg/kg/d given in two divided doses each day. However, cyclosporine has a number of side effects that can preclude its use, including hypertension, diabetes mellitus, tremor, renal impairment, and bone marrow suppression. Serum cyclosporine trough levels must be monitored periodically and dose adjustments made accordingly. Serum creatinine, blood pressure, and complete blood count monitoring is also required during cyclosporine use. Cyclosporine is associated with premature births and low birth weight, so use during pregnancy is only recommended if the benefit to the mother outweighs the fetal risks. Use during breastfeeding is contraindicated because the drug crosses into breast milk. Patients should avoid grapefruit juice because it can increase the absorption of cyclosporine and alter drug levels. Cyclosporine has a number of drug interactions, and a pharmacist can assist when medication changes are made to avoid harmful combinations.

Mycophenolate mofetil exerts its effects by inhibiting purine synthesis. The typical dose used for MG is 1000 mg PO bid. Mycophenolate mofetil has similar side effects to cyclosporine but is typically better tolerated. The most common side effects are nausea, vomiting, diarrhea, and bone marrow suppression. The drug is ideally administered on an empty stomach because food delays absorption; however, mycophenolate mofetil is often given with food to minimize GI adverse effects. Administration with antacids and cholestyramine can decrease drug levels and should be avoided. Monitoring of complete blood count should be done throughout therapy and use avoided in pregnancy and breastfeeding to avoid potential harm.

Intravenous Immune Globulin Therapy

Plasmapheresis and **IVIg** are treatment options for patients with severe MG or in myasthenic crisis who are resistant to other treatment options and need rapid improvement in their weakness. They are also used as a bridge therapy for patients starting immunosuppressive agents or undergoing thymectomy. The exact mechanism of action of IVIg is not clearly understood in MG, but it has been shown to have positive effects in many patients, with improvement beginning in 3 to 10 days and lasting for weeks to months. The typical dose of IVIg is 0.4 g/kg/d IV for 5 days or 1 g/kg/d IV for 2 days based on ideal body weight. Risk for adverse events is higher in patients with IgA deficiency and previous hypersensitivity to immune globulins. A number of different IVIg formulations are available and specific manufacturer guidelines should be followed. Of note, IVIg is very expensive and cost is an important consideration in the decision to use IVIg. An important nursing implication for IVIg use is to begin the infusion slowly, and if tolerated, the rate of infusion can be increased at 30-minute increments based on manufacturer information (e.g., Venoglobulin-I: initial infusion rate 0.01 to 0.02 mL/kg/min, maximum rate of 0.04 mL/kg/min). IVIg can be administered via a peripheral or central line and should not be mixed with other medications. The most common side effects are mild reactions such as arthralgia, cramps, headache, chills, and fever, which are often related to the rate of infusion. Rarely, renal failure, aseptic meningitis, and anaphylaxis have occurred.

Drugs that Worsen Myasthenia Gravis

A number of medications have been associated with clinical worsening of MG by disrupting the transmission of neural impulses to the resting muscle. It is important that patients consult a clinician before taking prescription or over-the-counter medications to avoid disease exacerbation. Drugs that are known to worsen MG include aminoglycoside antibiotics (e.g., gentamicin, tobramycin, amikacin), fluoroquinolone antibiotics (e.g., ciprofloxacin, moxifloxacin), macrolide antibiotics (e.g., erythromycin, azithromycin), clindamycin, D-penicillamine, phenytoin, lithium, beta blockers (e.g., metoprolol, atenolol, timolol), calcium channel blockers (e.g., verapamil, diltiazem), quinine, quinidine, procainamide, chloroquine, radiocontrast agents, neuromuscular blockers (e.g., vecuronium, cisatracurium, succinylcholine), and interferon alfa. If one of these medications is being considered for use in MG patients, it is important to consider alternative medications. In general, when any new medication is used in a patient with MG, careful monitoring for weakness and respiratory insufficiency is advised.

PHARMACOLOGIC TREATMENT OF PARKINSON'S DISEASE

Parkinson's disease (PD) is a degenerative disorder characterized by the progressive development of tremor, rigidity, bradykinesia, and postural instability, most commonly beginning in middle or late life. While the etiology of PD is unknown, the disease primarily affects the dopamine-containing neurons in the substantia nigra of the basal ganglia. No cure exists at this time for PD, and pharmacologic treatment options focus on providing symptomatic relief for patients. The decision when to begin drug therapy for PD is based on the severity of disability and the side effect profile of each drug. The drug classes available for symptomatic therapy for PD include monoamine oxidase B (MAO-B) inhibitors, levodopa, dopamine agonists, anticholinergic agents, catechol-O-methyltransferase (COMT) inhibitors, and amantadine.

Monoamine Oxidase B Inhibitors

In addition to symptomatic improvement in PD, the MAO-B inhibitor class of medications may offer possible neuroprotective effects that could postpone the need for levodopa. **Selegiline (Eldepryl)** is the most widely used MAO-B agent and is usually the first-line agent begun in the treatment of PD. When selegiline is added to levodopa/carbidopa therapy, a dose reduction of levodopa/carbidopa is usually required. Daily doses of 10 mg of selegiline should not be exceeded to avoid an interaction with tyramine-containing products (e.g., red wine, cheeses, aged food) in which sudden and severe high blood pressure can occur. Table 12-10 summarizes treatment options for PD.

Levodopa

The most effective pharmacologic agent available for PD is the dopamine precursor **levodopa**. Dopamine cannot be given orally because it is metabolized before it reaches the brain. However, levodopa crosses the blood–brain barrier and is centrally converted to dopamine by DOPA decarboxylase to replenish dopamine, which is deficient in the basal ganglia of PD patients. Because levodopa must be converted to dopamine within the brain, the addition of the peripheral DOPA decarboxylase inhibitor **carbidopa** blocks peripheral conversion of levodopa to dopamine, thus increasing the amount of levodopa available to the brain for conversion to dopamine. The addition of carbidopa also limits the peripheral side effects of levodopa such as nausea, vomiting, arrhythmias, and orthostatic hypotension. Therefore, the combination product **levodopa/carbidopa (Sinemet)** is the mainstay of PD drug therapy.

The decision when to initiate levodopa therapy can be difficult because the drug has a number of bothersome side effects including orthostatic hypotension, nausea, vomiting, sedation, dyskinesias (abnormal involuntary movements), nightmares, hallucinations, and anxiety. Treatment with levodopa is usually delayed until a patient has moderate disability and inadequate symptomatic control with alternate medications. Long-term levodopa therapy is associated with motor fluctuations and involuntary movements. The "on-off" phenomenon that occurs with long-term levodopa therapy involves rapid fluctuations from normal or dyskinetic "on" motor activity to bradykinetic "off" periods in which movement is difficult or impossible for patients, all within a

TABLE 12–10 PHARMACOLOGIC TREATMENT OPTIONS FOR PARKINSON'S DISEASE

DRUG CLASS	DRUG AND DOSE	ADVERSE EFFECTS
Monoamine oxidase B (MAO-B) inhibitor	Selegiline (Eldepryl) 5 mg bid with breakfast and lunch or 10 mg q$_{AM}$	Nausea, abdominal pain, dry mouth, confusion, hallucinations, insomnia, orthostatic hypotension, dyskinesias, nightmares
Carbidopa/ levodopa (Sinemet)	Regular-release product started at 10/100 mg or 25/100 mg 2–4 times/d; increase slowly to maximum of 200/2000 mg/d ***Regular-release*** tablet strengths available: • 10 mg carbidopa/100 mg levodopa • 25 mg carbidopa/100 mg levodopa • 25 mg carbidopa/250 mg levodopa ***Sustained-release*** tablet strengths available: • 25 mg carbidopa/100 mg levodopa • 50 mg carbidopa/200 mg levodopa	Nausea, vomiting, dyskinesias, dry mouth, orthostatic hypotension, hallucinations, constipation, dizziness, "on-off" phenomenon, dry mouth, depression
Carbidopa plus levodopa plus entacapone (Stalevo)	• 12.5 mg carbidopa, 50 mg levodopa, 200 mg entacapone • 25 mg carbidopa, 100 mg levodopa, 200 mg entacapone • 37.5 mg carbidopa, 150 mg levodopa, 200 mg entacapone	
Dopamine agonists	Bromocriptine (Parlodel) 1.25 mg bid increased by 2.5 mg/d in 2- to 4-wk intervals to usual dose range of 15–40 mg/d divided bid or tid Pramipexole (Mirapex) 0.125 mg tid increased by 0.75 mg/d qweek to usual dose of 1.5–4.5 mg/d divided tid Ropinirole (Requip) 0.25 mg tid increased by 0.75 mg/d qweek to usual dose of 3–12 mg/d divided tid	Nausea, headache, hallucinations, dyskinesias, somnolence, vomiting, postural hypotension, dizziness, fatigue, constipation, insomnia, vivid dreams, paranoid delusions
Anti-cholinergics	Benztropine (Cogentin) 0.5–1 mg/d increased in 0.5 mg/d increments q5–6d to max of 6 mg/d divided tid Trihexyphenidyl (Artane) 1 mg/d increased in 2 mg/d increments q3–5d to max of 12–15 mg/d divided tid (usual maintenance dose 3–10 mg/d)	Dry mouth, blurred vision, urinary retention, constipation, confusion, nervousness, nausea, sedation, forgetfulness
Catechol-O-methyl-transferase (COMT) inhibitors	Tolcapone* (Tasmar) 100–200 mg tid in combination with levodopa/carbidopa Entacapone (Comtan) 200 mg dose, up to max of 8 times/d in combination with levodopa/carbidopa	Nausea, dyskinesia, dizziness, fatigue, hallucinations, diarrhea, brown-orange urine discoloration Prolongs half-life of levodopa
Antiviral	Amantadine (Symmetrel) 100 mg/d increased by 100 mg/d q7–14d to max of 400 mg/d divided bid; dose adjustments necessary for renal impairment	Dry mouth, orthostatic hypotension, peripheral edema, insomnia, depression, anxiety, hallucinations, livedo reticularis (diffuse mottling of the skin), congestive heart failure, psychosis

*Use of tolcapone is restricted due to reports of fatal liver injury associated with use of this drug.

few minutes. End-of-dose deterioration or "wearing off" can occur with long-term levodopa use and may be lessened with more frequent dose administration or use of a controlled-release product.

Providing patients with information concerning levodopa is an important step for the health care provider. Patients should be counseled that while levodopa is best absorbed on an empty stomach, nausea is a common side effect; if nausea occurs, patients should take levodopa with food to minimize GI effects. High-protein foods (e.g., eggs, dairy products, nuts, meats, and soybean products) can inhibit the efficacy of levodopa and should be evenly distributed in moderation throughout the day to avoid fluctuations in levodopa absorption. Patients should be careful to rise slowly from a lying or sitting position because dizziness, lightheadedness, or fainting may occur. Consumption of alcohol can increase CNS depression when used with levodopa and should be avoided. **Pyridoxine (vitamin B$_6$)** and multivitamin prepara-

tions containing pyridoxine can decrease the efficacy of levodopa and concomitant use should generally be avoided. Also, patients should be instructed to avoid crushing or chewing sustained-release levodopa/carbidopa products.

Dopamine Agonists

The dopamine agonists currently available for the treatment of PD include **bromocriptine (Parlodel), pergolide (Permax), pramipexole (Mirapex), and ropinirole (Requip)**. Bromocriptine and pergolide are ergot-derived dopamine agonists, and pramipexole and ropinirole are non–ergot-derived dopamine agonists. There are three dopamine receptors (D1 to D3). Bromocriptine and pergolide stimulate D2 receptors and partially antagonize D1 receptors, while pramipexole and ropinirole act at D2 and D3 receptors but have no activity at the D1 receptor. The D2 receptors are thought to have a critical role in improving akinesia, bradykinesia, rigidity, and gait disturbances present in PD.

Dopamine agonists are useful in decreasing the frequency of "off" periods and providing a levodopa-sparing effect. Dopamine agonists are useful when added to levodopa therapy for patients with inability to tolerate higher doses of levodopa, patients with declining response to levodopa, and patients with fluctuations in their response to levodopa. While it is controversial and still under investigation, dopamine agonists may be used as initial therapy for PD, especially in younger patients. Older PD patients are more likely to have psychosis from dopamine agonists, and levodopa/carbidopa is typically the best first-line agent for elderly PD patients.

Side effects often limit the use of dopamine agonists in PD. The most common side effect is nausea/vomiting, and these drugs should be taken with food to minimize GI upset. Dopamine agonists may also cause dizziness, drowsiness, hypotension, and fainting, especially after the first dose; therefore, patients should use caution when driving, operating machinery, or performing tasks that require mental alertness. Alcohol should be avoided with the use of dopamine agonists due to increased CNS depression. Other common side effects are confusion, headache, lightheadedness, constipation, hallucinations, daytime sedation, vivid dreams, paranoid delusions, and dyskinesias.

Anticholinergic Agents

When tremor is the most prominent problem for PD patients, anticholinergic agents may be useful. Anticholinergic agents reduce the relative excess of cholinergic activity in the basal ganglia that develops because of dopamine deficiency in this area of the brain. The most commonly used anticholinergic medications for PD are **benztropine (Cogentin)** and **trihexyphenidyl (Artane)**. These agents can be used alone or in combination with levodopa and other antiparkinsonian agents. Side effects most commonly noted are dry mouth, blurred vision, constipation, and urinary retention. More concerning adverse effects include confusion, sedation, and memory impairment. Alcohol should be avoided with the use of anticholinergic agents. Elderly patients are more sensitive to the effects of anticholinergics, and lower doses are usually sufficient for symptomatic control.

Catechol-O-Methyltransferase Inhibitors

COMT inhibitors are a newer class of drugs that extend the effects of each levodopa dose. Two products, **tolcapone (Tasmar)** and **entacapone (Comtan)**, are currently available. These agents act as reversible and selective inhibitors of catechol-O-methyltransferase and have no effect on PD without levodopa. When taken with levodopa, COMT inhibitors alter the pharmacokinetics of levodopa by preventing the peripheral conversion of levodopa to 3-O-methyldopa, resulting in more sustained levodopa serum levels than levodopa taken alone. The resulting levodopa levels provide for increased concentrations available for absorption across the blood–brain barrier, thus prolonging the dopaminergic effects of levodopa. Tolcapone has been linked to three cases of fatal hepatotoxicity and is rarely prescribed for patients since an alternative is available in entacapone, which has not been reported to cause hepatotoxicity. At least a 25% reduction in the levodopa/carbidopa dose must typically take place upon initiation of COMT inhibitor therapy to manage dopaminergic side effects. Possible nausea, hallucinations, and a clinically irrelevant urinary discoloration may occur with the use of entacapone and tolcapone.

Amantadine

Amantadine (Symmetrel) is an antiviral drug that can be effective for symptomatic relief in mild PD. The exact mechanism of antiparkinsonian activity of amantadine is unknown, but the drug does block the reuptake of dopamine into presynaptic neurons, increase dopamine release from presynaptic fibers, and exert anticholinergic effects. The benefits obtained from amantadine are short lived, and loss of antiparkinson effects occurs in most patients after 6 to 12 weeks of therapy. The drug can be given alone or in combination with levodopa. Amantadine can be helpful for the "wearing-off" phenomenon with levodopa, and can also be especially useful against tremor due to its anticholinergic effects. Because amantadine is renally cleared, dose reduction is necessary in renal impairment. Common side effects include nausea, dizziness, insomnia, confusion, hallucinations, anxiety, restlessness, depression, irritability, peripheral edema, and orthostatic hypotension. Livedo reticularis, a diffuse mottling of the skin, is a common and reversible side effect of amantadine. Rare side effects include congestive heart failure, psychosis, urinary retention, and reversible elevations in liver enzymes.

Conclusion

Even though no cure is yet available for PD, a number of pharmacologic options exist for the symptomatic treatment of PD. While problems are associated with levodopa use, it remains the standard of therapy for PD. MAO-B inhibitors, dopamine agonists, anticholinergic agents, COMT inhibitors, and the antiviral amantadine are other agents available for PD. Drug-free periods or "drug holidays" have been investigated but are rarely recommended because of the associated risks and because limited gains have been observed for most patients. The goal of PD drug therapy continues to be maintaining acceptable symptomatic control with the minimum doses of antiparkinsonian drug(s) needed.

▌SUMMARY

This chapter is designed to be a quick reference for neuroscience nurses to assist them in understanding the neurological implications of the most commonly used pharmacologic interventions administered to the neuroscience patient population. For information on specific medications not included here, consult a pharmacist or standard references on the subject. By including the pharmacist in discussions regarding neurological pharmacotherapy, the neuroscience nurse enables them to become members of the team providing care to the neuroscience patient and increases opportunity for positive outcomes.

REFERENCES

1. Horn, E., & Jacobi, J. (2006). The critical care clinical pharmacist: Evolution of an essential team member. *Critical Care Medicine, 34,* 3(suppl.), S46–S51.
2. Janning, S. W., Stevenson, J. G., & Smolarek, R. T. (1996). Implementing comprehensive pharmaceutical services at an academic tertiary care hospital. *American Journal of Health-System Pharmacy, 53,* 542–547.
3. Kellum, J. A., & Decker, J. M. (2001). Use of dopamine in acute renal failure: A meta-analysis. *Critical Care Medicine, 29,* 1526–1531.
4. Bracken, M. B., Shepard, M. J., Collins, W. F., Holford, T. R., Young, W., Baskin, D. S., et al. (1995). A randomized, controlled trial of methylprednisolone or naloxone in the treatment of acute spinal cord injury. *New England Journal of Medicine, 322,* 1405–1411.
5. Bracken, M. B., Shepard, M. J., Holford, T. R., Leo-Summers, L., Aldrich, E. F., Fazl, M., et al. (1997). Administration of methylprednisolone for 24 or 48 hours or tirilazad mesylate for 48 hours in the treatment of acute spinal cord injury. *JAMA, 277,* 1597–1604.
6. Hurlbert, R. J. (2001). The role of steroids in acute spinal cord injury: An evidence-based analysis. *Spine, 26,* (suppl.), S39–S46.
7. Bennett, C. L., Connors, J. M., Carwile, J. M., Moake, J. L., Bell, W. R., Tarantolo, S. R., et al. (2000). Thrombotic thrombocytopenic purpura associated with clopidogrel. *New England Journal of Medicine, 342,* 1773–1777.
8. Toole, J. G. (1987). Use of hetastarch for volume expansion-response [letter]. *Journal of Neurosurgery, 66,* 636.
9. Cully, M. D., Larson, C. P., & Silverberg, G. D. (1987). Hetastarch coagulopathy in a neurosurgical patient [letter]. *Anesthesiology, 66,* 706–707.
10. *Hextend product information.* (2004). Lake Forest, IL: Hospira, Inc.

RESOURCES

Books

AHFS drug information 2006. (2005). Bethesda, MD: American Society of Health-System Pharmacists.
DiPiro, J. T., Talbert, R. L., Yee, G. C., Matzke, G. R., & Wells, B. G. (2005). *Pharmacotherapy: A pathophysiologic approach* (6th ed.). New York: McGraw-Hill.
Gahart, B. L., & Nazareno, A. R. (2005). *Intravenous medications* (21st ed.). St. Louis, MO: Mosby.
Drug facts and comparisons 2006. (2005). St. Louis, MO: Facts and Comparisons.
Lacy, C. F., Armstrong, L. L., Goldman, M. P., & Lance, L. L. (Eds.). (2005). *Drug information handbook* (13th ed.). Hudson, OH: Lexi-Comp.
Samuels, M. A. (Ed.). (1999). *Manual of neurologic therapeutics* (6th ed.). Philadelphia, PA: Lippincott Williams & Wilkins.

Periodicals

Allen, M. E., Kopp, B. J., & Erstad, B. L. (2004). Stress ulcer prophylaxis in the postoperative period. *American Journal of Health-System Pharmacy, 61,* 588–596.
Anonymous. (1999). ASHP therapeutic guidelines on stress ulcer prophylaxis. *American Journal of Health-System Pharmacy, 56,* 347–379.
Ballow, M. (2005). Clinical and investigational considerations for the use of IGIV therapy. *American Journal of Health-System Pharmacy, 62,* (Suppl. 3) S12–S18.
Choi, P. T., Yip, G., Quinonez, L. G., & Cook, D. J. (1999). Crystalloids vs. colloids in fluid resuscitation: A systematic review. *Critical Care Medicine, 27,* 200–210.
Drachman, D. B. (1994). Myasthenia gravis. *New England Journal of Medicine, 330,* 1797–1810.
Hirsch, J., Albers, G. W., Guyatt, G. H., Schunemann, H. J., et al. (2004). The seventh ACCP conference on antithrombotic and thrombolytic therapy: Evidence-based guidelines. *Chest, 126,* (suppl.), 163s–704s.
Jacobi, J., Fraser, G. L., Coursin, D. B., Riker, R. R., Fontaine, D., Wittbrodt, E. T., et al. (2002). Clinical practice guidelines for the sustained use of sedatives and analgesics in the critically ill adult. *Critical Care Medicine, 30,* 119–141.
Nasraway, S. A., Jacobi, J., & Murray, M. J. (2002). Sedation, analgesia, and neuromuscular blockade of the critically ill adult: Revised clinical practice guidelines for 2002. *American Journal of Health-System Pharmacy, 59,* 147–195.
Rascol, O., Goetz, C., Koller, W., Poewe, W., & Sampaio, C. (2002). Treatment interventions for Parkinson's disease: An evidence based assessment. *The Lancet, 359,* 1589–1598.
Siderowf, A., & Stern, M. (2003). Update on Parkinson disease. *Annals of Internal Medicine, 138,* 651–658.
Stangel, M., Hartung, H., Marx, P., & Gold, R. (1998). Intravenous immunoglobulin treatment of neurological autoimmune diseases. *Journal of Neurological Sciences, 153,* 203–214.
The SAFE Study Investigators. (2004). A comparison of albumin and saline for fluid resuscitation in the intensive care unit. *New England Journal of Medicine, 350,* 2247–2256.
Wagner, B. K. J., & D'Amelio, L. F. (1993). Pharmacologic and clinical considerations in selecting crystalloid, colloidal, and oxygen-carrying resuscitation fluids, part 1. *Clinical Pharmacy, 12,* 335–346.
Wagner, B. K. J., & D'Amelio, L. F. (1993). Pharmacologic and clinical considerations in selecting crystalloid, colloidal, and oxygen-carrying resuscitation fluids, part 2. *Clinical Pharmacy, 12,* 415–428.
Wittbrodt, E. T. (1997). Drugs and myasthenia gravis: An update. *Archives of Internal Medicine, 157,* 399–408.

Selected Websites

National Multiple Sclerosis Society: www.nationalmssociety.org
Myasthenia Gravis Foundation of America, Inc.: www.myasthenia.org

Section 4

Common Management Problems With Neuroscience Patients

Intracranial Hypertension: Theory and Management of Increased Intracranial Pressure

Joanne V. Hickey and DaiWai M. Olson

Intracranial hypertension is a clinically significant common pathophysiologic problem addressed daily by nurses and physicians who care for neuroscience patients. However, the specific sequence of pathophysiologic events leading to a sustained or unstable elevation in intracranial pressure (ICP) is still poorly understood. This chapter reviews the underlying physiologic cerebral hemodynamics and ICP concepts and applies this knowledge to the assessment and interventions for patient management.

CONCEPT OF INTRACRANIAL PRESSURE

Intracranial pressure is, literally, the pressure inside the cranium. As simple as it sounds, however, ICP represents a complex and dynamic constantly changing set of parameters. Pressure is determined by two variables, size and volume. The skull is a rigid bony structure incapable of changing in size during acute changes in ICP. Thus, within the cranial vault all components that occupy the intracranial space contribute to the ICP. Typically, we think of the three main space-occupying substances as being cerebrospinal fluid (CSF), blood, and tissue.

Under normal conditions, ICP is determined by changes in the intracranial blood volume and changes in the pressure exerted by the CSF that circulates around the brain and spinal cord and within the cerebral ventricles. Cardiac and respiratory components are superimposed on the ICP, which is referenced to atmospheric pressure. The normal range of ICP is generally 0 to 10 mm Hg, although 15 mm Hg is considered the upper limit of normal. In the clinical setting, ICP values are generally expressed as the average or mean ICP over a given unit of time. Abrupt change in ICP from a stable level in response to activity or to a sudden change in volume is called *transient increased ICP*. It is surmised that different physiologic mechanisms control steady and transient states of ICP.[1] With cerebral trauma or neurological disease, the normal homeostatic mechanisms controlling ICP may be disrupted, resulting in a sustained high ICP and eventual neurological and clinical death.

Because of the different compartments within the intracranial space, ICP can vary widely within different areas of the brain, especially with cerebral edema related to trauma or other disease entities. For example, the pressure in the tissue adjacent to an expanding, space-occupying lesion can be elevated, whereas the intraventricular pressure remains within a normal range. Additionally, elevated ICP is not always conveyed to the lumbar subarachnoid space where it would be reflected during a lumbar puncture. It is, therefore, more accurate to think in terms of ICP pressures, rather than a single, uniform ICP pressure.

Physiologic Considerations

Monro-Kellie Hypothesis

The average intracranial volume in the adult is approximately 1700 mL, composed of the brain (1400 mL), CSF (150 mL), and blood (150 mL). Basic to an understanding of the pathophysiologic changes related to ICP is the **Monro-Kellie hypothesis** (Box 13-1). It states that the skull, a rigid compartment, is filled to capacity with essentially noncompressible contents—brain and interstitial fluid (80%), intravascular blood (10%), and CSF (in the ventricles and subarachnoid space; 10%). The volume of these three components remains nearly constant in a state of *dynamic equilibrium.* If the volume of any one component increases, another component must decrease reciprocally for the overall volume and dynamic equilibrium to remain constant. If the volume of any one component increases with a reciprocal decrease in one of the other components, ICP will rise. This hypothesis applies *only* when the skull is fused (i.e., a closed box). Infants or very young children who have skulls with nonfused suture lines have some space for expansion of the intracranial space in response to increased volume, at least initially.

Volume–Pressure Relationship Within the Intracranial Cavity

According to the Monro-Kellie hypothesis, reciprocal compensation occurs among the three intracranial components—

brain tissue, blood, and CSF—to accommodate any alterations within the intracranial contents. The compensatory mechanisms that maintain the intracranial volume in a steady state include the following:

- Displacement of some CSF from the ventricles and cerebral subarachnoid space through the foramen magnum to the spinal subarachnoid space and through the optic foramen to the perioptic subarachnoid space (basal subarachnoid cisterns)
- Displacement of some blood by compression of the low-pressure venous system, especially the dural sinuses
- Decreased production of CSF
- Vasoconstriction of the cerebral vasculature, which results in a decrease in the intracranial blood volume

However, the amount of displacement of the brain, CSF, or blood that can occur through compensatory mechanisms is limited. After compensatory mechanisms have been exceeded, ICP rises and intracranial hypertension results. Specific medical therapies that have been used to maintain the intracranial volume in a steady state include the following:

- Displacement of some CSF from the cerebral ventricular system through an intraventricular shunt.
- Displacement of some blood by inducing arterial vasoconstriction. Vasoconstriction reduces the capacity of the artery to carry blood and thereby results in a net decrease in the volume of blood in the cranial vault.
- Displacement of some brain tissue volume through mechanisms to decrease intracellular volume. An example of this is seen when the increased osmotic pressure of the circulating blood draws off free water from brain cells and results in a net decrease in brain volume.

Compliance. Compliance is a measure of the adaptive capacity of the brain to maintain intracranial equilibrium in response to physiologic and external challenges to that system. It has been described as a measure of brain "stiffness." Compliance represents the ratio of change in volume to the resulting change in pressure. It is represented by the following formula, in which Δ represents the symbol for change, V volume, and P pressure:

$$Compliance = \frac{\Delta V}{\Delta P}$$

Applying this concept to intracranial dynamics, compliance is the ratio of change in ICP as a result of change in intracranial volume.

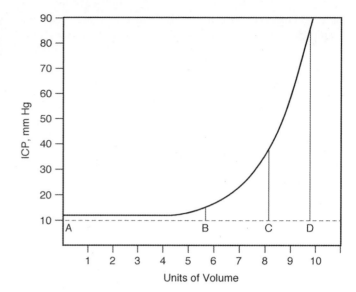

Figure 13-1 • Pressure–volume curve. From point A to just before B, the intracranial pressure (ICP) remains constant, although there is addition of volume (compliance is high). At point B, even though the ICP is within normal limits, compliance begins to change, as evidenced by the slight rise in ICP. From points B to C, the ICP rises with an increase in volume (low compliance). From points C to D, ICP rises significantly with each minute increase in volume (compliance is lost).

The intracranial dynamics are shown in Figure 13-1. The vertical axis represents pressure or ICP (measured in mm Hg). The horizontal axis represents intracranial volume. The shape of the curve demonstrates the effects on ICP when volume is added to the intracranial space. The ICP remains constant from point A to just before point B with the addition of volume. Compensatory mechanisms are adequate, and compliance is high. Point B is a threshold, so that even though the ICP is still within normal limits, compliance is decreased. From points B to C, the slope begins to increase, reflecting a decrease in compensatory mechanisms and low compliance. With even a small increment in volume (points C to D), the compensatory mechanisms are exceeded, compliance is lost, and a disproportionate elevation in ICP is noted.

Factors that influence compliance include the amount of volume increase, the time frame for accommodation of the volume, and the size of the intracranial compartments. Small volume increments made over long periods of time can be accommodated much more easily than a comparable quantity introduced within a short time interval. This concept helps to explain why a slow-growing tumor may become large (roughly equal to the size of a golf ball) without causing an elevation in ICP. The size of the intracranial compartments can vary because of cerebral atrophy, craniectomy, or immaturity of the cranium (i.e., suture lines are not fused). For example, an adult with an acute subdural hematoma, an enlarging lesion (typically over a few days), will develop increased ICP. Of note, in the elderly, some cerebral atrophy occurs with normal aging, thus creating a little more space in the cranial vault. Because of this extra intracranial space, a subdural hematoma in an older person may go unnoticed for days or weeks before there are signs and symptoms of a rise in ICP. However, a critical point is eventually reached beyond which physiologic compensation is exhausted, and there is a dramatic rise in ICP, regardless of how slowly minute-volume increments are added.

Estimating Compliance by Morphologic Changes in Intracranial Pressure Waveform.
Cerebral compliance can be estimated clinically by examining morphologic changes in ICP waveforms. This task requires astute observations of the ICP wave using a continuous real-time display monitor. The ICP pulse wave arises primarily from arterial pulsations and to a lesser degree from the respiratory cycle. In addition, effects from retrovenous pulsation and choroid plexus pulsations also influence the waveform.[2] Observing any variations in waveform during activities, treatments, or environmental changes allows one to determine the effects of these activities on patients and to protect them from risk, if necessary.

The ICP waveform has three peaks that are of clinical importance. These are aptly named P_1, P_2, and P_3. Other lesser peaks sometimes occur after P_3, but their significance is unknown.[3] The principal waveforms, in order of appearance, are:

- P_1, the percussion wave, which originates from pulsations of the arteries and choroid plexus, is sharply peaked and fairly consistent in amplitude.
- P_2, the tidal wave, is more variable and terminates in the dicrotic notch.
- P_3, the dicrotic wave, immediately follows the dicrotic notch.

Clinically, aligning the ICP waveform with an arterial pressure waveform demonstrates the association between systemic and cerebral hemodynamics. See Figure 13-2 for a comparison between ICP and arterial wave forms. Beginning with the ejection of blood from the left ventricle (cardiac ventricular systole), 10 to 15 mL of blood is pumped into the brain and provides the arterial influence of the ICP waveform. As the blood enters the brain, it produces a sudden increase in volume, which is transmitted through the choroid plexus to the ventricles and produces the characteristic sharp

up-slope of P_1. Throughout the remainder of ventricular cardiac systole, the amount of blood entering the brain tapers off and the ICP wave begins to fall.

The second upward trend in the ICP wave is the P_2 wave, which is also called the tidal wave. The presence of the P_2 wave is thought to be due to the reflexive compliance of the surrounding brain tissues as the effects of the P_1 wave are transmitted back through the skull. The size and shape of the P_2 wave and its relationship to P_1 most directly reflect compliance.[4] As compliance decreases, there is less absorption of the percussion wave and P_2 will increase. The end of the P_2 wave is marked by the presence of the dicrotic notch.

Physiologically, the dicrotic notch is associated with closure of the aortic valve and signals the end of ventricular systole.[5] Components of the ICP waveform that occur after the dicrotic notch cannot, therefore, be assumed to relate to arterial influence, but are related to changes in retrograde venous pressures. The dicrotic notch also signals the beginning of P_3 and the pressure tapers down to the diastolic position after P_3 unless retrograde venous pulsation creates additional waves.

Under stable conditions, the ICP waveform has a very predictable appearance. Changes in the ICP waveform that correspond to different points during the respiratory cycle likely reflect pressure changes in the intrathoracic cavity and will be discussed later in this chapter. At low ICP pressure, the pulse wave formation appears as a descending sawtooth pattern (Fig. 13-3). A rise in ICP is reflected as a progressive rise in P_2. The P_1 and P_3 waves rise to a much lesser degree so that the overall pulse wave has a rounded appearance (Fig. 13-4).

Clinical application of ICP waveform analysis is used to identify patients who exhibit low compliance as evidenced by an elevated P_2 wave. It is unclear whether the height of individual wave components indicates a continuum of compliance compromise from slight to severe. Because it is possible to observe responses to patient activities, treatments, and environmental factors immediately, it may be possible to use this information to develop an individual plan of care based on avoidance of individual risk factors. ICP waveform analysis should be a focus of more clinical research to explore its ramifications for integration into clinical practice.

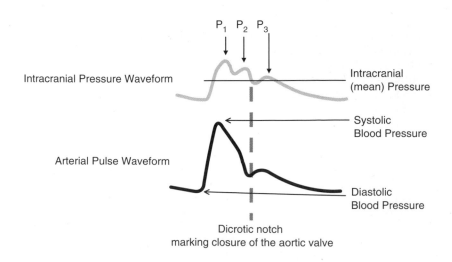

Figure 13-2 • Comparison of arterial and intracranial pressure waveforms.

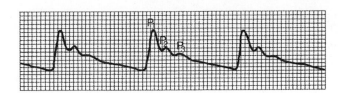

Figure 13-3 • Normal intracranial pressure waveform (ICP = 8 mm Hg).

Cerebral Hemodynamics

Several concepts related to cerebral hemodynamics are important to an understanding of the pathophysiology of increased ICP.

Cerebral Blood Volume. Cerebral blood volume (CBV) refers to the amount of blood in the brain at a given time. Normally, blood occupies about 10% of the intracranial space. Most blood is contained in the lower-pressure venous system. CBV is affected by the autoregulatory mechanisms that control cerebral blood flow (CBF). A limited compensatory mechanism is operational when ICP begins to rise. The mechanism responds by decreasing CBV. However, as the compensatory reserve is exhausted, pressure in the venous system rises, CBV increases, and ICP rises. Depending on the rate of decline in CBF and the duration of ischemia, cerebral infarction can occur.

Cerebral Blood Flow. Adequate blood flow and oxygenation are required to maintain normal neural function. At rest, the approximate **cerebral blood flow** through the brain is 45 to 65 mL/100 g brain per minute; given that a normal brain weighs between 1 and 1.5 kg, this translates into 450 to 1000 mL/min of blood flow for the whole brain.[6] Although the brain is only 2% of body weight, it receives 15% to 20% of total cardiac output and uses 20% of the oxygen consumed in the basal state. In normal conditions, the total oxygen consumed by the brain and CBF are almost constant. Local demand for blood can vary depending on different metabolic needs. Cortical gray matter receives about six times the amount of blood as white matter, and changes in blood flow respond to demands of varying neural activity.[7] A basic concept of any hemodynamic system is *the blood flow is directly proportional to the perfusion pressures and inversely proportional to the total resistance of the system.* CBF is represented by the following equation, in which MAP = mean arterial pressure, CVP = central venous pressure, CPP = cerebral perfusion pressure, and CVR = cerebrovascular resistance:

$$CBF = MAP - CVP/CVR \text{ or } CPP/CVR$$

Note: Under normal conditions CVP represents the resistance to venous outflow and CPP = MAP − CVP. Another common formula (CPP = MAP − ICP) incorporates the resistance to flow contributed from intracranial pressure.

If the CBF exceeds the amount of blood required for metabolism, a state of hyperemia is said to exist. **Hyperemia,** also called "luxury perfusion," is an excess of blood to a part of the body.

Factors That Modify Cerebral Blood Flow. Cerebral blood flow can be increased or decreased by several extracerebral and intracerebral factors.[8]

Extracerebral Factors These factors are primarily related to the cardiovascular system and include systemic blood pressure, cardiac function, and blood viscosity.

- **Blood pressure.** *The main force that maintains cerebral circulation is the pressure difference between the arteries and the veins.* In the brain, cerebral venous pressure is low (approximately 5 mm Hg) so that arterial blood pressure is the most important factor in maintaining CBF. Under normal circumstances, intrinsic regulatory mechanisms maintain CBF at a constant level even with systemic arterial blood pressure changes unless the MAP dips to less than 50 to 70 mm Hg.
- **Cardiac function.** Systemic arterial blood pressure is dependent on cardiac output and peripheral vasomotor tone (resistance), which are primarily under autonomic control from the vasomotor center of the medulla. Cardiac arrhythmias, altered myocardial function, circulating blood volume, and cardiac disease can affect cardiac output, thus influencing CBF. In addition, various carotid sinus and aortic arch reflexes assist in maintaining a constant blood pressure. Advanced age, atherosclerosis, and certain drugs can alter these reflexes, thus affecting arterial blood pressure and CBF secondarily.
- **Blood viscosity.** Blood viscosity is a measure of how thick the blood is. Blood viscosity is generally represented by hematocrit (Hct), where a higher Hct correlates with higher viscosity. Fluid replacement therapy and anemia are two primary causes of a sudden change in blood viscosity. Anemia may increase blood flow up to 30%, whereas polycythemia may decrease flow by more than 50%.

Intracerebral Factors. The primary intracerebral factors that influence CBF are widespread cerebrovascular artery disease and increased ICP.

Widespread cerebrovascular artery disease can increase cerebrovascular resistance (CVR), resulting in reduced CBF. Processes that rapidly shunt blood from arteries to veins (as in an arteriovenous malformation) result in a condition in which total CBF is increased but local tissue perfusion is decreased.

When **increased ICP** is present, it is transmitted to the low-pressure venous system, thus increasing cerebral venous pressure and decreasing CBF.

Regulation of Cerebral Blood Flow. Several other intracerebral regulatory mechanisms that can modify CBF include autoregulation, chemical-metabolic regulation, and neurogenic regulation.

Autoregulation. The ability of an organ (such as the brain) to maintain a constant blood flow despite marked changes in

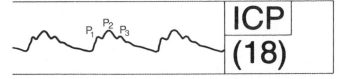

Figure 13-4 • Abnormal intracranial pressure (ICP) waveform (ICP = 18 mm Hg).

arterial perfusion pressure is called **autoregulation.** Autoregulation operates within limited parameters in healthy people— a mean arterial blood pressure of 60 to 150 mm Hg; below 60 mm Hg, CBF decreases, and above 150 mm Hg, CBF increases. In patients with chronic hypertension, the curve shifts to the right. Autoregulation generally operates with an ICP of less than 40 mm Hg.

Autoregulation is a major homeostatic and protective mechanism occurring in large and small arterioles. Autoregulation is achieved using myogenic, chemical-metabolic, and neurogenic mechanisms. Arterioles contain smooth muscles that respond to stretch receptors and intraluminal pressure causing vasoconstriction to increase intraluminal pressure and vasodilation to decrease intraluminal pressure. Specifically, *autoregulation is primarily a pressure-controlled myogenic mechanism that operates independently, yet synergistically, with other chemical-metabolic and neurogenic autoregulatory mechanisms.* Autoregulation provides a constant CBF, maintained within the normal range by adjusting the diameter of blood vessels.

Compensatory mechanisms to regulate CBF are limited. A critical point is reached when other forces overcome autoregulation, thereby causing local or global impairment in an unpredictable pattern. This pattern results from ICP that exceeds 40 to 50 mm Hg, local or diffuse injury, ischemia, inflammation, or cerebral perfusion pressure outside the range of 60 to 150 mm Hg. Note that both the upper and lower limits of autoregulation are elevated in patients with chronic hypertension.[8] There is a shift of the cerebral autoregulatory curve to the right. Without autoregulation, there is reduced cerebrovascular tone, known as **vasomotor paralysis,** and the CBF and CBV become passively dependent on changes in blood pressure.

Chemical-Metabolic Regulation. Chemical and metabolic regulation exert a strong influence on CBF; carbon dioxide, oxygen, and pH are important chemical regulators.

- **Carbon dioxide** (CO_2), found in the blood and locally in cerebral tissue as an end-product of cell metabolism, is the most potent agent that influences CBF. Cerebral blood vessels respond directly to changes in carbon dioxide ($PaCO_2$) levels. Increases in $PaCO_2$ result in vasodilation, thus increasing blood flow. Decreased $PaCO_2$ will cause vasoconstriction and result in a general decrease in blood flow. CBF generally changes by 2% to 3% for each change in $PaCO_2$ within the range of 20 to 80 mm Hg.
- **Oxygen** (O_2) has an opposite, but less profound, effect: reduction in local oxygen (PaO_2) produces vasodilation, and an increase in local PaO_2 produces vasoconstriction. The mechanism by which this is achieved is unclear.
- **H^+** ions are also powerful agents that influence CBF. In body fluids, CO_2 combines with water to form carbonic acid, with subsequent dissociation of hydrogen ions. Hydrogen ion concentration can also be increased by lactic acid, pyruvic acid, and other acids that result from cell metabolism. Excess hydrogen ions cause cerebral vessels to dilate, which results in a net increase in CBF.
- **pH** changes also have an effect on cerebral arterioles; a low pH (acidosis) results in vasodilation and increased CBF, and a high pH (alkalosis) results in vasoconstriction and a decreased CBF. A buildup of the metabolic end-products of cell metabolism (e.g., lactic acid, pyruvic acid, carbonic

acid) causes localized acidosis. An increase in the concentration of these acids will also increase CBF.

Neurogenic Regulation. Neurogenic factors play a lesser role in regulation of CBF than the chemical-metabolic regulators. Neurogenic regulation includes a rich neural network that is extrinsic and intrinsic to the brain.

- **Extrinsic neurogenic control.** Sympathetic innervation comes from postganglionic fibers of the superior cervical sympathetic ganglion that innervate the carotid and vertebral arteries and major intracranial branches. Norepinephrine, a vasoconstrictor, is released from the sympathetic fibers. Parasympathetic fibers come from the facial and superficial petrosal nerves to innervate large- and small-diameter cerebral blood vessels. They use acetylcholine as a neurotransmitter, which causes vasodilation.
- **Intrinsic neurogenic control.** The intrinsic pathways originate in the brainstem and interneurons in the cerebral cortex. Brainstem pathways course from the locus ceruleus (neurons use norepinephrine to produce microcirculatory vasodilation), raphe nuclei (neurons use serotonin, a vasoconstrictor), and fastigial nuclei of the cerebellum. Cortical interneurons contain both vasoconstrictor and vasodilator substances.

Other Factors. An increase in CBF and CBV can also result from pharmacologic agents, such as volatile anesthetic agents and those antihypertensives that cause vasodilation. Increased CBF and CBV is also associated with rapid eye movement (REM) sleep, arousal, pain, seizures, elevations in body temperature (about 6% per 1°C), and cerebral trauma.

Cerebral Perfusion Pressure. Cerebral perfusion pressure (CPP) is defined as the blood pressure gradient across the brain. An adequate CPP is necessary to maintain an adequate driving force for blood throughout the brain in order to prevent episodes of cerebral ischemia. The CPP found in a *normal* adult is in the range of 70 to 100 mm Hg. In the laboratory, ischemia is not seen until the CPP falls below 40 mm Hg.[9] In traumatic brain injury, however, the observations regarding global blood flow and ICP changes may not accurately reflect areas of severe regional ischemia. Therefore, in cerebral trauma, the lower limits of CPP are probably 60 to 70 mm Hg.

The decision to maintain a higher threshold for CPP remains controversial. Rosner and Daughton recommend a CPP of 70 to 80 mm Hg for patients with cerebral injury and intracranial hypertension.[10] Robertson et al., however, found no difference in 3-month and 6-month outcomes for patients treated to maintain CPP greater than 50 mm Hg versus patients treated to maintain CPP greater than 70 mm Hg.[11] Recently, a prospective study concluded that episodes of CPP less than 70 mm Hg are associated with a significant decrease in brain tissue oxygenation ($PbtO_2$), whereas this risk is markedly decreased when CPP is maintained greater than 70 mm Hg.[12] New technology enabling $PbtO_2$ monitoring may allow that CPP be targeted to a treatment goal rather than an absolute value. What is clear is that if CPP is inadequate, ischemia develops; if ischemia is not reversed, infarction results.

CPP is calculated as the difference between the incoming MAP and the opposing ICP. It is represented by the following formula:

$$CPP = MAP - ICP$$

CPP is an estimate of the adequacy of cerebral circulation. To calculate CPP, it is first necessary to compute the MAP. This is calculated as follows:

$$MAP = (systolic - diastolic)/3 + diastolic$$

Example: systolic = 130; diastolic = 82; ICP = 15

$$MAP = (130 - 82)/3 + 82 = 98$$

$$MAP - ICP = CPP$$

$$98 - 15 = 83$$

Cerebrovascular Resistance. Cerebrovascular resistance is the pressure across the cerebrovascular bed from the arteries to the jugular veins, which is influenced by inflow pressure, outflow pressure, the diameter of the vessels, and ICP. (The cerebral venous system does not have valves as do other veins in the body. Thus, any condition that obstructs or compromises venous outflow may also increase CBV because blood is backed up into the intracranial cavity.) CVR is the amount of resistance created by the cerebral vessels, and it is controlled by the autoregulatory mechanisms of the brain. The CVR increases with vasoconstriction, decreases with vasodilation, and varies inversely with CBV.

Cerebral Metabolism. Under normal circumstances, the brain depends almost exclusively on glucose to obtain its energy needs. Neural cells in the brain lack mitochondria and the ability to store energy. Therefore, a constant and critical supply of glucose must be transported to brain cells to produce energy in the form of adenosine triphosphate (ATP), which is synthesized through the glycolytic pathway, Krebs cycle, and respiratory chain (also called the electron transport chain). Both the Krebs cycle and the respiratory chain require oxygen, and this accounts for the brain's high and critical dependence on oxygen.

Aerobic metabolism is the usual pathway for glucose metabolism. Glucose is metabolized through the previously mentioned pathways to yield 38 moles of ATP per mole of glucose. However, if anaerobic metabolism occurs, Krebs' cycle and the respiratory chain cannot be activated because of lack of oxygen. In these circumstances, pyruvate derived from glycolysis is metabolized to lactate, yielding only 2 moles of ATP per mole of glucose. Therefore, much less ATP is available to fuel the ATP-dependent sodium-potassium pump of cell membranes.

PATHOPHYSIOLOGY

Pathophysiology: Cerebral Ischemia and Cerebral Infarction

Traumatic brain injury (TBI) can cause an immediate primary structural injury as a direct result of the injury. This is termed *primary injury*. *Secondary injury* occurs as a delayed effect of a primary injury or other cerebral pathology and can be caused by ischemia, inflammation, excitotoxicity, hypox-emia, metabolic insults, or other pathophysiologic processes that affect normal cerebral function. Both primary and secondary injuries can lead to increased ICP.[13]

When the brain is deprived of an adequate blood supply, a chain of events occurs called the *ischemic cascade*. The ultimate end-point of this process, unless reversed, is neuronal dysfunction and neuronal death. **Ischemia** is the state of *reversible* alteration in cell function caused by decreased oxygen supply (neuronal dysfunction). **Infarction** is the state of irreversible alteration in function resulting from lack of oxygen (neuronal death). Ischemia will always progress to infarction unless some reversal action is taken. The ischemic cascade, as outlined, includes the following:

- In the center of the ischemic area is a core of dead or dying cells surrounded by an area of minimally surviving cells. This area, called the ischemic **penumbra (halo around the infarction),** represents the cells at greatest risk for neuronal death. The cells of the penumbra receive marginal blood flow resulting in altered metabolic activities. However, these cells are *still alive and salvageable.*
- Local autoregulation, responsiveness to chemical-metabolic factors, and perfusion pressure are impaired or lost.
- The lack of an adequate supply of oxygen and glucose causes a switch to anaerobic metabolism, a decrease in ATP production, and an increase in lactate production.
- The decrease in ATP production, in turn, leads to ineffective cellular function and dysfunction of ATP-dependent neurotransmitter reuptake.
- Ischemic neurons release an excessive amount of the excitatory neurotransmitter glutamate; this results in increased neuronal necrosis.
  - Glutamate binds to *N*-methyl-D-aspartate (NMDA) receptors that are normally blocked by magnesium; this causes increased cell permeability to sodium and calcium ions.
  - Cellular swelling results primarily from the increased influx of sodium ions.
  - Cell lysis results from cellular swelling intracellular calcium-activated processes that lead to cell death.
  - Cellular lysis releases calcium ions into the postsynaptic neuron causing further neuronal ischemia and the release of more glutamate, which binds to NMDA receptors and increases cell membrane permeability to sodium and calcium, and the cycle of programmed cell death is perpetuated.
- The increase in intracellular calcium levels activates phospholipases and proteases, which generate oxygen-free radicals and nitric oxide. This leads to membrane, mitochondrial, and microtubular cellular damage and eventual death.
  - This cell death results in the release of glutamate, which binds to NMDA receptors and increases cell membrane permeability to sodium and calcium, and the cycle of programmed cell death is perpetuated.

Survival of the penumbral cells depends on successful re-establishment of an adequate circulation, the amount of end-products present, cerebral edema, and the alterations in local blood flow. If the cells of the penumbra die, the core of dead tissue enlarges, and the volume of surrounding tissue at risk increases.

With the breakdown in the blood–brain barrier, water content of the tissue increases, resulting in cerebral edema.

Cerebral Edema

Cerebral edema is an abnormal accumulation of water in the intracellular space, extracellular space, or both that is associated with an increase in brain tissue volume.[14] Cerebral edema can be a localized or generalized problem, and it is usually associated with increased ICP. Peak swelling usually occurs 2 to 4 days after initial brain injury.[13] Cerebral edema is serious and can be life threatening because the increase in brain bulk produces pressure on the tissue, resulting in neurological deficit and increased ICP. Severe cerebral edema can produce transtentorial herniation with progressive brainstem compression, herniation, and death. Three types of cerebral edema are recognized: *vasogenic*, *cytotoxic*, and *interstitial* edema.

Vasogenic edema is an extracellular edema of the white matter that results from increased permeability of the endothelial cells in the capillary beds as a result of the widening of tight junctions and increases in pinocytotic vesicles at the blood–brain barrier level. (*Pinocytes* are cells that ingest extracellular fluid and its content. *Pinocytosis* involves the formation of invaginations in the cell membrane, which close and break off to form fluid-filled vacuoles in the cytoplasm.) As a result, a plasma-like filtrate, including large molecules of protein, leaks into the extracellular space. Vasogenic edema is seen locally around brain tumors, although it can develop around a cerebral infarct or a cerebral abscess. Generalized vasogenic edema occurs with cerebral trauma or meningitis. There is disruption of the blood–brain barrier. Magnetic resonance imaging (MRI) or computed tomography (CT) imaging with contrast media can demonstrate parenchymal cerebral enhancement. Use of corticosteroids (dexamethasone) is effective only with brain tumors. An osmotic diuretic (mannitol) or hypertonic saline may be helpful in the acute phase.

Cytotoxic edema is an increase in fluid in the neurons, glia, and endothelial cells (i.e., intracellular space swelling) as a result of ATP-dependent sodium-potassium pump failure so that fluid and sodium accumulate within the cells, leading to diffuse brain swelling. Both gray and white matter can be involved. Development of cytotoxic edema is associated with a hypoxic or anoxic episode, such as a cardiac arrest or asphyxiation. It is also seen with hypo-osmolarity conditions, such as water intoxication, hyponatremia, and the syndrome of inappropriate secretion of antidiuretic hormone (SIADH). The goal of therapy for the patient with cytotoxic edema is to restore perfusion, ensuring an adequate oxygen supply to the neurons. Corticosteroids (dexamethasone) are not effective in treating cytotoxic edema. Osmotic diuretics may be beneficial in the acute stage when hypo-osmolarity is present.

Interstitial edema occurs with hydrocephalus. The edema is found in the periventricular white matter when the intraventricular pressure is greater than the ability of the ependymal cells to contain the CSF within the ventricle. This forces the CSF across the ependymal tissue into the periventricular white matter. It is associated with acute and subacute hydrocephalus and possibly with benign intracranial hypertension (pseudotumor cerebri). Corticosteroids or osmotic diuretics are ineffective; acetazolamide (Diamox) may be administered to decrease CSF production. Treatment options include the temporary drainage of CSF until the condition corrects itself or surgical placement of a shunt.

Summary. Vasogenic and cytotoxic edema may be seen concurrently. Cerebral edema is considered to be proportional to the severity of injury or insult and reaches its maximum level in approximately 2 to 4 days unless secondary injury exacerbates the process. It then gradually begins to subside, although it can persist, depending on the degree of injury and other circumstances such as secondary injury.

Intracranial Hypertension

Intracranial hypertension, more commonly called increased ICP, is a symptom rather than a distinct disease entity. **Intracranial hypertension** is a sustained elevated ICP of 15 mm Hg or higher. The term **malignant hypertension** has been used by some authors to describe a sustained ICP of 20 mm Hg or higher. **Refractory intracranial hypertension** describes a condition in which, following treatment, the ICP is sustained at greater than 50% of the maximum pretreatment value. Another common descriptor of refractory intracranial hypertension is that it is intracranial hypertension that does not respond to the usual treatment modalities. The underlying cause of increased ICP must be identified and treated to manage the problem effectively. Conditions that can cause intracranial hypertension can be classified as follows:

- Conditions that increase brain volume
  - Space-occupying masses (e.g., hematomas, abscesses, tumors, aneurysms)
  - Cerebral edema (e.g., brain injuries, Reye's syndrome)
- Conditions that increase blood volume
  - Obstruction of venous outflow
  - Hyperemia
  - Hypercapnia
  - Cerebral artery vasodilation
- Conditions that increase CSF volume
  - Increased production of CSF (e.g., choroid plexus papilloma)
  - Decreased absorption of CSF (e.g., communicating hydrocephalus, subarachnoid hemorrhage)
  - Obstruction to flow of CSF (e.g., noncommunicating hydrocephalus)

The rate of development and extent of involvement of increased ICP and intracranial hypertension are related to cellular dysfunction and its consequences. Several factors influence the process. After cerebral edema and increased ICP are established, a sequence of physiologic events contributes to the perpetuation of dysfunction at the cellular level. The sequence of events is as follows: ↓ Regional CBF → ↓ CPP in areas → ↑ CO_2 (hypercapnia) ↓ O_2 (hypoxia) → ↑ acidosis from end-products of cell metabolism → vasodilation → ↑ CBF → ↑ CBV → ↑ ICP → possible impairment of local autoregulation.

Moreover, decreased regional CBF and increased ICP activate the vasopressor ischemic response, resulting in increased

MAP and increased CBF. This, in turn, leads to increased edema and ICP.

This circular sequence continues until the autoregulatory mechanisms are inactivated. CBF passively responds to arterial blood pressure. CBF and CPP cannot be maintained in relationship to rising ICP. The CPP approaches zero, and the CBF ceases. Blood vessels and brain tissue are compressed, and herniation and death follow.

Summary of Factors Known to Increase Intracranial Pressure

Various factors known to increase ICP are included in Table 13-1. Many of these factors have been identified as a result of nursing research and are discussed further in the section on nursing management.

TABLE 13-1 FACTORS ASSOCIATED WITH INCREASED INTRACRANIAL PRESSURE

FACTORS AND DESCRIPTION	MECHANISMS
Hypercapnia	
$Pco_2 \geq 45$ mm Hg Excessive levels of CO_2 in the blood Potent cerebral vasodilator	Elevated CO_2 results in increased CBF, which leads to increased CBV and ICP Hypercapnia results from underventilation (decreased ventilatory volume or decreased ventilatory rate) of a patient in such circumstances as: • Sleep • Pulmonary diseases/conditions (e.g., atelectasis, pneumonia, COPD, neurogenic pulmonary edema, ARDS) • Oversedation • Shallow respirations, as seen with anxiety reactions, severe pain, undersedation, or ventilatory asynchrony • Pressure on brainstem respiratory centers • Improperly calibrated ventilator (e.g., rate, sensitivity)
Hypoxemia	
$PaO_2 < 50$ mm Hg Decreased O_2 in the blood Has much less effect as a vasodilator compared to CO_2	Decreased O_2 does not increase cerebral vasodilation until it is ~50 mm Hg or less. Hypoxemia results from: • Insufficient concentration of O_2 administered during O_2 therapy • Insufficient ventilation during and after suctioning • Inadequate ventilation during intubation • Partial or complete airway obstruction • Increased oxygen consumption
Respiratory Procedures	
Suctioning PEEP Asynchrony of respiratory rate when ambu bag is used Intubation	Suctioning decreases O_2, increases CO_2, and partially obstructs the airway with a catheter. PEEP increases intrathoracic pressure, which leads to increased central venous pressure, cerebral venous pressure, and ICP. Asynchronous use of the Ambu bag causes a response that is similar to the PEEP response. Same as suctioning
Vasodilating Drugs	
Anesthetic agents (halothane, enflurane, isoflurane, nitrous oxide) Some antihypertensives (nitroglycerine, Nipride) Some histamines	Vasodilation causes increased CBF, resulting in increased ICP.
Some Body Positions	
Trendelenburg's position (always contraindicated in neuroscience patients) Prone position (increased intra-abdominal and intrathoracic pressures; also, neck flexion impedes venous drainage) Extreme hip flexion (increased intra-abdominal pressure) Hip flexion on a pendulous abdomen (increased intra-abdominal pressure) Angulation of the neck; neck flexion, even from a small, improperly positioned pillow, or improper lateral positioning when turned (which impedes venous return from the brain)	Obstruction of venous return from the brain increases CBV, which results in increased ICP. The venous cerebrovascular system has no valves; thus, an increase in intra-abdominal, intrathoracic, or neck pressure is communicated as increased pressure throughout the open venous system, thus impeding drainage from the brain and increasing ICP It has been an accepted practice to elevate the head of the bed 30 degrees to facilitate drainage from the brain; current research is inconclusive as to what is the best degree of head elevation for promoting venous drainage from the brain.

(continued)

TABLE 13-1   FACTORS ASSOCIATED WITH INCREASED INTRACRANIAL PRESSURE (*Continued*)

Turning the patient laterally if the head of the bed is up and the knees are flexed on the abdomen (increased intraabdominal pressure)	

Pressure on Neck

Snug "track tape," soft collar, or other constricting material	These impede venous drainage from the brain.

Isometric Muscle Contractions

Increased muscle tension without lengthening of the muscle Examples: pushing against the bed with one's feet, as in pushing oneself up in bed; pulling on an extremity restraint; shivering; decortication; decerebration; other rigidity	Isometric muscle contractions increase systemic blood pressure and contribute to further elevation of increased ICP in the patient who is on the borderline of brain compliance or who already has increased ICP. Passive range of motion (PROM) exercises do not involve isometric contractions because the length of the muscle does change during contraction. Therefore, PROM exercises should be included in the plan of care. Chlorpromazine (Thorazine) has been used to control shivering; pancuronium bromide (Pavulon) and baclofen (Lioresal) have been used for decerebration in the patient at risk for ICP spikes.

Valsalva's Maneuver

Exhalation against a closed epiglottis Examples: straining at stool, moving in bed, sneezing	Increased intra-abdominal or increased intrathoracic pressure impede venous return from the brain, thereby increasing ICP. If the patient's ICP is already elevated or brain compliance is borderline, spikes in ICP may occur.

Coughing

Increases intra-abdominal and intrathoracic pressure as a result of muscle visceral contractions	Increased intra-abdominal and intrathoracic pressure impede venous drainage from the brain. Also, the increased pressure is transmitted through the spinal subarachnoid space to the intracranial subarachnoid space and through the veins that communicate with the dural venous sinuses and intracranial subarachnoid space. The venous return from the cranial vault is impeded, resulting in increased ICP.

Noxious Stimuli

e.g., invasive procedures, such as lumbar puncture, or painful nursing procedures, such as removal of tape from skin	Activation of the sympathetic nervous system is probably the major cause of increased blood pressure, increased CBF, and increased ICP, particularly in the patient who already has increased ICP.

Activities That Increase Cerebral Metabolism

Arousal from sleep REM phase of sleep Seizure activity Hyperthermia	A focal or generalized increase in cerebral metabolism results from these activities. There is regional or generalized increased CBF, which is reflected in increased CBV, which causes an increase in ICP.

Clustering of Activities

In a patient with already increased ICP, clustering of patient care activities (e.g., bathing, turning) and other activities known to increase ICP can cause dangerous elevations in ICP and plateau waves in the patient at risk. The impact of nursing activities may be compounded after having blood drawn or undergoing an invasive procedure. Note that suctioning is notorious for increasing ICP in the patient at risk.	The compounding effect of activities causes an increase in blood pressure, CBF, and ICP; elevations of ICP can be high enough to cause plateau waves and cerebral ischemia. Spacing of procedures allows the patient's ICP to return to a safe baseline level. Observing the effects and the return to baseline on an ICP monitor provides a guide for delivering safe care to the patient at risk.

CBF, cerebral blood flow; CBV, cerebral blood volume; ICP, intracranial pressure; COPD, chronic obstructive pulmonary disease; ARDS, acute respiratory distress syndrome; PEEP, positive end-expiratory pressure; PROM, passive range of motion; REM, rapid eye movement.

HERNIATION SYNDROMES OF THE BRAIN

Increased ICP that continues to develop will result in herniation. **Herniation** is defined as the abnormal protrusion of an organ or other body structure through a defect or natural opening in a covering membrane, muscle, or bone. Simply put, brain herniation is when one part of the brain moves beyond its normal border. It is important to note that there are different types of brain herniation. To understand the pathophysiology of these different cerebral mass lesions (Box 13-2), it is most important to understand the principles that govern herniation. The intracranial cavity is divided into several smaller compartments by folds of the fibrous, relatively rigid dura mater. The most important dural folds are:

- **Tentorium cerebelli** is a double fold of dura mater that forms a tent-like partition (higher in the middle) between the cerebrum and cerebellum. The area above the tentorium is the *supratentorial space*, and the area below the tentorium is the *infratentorial space*. To allow the brainstem, blood vessels, and accompanying nerves to pass through the tentorium, there is an oval opening in the tentorium called the **tentorial notch** or **incisura**.
- **Falx cerebri** is a double fold of dura mater that drops into the longitudinal fissure and is partially responsible for dividing the supratentorial space into the left and right hemispheres.
- **Falx cerebelli** is a double fold of dura mater that separates the cerebellum (in the infratentorial space) into a left and right side.

When cerebral edema or a mass lesion occurs within a compartment, the pressure exerted by the lesion is not evenly distributed. This uneven distribution of pressure results in shifting or herniation of the brain from a compartment of high pressure to one of lesser pressure. The shifting of cerebral structures resulting from pressure is called the **mass effect**. With mass effect, there is compression and traction of cerebral tissue that results in ischemia. Ischemia is potentially reversible, but without effective treatment, it will lead to infarction, which is irreversible.

In addition, the **foramen magnum** is the hole at the base of the skull (occipital bone) through which the spinal cord passes. If an elevated ICP resulting from a supratentorial lesion continues to expand unchecked, the uncus of the medial inferior temporal lobe will herniate through the tentorium, with resulting exertion of pressure on the brainstem. This will eventually result in cerebellar tonsillar herniation through the foramen magnum, the only opening in the closed cranial vault. Cerebellar tonsillar herniation is a sure cause of death because of pressure on the vital structures in the medulla.

An expanding mass lesion of the supratentorial space behaves differently than an expanding mass lesion in the infratentorial space. The intracranial pathologic changes radiate downward and away from the supratentorial lesion in a rostral-caudal pattern. (A **rostral-caudal pattern** means that the deterioration in function proceeds from the head to the tail.) Of particular importance is the clinical presentation of the Kocher-Cushing signs (more often referred to as *Cushing's response*) of a rising blood pressure, slowing pulse, and widening pulse pressure that *do not* occur with most supratentorial lesions. Cushing's response is most common with posterior fossa lesions. On rare occasions when these signs are associated with a supratentorial lesion, they usually indicate a rapidly expanding lesion such as an epidural hematoma or a massive hemorrhage that has *suddenly* increased the supratentorial and intraventricular pressure, transmitting its pressure effect directly to the posterior fossa and brainstem.[15]

Supratentorial Herniation

Progressive supratentorial lesions develop clinical signs and symptoms in a sequence of ocular, motor, and respiratory function. This pattern indicates the predictable continuum of rostral-caudal failure that proceeds from the diencephalon, to the midbrain, followed by the pons, and finally medullary function. The pattern of deterioration is predictable unless a significant hemorrhage occurs, an abscess ruptures into the ventricles, or a contraindicated lumbar puncture rapidly changes the intracranial dynamics resulting in compression of the medulla.

Three major patterns of herniation, described by Plum and Posner in their classic work, identify syndromes caused by expanding supratentorial lesions: (1) cingulate herniation, (2) central transtentorial herniation, and (3) uncal transtentorial herniation[15] (Fig. 13-5). Cingulate herniation usually has little clinical significance. A supratentorial developing cerebral lesion results in two distinct clinical syndromes, a *central syndrome* and an *uncal syndrome*. These two syndromes are the major clinical presentations encountered in practice. *Clinically, they are distinct patterns early in their course, but both*

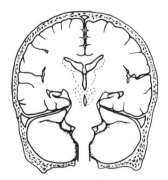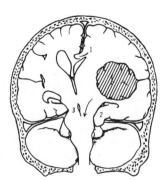

Figure 13-5 • Cross section of a normal brain (*left*) and a brain with intracranial shifts from supratentorial lesions (*right*). (1) Herniation of the cingulate gyrus under the falx. (2) Herniation of the temporal lobe into the tentorial notch. (3) Downward displacement of the brainstem through the notch. (From Plum, F., & Posner, J. [1972]. *Diagnosis of stupor and coma.* [2nd ed.]. Contemporary neurology series. Philadelphia: F.A. Davis.)

BOX 13–2   Lesion

The term **lesion** is often used in practice. This is a broad term that has several overlapping definitions. A lesion can be any of the following:
    An injury to an organ
    A pathological change in the tissue of some organ
    An area of infection

merge into a singular pattern once the pathophysiology begins to involve the midbrain level and below (brainstem structures).

Cingulate Herniation

An expanding lesion in one cerebral hemisphere can cause pressure medially so that the cingulate gyrus is forced under the falx cerebri, displacing it toward the opposite side. This displacement of the falx cerebri can compress the local blood supply and cerebral tissue, which causes edema and ischemia, which further increase the degree of ICP elevation. Cingulate herniation (also called a subfalcine herniation) is common, but little is known about its clinical signs and symptoms, except in those instances when the blood supply of the anterior cerebral artery is compromised as a result of the subfalcine shift.

Central Transtentorial Herniation (Central Syndrome)

The usual causes of rostral-caudal downward displacement of central transtentorial herniation follow:

- A lesion located on the central neural axis
- An extracerebral lesion located around the central apex of the cranium
- Bilaterally positioned lesions in each hemisphere
- Unilateral cingulate herniation

The lesion produces a downward displacement of the cerebral hemispheres, basal ganglia, diencephalon, and midbrain through the tentorial incisura. The diencephalon can be compressed tightly against the midbrain with such force that edema and hemorrhage result. Often, anterior choroidal artery depression is noted on the cerebral arteriogram. Central herniation may or may not be accompanied by uncal herniation. The *early* symptoms of the central syndrome include:

- Deterioration in the level of consciousness (LOC) (confusion and restlessness)
- *Bilateral small*, reactive pupils (in early diencephalic stage)
- Gradual loss of upward (vertical) gaze
- Contralateral monoplegia or hemiparesis to hemiplegia

The progression of signs and symptoms with continued pressure is detailed in Table 13-2. There is clinical importance to the signs and symptoms caused by the diencephalic stage of progression. If the supratentorial process can be alleviated *before* midbrain signs and symptoms occur, there is a good possibility of complete recovery. However, after the area of pathophysiology has expanded *beyond* the diencephalon and into the brainstem, the process is generally irreversible and prognosis poor. The underlying pathophysiology is that ischemia and compression, both reversible conditions, are the basis for the signs and symptoms of diencephalic involvement. Once the midbrain becomes involved, infarction has begun and the condition is most likely irreversible.[15]

Uncal Transtentorial Herniation (Uncal Syndrome)

The most common cerebral herniation syndrome is the *uncal syndrome*. An expanding lesion of the uncus of the hippocampal gyrus of the inferior, medial temporal lobe herniates through the incisura of the tentorium. The diencephalon and midbrain are compressed and displaced to the opposite side by the uncal herniation. With this lateral displacement, the cerebral peduncle (contralateral to the primary uncal herniation) may be compressed against the firm, unyielding edge of the tentorium incisura, producing **Kernohan's notch**. This finding is important because it results in hemiparesis ipsilateral to the expanding supratentorial lesion (Fig. 13-6).[16]

Evaluating changes in pupillary findings and level of consciousness is an important tool in differentiating central and uncal herniation syndromes. In the case of uncal herniation, the diencephalon, associated with consciousness, may not be the first anatomic area affected, so that *impaired consciousness is not consistently an early sign of impending uncal herniation.* The oculomotor nerve (cranial nerve [CN] III) and the posterior cerebral artery on the same side of the expanding temporal lobe lesion are frequently caught between the overhanging edematous uncus and the free edge of the tentorium. The entrapment of the oculomotor nerve results in ipsilateral pupillary dilation. *Unilateral pupillary dilation is the earliest and consistent sign of uncal herniation.* The progression of signs and symptoms is outlined in Table 13-3. The signs of uncal herniation include:

- Gradual ipsilateral (to primary lesions) pupillary dilation, sluggish pupillary reaction to light (earliest sign), and possible development of an ovoid pupil (CN III)
- Paralysis of the oculomotor extraocular muscles (CN IV, VI)
- Restlessness, then LOC deteriorating from stupor to coma (frontal lobe and diencephalon)
- Contralateral hemiparesis or hemiplegia (motor strip of frontal lobe)
- Most often, progression to decerebrate posturing; note that decorticate posturing is unusual (red nucleus lesion)
- Positive Babinski's signs (upper motor neuron lesion)
- Respiratory changes (e.g., hyperventilation) (pontine lesion)
- Finally, dilated, fixed pupils; flaccidity; and respiratory arrest (brainstem infarction)

As noted during early development of the uncal syndrome, the unilateral dilating, sluggish pupil is usually the *only sign noted for several hours before other signs occur.* There are no abnormal changes in extraocular movement, motor function, or respirations. Any motor deficits present are those specific to the supratentorial lesion. However, after any signs of herniation or brainstem compression appear, deterioration may proceed rapidly in a time line of only a *few hours* in which a fully conscious patient deteriorates to deep coma. This means that unless uncal herniation is recognized early and interventions effective, after midbrain (upper portion of the brainstem) involvement is noted, the process is most likely irreversible and the outcome poor.

Effects of Supratentorial Herniation

Any supratentorial herniation syndrome can initiate vascular and obstructive complications that can further exaggerate the neurological deterioration. Compression of the aqueducts of the ventricular system can cause CSF circulation to be interrupted. As a result, major spikes in ICP and obstructive

TABLE 13-2   PROGRESSION OF SIGNS AND SYMPTOMS OF THE CENTRAL SYNDROME*

ASSESSMENT	EARLY DIENCEPHALON	LATE DIENCEPHALON	MIDBRAIN UPPER PONS	LOWER PONS/ UPPER MEDULLA	MEDULLA
Outcome	Potentially Reversible		Irreversible—Poor Prognosis		
Level of consciousness	Pattern varies from decreased alertness and behavior with difficulty to concentrate Some become agitated; others become drowsy	Stupor to coma	Deep coma	Deep coma	Deep coma
Ocular					
Pupillary size and reaction to light	Small (1–3 mm) reactive, but contraction difficult to see; examine using bright light	Small (1–3 mm), reactive but range of contraction slight; difficult to see	Midpoint (3–5 mm) nonreactive Often irregularly shaped	Midpoint (3–5 mm) nonreactive Often irregularly shaped	Dilated and nonreactive
Extraocular movement Oculocephalic (OC) and oculovestibular (OV) response	Oculocephalic (OC) and oculovestibular (OV) response Conjugate or slightly dysconjugate at rest; may note roving eyes OC and OV intact	— Brisk lateral OC; impaired upward conjugate on vertical OC Full lateral OV response	— Impaired OC OV difficult to elicit; dysconjugate with limited horizontal movement	Absent OC and OV	— Absent OC and OV
Motor					
Function	Pre-existing hemiparesis or hemiplegia develop to bilateral signs in early diencephalic stage Hemiparesis or hemiplegia worsens and paratonic rigidity develops homo-lateral to lesion[†] Purposeful response to painful stimuli	Decortication first contralateral to primary lesion in response to painful stimuli then bilateral May see a pattern of decortication ipsilateral and decerebration contralateral to primary lesion	Decortication to bilateral decerebration in response to painful stimuli or sometimes spontaneously	Flaccid at rest Occasional flexor response of lower extremities to painful stimuli	Flaccid at rest Occasional flexor response of lower extremities to painful stimuli
Reflexes	Babinski's sign absent	Bilateral Babinski's sign less vigorous ipsilateral to lesion Grasp reflex present	Bilateral Babinski's sign present	Bilateral Babinski's sign present	—
Respirations					
	Deep sighs, yawns, and occasional pauses	Cheyne-Stokes syndrome	Gradual change to sustained hyperventilation	Normal pattern of respirations, but more rapid (20–40/min) and shallow	Slow and irregular rate and amplitude (ataxic respirations); interrupted by deep sighs, gasps, and periods of apnea
Other					
			Diabetes insipidus Fluctuation in temperature; hyperthermia	Often hyperthermia Cushing's triad	Often hyperthermia Cushing's triad

*An important point to keep in mind when observing a patient with a possible herniation syndrome is that there is predictable order to the development of signs and symptoms. The neurological deterioration in both central and uncal syndromes proceeds in an orderly rostral-caudal direction; the diencephalon, midbrain, pons, and finally, the medulla are affected from the increasing pressure. Signs and symptoms characteristic of each area can be identified. Notice that the last stages of central and uncal herniation are the same.

[†]Often there is an original hemispheric lesion that results in contralateral hemiparesis or hemiplegia. With diencephalic involvement, hemiparesis or hemiplegia worsens and extremities ipsilateral to the lesion develop paratonic resistance (an intermittent abnormal increase in resistance to passive movement in a comatose patient). Table based on classic work of Plum, F., & Posner, J. B. (1982). *The diagnosis of stupor and coma* (3rd ed., pp. 103–108). Philadelphia: FA Davis.

TABLE 13-3   PROGRESSION OF SIGNS AND SYMPTOMS OF THE UNCAL SYNDROME*

ASSESSMENT	EARLY DIENCEPHALON	LATE DIENCEPHALON	MIDBRAIN UPPER PONS	LOWER PONS/ UPPER MEDULLA	MEDULLA
Outcome	**Potentially Reversible**		**Irreversible—Poor Prognosis**		
Level of consciousness	May not be impaired initially	After deterioration begins, quick progression to deep stupor and coma	Deep coma	Deep coma	Deep coma
Ocular					
Pupillary size, reaction to light, and shape	Unilateral dilating pupil ipsilateral to primary lesion Sluggish response Round to ovoid	Fully dilated pupil ipsilateral to lesion Nonreactive Round to ovoid Other pupil dilates	Two possibilities for pupil contralateral to lesion: Fully dilated and fixed *or* Enlarged to midpoint (5–6 mm) and fixed	Bilateral midpoint (5–6 mm) pupils Often irregularly shaped	Bilateral fully dilated and nonreactive
Extraocular movement	Full movement	Paralysis of oculomotor soon after dilated pupil	—	—	—
Oculocephalic (OC) and oculovestibular (OV) response	OC and OV intact or contralateral eye of OV on cold calorics, may not move medially	OC and OV sluggish, then absent	OC and OV absent	OC and OV absent	OC and OV absent
Motor					
Function	No abnormalities may be present; if present, related to primary supratentorial lesion	• Contralateral intermittent abnormal increase in resistance to passive movement • *Ipsilateral* hemiplegia • Decerebrate posturing of limbs (decortication is uncommon)	Bilateral decerebration	• Flaccid at rest • Occasional flexor response of lower extremities to painful stimuli	• Flaccid at rest • Occasional flexor response of lower extremities to painful stimuli
Reflexes	Babinski's sign	Bilateral positive Babinski's sign	Bilateral positive Babinski's sign	Bilateral positive Babinski's sign	
Respirations	Normal pattern and rate	Most often hyperventilation (20–40/min), rarely Cheyne-Stokes reaction	Hyperventilation (20–40/min)	Normal pattern of respirations, but more rapid (20–40/min) and shallow	Slow and irregular in rate and amplitude (ataxic respirations); interrupted by deep sighs, gasps, and periods of apnea
Other					
	—	Possible ptosis ipsilateral to primary lesion	—	Often hyperthermia Cushing's triad	Often hyperthermia Cushing's triad

*An important point to keep in mind when observing a patient with a possible herniation syndrome is that there is predictable order to the development of signs and symptoms. Neurological deterioration in both central and uncal syndromes proceeds in an orderly rostral-caudal direction; the diencephalon, midbrain, pons, and, finally, medulla are affected from the increasing pressure. Signs and symptoms characteristic of each area can be identified. Notice that the last stages of central and uncal herniation are the same.

Table based on classic work of Plum, F., & Posner, J. B. (1980). *The diagnosis of stupor and coma* (3rd ed., pp. 109–111). Philadelphia: FA Davis.

hydrocephalus can develop. Cingulate herniation can compress both arterial and venous vessels (portions of the anterior cerebral artery and the great cerebral vein), causing exacerbation of already present ischemia and edema.

With uncal herniation, the herniated tissue through the tentorial incisura compresses the posterior cerebral artery,

resulting in partial occipital lobe infarction and edema. Brainstem edema, ischemia, and hemorrhage can develop from the diencephalon to the pons-medulla area secondary to the downward displacement from central herniation.

The result of progressive, unresolved downward displacement from any of the supratentorial herniation syndromes is

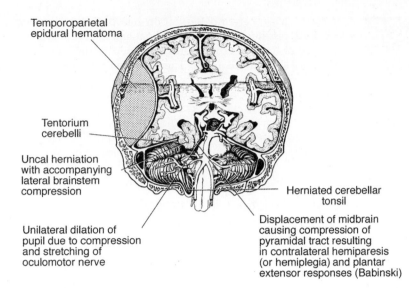

Temporoparietal epidural hematoma

Tentorium cerebelli

Uncal herniation with accompanying lateral brainstem compression

Unilateral dilation of pupil due to compression and stretching of oculomotor nerve

Herniated cerebellar tonsil

Displacement of midbrain causing compression of pyramidal tract resulting in contralateral hemiparesis (or hemiplegia) and plantar extensor responses (Babinski)

Figure 13-6 • Cross section of the brain showing herniation of part of the temporal lobe through the tentorium as a result of a temporoparietal epidural hematoma. (Kentzel, K. C. [1997]. *Advanced concepts in clinical nursing* [2nd ed.]. Philadelphia: J. B. Lippincott.)

brainstem herniation, in which the medulla herniates into the foramen magnum. Brain death is immediate and is attributable to medullary compression, ischemia, and infarction. The medulla controls vital functions, such as respiration, blood pressure, cardiac function, and vasomotor tone, all of which are absolutely necessary to sustain life.

Infratentorial Herniation

Lesions of the infratentorial compartment contributing to herniation are much less frequent than those involving the supratentorial region. The infratentorial compartment includes the brainstem and cerebellum. The three possible effects of an expanding lesion in the infratentorial compartment include:

- *Direct compression* of the brainstem, cerebellum, or their vascular supply
- *Upward transtentorial herniation* of the brainstem and cerebellum through the tentorial incisura, resulting in maximal pressure on the midbrain
- *Downward herniation* of both or one cerebellar tonsil through the foramen magnum to the cervical spine with compression of the medulla, an immediate cause of death (Fig. 13-7)

An expanding lesion causes compression and ischemia to selected structures. The increased pressure interferes with the normal function of the involved tissue and causes edema, ischemia, infarction, and necrosis if the process is not reversed. As the lesion continues to enlarge, the only egress from the infratentorial compartment is through the tentorial incisura (above) to the supratentorial compartment or through the larger orifice, the foramen magnum (below), into the cervical spine. In either case, neurological demise is rapid with high mortality.

The brainstem structures, particularly the medulla oblongata, contain centers for vital functions. If medullary compression develops, immediate death occurs as a result of respiratory and cardiac arrest. Infratentorial expanding lesions can also encroach on a portion of the ventricular system (third or fourth ventricle), resulting in acute hydrocephalus. The signs and symptoms noted with an infratentorial herniation vary widely depending on the brainstem area most involved. It is unclear whether posterior fossa lesions

causing upward transtentorial herniation produce a consistent syndrome.[17] The most prominent signs associated with upward herniation include:

- Immediate onset of deep coma
- Conjugate downward deviation of the eye to failure of upward voluntary or reflex movement (pretectal compression)
- Small, equal, fixed pupils (pontine compression) to unequal, midpoint fixed pupils
- Decerebration
- Abnormal respiratory patterns (e.g., slow rate with intermittent deep sighs or ataxia)
- Vital sign abnormalities (Cushing's signs)

In summary, herniation syndromes are life-threatening occurrences that can progress rapidly. Early recognition of signs and symptoms (Chart 13-1) is important for prompt intervention to prevent neurological demise.

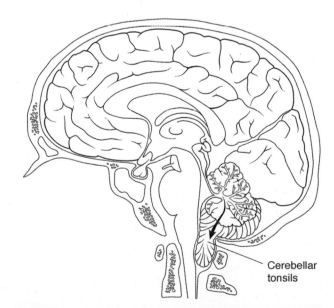

Cerebellar tonsils

Figure 13-7 • Herniation of the cerebellar tonsils into the foramen magnum is the final outcome of increased intracranial pressure. Respiratory centers within the medulla oblongata are compressed, and apnea leads to cardiac arrest and death.

CHART **13-1** **Signs and Symptoms of Impending Herniation**

- Decreased level of consciousness (coma)
- Pupillary abnormalities
- Motor dysfunction (hemiplegia, decortication, or decerebration)
- Impaired brainstem reflexes (corneal, gag, swallowing)
- "Cushing's triad" of alterations in vital signs (bradycardia, hypertension, and respiratory irregularity)

SIGNS AND SYMPTOMS OF INCREASED INTRACRANIAL PRESSURE

Perspective

Increased ICP is a syndrome with multiple patterns (central syndrome, uncal syndrome), not a specific disease entity. A large percentage of neuroscience patients are at risk for developing increased ICP. Nursing assessment of neurological signs is directed at detecting *early* signs and symptoms of increased ICP when nursing and medical interventions are still effective. The conduct and interpretation of the neurological exam by knowledgeable clinicians remains the most sensitive indicator of neurologic change. The astute clinician must continually evaluate a comparison between the baseline neurological assessment and ongoing assessments to interpret the evolving relationship of these changes to changes in ICP. When *late* signs appear (brainstem signs of changes in vital signs or respiratory pattern), it may be too late for effective interventions to reverse cerebral deterioration, herniation, or even death.

As discussed previously, several cerebral *compensatory mechanisms* provide adequate CBF, CPP, and substrates for cerebral metabolism. These compensatory mechanisms act even when there is evidence of increased ICP. **Cushing's response** is a compensatory response that attempts to provide adequate CPP in the presence of rising ICP. The signs associated with a Cushing's response include the following:

- A rising systolic pressure
- A widening pulse pressure
- Bradycardia

These signs profile late brainstem dysfunction resulting from rising ICP and correlate with decreasing brain compliance.

Cushing's triad (also called Cushing's sign) has subtle yet important differences from Cushing's response. Whereas Cushing's response is a compensatory response, Cushing's triad represents a loss of compensatory mechanisms and is a presentation of brainstem dysfunction, which correlates with low or loss of brain compliance. Cushing's triad, which is a late finding and may not be present in all cases of herniation, includes the following:

- Hypertension, usually with a widened pulse pressure
- Bradycardia
- Abnormal/irregular respiratory patterns

In such cases, cerebral herniation has probably already occurred, resulting in a critically ill patient. Interventions are directed at life-saving measures; cerebral dysfunctions may be irreversible at this point. Therefore, neurological assessment is directed toward *early* identification of neurological alterations so that interventions can be instituted when the chances of control and reversal are good.

Before discussing the traditional signs and symptoms associated with increased ICP, it may be helpful to consider a few points about ICP and how it can be masked or misinterpreted.

Clinical Variations in Increased Intracranial Pressure

Although the neurological examination is a valid and effective method of monitoring ongoing changes in brain function, what are the limitations of this examination? The overriding principle in explaining the physiologic dynamics is the *degree of compliance in the brain,* as explained by the pressure–volume curve (see Fig. 13-1). Clinicians rely on clinical assessment for detection of the signs and symptoms of increased ICP and compromised CPP, but the related physiologic basis is not necessarily apparent on clinical assessment of neurological function. One cannot determine by clinical inspection where the patient is in relation to the pressure–volume curve. The patient's brain may be at the *high compliance* end of the curve or at the *low compliance* end when the slightest increase in ICP will result in decompensation and a significant elevation in ICP.

Direct Brainstem Injury

Many of the signs and symptoms of increased ICP often cited (e.g., decerebration, loss of the corneal reflex, changes in vital signs) relate to brainstem dysfunction. However, direct primary brainstem injury can also produce these signs and symptoms in the absence of increased ICP.

Transient Pressure Signs

The ICP is dynamic rather than constant. Certain activities, such as straining and coughing, can elevate ICP. In a patient at risk who already has an elevated ICP, initiating an activity known to increase ICP can precipitate *transient signs of increased ICP,* also known as *transient pressure signs* or *transient ischemic signs* (Chart 13-2). At the time of such a transient episode, the nurse may observe the onset of new deficits in patients whose previous neurological assessment produced normal results. Reassessment within 5 to 20 minutes may reveal reversal of all symptoms. A transient elevation in ICP caused by a temporary interference with CPP resulting in transient ischemia is responsible for the clinical deterioration noted.

Specific Signs and Symptoms of Increased Intracranial Pressure

The presenting signs and symptoms of increased ICP observed will vary, depending on the following:

- The compartmental location of the lesion (supratentorial or infratentorial)

CHART 13-2   Transient "Pressure Signs"

The following signs and symptoms are associated with transient elevations in ICP and cerebral hypoxia whereby there is temporary interference with CPP, resulting in transient ischemia. The signs and symptoms last a few minutes, occurring most often at the peak of plateau waves and then disappearing as the pressure decreases and CPP is once again re-established. The signs and symptoms of transient "pressure signs" include:

• Decreased level of consciousness (e.g., confusion, lethargy)
• Pupillary abnormalities
• Visual disturbances
• Motor dysfunction (hemiparesis or hemiplegia)
• Headache
• Aphasia (new-onset aphasia and/or change from baseline)
• Changes in respiratory pattern (e.g., Cheyne-Stokes)
• Changes in vital signs

ICP, intracranial pressure; CPP, cerebral perfusion pressure.

• The specific location of the mass (e.g., diencephalon, brainstem, or cerebellum)
• The mass effect of the lesion including edema
• The degree of intracranial compensation (compliance)

The following signs and symptoms associated with increased ICP are discussed to clarify their relationship to the cluster of clinical observations found in increased ICP. Guidelines for neurological assessment are found in Chapter 7.

Deterioration in Level of Consciousness

Changes in the LOC, although an important clinical sign, may vary from an early to a late sign depending on the lesion and progression of illness. As has been noted in the discussion of the uncal syndrome, many patients with early uncal herniation demonstrate near wakefulness. Because LOC may not be affected early in the process, it is *not the earliest sign* of herniation with the uncal syndrome. In the case of the central syndrome, some changes in LOC are part of the constellation of early signs. When LOC is affected, the earliest changes in a deteriorating LOC are confusion, restlessness, and lethargy. Generally, disorientation is noted, first to time, then to place, and finally to person. As the ICP continues to rise, the patient becomes lethargic, stuporous, and finally comatose. In the terminal stages, there is no response to painful stimuli, and the patient is deeply comatose. After the patient becomes comatose, LOC is less useful as a localizing sign and has little value in determining whether the patient is improving or getting worse. The ocular, motor, and respiratory signs become more useful for localization and prognosis.

Pupillary Dysfunction

Pupillary reaction to light is an upper brainstem function (oculomotor nerve [CN III]) and provides data about brainstem function that are especially helpful when assessing the unconscious patient. Compression of the oculomotor nerve against the base of the skull results from mass effect and produces changes in pupillary size, shape, and reaction to light. Different pupillary patterns are noted with uncal and central syndromes.

Uncal Syndrome. Unilateral, pupillary dilation is the *most consistent early finding* with uncal herniation. In addition, the pupillary response to light becomes sluggish and the pupil may become slightly ovoid. The Hippus response (see Chap. 7) to light may be observed with the beginning of pressure on the oculomotor nerve. Because the source of the rising ICP (e.g., edema, space-occupying lesion) tends to be compartmentalized in the early stages, the pupillary dysfunction is ipsilateral to the lesion. In the later stages of increased ICP, both pupils become dilated to midpoint and nonreactive (fixed) to light. Finally, in the terminal stages with herniation, both pupils become bilaterally maximally dilated and fixed.

Central Syndrome. In contrast, bilateral small (1 to 3 mm) reactive pupils are seen with early central herniation. As the process progresses to involve the midbrain, pupils dilate to 3 to 5 mm. Further pathophysiologic advancement is indistinguishable from that associated with uncal syndrome.

Visual and Extraocular Movement Abnormalities

Visual deficits that can develop in the early stages of increasing ICP include decreased visual acuity, blurred vision, diplopia, and field cuts, all of which are subjective signs. These subjective symptoms require a conscious, conversant patient to provide this information to the examiner. Extraocular motor (EOM) assessment can be conducted with a conscious, cooperative patient or by using the oculocephalic or oculovestibular responses in the unconscious patient.

Decreased acuity and blurring are probably associated with early hemispheric pressure because the visual pathways transect all of the lobes of the cerebral hemisphere. Diplopia is associated with paresis or paralysis of one or more extraocular muscles. With an attempt to focus in one direction, the images from both eyes will not fall on the same point on each retina, resulting in double vision. Visual fields and field cuts can be assessed by confrontation testing, again, requiring a cooperative, conscious patient.

EOM assessments can be tested by directing the patient to follow the examiner's finger through the full range of movement, or in an unconscious patient, the oculocephalic or oculovestibular reflex can be assessed. The oculocephalic reflex provides data on the reflex ability of the eyes to cross midline. Dysfunction may result from pressure from intracranial bulk that affects any EOM pathway. EOM function is innervated by CNs III, IV, and VI with nuclei located in the brainstem; they provide data about brainstem function that is especially helpful when assessing the unconscious patient. See Tables 13-2 and 13-3 for variations in uncal and central syndrome patterns.

When conducting EOM assessments, it is often helpful to note any gaze preference. In the case of localized lesions to the cerebral cortex, the eyes will deviate in the ipsilateral direction. Interestingly, a lesion that produces seizure activity will result in a contralateral gaze preference; this gives rise to the mnemonic that the brain-injured patient will "look at an injury" and "look away from a seizure."

Deterioration of Motor Function

In the early stages, monoparesis or hemiparesis develops contralateral to the intracranial lesion owing to pressure on the pyramidal tracts. In the later stages, hemiplegia, decortication, or decerebration develops because of increasing pressure on the brainstem. Decortication or decerebration may be unilateral or bilateral. In the terminal stages, the patient becomes bilaterally flaccid.

Clinically, there may be confusion about one of the most primitive flexion reflexes, sometimes called **triple flexion**, seen in the late stages. Flexor motor neuron activation is widespread, and the reflex results in flexor muscle contraction away from the source of the stimuli. This means that the flexor muscles at the ankle, knee, and hip contract to withdraw the whole limb. The clinical significance of this sign is that it is a primitive spinal reflex.

Headache

In the early stages of rising ICP, some patients complain of a slight headache. Headaches are not as common as one might expect. The following hypothesis of headaches and intracranial pathophysiology may be helpful. The intracranial structures that are sensitive to pain are the middle meningeal arteries and branches, the large arteries at the base of the brain, the venous sinuses, the bridging veins, and the dura at the base of the skull. The brain is normally cushioned by CSF. When the volume of CSF is reduced, the cushion is decreased or eliminated. When the head is in the erect position, the brain sinks. In the horizontal position, the brain shifts to one side. To compensate for the decrease in CSF and to provide an adequate cerebral blood supply, the cerebral vessels dilate, particularly in the venous components. Dilation of the vessels, traction on the bridging veins, and stretching of the arteries at the base of the brain cause pain and headache.

Headache associated with increased ICP is worse on arising in the morning. This can be explained by noting that ICP rises to high levels during the REM phase of sleep, which increases metabolism and produces CO_2 as an end-product. Associated hypercapnia causes vasodilation; this results in traction on proximal venous vessels and arterial stretching at the base of the skull. The result is headache.

Vomiting

Vomiting caused by increasing ICP is associated with infratentorial lesions or direct pressure on the vomiting center, the vagal motor centers located in the floor of the fourth ventricle in the medulla. The vagal motor center also mediates the motility of the gastrointestinal tract. An increase in ventricular pressure transmitted to these centers probably accounts for vomiting. When the vomiting mechanism is directly affected by a neurological lesion, the afferent limb is short circuited to produce vomiting without nausea. Without the warning of nausea, vomitus is ejected with undiminished force because of the suddenness with which the thoracic and abdominal muscles contract.[15] The term *projectile vomiting* is used to describe the forceful character of the vomiting.

Changes in Vital Signs

Blood Pressure. Blood pressure and pulse remain relatively uninfluenced by ICP during the early stages of intracranial hypertension. Only in the later stages, as rising ICP exerts pressure on the brainstem, do changes in blood pressure occur as a result of changes in ICP. These changes occur because ischemia in the medullary vasomotor center triggers an *ischemic reflex*, which causes an increase in systemic arterial pressure. The intraluminal arterial pressure must be greater than the ICP for continued blood flow. As ICP rises, the blood pressure rises reflexively to compensate. Cushing's response is activated. The resultant elevation in blood pressure increases cardiac output so that the heart pumps with greater force, thus widening the pulse pressure. Increasing systemic blood pressure with a widening pulse pressure is the compensatory phase of increasing ICP. With deterioration, the decompensation phase begins and blood pressure decreases.

Pulse. In the early stages of intracranial hypertension, the pulse rate also remains relatively unaffected by increasing ICP; changes in pulse rate are associated with brainstem involvement. Bradycardia probably results from pressure on the vagal control mechanism in the medulla. With a continued rise in pressure, the pulse drops to 60 per minute or less and becomes full and bounding. The decreased rate and bounding quality are compensatory to pump blood upward into vessels on which pressure is being exerted from expanding intracranial bulk. In the decompensatory stage, the pulse becomes irregular, rapid, and thready and then ceases.

Respirations. Alterations in the respiratory pattern are associated with direct pressure on the brainstem respiratory centers of the pons and medulla. The various patterns and associated anatomic levels are discussed in Chapter 7. In addition, an acute increase in ICP can trigger development of acute neurogenic pulmonary edema in the absence of cardiac disease. Other possible acute respiratory complications include acute respiratory distress syndrome and disseminated intravascular coagulopathy.

Temperature. Variations in temperature are usually associated with hypothalamic dysfunction either by direct injury or as a result of traction on connecting tracts. During the compensatory phase of increasing ICP, body temperature will probably remain within normal limits. During the decompensatory phase, high temperatures are frequently observed. Elevations in either phase need to be evaluated and differentiated between neurogenic hyperthermia and a temperature elevation due to an infection such as pneumonia.

Advances in technology have now made it possible to directly monitor the temperature of brain tissues. The temperature of brain tissue is generally $0.5 \pm 0.2°C$ higher than core body temperature in the normal adult.[18] A sudden and profound shift to cerebral hypothermia has been associated with poor patient outcomes.[19] This is most likely associated with a sudden decrease in CBF and consequent decrease in tissue perfusion. Monitoring for changes in both the absolute and the relative change in body and brain temperature will provide the nurse with a stronger comprehension of the intracranial pathology.

CLINICAL PEARLS: Don't ignore the basics: changes in heart rate, blood pressure, and temperature may be cause and effect of changes in ICP.

Loss of Brainstem Reflexes

In the late stages of rising ICP, pressure on the brainstem causes loss or dysfunction of reflexes mediated by the brainstem. These reflexes include the pupillary, corneal, gag, swallowing, oculocephalic, and oculovestibular reflexes (see Chap. 7). The prognosis is poor for patients who have lost their brainstem reflexes.

Papilledema

Papilledema, discussed in Chapter 7, is a blurring of the optic disc margin as noted during an ophthalmoscopic examination. Because the subdural and subarachnoid spaces continue along the optic nerve, increased pressure within the intracranial cavity is transmitted along the nerve. The result is edema of the head of the optic nerve, which can be seen when viewing the optic disc with an ophthalmoscope.

Depending on circumstances, papilledema may be a late finding with increased ICP. It does not occur until ICP has reached markedly elevated levels. Papilledema is not a universal observation made in all patients with increased ICP. In some patients, this may be the first sign observed if an elevated ICP has developed gradually.

MANAGEMENT OF PATIENTS WITH INTRACRANIAL HYPERTENSION: A COLLABORATIVE PROBLEM

Management of patients with intracranial hypertension is a collaborative problem in which all members of the interdisciplinary team share responsibilities for patient outcomes. In addition to intracranial hypertension, other possible collaborative problems associated with intracranial hypertension must be kept in mind (Box 13-3).

BOX 13-3 Major Collaborative Problems Associated With Increased Intracranial Pressure and Intracranial Hypertension

- Hypovolemic shock
- Cardiogenic shock
- Dysrhythmias
- Hypotension
- Hypertension
- Deep vein thrombosis/pulmonary embolism
- Disseminated intravascular coagulation
- Neurogenic pulmonary edema
- Atelectasis/pneumonia
- Ventilator dependency
- Electrolyte imbalances
- Hypoglycemia/hyperglycemia
- Diabetes insipidus
- Sepsis
- Acidosis/alkalosis
- Hyperthermia
- Stroke
- Seizures
- Gastric ulcer (Cushing's ulcer) with gastrointestinal bleeding
- Renal failure

BOX 13-4 Major Patient Problems Associated With Increased Intracranial Pressure and Intracranial Hypertension

- Altered Cerebral Tissue Perfusion
- Ineffective Respiratory Function
- Ineffective Airway Clearance
- Risk for Aspiration
- Risk for Infection
- Risk for Injury
- Hyperthermia
- Total Incontinence
- Constipation

Medical and nursing management of the patient with intracranial hypertension is directed toward the prevention of secondary brain injury.[20] Therapy includes the early diagnosis and treatment of the underlying cause(s), management of factors known to increase ICP, control and management of intracranial hypertension, support of all body systems, and prevention of complications. Most patients will be admitted to an acute care unit or an intensive care unit (ICU) where technological and other resources are available to support the patient. These are vulnerable patients at high risk for complications and thus need expert assessment, monitoring, and treatment through a collaborative effort of the entire team for optimal patient outcomes. Nurses may also wish to consider patient problems to guide care. Box 13-4 shows the major patient problems associated with increased ICP and intracranial hypertension.

Assessment, Management Strategies, and Interventions for Intracranial Hypertension

Neurological Assessment

Baseline and ongoing neurological assessments are the foundation of patient management. Frequent assessment (every 15 minutes to every 1 hour), depending on stability of neurological signs, provides information on changes in neurological status. This includes:

- LOC (i.e., deterioration in LOC)
- Pupillary size and reaction to direct light (unilateral or bilateral pupillary dilation)
- Motor function (weakness, paralysis, or abnormal posturing)
- Respiratory pattern

The most convincing evidence of the development of intracranial hypertension is the evolving presence of one or more of these signs.[21] Changes in findings are often subtle and may be detected only by performing serial assessments and comparing serial data. For example, if the nurse notices that a previously alert and oriented patient is now confused, this is a significant finding. The nurse may need to consider other explanations of confusion, such as response to drugs, but alteration in consciousness is often apparent *before* changes in pupillary size or reaction to light, eye movement, or motor or sensory function occur. Vigilant nursing assessment and monitoring are the most sensitive means to detect early change.

Early recognition of deterioration allows definitive action to be taken while treatment strategies can still be effective. However, after pupillary and other brainstem signs become apparent, the downhill course of events can occur rapidly, and the effectiveness of treatment limited. Noting trends of subtle changes applies not only to the LOC, pupillary size and reaction, and motor function, but also to vital signs.

Trends in vital signs must be noted because deterioration in neurological status can herald a change from a compensatory neurological state to one of decompensation. Slowing of the pulse, widening pulse pressure, and an elevating systolic pressure are *late signs* of neurological deterioration. The nurse should not wait until these signs are present before intervening. Therefore, serial neurological assessments are the basis for identifying neurological change.

Management Strategies and Interventions

There are many brain-specific and general supportive strategies and interventions to manage patients with intracranial hypertension. This section is divided into brain-specific strategies and interventions for intracranial hypertension and cardiopulmonary supportive strategies and interventions. Evidence-based practice guidelines published in 2007 provide an excellent foundation for patient care and examining the efficacy of specific treatment strategies.[22]

Brain-Specific Strategies and Interventions for Intracranial Hypertension.

In this section head elevation, hyperventilation, blood pressure and oxygenation, CPP, CSF drainage, mannitol and corticosteroids, analgesia/sedation, neuromuscular blockade, fluid management, temperature control, seizure control, hypothermia, barbiturate coma, and surgery are discussed.

Elevation of Head of Bed. Elevation of the head of the bed to 30 degrees has been employed to improve jugular venous drainage, thereby lowering ICP.[21,23–26] Venous drainage from the brain has no valves and thus the use of gravity facilitates drainage with concurrent lowering of ICP. This is considered safe so long as the patient is *not hypovolemic*, a condition that could threaten adequate CPP. Therefore, maintaining adequate intravascular volume is necessary to elevate the head of the bed safely.

Chesnut points out one disadvantage of head elevation.[27] Patients must be placed flat for transport, CT scanning, and other procedures. This flat position often results in intracranial hypertension. This effect should be anticipated, so that Chesnut recommends lowering the bed to the flat position 15 to 30 minutes before transport so that alterations in ICP and other physiologic parameters can be corrected in the ICU rather than during transport.

Hyperventilation. Use of **hyperventilation** to reduce increased ICP has been controversial, but clearer guidelines are now available.[28] To understand this controversy it is necessary to have a firm understanding of how CO_2 affects intracranial dynamics. CO_2 is a potent cerebral vasodilator, and lowering cerebral CO_2 can cause rapid cerebral vasoconstriction resulting in decreased CBF; this decrease in blood flow decreases the intracranial blood volume and thereby decreases the ICP. Change in the pH of the serum and CSF results in alkalosis, thus causing cerebral vasoconstriction and a reduced intracranial volume and decreased ICP. In traumatic brain-injured patients, CBF is lowest in the first day after TBI and slowly increased over the next 3 to 4 days.[29,30] Aggressive lowering of $PaCO_2$ by hyperventilation to levels of 25 mm Hg can rapidly reduce ICP, but the abrupt cerebral vasoconstriction can lead to a decrease in CBF and ischemia.[31]

A prospective study of patients with severe TBI randomized to prophylactic hyperventilation for 5 days after injury with a PCO_2 of 25 mm Hg was compared with findings in a control group without hyperventilation and a PCO_2 of 35 mm Hg. At 3-month and 6-month follow-up, those treated with hyperventilation with a Glasgow Coma Score of 4 or 5 had significantly worse outcomes than the control group.[32]

Monitoring jugular oxygen concentration has demonstrated a relationship between hyperventilation and decreased CBF and decreased cerebral oxygen delivery in two studies.[33,34] In both groups, there was a rapid improvement in jugular venous oxygen concentration following the return to normocapnia, which suggested improved CBF and oxygenation of cerebral tissue.[28] Given these data, which evidence-based guidelines assist the clinician in the use of hyperventilation as a treatment option in managing increased ICP? In a 2002 study, Oertel et al.[35] concluded that hyperventilation may be an effective means of lowering ICP, but only when brain oxygen monitoring is employed during episodes of hyperventilation.

Hyperventilation has an important role in rapidly reducing *acute episodes* of increased ICP when a patient has an *acute onset* of "pressure signs" (e.g., deteriorating LOC, dilated or ovoid pupil) and needs rapid reduction of ICP. By inducing hypocarbia, cerebral vasoconstriction and reduced CBF result. As a result, the ICP drops almost immediately. The patient can be hyperventilated using a manual resuscitation (Ambu) bag when a ventilator is not present. This urgent intervention lasts minutes to lower the ICP rapidly so that definitive treatment can be started. In a mechanically ventilated patient, increasing the ventilatory rate while maintaining a tidal volume of 12 to 15 mL/kg provides hyperventilation. The target level of PCO_2 is 30 to 35 mm Hg. The effectiveness of hyperventilation appears to be time limited and thus transient.

Evidence-based guidelines for hyperventilation offer the following recommendations.[22] Hyperventilation is useful as an adjunct to osmotic therapy.[36] Neither prophylactic nor prolonged hyperventilation is recommended. *Prophylactic hyperventilation* ($PaCO_2$ of 35 mm Hg or less) during the first 24 hours after severe TBI should be avoided. Hyperventilation may be used for intracranial hypertension for longer periods of time if the ICP does not respond to usual treatment strategies (e.g., sedation, CSF drainage). When hyperventilation is discontinued, it should also be withdrawn gradually over 12 to 24 hours. Hyperventilation is useful and recommended only for brief periods to reverse *acute* neurological deterioration.

To prevent complications from hyperventilation, maintain adequate intravascular volume and systemic blood pressure. A central line is helpful to monitor hemodynamics. End-tidal carbon dioxide ($ETCO_2$) can be used to monitor trends in CO_2, although arterial gases are more accurate gauges. Review blood gas to determine achievement of target levels. A jugular venous catheter is useful to monitor jugular venous oxygen concentration (SjO_2) and arterial-jugular venous oxygen content differences ($AvDO_2$) to identify cerebral ischemia. If available, direct brain tissue oxygen monitoring ($PbtO_2$) is helpful in monitoring the adequacy of brain perfusion and preventing episodes of ischemia associated with decreased CBF.[37] If the patient is agitated or is fighting the ventilator, try to determine the cause and treat it; if the agitation continues, the physician may order sedation or neuromuscular blockade drugs to synchronize the patient with the ventilator. Finally, there is a role for hyperventilation with increased ICP, but specific guidelines must be followed.

Oxygenation and Blood Pressure Control. Managing blood pressure is an important concern because of the serious consequences related to extremes in blood pressure. **Hypotension** is directly related to cerebral ischemia and secondary brain injury, whereas **hypertension** has little effect on CBF and ICP. Maintaining adequate CPP is critical in preventing ischemia; this important point will be further discussed. The guidelines for traumatic brain injury treatment are clear for hypotension (systolic blood pressure below 90 mm Hg). These guidelines state that hypotension or hypoxia (apnea, cyanosis, or a PaO_2 below 60 mm Hg) must be avoided, or if it occurs, must be corrected immediately. The mean arterial blood pressure should be maintained above 90 mm Hg at all times to maintain a CPP above 70 mm Hg.[22] If a hypotensive event occurs, a fluid bolus and a vasoactive drug are indicated (see Chap. 11). The prevention and treatment of hypoxia should begin with airway management and may require increased ventilatory support.

The patient must be carefully monitored to prevent hypotensive episodes. An adequate intravascular volume (euvolemia) must be maintained. In addition to careful clinical assessment, review of arterial blood gases, ongoing data from the pulse oximetry (SpO_2), and invasive monitoring data assist in clinical reasoning. Alarms on the ventilator must be kept on at all times to alert the nurse to any situation that compromises adequate oxygenation.

Cerebral Perfusion Pressure. Cerebral perfusion pressure is the mean arterial blood pressure minus ICP. It is the pressure gradient responsible for CBF and metabolite delivery and is directly related to ischemia. Cerebral ischemia is considered the most important secondary event affecting poor outcome. Therefore, it is critical to maintain an adequate CPP, a minimum of 70 mm Hg. According to the most recent guidelines,[22] the following recommendations are made: aggressive attempts to maintain CPP above 70 mm Hg with fluids and pressors should be avoided because of the risk of acute

respiratory distress syndrome; CPP of less than 50 mm Hg should be avoided; the CPP value to target lies within the range of 50 to 70 mm Hg; patients with intact pressure autoregulation tolerate higher CPP values; and ancillary monitoring of cerebral indicators that include blood flow, oxygenation, or metabolism facilitates CPP management.

In summarizing the underpinnings of CPP management, the guidelines distinguish between physiologic thresholds representing potential injury from clinical thresholds to treat. Much of the information about physiologic thresholds can come from simple physiologic monitoring, whereas clinical thresholds come from clinical evidence from controlled trials using outcome as the dependent variable. The critical threshold for cerebral ischemia is somewhere in the range of 50 to 60 mm Hg. It can be further fine-tuned in a particular patient with ancillary monitoring. Clifton et al. suggest that a CPP target threshold should be set approximately 10 mm Hg above what is determined to be a critical threshold in order to avoid dips below the critical level.[38] The rationale for maintaining a CPP of 70 mm Hg or above is based on evidence that CBF is usually very low after TBI, often near the ischemic threshold.[29,39–41] Further, CBF adjacent to contusions and subdural hematomas is reduced even more than global CBF.[42,43] A 2005 review article summarizing the available literature on various CPP treatment thresholds has concluded that the present level of 70 mm Hg remains the current standard.[44]

Evidence about hypertension has equally evolved. Concerns have been raised about adverse effects from hypertensive therapy used in some patients with severe TBI to maintain adequate CPP. The concern focuses on an increase in ICP in response to therapy with subsequent poor outcomes.[22] The evidence does not support this concern. For example, the effects on ICP and CBF in response to artificial hypertension were studied by Bouma and Muizclaar in 35 patients with severe TBI.[45] Elevating the mean arterial blood pressure from 92 ± 10 to 123 ± 8 mm Hg resulted in only a slight increase (<1%) in ICP in patients with an intact autoregulation. In those with loss of autoregulation, there was a decrease in mean ICP. This study and others demonstrate that ICP usually changes very little when blood pressure is increased by as much as 30 mm Hg in TBI patients regardless of the status of autoregulation (defined as an increase in CBF when the blood pressure is increased). Therefore, there is no direct relationship between CBF and ICP. A moderate increase in blood pressure, such as might be initiated to maintain adequate CPP, should not cause an increase in ICP in most TBI patients.[22] If antihypertensive drugs are indicated, those most often used are intravenous beta blockers or the combined alpha and beta blocker labetalol (see Chap. 12).

Cerebrospinal Fluid Drainage. The insertion of a catheter into a lateral ventricle through a burr hole made in the skull for CSF drainage is called a **ventriculostomy**. Drainage of CSF from a ventriculostomy is a temporary method to reduce ICP rapidly and can sustain the patient through spikes in ICP or during acute hydrocephalus associated with subarachnoid hemorrhage. The ventriculostomy catheter may be inserted exclusively for periodic CSF drainage, or the catheter may be connected to an external drainage and pressure monitoring system that is capable of providing periodic CSF drainage and ICP monitoring (Fig. 13-8).

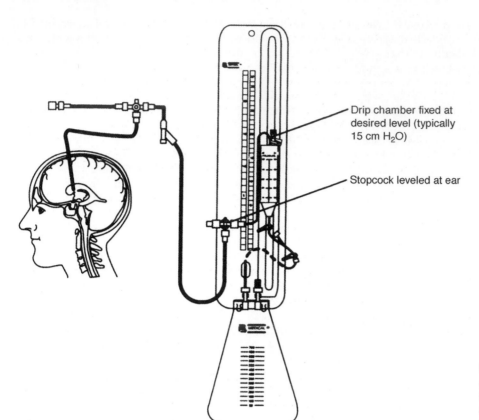

Drip chamber fixed at desired level (typically 15 cm H_2O)

Stopcock leveled at ear

Figure 13-8 • Becker intraventricular external drainage and landmarks for calibration. (Widjicks, E. [1997]. *The clinical practice of critical care neurology.* Philadelphia: Lippincott-Raven.)

The most recent guidelines[22] state that treatment should be initiated with intracranial pressure thresholds above 20 mm Hg. One intervention is drainage of CSF. When CSF drainage is desired via a ventriculostomy, the nurse can periodically drain the CSF according to a physician's order. Although there is not an exact target point at which treatment is necessary to decrease ICP, current data support greater than 20 mm Hg as an upper threshold above which ICP lowering therapy should be initiated.[22] When the ICP reaches or exceeds the given threshold set by the physician (e.g., 20 or 25 mm Hg), the stopcock is opened and CSF drained according to the physician's order (e.g., 5 minutes). There are specific management points that must be followed: the stopcock of the drainage system should be leveled to an anatomic reference point such as the level of the ear; to decrease the risk of overdrainage, a ventriculostomy system should not be left open to drainage without supervision; current systems do not permit accurate recording of the ICP during periods of drainage; and the nurse should periodically assess the ICP with the stopcock turned off to drainage. Insertion of a ventricular catheter is associated with an increased risk of infection.

CLINICAL PEARLS: Do not leave an unattended ventriculostomy open to drainage. This may result in a sudden excess of CSF drainage if the patient changes position, coughs, or has episodes of spontaneous Valsalva's maneuver.

Mannitol and Corticosteroids (see also Chap. 12). Mannitol, an osmotic diuretic, works on the principle of establishing a

high osmotic gradient to draw water from the extracellular space of the edematous cerebral tissue into the plasma. Mannitol (Osmitrol), because it does not cross the blood–brain barrier, is the mainstay of hyperosmolar therapy. The osmotic effect of hyperosmolar therapy causes water to be drawn from the extracellular space of the edematous brain into the plasma, thereby reducing brain volume and decreasing ICP. The free water in the plasma is then excreted via the kidneys.

Mannitol (20% to 25%) is considered relatively safe and is administered intravenously through a filter. The filter is necessary because of the risk of crystallization of the drug. The current practice is to give mannitol as a bolus at a dose of 0.25 to 0.5 g/kg or up to 1g/kg every 3 to 6 hours, infused rapidly.[22] The ICP, CPP, and serum osmolality are monitored frequently. Therapy is directed at keeping the serum osmolality at approximately 310 to 315 mOsm. Serum osmolalities above 320 mOsm/L and hypovolemia should be avoided.[22] The maximal effect of mannitol should be noted within 15 to 30 minutes and can last for 1 to 3 hours. In some patients, a rebound effect, observed as a rise in ICP, may occur after administration.

Mannitol can result in dehydration, hypoosmolality, electrolyte imbalance (e.g., hypokalemia, hyponatremia), or renal failure. Serum osmolality, electrolytes, blood urea nitrogen, creatinine, and the intake and output record must be monitored. An indwelling catheter is necessary to monitor urinary diuresis. Electrolyte balance should be carefully monitored and replaced as needed (see Chap. 9). Mannitol is not administered to patients with hypovolemic shock, congestive heart failure, dehydration, or kidney disease. Furosemide, a loop diuretic, may be used to manage the rebound effect from mannitol, but it is not a mainstay drug for the primary management of increased ICP.

Corticosteroids have *no* demonstrated benefit for treatment of increased ICP in cerebral infarction with edema or TBI and are, therefore, *not* a standard of care.[46]

Analgesia and Sedation. Pain, restlessness, and agitation are known to exacerbate existing increased ICP. Analgesics with or without sedation can be useful.[19] The Society of Critical Care Medicine has developed and published practice guidelines for intravenous analgesia and sedation for the adult patient in the ICU.[47] Narcotic analgesics can be effective in controlling pain and providing sedation. These recommendations apply to critically ill adults in the ICU and are summarized in an executive summary.[48] Morphine sulfate is the preferred analgesic agent for critically ill patients. Fentanyl is the best choice if the patient is hemodynamically unstable, demonstrating histamine release with morphine, or allergic to morphine. Hydromorphone can be used as an alternative to morphine.

While sedation may play an important part in decreasing episodes of increased ICP, caring for neurologically injured patients often requires that the patient be awakened from sedation such that the nurse may obtain a comprehensive neurologic assessment. This creates the sedation-assessment conundrum, described by Olson et al.,[49] in which nurses must quickly and carefully interrupt sedation while attending to the risk of secondary brain injury from ICP changes. Midazolam (Versed) and propofol (Diprivan) are the preferred choices only for short-term (i.e., <24-hour) treatment of anxiety.[50] Lorazepam (Ativan) is the drug of choice for prolonged treatment of anxiety, and haloperidol is preferred for delerium.[48] The updated guidelines promote an environment wherein sedation goals are defined by the needs of the patient and regularly reassessed by the medical team.[47] Pharmacologic sedation of this population requires careful consideration of the underlying neurophysiologic disturbances and potential adverse effects introduced by sedative drugs (see Chap. 12).[51]

Neuromuscular Blockade (Paralysis). Paralysis (neuromuscular blockade) and sedation are used as chemical restraints to control restlessness and agitation that increase cerebral metabolism, blood pressure, and ICP. Some motor activities such as dyssynchrony with a ventilator (i.e., "bucking" or fighting the ventilator) or abnormal posturing (e.g., decortication, decerebration) also contribute to increased ICP by increases in intrathoracic pressure and central venous pressure. The Society of Critical Care Medicine has developed and published practice parameters for sustained neuromuscular blockade in the adult critically ill patient. They are summarized in an executive summary.[48] Three recommendations have been made. Pancuronium is the preferred neuromuscular blockade (NMB) for most critically ill patients. Vecuronium is preferred for patients with cardiac disease or hemodynamic instability when tachycardia could have a negative effect. All patients receiving neuromuscular blockade should be appropriately assessed for the degree of blockade achieved. Side effects may be minimized by careful monitoring of the degree of muscle blockade and the drug dosage.

Using a peripheral nerve stimulator and monitor of muscle movement are safe ways to periodically monitor the degree of blockade.[52] The peripheral nerve stimulator delivers electrical current to the nerve through electrodes. Before the patch electrodes can be applied, the skin must be hairless, clean, and dry. The terminal outputs of the peripheral nerve stimulator include the positive (anode) and negative (cathode) terminals. The active electrode concentrates the electrical current and is placed near the nerve. The inactive electrode is located farthest from the nerve and is used to complete the circuit (Fig. 13-9). The ulnar, facial, posterior tibial, or peroneal nerve can be used for monitoring. The ulnar nerve is most commonly used because it is superficial and easy to locate. The ulnar nerve innervates the adductor pollicis muscle in the thumb. Various configurations can be used to apply the electrodes. The most accessible part of the ulnar nerve is between the tendon flexor carpi ulnaris medially and the ulnar artery laterally about 2 to 3 inches proximally from the crease of the wrist.[53] Proper positioning of the electrodes along the nerve is necessary for a response (see Fig. 13-9).

The train-of-four (TOF) stimulation is the best and most common method of peripheral nerve stimulator monitoring to assess the level of neuromuscular blockade. Four electrical stimuli of 2 Hz each are delivered at 0.5-second intervals, for a total of four pulses. The number of responses to TOF stimuli indicates the degree of the neuromuscular blockade. As the depth of the blockade increases, the number of elicited responses decreases. The hand on the stimulated limb is positioned palm up. Observe or palpate for thumb adduction with each stimuli. If you see three twitches, it indicates a blockade of 80%; two equal 85%; and one 90%. An absence of twitches is equivalent to 100% blockade.[54] The frequency of TOF depends on whether the drug is being titrated to a set TOF, commonly two of four, or whether an infusion is being maintained. Generally, TOF should be assessed at least every 4 hours. The nurse titrates the drug to a prescribed response such as two adductions out of four stimuli on the TOF.[52]

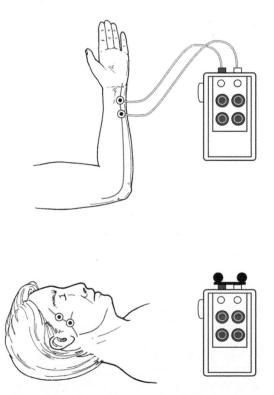

Figure 13-9 • Train-of-four peripheral stimulator.

TABLE 13-4   RAMSAY SCALE FOR ASSESSING LEVEL OF SEDATION

LEVEL OF SEDATION	RESPONSE
1	Patient anxious and agitated, restless, or both
2	Patient cooperative, oriented, and tranquil
3	Patient responds to commands only
4	Patient asleep; brisk response to light glabellar tap or loud auditory stimuli
5	Patient asleep; sluggish response to light glabellar tap or loud auditory stimulus
6	Patient does not respond to painful stimulus

From Ramsay, M. A., Savege, T. M., Simpson, B. R., & Goodwin, R. (1974). Controlled sedation with alphaxalone-alphadolone. *British Medical Journal, 2*(920), 656–659.

It is fundamentally important to distinguish between paralysis and sedation. The use of neuromuscular blockers such as pancuronium results in muscular paralysis, but does not impair the patient's consciousness; nor does paralysis impair the ability to recall unpleasant events. Observational sedation assessment tools such as the Ramsay Scale (Table 13-4) have limited use because they require the paralyzed patient to respond (physically) to a stimulus.[55] Recently, the bispectral index (BIS) monitor has been explored as a means of providing information about the paralyzed patient's level of sedation.[56]

Fluid Management and Euvolemia. The use of hypertonic solutions is gaining use in clinical practice. The principal effect of hypertonic saline on ICP is possibly due to osmotic mobilization of water across the intact blood–brain barrier, which reduces cerebral water content.[57] A number of studies have been conducted to evaluate the use of hypertonic saline solutions from normal saline to 23.4% sodium chloride solutions to reduce intracranial pressure.[58–60] According to the 2007 guidelines,[22] there is not strong enough evidence to make recommendations for the use, concentration, and method of administration of hypertonic saline for the treatment of traumatic intracranial hypertension at the current time.[61] More research is needed to determine the efficacy of hypertonic solutions.

Hypotension and dehydration are dangerous and can result in decreased CPP and cerebral ischemia. The concurrent hypoxemia and cerebral hypoxia can result in further increases in ICP. The fluid management goal in the treatment of increased ICP is euvolemia; adequate fluid management with *saline* is the preferred treatment for preventing hypotension and dehydration. Glucose solutions are avoided because of the potential to increase cerebral edema. Monitoring of serum osmolality, electrolytes, urine specific gravity, daily weight, and glucose is necessary to guide clinical decisions regarding electrolyte replacement, selection of saline concentration of fluids, rate of fluid administration, and glucose management.

Hypoglycemia and hyperglycemia can result in neurological changes, so they are to be avoided. Hypotonic glucose intravenous solutions are avoided. Recent literature suggests that aggressive management to control serum blood sugar is associated with improved outcomes following neurologic injury.[62,63] Hyperglycemia is controlled with a sliding scale of regular insulin according to periodic fingersticks and, if needed, a regular insulin intravenous drip can be started.

Temperature Control. CBF increases approximately 5% to 6% for each 1°C increase. The cerebral metabolic rate increases 5% to 7% for each 1°C increase.[64] An increased metabolic rate produces more end-products of cellular metabolism (CO_2 and organic acids, such as lactic acid). In the patient with existing cerebral hypertension, the increase in systemic blood pressure and CBF exacerbates the existing increase in ICP. Therefore, it is important to treat hyperthermia aggressively. This is accomplished with antipyretic drugs such as acetaminophen, poikilothermic drugs such as propofol, and neuromuscular blockers. Pharmacotherapy may be used alone or in combination with a variety of mechanical temperature control devices. These devices may be invasive (e.g., the placement of an intravenous cooling device) or noninvasive (e.g., devices that circulate a coolant through pads or blankets that are wrapped around the patient's body). If a cooling device is used, cool the patient slowly and attempt to prevent shivering because this will increase ICP. If shivering does occur, ICP will increase; thus, the patient must be monitored closely to prevent this adverse effect. Some sedatives, such as propofol and Thorazine, are useful to control shivering.[36] Buspirone (BuSpar) may aid in the reduction of the shivering response.[65]

Recent publications address the importance of maintaining normothermia in the neuroscience patient.[66,67] To maintain normothermia, the nurse should:

- Monitor the core body temperature hourly (axillary and oral temperatures are unreliable).
- Administer antipyretics as ordered.
- Monitor the skin for impaired circulation (including the dorsal surfaces) every 2 hours.
- If a cooling blanket is used, turn off the blanket when the temperature is approximately 1°C above the desired level. (Temperature will continue to drift downward because the blanket will remain cool.*)
- If a cooling blanket is used, lower the temperature gradually to prevent shivering.*
- Monitor intravascular cooling insertion sites for bleeding or infection.

Seizure Control. Cerebral metabolic rates are increased with seizures; this results in increased CBF, CBV, and ICP. Posttraumatic seizures are classified as early (i.e., occurring within 7 days of injury) or late (i.e., occurring 7 days after injury). Seizure prophylaxis should be instituted for patients who are high risk for *early* seizures (e.g., penetrating injury). Routine seizure prophylaxis after 7 days following head injury is not recommended.[22] Both phenytoin (Dilantin) and

---

*Many cooling devices (such as body-wrap and intravascular cooling systems) now come with computerized feedback algorithms and it is not necessary to turn the device off, nor to slow down the rate of cooling.

levetiracetam (Keppra) are effective in preventing early post-traumatic seizures. A loading dose of phenytoin can be given intravenously over 1 hour for the seizing patient. The average maintenance dosage of phenytoin is 100 mg orally or through a nasogastric tube, three to four times daily. See Chapter 12 for further discussion of anticonvulsants. The nursing responsibilities involved in seizure control include:

- Monitoring serum levels to ensure therapeutic drug levels
- Because phenytoin binds to albumin, monitoring albumin level if serum values drop
- Once tube feedings are started, the protein may decrease a previously therapeutic phenytoin level, thus requiring a bolus dose and higher maintenance dose.

Hypothermia. In laboratory animal studies, treatment with moderate, systemic hypothermia reduced the rate of cerebral edema and death after cerebral cortex injury.[68–70] This work was followed by early studies of hypothermia in humans that were inconclusive.[71,72] In two trials of patients with brain injury, moderate hypothermia maintained for 48 and 24 hours resulted in 15% and 18% increases, respectively, in the patients who had good outcomes compared with others in their cohort group.[73,74] Early use of moderate hypothermia (core temperature 32 to 33°C) for 24 hours was tried to decrease central metabolism and oxygen consumption to preserve neuronal tissue and improve outcomes.[75] Cooling blankets were placed above and below a chemically paralyzed and sedated, mechanically ventilated patient. Side effects of treatment included myocardial suppression, arrhythmias, and renal dysfunction. A large multicenter trial was conducted from 1994 through May 1998. The conclusion of the study was that treatment with hypothermia, with the body temperature reaching 33°C within 8 hours after injury, is *not* effective in improving outcomes in patients with severe brain injury.[76]

The use of induced hypothermia as treatment for traumatic brain injury continues to be controversial. Recent studies have found that hypothermia is associated with a decrease in ICP and improved outcomes for select patients with extradural trauma.[77] Other studies have concluded that the duration of hypothermia and goal temperature are focal in developing effective hypothermia treatment.[78] The Guidelines for the Management of Severe Traumatic Brain Injury,[22] in providing level III recommendations, cite pooled data indicating that prophylactic hypothermia is not significantly associated with decreased mortality when compared with normothermic controls. However, preliminary findings suggest that a greater decrease in mortality risk is observed when target temperatures are maintained for more than 48 hours. They go on to say that prophylactic hypothermia is associated with significantly higher Glasgow Outcome Scale scores when compared to scores for normothermic controls. The use of hypothermia in treating increased ICP is still being determined.

The use of hypothermia after cardiac arrest (HACA) to prevent neurocognitive complications following the return of spontaneous circulation after cardiac arrest is now a class IIa (following ventricular fibrillation [VF] cardiac arrest) or class IIb (following non-VF cardiac arrest) recommendation.[79]

High-Dose Barbiturate Coma. High-dose barbiturate coma therapy has been used for many years. It is a second-tier intervention

to manage intractable intracranial hypertension resistant to conventional medical and surgical therapies in hemodynamically stable patients.[22] It has been useful in reducing increased ICP in selected salvageable patients with TBI, Reye's syndrome, encephalitis, and cerebral hemorrhage. The underlying therapeutic of the drug is a vasoconstricting effect and a rapid decrease in cerebral metabolism and CBF, which leads to a decrease in CBV and ICP.

Barbiturate coma therapy consists of administering a loading dose and maintenance doses of a short-acting barbiturate—most often pentobarbital (Nembutal), although some physicians prefer thiopental.[80] After barbiturate coma has been induced, the usual parameters of neurological assessment, such as the pupillary, gag, and swallowing reflexes, are lost.[81] Cortical activity, as measured by electroencephalogram, is depressed, although brainstem–evoked responses may remain intact.[82] Continuous invasive monitoring of ICP and of cardiac and pulmonary functions is necessary. Peripheral and central lines for fluid and drug administration are required. The patient must remain intubated and mechanically ventilated. Induction of coma is accomplished by administering a loading dose of intravenous pentobarbital, 10 mg/kg, over 30 minutes followed by 5 mg/kg every hour for three doses.[9] A maintenance dose of 1 to 3 mg/kg/hour by continuous intravenous infusion is adjusted to maintain control of ICP.[9,20] Control of ICP can generally be achieved with serum barbiturate levels in the range of 30 to 40 mg/dL, which will also cause burst suppression on the electroencephalogram.

Barbiturate coma may have almost an immediate effect of lowering the ICP. After the patient has maintained an ICP of less than 20 mm Hg (or the level prescribed by protocol) for 24 to 48 hours, the drug is gradually tapered. If there is no response to therapy, the physician must decide how long the trial period should continue before the therapy is declared unsuccessful. The major problems associated with barbiturate coma are hypotension, dehydration, myocardial depression, and erratic dose response. Vasopressors such as phenylephrine hydrochloride or dopamine are administered to maintain blood pressure within targeted ranges. Albumin and other fluids are given to provide adequate volume and to prevent dehydration. Other conventional drugs used in the management of increased ICP such as mannitol are also continued.

Barbiturates are stored in body fat. This can create a problem when brain-death criteria are considered because of elevated barbiturate blood levels that could explain loss of spontaneous respirations and brainstem reflexes. Therefore, brain-death criteria cannot be met until the drug is cleared from the body. It can be difficult to wait, especially if organ donation is a consideration. However, there are serious medicolegal implications if all components of brain-death criteria are not met.

Surgery. If there is a localized mass, such as a hematoma, tumor, or abscess, removal or debulking of the lesion should help to reduce intracranial hypertension. In addition, a decompressive hemicraniectomy (in which a large portion of the skull is removed to allow for expansion of the brain due to cerebral edema) has gained support to improve control of intracranial hypertension (Box 13-5). After the ICP has subsided, the bone flap can be reinserted.

Cardiovascular and Pulmonary Strategies and Interventions for Increased Intracranial Pressure and Intracranial Hypertension

Although this chapter has addressed increased ICP and intracranial hypertension as a collaborative problem, cardiopulmonary management deserves additional comments, especially for the nurse. The brain requires a continuous and adequate supply of oxygen through the cardiac and respiratory systems. The interrelatedness of these systems to cerebral function is critical to patient outcomes.

Cardiovascular Management. Cardiac dysfunction in acute neurological conditions is common. The negative effects of hypertension and especially hypotension have been addressed in a previous section. Cardiac arrhythmias, left ventricular dysfunction, and cardiac disease or injury are briefly discussed in this section. Cardiac problems associated with specific neurological conditions, such as cerebral aneurysms, are discussed in other chapters.

Cardiac arrhythmias are common and often seen in patients who are at risk for intracranial hypertension and secondary brain injury. These arrhythmias are associated with sympathetic hyperactivity and preponderance, underlying heart disease, pulmonary disease, electrolyte imbalance, hypoxia, and response to therapy (drugs and fluid). Some arrhythmias may be easily corrected and will not impact the patient's outcome if treated promptly. One such example is the increase in premature ventricular contractions (PVCs) that may be noted when fluid resuscitation does not provide adequate replacement of potassium.

Some arrhythmias are life threatening, and all arrhythmias should be evaluated with an understanding of the patient's underlying health status. Left ventricular dysfunction, as a result of various acute neurological conditions, can lead to life-threatening arrhythmias and heart failure. The possibility of underlying coronary artery disease that can lead to myocardial infarction (MI) must be kept in mind. The physiologic stress of catastrophic acute neurological illness with sympathetic predominance and side effects of treatments can precipitate an MI. Additionally, in trauma patients, the possibility of direct injury to the heart or major blood vessels can result in various problems such as pericardial effusion or aortic dissection. Therefore, early detection of the cardiac dysfunction, identification of the underlying cause, and prompt treatment are critical to prevention of secondary cerebral injury. Secondary cerebral injury results from hypoxia and cerebral ischemia that can lead to irreversible infarction.

Nursing Management. Patients with acute neurological problems often need common technologies such as electrocardiography (ECG), pulmonary catheter, arterial line, and pulse oximetry for ongoing monitoring. Most continuous ECG monitoring systems are designed to recognize and print tracings of arrhythmias in addition to triggering an alarm. Many systems include an interface of multiple parameters to provide a composite of data.

The focus of nursing management is directed at vigilant ongoing monitoring of cardiovascular function for early identification of cardiac problems for prompt intervention and treatment. Assessing cardiac function includes:

- Monitoring vital signs, which include heart rate and blood pressure, hourly
- Auscultating for heart sounds (e.g., S_3, S_4, murmurs, clicks)
- Monitoring ongoing ECG leads for sinus rhythm, rate, arrhythmias, and other ECG abnormalities
- Analyzing cardiac waveform components hourly
- Recording periodic 12-lead ECG as necessary
- Maintaining alarms on all systems to alert health care providers that settings have been exceeded
- Monitoring periodic blood gases
- Monitoring hemoglobin for evidence of anemia
- Monitoring cardiac output data (with a pulmonary catheter) for evidence of dysfunction
- Monitoring mean arterial pressure (MAP)
- Calculating CPP hourly for patients with ICP monitors in place
- Monitoring the pulse oximeter (which has been placed on a finger or earlobe)
- Monitoring the $ETCO_2$ level in patients who are mechanically ventilated
- Monitoring the jugular venous catheter data for adequacy of cerebral oxygen utilization
- Recognizing high risk for deep vein thrombosis development and monitoring for signs and symptoms

Use of technologies requires that the nurse be competent in the use of the equipment and interpretation of the data produced. The target range for physiologic parameters must be known and maintained. The physician should be consulted when deviations from normal or targeted ranges occur. Based on abnormal findings, diagnostics such as an echocardiogram or chest radiograph may be ordered.

Interventions. There are often standing orders for treatment of abnormal cardiac findings available to the nurse. Follow the protocol and report unusual findings or trends to the physician.

Respiratory Management. Adequate oxygen and gas exchange, a patent airway, and ability to protect one's airway are necessary for all patients. If a patient is unable to protect his or her airway, an endotracheal tube will need to be inserted and oxygen therapy and possibly ventilatory support will need to be provided. Most patients with intracranial hypertension are intubated and ventilated. If use of a ventilator is indicated, pressure support mode and positive end-expiratory pressure (PEEP) may be used within limitations. Many will receive PEEP.[83]

The controversial effects of PEEP on ICP stem from two competing schools of thought. The concern that PEEP as a component of ventilatory support will result in increased ICP stems from the effects of PEEP on cerebral venous outflow. Positive airway pressure, which includes the effects of PEEP from mechanical ventilation, is thought to impede venous return from the brain, thus contributing to an increase in ICP. As the amount of PEEP is increased, this effect is magnified. A newer school of thought finds that PEEP elevates the mean airway pressure and thus decreases systemic mean arterial blood pressure by inducing arterial vasodilation. The decrease in systemic arterial pressure can decrease CPP (a potentially dangerous sequela). However, neurogenic pulmonary edema, the chief reason for providing PEEP, decreases pulmonary compliance and attenuates the transmission of positive airway pressure through the lungs to the mediastinal cavity. As a result, PEEP has less of an effect on ICP than previously thought. PEEP of 5 to 15 cm H_2O is well tolerated in patients with increased ICP.[84] Higher levels of PEEP (15 to 20 cm H_2O) may not significantly affect cerebral venous return.[36]

Nursing Management. The focus of nursing management is directed at maintaining a patent airway, supporting adequate ventilation, and preventing complications such as atelectasis, pneumonia, and barotrauma. Assessing the patency of the airway and ventilation adequacy can be determined by:

- Observing the airway for mucus or other drainage
- Auscultating the lungs for breath sounds
- Observing the respiratory pattern
- Observing the chest and abdominal movement for evidence of respiratory distress
- Observing synchrony with the ventilator
- Noting presence of restlessness or a change in color of the skin (slight cyanosis)
- Reviewing and monitoring blood gases, hemoglobin, hematocrit, pulse oximetry, $ETCO_2$, and other invasive data
- Determining necessary interventions

Oxygen Therapy. Oxygen therapy is provided to a patient whose airway is often maintained with an endotracheal tube. Suctioning is necessary to maintain patency of the airway. Chest physical therapy should be provided for all patients. The goal is to prevent hypercapnia and hypoxemia, which contribute to increased ICP and cerebral ischemia. The following summarizes respiratory management in the patient with intracranial hypertension. *For ventilated patients,* the following points should be considered:

- Patients who are not synchronized with their ventilator are not being ventilated properly; additionally, their intrathoracic pressure is raised, which impedes venous drainage from the brain and raises ICP.
- Patients who are "bucking" the ventilator (asynchrony) may have to be medicated to decrease the respiratory drive or paralyze the respiratory muscles. See previous discussion on sedation and neuromuscular blockade.
- Maintain mode, pressure support, and PEEP according to physician's orders.

Suctioning. Suctioning can cause elevations in ICP and sometimes plateau waves in patients who already have an elevated ICP. Endotracheal suctioning should be undertaken with great care and gentleness with risk balanced by therapeutic goals. The need to suction is determined by observing the patient's color, chest and abdominal movement, presence of secretions within the upper respiratory pathways, and chest auscultation. Listen for adventitious lung sounds or decreased lung sounds in each lobe, and particularly in the bases of the lungs. The rasping sound of mucus in the upper respiratory tract is obvious to the ear without auscultation. It is critical for the nurse to be alert for the subtle signs of respiratory distress, which can be caused by partial obstruction of the respiratory tract. These subtle symptoms include an increase in pulse rate, perspiration, and restlessness.

Evaluate the patient frequently for any obvious or subtle indications of the need for suctioning. The usual protocol for suctioning includes the following:

- Preoxygenate the patient with 100% oxygen for 20 to 30 seconds before and after suctioning (most ventilators can do this with a manual control) because this helps to maintain levels of oxygen.
- Suction as necessary to remove secretions and maintain a patent airway; suction gently. Limit catheter insertion to **no more than 10 seconds** for each insertion, oxygenate between each catheter insertion, and limit attempts to suction to two insertions.[85,86]

CLINICAL PEARLS: When performing endotracheal suctioning, a patient may require hyperoxygenation, but not necessarily hyperventilation. They should be considered two mutually exclusive nursing interventions.

Positioning to Enhance Respiratory Function. In addition to suctioning, respiratory function can be enhanced by changing the patient's position periodically (i.e., by turning patient every 2 hours). Positioning on the side facilitates drainage of oral secretions to promote a patent airway and prevents aspiration. Turn from side to side at least every 2 hours to prevent pooling of secretions. The use of continuous lateral rotation therapy (CLRT) has been explored in the literature and found to be beneficial in select patients.[87] However, study sample sizes are small and many lack statistical significance.[88] Therefore, CLRT should be used judiciously and carefully monitored by the nursing staff. The head of the bed is elevated and the neck maintained in a neutral position to facilitate cerebral venous drainage.

Managing Factors Known to Increase Intracranial Pressure

Several nurse researchers have contributed to the body and knowledge for evidence-based practice for patients with increased ICP. These studies have identified relationships between independent nursing activities (e.g., turning, positioning) and changes in ICP. Although many questions are unanswered, the body of knowledge for evidence-based practice continues to grow. Table 13-1 summarizes factors known to cause an increase in ICP. The nurse can apply this knowledge to assist in managing activities that have the potential to increase ICP, some of which are described in the next section.

Positioning and Turning. Valsalva's maneuver is the forceful expiration of air against a closed glottis, which increases intra-abdominal and intrathoracic pressure, impedes venous return from the brain, and impedes venous return to the heart. Changing a patient's position may precipitate Valsalva's maneuver. To avoid stimulating Valsalva's maneuver, the patient is turned and positioned in proper body alignment, avoiding angulation of body parts. The proper technique can be compared with rolling a log, which actually facilitates alignment when turning. Special attention must be given to the neck and hips. The neck is maintained in the neutral position at all times. A soft collar, towel roll, or small pillow may be helpful if the patient cannot maintain the neutral position independently. The following positions should be avoided:

- Lateral flexion of the neck
- Trendelenburg's or prone position
- Extreme hip flexion or flexion of the upper legs on a pendulous abdomen

The head of the bed is elevated 30 degrees to facilitate cerebral venous drainage. In recent years, there has been discussion about elevation of the head and its effect on CPP. Some physicians prefer to keep the head of the bed flat, arguing that this position better facilitates adequate CPP.[89] The flat position is maintained within preset ICP and CPP parameters; after these parameters have been exceeded, the decision may be made to elevate the head of the bed. The majority of recent studies have found that head elevation is associated with a decrease in ICP but no change in CPP.[90] Elevation of the head of the bed to 30 degrees is the general practice by most physicians. The patient should be positioned in good body alignment in the lateral position. This also facilitates oropharyngeal drainage. Pillows are useful to position the patient properly. If able to follow instructions, the patient should be instructed to exhale when being turned.

Bowel Management. A bowel program should be initiated to prevent constipation, which increases intra-abdominal pressure and causes straining at stool, both of which increase ICP. Stool softeners are usually administered once the patient is stabilized and able to tolerate intake through a feeding tube. Chapter 11 covers the components of a bowel program.

Isometric Muscle Contractions. An **isometric muscle contraction** is characterized by an increase in muscle tension without changes in the length of the muscle. With this in mind, footboards are not used. Canvas or running shoes or other commercially available foot positioners can be applied to maintain foot position. Other activities that cause isometric contractions include:

- Pushing oneself up using the feet or elbows to push against the mattress
- Pulling on arm restraints
- Decortication or decerebration
- Shivering

Emotional Upset and Noxious Stimuli. Conversations that may be emotionally stimulating to the patient, such as a discussion of prognosis, deficits, legal proceedings,

restraints, or pain, should not be conducted within the patient's hearing range. One study found that such conversations, when overheard by the patient, caused an elevation in ICP.[91] Families should also be cautioned about refraining from unpleasant or stimulating conversations.

Soft stimuli are useful, such as a soft, soothing voice; pleasant conversation; soft music; the voices of loved ones being played on a tape recorder; or gentle therapeutic touching of the skin. The nurse should guard the patient from emotional upset. Even though certain patients may be classified as comatose, there is no way of knowing whether their hearing is intact or whether they can understand what is being said. The most reasonable approach for the nurse and others to take is to assume that patients can hear and understand.

Noxious stimuli, which are unpleasant or painful stimuli, increase ICP. Common noxious stimuli that the patient might experience include:

- Plugging in a drainage tube (e.g., urinary catheter), which causes pressure and pain from bladder distention
- Painful nursing or medical procedures (e.g., removing tape from the skin)
- Loud noises (e.g., television, monitor alarms)
- Sudden jarring of the bed
- Bright overhead lights
- Parts of the neurological examination, especially motor response to painful stimuli

Noxious stimuli should be prevented, if possible, or minimized by technique or by avoiding the need to perform multiple uncomfortable procedures. Soft stimuli, such as those mentioned previously, are useful to decrease the input of noxious stimuli when an uncomfortable procedure must be performed. The value of therapeutic touch cannot be overemphasized.

Clustering of Nursing Activities. In patients at risk, clustering of activities and procedures known to increase ICP often has a cumulative effect, causing spikes in ICP that can result in ischemia. For example, bathing, turning, and other common activities involved in routine care when clustered together may increase ICP. Even arousing the patient to assess neurological signs increases ICP. Suctioning and other respiratory procedures that are provided frequently for the acutely ill patient are notorious for their effect of increasing ICP. The nurse should plan care to avoid clustering of activities.[92] In patients who are undergoing continuous ICP monitoring, the nurse should watch the monitor to determine the effect each activity has on ICP. Rest periods between procedures should be planned so that the ICP is allowed to return to the baseline level. If an ICP monitor is in place, it should be observed to determine responses.

CLINICAL PEARLS: Find the balance between what must be done and what can wait. Nurses often feel the need to get "everything done" as soon as possible. Clustering nursing interventions in this way may result in more harm than good.

▨ MONITORING INTRACRANIAL PRESSURE

Continuous ICP monitoring has become common in neurological ICUs for patients with intracranial hypertension associated with conditions such as severe TBI (Glasgow Coma

Scale ratings of 3 to 8), Reye's syndrome, subarachnoid hemorrhage, and herpes encephalitis. A large body of literature and clinical experience identifies that ICP monitoring:

1. Helps in the earlier detection of intracranial mass lesions
2. Can limit indiscriminate use of therapies to control ICP, which themselves can be potentially harmful
3. Can reduce ICP by CSF drainage and thus improve cerebral perfusion
4. Can help in determining prognosis
5. May improve outcomes

When ICP monitoring is indicated, selection of the type of monitoring device must be made. The optimal ICP monitoring device is one that is accurate, reliable, and cost effective, and causes minimal patient discomfort.

There are primarily two types of ICP monitoring devices based on the location of the transducer.[60] The first includes an external strain gauge transducer that uses a fluid-filled line to couple the *extracranial transducer* to the patient's intracranial space. Traditional ventricular catheters, subarachnoid bolts, and subdural catheters are included in this group. The intraventricular catheter is the most common and least expensive method of monitoring ICP; it also allows for therapeutic drainage of CSF. The second type includes a catheter-tip–strain device that directly monitors ICP using an *intracranial transducer* located in the tip of the catheter. Included in this group are fiberoptic and pneumatic systems. Potential sites for placement of an ICP monitoring catheter is the intraventricular space, subarachnoid space, intraparenchymal space, epidural space, or subdural space.

A newer type of multimodal monitoring now exists, which utilizes both strain gauge and fiberoptic monitoring technology. These devices can be placed into the intraventricular space to allow for venous drainage and have a fiberoptic pressure sensor at the catheter tip but also allow for an extracranial transducer to be linked to the system. The current version of this hybrid type of device also contains a thermistor to allow for direct brain temperature monitoring.

Calibration

Regardless of the type of ICP monitoring system used (i.e., external or internal transducer), it is necessary to calibrate or "zero" the system. Calibration is always to an atmospheric reference point called the "zero" point, and the referencing of the transducer to atmospheric pressure is referred to as "zeroing the transducer." This process differs for an external and internal transducer.[93]

External Transducer

When an external transducer is used with a fluid-coupled system, the hydrostatic dynamics of the fluid require that the transducer must be leveled to a consistent anatomic reference point and zero-balanced to account for variations in the patient's head position. The most common *reference points* used are the top of the ear, external auditory meatus, or outer canthus of the eye. All these points approximate the location of the catheter tip at the foramen of Monro. Regardless of the reference point chosen, it is important to *use the same point for all readings consistently* to ensure accuracy. Therefore, whenever there is a change in the position of the patient's head in relation to the transducer, the transducer must be releveled to the consistent anatomic reference point before reading the ICP pressure. For accuracy, a carpenter's level or a laser leveling device is used to level the transducer to the anatomic reference point.[94]

Internal Transducer

Calibrating an ICP monitoring system that uses an intracranial transducer is simpler. A fiberoptic transducer-tipped catheter (FTC) is calibrated by the manufacturer before shipping. Just before insertion, the catheter is zero (atmospherically) balanced. There is no further recalibration possible during use (without an associated ventricular catheter). Therefore, there is no need to level the transducer to an external site, which is a time saver for the nurse. However, if there is drift and if recalibration is not possible, then measurement error will result. With some monitors, in vivo calibration is possible. The advantage of this option is that it allows for in vivo calibration to be performed to counteract the slight drift of the reference point over time that can affect accuracy.[94]

Intracranial Pressure Monitoring Systems: External Transducer and Internal Transducer Systems

External Transducer Systems

Three types of external transducer systems are discussed in this section: the ventricular catheter, the subarachnoid bolt or screw, and the subdural catheter (Fig. 13-10). Although epidural placement is possible, it is rarely used.

Intraventricular Catheter. The intraventricular catheter (IVC) was pioneered by Lundberg in 1960 and remains the standard criterion with which all other catheters and ICP monitoring systems are compared.[95] The soft, Silastic, radiopaque IVC is inserted through a small burr hole made with a twist drill usually into the anterior horn of the nondominant lateral ventricle (see Fig. 13-10A). The IVC is connected to a closed fluid-filled system. Several systems are available, all based on the same principles and components. These components include a proximal stopcock or sampling port and a more distal stopcock that interfaces with either an external transducer for ICP monitoring or a collection system for CSF drainage.[85] For example, the Becker intraventricular external drainage and monitoring system (PS Medical, Goleta, CA) is a commonly used system in many centers (see Fig. 13-8). It consists of a side port that is used for continuous drainage and sampling of CSF. The external pressure transducer can be connected to the main system stopcock, which is leveled to the reference point on the patient's head (e.g., external auditory meatus). The drip chamber can be moved up and down and placed at a desired level against the zero-reference-level stopcock. The drip chamber at the end of the drain line is typically fixed by a 15-cm length of pressure tubing to secure drainage in the drip chamber when ICP rises above a predetermined level, typically 15 or 20 mm Hg.[36] Using

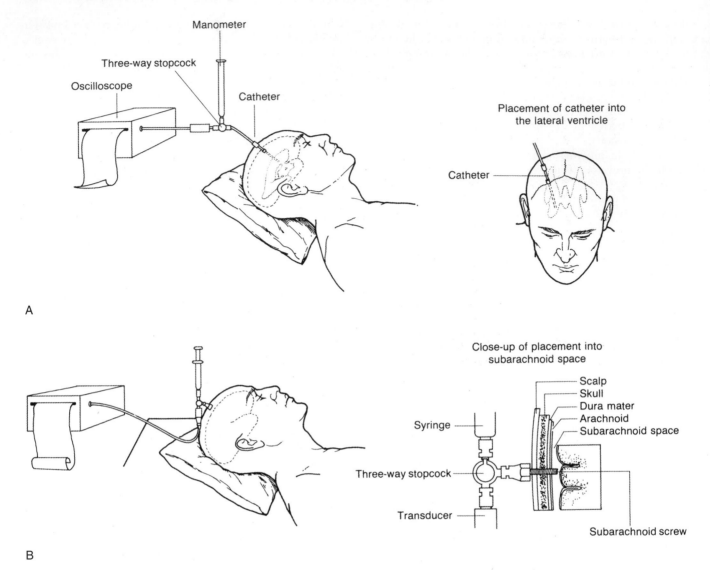

Figure 13-10 • Major intracranial pressure monitoring devices. (*A*) Ventricular catheter monitor. (*B*) Subarachnoid screw or bolt monitor. (From Smeltzer, S., & Bare, B. [1996]. *Brunner and Suddarth's textbook of medical-surgical nursing* [8th ed.]. Philadelphia: Lippincott-Raven Publishers.)

the shortest possible length of tubing between the catheter and the transducer and eliminating air bubbles from the system are necessary for accuracy of ICP readings.

The *advantages* of the IVC are the ability to drain CSF fractionally to reduce ICP, to collect CSF for laboratory analysis, and to inject contrast media to visualize the ventricle, as well as its accuracy and low cost. The *disadvantages* include difficulty of insertion into a small ventricle because of lateral mass shift; CSF leakage around insertion site; plugging of the catheter with blood or cerebral tissue; higher risk of infection; and need to zero and recalibrate frequently.

Subarachnoid Bolt or Screw. The subarachnoid (SA) bolt was developed by Vires in 1973 as an option to decrease infections and insertion limitations associated with IVCs. The insertion is similar to that of an IVC except that there are more options for placement because the brain parenchyma is not penetrated.[96] The bolt consists of a hollow metal shaft or screw that is threaded at one end

through a burr hole and dura into the subarachnoid space (see Fig. 13-10*B*). The bolt is hydrostatically coupled to fluid-filled pressure tubing, a stopcock, and an external transducer. The transducer is leveled to the anatomic reference point. The subarachnoid bolt is only a monitoring device; CSF cannot be readily withdrawn from it, and may lead to bolt occlusion.[96]

The *advantages* of the bolt are the simplicity of the bolt; the ease of rapid insertion; that it is usable in patients who fail use of the IVC or are not candidates for IVC placement; and that it does not penetrate the brain parenchyma (less invasive), therefore decreasing the possibility of hemorrhage and infection. The *disadvantages* include plugging of the bolt with blood, debris, or obliteration from an edematous brain; that it may underestimate ICP when it is elevated; its inaccurate ICP readings because of different compartmental pressures; risk of infection, although this is lower than with IVCs; and the need to zero and recalibrate frequently. If plugging is suspected because of a dampened waveform or low ICP pressure, the bolt can be flushed by the physician with 0.1 to 0.2 mL of preservative-free (non-bacteriostatic) saline to restore accurate ICP reading.[97] In most situations, this small amount of saline does not cause dangerous ICP elevations.[96]

> **CLINICAL PEARLS:** Always use preservative-free saline when flushing any intracranial monitoring device or tubing.

Subdural Catheters. Another method of monitoring ICP with an external transducer involves placement of a catheter in the subdural space. Currently this method is not used often because of an underestimation of ICP and dampening of waveforms, especially with high ICP pressures.[90] The infection rate and risk of hemorrhage are about the same as with the subarachnoid bolts.

Internal (Intracranial) Transducer Systems

An FTC is available for ICP monitoring and uses a different technology, in part, to overcome some of the disadvantages of external transducer systems. A miniature transducer in the catheter tip is coupled by a long, continuous wire or fiberoptic cable to an external electronic module. One of the better-known fiberoptic systems (Camino, Integra Lifesciences Corporation, Plainsboro, NJ) operates according to the following principle. Light fibers within the catheter convey light impulses created by movement of a mirrored diaphragm, which reflects pressure changes. The light signal is converted into electrical signals in the amplifier connector. Systolic, diastolic, and mean pressures are displayed on a digital monitor that can interface with an additional analog monitor for display of continuous waveforms (Fig. 13-11A). The FTC can be inserted easily into the lateral ventricle, subarachnoid space, subdural space, or brain parenchyma, or under a bone flap. A scalp stab wound is made, and a small twist drill is used to drill a small burr hole through bone. A housing device (a small bolt) is then screwed into place. The dura is perforated, and the transducer probe is threaded through the housing device to the desired depth and fixed in position by tightening the ring unit over the housing device. Finally, a protective sheath is snapped into position. If the intraventricular monitoring technique is used, it can be configured to both monitor ICP and to drain CSF (see Fig. 13-11B).

This technology is more expensive than fluid-coupled monitoring systems. There is the cost of the disposable catheter and initial expense and maintenance of the cable and compatible monitor. It does have its own portable monitor that is transportable so that continuous ICP monitoring is possible during transport. That the catheter is calibrated by the manufacturer and is zero-balanced only once at the time of insertion is both a benefit and a drawback of this system. Because the transducer is internal, it does not need to be zero-referenced to an anatomic point while in use. Because there is no coupling with fluid, there are no problems of dampening waveforms resulting from catheter occlusion or air bubble entrapment. This is a time saver for the nurse. It is also neither possible to assess for drift that occurs over time nor to recalibrate if drift is suspected. Drift is a source of measurement error associated with both external and internal transducer systems,[99–101] but the lack of ability to identify

and correct drift with the FTC system is a disadvantage. Finally, nurses who work directly with the fiberoptic cable must take care to prevent bending the cable, which can result from patient movement, transport, or care. After clinicians have become accustomed to working with the equipment, breakage is not a significant problem.[93] In summary, the *advantages* of the FTC are ease of insertion; options for multiple insertion sites; no need to zero to an anatomic point every time the position of the head changes; decreased risk of infection; and continuation of monitoring during transport. Disadvantages include increased expense as compared to fluid-coupled systems; fragile fiberoptic cable that can break; and inability to identify and correct drift.

Pressure Waves

With continuous ICP monitoring, the fluctuations in waveforms correlate with both respirations and the cardiac cycle. Positive deflections of 2 to 10 mm H_2O can be observed in the patient who is not receiving ventilatory support with positive pressure. These deflections are noted immediately after systole and exhalation. Waveforms, which can be examined individually or in trend recordings, are helpful in identifying changes in the patient's condition. The morphology of each waveform has been discussed previously in relation to compliance. Trend recordings compress continuous ICP recording data into time periods (e.g., 5- to 60-minute blocks) to reflect general trends in ICP over longer periods.

Three distinct pressure waves have been identified by Lundberg[95]: A waves (plateau), B waves, and C waves (Fig. 13-12). Since their identification over 40 years ago, no new wave patterns have been added, although interpretation of their meaning has evolved. It may be impossible to identify these very low-frequency waves unless the sampling frequency is adequate (i.e., more than once per second) to capture these changes.[96] The following sections describe each of the waveforms.

A Waves (Plateau Waves)

These waves derive their name from the "plateau" shape of the trended waveforms. This is best noted when the ICP trend is viewed over a longer period of time (e.g., 30 to 60 minutes). Plateau waves consist of sudden, transient waves that begin from an *already* elevated ICP—20 mm Hg or more to levels of 50 to 100 mm Hg—and persist 5 to 20 minutes before terminating with a rapid decline to the level of or below the baseline ICP. Plateau waves are often not accompanied by a corresponding elevation of mean arterial blood pressure, which leads to a drop in CPP that is often associated with this waveform. Therefore, there is sustained low CPP with concurrent cerebral ischemia and transient or paroxysmal symptoms, sometimes called *pressure signs* (see discussion that follows), that are seen in patients with *already* elevated ICP who have *decreased cerebral compliance.*

Plateau waves are precipitated by a chain of physiologic and pathophysiologic events.[63] A gradual rise from the baseline ICP begins to compromise CPP, causing incomplete ischemia. The ischemia initiates a concurrent vasodilator response and increase in CBV in the cerebral hemispheres.[102–104] Increased CBV rapidly increases ICP, which

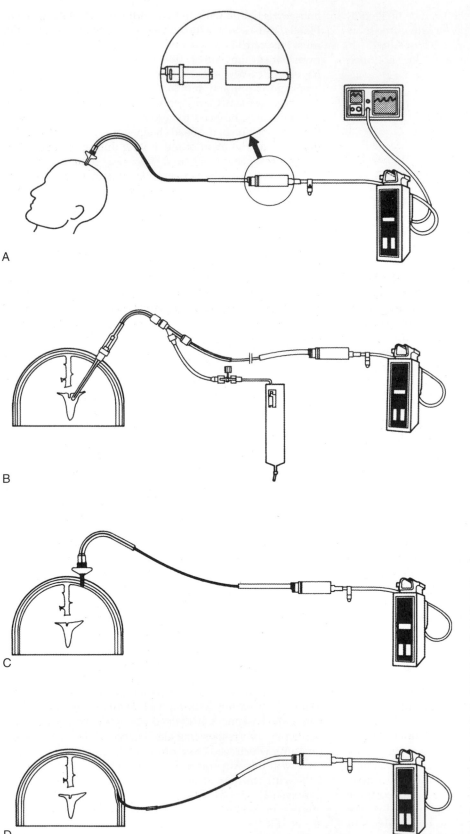

Figure 13-11 • Fiberoptic transducer-tipped catheter (FTC) developed by Camino Laboratories, San Diego, CA. (*A*) Major components of the FTC monitoring system and interface to monitors. The upper monitor provides a continuous digital readout of intracranial pressure (ICP). The circular inset illustrates the connection between the FTC and the pre-amplifier cable. (*B*) Ventriculostomy ICP monitoring via FTC and cerebrospinal fluid (CSF) drainage. An A–Y connector at the proximal end of the catheter is attached to a CSF drainage bag, allowing for CSF drainage. (*C*) The FTC is placed in the subdural space for ICP monitoring. (*D*) The FTC is placed beneath the bone flap for postcraniotomy ICP monitoring. (Courtesy of Camino Laboratories, San Diego, CA.)

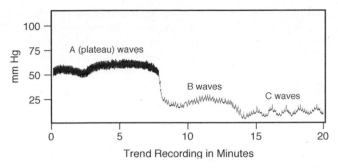

Figure 13-12 • Intracranial pressure waves. Composite diagram of A (plateau) waves, B waves, and C waves.

further reduces CPP and CBF. The plateau waves continue until the intracranial volume is reduced, usually by reduction in the volume of CSF or by reduction of blood volume with hyperventilation. Research has shown that plateau waves are related to poorer outcomes and herniation.[105] Although the patient tolerates the specific event, it suggests a need for expansion of ICP therapies (e.g., CSF drainage, mannitol). Williams and Hanley call attention to a practical clinical point.[96] They note that the rising phase of a plateau wave (which the patient might conceivably survive) cannot be differentiated clinically *as it is happening* from sudden ICP elevation associated with herniation. Therefore, given the clinical picture, the clinician would treat the patient as herniation and institute expanded ICP therapies. Only on retrospective ICP trend analysis is it apparent that a plateau wave did occur.

B Waves

Sharp, rhythmic spikes occurring every 30 seconds to 2 minutes characterize B waves. The ICP peaks to 20 to 50 mm Hg, although these elevated levels are not sustained. In a spontaneously breathing patient, B waves may be seen with Cheyne-Stokes respirations or with brief episodes of decreased respirations or apnea. B waves are probably caused by variations in CVR or reactivity.[95] They indicate a decreased cerebral adaptive capability and may be a warning sign of A waves.[106] They are an indication for initiation of therapy to reduce ICP.

C Waves

These low-amplitude, transient, rhythmic oscillations occur four to eight times per minute, reaching pressures of up to 20 mm Hg.[95] C waves are related to normal changes of the systemic arterial blood pressure and ventilation. The clinical significance of these waves is unknown; therefore, there is currently no indication for a change in therapy.

Clinical Implications of Plateau Waves

Plateau waves are clinically significant because they peak to levels of 50 to 100 mm Hg from an **already elevated baseline ICP**. Plateau waves correlate physiologically with cerebral hypoxia, ischemia, and possible infarction to selected areas. Clinically, plateau waves are associated with changes in mean arterial blood pressure; however, the exact relationship

between MAP and ICP in the presence of plateau waves remains somewhat controversial. It is difficult to determine whether MAP changes in response to ICP or is the cause of ICP changes.[6] Some evidence now exists to support that the sharp increase in ICP is caused by vasodilation (which is seen clinically as a drop in MAP), and resolved by a compensatory increase in MAP (vasoconstriction).[107] Because cerebral tissue is sensitive to decreased O_2, symptoms of cerebral dysfunction may be evident.

The degree of dysfunction may be subtle (e.g., confusion, restlessness) or pronounced (e.g., hemiplegia, posturing). **Pressure signs** may include deterioration in LOC; decreased pupillary reaction; paresis, paralysis, decortication, or decerebration; aphasia; headache; changes in respiratory pattern (e.g., Cheyne-Stokes); and other changes in vital signs. Although pressure symptoms are paroxysmal transient manifestations, they may last for a prolonged period after the plateau waves have subsided. Early recognition of a tendency toward plateau waves or the presence of factors that trigger plateau waves should be followed by early intervention to prevent or control these dangerous waves.

Infection Control and the Intracranial Pressure Monitor

Infections are the primary complication encountered with ICP monitoring. The Centers for Disease Control and Prevention have defined CSF infections.[108] The range of CSF infections reported in patients undergoing ICP monitoring was 0% to 40%, with an average of 10%.[109–114] In a study by Rebuck et al., 7.4% of 215 ICP monitored patients developed CSF infection.[115] Risk factors for CSF infection were also examined. They included duration of monitoring longer than 5 days; presence of ventriculostomy; CSF leakage; concurrent systemic infection (e.g., pneumonia, urinary tract infection); and replacement of ICP monitoring device. Patients with subarachnoid hemorrhage, intraventricular hemorrhage, and open craniotomy are more susceptible to ventriculostomy-related infections than patients with closed head trauma not resulting in hemorrhage.[116] Patients with intraventricular placement compared with intraparenchymal placement had a higher incidence of infections. Use of prophylactic antibiotics was examined. Although not a standard of practice, antibiotics were administered to 63% of infected and 59% of noninfected patients. Poon et al. reported a decreased incidence of infection in patients randomized to prophylaxis for the duration of ICP monitoring.[117] Rebuck et al. concluded that duration of prophylaxis has no significant influence on development of infection. When antibiotics were given, vancomycin followed by cefazolin were the drugs of choice.[99]

One can conclude that there are variations in reported incidence and identification of risk factors. More randomized control trials are needed to establish evidence-based practice. Table 13-5 lists the most commonly identified risk factors. However, recommendations do exist to assist the clinician. Ventriculostomy catheters for ICP monitoring should be removed as quickly as possible, and in circumstances in which prolonged monitoring is required, there appears to be no benefit from catheter exchange.[114] With the new onset of fever in a patient with an intracranial device, CSF should be

TABLE 13-5 RISK FACTORS FOR INFECTIONS IN PATIENTS UNDERGOING ICP MONITORING

- Use of intraventricular catheter
- ICP monitoring longer than 5 days
- Flushing of the system
- CSF leakage
- Concurrent systemic infection
- Serial ICP monitoring catheters (e.g., replacing a catheter)
- ICP catheters placed outside of OR setting

ICP, intracranial pressure; CSF, cerebrospinal fluid; OR, operating room.

obtained for analysis from the CSF reservoir for a Gram stain and culture.[118] Guidelines[22] made level III recommendations related to ventricular catheters. They recommend that routine ventricular catheter exchange or prophylactic antibiotic use for ventricular catheter placement is not recommended to reduce infection.

CLINICAL VIGNETTE: Ms. RB is a 59-year-old black female admitted with the diagnosis of SAH secondary to a ruptured anterior communicating (A-comm) artery aneurysm. Her history is positive for alcohol abuse, cocaine use, and poor compliance with prescribed antihypertensives. On admission she was intermittently conscious and a noncontrasted CT scan showed blood in her ventricles. A ventriculostomy was placed to facilitate ICP management and Ms. RB was taken to the radiology suite where she underwent endovascular coiling of her aneurysm. Upon return from radiology, her ICP was consistently 15 to 20 mm Hg and was controlled with CSF drainage for ICP sustained over 20 mm Hg and osmotic therapy (mannitol and hypertonic saline).

On day 3 Ms. RB began having profound spikes in her ICP with pressures often reaching 35 to 40 mm Hg. These spikes were refractory to osmotic therapy, appeared to be short term, and did not correlate to a change in her level of consciousness. A repeat of her CT scan showed only slight worsening of her cerebral edema. The staff modified the ICU monitor to display her ICP waves at a sweep speed of 6.25 mm/sec instead of the standard 25 mm/sec. This manipulation allowed the team to view the ICP waveform over a greater period of time and it was noted that each ICP spike lasted approximately 45 seconds, after which the ICP returned to baseline. The attending neurosurgeon was notified that the ICP waveform was consistent with Lundberg B waves.

Nursing Management of the Patient During Intracranial Pressure Monitoring

As outlined earlier in this chapter, ICP monitoring has several well-established purposes. From the nurse's perspective, monitoring of ICP provides data that augment serial neuro-

logical assessment, data for making treatment decisions, data for gauging progress, and a means of observing intracranial responses to nursing interventions and medical treatment. Most patients who are undergoing ICP monitoring also have central lines for hemodynamic monitoring and arterial lines that supply continuous data on MAP. These data are used to calculate CPP. Normal range is 60 to 90 mm Hg, although the target goal may be set higher than minimum for certain patients, such as those with severe TBI (i.e., 70 mm Hg or above). Generally, elevated CPP targets are not recommended unless there is a means of evaluating the effect on CBF and tissue perfusion (e.g., intracranial oxygen tissue monitoring). CPP is a direct indicator of the adequacy of cerebral perfusion, so monitoring the CPP is as important as monitoring the ICP. The ability to interpret continuous waveforms, trends in waveforms (previously discussed in this chapter), and CPP accurately assists the nurse in data-based clinical decision making.

The American Association of Neuroscience Nurses has published a clinical guide about ICP monitoring that is helpful.[119] There are several specific considerations in the nursing management of a patient with an ICP monitor.[120] For troubleshooting, follow the manufacturer's specific instructions for use of the monitoring system and the treating hospital's policy. The following section outlines key points related to data collection, accuracy of ICP and waveform, and infection prevention:

- Data collection
  - Collect and interpret waveforms.
  - Alert the physician as necessary to evidence of increasing ICP.
  - Monitor waveforms for dampening effect.
  - Calculate CPP at least hourly (CPP = MAP − ICP).
- Accuracy of ICP and waveforms
  - Rezero and recalibrate the device according to manufacturer's instruction and hospital policy.
  - Recognize that a certain amount of drift will occur each day that the catheter is in place; take this into consideration in determining the validity and reliability of the data with other clinical data.
- For systems with external transducers
  - Zero to the same anatomic reference point each time.
  - Relevel the transducer each time the position of the head changes and at least every 2 to 4 hours.
  - If a dampened waveform occurs:
    - Observe fluid lines for leakage or disconnection of components; if either occurs, the system is no longer sterile; the physician must be notified; and the system will need to be replaced according to hospital policy.
    - Observe for air bubbles or debris in the tubing; air bubbles and debris will cause error in the transduced pressure. If found, flush the line, being sure to close the stopcock to the catheter and patient (follow hospital policy).
- For systems with internal transducers
  - Recalibration after insertion is not possible.
  - With FTCs, do not bend the cable as a precaution in preventing breakage.
  - Notify the physician if the waveform becomes dampened.

- Decreasing the risk of infection
  - Maintain an occlusive dry sterile dressing around the insertion site, and change it on a prescribed schedule according to hospital policy (usually, a sterile dressing change performed every 24 to 72 hours).
  - Monitor the insertion site for signs of infection, drainage, or CSF leakage.
  - Keep all connections tightly connected to maintain the integrity and sterility of the system.
  - Avoid leaving external drainage devices open for prolonged periods.
- Ventricular catheter to CSF drainage bag
  - Monitor height of collection chamber and clamps (based on order to open or close) every 2 hours.
  - Adjust height of collection chamber to be level with or above the transducer according to physician's order.
  - **Do not** position the top of the collection chamber **below** the level of the anatomic reference point to prevent siphoning of CSF when the drain is opened.
  - Monitor the color, clarity, and amount of CSF drainage (lack of drainage will occur with obstruction of the catheter or connecting tubing; this should be reported and discussed with the physician).
  - Collection of CSF is done under strict aseptic technique and according to manufacturer's instruction and hospital policy.

SPECIAL SYNDROMES: BENIGN INTRACRANIAL HYPERTENSION AND HYDROCEPHALUS

Two special syndromes associated with increased ICP and CSF flow are benign intracranial hypertension and hydrocephalus.

Benign Intracranial Hypertension (Pseudotumor Cerebri)

Pseudotumor cerebri, now commonly called *benign intracranial hypertension*, is seen most often in obese adolescent girls and young women.[121] The chief complaint is headache and, in some instances, blurred vision, diplopia, slight numbness in the face, or dizziness. On physical examination, the patient is alert, aware, and conversant, and seems otherwise well. The only abnormal finding is papilledema. On lumbar puncture, CSF pressure is usually about 250 to 450 mm H_2O. On CT scan or MRI, ventricles are of normal size, and there is no evidence of an intracranial mass or obstruction of CSF. Visual testing may find slight peripheral deficits. The immediate management focus is to reduce the papilledema to prevent visual impairment. Treatment options include:

1. Serial lumbar puncture to remove CSF until normal pressure is maintained (performed daily and then at increasing intervals)
2. Drug therapy if CSF pressure continues to be elevated and papilledema persists

- Prednisone 40 to 60 mg/d
- Acetazolamide (Diamox); 750 mg to 1.0 g/d in two to four divided doses; carbonic anhydrase inhibitors that decrease CSF production

3. In the approximately 10% of patients who do not respond to these treatments, a trial of lumbar drainage, followed by placement of a lumbar peritoneal shunt, may be necessary.

Hydrocephalus

Hydrocephalus refers to a progressive dilatation of the ventricular system because the production of CSF exceeds the absorption rate. Hydrocephalus is a clinical syndrome rather than a disease entity. Abnormalities in overproduction, circulation, or reabsorption of CSF can result in hydrocephalus. (See Chap. 4 for a review of CSF and circulation.)

Classification

Hydrocephalus can be subdivided into noncommunicating and communicating hydrocephalus:

- **Noncommunicating hydrocephalus** is a condition in which CSF in the ventricular system does not communicate properly within the subarachnoid space and therefore cannot be reabsorbed by the arachnoid villi. The net result is an increase in the amount of CSF in the ventricles. Obstruction can be caused by a mass, such as a tumor within or adjacent to the ventricular system; a congenital obstruction; debris, such as blood clogging the aqueduct of Sylvius; or an obliteration from an inflammatory process.
- **Communicating hydrocephalus** is a condition in which too few, or poorly functioning, arachnoid villi are unable to reabsorb CSF sufficiently. Subarachnoid hemorrhage secondary to aneurysmal rupture or a TBI can produce transient or lasting communicating hydrocephalus. The arachnoid villi become plugged and cannot reabsorb CSF. Plugging can occur from the end-products of blood cell breakdown or the exudate from meningitis.

The signs and symptoms of hydrocephalus depend on the type of hydrocephalus and the age of the patient. For noncommunicating hydrocephalus, treatment of the primary problem is necessary, usually with surgery. In communicating hydrocephalus, CSF drainage may be attempted to clear the arachnoid villi of exudate so that normal function will be resumed in the future. If this is ineffective, a surgical shunting procedure will be necessary. Selection of the particular procedure depends on the age of the patient and any preexisting health problems.

Because the scope of this text is limited to adult problems, no discussion of hydrocephalus in the infant or child is included. The reader is directed to a pediatric text for discussion of this topic.

Normal-Pressure Hydrocephalus

An important type of communicating hydrocephalus seen in older adults is called **normal-pressure hydrocephalus**; it is usually reversible. (This syndrome is also called *occult hydrocephalus*, *low-pressure hydrocephalus*, and *normotensive* *hydrocephalus.*) In normal-pressure hydrocephalus, there is ventricular enlargement with compression of the cerebral tissue, but normal CSF pressure is noted on lumbar puncture. Various circumstances have been associated with the development of normal-pressure hydrocephalus:

- Plugging of the arachnoid villi secondary to subarachnoid hemorrhage
- Thrombosis of the superior sagittal sinus
- Injury from brain trauma or related to surgery, in which scarring of the basal cistern is thought to occur
- Bacterial meningitis, in which there is plugging and possible fibrotic changes of the arachnoid villi

After careful evaluation of some patients, particularly those between 60 and 70 years old, if no associated precipitated condition has been found, the diagnosis is **idiopathic normal pressure hydrocephalus.**

Signs and Symptoms. The onset of normal-pressure hydrocephalus (when not associated with acute brain injury) is insidious and slow to develop (over weeks or months). Changes occur so slowly that they can easily be overlooked by the patient and family, or they may be attributed to the aging process when an older patient is involved.

The cardinal symptoms include mental changes, urinary incontinence, and disturbances in gait. Mental changes may begin as mild forgetfulness along with a diminished level of generalized cognitive function and progress to severe impairment. In advanced cases, mutism and hypokinesia may be apparent. Gait disturbances begin with a slowed pace that includes wide-based, zigzag steps; subsequently, gait is unsteady, and falling is common. Upper extremity movement may be unaffected or slowed. With progression, the ability to maintain independent ambulation is lost.

Urinary incontinence is not an early sign; it appears later. Lost social inhibition and forgetfulness caused by cerebral atrophy are the probable causes. No headache or papilledema is noted, although unexplained nystagmus is apparent in many patients. Tendon reflexes, particularly in the lower extremities, are increased. In advanced cases, Babinski's, grasping, and sucking reflexes may be present.

Diagnostic Studies. The most common diagnostic studies are CT and MRI. Atrophy and enlarged ventricles are noted. A positive history of a slowly developing progression of symptoms is essential in establishing the diagnosis. Normal CSF pressure is noted on lumbar puncture.

Treatment. The accepted treatment for normal-pressure hydrocephalus is a ventricular shunt. When cerebral atrophy has occurred, reversal of symptoms is minimal. Often, an externalized ventriculostomy drain is first placed as a trial to assess the potential benefits of an indwelling ventricular shunt. The following describes optimal outcomes from successful ventricular shunting:

- The most dramatic improvement that may be apparent almost immediately is in mental status. The patient will become much more alert, oriented, and manageable. Others, however, will show more gradual improvement.
- Incontinence may be quickly reversed.
- Reversal of gait disturbance takes longer; a permanent residual deficit may result.

SUMMARY

Management of ICP and preventing episodes of intracranial hypertension are fundamental components of clinical neuroscience practice. A review of the physiologic basis for ICP, independent and collaborative nursing roles, and major management concerns has been provided. Evidence-based practice is growing, and current evidence has been incorporated into this discussion.

REFERENCES

1. Marmarou, A., & Tabaddor, K. (1993). Intracranial pressure: Physiology and pathophysiology. In P. R. Cooper. (Ed.). *Head injury* (3rd ed., pp. 203–224). Baltimore: Williams & Wilkins.
2. Germon, K. (1988). Interpretation of ICP pulse waves to determine intracerebral compliance. *Journal of Neuroscience Nursing, 20*(6), 344–351.
3. Cardosa, E. R., Rowan, J. O., & Galbraith, S. (1983). Analysis of cerebrospinal fluid pulse wave in intracranial pressure. *Journal of Neurosurgery, 59*, 817–821.
4. Citerio, G., & Andrews, P. J. (2004). Intracranial pressure. Part two: Clinical applications and technology. *Intensive Care Medicine, 30*(10), 1882–1885.
5. Alspach, J. (1998). *AACN core curriculum for critical care nursing* (5th ed., pp. xxi, 936). Philadelphia: Saunders.
6. Greenberg, M. S. (1999). *Handbook of neurosurgery* (5th ed., p. 974). Lakeland, FL: Thieme.
7. Benarroch, E. E., Westmoreland, B. F., Daube, J. R., et al. (1999). *Medical neurosciences: An approach to anatomy, pathophysiology, and physiology by systems and level* (4th ed., pp. 136–150, 326–333). Boston: Little, Brown.
8. Ropper, A. H., & Kennedy, S. K. (1993). Physiology and clinical aspects of raised intracranial pressure. In A. H. Ropper (Ed.). *Neurological and neurosurgical intensive care* (3rd ed., pp. 11–28). New York: Raven Press.
9. Eisenberg, H. M., Frankowski, R. F., Contant, L. P., Marshall, L. F., & Walker, M. D. (1988). High dose barbiturate control of elevated intracranial pressure in patients with severe head injury. *Journal of Neurosurgery, 69*, 15–23.
10. Rosner, M. J., & Daughton, S. (1990). Cerebral perfusion pressure management in head injury. *Journal of Trauma, 30*(8), 933–941.
11. Robertson, C. S., Valadka, A. B., Hannay, H. J., Contant, C. F., Gopinath, S. P., Cormio, M., et al. (1999). Prevention of secondary ischemic insults after severe head injury. *Critical Care Medicine, 27*(10), 2086–2095.
12. Marin-Caballos, A. J., Murillo-Cabezas, F., Cayuela-Dominguez, A., Dominguez-Roldan, J. M., Rincon-Ferrari, M. D., Valencia-Anguita, J., et al. (2005). Cerebral perfusion pressure and risk of brain hypoxia in severe head injury: A prospective observational study. *Critical Care, 9*(6), R670–676.
13. Firlik, A. D., & Marion, D. W. (2000). Intracranial pressure: Physiology and pathophysiology. In P. R. Cooper & J. G. Golfinos (Eds.). *Head injury* (4th ed., pp. 221–228). New York: McGraw-Hill.
14. Klatzo, I. (1967). Neuropathological aspects of brain edema. *Journal of Neuropathology and Experimental Neurology, 20*, 1.
15. Plum, F., & Posner, J. B. (1982). *The diagnosis of stupor and coma* (3rd ed.). Philadelphia: F. A. Davis.
16. Kernohan, J. W., & Woltman, H. W. (1929). Incisura of the crus due to contralateral brain tumor. *Archives of Neurology & Psychiatry, 21*, 274–287.
17. Knupling, R., Fuchs, E. C., Aschenbrenner, C. A., Gerull, G., Giesen, M., & Mrowinski, D. (1979). Chronic and acute transtentorial herniation with tumors of the posterior cranial fossa. *Neurochirurgia, 22*, 9–17.

18. Verlooy, J., Heytens, L., Veeckmans, G., & Selosse, P. (1995). Intracerebral temperature monitoring in severely head injured patients. *Acta Neurochir (Wien), 134*(1–2), 76–78.

19. Soukup, J., Zauner, A., Doppenberg, E. M., Menzel, M., Gilman, C., Bullock, R., et al. (2002). Relationship between brain temperature, brain chemistry and oxygen delivery after severe human head injury: The effect of mild hypothermia. *Neurological Research, 24*(2), 61–68.

20. Wong, F. W. (2000). Prevention of secondary brain injury. *Critical Care Nurse, 20*(5), 18–27.

21. Shapiro, H. M. (1973). Intracranial hypertension: Therapeutic and anesthetic considerations. *Anesthesiology, 43*, 445–471.

22. Brain Trauma Foundation, American Association of Neurological Surgeons, Congress of Neurological Surgeons, & AANS/ CNS Joint Section on Neurotrauma and Critical Care. (2007). Guidelines for the management of severe traumatic brain injury, 3rd ed. *Journal of Neurotrauma, 24*(Suppl. 1), S1–S106.

23. Hulme, A., & Cooper, R. (1976). The effects of head position and jugular vein compression on intracranial pressure. In J. Beks, D. A. Bosch, & M. Brock (Eds.). *Intracranial pressure III* (pp. 259–263). Berlin: Springer-Verlag.

24. Ropper, A. H., Marshall, L. F., & Shapiro, H. M. (1979). High-dose barbiturate therapy in humans: A clinical review of 60 patients. *Annals of Neurology, 6*, 194–199.

25. Durward, Q. J., Amacher, A. L., Delmaestro, R. F., & Sibbald, W. J. (1983). Cerebral and cardiovascular responses to changes in head elevation with intracranial hypertension. *Journal of Neurosurgery, 59*, 15–23.

26. Feldman, Z., Kanter, M. J., Robertson, C. S., Contant, C. F., Hayes, C., Sheinberg, M. A., et al. (1992). Effect of head elevation on intracranial pressure, cerebral perfusion pressure, and cerebral blood flow in head injured patients. *Journal of Neurosurgery, 76*, 207–211.

27. Chesnut, R. M. (2000). Medical management of intracranial pressure. In P. F. Cooper & J. G. Golfinos (Eds.). *Head injury* (4th ed., pp. 259–263). New York: McGraw-Hill.

28. Allen, C. H., & Ward, J. D. (1998). An evidence-based approach to management of increased intracranial pressure. *Critical Care Clinics, 14*(3), 485–495.

29. Bouma, G. J., Muizelaar, J. P., Choi, S. C., Newlon, P. G., & Young, H. F. (1991). Cerebral circulation and metabolism after severe traumatic brain injury: The elusive role of ischemia. *Journal of Neurosurgery, 75*, 685–693.

30. Robertson, C. S., Constant, C. F., Gokaslan, Z. I., Narayan, R. K., & Grossman, R. G. (1992). Cerebral blood flow, arteriovenous oxygen difference, and outcome in head injured patients. *Journal of Neurology, Neurosurgery, and Psychiatry, 55*, 594–603.

31. Raichle, M. E., & Plum, F. (1972). Hyperventilation and cerebral blood flow. *Stroke, 3*, 566–575.

32. Muizlaar, J. P., Marmarou, A., Ward, J. D., Kontos, H. A., Choi, S. C., Becker, D. P., et al. (1991). Adverse effects of prolonged hyperventilation in patients with severe head injury: A randomized clinical trial. *Journal of Neurosurgery, 75*, 731–739.

33. Cruz, J., Miner, M. E., Allen, S. J., Alves, W. M., & Gennarelli, T. A. (1991). Continuous monitoring of cerebral oxygenation in acute brain injury: Assessment of cerebral hemodynamic reserve. *Neurosurgery, 29*, 743–749.

34. Sheinberg, M., Kaner, M. J., Robertson, C. S., Contant, C. F., Narayan, R. K., & Grossman, R. G. (1992). Continuous monitoring of jugular venous oxygen saturation in head-injured patients. *Journal of Neurosurgery, 76*, 212–217.

35. Oertel, M., Kelly, D. F., Lee, J. H., McArthur, D. L., Glenn, T.C., Vespa, P., et al. (2002). Efficacy of hyperventilation, blood pressure elevation, and metabolic suppression therapy in controlling intracranial pressure after head injury. *Journal of Neurosurgery, 97*(5), 1045–1053.

36. Wijdicks, E. F. M. (1997). *The clinical practice of critical care neurology* (pp. 76–87). Philadelphia: Lippincott-Raven.

37. Littlejohns, L. R., Bader, M. K., & March, K. (2003). Brain tissue oxygen monitoring in severe brain injury, I. Research and usefulness in critical care. *Critical Care Nurse, 23*(4), 17–25; quiz 26–27.

38. Clifton, G. L., Miller, E. R., Choi, S. C., & Levin, H. S. (2002). Fluid thresholds and outcome from severe brain injury. *Critical Care Medicine, 30*, 739–745.

39. Bouma, G. J., Muizelaar, J., Stringer, W., Choi, S. C., Fatouros, P., & Young, H. F. (1992). Ultra early evaluation of regional cerebral blood flow in severely head-injured patients using xenon enhanced computed tomography. *Journal of Neurosurgery, 77*, 360–368.

40. Marion, D. W., Darby, J., & Yonas, H. (1991). Acute regional cerebral blood flow changes caused by severe head injuries. *Journal of Neurosurgery, 74*, 407–414.

41. Robertson, C. S., Contant, C. F., Narayan, R. K., & Grossman, R. G. (1992). Cerebral blood flow, Avdo2, and neurological outcome in head-injured patients. *Journal of Neurotrauma, 9*, S349–S358.

42. McLaughlin, M. R., & Marion, D. W. (1996). Cerebral blood flow and vasoresponsivity within and around cerebral contusions. *Journal of Neurosurgery, 85*(5), 871–876.

43. Salvant, J. B., & Muizellar, J. P. (1993). Changes in cerebral blood flow and metabolism related to the presence of subdural hematoma. *Neurosurgery, 33*, 387–393.

44. Ling, G. S., & Neal, C. J. (2005). Maintaining cerebral perfusion pressure is a worthy clinical goal. *Neurocritical Care, 2*(1), 75–81.

45. Bouma, G. J., & Muizelaar, J. P. (1990). Relationship between cardiac output and cerebral blood flow in patients with intact and with impaired autoregulation. *Journal of Neurosurgery, 73*(3), 368–374.

46. Kelley, D. F. (1995). Steroids in head injury. *New Horizons, 3*(3), 453–455.

47. Jacobi, J., Fraser, G. L., Coursin, D. B., Riker, R. R., Fontaine, D., et al. (2002). Clinical practice guidelines for the sustained use of sedatives and analgesics in the critically ill adult. *Critical Care Medicine, 30*(1), 119–141.

48. Shapiro, B. A., Warren, J., Egol, A. B., Greenbaum, D. M., Jacobi, J., Nasraway, S. A., et al. (1995). Practice parameters for intravenous analgesia and sedation for adult patients in the intensive care unit: An executive summary. *Critical Care Medicine, 23*(9), 1596–1600.

49. Olson, D. M., Graffagnino, C., King, K., & Lynch, J. R. (2005). Toward solving the sedation-assessment conundrum: Bispectral index monitoring and sedation interruption. *Critical Care Nursing Clinics of North America, 17*(3), 257–267.

50. Covington, H. (1998). Use of propofol for sedation in the ICU. *Critical Care Nurse, 18*(4), 34.

51. Mirski, M. A., Muffelman, B., Ulatowski, J. A., & Hanley, D. F. (1995). Sedation for the critically ill neurologic patient. *Critical Care Medicine, 23*(12), 2038–2053.

52. Ford, E. V. (1995). Monitoring neuromuscular blockade in the adult ICU. *American Journal of Critical Care, 4*(2), 122–130.

53. Muzelaar, J. P., & Obrist, W. D. (1985). Cerebral blood flow and brain metabolism with brain injury. In D. P. Becker & J. T. Povlishock (Eds.). *Central nervous system trauma report* (p. 123). Washington, DC: NINCDS.

54. Hudes, R., & Lee, L. (1987). Clinical use of peripheral nerve stimulator in anesthesia. *Canadian Journal of Anesthesiology, 34*, 525–534.

55. Ramsey, M. A. E., Savage, T. M., Simpson, B. R. J., & Goodwin, R. (1974). Controlled sedation with alphaxalone/alphadolone. *British Journal of Medicine, 2*, 656–659.

56. Arbour, R. B. (2003). Continuous nervous system monitoring, EEG, the bispectral index, and neuromuscular transmission. *AACN Clinical Issues, 14*(2), 185–207.

57. Berger, D. P., Schurer, L., Hartl, R., Messmer, K., & Baethmann, A. (1999). Reduction of post-traumatic intracranial hypertension by hypertonic/hyperoncotic saline/dextran and hypertonic mannitol. *Neurosurgery, 37*, 98–107.

58. Bhardway, A., & Ulatowski, J. A. (2004). Hypertonic saline solutions in brain injury. *Current Opinions in Critical Care, 10,* 126–131.

59. Qureshi, A. I., & Suarez, J. I. (2000). Use of hypertonic saline solutions in treatment of cerebral edema and intracranial hypertension. *Critical Care Medicine, 28*(9), 3301–3313.

60. Ware, M. L., Nemani, V. M., Meeker, M., Lee, C., Morabito, D. J., & Manley, G. T. (2005). Effects of 23.4% sodium chloride solution in reducing intracranial pressue in patients with traumatic brain injury: A preliminary study. *Neurosurgery, 57*(4), 727–736.

61. Bratton, S. L., Chestnut, R. M., Ghajar, J., McConnell Hammond, F. A., Harris, O. A., Hartl, R., et al. (2007). Guidelines for the management of severe traumatic brain injury, 3rd ed., II. Hyperosmolar therapy. *Journal of Neurotrauma, 24*(Suppl. 1), S14–S20.

62. Van den Berghe, G., Schoonheydt, K., Becx, P., Bruyninckx, F., & Wouters, P. J. (2005). Insulin therapy protects the central and peripheral nervous system of intensive care patients. *Neurology, 64*(8), 1348–1353.

63. Zygun, D. A., Steiner, L. A., Johnston, A. J., Hutchinson, P. J., Al-Rawi, P. G., Chatfield, D., et al. (2004). Hyperglycemia and brain tissue pH after traumatic brain injury. *Neurosurgery, 55*(4) 877–881.

64. Vandam, L. D., & Burnap, T. K. (1959). Hypothermia. *New England Journal of Medicine, 231,* 595–603.

65. Mokhtarani, M., Mahgoub, A. N., Morioka, N., Doufas, A. G., Dae, M., Shaughnessy, T. E., et al. (2001). Buspirone and meperidine synergistically reduce the shivering threshold. *Anesthesia & Analgesia, 93*(5), 1233–1239.

66. Thompson, H. J., Kirkness, C. J., & Mitchell, P. H. (2007). Fever management practices of neuroscience nurse: National and regional perspectives. *Journal of Neuroscience Nursing, 39*(3), 151–162.

67. Thompson, H. J., Kirkness, C. J., & Mitchell, P. H. (2007). Fever management practice of neuroscience nurse, part II: Nurse patient, and barriers. *Journal of Neuroscience Nursing, 39*(4), 196–201.

68. Clasen, R. A., Pandolfi, S., Russell, J., Stuart, D., & Hass, G. M. (1968). Hypothermia and hypotension in experimental cerebral edema. *Archives of Neurology, 19,* 472–486.

69. Laskowski, E. J., Klatzo, I., & Baldwin, M. (1960). Experimental study of the effects of hypothermia on local brain injury. *Neurology, 10,* 499–505.

70. Rosomoff, H. L., & Gilbert, R. (1955). Brain volume and cerebrospinal fluid pressure during hypothermia. *American Journal of Physiology, 183,* 19–22.

71. Drake, C. G., & Jory, T. A. (1962). Hypothermia in the treatment of critical head injury. *Canadian Medical Association Journal, 87,* 887–891.

72. Shapiro, H. M., Wyte, S. R., & Loeser, J. (1974). Barbiturate-augmented hypothermia for reduction of persistent intracranial hypertension. *Journal of Neurosurgery, 40,* 90–100.

73. Clifton, G. L., Allen, S. J., Barrodale, P., Plenger, P., Berry, J., Koch, S., et al. (1993). A phase II study of moderate hypothermia in severe brain injury. *Journal of Neurotrauma, 10,* 263–271.

74. Marion, D. W., Obrist, W. D., Carlier, P. M., Penrod, L. E., & Darby, J. M. (1993). The use of moderate hypothermia for patients with severe head injuries: A preliminary report. *Journal of Neurosurgery, 79,* 354–362.

75. Clifton, G. L. (1995). Hypothermia and hyperbaric oxygen as treatment modalities for severe head injury. *New Horizons, 3*(3), 474–478.

76. Clifton, G. L., Miller, E. R., Choi, S. C., Levin, H. S., McCauley, S., Smith, Jr., K. R., et al. (2001). Lack of effect on induction of hypothermia after acute brain injury. *New England Journal of Medicine, 344*(8), 556–563

77. Smrcka, M., Vidlak, M., Maca, K., Smrcka, V., & Gal, R. (2005). The influence of mild hypothermia on ICP, CPP and outcome in patients with primary and secondary brain injury. *Acta Neurochirurgica Supplement, 95,* 273–275.

78. Jiang, J. Y., Xu, W., Li, W. P., Gao, G. Y., Bao, Y. H., Liang, Y. M., et al. (2006). Effect of long-term mild hypothermia or short-term mild hypothermia on outcome of patients with severe traumatic brain injury. *Journal of Cerebral Blood Flow Metabolism, 26*(6), 771–776.

79. 2005 American Heart Association guidelines for cardiopulmonary resuscitation and emergency cardiovascular care. (2005). *Circulation, 112*(24 Suppl.), IV1–203.

80. Wilberger, J. E., & Cantella, D. (1995). High-dose barbiturates for intracranial pressure control. *New Horizons, 3*(3), 469–473.

81. Bader, M. K., & Palmer, S. (2000). Keeping the brain in the zone. Applying the severe head injury guidelines to practice. *Critical Care Nursing Clinics of North America, 12,* 413–427.

82. Bader, M. K., Arbour, R., & Palmer, S. (2005). Refractory increased intracranial pressure in severe traumatic brain injury: Barbiturate coma and bispectral index monitoring. *AACN Clinical Issues, 16,* 526–541.

83. Borel, C. O., & Guy, J. (1995). Ventilatory management in critical neurologic illness. *Neurologic Clinics, 13*(3), 627–645.

84. Frank, J. (1993). Management of intracranial hypertension. *Medical Clinics of North America, 77*(1), 63.

85. Kerr, M. E., Rudy, E. B., Brucia, J., & Stone, K. S. (1993). Head-injured adults: Recommendations for endotracheal suctioning. *Journal of Neuroscience Nursing, 25,* 86–91.

86. Rudy, E. B., Turner, B. S., Baun, M., Stone, K. S., & Brucia, J. (1991). Endotracheal suctioning in adults with head injury. *Heart & Lung, 20,* 667–674.

87. Washington, G. T., & Macnee, C. L. (2005). Evaluation of outcomes: The effects of continuous lateral rotational therapy. *Journal of Nursing Care Quality, 20,* 273–282.

88. Martin, A. H. (2001). Should continuous lateral rotation therapy replace manual turning? *Nursing Management, 32,* 41–45.

89. Rosner, M. J., & Coley, I. B. (1986). Cerebral perfusion pressure, intracranial pressure, and head elevation. *Journal of Neurosurgery, 65,* 636–641.

90. Fan, J. Y. (2004). Effect of backrest position on intracranial pressure and cerebral perfusion pressure in individuals with brain injury: A systematic review. *Journal of Neuroscience Nursing, 36,* 278–288.

91. Johnson, S. M., Omery, A., & Nikas, D. (1991). Effects of conversation on intracranial pressure in comatose patients. *Heart & Lung, 18,* 56–63.

92. Yanko, J. R., & Mitcho, K. (2001). Acute care management of severe traumatic brain injuries. *Critical Care Nursing Quarterly, 23,* 1–23.

93. McNair, N. D. (1996). Intracranial pressure monitoring. In J. M. Clochesy, C. Breu, S. Cardin, A. A. Whittaker, & E. B. Rudy (Eds.). *Critical care nursing* (2nd ed., pp. 289–307). Philadelphia: W. B. Saunders.

94. Bisnaire, D., & Robinson, L. (1997). Accuracy of leveling intraventricular collection drainage systems. *Journal of Neuroscience Nursing, 29*(4), 261–268.

95. Lundberg, N. (1960). Continuous recording and control of ventricular fluid pressure in neurosurgical practice. *Acta Psychiatrica et Neurologica Scandinavia, 36*(Suppl. 149), 1–193.

96. Williams, M. A., & Hanley, D. F. (1998). Monitoring and interpreting intracranial pressure. In M. J. Tobin (Ed.). *Principles and practice on intensive care monitoring* (pp. 995–1009). New York: McGraw-Hill.

97. Doyle, D. J., & Mark, P. W. S. (1992). Analysis of intracranial pressure. *Journal of Clinical Monitoring, 8,* 81–90.

98. Barlow, P., Mendelow, A. D., Lawrence A. R., Barlow, M., & Rowan, J. O. (1985). Clinical evaluation of two methods of subdural pressure monitoring. *Journal of Neurosurgery, 63,* 578–582.

99. Piek, J., & Beck, W. J. (1990). Continuous monitoring of cerebral tissue pressure in neurosurgical practice-experiences with 100 patients. *Intensive Care Medicine, 16,* 184–188.

100. Piek, J., Kosub, B., Kuch, F., & Bock, W. J. (1987). A practical technique for continuous monitoring of cerebral tissue pressure in neurosurgical patients: Preliminary results. *Acta Neurochirurgica (Wien) 87,* 144–149.

101. Ostrup, R. C., Luerssen, T. G., Marshall, L. F., & Zornow, M. H. (1987). Continuous monitoring of intracranial pressure with a miniaturized fiberoptic device. *Journal of Neurosurgery, 67,* 206–209.

102. Hayashi, M., Kobayashi, H., Handa, Y., Kawano, H., & Kabuto, M. (1985). Brain blood volume and blood flow in patients with plateau waves. *Journal of Neurosurgery, 63,* 556–561.

103. Lundberg, N., Cronqvist, S., & Kjallquist, A. (1968). Clinical investigations on interrelations between intracranial pressure and intracranial hemodynamics. *Progress in Brain Research, 30,* 69–75.

104. Risberg, J., Lundberg, N., & Ingvar, D. H. (1969). Regional cerebral blood volume during acute transient rises of the intracranial pressure (plateau waves). *Journal of Neurosurgery, 31,* 303–310.

105. Tsementzis, S. A., Gordon, A., & Gillingham, F. J. (1979). Prognostic signs during continuous monitoring of the ventricular fluid pressure in patients with severe brain injury. *Acta Neurochirurgica Supplement, 28,* 78–84.

106. McQuillan, K. A. (1991). Intracranial pressure monitoring: Technical imperatives. *AACN Clinical Issues in Critical Care, 2,* 623–639.

107. Bota, D. P., Lefranc, F., Vilallobos, H. R., Brimioulle, S., & Vincent, J. L. (2005). Ventriculostomy-related infections in critically ill patients: A 6-year experience. *Journal of Neurosurgery, 103,* 468–472.

108. Garner, J. S., Jarvis, W. R., Emori, T. G., Horan, T. C., & Hughes, J. M. (1988). CDC definitions for nosocomial infections. *American Journal of Infection Control, 16,* 128–140.

109. Aucoin, P. J., Kotilainen, H. R., Gantz, N. M., Davidson, R., Kellogg, P., & Stone, B. (1986). Intracranial pressure monitoring: Epidemiological study of risk factors and infections. *American Journal of Medicine, 80,* 369–376.

110. Bader, M. K., Littlejohns, L., & Palmer, S. (1995). Ventriculostomy and intracranial pressure monitoring: In search of a 0% infection rate. *Heart & Lung, 24,* 166–172.

111. Bogdahn, V., Lau, W., Hassel, W., Gunreben, G., Mertens, H. G., & Brawanski, A. (1992). Continuous pressure controlled external ventriculostomy drainage for treatment of acute hydrocephalus: Evaluation of risk factors. *Neurosurgery, 31,* 898–904.

112. Mayhall, G. C., Archer, N. H., Lamb, V. A., Spadora, A. C., Baggett, J. W., Ward, J. D., et al. (1984). Ventriculostomy related infections: A prospective epidemiological study. *New England Journal of Medicine, 310,* 553–559.

113. Winfield, J., Rosenthal, P., Kanter, R., & Casella, G. (1993). Duration of intracranial pressure monitoring does not predict daily risk of infectious complications. *Neurosurgery, 33,* 424–431.

114. Holloway, K. L., Barnes, T., Choi, S., Bullock, R., Marshall, L. F., Eisenberg, H. M., et al. (1996). Ventriculostomy infections: The effect of monitoring duration and catheter exchange in 584 patients. *Journal of Neurosurgery, 85,* 419–424.

115. Rebuck, J. A., Murry, K. R., Rhoney, D. H., Michael, D. B., & Coplin, W. M. (2000). Infection related to intracranial pressure monitors in adults: Analysis of risk factors and antibiotic prophylaxis. *Journal of Neurology, Neurosurgery, & Psychiatry, 69,* 381–384.

116. Bota, D. P., Lefranc, F., Vilallobos, H. R., Brimioulle, S., & Vincent, J. L. (2005). Ventriculostomy-related infections in critically ill patients: A 6-year experience. *Journal of Neurosurgery, 103,* 468–472.

117. Poon, W. S., Ng, S., & Wai, S. (1998). CSF antibiotic prophylaxis for neurosurgical patients with ventriculostomy: A randomized study. *Acta Neurochirurgica Supplement (Wien), 71,* 281–286.

118. O'Grady, N. P., Barie, P. S., Bartlett, J., Bleck, T., Garvey, G., Jacobi, J., et al. (1998). Practice parameters for evaluating new fever in critically ill adult patients. *Critical Care Medicine, 26*(2), 392–408.

119. American Association of Neuroscience Nurses. (1997). *Intracranial pressure monitoring.* Chicago, IL: Author.

120. Wisinger, D., & Mest-Beck, L. (1990). Ventriculostomy: A guide to nursing management. *Journal of Neuroscience Nursing, 22,* 365–369.

121. Adams, R. D., Victor, M., & Ropper, A. H. (1997). *Principles of neurology* (6th ed., pp. 634–637). New York: McGraw-Hill.

Management of Patients Undergoing Neurosurgical Procedures

Joanne V. Hickey and Jamie L. Zoellner

THE PREOPERATIVE PHASE

For the patient undergoing a neurosurgical procedure, the circumstances of admission influence preoperative preparation. Unplanned emergency hospital admissions are often related to trauma or a sudden, life-threatening event such as an aneurysmal rupture. Immediate surgery may be a necessary life-saving measure. The urgency of the surgery compresses all preoperative preparations. With elective or delayed surgery, there is time for preoperative teaching. For the patient who is conscious and oriented, the prospect of a neurosurgical procedure is often associated with overwhelming anxiety and fear. Paramount is the fear of loss of life, cognitive and physical abilities, self-control, personality, and independence. In addition, concerns about permanent disability and chronic illness create concerns about their effects on relationships with family and friends and about burden on loved ones. In contrast, patients with an altered level of consciousness or impaired cognitive function may be unable to grasp the seriousness of the situation and appear apathetic. The crisis and the related high-stake uncertainty are experienced by the family and friends. The impact on each family member and friend will vary depending on the pre-event relationship with the patient. A family member or significant other may become the surrogate decision maker for the unconscious or impaired patients.

Informed Consent

In obtaining informed consent, the physician discusses the purpose of surgery, alternative treatments, potential risks, and expected outcomes. Discussing these points honestly and answering all questions can reduce the possibility of misunderstandings and litigation. Because altered consciousness, impaired cognition, or both can severely influence comprehension, a responsible family member should be present during the discussion. In some instances, it will be necessary for the next of kin or guardian to consent for surgery. This is an awesome responsibility for which most people are not prepared. The nurse has an important role as a patient advocate and coach for the decision maker.

Where does the nurse begin in supporting the surrogate decision maker? First, frame the responsibility being assumed. The surrogate decision maker is asked to make decisions that he or she believes the patient would make if he or she were able to speak for him- or herself. The nurse can help to ask probe questions such as, "Has your loved one ever made statements about what he or she would want done if he or she was critically ill?" "What was the quality of life that your loved one expected?" and "What quality of life would not be acceptable?" Probe questions help the surrogate decision maker to recall conversations that provide insights about the patient's wishes.

Second, help the surrogate decision maker gather necessary information to make an informed decision. Helping the person ask questions of the physician is critical. Such questions include, "What is the best- and worse-case scenario?" "What can be expected if the surgery is performed?" "What is the best- and worst-case scenario if the surgery is not performed?" "How will the patient be on a day-to-day basis in terms of independence in activities of daily living and cognitive functions?" and "Are there other options to surgery and, if so, what are the advantages and disadvantages?" With sufficient information, the surrogate decision maker can better weigh what he or she believes would be the patient's wishes against each option.

Third, the nurse supports the decision maker in whatever choices are made. He or she also supports the decision maker in sharing that decision with care providers, family, and friends. The support continues through the postdecision time period when the decision maker may have second thoughts about the soundness of the decision made. The advocate, couch, and supportive role of the nurse provide the professional care and healing that has ramifications not only for the present, but also for how the decision maker feels about the experience in the future.

Preoperative Teaching and Support

The nurse is tasked with the major responsibility for patient and family preparation and for provision of emotional support throughout the experience. The teaching plan is individualized and directed toward providing information and anticipatory guidance about activities associated with the

TABLE 14-1	GENERAL PREOPERATIVE TEACHING PLAN FOR NEUROSURGICAL PROCEDURES

Patient and Family*

- Clarify and reinforce information provided by the physician.
- Provide printed material about the specific type of surgery and review it with the patient/family.
- Describe preparatory events before surgery (e.g., blood work, electrocardiogram, chest radiograph, application of thromboembolic (TED) stockings and sequential compression device, visit from anesthesiologist, NPO before surgery).
- Discuss the need to cut/shave some hair from the scalp for the procedure.

Patient

- Teach any special activities, such as leg exercises or deep breathing exercises.
- Review what to expect throughout hospitalization and after.

Family

Discuss:
- Location of the waiting area and amenities (e.g., telephones, restrooms, food)
- Location of where the neurosurgeon will talk to the family after the surgery
- If not physically present, how the family can be reached by telephone
- Provisions for periodic updates if the surgery time is extended
- Unit to which the patient will go after surgery (e.g., recovery room; intensive care unit [ICU])
- Visiting hours before surgery and in the ICU
- Estimated length of intracranial surgery (may take several hours and this is not unusual)
- What to expect in the ICU (e.g., tubes, monitors, intravenous lines, change in appearance for dressings or ecchymosis)

*Be prepared to repeat and reinforce information (people under stress often have difficulty retaining information).

neurosurgical procedure (Table 14-1). In addition, printed material is helpful and is a tangible resource that can be reviewed. If slight to moderate cognitive deficits are present, provide a more simplified explanation. With severe deficits, the family assumes a greater decision-making role and often becomes the major focus of teaching. Encourage family members to take care of themselves with adequate rest, nutrition, and support. The expected outcomes of the teaching plan include control of fear and anxiety and maximization of patient and family coping strategies. Common related patient problems include knowledge deficit, anxiety, fear, and family dysfunction.

Preoperative Preparations

For planned admissions, routine tests for any surgical patient are often completed on an outpatient basis. Specific neurological diagnostics that lead to the decision for neurosurgical intervention are typically performed prior to admission. Additional tests may be required upon admission. Because many patients are now admitted on the day of surgery, any preoperative home preparation must be discussed ahead of time and expectations clearly specified (i.e., nothing by

mouth after the specified hour, time to arrive at the registration desk prior to procedure, which home medications to take the morning of surgery and which should be withheld). Other preoperative activities are completed on admission such as verifying nothing by mouth (NPO) status, review of procedure and permit completion, obtaining intravenous (IV) access, and preoperative antibiotic administration if ordered.

CLINICAL PEARLS: Completion of a preoperative checklist enables the nurse to ensure that all preparations for surgery have been completed prior to transporting the patient to the operating room, and that the pertinent data are included in the chart.

Additional preoperative preparations are related to the specific surgical procedure and operative site. For intracranial surgeries, hair should be clean and long hair neatly secured in a manner that will not cause pressure or tension, such as loosely braided. Skin preparation, including hair clipping or shaving, is completed in the operating room (OR). Because neurosurgical procedures are often long, the risk of deep vein thrombosis (DVT) and pulmonary embolus (PE) is high.[1] Thigh-high support (TED) stockings and/or sequential compression devices (SCDs) should be applied preoperatively and used intraoperatively with most neurosurgical patients. The final preoperative neurological assessment and vital signs are recorded and sent with the medical record to the OR with the patient.

Depending on the circumstances, the family may visit briefly before surgery (see Table 14-1 for family support and needs). Any other special preoperative orders are completed, and the patient is transported to the OR.

THE INTRAOPERATIVE PHASE

Arrival in the Operating Room Suite

Once in the OR suite, monitoring equipment is attached and IV anesthetic induction is begun. Other preparation includes:

- General monitoring
  - Various devices for ongoing intraoperative monitoring are connected. Such equipment may include continuous electrocardiogram, esophageal or tympanic temperature probe to gauge cooling efforts, arterial line for continual monitoring of arterial blood pressure, central venous catheter, precordial Doppler placed over the right atrium (to detect venous air emboli, especially if the sitting position is used), pulse oximeter, and other devices as necessary. In addition, end-tidal carbon dioxide ($ETCO_2$) and other respiratory parameters may be monitored.
- General points
  - The anesthesia team intubates the patient and connects respiratory support equipment.
  - If not already present, an indwelling urinary catheter may be inserted.
  - To protect the eyes from corneal abrasions, a bland eye ointment is applied and the eyelids are taped closed; sterile eye pads may be applied.

- Surgical clippers are used to remove hair from the operative site. The hair may be saved in a labeled envelope and sent with the patient postoperatively.
- SCDs may be activated to prevent pooling of blood in the lower extremities (can lead to DVTs).
- Positioning
  - Optimal positioning to facilitate surgery is selected by the surgeon. Common positions include sitting, lateral, or prone positions. For example, the sitting position may be used for posterior fossa surgery because it affords optimal visualization of the operative field.
  - Various support devices, such as a headrest and armrests, are carefully positioned and adjusted; areas of potential pressure are padded to prevent pressure ulcer and ischemic pressure injury to peripheral nerves. Positioning is often complex and may take an hour or more to complete.

Ongoing Neurophysiological Monitoring

Patients undergoing neurosurgical procedures have an inherent increased risk of ischemic/hypoxic damage or direct injury to the central nervous system (CNS). Patient outcomes may be improved by the use of intraoperative neurophysiological monitoring in two ways[2]:

1. Allows early detection of cerebral ischemia so that care providers can intervene before irreparable damage occurs
2. Assists the surgeon to optimize treatment as dictated by monitoring parameters and their indication of the patients' tolerance or response to surgical manipulation

The major categories of neurophysiological cerebral monitoring are function, blood flow/pressure, and metabolism. *Functional parameters* include electroencephalography (EEG), bispectral analysis, evoked potentials, and electromyography (EMG). *Cerebral blood flow* is most commonly estimated in the OR by indirect or relative measurements using laser Doppler blood flow and transcranial Doppler sonography. *Intracranial pressure* (ICP) data are collected with a catheter placed in the intraventricular, intraparenchymal, subarachnoid, or epidural spaces. *Metabolism* can be monitored invasively and noninvasively. Invasive monitoring is done with a brain tissue PO_2 electrode or jugular bulb venous oximetry, whereas noninvasive monitoring uses transcranial cerebral oximetry (near-infrared spectroscopy).[2]

Neuroanesthesia

Preoperative assessment is important to determine the general physical and neurological status of the patient. The American Society of Anesthesiologists has developed a five-point grading scale to estimate anesthetic risk for any type of surgery based on physical status.[3] Class 1 includes healthy people without any organic disturbances, whereas Class 5 includes moribund patients for whom surgery is a last effort for survival. Physical status and acuity are factors considered in providing anesthesia. Anesthetic management of neurosurgical patients is based on how the selected agents affect CNS physiology. Neuroanesthesia combines agents that

TABLE 14–2 EFFECTS OF ANESTHETIC AGENTS ON CEREBRAL BLOOD FLOW, CEREBRAL METABOLIC OXYGEN CONSUMPTION, AND INTRACRANIAL PRESSURE

ANESTHETIC	CBF	CMRO$_2$	ICP
Thiopental	Decrease	Decrease	Decrease
Etomidate	Decrease	Decrease	Decrease
Propofol	Decrease	Decrease	Decrease
Fentanyl	0/Decrease	0/Decrease	0/Decrease
Alfentanil	0/Decrease/increase	0/Decrease	0/Decrease/increase
Sufentanil	0/Decrease/increase	0/Decrease	0/Decrease/increase
Ketamine	Increase	0/Increase	Increase
Midazolam	Decrease	Decrease	0/Decrease
Nitrous oxide	Increase	0/Increase	Increase
Halothane	Increase	Decrease	Increase
Enflurane	Increase	Decrease	Increase
Isoflurane	Increase	Decrease	Increase
Desflurane	Increase	Decrease	Increase
Sevoflurane	Increase	Decrease	Increase

CBF, cerebral blood flow; CMRO$_2$, cerebral metabolic oxygen consumption; ICP, intracranial pressure.

From Neufield, P., & Cottrell, J. C. (Eds.). (1999). *Handbook of neuranesthesia.* Philadelphia: Lippincott Williams & Wilkins.

favorably affect cerebral hemodynamics, cerebral metabolism, and ICP with goals of providing optimal operating conditions (i.e., hemostasis and adequate brain relaxation) and promoting the best possible outcome. Of particular interest when choosing an anesthetic agent is its effect on cerebral blood flow (CBF), cerebrospinal fluid volume, and cerebral metabolic oxygen consumption (CMO$_2$) in addition to the ICP (Table 14-2). These criteria are used for evaluating the usefulness and safety of new drugs.[4]

For neurosurgical procedures, a combination of inhalants and IV drugs are used. Common combinations of drugs include[4,5,6]:

- IV agents
  - Barbiturates (thiopental)
  - Benzodiazepines (midazolam, lorazepam)
  - Sedatives (etomidate primarily for induction; dexmedetomidine)
  - Sedative hypnotic (propofol)
  - Narcotics (fentanyl, sufentanil)
  - Paralytics (succinylcholine primarily for induction; vecuronium, pancuronium)
  - Other (e.g., lidocaine suppresses laryngeal reflexes during intubation to blunt increases of ICP)
- Inhalation agents that may impart some degree of cerebral protection
  - Isoflurane
  - Desflurane
  - Sevoflurane
  - Oxygen

IV mannitol is given to reduce brain volume. Cerebrospinal fluid (CSF) may be removed to facilitate an optimal operative site using a ventricular or lumbar drain.[6] Other drugs administered during the procedure include dexamethasone to control cerebral edema, phenytoin to control seizure activity, and antibiotics as prophylaxis against infection. Vasoactive medications are often required to maintain strict blood pressure parameters.

Cerebral Protection

During surgery, goals include preservation of CBF, as well as avoiding hypoxemia (insufficient oxygenation of arterial blood) and hypoxia (inadequate oxygen supply to the tissues). Interventions are directed at maximizing oxygenation by increasing oxygen supply and decreasing oxygen demand.[7] Controlled hypothermia, induced hypotension, and mild hyperventilation are useful.

Hypothermia. Many neurosurgical patients are candidates for hypothermia therapy. However, recent research has made the routine use of intraoperative hypothermia controversial.[8] Candidates for hypothermia therapy include patients with: [7]

- Space-occupying lesions with or without increased ICP
- Cerebral aneurysm, arteriovenous malformation, or cavernous angioma requiring clipping or excision
- Carotid occlusion requiring extracranial vascular procedures, such as carotid endarterectomy or superficial temporal artery to middle cerebral artery bypass
- Traumatic brain injury

CLINICAL PEARLS: Controlled hypothermia is now employed in neurological intensive care units to assist in cerebral protection during the acute phase of injury as well as to assist in control of intractable ICP.

Hypothermia is useful to decrease metabolic and functional activities of the brain by reducing the cerebral metabolic rate for oxygen consumption ($CMRO_2$) by 6% to 7% for each 1°C decline. Small decreases in temperature result in substantial reductions in the tissue effects of cerebral ischemia. Thus far, no drugs are available that mimic hypothermic ability to reduce neuronal maintenance energy. Current therapeutic recommendations for hypothermic protection are mild hypothermia with a brain temperature of 32 to 35°C, or the more commonly measured core temperature of as low as 32°C. If the temperature drops below 28°C (82.4°F), cardiac irritability increases and extracorporeal support of the systemic circulation becomes necessary. Equally important, hyperthermia must be avoided to avert increases in cerebral oxygen consumption and exacerbation of ischemic injury.[7,9]

Hypotension. Induced hypotension is the intentional reduction of mean arterial blood pressure (MAP) to a level of 50 to 65 mm Hg in baseline normotensive patients. Lowering the MAP during neurosurgery decreases blood loss, optimizes the surgical field, and decreases the need for blood transfusions. In cerebral aneurysm clipping procedures, induced hypotension is employed after dissection and identification of the aneurysm, just prior to clip applica-

tion. By decreasing systemic pressure, hypotension within the aneurysm itself is induced, thereby decreasing the risk of rupture during manipulation as well as facilitating clip application. Significant risks associated with induced hypotension include myocardial and cerebral ischemia, which are exacerbated if underlying anemia or hypovolemia are not corrected prior to MAP manipulation. A uniform safe level of hypotension has not been established and is case specific. Close monitoring guides individual response and optimal parameters.[9,10]

Hyperventilation. Controlled hyperventilation is often maintained during neurosurgical procedures. Mildly reduced PCO_2 blood levels (30 to 35 mm Hg) result in vasoconstriction and a reduction in cerebral blood volume, causing a reduction in brain bulk and ICP. These effects are self-limited until CSF pH metabolically normalizes. Hyperventilation for prolonged periods or excessive PCO_2 reduction results in diffuse cerebral oligemia and hypoxia as well as lactic acid buildup, which are counterproductive. Reductions in coronary artery perfusion, venous blood return, and hypokalemia also occur with hyperventilation.[11,12]

SITTING POSITION

A potentially life-threatening problem associated with the sitting operative position is a venous air embolism (VAE). It is uncommon when the head is raised 20 degrees or less. The head is higher than the heart in the sitting position, and negative pressure is created in the dural venous sinuses and veins draining the brain and head. If air is introduced into the venous system, through the venous sinuses and/or cerebral veins, it is quickly carried to the right side of the heart, resulting in transient cardiovascular deficits or insufficiencies. Early signs of VAE are precordial Doppler sounds, increased end-tidal nitrogen (ETN_2), and increased $ETCO_2$. Late signs include a rise in CVP, pulmonary artery pressure, and pulse oximetry desaturation. Final signs are hypotension, tachycardia, cyanosis, and a mill-wheel murmur.[6]

When an air embolus is suspected, the surgeon is notified so that an attempt can be made to identify and occlude the possible site of air entry. When the problem site has been occluded, the anesthesiologist can aspirate air through the central venous catheter using a 20-mL syringe and an airtight stopcock. If the entry site cannot be located, the patient is placed in the supine position, and the surgery is terminated.

NEUROSURGICAL PROCEDURES AND OTHER RELATED THERAPEUTIC TECHNIQUES

Refinement of instrumentation, lasers, and radiation therapy has increased the options offered to neurosurgical patients. A craniotomy may be combined with laser treatment for some conditions previously managed by craniotomy alone. Other nonsurgical treatment modalities have been introduced that may decrease the need for conventional surgery.

Below are explanations of several common terms and neurosurgical procedures:

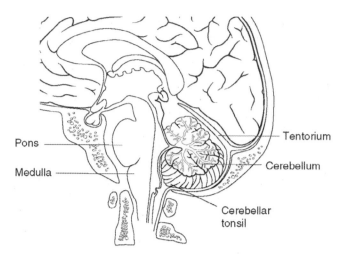

Pons

Medulla

Tentorium

Cerebellum

Cerebellar
tonsil

Figure 14-1 • Surgery on the area of the brain above the tentorium is called *supratentorial;* surgery below the tentorium is *infratentorial.*

- **Surgery** can be classified by anatomic location. Two terms differentiate the areas of the brain on which surgery is performed (Fig. 14-1):
  - **The supratentorial area** is above the tentorium and includes the cerebral hemispheres. The tentorium cerebelli is a double fold of dura mater that forms a partition between the cerebral hemispheres and the brainstem and cerebellum. The supratentorial approach is used to gain access to lesions of the frontal, parietal, temporal, and occipital lobes.
  - **The infratentorial area** is below the tentorium in the posterior fossa and includes the brainstem (midbrain, pons, medulla) and cerebellum. The infratentorial approach is used to gain access to lesions of the brainstem or cerebellum. Occasionally, temporal or occipital lobe lesions located close to the tentorial margin may be excised through the infratentorial approach.
- A **burr hole** is created in the skull with a special drill that permanently removes a small circular area of bone. The burr hole may be used to evacuate an extracerebral clot, to introduce a biopsy probe for isolated tissue sampling, or in preparation for craniotomy. In the case of a craniotomy, a series of burr holes are made for introduction of a special saw that cuts between the holes, allowing removal of the piece of bone or creation of a flap.
- A **craniotomy** is a surgical opening of the skull to provide access to the intracranial contents for reasons such as removal of a tumor, clipping of an aneurysm, or repair of a cerebral injury. It involves creating a bone flap at the area over the lesion. The flap created is either a free flap or an osteoplastic flap. With a **free flap**, the bone is completely removed and preserved for replacement prior to completion of the case. With a **bone flap**, the muscle is left attached to the skull to maintain the vascular supply (Fig. 14-2).
- A **craniectomy** is excision of a portion of the skull without replacement. This may be a permanent removal, such as with a suboccipital craniectomy where the bony skull is so thick that it requires meticulous chipping away of small pieces of bone while avoiding the underlying dura until

an opening is created. There is no remaining bone flap to replace. A craniectomy may also involve saving the created free bone flap for replacement at a later date. The bone may be surgically implanted in the patients' abdominal fat, or stored frozen in the hospital lab. Craniectomies are performed to achieve decompression after cerebral debulking, as a life-saving measure during periods of maximal cerebral swelling to oppose herniation (i.e., following cerebral trauma, high-grade subarachnoid hemorrhage [SAH], or massive cerebrovascular accident [CVA]), or for removal of bone fragments from skull fracture.

- **Cranioplasty** is repair of the skull to re-establish the contour and integrity of the cranial vault. This procedure involves replacement of a skull defect with synthetic material or replacement of the original craniectomy bone flap.
- **Microsurgery** is defined as any surgery performed with the assistance of an operating microscope that provides magnification of small and delicate tissues. The surgical technique (micro-operative technique), instruments (microinstrumentation), illumination for visualization, and magnification (operating microscopes), along with a host of other equipment, are specifically designed for this use. **Surgical microscopes** continue to evolve with new technology. Advances in optical, electrical, and mechanical technology have made it possible to design microscopes with enhanced precision and maneuverability. Figure 14-3 shows a surgical microscope that also allows the assistant to directly observe the operative field in three dimensions. Many microscopes attach to a television monitor, allowing others assisting in the operating room to view the operative field.
- An **ultrasonic surgical aspirator** may be used during a craniotomy. Larger solid lesions with a capsule or pseudocapsular membrane border that are noninfiltrating can be removed with the ultrasonic surgical aspirator. Pulsatile ultrasonic waves disintegrate the mass into pieces, and gentle concurrent irrigation and suction "vacuum" the tumor fragments with minimal or no damage to the surrounding healthy tissue and vessels.[13]
- **Stereotaxis** pertains to precise localization of a specific target point based on three-dimensional coordinates derived with the use of a stereotaxis frame and computed tomography (CT) scanner. It operates according to a target-centered arc principle, which means that all arc paths intersect at the target lesion (Fig. 14-4). A stereotactic frame, such as the CRW, is applied to the patient's head prior to the preoperative CT scan; utilizing skull pins to hold the frame in a fixed position around the head. The target site within the brain is located by determining the X (anteroposterior), Y (superior-inferior), and Z (left to right) coordinates on the CT scan in relation to the stereotactic frame (Fig. 14-5). The point of intersection of all three coordinates identifies the target tissue. Once geometric equipment is attached to the stereotactic head frame in the operating room, the coordinates are used to position the probe guide. The probe is then introduced through a burr hole into the brain to the coordinate depth, allowing the surgeon to directly access the desired tissue for specimen without having to dissect through or unnecessarily manipulate surrounding tissues (Fig. 14-6). Image-guided stereotactic surgery can be performed under local anesthesia

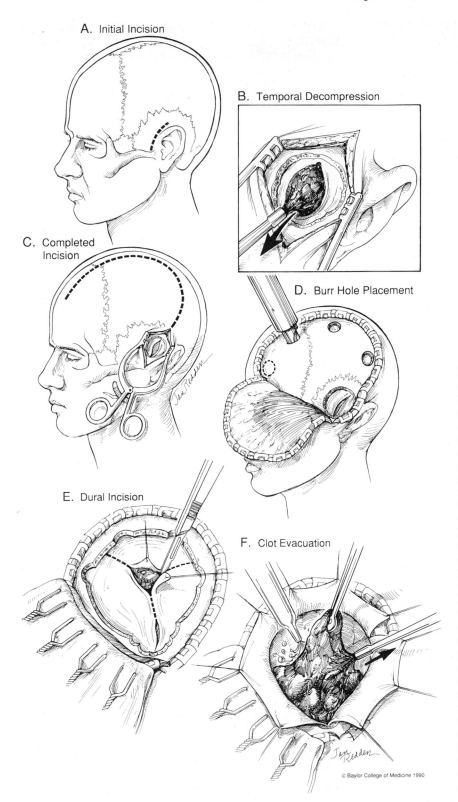

A. Initial Incision

B. Temporal Decompression

C. Completed Incision

D. Burr Hole Placement

E. Dural Incision

F. Clot Evacuation

© Baylor College of Medicine 1990

Figure 14-2 • Craniotomy. The procedure is directed at the removal of an acute subdural hematoma. A number of steps are involved in a craniotomy to gain access to the brain. (*A*) With clinical evidence of rapid neurological deterioration secondary to herniation, temporal decompression is recommended as the first step. An incision is made just anterior to the ear and taken down to the zygoma, which marks the floor of the temporal fossa. (*B*) A burr hole is made, followed by a quick craniectomy. The dura is incised, and as much of the blood clot as possible is aspirated. (*C*) The incision is then extended upward to form a large question mark, the medial extent of which follows the midline. (*D*) Additional burr holes are then made, the medial ones 1.5 cm off the midline to avoid injury to the major venous structures and granulations. A flap is created. The anterior burr hole is placed above the frontal sinus, the size of which can be estimated from preoperative radiographs. (*E*) The dura can be opened with a Y-shaped and X-shaped incision, with a flap being based on the superior sagittal sinus. (*F*) The subdural hematoma is gently evacuated with suction, irrigation, and other mechanical means. Sources of bleeding are identified and cauterized. Contused brain is debrided, and pial edges are carefully cauterized. Ultrasound may be used to rule out the presence of occult intracerebral or contralateral hematomas.

with conscious sedation or general anesthesia depending on the surgeon's preference and planned procedural time.

Stereotactic surgery can assist in multiple procedures, including:

• Biopsy of deep lesions or multiple lesions
• Evacuation of intracerebral hemorrhage

• Catheter placement for drainage of deep lesions or administration of medications or radioactive implants directly into the brain lesion
• Placement of electrodes for epilepsy
• Ablative procedures for extrapyramidal diseases such as Parkinson's disease (tremors, rigidity, and others)

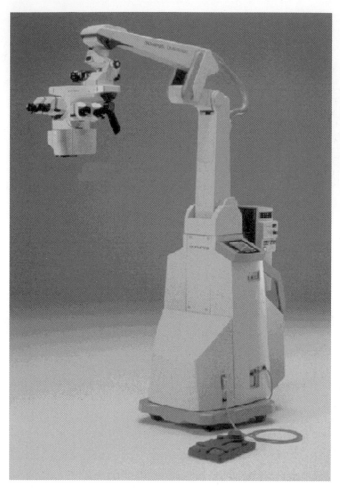

Figure 14-3 • Olympus OME-8000 surgical microscope with enhanced ease of use and precision. In addition, it provides for three-dimensional viewing by the assistant. (Courtesy of Olympus America, Inc., Melville, NY.)

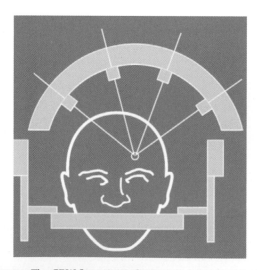

Figure 14-4 • The CRW Stereotactic Systems Arc-Center Principle is a target-centered approach, which means all arc paths pass to the target lesion. (Courtesy of Radionics, Burlington, MA.)

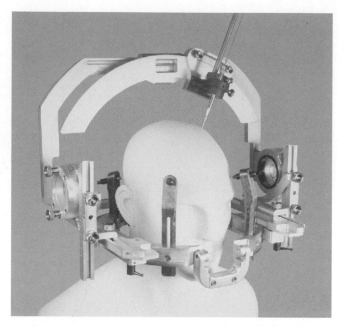

Figure 14-5 • With the CRW equipment, all approaches needed to treat various lesions are easily achieved, including transsphenoidal, full lateral, posterior fossa, and standard approaches (shown in picture). (Courtesy of Radionics, Burlington, MA.)

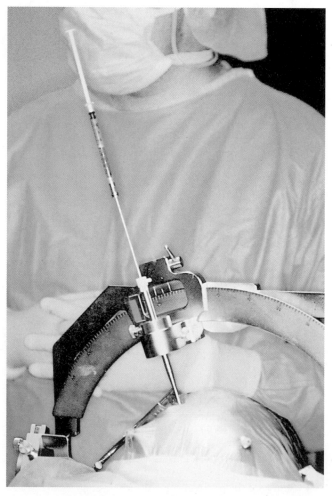

Figure 14-6 • The CRW attached to a patient's head with the probe in place. (Courtesy of Radionics, Burlington, MA.)

- Chronic pain control either with placement of a deep brain stimulator or surgical treatment
- **Neuronavigation.** Navigational guidance systems (e.g., StealthStation, Medtronic Sofamor Danek; BrainLab) have advanced stereotactic surgery into virtual reality computer imaging. This technology replaces skull pins and the bulky head frame with adhesive skin markers and a magnetic resonance imaging (MRI) scan, which are entered into a computer and utilized to create the X, Y, and Z axes. Intra-operative instrumentation movements are tracked by infrared beams from a frameless system and fed into a computer where the patients' MRI scan has been stored. Digitizers transfer the information onto the computer screen's multidimensional image. This enables the surgeon to visually track placement and positioning of instruments and provides real-time calculated and indirect image guidance for advancing the instruments precisely into the desired surgical site. Newer developments include a contour laser that scans anatomy into the computer, negating the need for skin markers and preoperative MRI input to create the virtual image. A neuronavigation guidance system offers precision treatments of lesions deep within the brain or in close proximity to functionally important areas of the brain, as well as the spine and other operative sites.[14]
- **Lasers.** Surgical lasers were first introduced in the early 1960s, but it was not until 1979 that laser neurosurgery gained attention in the United States. The word **laser** is an acronym for **l**ight **a**mplification by **s**timulated **e**mission of **r**adiation. Laser is a device that concentrates a single wavelength of light into an intense, narrow beam of coherent monochromatic light energy that can be accurately focused on specific tissue. The selected body tissue absorbs the laser beam. The laser beam is transformed into immense heat energy, and the thermal energy allows simultaneous surgical dissection and coagulation. The beam can be applied directly to tissue, or it can be used to heat microprobes, which are then applied to tissue. Lasers dissect tissue by vaporization (while leaving adjacent tissue uninjured), coagulate blood vessels, and in some instances, shrink tumors. Patients with tumors that are extrinsic to brain tissue but proximal to delicate cerebral tissue are considered good candidates for laser surgery. Acoustic neuromas, craniopharyngiomas, certain brain-stem gliomas, pinealomas, ventricular tumors, and meningiomas have been removed successfully with laser surgery. Removal of selected intradural and extradural spinal cord tumors has also been successful.
- **Radiosurgery**
  - The gamma knife, which is not actually a knife at all, was developed in 1968 (Fig. 14-7). It consists of a heavily shielded helmet containing 201 radially distributed, sealed, radioactive sources containing curies of cobalt-60. These are focused with precision on a central common target for the purpose of delivering high-dose radiation while minimizing damage to surrounding tissue. Stereotaxis is used to focus the point of radiation. Unlike conventional radiation therapy, stereotactic radiosurgery is capable of destroying deep and inaccessible lesions in a single treatment session, offering treatment options to some for whom treatment previously did not exist. The gamma knife can be used for arteriovenous malformations (AVMs), deep and difficult-to-access brain tumors

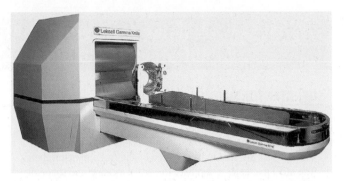

Figure 14-7 • Gamma knife. (Courtesy of Elekta Instruments, Norcross, GA.)

(e.g., acoustic neuromas), and various other intracranial conditions for which conventional surgery is inappropriate, including numerous brain metastases and intracranial cavernous hemangiomas. The cost–benefit ratio associated with the gamma knife is attractive.[15]
  - LINAC or stereotactic linear accelerator is another method of radiosurgery. It utilizes a specialized stereotactic head frame to guide multiple beams of high-dose radiation precisely onto the target tissue. Minimal amounts of radiation reach normal brain structures, unlike conventional radiation therapy. Also a single-treatment therapy, LINAC may be performed on an outpatient basis because there is no recovery phase. Indications are similar to gamma knife, as LINAC offers treatment of intracranial disorders too high risk for conventional brain surgery.[16]
  - Note that there are other vendors of this technology such as Novalis, Cyberknife, and others.

POSTOPERATIVE PHASE

After surgery, the patient is taken to the postanesthesia care unit (PACU) or, at some hospitals, immediately to the neurological intensive care unit (ICU). A stay in an ICU allows for close observation and extensive physiologic monitoring (see Chap. 16 for discussion of critical care management).

Admission to the Intensive Care Unit

During transfer to the ICU, the nurse should expect a complete report, including:

- Overview of surgery (reason for surgery, anatomic approach, length of surgery, and specific area of the brain involved)
- History of preoperative neurological deficits
- Pre-existing medical problems
- Current baseline neurological signs
- Information provided to the family
- Review of the postoperative orders

This report is a basis for planning care. The approach to care depends on whether the patient has undergone supratentorial or infratentorial surgery. A comparison of the nursing focus associated with each approach is found in Chart 14-1.

CHART **14-1** Nursing Management After Supratentorial and Infratentorial Surgery

SUPRATENTORIAL	INFRATENTORIAL

INCISION

- The scalp incision is made within the boundaries of the hairline, directly over the area to be explored on the cerebral hemisphere. The incision creates a skin flap. The actual location and shape of the skin flap can vary from one that appears horseshoe shaped to one that follows the hairline in the frontal region.
- Sutures are usually removed within 7–10 days.

- The incision (skin flap) is made above the nape of the neck around the occipital area or posterolaterally in the occipitotemporal region.
- Sutures are usually removed 7–10 days after surgery.

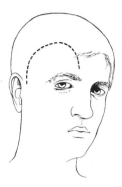 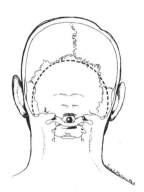

(Figures above are from Smeltzer, S., & Bare, B. [1996]. *Brunner and Suddarth's textbook of medical-surgical nursing* [8th ed.]. Philadelphia: Lippincott-Raven Publishers.)

HEAD DRESSING

- A turban-style dressing is applied initially.
- Many physicians remove the dressing completely after 24 hours.
- The dressing is monitored for evidence of blood or cerebrospinal fluid (CSF) drainage.
- The incision is monitored for redness, drainage, or signs of wound infection.

- A turban-style dressing is applied initially.
- Many physicians remove the dressing completely after 24 hours.
- The dressing is monitored for evidence of blood or CSF drainage.
- The incision is monitored for redness, drainage, or signs of wound infection.

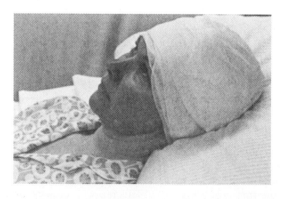

(continued)

CHART 14-1 | **Nursing Management After Supratentorial and Infratentorial Surgery** (Continued)

POSITIONING OF THE HEAD OF THE BED

The position of the head of the bed (HOB) depends on the specific surgical procedure and the physician's preference. Review the doctor's order sheet for any specific instructions. If there are any position restrictions for the HOB, a sign should be posted conspicuously at the HOB and in the nursing care plan.

Some physicians follow a protocol of gradual elevation of the HOB for postoperative management of ventricular shunts and chronic subdural hematomas to prevent cerebral hemorrhage. An example of a protocol followed for postoperative management of both shunts and evacuation of a chronic subdural hematoma is as follows: keep the HOB flat for 24 hours; then elevate the HOB 15 degrees for the next 24 hours; then elevate the HOB 30 degrees for the next 24 hours; then elevate the HOB 45 degrees for the next 24 hours; finally elevate the HOB to 90 degrees.

SUPRATENTORIAL

- The HOB is elevated 30 degrees. (This position facilitates venous blood return from the brain and promotes a decrease in intracranial pressure [ICP].)
- A pillow may be placed under the patient's head and shoulders. The neck should be maintained in a neutral position.

INFRATENTORIAL

- The HOB may be elevated at a 30-degree angle or lowered flat, depending on the preference of the physician.
- *Do not angulate the neck anteriorly or laterally.* A small pillow is placed under the head for comfort.
- For the patient who experiences dizziness or orthostatic hypotension, the HOB is elevated gradually while concurrently monitoring vital signs.

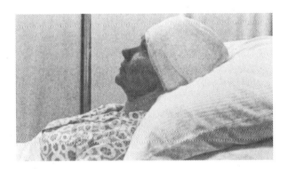

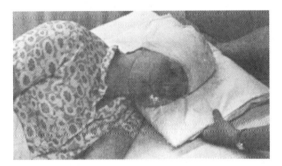

TURNING AND POSITIONING

- There is usually no restriction on turning.
- If a large tumor has been removed from a cerebral hemisphere, the physician may write an order to avoid positioning on the operative site to prevent shifting of cranial contents secondary to gravity.
- Positioning an unconscious patient or one who is recovering from anesthesia on the side facilitates drainage of oral secretions and promotes a patent airway.
- When positioning a patient, avoid extreme flexion of the upper legs or lateral or anterior flexion of the neck. A soft collar may be applied to keep the neck in a neutral position.

AMBULATION

The patient is allowed out of bed as soon as tolerated, which will depend on the specific procedure, invasive equipment, general patient condition, and the judgment of the physician and nurse.

TURNING AND POSITIONING

- There is usually no restriction on turning.
- If a large tumor has been removed from a cerebral hemisphere, the physician may write an order to avoid positioning on the operative site to prevent shifting of cranial contents secondary to gravity.
- Positioning an unconscious patient or one who is recovering from anesthesia on the side facilitates drainage of oral secretions and promotes a patent airway.
- When positioning a patient, avoid extreme flexion of the upper legs or lateral or anterior flexion of the neck. A soft collar may be applied to keep the neck in a neutral position.

AMBULATION

The patient is allowed out of bed as soon as the vertical position can be tolerated. Patients undergoing infratentorial procedures are often maintained on bed rest longer than those undergoing supratentorial procedures because of the frequency of dizziness experienced by these patients. This dizziness is caused by transient edema in the area of cranial nerve VIII.

(continued)

CHART **14-1** Nursing Management After Supratentorial and Infratentorial Surgery (Continued)

SUPRATENTORIAL	**INFRATENTORIAL**

NUTRITION

SUPRATENTORIAL

- The patient is given nothing by mouth (NPO) for 24 hours; IV fluids are administered slowly.
- If the patient is not experiencing nausea or vomiting and can protect his or her airway, clear fluids are started.

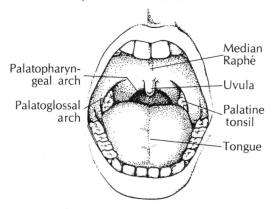

- The diet is progressed as tolerated.
- If fluid restriction is ordered, the daily allowance is strictly maintained.

INFRATENTORIAL

- The patient is kept NPO for at least the first 24 hours; IV fluids are administered slowly. Nausea tends to be more of a problem with surgery in this region than in the supratentorial area. Presence of the gag reflex and ability to protect the airway must be evident before food and fluids are given.
- Edema of cranial nerves IX and X may affect the swallowing and gag reflexes.
- If no nausea or vomiting is noted, and the gag and swallowing reflexes are present, the patient may sip water using a straw. Ask the patient to take a small sip and swallow it.
- The gag reflex is checked by touching the posterior wall of the pharynx. The normal response is contraction of the pharynx.
- If nausea or vomiting occurs, continue the patient's NPO status and IV therapy; after nausea or vomiting has subsided, ingestion of oral fluids may be attempted again.
- Once the patient is able to tolerate fluids, progress from clear liquids to a diet as tolerated.
- If fluid restriction is ordered, the daily allowance is adhered to strictly.

ELIMINATION

SUPRATENTORIAL

- An indwelling urinary catheter is inserted for most neurosurgical procedures. The catheter is removed as soon as possible. If there is difficulty with voiding, a bladder retraining program is begun.
- Constipation can occur as a result of diuretics, pain medication, immobility, and dietary alterations. Undesirable straining at stool initiates the Valsalva's maneuver, which can increase ICP. A bowel program is begun to avoid straining at stool and/or constipation.

INFRATENTORIAL

- An indwelling urinary catheter is inserted for most neurosurgical procedures. The catheter is removed as soon as possible. If there is difficulty with voiding, a bladder retraining program is begun.

FLUID AND ELECTROLYTE BALANCE

SUPRATENTORIAL

- Most patients are maintained euvolemic. Intake is balanced with output.
- An intake and output record is maintained, and the fluid restriction is adhered to strictly.
- Serum electrolyte and osmolarity levels are monitored.
- If surgery is performed in the area of the pituitary gland or hypothalamus, transient diabetes insipidus may develop. Urinary output and specific gravity are monitored every 1–4 hours.

INFRATENTORIAL

- Most patients are maintained euvolemic. Intake is balanced with output.
- An intake and output record is maintained, and the fluid restriction is adhered to strictly.
- Serum electrolyte and osmolarity levels are monitored.

SPECIAL FOCUS OF NEUROLOGICAL ASSESSMENT

The nurse monitors the patient's neurological status, performing an assessment at frequent intervals. Based on an understanding of specific neurological functions controlled by the supratentorial region and infratentorial region, the nurse places special emphasis on the following areas of assessment:

(continued)

CHART 14-1	Nursing Management After Supratentorial and Infratentorial Surgery (Continued)

SUPRATENTORIAL	INFRATENTORIAL

• Potential cranial nerve (CN) dysfunction
  Optic (CN II): visual deficits, homonymous hemianopia
  Oculomotor (CN III): ptosis
  Oculomotor, trochlear, abducens (CNs III, IV, VI): deficits in extraocular movement
	• Potential CN dysfunction
	  Oculomotor, trochlear, abducens (CNs III, IV, VI): deficits in extraocular movement
	  Facial (CN VII): lower lid deficit, absent corneal reflex, weakness or paralysis of the facial muscles
	  Acoustic (CN VIII): decreased hearing, dizziness, nystagmus
	  Glossopharyngeal, vagus (CN IX, X): diminished or absent gag or swallowing reflex, orthostatic hypotension
	• Potential cerebellar dysfunction
	  Ataxia, difficulty with fine motor movement, difficulty with coordination

The basic maintenance and supportive nursing care provided, regardless of procedure or anatomic location, are summarized in Chart 14-2. See Chapter 12 for information pertinent to postoperative drug therapy.

Assessment and Monitoring in the Neurological Intensive Care Unit

Hemodynamic, respiratory, metabolic, and neurological assessment and monitoring are frequent and ongoing. Knowledge that the patient has recently undergone surgical insult is reason enough to draw the conclusion that increased ICP may be present. When assessing the neurological signs, the nurse must identify changes in condition that may be obvious or subtle. Current findings are compared with baseline findings to determine trends that may indicate deterioration. Rapid notification and activation of the neurosurgical team in the face of a worsening clinical exam may prevent irreversible damage to the brain.

CLINICAL PEARLS: Due to the finite amount of space available for brain tissue, blood, and CSF within the closed skull, any increase in one of the three contents can only be tolerated by displacing another of the contents (i.e., CSF shunts to the spine when brain edema occurs). Decompensation and subsequent clinical deterioration occurs rapidly when volume in the skull increases. Thus, the nurse must perform frequent neurological exams postoperatively for early recognition and intervention.

The frequency with which assessments are conducted depends on how stable the patient's condition is and how soon after surgery they are performed. Neurological signs should be assessed every 15 to 30 minutes for the first 8 to 12 hours postoperatively, then every hour for the next 12 hours.

As the patient stabilizes, the frequency of assessment can eventually be reduced to every 4 hours. Blood chemistries, complete blood counts, and other laboratory monitoring are frequent. Chest radiographs, CT scans, electroencephalogram monitoring, and other diagnostic modalities may be necessary to monitor progress.

Transfer from the Intensive Care Unit to an Acute Care Unit

After the patient is physiologically stable and discharge criteria have been met, transfer from the ICU occurs. To maintain continuity of care, the ICU nurse should communicate with the nurse accepting the patient to ensure a smooth transition, as well as perform a neurological exam on the patient with the receiving nurse so that he or she is clear about the baseline exam.

CLINICAL PEARLS: The off-going nurse and oncoming nurse should perform a neurological examination of the patient together. This ensures accuracy of the baseline exam for the oncoming nurse. This procedure should also be followed when a patient is transferred from one unit to another care area. This decreases the chance of miscommunication of important neurological details and oversight of subtle neurological deterioration.

The patient and patient's family need reassurance that the patient is stable and ready for this transfer. If possible, it is helpful for the receiving nurse to meet the patient and family before the transfer to relieve anxiety and fear. Once transferred from the ICU, the family may be offered the opportunity to increasingly and actively participate in the patient's care to an extent not available in the ICU environment because of its inherent monitoring equipment, need for decreased stimulus, and instability of the patient.

CHART 14–2   Basic Nursing Management After Cranial Surgery

NURSING MANAGEMENT

- Give basic hygienic care until the patient is able to participate in self-care (e.g., bath, oral hygiene, hair combing, nail cutting).
- Apply thigh-high elastic stockings and sequential compression air boots, and inspect legs daily. Note any signs of thrombophlebitis (redness, tenderness, warmth, swelling).
- Provide skin care every 4 hours.

- Turn patient every 2 hours, being careful to maintain the patient's body alignment. (It may be necessary to use pillows and other similar devices to maintain good body alignment.)
- Carry out range-of-motion exercises four times daily.
- Provide urinary catheter care daily using soap and water. Pin the catheter to prevent undue traction on the meatus. Remove the catheter as soon as possible.
- Apply warm or cold moist compresses to the eye area.
- Inspect eyes every 4 hours for signs of irritation or dryness. Lubricate the eye with normal saline; commercially prepared eye lubricant, or ointment, as prescribed by the physician. To protect the eye from injury (corneal ulcerations or abrasions) if the lids do not tightly cover the eye, use an eye shield, or tape the eye closed.
- Pull up the side rails of the bed, and apply restrains as necessary.
- Evaluate periods of restlessness for an underlying cause (check for patency of the airway, evidence of pain, or distention of the bladder).

- Administer analgesics as ordered (the drug selected should not mask neurological signs).

> - Do not combine nursing activities that are known to increase intracranial pressure (ICP) in the patient at risk.

- Monitor routine vital signs.
- Assess neurological signs at prescribed intervals:
    Level of consciousness and orientation
    Pupillary reaction
    Eye movement
    Motor function
    Sensory function
- Review laboratory reports. Conventional normal values for some studies are as follows:
    Hemoglobin: 12.0–16.0 g in females
                        13.5–18.0 g in males
    Hematocrit: 37%–48% in females
                        42%–50% in males
    BUN: 8–25 mg
    Potassium: 3.5–5.0 mEq
    Calcium: 8.5–10.5 mg
    Sodium: 135–145 mEq
    Fasting blood sugar: 70–110 mg
    Creatinine: 0.6–0.9 mg/dL in females
                        0.8–1.2 mg/dL in males
    Serum osmolarity: 275–295 mOsm/L

RATIONALE

- Maintains cleanliness and encourages independence in activities of daily living
- Improves blood return to the heart and decreases the risk of thrombophlebitis

- Cleanses, lubricates, and provides the opportunity for an inspection of the skin to note irritation or skin breakdown
- Prevents prolonged pressure on specific areas of the skin, pooling of secretions, and development of musculoskeletal abnormalities; decreases the risk of pneumonia and atelectasis
- Maintains muscle tone to prevent atrophy and contractures
- Reduces the incidence of urinary tract infection

- Relieves periorbital edema
- Decreases the risk of corneal ulceration, eye infections, or injury

- Provides for patient's safety
- In a neurological patient, restlessness may be caused by an obstructed airway, pain, or a distended bladder; the nurse should identify the underlying cause and provide the appropriate intervention.
- Provides for the comfort of the patient and helps to control restlessness

- Prevents dangerous spikes in ICP

- Provides baseline data and data for comparison
- Provides data about the patient's neurological condition and allows comparison with previous signs to detect any change in the patient's condition

- Identifies abnormal levels that signal the need for intervention. Also, some medical orders may set parameters for treatment (e.g., maintain the serum osmolarity at 305–310 mOsm/kg). A review of the laboratory data also provides guidelines for interventions.

POSTOPERATIVE MANAGEMENT AND PREVENTION OF COMPLICATIONS

Numerous complications can develop after brain surgery. Some complications are related to the surgical site; for example, patients who undergo posterior fossa surgery are at high risk for lower cranial nerve dysfunction that results in inability to protect the airway. Complications may be time dependent in that some complications occur earlier in the postoperative periods (i.e., anesthetic-related nausea and vomiting, cerebral edema), whereas others, such as wound infection, appear later. Other complications can occur at any time, such as rebleeding or pneumonia. The nurse is responsible for providing general management and care with particular attention to the prevention of complications.

> **CLINICAL VIGNETTE:** A 43-year-old previously healthy male fell 15 feet from scaffolding, hitting his head in the fall. He suffered a right temporal skull fracture with underlying bilateral subdural contusions and a midline shift on CT scan. He was intubated upon arrival in the emergency room because of rapidly deteriorating mental status and a Glasgow Coma Score of 5. He was taken emergently to the OR for a right hemicraniectomy. A ventriculostomy was placed postoperatively to monitor ICP; it was 45 mm Hg. Serum osmolarity was 316 mEq/L and serum sodium was 152 mEq/L so that use of hyperosmolar therapy was excluded. Mild hypothermia was used; he was cooled to 35.6°C (96°F), paralyzed to prevent shivering, and sedated. His ICP dropped to a range of 12 to 15 mm Hg.

Cardiopulmonary and Cardiovascular Management

There exists a close relationship between the CNS and the cardiovascular system. Sympathetic and parasympathetic nerve fibers within the CNS regulate the autonomic nervous system (ANS) and may cause cardiovascular dysfunction. Likewise, a host of respiratory disorders may be a result of CNS dysfunction, which may lead to arterial hypoxemia (i.e., respiratory depression, neurogenic respiratory patterns, aspiration from altered mental status, neurogenic pulmonary edema). The goal of cardiopulmonary monitoring is to ensure the adequacy of oxygenation, cardiac output, and tissue perfusion. Oxygenation is monitored in several ways, including the physical examination, pulse oximetry, and arterial blood gases. $ETCO_2$ may be helpful in a mechanically ventilated patient. Cardiac function is monitored with ongoing blood pressure monitoring and ECG monitoring with waveform analysis to detect changes in rate or rhythm and identify arrhythmias. In addition, hemodynamic monitoring of central venous pressure and hemodynamics derived from the use of a pulmonary artery catheter such as pulmonary wedge pressure, left ventricular end-diastolic pressure, and cardiac output may provide ongoing data on cardiac function. Because adequate cerebral oxygenation is a goal in management, a jugular bulb catheter may be used to monitor arteriojugular differences of global cerebrovenous oxygenation (see Chap. 16).[17,18,19]

Hypovolemic Shock. Hypovolemic shock results from general fluid loss (blood, plasma, or water), particularly if osmotic diuretics have been used. Signs and symptoms include decreased CVP; tachycardia; decreasing blood pressure; shallow and rapid respirations; cool, pale skin; low urinary output (0 to 25 mL/hour); and restlessness to coma. Hemodynamics (e.g., CVP, cardiac output), oxygenation (arterial blood gases [ABGs], SaO_2) and vital signs should be monitored frequently. Treatment is directed toward fluid replacement using a bolus of isotonic crystalloid solutions such as normal saline (0.9%) or lactated Ringer's, colloid solutions such as Plasmanate and albumin (5% to 25%), or blood products. Vasopressors (e.g., phenylephrine hydrochloride, norepinephrine, vasopressin, or dopamine) may be given as an adjunct to fluid replacement.

Cardiac Arrhythmias. Cardiac arrhythmias are not unusual, especially after posterior fossa surgery or if blood has entered the CSF. Acute elevations of ICP result in a catecholamine release, which can cause myocardial dysfunction and arrhythmias. Bradyarrhythmias are commonly seen with increased vagus nerve stimulation.[18] Continuous cardiac monitoring is important in the immediate postoperative period and throughout episodes of critical neurological dysfunction. Periodically observe the rate, rhythm, and pattern on the monitor to determine the presence of an arrhythmia. If a monitor is not available (e.g., after ICU discharge), the apical pulse should be checked during the postoperative period to identify abnormalities in the heart rate or rhythm. Treatment is arrhythmia specific and will depend on the etiology as well as resulting hemodynamic effects. In addition, serum potassium levels should be monitored for depletion secondary to diuresis, which can also cause arrhythmias.

Airway Obstruction. Partial or complete obstruction of the airway can result from improper positioning or accumulation of mucus or other drainage.

- Unconscious patients should not be positioned on their backs with the head of bed flat (unless specifically ordered) because the tongue can easily slip backward and obstruct the airway.
- Maintain the neck in neutral position.

If an unconscious patient begins to snore, it is most likely a partial obstruction of the airway. This situation must be corrected immediately to prevent respiratory failure, secondary brain injury from cerebral hypoxia, and an increase in ICP. If obstruction is suspected, the jaw is pulled forward and downward to relieve the obstruction and the patient positioned laterally. Elevating the head of the bed to 30 degrees helps promote a patent airway and facilitate drainage of secretions.

> **CLINICAL PEARLS:** A partially occluded airway will result in $PaCO_2$ buildup with subsequent elevation of ICP, as well as decreased PaO_2, which further insults edematous brain tissue in the postoperative period. Careful attention to patent airway maintenance is fundamental.

Aspiration. Edema involving the lower cranial nerves following infratentorial surgery or from generalized cerebral edema from supratentorial surgery, or an altered mental status can result in inability to protect one's airway. Endo-tracheal intubation may be necessary to protect the airway. Aspiration can be minimized by properly positioning the patient and frequent oral care to minimize pooling of secretions. Additionally, oral intake should be withheld until the presence of the gag and swallowing reflexes has been verified and the patient is able to protect his or her own airway.

Neurogenic Pulmonary Edema. A sudden, massive increase in ICP can trigger a catecholamine surge, which results in the development of neurogenic pulmonary edema. Signs and symptoms are similar to those associated with acute pulmonary edema caused by cardiac decompensation, although there may not be underlying cardiac disease to which acute pulmonary edema can be attributed. Treatment involves supportive measures including positive pressure ventilation, controlling elevated ICP, blood pressure support, and diuresis.[20]

CLINICAL VIGNETTE: CJ is a 43-year-old previously healthy black male who fell 15 feet off scaffolding onto his head, suffering a right temporal skull fracture with underlying subdural hematoma (SDH) and bilateral temporal contusions with midline shift. Upon arrival to the emergency department, CJ is intubated for a rapidly deteriorating mental status to a Glasgow Coma Score of 5 and taken emergently to the OR for a right hemi-craniectomy with evacuation of the SDH. Postoperatively, the external ventricular drainage device is transduced for ICP monitoring and reveals an ICP of 45 mm Hg. Elevated lab values of serum osmolarity of 316 mOsm/L and sodium of 152 mmol/L leave no room for hyperosmolar therapy. Alternatively, CJ is managed with a hypothermia protocol for control of his intracranial hypertension. He is appropriately sedated, actively cooled to 35.6°C (96.0°F), and chemically paralyzed to prevent shivering with resulting ICP of 12 to 15 mm Hg. Critical nursing management includes maintaining neutral head alignment to increase venous return, posting a notice above the head of CJ's bed that says "No right bone flap" to warn other care providers of loss of skull protection, and careful attention to prevent pressure points as chemical paralysis results in forced immobility and hypothermia leads to decreased skin perfusion. Also important is ABG surveillance after paralytic initiation as an obliterated respiratory drive can result in undesirable hypercarbia, which contributes to elevated ICP. The nurse will also be concerned with serum potassium levels as cooling shifts potassium intracellularly, resulting in low to low-normal serum levels during hypothermia. If the potassium is replaced to a normal level during hypothermia, when the patient's potassium moves back out of the cell during rewarming, the patient may develop a dangerous level of hyperkalemia.

Neurological Complications

Cerebral Hemorrhage. Hemorrhage is a serious postoperative complication that can occur in the subdural, epidural, intracerebral, or intraventricular space. Unlike bleeding that is visible externally, occult bleeding within the cranial vault is characterized by signs and symptoms of rapidly

increasing ICP that requires early recognition and immediate intervention. Postoperative hemorrhage can also be determined by a sudden and sustained increase in bloody drainage from an external ventricular drainage device (EVD, ventriculostomy) or subdural drain if present. Cerebral hemorrhage is suspected on a clinical basis and confirmed by emergent CT scan. Treatment depends on CT findings and may require coagulopathy diagnosis and correction, control of hypertension (HTN), or even emergency surgery.

Increased Intracranial Pressure. Although some elevation of ICP is expected (peak cerebral swelling occurs within 72 hours after surgery), acute spikes in ICP or persistent elevations above 20 mm Hg are brain threatening. Postoperative increases in ICP can result from cerebral edema, hemorrhage, meningitis, surgical trauma, volume overload, loss of cerebral autoregulation, hydrocephalus, hypercarbia, pneumocephalus, fever, shivering, or patient stimulation and agitation. Treatment includes management of the underlying cause, judicious use of osmotic diuretics, and possible ventricular drainage. See Chapter 13 for a more detailed discussion of increased ICP.

Pneumocephalus. Pneumocephalus is entry of air into the subdural, extradural, subarachnoid, intracerebral, or intraventricular compartments. If the pneumocephalus expands and becomes large enough to cause mass effect and midline shift, which is diagnosed by emergent CT scan, this is a surgical emergency known as tension pneumocephalus. Pneumocephalus can be a postoperative complication associated with craniotomy, burr holes, shunt insertion, and transsphenoidal surgeries. The sitting position assumed during posterior fossa surgery is a risk factor. During hypophysectomy, air enters the subarachnoid space through the pituitary fossa and is gradually absorbed. However, in the presence of CSF rhinorrhea, additional air can enter the intracranial space, creating a pneumocephalus.

The trapped air, when warmed within the body, expands. A small amount of air within the skull can usually be reabsorbed and does not require aggressive treatment. However, if the air pocket is of sufficient volume acting as a space-occupying lesion causing neurological deterioration, or if there is a tension pneumocephalus, immediate surgical evacuation is required. Common time frames for pneumocephalus to develop are either early (within 24 hours after surgery) or late (1 week following surgery), depending on dural integrity. Signs and symptoms include headache, nausea and vomiting, drowsiness, decreased level of consciousness, focal or lateral deficits, and possibly seizures. The diagnosis is established by CT scan. Treatment includes surgical evacuation of the air.

Hydrocephalus. Hydrocephalus can develop at any time during the postoperative course. Intraventricular blood can interfere with the normal absorption of CSF by plugging the arachnoid villi. Such plugging is also associated with a ruptured cerebral aneurysm or head trauma. Scarring or obstruction in the ventricular system can also lead to hydrocephalus. The signs and symptoms of hydrocephalus are outlined in Chapter 13. The usual treatment is a ventriculostomy to drain CSF temporarily. If the hydrocephalus does not resolve, a surgical shunting procedure is warranted. This is necessary to relieve the brain of excessive CSF and to prevent cerebral atrophy.

Seizures. Seizures following intracranial surgery may take the form of generalized convulsions or focal seizure activity, and may be brief and self-limiting or prolonged, requiring treatment. Seizures can occur at any time postoperatively, although seizures within the first 7 days are more common. Focal seizures in the form of twitching of selected muscles, particularly of the face or hand, are common because both occupy large areas on the motor strip of the cerebral cortex; therefore, irritation from surgery or cerebral edema can easily initiate such seizure activity. Patients undergoing craniotomy often receive prophylactic anticonvulsants, most commonly phenytoin, to prevent seizure activity. Drug blood levels must be monitored to maintain a therapeutic range. Patient management during seizure activity is directed at adequate oxygenation, preventing aspiration and injury from motor activity, monitoring vital signs, and possible administration of a benzodiazepine to break the seizure activity if sustained (see Chap. 29 for seizure treatment details). A follow-up CT scan may be ordered to rule out postoperative hemorrhage as a cause of the seizure.

Cerebrospinal Fluid Leakage. Leakage of CSF can occur at any time in the postoperative course and is caused by an opening in dura to the subarachnoid space. It is often seen as CSF leakage from the operative site, but may be noted as clear, watery drainage from the ears (otorrhea) or nose (rhinorrhea). A CSF leak can also be associated with head trauma, especially a basal skull fracture. If CSF is present in nasal drainage, nasal suctioning or blowing of the nose is prohibited. The neurosurgical team should be notified at once if there is evidence of a CSF leak. To determine whether the drainage is CSF, a Dextrostix can be used to test the fluid. If the drainage is CSF, the fluid will test positive for glucose. Mucus does not contain glucose, although blood does contain glucose. If more conclusive evidence is required and CSF can be collected, it should be sent to the laboratory to be checked for chloride. CSF will show a glucose level that is approximately 60% to 80% that of the blood level and a chloride level greater than the serum level.

A CSF leak will often seal spontaneously. Serial lumbar punctures or a lumbar drain may be necessary to keep CSF pressure low. If these measures are not successful, surgical repair may be indicated. Prophylactic antibiotics are ordered to prevent infection when a CSF leak is discovered.

Meningitis. Microorganisms that cause meningitis can be introduced into the meninges or CSF by spreading from a wound infection, from a head injury in which the dura mater has been punctured, by contamination during surgery, by contamination of an EVD or subdural drain, or by a contaminated dressing on a head wound. Presence of a dural tear, which is a prime site for entrance of microorganisms, is a risk factor for meningitis. Meningitis is treated with antibiotics, fever control, fluid and electrolyte management, pain control, and a quiet environment (see Chap. 30 for more details).

Prevention measures such as strict aseptic technique should be followed in the management of the surgical site. Most neurosurgeons routinely order prophylactic antibiotics during and after intracranial surgeries to prevent meningitis. Part of the nursing responsibility is checking for drainage on the dressing and observing its character. A wet dressing should be reinforced immediately and the physician notified. A wet dressing is an ideal medium on which organisms can grow. The gauze used in most dressings absorbs drainage by capillary wicking action, which helps to remove drainage from the skin. A wet dressing on the incision can result in wound contamination by organisms in the air or on the bedclothes by the wicking action of the moist dressing.

When head dressings are changed, a strictly aseptic technique must be followed. Usually, the initial dressing is not touched until the neurosurgery team discontinues it or unless it has become wet. The wound should be kept dry until stitches or staples are removed. Some physicians remove the dressing completely after 24 hours. The policy of the treating hospital and physician preference should be followed.

Other Complications

Wound Infection. Wound infections can result from compromised aseptic technique during surgery or dressing changes. Infection can also result from the patient touching the incision. Patients must be cautioned against such action and restrained if necessary. The most frequent causative organisms for wound infections are various staphylococcal organisms. Observe the dressing for evidence of drainage and the incision for redness, edema, or drainage. Fever, a foul odor from the wound, or an elevated white blood cell count raises suspicion of a wound infection. Treatment includes antibiotics, fever management, and wound care. Severe wound infections may require incision and drainage.

Gastric Ulceration/Hemorrhage. Neurological procedures and acute and chronic CNS disease (e.g., craniocerebral trauma, tumors) are often associated with gastritis, gastric ulcerations, and symptoms of active gastric bleeding. An increased incidence of gastric ulcers is associated with posterior fossa injury or surgery. Some of the drugs used in neurological treatment protocols (dexamethasone, phenytoin, and certain antibiotics) also contribute to gastric irritation. Monitor hematocrit and hemoglobin trends and be alert to significant decreases without an obvious source. Assess for abdominal tenderness, increasing distension, and firmness. Nasogastric output and stools should be closely monitored for black, burgundy, or bright red color changes indicating bleeding in the gastrointestinal (GI) tract. Acetaminophen (Tylenol) is preferred over ibuprofen or aspirin (known to impair mucosal defense and platelet function) for the treatment of mild discomfort or as an antipyretic drug. Magnesium hydroxide, sucralfate, an H_2 receptor antagonist, or a proton pump inhibitor may be used to reduce gastric irritation and protect against gastric hemorrhage.

Deep Vein Thrombosis. Neurosurgical patients are at high risk for upper and lower extremity DVT, which may lead to PE because of the longer surgery, positioning during surgery, coagulopathies, and therapies such as hypothermia, indwelling vascular catheters, and bed rest. Half of the patients with DVT may not exhibit the classic findings of tenderness, swelling, and redness of the extremity, requiring the clinician to be particularly vigilant for subtle changes. Duplex ultrasonography is commonly employed to assess for the presence of DVT. Preventative measures are the mainstay. Elastic TED stockings and/or SCDs are applied early in the admission and should be used on a continuous basis in the postoperative period until the patient is ambulatory or anticoagulation can safely be instituted. In the patient who develops a lower extremity DVT during a time when anticoagulation is contraindicated (i.e., recent severe head injury or craniotomy, GI bleeding), placement of an inferior vena cava filter may be indicated to prevent clot migration into a PE. Conventional treatment of DVTs includes bed rest, elevation of the affected extremity, anticoagulation, ambulation after 7 to 10 days, and continuous prophylaxis for the risk of recurrent DVT.[21,22] See guidelines for DVT prophylaxis of neurosurgical patients in Chapter 15.[23]

Metabolic Imbalances. The most common metabolic and fluid imbalances result from cerebral salt wasting, hyperglycemia, electrolyte imbalances, and diabetes insipidus (DI) (see Chap. 10 for detailed discussion).

- **Diabetes Insipidus.** Patients with severe brain injury, significant cerebral edema, or hypothalamic-pituitary axis damage frequently exhibit central DI. The posterior lobe of the pituitary gland produces antidiuretic hormone (ADH). If this hormone is not secreted in sufficient quantity, the patient excretes large amounts (>250 mL/hr) of dilute urine with a low specific gravity (<1.005). Loss of free water leads to hypernatremia and hyperosmolarity. Use of mannitol in the at-risk patient population may impair early diagnosis of DI. Development of DI is often a transient problem that frequently resolves within 12 to 36 hours following surgery, requiring no specific treatment other than adjusting IV therapy to correlate with urinary output. An indwelling urinary catheter is placed in the early postoperative period when DI is most apt to appear. An accurate intake and output record must be kept and serial serum sodium checks monitored. The specific gravity of urine is monitored every 1 to 4 hours. If the condition does not correct itself or there is difficulty maintaining euvolemia, desmopressin (DDAVP) is used to reduce urine output.[24,25]

- **Cerebral Salt Wasting.** Hyponatremia is common in the neurosurgical population, particularly after subarachnoid hemorrhage, and may result from cerebral salt wasting (CSW). The kidneys fail to retain sodium, resulting in hyponatremia and intravascular volume deficits, thought to be due to the release of atrial natriuretic peptide (ANP) from the injured brain. Assess for signs and symptoms of dehydration and hyponatremia (confusion, lethargy), and monitor sodium trends. Treatment is saline solution to correct fluid balance and low sodium levels. Hypertonic saline, oral salt supplementation, or fludrocortisone may be added to promote renal sodium retention if CSW persists (see Chap. 12 for further details).[24, 25]

CLINICAL PEARLS: Differentiation between CSW and the syndrome of inappropriate secretion of antidiuretic hormone (SIADH) can be difficult, although it is imperative for appropriate treatment. CSW involves hypovolemia, requiring salt and fluid replacement to prevent neurological deterioration and hemodynamic instability. In opposition, SIADH involves fluid overload, requiring fluid restriction and perhaps diuresis to control cerebral edema.

- **Syndrome of Inappropriate Antidiuretic Hormone Secretion.** Another cause of hyponatremia in the neurosurgical population is SIADH. Although SIADH may mimic CSW, the physiology and management greatly differ. SIADH is typically seen following neurotrauma or with intracranial infections such as meningitis. Excessive ADH is secreted and the patient retains too much free water, leading to dilutional hyponatremia and hypo-osmolarity. The patient is assessed for confusion, decreased mental status, nausea, and vomiting related to hyponatremia, which if severe can lead to seizures and coma. Signs of fluid overload (generalized edema, pulmonary edema) may not be present. Treatment is fluid restriction. Monitor serial sodium to gauge correction rate and success. If hyponatremia is compromising the patient's mental status, hypertonic saline and diuresis may be added to slowly correct the salt balance.[24, 25]

- **Hyperglycemia.** Hyperglycemia is a stress response and should be avoided as it is related to poorer outcomes. Neuronal metabolism is increased with hyperglycemia, creating anaerobic metabolism and its by-products within the nerve cells, further increasing cell stress and ischemic risk. Steroid use further exacerbates hyperglycemia. Monitor glucose periodically and treat with regular insulin to avoid aggravation of cerebral edema.[26,27]

NEUROLOGICAL DEFICITS IN THE POSTOPERATIVE PERIOD

As a result of surgery, various transient neurological deficits may be noted. Particular deficits depend on preoperative deficits, the type of surgical procedure, and the amount of edema present. Many of these deficits resolve completely in the postoperative period. Others may require rehabilitation. The nurse assesses and monitors the patient for changes. Independent nursing and collaborative interventions may be implemented to manage the various problems.

Diminished Level of Consciousness. As cerebral edema subsides postoperatively, ICP decreases and the level of consciousness (LOC) improves. A patient who is fully alert and well oriented immediately after surgery likely has minimal to no cerebral edema. Debulking of a cerebral mass, such as a brain tumor, can make a significant difference in the expected postoperative edema because of tissue manipulation. For these patients, improvement in the LOC occurs slowly as cerebral edema gradually subsides.

Communication Deficits. The postoperative ability to express oneself verbally and to understand the spoken word depends on deficits present before surgery and which part of the brain was subject to surgical manipulation. Recovery will be slower if the deficit was prominent before surgery or if surgical dissection was close to the language area. Referral to a speech therapist will be helpful. Evaluate the type of communication deficit present and develop alternative methods of communication. If these adjustments are consistently carried out by all personnel, it will greatly reduce frustration of the patient and staff when communicating.

Motor and Sensory Deficits. As with other deficits, a decrease in cerebral edema results in improved motor and sensory function. For patients with motor deficits, a physical therapy evaluation and treatment plan are implemented to facilitate return of motor function. The nurse must be aware of specific deficits experienced by the patient and should participate in and support the principles of the physiotherapeutic program, thereby promoting continuity of care. The nurse encourages the patient to use a weak limb in the activities of daily living (ADLs), administers range-of-motion (ROM) exercises, ensures proper positioning, applies prescribed braces and splints, and helps the patient ambulate. Enlist family and friends to participate in physiotherapy. The nurse provides emotional support as the patient deals with loss of body function and alterations in body image.

CLINICAL PEARLS: Exercising and ROM are not just for the physical therapists to perform. When not interfering with ICP control, ROM should be provided often throughout the nursing shift. Enlisting family and friends to assist with passive ROM after appropriate instruction is good for all involved. In addition to desirable effects on patient mobility, family and friends are offered an opportunity to participate in their loved one's care in what often appears as a helpless situation.

Headache. Postoperatively, headache is expected in the first few days, and may be moderate to severe. Much of the pain originates from surgical stretching or irritation of the nerves of the scalp. Pain can also result from traction on the dura or large blood vessels within the intracranial space. Headache can be intensified by a head dressing that has been applied tightly to control scalp bleeding or that has become tight from tissue edema. The snugness of the dressing should be assessed for comfort. A cool pack can be applied to decrease edema and topical pain. Narcotic pain relievers are commonly ordered to control headache. A quiet environment with limited direct light or a dimly lit room can be soothing.

Elevation in Temperature. A modest elevation in temperature is common in the early postoperative period. Fever may indicate the presence of infection or an irritation of the hypothalamus, the area of the brain responsible for regulation of the body temperature. Determining the specific cause of fever in the postoperative period is challenging. Nearly three quarters of fevers within the first 48 hours postoperatively are noninfectious. No correlation has been established between the severity of the temperature and the presence of infections. The most common noninfectious etiology of fever is atelectasis. Less common considerations include hematoma, tissue trauma, drug reactions, DVT, PE, tumors, phenytoin (Dilantin), and blood product reactions. Fevers due to infection may be a result of wound infections, urinary tract infection, or respiratory tract processes and are more commonly seen on or after the third postoperative day. Regardless of the etiology, temperature elevation is associated with an increase in heart rate, blood pressure, cerebral blood flow, and cerebral oxygen consumption. As cerebral metabolism increases, production of the metabolic by-products carbon dioxide and lactic acid increases, both of which are potent vasodilators that contribute to increased ICP. Fever also lowers the seizure threshold. An elevation in temperature is treated with antipyretic drugs, such as acetaminophen. Adjunct therapies, such as a hypothermia blanket, control-

ling the environmental temperature, removal of excess bedclothes, and cool water sponging, may be utilized. Shivering can increase ICP, further increasing hypermetabolism from the muscle activity, and counteract fever reduction measures. If shivering occurs, meperidine (Demerol) or chlorpromazine (Thorazine) may be ordered.[28]

CLINICAL VIGNETTE: JK is a 28-year-old computer programmer with an 8-week progressive weakness of her left hand and "clumsiness" of her left leg. She does not seek medical attention until she is brought to the emergency department following new-onset seizure activity that is self-limiting. Head CT scan shows a right hemispheric mass that is further evaluated by MRI of the brain with and without contrast. A 2.5 × 3 cm ring-enhancing lesion is demonstrated, suspicious for malignant tumor. JK undergoes a right craniotomy for tumor resection. Preliminary pathology indicates a low-grade glioma, and it is felt the entire tumor has been resected. JK is extubated in the operating room and arrives to the neurological ICU with stable vital signs, pupils equal and reactive, Glasgow Coma Score of 14, and moving all extremities without difficulty. Thirty minutes later, a routine neurological check reveals sudden deterioration to Glasgow Coma Score of 11 (opens eyes to pain, inappropriate verbal response, obeys commands only with persistent stimulus). The nurse recognizes this critical change and immediately summons the neurosurgical team, and the patient is taken for a STAT head CT, which shows bleeding into the tumor bed (the area of recent tumor evacuation) with surrounding edema. JK returns emergently to the operating room where the blood clot is evacuated and an arteriole bleed is cauterized. One hundred grams of mannitol is given for cerebral edema. JK returns to the neurological ICU intubated, with stable vital signs, Glasgow Coma Score of 8 (opens eyes to pain, intubated—no verbal, localizes pain), and weak left upper extremity movement. Frequent neurological exams overnight show a steady improvement in level of consciousness and left arm strength. Although the nurse implements seizure precautions, no further seizure activity is noted. The next morning, JK is alert to speech, follows commands, and is successfully extubated. Her follow-up routine head CT scan shows no additional rebleeding. JK's remaining hospital course is uneventful.

Diminished Gag/Swallowing Reflexes. Gag and swallowing reflexes are controlled by cranial nerves (CNs) IX, X, and XII, located in the lower brainstem at the medulla. Surgery in the posterior fossa (infratentorial area) may cause edema, which can transmit pressure onto the CNs, resulting in temporary loss or diminished response of these reflexes. The danger of an inability to protect the airway lies in aspiration leading to laryngospasm, pneumonitis, or pneumonia. Therefore, oral intake should not be started until the patient is able to protect his or her airway. Suction equipment should be readily available. As edema subsides, the reflexes return.

Periorbital Edema. Swelling around one or both eyes is common after cranial surgery because of the manipulation of scalp, skull, and intracranial contents. It is usually accompanied by discoloration and ecchymosis, and peaks about 48 to 72 hours postoperatively. Cold compresses help reduce edema. Gently cleanse the eyes to prevent crusting and lubricate the eye with saline drops as the blinking mechanism may be impaired by the edema. Periorbital edema dissipates within 5 to 6 days. Ecchymosis may take 10 to 14 days to resolve.

Visual Disturbances. Diplopia and field cuts can be assessed in the patient who is sufficiently conscious to provide information. If diplopia is present, a unilateral eye patch can be worn to control the symptoms. In noncommunicative patients, the nurse can often draw a presumptive conclusion about visual deficits by observation. For example, the patient may not notice objects on one side of the bed or may react only when someone approaches from a particular side. Both situations suggest visual deficits and should be considered during care planning.

Loss of Corneal Reflex. If the corneal reflex is absent, the affected eye must be protected from injury. Corneal abrasion and ulceration can develop from direct injury or from depriving the eye of proper lubrication. Blindness can be the unfortunate and permanent consequence of corneal ulceration. Applying an eye shield or taping the lids closed can prevent corneal abrasion. Periodic inspection and administration of artificial tears or saline solution can moisten the eye and prevent drying of the cornea.

Personality Changes. Changes in baseline personality may be temporary or permanent. Permanent changes can occur from cerebral anoxia or surgery in the frontal area. Temporary personality changes can result from cerebral edema, surgery, drugs, or emotional stress and resolve in the postoperative period. Personality changes, although common after cranial surgery, are among the most disturbing sequelae for the patient and the family.

NURSE'S ROLE IN REHABILITATION AND DISCHARGE PLANNING

Craniotomy is a conventional neurosurgical treatment for many underlying problems. The degree and time of recovery and the need for further treatment and rehabilitation are individual. For example, the discharge planning for a young patient who has had a craniotomy for a benign pituitary tumor will be different from the plan for an elderly person undergoing craniotomy for a malignant tumor. Neurological deficits in these two patients will be different, as is the impact of surgery on the patients and their families. The need for individual planning thus becomes apparent. As cerebral edema subsides, a more accurate profile of neurological deficits emerges. Some deficits recover spontaneously with time, whereas other deficits need treatment and rehabilitation to achieve the optimal level of recovery. The human impact is assessed by talking to the patient and family and assessing their responses.

Independent Nursing Role

As part of the independent nursing role, the nurse assesses the patient's functional level and collects the following data,

which will be used for planning nursing care and for discharge planning:

- Level of consciousness and cognitive function (important for patient teaching)
- Presence of neurological deficits
- Verbal communication skills (ability to participate in a conversation, any word-finding difficulty)
- Independence in performing ADLs
- Emotional response to surgery and underlying problems (e.g., depression)
- Safety concerns (is the patient at risk for injury or falls?)
- Previous family role and responsibilities
- Support systems and living situation (could the patient manage at home safely? If the patient needs assistance, will a family member be available to assist the patient?)

Integration of the principles of rehabilitation into the plan of nursing care is directed at helping the patient achieve the highest level of independence possible. Involve the patient with the environment and ADLs as much as possible. Many patients are easily fatigued after surgery. Plan rest to prevent exhaustion and increase endurance. Support the patient and family throughout the hospitalization and prepare them for discharge. Patient and family teaching begun earlier in the course of hospitalization is now expanded. The family is encouraged to participate in basic care and ADL routines to develop skill and confidence in posthospital care.

Anxiety, ambivalence, hostility, and depression are common in the postoperative period and continue even after transition to the home. One interesting cause of depression relates to the degree of progress made postoperatively. During the hospital stay and initially after discharge, recovery and improvement are often rapid. If one were to chart this on a graph, it would be represented initially by a steeply ascending line; a plateau would then be reached, marking a period of small improvements or no apparent improvement. If patients are unable to perform activities that they believe are realistic and feasible, they may become upset. Discouragement is further augmented by fatigue, which causes these patients to abandon certain activities. This sequence of events reinforces discouragement, depression, and complaints of constant fatigue. In these circumstances, the patient needs help to set more realistic goals. A sympathetic approach and explanation of the postoperative course is helpful.

Collaborative and Interdisciplinary Role

Early in the postoperative period, the nurse, physician, and other health professionals collaboratively identify neurological deficits that need further evaluation by other health care professionals. Although the needs of each patient vary, the most frequent referrals are made to physical therapy, occupational therapy, speech therapy, social services, and sometimes psychiatry. The physician may also make a referral to another physician, such as the neuro-oncologist or neuroradiologist. After the patient has been evaluated and patient needs are identified in concrete terms, a discharge plan is formalized and implemented.

It is impossible to generalize about typical responses to a craniotomy. For some patients, a craniotomy provides a cure for a treatable condition, such as a subdural hematoma. For others, intracranial surgery ameliorates symptoms of cerebral compression so that an extension of time can be offered for patients with a terminal prognosis. The implications of the craniotomy in terms of the patient's life can only be assessed individually. Depending on the reason for surgery and the prognosis, the patient or family may need to make major decisions about postacute care facilities and choice of treatment.

SELECTED NEUROSURGICAL PROCEDURES

Four additional surgical procedures are presented in this section: transsphenoidal surgery, carotid endarterectomy, endovascular carotid artery interventions (carotid stenting and angioplasty) and placement of a ventricular shunt.

Transsphenoidal Surgery

Pituitary adenomas, craniopharyngiomas, CSF rhinorrhea control, tumors extending into the sphenoid sinus, and a complete hypophysectomy for control of bone pain in metastatic cancer are conditions for which a transsphenoidal surgical approach are used. Microsurgical techniques and equipment are utilized due to the deep and narrow operative field (Fig. 14-8). For the transsphenoidal surgical approach, an incision is made inside the superior upper lip, above the hard palate. After the sphenoid sinus floor is dissected, the sella turcica is visible. A portion of the sella floor is removed, and the dura incised. With the aid of a surgical microscope, the pituitary is partially or completely removed or the impinging tumor excised while the pituitary gland remains intact, depending on the reason for the surgery. A fat pad taken from the abdomen is applied to the surgical site as a patch to prevent CSF leakage. Nasal Vaseline packings may be inserted to control bleeding and protect septal mucosa. A dry, sterile dressing is firmly applied to the donor site on the abdomen. The

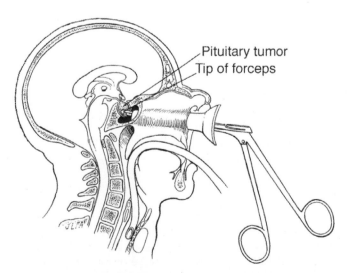

Figure 14-8 • Transsphenoidal approach in pituitary surgery. (From Smeltzer, S. C., & Bare, B. G. [1996]. *Brunner and Suddarth's textbook of medical-surgical nursing* [8th ed., p. 1738]. Philadelphia: Lippincott-Raven Publishers.)

transsphenoidal approach requires no brain retraction, and therefore should not result in cerebral edema and its sequelae. There is no external scar on the head or the face.

Palliative Surgery for Pain Secondary to Cancer. Palliative hypophysectomy for cancer necessitates total removal of the pituitary. The surgeon attempts to excise the pituitary in one piece, because cells left at the surgical site continue to secrete hormones and decrease the anticipated relief of pain. It is unclear why a hypophysectomy can alleviate pain or further slow metastasis. Removal of the anterior lobe, with the resultant cessation of prolactin and the growth-stimulating hormone, helps to control breast and prostate cancer. Preoperative preparation begins with patient and family teaching. The patient needs realistic expectations of outcome and the need for drug replacement therapy.

Postoperative Complications. Urine output is often replaced equally with the appropriate intravenous fluid to prevent dehydration. The patient is cautioned against blowing the nose, sneezing, using a straw, and no incentive spirometry as each of these activities create high-pressure flows through the sphenoid sinus, which could dislodge the fat graft. The patient is monitored for development of major complications associated with transsphenoidal surgery, including CSF leakage (rhinorrhea), DI, sinusitis, hormonal imbalance, visual impairment, and delayed epistaxis. Of these complications, only DI is discussed.[29]

Central DI is defined as the cessation of ADH secretion by the pituitary gland as a result of damage from disease or injury of the hypothalamus, the supraoptic hypophyseal tract, or the posterior pituitary. Postsurgical DI can occur up to 2 weeks postoperatively. Monitoring for the development of DI is a major postoperative nursing responsibility (see previous discussion in this chapter as well as Chap. 12 for further discussion). Urine specific gravity and serum osmolarity need to be checked every 1 to 2 hours as ordered in expectation of the onset of DI as a result of surgical manipulation of or around the pituitary gland. If the patient is able to drink enough fluid to quench thirst and maintain fluid and electrolyte balance, no medical treatment is indicated. Some patients may experience a period of low urinary output 2 or 3 days postoperatively before permanent DI develops. In the case of a total hypophysectomy, permanent DI is expected and replacement therapy begun. With partial pituitary resection, DI is not permanent. In the immediate postoperative period, aqueous vasopressin or DDAVP should be instituted (see Chap. 12). After the nasal packings have been removed, intranasal DDAVP can be used.[29] The patient must be instructed in safe use of the drug:

- Nasal mucosa irritation may occur; this will interfere with absorption of the drug.
- Overuse of the drug will cause water intoxication (mental confusion, drowsiness).
- Daily weight must be monitored.
- Oral intake must be balanced with daily output.

Postoperative Nursing Management After Transsphenoidal Surgery. Specific points regarding the nursing management of the patient undergoing surgery by the transsphenoidal approach are outlined in Chart 14-3. After

CHART 14-3   Nursing Management After Transsphenoidal Surgery

NURSING MANAGEMENT	RATIONALE
EARLY POSTOPERATIVE MANAGEMENT	
• Frequently monitor vital and neurological signs.	• Provides information for baseline comparisons to indicate trends, deterioration, or complications
• Maintain the head of bed at 30 degrees.	• Promotes venous drainage from the brain, controls intracranial pressure, and prevents hemorrhage at the operative site
• Check the dressing at the donor site.	• Detects bleeding for early intervention
• Frequently check nasal drains and packing; observe for hemorrhage or cerebrospinal fluid (CSF) drainage from the operative site; the mustache dressing should be observed and changed as necessary.	• Promotes early detection of hemorrhage or CSF and subsequent early intervention
PREVENTION OF COMPLICATIONS	
• Monitor urinary output and specific gravity frequently.	• Monitors for evidence of diabetes insipidus
• Monitor electrolyte and osmolarity laboratory values for abnormally high or low readings (serum and urine osmolarity, serum sodium). Normal values are as follows: Serum osmolarity: 280–295 mOsm/L Urine osmolarity: 500–800 mOsm/L Serum sodium: 135–145 mEq/L	• In diabetes insipidus, the serum sodium level is increased, serum osmolarity is increased, and urine osmolarity is decreased; also, serum electrolyte testing can indicate an electrolyte imbalance.
• Give frequent mouth care, but do not allow the patient to brush teeth if the oral approach was used.	• Prevents injury at the suture line, yet allows the mouth to be refreshed and cleansed
• Progress diet from liquid to soft as necessary.	• Prevents injury to the suture line
• After packings are removed, caution the patient against blowing the nose or sneezing for at least 1 month.	• Prevents hemorrhage from fragile nasal tissue at operative site
SUPPORTIVE CARE	
• Provide for routine hygienic care, such as bathing, hair combing, and nail cutting.	• Maintains general well-being
• Offer fluids frequently, as ordered.	• Maintains hydration and moistens the oral mucous membrane, which becomes dry from mouth breathing (required when nasal packings are in place)
• Provide eye care (clean and lubricate).	• Prevents infection, inflammation, and drying of the cornea
• Apply compresses to the periorbital region if periobital edema occurs.	• Controls and alleviates periobital edema
PATIENT TEACHING	
• Prepare and implement a patient teaching plan to outline any adjustments in lifestyle, precautions necessary with the drug protocol, and general information about the patient's health problem.	• Provides for the safety and well-being of the patient and includes the patient as an involved, informed participant in health management
• Provide written material to summarize the major points of home management for the patient.	• Reinforces the major points of the teaching plan and reduces the possibility of confusion or questions about home protocol
• Include the family in the teaching plan.	• Includes the family in the plan of care so that they can become a knowledgeable support system for the patient

surgery, minimal pain is noted at the oronasal suture line because pain receptor fibers have been cut, resulting in loss of pain perception. Headache or ear discomfort as a result of sinus congestion is common. Nasal packings are removed in 3 to 4 days. Nasal mucosa healing requires at least 1 month. Senses of smell and taste typically return in 2 or 3 weeks.

If the hypophysectomy was performed to control metastasis and bone pain, relief may be evident within hours after surgery; in other patients, it may take days to a few

weeks. The surgery is a "last chance" effort to control severe pain that has made ADLs impossible. Many patients express a desire for their families to see them comfortable without the use of drugs and to fulfill certain life goals before death. The nurse's role in such cases is supportive.

Hormonal Replacement. In the case of total hypophysectomy, other hormonal replacement is necessary. An endocrinology team will join the neurosurgical team for long-term care of this patient population. Typical drugs ordered include cortisone acetate continued postoperatively at a lower dose than preoperatively prescribed and adrenocorticotropic hormone (ACTH) beginning immediately after surgery. Thyroid replacement therapy is delayed for 3 to 4 weeks following surgery.

Patient Teaching for Drug Replacement. If lifelong replacement drug therapy is necessary, it is most important that the patient and family understand the purposes of drug therapy. The nurse should begin with a basic overview of the pituitary gland to foster an understanding of the rationale for drug replacement therapy. To reinforce verbal explanations, written and visual aids are helpful. The teaching plan should include:

- Specific information to record and submit to the physician, such as daily weight
- Signs and symptoms of undermedication or overmedication
- Side effects of drugs
- Lifestyle alterations necessitated as a result of drug therapy, such as learning new coping mechanisms to balance physical and emotional stresses and when increases in cortisol dosing to prevent addisonian crisis will be required (i.e., future surgery or major illnesses).

The patient receiving **cortisone therapy** should know the following:

- The drug must be taken daily as ordered; failure to take the drug can be life threatening.
- The dosage must be increased during periods of emotional stress, illness, excessive exercise, major changes in daily routine, exposure to high altitudes, tooth extraction, fever, or infection.
- Gastric irritation, a side effect of steroid therapy, can be minimized by taking an antacid with each dose of the drug or dosing with meals.
- The presence of tarry stools indicates gastrointestinal hemorrhage, which should be reported to the physician immediately.
- Check blood pressure periodically for HTN. An elevation in blood pressure is common with cortisone therapy. If the patient is already taking antihypertensives, adjustments in the dosage may be necessary.
- Check for hyperglycemia; ACTH is associated with diabetes mellitus.
- Behavioral changes such as euphoria, restlessness, sleeplessness, agitation, and depression are common with cortisone therapy.
- The following are signs and symptoms of *undermedication* (addisonian crisis), which is a medical emergency, and the patient should seek immediate medical attention:
  - Weakness, dizziness, orthostatic hypotension
  - Confusion, lethargy, agitation
  - Nausea and vomiting, diarrhea, abdominal pain
  - Hyponatremia, hyperkalemia, hypoglycemia, metabolic acidosis
  - Extracellular volume depletion, decreased blood pressure[30,31]
- Management of cortisone insufficiency requires parenteral Solu-Cortef and intravenous fluid hydration. Failure to treat will lead to circulatory collapse.
- The following are signs and symptoms of *overmedication* (Cushing's syndrome):

- Cushingoid signs (moon face, fat pads, buffalo hump, acne, hirsutism, hyperpigmentation, and weight gain)
- HTN
- Hyperglycemia, hypokalemic alkalosis, hypernatremia
- Psychiatric disturbances (depression, emotional lability, dementia)[32]
- A medical alert bracelet must be worn at all times.

Carotid Endarterectomy

Cerebrovascular insufficiency can result from stenosis of the carotid artery secondary to atherosclerosis, a progressive disease that begins around 20 years of age. If significant stenosis remains untreated, this can lead to transient ischemic attacks (TIAs). In some instances, even though the internal carotid artery is occluded, the external carotid artery will remain patent as a result of collateral blood flow from the contralateral external carotid artery. In this event, the external carotid artery becomes extremely important in maintaining an adequate blood supply to the brain. Thus, a patient with occlusion of a carotid artery may be asymptomatic because of continued collateral circulation.[33]

Carotid Atherosclerosis. Atheromas (atherosclerotic plaques) commonly form in the larger cerebral arteries such as the common carotid artery, especially at the bifurcation of the internal and external carotid arteries. The atheroma gradually narrows the blood vessel lumen, compromising adequate cerebral blood flow. The atheroma can break off and act as an embolus, or its irregular surface can become the site for the formation of a thrombus. Both processes can lead to cerebral ischemia and stroke (cerebral infarction).

Diagnosis and Treatment. An arterial angiogram is the "gold standard" for diagnosing cerebrovascular disease, although cost and risks from the invasive procedure prohibit its use as a screening tool. Less invasive studies include magnetic resonance angiography (MRA), which is useful in mapping cerebrovascular irregularities, although it may overestimate stenosis. CT angiogram (CTA) provides information similar to an MRA much more quickly. Angiography and CTA each involve intravascular dye injection, which is excreted by the kidneys, raising concern for renal protection in the face of renal insufficiency or repetitive studies requiring recurring dye loads (although gadolinium used in MRA is not nephrotoxic). Carotid Doppler ultrasound is a noninvasive analysis of blood flow up to the level of the mandible. Transcranial Doppler sonography measures CBF velocities and resistance of the major vessels in the circle of Willis. Based on the degree of stenosis, patient symptoms, and comorbidities, appropriate treatment options are offered. Treatment alternatives include medical management, carotid endarterectomy (CEA), and endovascular techniques (stenting).[33] The most common surgical procedure for stroke prevention is CEA.[34]

Symptomatic Carotid Artery Disease. The results of a landmark study, the North American Symptomatic Carotid Endarterectomy Trial (NASCET), were reported in 1991. TIA or mildly disabled stroke patients with 70% to 99% narrowing of the symptomatic internal carotid artery were randomized to either medical management or surgery. The CEA group had a clear benefit in reducing

TABLE 14-3   RECOMMENDATIONS FOR PATIENTS WITH ASYMPTOMATIC CAROTID ARTERY DISEASE BASED ON SURGICAL RISK

INDICATIONS/RISK	PROVEN	ACCEPTABLE/NOT PROVEN	UNCERTAIN
Surgical risk: <3% and life expectancy of at least 5 years	Ipsilateral carotid endarterectomy (CEA) for stenotic lesions (≥60% diameter reduction of distal outflow tract with or without ulceration and with or without antiplatelet therapy, irrespective of contralateral artery status, ranging from no disease to occlusion)	Unilateral CEA simultaneous with coronary artery bypass graft for stenotic lesions (≥60% diameter reduction with or without ulcerations with or without antiplatelet therapy, irrespective of contralateral artery status)	Unilateral CEA for stenosis >50% with B or C ulcer irrespective of contralateral internal carotid artery status
Surgical risk: 3%–5%	None	Ipsilateral CEA for stenosis ≥75% with or without ulcerations but in the presence of contralateral internal carotid artery stenosis ranging from 75% to total occlusion	See guidelines
Surgical risk: 5%–10%	None	None	See guidelines

From Biller, J., Feinberg, W. M., Castoldo, J. E., Whittemore, A. D., Harbaugh, R. E., Dempsey, R. J., et al. (1998). Guidelines for carotid endarterectomy: A statement for healthcare professionals from a special writing group of the Stroke Council, American Heart Association. *Circulation, 97,* 501–509.

the overall risk of fatal and nonfatal ipsilateral stroke when compared to the medically managed group. For symptomatic patients with 70% stenosis or more, CEA is *three times* as effective as medical therapy alone in reducing incidence of stroke. CEA is not deemed beneficial for symptomatic patients with 0% to 29% stenosis. Uncertainty remains about the potential benefit of CEA for symptomatic patients with 30% to 69% stenosis.[34–38] In 2005, CEA practice guidelines were updated by the Therapeutics and Technology Assessment Subcommittee of the American Academy of Neurology based on a literature review from 1990 to 2004, again recommending CEA for symptomatic stenosis. The NASCET plus the 1998 report of the European Carotid Surgery Trial (ECST) remain the "gold standard" trials[34] (Table 14-3).

Asymptomatic Carotid Artery Disease. The Asymptomatic Carotid Atherosclerosis Study (ACAS) clarified indications for surgery in the asymptomatic carotid artery disease population. In the ACAS trial, patients were randomly assigned to a surgical group or medical group. Knowledge gained from the ACAS study was initially reflected in the updated American Heart Association (AHA) 1998 guidelines for CEA.[39] Recommendations are organized around surgical risk graded from I to IV based on neurological stability, comorbidity, and angiographic risk. Grade I includes patients who are neurologically stable with no medical or angiographic risks, whereas grade IV comprises neurologically unstable patients with or without medical or angiographic risks.[33] Similarly, the Asymptomatic Carotid Surgery Trial (ACST) studied immediate CEA versus basic medical management (BMM) in patients with at least 60% carotid artery stenosis. These notable studies support CEA for asymptomatic patients with 60% or greater stenosis.[34]

Carotid Endarterectomy. CEA is the most frequently performed noncardiac vascular procedure today (Fig. 14-9).[39] The first successful CEA dates back to 1953. Patient selection and the skill of the surgeon and surgical team are important factors in maintaining low surgical complications. In addition, the quality of nursing care is critical in prevention and early recognition of complications and in

supporting optimal outcomes. Unfortunately, atherosclerosis is a progressive systemic disease that continues in these patients, and CEA is a focal intervention to minimize stroke rates. Reocclusion at the surgical site or distal occlusions may still occur postoperatively. Patients must understand that long-term medical management with antithrombotic agents (clopidogrel, aspirin), cholesterol-lowering agents (particularly statin drugs), and certain antihypertensive agents (angiotensin-converting enzyme inhibitors [ACE-Is], angiotensin receptor blockers [ARBs]) may decrease risks of recurrent cerebrovascular events as well as cardiovascular events from systemic atherosclerotic disease. CEA should not be a stand-alone therapy.[40]

Preoperative Concerns. Many patients who have cerebrovascular atherosclerosis also have concurrent conditions and risk factors, such as coronary artery disease, peripheral vascular disease, renal disease, diabetes mellitus, hyperlipidemia, and HTN. Treatment and stabilization of these and other medical conditions plus attention to risk factors are necessary before surgery. In particular, HTN must be controlled before surgery. Table 14-4 lists these risk factors.

Perioperative and Postoperative Complications. Perioperative complications of CEA include stroke, myocardial infarction, and death. Postoperative complications include HTN, hypotension, hyperperfusion syndrome, intracerebral hemorrhage, seizures, nerve injury, stroke, and wound hematoma.

• **Postoperative HTN.** Preoperative HTN is the single most important determinant for the development of postoperative HTN. Poorly controlled HTN increases the risk of wound hematoma and hyperperfusion syndrome. In addition, neurological deficits, intracerebral hemorrhage, and death are more common in patients who develop postoperative HTN. The first 48 hours after the CEA is the peak time for postoperative HTN. About 21% of normotensive patients may have increased blood pressure after CEA.[41] Unstable blood pressure is common during the first 24 hours after CEA and may be related to surgically induced changes in

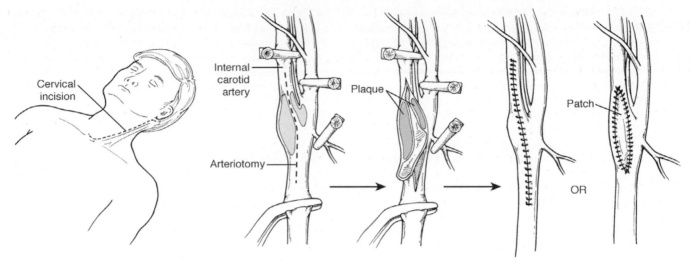

Figure 14-9 • Carotid endarterectomy. An oblique cervical incision allows dissection of the carotid bifurcation. Following heparinization, the arteries of the bifurcation are cross-clamped and an arteriotomy is performed. The plaque is dissected precisely in the subintimal plane, with a subsequent closure (primary or via patch reconstruction) of the arteriotomy. Other aspects of the surgery include intraoperative monitoring during cross-clamping, microsurgical technique allowing optimal lighting and magnification, patch angioplasty, shunting, and verification of patency.

carotid body baroreceptor sensitivity. Avoidance of long-acting pharmacologic agents during this time may avert rebound hypotension or hypertension.[33] Frequent monitoring of blood pressure is very important in the postoperative period. Blood pressure must be maintained within a target range to prevent complications previously mentioned.

CLINICAL VIGNETTE: BC is a 62-year-old white female with a history of hypercholesterolemia and diet-controlled diabetes who has undergone an elective left CEA for 85% asymptomatic stenosis. She arrives to the recovery room with a blood pressure (BP) of 186/80 mm Hg by arterial line measurement and confirmed with a blood pressure cuff. The nurse initially tries pain control measures, which

TABLE 14-4 STROKE RISK FACTORS, MANAGEMENT, AND RELATIONSHIP TO OUTCOMES AFTER CAROTID ENDARTERECTOMY (CEA)

RISK FACTOR FOR STROKE	EFFECT AFTER CEA	TREATMENT
Hypertension (HTN)	↑ risk of hyperperfusion syndrome ↑ risk of intracerebral bleeding	Control blood pressure according to JNC VII standards*
Cigarette smoking	Risk factor for restenosis	Smoking cessation program
Hyperlipidemia	Risk factor for restenosis Drug Rx ↓ stroke by 30%[†]	Follow NCEP guidelines[‡]
Alcohol consumption	High consumption = ↑ risk of stroke Moderate consumption = no effect or slight protection	Avoid high consumption of alcohol
Postmenopausal estrogen	No effect or slight ↓ risk	Unclear; individual decision at this time
Antiplatelet drugs	23% ↓ for nonfatal stroke 22% ↓ for all vascular events (nonfatal stroke, nonfatal myocardial infarction, and vascular death)[§]	81 or 325 mg/d aspirin at least 3 mo postoperatively; indefinitely if not contraindicated. Insufficient data on other antiplatelet agents[‖]

*The Seventh Report of the Joint National Committee on Prevention, Detection, Evaluation, and Treatment of High Blood Pressure. (2003). *JAMA, 289,* 2560–2572.

[†]Scandinavian Simvastatin Survival Study Group. (1994). Randomized trial of cholesterol lowering in 4444 patients with coronary heart disease: The Scandinavian Simvastatin Survival Study (4S). *Lancet, 344,* 1383–1389.

[‡]National Cholesterol Education Program (NCEP) Expert Panel. (2002). Third report of the National Cholesterol Education Program (NCEP) Expert Panel on detection, evaluation and treatment of high blood cholesterol in adults (Adult Treatment Panel III): Final Report. *Circulation, 106,* 3143–3421.

[§]Antiplatelet Trialists' Collaboration. (1994). Collaborative overview of randomized trials of antiplatelet therapy I: Prevention of death, myocardial infarction, and stroke by prolonged antiplatelet therapy in various categories of patients. *BMJ, 308*(6921), 81–106.

[‖]Chaturvedi, S., Bruno, A., Feasby, T., Holloway, R., Benavente, O., Cohen, S. N., Cote, R., et al. (2005). Carotid endarterectomy—An evidence-based review: Report of the Therapeutics and Technology Assessment Subcommittee of the American Academy of Neurology. *Neurology, 65,* 794–801.

fail to control the HTN. BC has no prior history of HTN, but the care team is not surprised by the current elevation as nearly one fourth of normotensive patients suffer HTN postoperatively. A short-acting vasodilator is initiated by intravenous drip to maintain BP parameters prescribed by the surgeon. Close observation of the surgical wound is made to ensure that no hematoma develops, a rare and critical complication occurring when BP elevation causes a disruption of the anastomosis (vascular suture line). Continuous BP monitoring and frequent vasodilator titration is required for BC during the first 28 hours postoperatively, when BP parameters are maintained without further treatment. During this time, the nurses perform frequent neurological checks with specific concerns for hyperperfusion syndrome. BC demonstrates no focal neurological deficits. Her headache is intermittently moderate and generalized in nature (not severe and unilateral). No seizure activity is observed. Her remaining postoperative course is uneventful and BC is discharged home in stable condition on postoperative day 3.

- **Postoperative Hypotension.** Postoperative hypotension (i.e., systolic blood pressure <120 mm Hg) occurs in approximately 5% of patients.[42] A fluid bolus and low-dose vasopressor infusion are usually effective. Hypotension usually resolves in 24 to 48 hours. If significant hypotension persists, a myocardial infarction must be ruled out through serial electrocardiograms and cardiac enzyme measurements. Possible consequences of hypotension include cerebral hypoxia and ischemic stroke. Adequate blood pressure within a targeted range must be maintained. Monitoring central venous pressure in the early postoperative period may be helpful.

- **Hyperperfusion Syndrome.** Patients at risk for hyperperfusion syndrome are those with high-grade stenosis of the internal carotid, chronic HTN, and severe contralateral stenosis. Return of unrestricted blood flow to an area with impaired autoregulation is the basis for the syndrome. As a result of high-grade stenosis, a chronic state of hypoperfusion exists in the hemisphere distal to the stenosis. The smaller blood vessels are in a chronic state of maximal dilation to provide adequate blood flow, eventually resulting in loss of autoregulation. After the stenosis has been corrected, the hypoperfused hemisphere receives blood at a normal or elevated perfusion pressure. If autoregulation is impaired, vasoconstriction cannot occur to protect the capillaries. This results in edema and hemorrhage. Clinically, hyperperfusion syndrome is characterized by a severe unilateral headache, altered mental status, focal neurological deficits, or seizures. Raising the head of the bed will often improve the headache. Strict control of blood pressure is crucial to prevent or to limit the severity of hyperperfusion syndrome.[39,42,43]

- **Intracerebral Hemorrhage.** The potential exists for intracerebral hemorrhage secondary to hyperperfusion syndrome. This is often fatal (60%); less frequently, it results in poor patient outcomes (25%). Risk factors for hemorrhage are the same as for hyperperfusion syndrome, with the addition of advanced age and poor collateral flow on angiography. Control of blood pressure is critical to avoid or control hemorrhage.[33,44]

- **Seizures.** Generally a late postoperative complication with onset 5 to 13 days postoperatively, up to 1% of the CEA population will experience seizure activity. This may be due to hyperperfusion syndrome, emboli, or intracerebral hemorrhage. Control of seizures may initially be difficult. Lorazepam and phenytoin are the treatments.[33]

- **Nerve Injury.** The transverse cervical nerve and the greater auricular nerve are frequently severed or injured during the course of CEA. What may result is a permanent ipsilateral numbness of the upper neck, lower face, and lower ear that is generally well tolerated. Damage to the cervical sympathetic chain can result in a complete or incomplete Horner's syndrome.[45] Injury to the cranial nerves is a potential complication, although infrequent. The cranial nerves that are most vulnerable are the facial, glossopharyngeal, vagus, spinal accessory, and hypoglossal.[33, 45] The surgeon's skill is critical to a good outcome. Postoperative neurological assessment is important for early identification of potential deficits.

- **Wound Hematoma.** In the NASCET study, a wound hematoma occurred in about 5.5% of patients.[38] Most hematomas are small and not uncomfortable. Larger hematomas can expand quickly and may necessitate emergency surgical evacuation. If the airway is compromised by pressure from an expanding hematoma, the surgical team may need to emergently open the wound at the bedside. Intraoperatively, meticulous hemostasis and reversal of anticoagulation is important to prevention. Postoperatively, control of HTN is the primary preventative measure. Frequently monitor the incision for development of a hematoma, noting any dysphagia or tracheal deviation.[33]

Postoperative Management. Many potentially life-threatening cardiovascular and cerebrovascular complications exist following CEA. Frequent neurological and vital sign monitoring and close medical management of these patients are critical for optimal outcomes. Throughout the country, patients are admitted to areas offering various levels of care including a PACU, ICU, an intermediate unit or general floor care. Questions have been raised about the need for ICU admission. One study reported that only a few patients benefit from ICU care.[46] These patients are at high risk for serious complications as a result of the procedure itself, as well as pre-existing comorbidities. Appropriate monitoring and care must be provided regardless of clinical setting selected.

Ongoing Nursing Assessment and Monitoring. Frequent vital signs, neurological, and wound assessment should be conducted for the CEA population. Some physicians insert a Jackson-Pratt drain at the operative site to manage drainage and prevent hematoma development, which could compress the new graft, airway, or both. If a venous graft is used, the donor site is also monitored (i.e., saphenous vein graft from the leg). The physician sets target parameters for maintenance of blood pressure based on a reasonable baseline before surgery. Vasopressors or vasodilators may be ordered to maintain BP parameters.

Frequent monitoring of neurological signs is necessary to determine any neurological changes associated with cerebral ischemia or stroke. Cranial nerves, especially V, VII, IX, X, XI, and XII, are assessed for deficits (facial drooping, hoarseness, diminished/lost gag and/or swallowing reflexes, and weakness of the tongue). Note presence of a small unilateral pupil, ptosis, and flushing of the skin, which may suggest development of Horner's syndrome caused by pressure on the nerve plexus around the internal carotid artery.[33]

In the immediate postoperative period, the head of the bed may be flat or elevated, depending on physician preference. The patient is positioned off the operative site. A central venous line, peripheral IV line, arterial line, urinary catheter, cardiac monitor, and oxygen therapy may be used. After the patient demonstrates ability to protect the airway, clear liquids may be given and the diet advanced as tolerated.

Most patients are discharged from the hospital in a day or two with a prescription for antiplatelet agents (aspirin, ticlopidine, clopidogrel) unless contraindicated. Patient education should include what to report immediately to the physician. This includes new onset of unilateral headache, neurological deficits, or seizure activity. The importance of maintaining good blood pressure control and monitoring of blood pressure is stressed. Other risk modification, with the assistance of the primary care provider, is also discussed—such as smoking cessation, cholesterol and glucose control, and BP management.

Endovascular Carotid Artery Interventions

Carotid Stenting and Angioplasty. Carotid artery stenting (CAS) is a proven alternative to CEA, particularly for those patients whose comorbidities place them at high risk for surgical intervention. The landmark Stenting and Angioplasty with Protection in Patients at High Risk for Endarterectomy (SAPPHIRE) Trial helped solidify CAS as a viable option to CEA primarily for asymptomatic stenosis, with comparable complication rates to the more invasive CEA. As of this writing, interventional radiologists, vascular surgeons, and neurosurgeons, as well as neurologists, eagerly await completion of the Carotid Revascularization Endarterectomy versus Stent Trial (CREST), which is an ongoing trial studying CAS versus CEA for symptomatic carotid artery stenosis greater than 50%.[47,48]

Advantages of CAS over CEA include lack of a cervical incision (with its inherent potential for wound complications, cranial nerve injuries, and anesthesia risks) and potentially shorter lengths of stay. Currently, there exists no published consensus or guidelines directing the medical management of CAS patients. Many centers take direction from published cardiology/coronary artery stenting guidelines, which include postintervention glycoprotein (GP IIb/IIIa) inhibitor intravenous infusions such as abciximab or eptifibatide for 12 to 24 hours, followed by 4 to 6 weeks of aspirin plus clopidogrel antiplatelet therapy, then reduction to long-term clopidogrel therapy alone. Neurological complications of CAS include TIA, CVA, myocardial infarction (MI), hemorrhage (from the femoral access site or intracerebral due to cerebral hyperperfusion), and death.[47,49]

Similar to coronary artery interventions, CAS involves introduction of an arterial sheath, most commonly via the femoral artery, through which a guidewire is advanced under fluoroscopy through the aorta into the affected carotid artery. Because of the risk of distal embolization of clots and disrupted atherosclerotic debris during arterial manipulation, a cerebral protection device is deployed just distal to the stenotic area prior to angioplasty and/or stenting. Two common protection devices include (1) an umbrella filter that collects debris and clots throughout the procedure while still allowing blood flow, and that is closed to envelop and remove the debris at the end of the procedure, and (2) a distal occlusion balloon that occludes blood flow during the procedure (much like the cross-clamp applied during CEA); following angioplasty and stent deployment, blood is aspirated proximal to the balloon to remove loosened debris and clot prior to balloon deflation and removal. Studies have shown a reduction in stroke and death rates at 30 days postprocedure from 5.5% down to 1.8% since implementation of cerebral protection devices.[47]

Restenosis rates following carotid angioplasty have declined since the addition of stenting. Other complication rates have similarly declined as operators become more experienced with the greater acceptance and increased performance of CAS and with improvements in endovascular techniques and equipment.[47] CAS is being considered for symptomatic traumatic carotid artery dissection when the standard treatment of anticoagulation and antiplatelet agents is contraindicated based on coexisting multitrauma and hemorrhage.[48]

An illustration of CAS can be seen in the *Annals of Vascular Surgery* (2005), 19(3), p. 436.

Cerebral Ventricular Shunting

Ventricular Shunts. A ventricular shunt is used to treat hydrocephalus. It consists of a primary catheter, a reservoir, a one-way valve, and a terminal catheter, which are implanted surgically to provide drainage of excessive CSF from the brain to decrease or prevent increased ICP. A small incision is made behind the ear. The primary catheter is implanted into the lateral ventricle through a burr hole. The ventricular catheter is connected to a reservoir that rests on the mastoid bone. CSF flows from the catheter to the reservoir, in which the CSF collects. A one-way valve on the reservoir prevents CSF reflux. A special instrument is used to tunnel the terminal catheter under the skin to the terminal point, such as the peritoneum or vena cava. The shunt is left in place permanently unless it becomes dislodged, plugged, or infected. In these situations, the shunt is removed surgically and replaced.

Depending on the type of shunt placed, the surgical team may write an order to pump the shunt a given number of times at prescribed intervals (e.g., three times every 6 hours). The purpose of pumping a shunt is to flush the system of exudates that could plug the small tubing. To pump the shunt, lightly palpate the mastoid process with the index and middle fingers until the reservoir is palpated. Compress and gently release the reservoir the prescribed number of times. If functioning correctly, the reservoir will refill with CSF from the ventricle following each compression. Documentation of pump function and any changes in neurological function are recorded in the patient's chart.

CLINICAL PEARLS: Caution—pumping a shunt may also cause shunt failure in some circumstances. Do not routinely pump shunts without an order.

FUTURE TRENDS

Much of the future in neurosurgery is directly related to the rapid advances in computer technology, intraoperative CT scanning, and progression of endovascular techniques. The explosion of computer technology is responsible for the introduction and improvements in real-time intraoperative imaging and navigation systems such as the previously discussed StealthStation.

Helical three-dimensional CT scanning data may now be entered into image-guiding systems, which provide more details for the surgeon, such as volume, morphology, and relationship of the operative lesion to bone anatomy, making surgical planning and localization of the lesion much more precise. Three-dimensional CT angiography data entry into the intraoperative imaging program provides more detail for cerebral aneurysm repair than previously available, giving the surgeon a real-time navigational map of the aneurysmal structure, position, and spatial orientation, as well as additional details of the aneurysm sac, neck, and arterial branching—previously not available during the surgical procedure.[50] The MRI has also developed to produce exquisite-quality films in shorter periods of time. Its use with neuronavigation systems has already been addressed. The newer open models have significantly decreased the feeling of confinement, thus making MRI technology more acceptable to patients with claustrophobia.

Intracranial endoscopic surgery continues to evolve. For example, conventional open surgery for ventricular tumors has been associated with significant morbidity and mortality. Minimally invasive neuroendoscopy is showing great promise for resection of ventricular lesions in the face of hydrocephalus. This technique reduces surrounding tissue trauma during dissection and increases anatomic visualization through the use of directional endoscopes of structures that would have been obscured to the microsurgical field. Compared to conventional craniotomy, the skin incision is reduced to approximately 4 to 6 cm. The "keyhole" craniotomy or skull opening is typically 1.5 to 2 cm in diameter. Brain tissue dissection and retraction, known as the surgical corridor, can be as small as 1 cm in diameter. Microscopic or image guidance can be added to neuroendoscopy for further precision. Overall, neuroendoscopy offers a select patient population a more comfortable surgical option with less tissue manipulation and subsequent complications from tissue trauma.[51]

Endovascular treatments for cerebral artery disease continue to expand as previously discussed. Interventional radiologists are performing intra-arterial injection of thrombolytics directly into the occluded cerebral artery at the time of stroke to improve cerebral blood flow.

Recent improvements of aneurysm coiling material combined with deployment of stents across the aneurysm neck are improving treatment of wide-necked aneurysms, previously deemed more appropriate for surgical treatment. Liquid embolic agents are also emerging as an endovascular means of obliterating aneurysms.[50,52]

The advancements and trends for neurosurgery provide many new options for patients with intracranial and cerebrovascular lesions. Fewer lesions are deemed "inoperable." High-risk surgeries are becoming more precise with less injury to surrounding tissues. The future of neurosurgery is exciting, bright, and full of promise for the patient population whose diagnosis is often full of dread, anxiety, debilitation, and even death.

REFERENCES

1. Hamilton, M. G., Hull, R. D., & Pineo, G. F. (1994). Venous thromboembolism in neurosurgery and neurology patients: A review. *Neurosurgery, 34,* 280–296.
2. Lam, A. M. (1999). Neurophysiological monitoring. In P. Newfield & J. C. Cottrell (Eds.). *Handbook of neuroanesthesia* (3rd ed., pp. 34–52). Philadelphia: Lippincott Williams & Wilkins.
3. American Society of Anesthesiologists. (1963). New classification of physical status. *Anesthesiology, 24,* 111.
4. Hickey, R. (1999). Effects of anesthesia on cerebral and spinal cord physiology. In P. Newfield & J. C. Cottrell (Eds.). *Handbook of neuroanesthesia* (3rd ed., pp. 20–33). Philadelphia: Lippincott Williams & Wilkins.
5. Greenberg, M. S. (2006). *Handbook of neurosurgery* (6th ed., pp. 1–3). New York: Thieme.
6. Carras, D., Farrell, S., & Todd, M. M. (1999). Neuroanesthesia. In R. G. Grossman & C. M. Loftus (Eds.). *Principles of neurosurgery* (2nd ed., pp. 15–30). Philadelphia: Lippincott-Raven.
7. Pittman, J., & Cottrell, J. E. (1999). Cerebral protection and resuscitation. In P. Newfield & J. C. Cottrell (Eds.). *Handbook of neuroanesthesia* (3rd ed., pp. 53–73). Philadelphia: Lippincott Williams & Wilkins.
8. Todd, M. M., Hindman, B. J., Clarke, W. R., & Torner, J. C. (2005). Mild intraoperative hypothermia during surgery for intracranial aneurysm. *New England Journal of Medicine, 352*(2), 121–124.
9. Greenberg, M. S. (2006). *Handbook of neurosurgery* (6th ed., p. 807). New York: Thieme.
10. Gorarten, W., & Van Aken, H. (1999). Induced hypotension. In P. Newfield & J. C. Cottrell (Eds.). *Handbook of neuroanesthesia* (3rd ed., pp. 299–309). Philadelphia: Lippincott Williams & Wilkins.
11. Ravussin, P. A., & Wilder-Smith, O. H. G. (1999). Anesthesia for supratentorial tumors. In P. Newfield & J. C. Cottrell (Eds.). *Handbook of neuroanesthesia* (3rd ed., pp. 146–164). Philadelphia: Lippincott Williams & Wilkins.
12. Bolognese, P. (1999). Disruption of the blood-brain barrier. In P. Newfield & J. C. Cottrell (Eds.). *Handbook of neuroanesthesia* (3rd ed., pp. 226–233). Philadelphia: Lippincott Williams & Wilkins.
13. Walker, M. L., Emadian, S. M., & Honeycutt, Jr., J. H. (1999). Diagnosis and management of primary pediatric brain tumors. In R. G. Grossman & C. M. Loftus (Eds.). *Principles of neurosurgery* (2nd ed., pp. 33–46). Philadelphia: Lippincott-Raven.
14. Scherer, R., & McGrath, J. (2001). Medtronic introduces StealthStation® Treon™ system, further reducing guesswork in high-risk surgery. Retrieved March 8, 2006, from http://wwwp.medtronic.com/Newsroom/NewsReleaseDetails.do?itemId=1095955401014.
15. Somaza, A., Lunsford, L. D., Kondziolka, D., Flickinger, J. C., & Maitz, A. (1999). Gamma knife radiosurgery. In R. G. Grossman & C. M. Loftus (Eds.). *Principles of neurosurgery* (2nd ed., pp. 721–736). Philadelphia: Lippincott-Raven.
16. The University of Florida Linac scalpel. Retrieved March 8, 2006, from http://ufbi.ufl.edu/patient/linacscalpel.html.
17. Arab, D., Kirmani, J. F., Xavier, A. R., Yahia, A. M., Suarez, J. I., & Qureshi, A. I. (2004). Cardiac monitoring in the neurosciences critical care unit. In J. I. Suarez (Ed.). *Critical care neurology and neurosurgery* (pp. 137–150). Totowa, NJ: Humana Press.
18. Andrews, B. T. (1999). General management and intensive care of the neurosurgical patient. In R. G. Grossman & C. M. Loftus (Eds.). *Principles of neurosurgery* (2nd ed., pp. 3–14). Philadelphia: Lippincott-Raven.
19. Domino, K. B. (1999). Respiratory care of the neurosurgical patient. In P. Newfield & J. C. Cottrell (Eds.). *Handbook of*

neuroanesthesia (3rd ed., pp. 337–353). Philadelphia: Lippincott Williams & Wilkins.

20. Greenberg, M. S. (2006). *Handbook of neurosurgery* (6th ed., pp. 7–8). New York: Thieme.

21. Greenberg, M. S. (2006). *Handbook of neurosurgery* (6th ed., pp. 21–27). New York: Thieme.

22. Diaz, J. L., Granados, M., & Suarez, J. I. (2004). Management of medical complications in the neurosciences critical care unit. In J. I. Suarez (Ed.). *Critical care neurology and neurosurgery* (pp. 193–219). Totowa, NJ: Humana Press.

23. Geerts, W. H., Pineo, G. F., Heit, J. A., Bergqvist, D., Lassen, M. R., Colwell, C. W., et al. (2004). Prevention of venous thromboembolism. *Chest, 126*, 338S–400S.

24. Rodrigue, T., & Selman, W. R. (2004). Postoperative management in the neurosciences critical care unit. In J. I. Suarez (Ed.). *Critical care neurology and neurosurgery* (pp. 433–448). Totowa, NJ: Humana Press.

25. Greenberg, M. S. (2006). *Handbook of neurosurgery* (6th ed., pp. 12–19). New York: Thieme.

26. Greenberg, M. S. (2006). *Handbook of neurosurgery* (6th ed., p. 658). New York: Thieme.

27. Kuniyoshi, S., & Suarez, J. I. (2004). Traumatic head injury. In J. I. Suarez (Ed.). *Critical care neurology and neurosurgery* (p. 410). Totowa, NJ: Humana Press.

28. Holman, R. G., & Dellinger, E. P. (1996). Fever, infection, and antibiotics. In J. A. Weigelt & F. R. Lewis, Jr. (Eds.). *Surgical critical care* (pp. 151–170). Philadelphia: W.B. Saunders.

29. Greenberg, M. S. (2006). *Handbook of neurosurgery* (6th ed., pp. 454–455). New York: Thieme.

30. Greenberg, M. S. (2006). *Handbook of neurosurgery* (6th ed., p. 11). New York: Thieme.

31. Williams, G. H., & Dluhy, R.G. (2005). Diseases of the adrenal cortex. In D.L. Kasper, E. Braunwald, A.S. Fauci, S. L. Hauser, D. L. Longo, & J. L. Jameson (Eds.). *Harrison's principles of internal medicine* (16th ed., pp. 2127–2148). New York: McGraw-Hill.

32. Greenberg, M. S. (2006). *Handbook of neurosurgery* (6th ed., p. 440). New York: Thieme.

33. Greenberg, M. S. (2006). *Handbook of neurosurgery* (6th ed., pp. 869–886). New York: Thieme.

34. Chaturvedi, S., Bruno, A., Feasby, T., Holloway, R., Benavente, O., Cohen, S. N., et al. (2005). Carotid endarterectomy—An evidence-based review: Report of the Therapeutics and Technology Assessment Subcommittee of the American Academy of Neurology. *Neurology, 65*, 794–801.

35. Steering Committee of NASCET. (1991). North American Symptomatic Carotid Endarterectomy trial: Methods, patients' characteristics and progress. *Stroke, 22*, 711–720.

36. European Carotid Surgery Trialists' Collaborative Group. (1991). MRC European Surgery Trial: Interim results for symptomatic patients with severe (70–99%) or with mild (0–29%) carotid stenosis. *Lancet, 337*, 1235–1243.

37. European Carotid Surgery Trialists' Collaborative Group. (1996). Endarterectomy for moderate symptomatic carotid stenosis: Interim results form the MRC European Surgery Trial. *Lancet, 347*, 1591–1593.

38. North American Symptomatic Carotid Endarterectomy Trial Collaborators. (1991). Beneficial effect of carotid endarterectomy in symptomatic patients with high-grade carotid stenosis. *New England Journal of Medicine, 325*, 445–453.

39. Biller, J., Feinberg, W. M., Castoldo, J. E., Whittemore, A. D., Harbaugh, R. E., Dempsey, R. J., et al. (1998). Guidelines for carotid endarterectomy: A statement for healthcare professionals from a special writing group of the Stroke Council, American Heart Association. *Circulation, 97*, 501–509.

40. Betancourt, M., Van Stavern, R. B., Share, D., Gardella, P., Martus, M., & Chaturvedi, S. (2004). Are patients receiving maximal medical therapy following carotid endarterectomy? *Neurology, 63*, 2011–2015.

41. Benzel, E. C., & Hoppens, K. D. (1991). Factors associated with postoperative hypertension complicating carotid endarterectomy. *Acta Neurochirurgica (Wien), 112*, 8–12.

42. Zabramski, J. M., Greene, K. A., Marciano, F. F., & Spetzler, R. F. (1994). Carotid endarterectomy. In L. P. Carter, R. F. Spetzler, & M. G. Hamilton (Eds.). *Neurovascular surgery* (pp. 325–357). New York: McGraw-Hill.

43. Bernstein, M., Fleming, J. F. R., & Deck, J. H. N. (1984). Cerebral hyperperfusion after carotid endarterectomy: A cause of cerebral hemorrhage. *Neurosurgery, 15*, 50–56.

44. Piepgras, D. G., Morgan, M. K., Sundt, T. M., Yanagihara, T., & Mussman, L. M. (1988). Intracerebral hemorrhage after carotid endarterectomy. *Journal of Neurosurgery, 68*, 532–536.

45. Clagett, G. P., & Robertson, J. T. (1998). Surgical considerations in symptomatic disease. In H. J. M. Barnett, J. P. Mohr, B. M. Stein, & F. M. Yatsu (Eds.). *Stroke: Pathophysiology, diagnosis, and management* (pp. 1209–1228). New York: Churchill Livingstone.

46. O'Brien, M. S., & Ricotta, J. J. (1991). Conserving resources after carotid endarterectomy: Selective use of the intensive care unit. *Journal of Vascular Surgery, 14*, 796–800.

47. Rabe, K., & Sievert, H. (2004). Carotid artery stenting: State of the art. *Journal of Interventional Cardiology, 17*, 417–426.

48. Fateri, F., Groebli, Y., & Rufenacht, D. A. (2005). Intraarterial thrombolysis and stent placement in the acute phase of blunt internal carotid artery trauma with subocclusive dissection and thromboembolic complication: Case report and review of the literature. *Annals of Vascular Surgery, 19*, 434, 437.

49. Wholey, M. H., Wholey, M. H., Tan, W. A., Toursarkissian, B., Bailey, S., Eles, G., et al. (2001). Management of neurological complications of carotid artery stenting. *Journal of Endovascular Therapy, 8*, 341–353.

50. Benvenuti, L., Chibbaro, S., Carnesecchi, S., Pulera, F., & Gagliardi, R. (2005). Automated three-dimensional volume rendering of helical computed tomographic angiography for aneurysms: An advanced application of neuronavigation technology. *Neurosurgery, 57 (ONS Supplement 1)*, 69–77.

51. Charalampaki, P., Filippi, R., Welschehold, S., Conrad, J., & Perneczky, A. (2005). Tumors of the lateral and third ventricle: Removal under endoscope-assisted keyhole conditions. *Neurosurgery, 57 (ONS Supplement 1)*, 302–311.

52. Lanzino, G., Kanaan, Y., Perrini, P., Dayoub, H., & Fraser, K. (2005). Emerging concepts in the treatment of intracranial aneurysms: Stents, coated coils, and liquid embolic agents. *Neurosurgery, 57*, 449–459.

RESOURCES

Professional

Greenberg, M. S. (2006). *Handbook of neurosurgery* (6th ed.). New York: Thieme.

Grossman, R. G., & Loftus, C. M. (Eds.). (1999). *Principles of neurosurgery* (2nd ed.). Philadelphia: Lippincott-Raven.

Ojemann, R. G., Ogilvy, C. G., Crowell, R. M., & Heros, R. C. (1995). *Surgical management of cerebrovascular disease* (3rd ed.). Baltimore: Williams & Wilkins.

Patient and Family

StayWell Company (1999). *Craniotomy: Understanding your care*. San Bruno, CA: Author (Telephone: 1-800-333-3032).

Nursing Management of Patients With a Depressed State of Consciousness

Joanne V. Hickey and Mary Bray Powers

Unconsciousness or **depressed state of consciousness** is a physiologic state in which the patient generally is unresponsive to sensory stimuli and lacks awareness of self and the environment. Myriad central nervous system conditions and dysfunction of other body organs can result in unconsciousness. The depth and duration of unconsciousness or depressed state of consciousness span a broad spectrum of presentations from fainting, with momentary loss of consciousness, to prolonged depressed states of consciousness lasting weeks or months. The term *coma* is reserved for a clinical presentation in which the state of unconsciousness is maintained for a prolonged period, from hours to months. The pathophysiologic basis for coma is direct structural injury or physiologic dysfunction in *both* cerebral hemispheres, the brainstem, or both hemispheres and brainstem. Coma is typically a transient state evolving toward the recovery of consciousness, persistent vegetative state, or brain death.[1] See Chapter 7 for a discussion of depressed states of consciousness. In addition, the multiple causes of a depressed state of consciousness, including central nervous systems lesions and metabolic causes, are also discussed in Chapter 7. An in-depth discussion of impairment in consciousness and approach to the patient can be found in selected references.[2-4]

In neuroscience nursing practice, the nurse often cares for patients who are experiencing depressed states of consciousness for prolonged periods of time. These patients lack voluntary movement and are usually bedridden. The physiologic consequences of short- and long-term immobilization, well described in the literature, contribute to poor outcome and disability. Not only does patient survival directly depend on the quality of care provided, but also the realization of optimal rehabilitation potential hinges on the quality of nursing care. In addition to managing the primary neurological problem, the nurse must also incorporate a rehabilitation framework to maintain intact function; prevent secondary brain injuries, complications, and disabilities; and restore lost function to the highest degree possible.

The purpose of this chapter is to provide a basic physical-psychosocial nursing care framework for neurological patients with depressed states of consciousness. Care is designed to achieve optimal outcomes and to include specific points of care relative to the management of the neuro-science patient. *Because depressed consciousness can be caused by many neurological problems, there may be variations in care related to the primary diagnosis.* The basic standard of care for patients with depressed states of consciousness is outlined in this chapter. (Chart 15-1 gives a sample nursing care plan.)

IMMOBILITY

Kinesis, a word of Greek origin, means motion or to move. The human body is designed for physical activity and movement. Even at rest, the normal healthy adult changes position on average every 11.6 minutes during sleep; this physiologic requirement for movement is termed the **minimal physiologic mobility requirement**.[5] Exercise contributes to health, whereas lack of exercise, regardless of reason, leads to a continuum of multisystem deconditioning and anatomic and physiologic changes. Deconditioning is a complex process of physiologic change due to a period of inactivity, bed rest, or sedentary lifestyle. It results in functional losses in such areas as activities of daily living and mental status.[6] Depending on the degree of inactivity, deconditioning can occur gradually or acutely.

Bed rest was first recognized as a therapeutic modality in the 1860s. The therapeutic value of bed rest includes decreased oxygen consumption, prevention or reduction of trauma to a body part, and redirection of energy resources toward healing.[7] However, this belief is balanced by the recognition that immobility has also been described as the most potentially dangerous treatment prescribed today.[8] Bed rest deconditioning, independent of disease effects, contributes significantly to the reduced reserve capacity to perform regular physical activity during periods of relative immobility. The fact that bed rest deconditioning can be partly explained independent of disease highlights the need for physical activity directed at limitation of the debilitating effects of bed rest.[9] This is challenging in patients with altered states of consciousness, but a collaborative interdisciplinary approach can provide effective clinical interventions.

Immobility produces a *disuse phenomenon* that results in physiologic as well as psychosocial effects. The morbidity of immobility is directly associated with the length of time of

(text continues on page 340)

CHART 15-1	Nursing Care Plan for the Patient With a Decreased Level of Consciousness

PATIENT PROBLEMS/EXPECTED OUTCOMES	NURSING INTERVENTIONS

Self-Care Deficit: R/T immobility and unconsciousness*
 	
• Basic self-care needs will be provided by the nursing staff.
• Self-care deficit syndrome:
    Bathing/hygiene
    Dressing/grooming
    Feeding
    Toileting
	• Provide basic hygiene care.
	• Dress and groom patient.
	• Provide nutritional support by alternate means, as ordered.
	• Provide for the elimination needs of the patient.
	• Ensure patient safety—proper identification, falls prevention, privacy.

RESPIRATORY FUNCTION	
Risk for Altered Respiratory Function: R/T immobility • Adequate respiratory function will be maintained.	• Conduct a risk assessment of respiratory function. • Apply preventive strategies to prevent complications.
Risk for Aspiration • Patient will not aspirate.	• Keep NPO until a risk assessment is completed. • Do not feed if airway protection or swallowing is compromised. • Position to facilitate oral drainage; position in lateral recumbent position, unless contraindicated. • Elevate head of bed to 30 degrees, unless contraindicated. • Follow precautions to prevent enteral feeding aspiration.
Ineffective Airway Clearance: R/T altered consciousness and ineffective cough reflex • A patent airway will be maintained. • Drainage of secretions from the oropharynx will be facilitated.	• Keep the neck in a neutral position. • Limit suctioning to 10 seconds or less and one insertion per attempt. • If a tracheostomy tube in place, administer tracheostomy care every 4 hours. • Suction oropharyngeal airway or via endotracheal or tracheostomy tube every 1–2 hours to clear airway of drainage. • Position in the lateral recumbent position; reposition every 1–2 hours. • Elevate the head of the bed 30 degrees, unless contraindicated.
Ineffective Breathing Pattern: R/T immobility and underlying neurological problem(s) • An effective breathing pattern will be maintained.	• Monitor the rate, depth, and pattern of respirations frequently. • Monitor tidal volume and blood gas levels. • Observe frequently for signs and symptoms of respiratory distress. • Auscultate the chest frequently. • Elevate the head of the bed 30 degrees, unless contraindicated. • Position to facilitate respirations. • For patients maintained on a ventilator, monitor for synchrony with the ventilator; report asynchrony to the physician; administer ordered drug therapy.
Impaired Gas Exchange: R/T immobility • Adequate gas exchange will be facilitated.	• Auscultate the chest every 2 hours for adventitious sounds. • Monitor period blood gases and continue pulse oximetry. • Monitor for cyanosis and respiratory distress. • Turn patient side to side at least every 2 hours. • Provide for periodic chest physiotherapy. • Preoxygenate with 100% oxygen before and after suctioning. • Administer oxygen as ordered.

(continued)

CHART 15-1   **Nursing Care Plan for the Patient With a Decreased Level of Consciousness** (Continued)

PATIENT PROBLEMS/EXPECTED OUTCOMES	NURSING INTERVENTIONS
Risk of Developing Infection: R/T artificial airway • Patient will not develop ventilator- or hospital-acquired pneumonia.	• Elevate head of bed 30 degrees, unless contraindicated. • Provide mouth care every 2–4 hours with brushing of teeth every 8 hours. • If patient is mechanically ventilated, use "sedation vacation" with spontaneous breathing trial. • Use peptic ulcer prophylaxis (ordered by physician). • Use deep vein thrombosis prophylaxis. • Apply TED hose and sequential compression devices.

CARDIOVASCULAR FUNCTION

Cardiac Output, Altered: R/T immobility • Cardiac output will be maintained within targeted limits.	• Monitor vital signs frequently. • Monitor the rate, rhythm, and quality of the radial and apical pulses. • Document any arrhythmias. • Observe monitor every 30 minutes–1 hour; maintain alarms at all times.
Altered Peripheral Tissue Perfusion: R/T immobility • Adequate peripheral perfusion will be maintained. • Dependent edema will not develop in the arms.	• Apply thigh-high elastic stockings and sequential compression air boots. • When placing patient in the lateral recumbent position, position upper leg so that it does not cause pressure on the lower leg. • Do not use the foot gatch under the patient's knees or place constricting objects to the backs of the knees. • Position so that each joint is higher than the previous joint so that the distal joints are highest. • Monitor for signs of deep vein thrombosis (DVT). • Administer pharmacologic agents as ordered for DVT prevention.
Altered Cerebral Tissue Perfusion: R/T immobility • Adequate cerebral perfusion pressure will be maintained.	• Maintain patient's head and neck in a neutral position. • Elevate the head of the bed at 30 degrees unless contraindicated. • Avoid positions known to increase intracranial pressure (e.g., hip flexion, prone; see Chap. 13). • If an intracranial pressure monitor is being used, observe monitor every 30–60 minutes for a rise in pressure and any correlation to care or other activities. • Do not cluster nursing activities; allow pressure fall before beginning another procedure. • Maintain normothermia. • Provide "soft" stimuli (e.g., soft music, family voices).

INTEGUMENTARY SYSTEM

Risk for Impaired Skin Integrity: R/T immobility • Skin will remain intact.	• Assess skin integrity daily. • Provide pressure-relieving devices. • Avoid donut pressure-type devices. • Utilize protective barriers on fragile/irritated skin. • Utilize lifting devices and avoid dragging. • Avoid massage over bony or reddened areas. • Utilize Braden/Norton Scales. • Provide skin care frequently (daily baths; mouth, back, and perineal care). • Lubricate dry lips with water-based moisturizer and skin with lanolin. • Monitor skin for redness and pressure ulcers frequently. • Do not position patient on reddened areas of skin. • Provide clean tape for securing of nasogastric or endotracheal tube daily, wash the skin, and do not apply new tape in the same place. • Keep the heels off the bed at all times. • Cut and file fingernails and toenails. • Turn and reposition at least every 2 hours.

CHART 15-1	**Nursing Care Plan for the Patient With a Decreased Level of Consciousness** (Continued)

PATIENT PROBLEMS/EXPECTED OUTCOMES	NURSING INTERVENTIONS
Risk for Impaired Tissue Integrity (corneal): R/T immobility • The eye will be maintained infection and injury free.	• Inspect the eyes for signs of irritation and cleanse them every 4 hours. • Position patient to protect the eyes; apply shield or tape eyelids as ordered. • Instill methylcellulose drops or other lubricating solution as ordered.
Altered Oral Mucous Membrane: R/T dryness, decreased saliva • The oral mucosa will remain intact and free of dryness, lesions, and exudate.	• Provide mouth care frequently. • Brush patient's teeth every 6–8 hours. • Monitor patient's mouth for lesions, dryness, or bleeding.

MUSCULOSKELETAL FUNCTION

Impaired Physical Mobility: R/T altered consciousness and underlying neurological problem(s) causing immobility (e.g., paresis, paralysis, or rigidity) • Range of motion will be maintained and deformities/contractures prevented.	• Administer passive range-of-motion exercises at least four times daily. • Position in proper body alignment; reposition every 2 hours. Use trochanter roll, splints, slings, pillows, and foot positioners/athletic shoes, as needed. • Reposition decorticate or decerebrate patients every hour; control noxious stimuli that may affect abnormal positioning. • Collaborate with the physical therapist.
Risk for Trauma Injury: Stress fracture and joint dislocation • No stress fractures or joint dislocations will occur.	• Do not pull or tug on joints. • Administer passive range-of-motion exercises at least four times daily. • Position in proper body alignment. • Provide rolls and pillows to maintain desired position.
Altered Urinary Elimination: R/T immobility: incontinence, retention, or large residual urine • Adequate urinary elimination will be maintained.	• Monitor intake and output. • Remove the urinary catheter as soon as possible. • Consider an intermittent catheterization program. • Provide perineal care. • Palpate the bladder for distention.
Risk for Infection: R/T immobility: urinary tract infection • Factors contributing to infection will be controlled.	• Follow strict aseptic technique in the care of the patient's urinary drainage catheter. • Remove the urinary catheter as soon as possible. • Monitor urinalysis and urine culture and sensitivity for signs and symptoms of infection.

GASTROINTESTINAL FUNCTION

Altered Bowel Elimination: R/T immobility • Stool will be soft and formed. • The bowel will be evacuated every 1–3 days.	• Monitor and record character and frequency of bowel movements. • Auscultate abdomen for bowel sounds. • Initiate a bowel program.

NEUROLOGICAL FUNCTION

Elevated Body Temperature: R/T underlying neurological problem(s) or infection • Normothermia will be maintained.	• Monitor patient's temperature periodically. • If temperature elevated, remove excess clothing and top linen; provide a sponge bath, as necessary. • Consider the underlying reasons for elevated body temperature; implement appropriate interventions. • Administer antipyretics and other cooling interventions (e.g., cooling blanket) as indicated.

(continued)

CHART 15-1   **Nursing Care Plan for the Patient With a Decreased Level of Consciousness**   (Continued)

PATIENT PROBLEMS/EXPECTED OUTCOMES	NURSING INTERVENTIONS
Sensory/Perceptual Alterations: R/T unconsciousness • Multisensory stimuli will be provided throughout the day.	• Provide sensory stimuli by talking to the patient; describe surroundings, treatments, etc. • Stimulate as many senses as possible. • Turn on the radio, TV, or tape recorder when no one is with the patient. • Encourage family to touch and talk to the patient. • After patient begins to awaken, use orientation instruments, such as a clock, calendar, window, favorite objects, or family pictures.
Pain: R/T immobility, physiologic dysfunction, or injury • Patient will report being pain free or rate it at 1–3 on a 1 to 10 scale.	• Assess for nonverbal pain indicators (i.e., grimacing, crying, increased respiratory and heart rate, brow furrowing, diaphoresis). • Position in proper body alignment. • Assess for distended bladder. • Assess for fecal impaction. • Assess for foreign object on or under skin (e.g., in bed linen). • Treat with analgesics, as ordered. • Provide alternatives to analgesics (e.g., massage therapy, aromatherapy, music, therapeutic touch).
NUTRITION AND HYDRATION	
Altered Nutrition: Less than Body Requirements: R/T unconsciousness • Adequate nutrition will be provided. • An appropriate weight level will be maintained.	• Monitor the patient's weight at least twice weekly. • Request a nutritional consultation. • Collaborate with the clinical dietician for a nutrition consultation and orders. • Maintain an accurate intake and output record; include a daily calorie count.
Fluid Volume Deficit: R/T unconsciousness • Adequate fluid volume will be maintained.	• Maintain accurate intake and output record. • Monitor skin turgor and mucous membranes for dryness. • Monitor vital signs, specific gravity of urine, and serum osmolality values. • Provide hydration as ordered. • Weigh daily. • Elevate electrolytes.

*R/T = related to.

immobilization and patient-specific risk factors. Some physiologic effects occur almost immediately on the institution of bed rest, whereas other physiologic and pathophysiologic changes occur over a longer period of time. Although there are physiologic changes with short periods (e.g., 1–3 days) of immobility, they are generally less severe and may be reversible. Prolonged periods of immobility, which often occur with coma, spinal cord injury, or Guillain-Barré syndrome, result in pathophysiologic changes associated with serious morbidity and permanent disabilities. Risk factors that increase the probability of complications from immobility include length and degree of immobility, incontinence, poor nutrition, hypotension, infection, altered motor or sensory function, multiorgan failure, underweight or obesity, advanced age, and comorbidity. The effects of immobility give rise to many of the complications in the unconscious patient, hence the need for the implementation of a broad range of nursing skills.[10] Elderly people are particularly vulnerable to the deleterious effects of immobility resulting from concurrent age-related factors.[11] Immobility and

its consequences to each body system are well known. Yet, risk assessment and preventive strategies to address this complex, multidimensional problem continue to be challenging. The use of evidence-based practice and best practices should guide nurses in providing the best-quality care.

SPECIALTY BEDS AND SUPPORT SURFACES

Various types of specialty beds and support surfaces are used to prevent skin irritation and decubitus ulcers and other complications of immobility in high-risk patients. A wide range of mattress overlays and mattresses are available, and each manufacturer offers special features that may be of particular value to patients depending on their individual needs. On admission, a risk assessment for pressure ulcers should be conducted using a standardized scale such as the Braden Scale. Based on the score, there are algorithms and clinical practice guidelines that guide bed selection as well as other treatment options that must be implemented. Risk assessment of the skin using the Braden Scale is conducted upon admission and weekly thereafter, or more frequently if the patient's conditions changes dramatically to suggest changes in risk or treatment needs. The cost effectiveness of ordering a special bed must be considered. Health care facilities and managed care plans often have established criteria for identifying high-risk patients for whom special beds will be helpful and cost effective. Institutional guidelines should be followed in the selection and use of specific beds.

CLINICAL PEARLS: Specialty beds are not a substitute for frequent repositioning of patients.

THE CONSEQUENCES OF IMMOBILITY: NURSING MANAGEMENT OF THE PATIENT WITH DEPRESSED CONSCIOUSNESS

Meticulous nursing care has a direct impact on patient outcomes. Clinical reasoning, based on a systematic ongoing assessment of all body systems, alerts the nurse to signs and symptoms of complications. The nurse should implement preventive strategies as well as treatment protocols according to the best practices related to optimal outcomes. Ongoing assessment is the basis for identifying patient, nursing, and collaborative problems. Several collaborative problems that are common to most patients with depressed consciousness are listed in Chart 15-2. Because the patient is immobilized and multiple body systems are threatened, the patient problems of *disuse syndrome* encompassing all systems and *total self-care deficit syndrome* addressing the total depend-

ency are prominent concerns for the nurse in providing care. The remaining content of this chapter is organized according to body systems and related treatment implications.

Respiratory Function

The supine position and horizontal plane cause physiologic changes in the mechanics of breathing and in lung volumes. Mechanical restriction results from decreased overall respiratory muscle strength and from reduced intercostal, diaphragmatic, and abdominal muscle excursion with a consequent decrease in thoracic volume. Normally, tidal breathing in the upright position predominantly results from rib cage movement, whereas in the supine position, abdominal muscles predominate. Maximal inspiration capacity is decreased, resulting in decreased vital and functional respiratory capacities.[12]

All lung volumes decrease except for tidal volume. The decrease in thoracic size and increase in intrathoracic blood volume associated with the supine position cause a decrease in residual volume and functional residual capacity (FRC). Normally, FRC exceeds closing volume through maintaining an open airway. When the FRC is exceeded by the closing volume, the partial or complete collapse of lung units causes atelectasis, regional differences in ventilation-perfusion ratio (V/Q mismatch), poorly ventilated and overly perfused areas, and arteriovenous shunts. If increased metabolic demands occur, hypoxia results.[13] In addition, impaired mucociliary function causes mucous secretions to accumulate in the dependent respiratory bronchiole, which contributes to the development of atelectasis and hypostatic pneumonia.

Assessment

Respiratory function is assessed using a number of parameters: airway patency; rate, quality, and pattern of respirations; chest auscultation; and objective signs of oxygenation (i.e., pulse oximetry). The highest priority in managing a patient is assigned to **airway patency**, which is the openness of the upper airway (nose, mouth, pharynx, trachea, bronchi) that provides the route for air exchange. Obstruction of the airway may be caused by injury, edema, mucus, or other drainage. Airway patency must be assessed frequently.

Clinical evidence of an ineffective breathing pattern includes apnea, dyspnea, shortness of breath, stridor, rapid or shallow respirations, Cheyne-Stokes pattern, a prolonged expiration or inspiration phase, nasal flaring, pursed lips, intercostal or substernal retraction, abdominal breathing, and altered chest expansion.

Assess and monitor the following:

- Airway patency
- Rate, quality, and pattern of respirations
- Adventitious breath sounds by chest auscultation of both lungs
- Correlation of findings of recent chest radiograph with clinical findings
- Amount and characteristics of airway secretions
- Capillary refill and subtle cyanosis or dustiness in periorbital area, ear lobes, and fingernails
- Oxygen saturation levels with pulse oximetry
- Periodic blood gases

CHART 15-2 **Common Collaborative Problems for the Patient With a Depressed Level of Consciousness**

- Atelectasis/pneumonia (aspiration, bacterial pneumonia)
- Deep vein thrombosis/pulmonary embolism
- Ventilator dependency
- Tracheal ulceration or necrosis
- Anemia
- Pressure ulcers (decubitus ulcers)
- Acute urinary retention
- Paralytic ileus
- Gastric ulcer
- Electrolyte imbalance
- Negative nitrogen balance
- Peripheral nerve impairment/neuropathies
- Corneal ulceration
- Stress fractures, contractures
- Osteoporosis
- Joint dislocation
- Pain

- Lung volumes and respiratory mechanics
- Overall work of breathing
- Cough reflex
- Gag reflex

Respiratory Problems

The patient with depressed consciousness is at high risk for developing respiratory problems. A secondary effect of compromised respiratory function is cerebral hypoxia, which leads to secondary brain injury unless the early signs and symptoms of respiratory insufficiency are recognized and interventions initiated expeditiously. Respiratory problems to be considered include airway obstruction, aspiration, atelectasis, and pneumonia. Other conditions seen in relation to trauma and intracranial hemorrhage are neurogenic pulmonary edema, adult respiratory distress syndrome, and disseminated intravascular coagulation; these conditions are discussed in other chapters.

Airway Obstruction. In the patient with depressed consciousness, a partially or completely obstructed airway can occur because of mucous accumulation or plugging by other foreign materials or through posterior displacement of oropharyngeal soft-tissue structures, particularly the tongue, as a result of improper positioning of the head and neck.[14] A patient lacking the ability to protect his or her airway is unable to reposition his or her head and neck to maintain airway patency. Other mechanical deficits that affect respiratory structures include postanesthesia recovery, airway edema following extubation, and diaphragmatic or intercostal muscle paralysis related to spinal cord injury or neuromuscular diseases. Results of partial airway obstruction include alveolar hypoventilation, hypoxia, hypercarbia, increased respiratory rate, and atelectasis. The early signs and symptoms observed are shallow and noisy respirations, increased secretions, and restlessness.

Aspiration. The patient with depressed consciousness is unable to protect his or her airway and therefore is at high risk for aspiration. Regurgitation and microaspiration, as well as actual vomiting of gastric contents, may occur, resulting in a nosocomial pneumonia.[15,16] Aspiration of tube feedings from a dislodged feeding tube or vomiting from a distended stomach can also lead to aspiration pneumonia.

CLINICAL PEARLS: Increased respirations, heart rate, and temperature with decreasing oxygen saturation may indicate acute aspiration—evaluate further.

Atelectasis and Pneumonia. Atelectasis, a state of alveolar collapse in a segment or lobe, has long been known to be a consequence of prolonged bed rest and immobility. The concurrent stasis and pooling of secretions collected in the dependent position leads to hypostatic pneumonia and a medium ripe for bacterial growth.[17] If the patient is dehydrated or receiving drugs that affect the tenacity of the secretions, bacteria can rapidly develop. In addition, patients are at high risk for nosocomial infections as a result of a compromised immunologic state and potential for colonization of the endotracheal tube.

Common related patient problems include *ineffective airway clearance, risk for aspiration, ineffective breathing pattern, impaired gas exchange, risk for altered respiratory function, dysfunctional ventilatory weaning response, and risk for infection.*

Nursing Interventions

Nursing interventions are aimed at maintaining a patent airway and facilitating adequate respirations.

Airway Patency. Maintaining a patent airway is the highest priority. The patient with depressed consciousness is defenseless against threats to a patent airway, particularly if the cough reflex is absent. In these patients and in conscious patients who do not have an intact cough reflex and are therefore at high risk for aspiration, suctioning will be necessary (see below). If there is evidence of inability to protect the airway, the physician may insert an endotracheal tube on an emergency basis to prevent aspiration and the risk of aspiration-related infection. If depressed consciousness is prolonged and the patient continues to need an artificial airway, a tracheotomy tube will be needed.

Prevention of Nosocomial Pneumonia. The Centers for Disease Control and Prevention as well as the American Thoracic Society have provided guidelines for the prevention of nosocomial pneumonia.[18–20] These guidelines should be followed in administering care.

Positioning. The lateral recumbent position promotes drainage of secretions, facilitates respirations, prevents pooling of secretions, and prevents the tongue from obstructing the airway. Turn the patient from side to side every 2 hours to prevent pooling of secretions.[15,21] Patients with depressed consciousness are cautiously positioned on their backs because of the risk of soft-tissue obstruction of the airway and the threat of aspiration. Unless contraindicated, the head should be elevated and turned to the side to facilitate drainage of secretions when lying in bed.

Mouth Care. Based on accumulating research, it is clear that the flora of the oral cavity has a relationship to the development of pneumonia, especially in ventilated patients. Mouth care, considered a comfort measure in the past, has gained new importance as an intervention to decrease the risk of pneumonia, especially in ventilator-associated pneumonia.[22]

Ventilator-associated pneumonia (VAP) is associated with increased morbidity and mortality. One important preventive strategy is frequent mouth care based on current standards.[16,23,24] There are no current evidence-based guidelines that define the optimal method and frequency of oral care, but best practices are available in the literature. In discussing mouth care, the literature elucidates a number of components for comprehensive oral care for patients on mechanical ventilation.[25] These same principles apply to patients with depressed levels of consciousness who are not mechanically ventilated. These principles include[19,26,27]:

- Daily assessment of the oral cavity
- Routine brushing of teeth to prevent the formation of dental plaque
- Oral care every 2 to 4 hours and as needed to promote healing and maintenance of the oral cavity

- Use of alcohol-free antiseptics to prevent or reduce bacterial load and colonization of the oropharyngeal area
- Routine suctioning of the mouth and pharynx to remove secretions and minimize aspiration
- Applying a water-based moisturizer to the lips and oral mucosa
- Avoiding the use of lemon glycerin swabs, which have no moisturizing properties, irritate the oral mucosa, decalcify teeth, and dry the mucous membrane from the citric acid and glycerin[28]

Suctioning. Periodic oropharyngeal or tracheal suctioning may be necessary to clear the airway of mucus, blood, or other drainage. Do not suction nasally if there is any possibility of a basal skull fracture or cerebrospinal fluid drainage from the nose or ear. With increased intracranial pressure (ICP), suctioning is limited to 10 seconds or less and catheter insertion is limited to only two times to prevent hypoxia. The lungs are oxygenated (using an Ambu bag) with 100% oxygen with a few breaths before and after suctioning to control hypoxemia. (A patient with chronic obstructive lung disease should not receive 100% oxygen; a lower concentration must be used.) Suction equipment must be checked at the beginning of every shift and maintained in a ready state for immediate use.

CLINICAL PEARLS: Nasopharyngeal airways facilitate suctioning of patients without endotracheal tubes or tracheostomies.

Other. A consultation with the respiratory therapist is helpful. Chest physical therapy may be recommended. Chest physical therapy consists of percussion and vibration, oropharyngeal stimulation of coughing, suctioning, and possible use of bronchodilators or mucolytic agents to facilitate movement of secretions. Managing a patient on a ventilator and ventilator weaning require skilled nursing care and are discussed in Chapter 16.

Cardiovascular Function

Maximal oxygen uptake (VO_{2max}) is a useful indicator of cardiovascular function in health and disease. Convertino et al. have provided excellent information on the effect of bed rest on cardiovascular function; this is summarized below.[29] During bed rest VO_{2max} is reduced, and the degree of loss is dependent on the duration of bed rest and baseline aerobic fitness (VO_{2max}). Bed rest causes an elevation in maximal heart rate, which is associated with decreased cardiac vagal tone, increased sympathetic catecholamine secretion, and greater cardiac (beta) receptor sensitivity. Despite the elevation in heart rate, VO_{2max} is reduced primarily from decreased maximal stroke volume, cardiac output, and venous return associated with lower circulating blood volume, reduced central venous pressure, and higher venous compliance in the lower extremities. Reductions in baseline and maximal muscle blood flow, red blood cell volume, and capillary function in working muscles represent peripheral mechanisms that may contribute to limited oxygen delivery and, subsequently, lowered VO_{2max}. Thus, alterations in cardiac and vascular functions induced by prolonged bed rest contribute to a decrease of maximal oxygen uptake and reserve capacity to perform physical work, and will impact on recovery.

Physiologic changes in cardiovascular function associated with immobility include increased cardiac workload and heart rate, decreased cardiac output, decreased stroke volume, increased peripheral vascular resistance, and decreased blood.

Cardiac workload is affected by Valsalva's maneuver. The **Valsalva's maneuver** is defined as a forced expiration against a closed epiglottis. Physiologic alterations include a period of thoracic fixation without expiration, which elevates intrathoracic pressure, thereby impeding venous blood from entering the large veins. When the patient exhales, there is a significant decrease in intrathoracic pressure, and a surge of blood is injected into the heart, thus increasing the workload of the heart. Neuroscience nurses are well aware of the effect of ICP rapid elevations that result from initiation of the Valsalva's maneuver. Significant spikes in ICP are potentially dangerous to patients with already elevated ICP.

Assessment

Assessment of cardiovascular function in the unconscious patient includes:

- Rate, rhythm, and quality of the apical and radial pulses
- Chest auscultation of heart sounds
- Quality of peripheral pulses
- Skin color, turgor, and edema
- Blood pressure, including ranges of systolic and diastolic over time
- Evidence of orthostatic hypotension with head elevation
- Periodic review of electrolytes
- Complete blood count, including hematocrit and hemoglobin
- Other hemodynamic parameters such as cardiac output, peripheral vascular resistance, and pulmonary artery wedge, all data available if the patient is centrally monitored

Cardiovascular Problems

Various cardiovascular problems result from cardiac deconditioning, deep vein thrombosis, pulmonary emboli, and orthostatic hypotension. Deconditioning of the cardiovascular system occurs within days; fluid shift, fluid loss, decreased cardiac output, decreased peak oxygen uptake, and increased resting heart rate result.[30]

Cardiac Deconditioning. Central fluid shifts occur with immobilization from the upright to supine position. The physiologic effect is an 11% total blood volume shift from the legs to other parts or the body, of which 80% moves to the thorax and 20% to the head.[31,32] The result is an increased central venous (CVP), left ventricular end-diastolic pressure (LVEDP), and stroke volume. In a patient with increased ICP, elevation of the head to 30 degrees is directed at improving venous return to the heart, which is impaired by the increased CVP. In response to the supine position, volume receptors are stimulated and diuresis occurs. As a result, there is an eventual reduction of plasma volume, total blood volume, and end-diastolic filling pressure and volumes; this is independent of total fluid intake.[7] With prolonged bed rest, there is an initial decrease in interstitial volume, although plasma volume remains low.[31]

Alterations in blood pressure and pulse may be the result of cardiac reconditioning or may be related to the primary neurological problem. A brief discussion of cardiovascular dysfunction is included here for the nurse to consider when evaluating the patient. Hypotension or hypertension should be viewed in relation to the patient's pulse rate, pulse quality, and pulse pressure.

- **Hypotension and pulse variations.** Hypotension is attributable to a number of possibilities. Hypotension associated with severe cerebral injury may be seen in the early phases of injury or in the terminal stage when compensatory mechanisms have been exhausted. The concurrent findings of *hypotension and tachycardia* should raise suspicion of occult internal hemorrhage (intra-abdominal, intrathoracic, pelvic, or long bone injury) or hypovolemic shock. Other signs of hypovolemic shock include restlessness, tachycardia, ashen skin color, cold and clammy skin, and a rapid, thready pulse. The combination of *hypotension and bradycardia* may be secondary to cervical spinal cord injury and related to interruption of descending sympathetic pathways. Hypotension and tachycardia can also be a hemodynamic response to prolonged bed rest. A cerebral perfusion pressure (CPP) of 60 to 70 mm Hg is required to provide an adequate cerebral blood flow (CBF); current practice is aimed at maintaining adequate CPP to overcome raised ICP.[33]
- **Hypertension and pulse variations.** Hypertension may occur with increases in intracranial pressure related to various cerebral problems, such as ischemic stroke or subarachnoid hemorrhage. The combination of *an elevated blood pressure, widening pulse pressure, and bradycardia* is called *Cushing's response* (see Chap. 7). Hypertension may also be attributable to pre-existing hypertension or presence of acute pain. Drug therapy may be instituted to control and maintain the blood pressure within a target range according to parameters ordered by the physician. These parameters may be set in a hypertensive range to maintain cerebral perfusion pressure if increased intracranial pressure is present.

Deep Vein Thrombosis and Pulmonary Embolism. Immobilization is a major risk factor for the formation of a deep venous thrombus (DVT) with the potential for the complication of a pulmonary embolism (PE). Thrombus formation is caused by venous stasis, decreased vasomotor tone, pressure on the blood vessels, and hypercoagulable state.[34] Several factors place the neurolgical patient at higher risk for the development of DVTs:

- Muscle contraction of the legs ordinarily promotes venous blood return to the heart, but in the case of the immobilized unconscious patient, the blood pools and venous stasis results.
- Paresis and paralysis of a limb or limbs contribute to poor venous blood return to the heart.
- Hypercoagulability states are a common finding in neurological patients. Immobility is often associated with dehydration and resulting hemoconcentration. Dehydration and a state of hypercoagulability, common in

these patients, contribute to venous thrombosis.[35] In addition, increased serum calcium contributes to hypercoagulation. (Calcium is liberated from the bones of any non–weight-bearing person.)
- Prolonged external pressure leads to intimal layer injury of blood vessels. Platelets collect at the injured intimal site, forming a layer that can become the foundation for clot formation. External pressure commonly results from pillow placement under the knees, from the upper leg resting on the lower leg in the lateral recumbent position, and from continual resting of the heels on the bed.

Orthostatic Hypotension. The third major effect of immobility on cardiovascular function is **orthostatic hypotension**, which is the inability of the autonomic nervous system to maintain an adequate blood supply to the upper regions of the body when the patient is placed upright in bed. In the immobilized patient, orthostatic hypotension is attributable to a loss of general motor tone and decreased efficiency of the orthostatic neurovascular reflexes (which normally cause contraction of the blood vessels so that blood can flow upward against gravity). Common related patient problems include *decreased cardiac output, peripheral neurovascular dysfunction, altered peripheral tissue perfusion, altered cerebral tissue perfusion, and activity intolerance.*

Interventions

Appropriate nursing interventions and nursing management designed to support cardiovascular function in the unconscious immobilized patient include the following:

- Turn and reposition the patient frequently, usually every 1 to 2 hours.
- When positioning the patient in the lateral recumbent position, position the upper leg to prevent pressure ulcers on the lower leg. Use a pillow to separate the legs.
- Apply thigh-high elastic stockings and sequential compression air boots to improve blood return to the heart and minimize venous stasis.
- Monitor the patient for signs and symptoms of deep vein thrombosis or thrombophlebitis (i.e., comparison of leg circumference, distal pulses, Homan's sign).
- Periodically, sit the patient in a chair, if at all possible; this alters intravascular pressure and stimulates the orthostatic neurovascular reflexes.
- Review the patient's hemodynamic profile and trends over time.
- Maintain blood within targeted range.
- Evaluate lower extremity Doppler studies.

The nurse must assess the risk factors for the development of venous thromboembolism. These include advanced age, known malignancy, presence of a neurological deficit, or a previous DVT. The most common evidence-based guidelines cited for the prevention of venous thromboembolism are published by the American College of Chest Physicians and updated periodically.[36] They include the following:

- Neurosurgery: DVT prophylaxis should be routinely used for patients undergoing major neurosurgery.

- Use intermittent pneumatic compression (IPC) boots with or without graduated compression (elastic) stockings (GCS).
- An acceptable alternative to the above is prophylaxis with low-dose unfractionated heparin (LDUH).
- Elective spine surgery
  - With no addition risk, no prophylaxis is recommended other than early mobilization.
  - With additional risk such as advanced age, known malignancy, etc., some form of prophylaxis is recommended.
  - With high-risk patients, prophylaxis is recommended with a variety of options that should be matched to the patient profile.
- Spinal cord injury
  - DVT prophylaxis is recommended for all patients with spinal cord injury.
  - The guidelines recommend *against* the use of LDUH, GCS, or IPC as a *single* modality. Therefore, the nurse should expect to provide a combination of interventions to prevent DVTs.

The Skin and Related Structures

The skin is an important barrier to infection; it assists in heat regulation through sweating to release heat and pilo-erection to retain heat as well as cushioning the bony prominences. Sustained immobilization is the most important cause of skin breakdown. Pressure transmitted to the skin, subcutaneous tissue, and muscles, particularly over bony prominences, can result in ischemia and necrosis. Shearing forces and friction related to moving patients can cause direct injury to the skin, which results in pressure ulcers. In addition, incontinence, profuse perspiration, poor nutrition, and obesity are factors related to pressure ulcer development. Immobilized patients are at high risk for developing pressure ulcers.

Assessment

The skin and related structures (hair, fingernails, toenails, scalp, hair, eyes, and oral cavity) should be assessed according to the following guidelines.

Skin

- Identify all risk factors present for skin breakdown.
- Assess the risk of skin breakdown using the Braden Scale or Norton Scale upon admission and discharge as well as weekly during the hospitalization.
- Assess the skin for color, temperature, edema, dryness, redness, abrasions, and pressure ulcers.
- Every square inch of skin should be observed every shift (many areas are observed more frequently).
- Bony prominences, such as the elbows, iliac crest, or outer aspect of the ankle, can become irritated and red; assess all bony prominences for redness, irritation, or tears.
- Do *not* position the patient on an area with reddened or broken skin.
- Assess fingernails and toenails for length and cleanliness.
- Assess the nose for signs of skin breakdown resulting from irritation caused by a nasal cannula, nasogastric tube, or endotracheal tube inserted nasally.

Other

- As previously discussed, assess the mucous membranes of the oral cavity for dryness, irritation, signs of oral infections (yeast and others), and broken areas; the tongue may be coated daily.
- Assess eyes for edema, redness, and drainage daily.
- Assess scalp and hair for reddened areas (especially at occiput), abrasions, and pediculosis.

Abnormal findings may include redness of the skin, broken skin, pressure ulcers, dry lips and oral cavity, cracked lips, oral infection, eye infection, dryness of the eye, drainage from the eye, inability to close the eye, matted hair, pediculosis, long fingernails that cut into the palms of the hand, and long toenails that scratch the skin. Common related patient problems include *risk for impaired skin integrity, altered oral mucous membrane, risk for infection, and risk for impaired tissue integrity (corneal).*

Nursing Interventions

Evidence-based practice guidelines are available to predict, prevent, and treat pressure ulcers. These are outlined in the Clinical Practice Guideline *Pressure Ulcers in Adults: Prediction and Prevention.*[37] Follow your institutional evidence-based practice guidelines to prevent pressure ulcers.

The following section lists additional points for nursing care.

Skin Care

- Keep the skin clean and dry; provide frequent skin care.
- Male patients should be shaved daily. If the patient is receiving anticoagulation therapy, an electric razor should be used.
- Trophic skin changes, such as dryness, can occur with some neurological conditions; lubricate the skin with lotion to prevent skin breakdown.
- Provide frequent skin care.
- Turn and reposition the patient every 1 to 2 hours; be sure the heels are off the bed and other vulnerable areas are positioned and protected to prevent pressure ulcers.
- Do not use donut appliances, which simply reposition areas of breakdown.
- When moving the patient, turn and lift rather than pull, which results in shearing and friction on skin.
- Consider using a special bed to prevent skin breakdown in high-risk patients.
- Retape and reposition the nasogastric and endotracheal tubes daily to prevent skin necrosis from the tube.

Mouth Care

- Cleanse and lubricate the mouth, gingiva, and tongue frequently (e.g., q4h) to prevent dryness, oral infections, and gum disease.
- Brush the teeth three to four times daily with the aid of a suction catheter to remove drainage from mouth.
- Lubricate the lips and oral cavity with a water base moisturizer to prevent dryness and cracking.
- Follow research-based best-practice protocols for mouth care.

Eye Care

- Inspect eyes for signs of edema, ecchymosis, eye drainage, irritation, or abrasions.
- Cleanse eyes to remove exudate with cotton balls and saline; the eyes should then be lubricated with methylcellulose or normal saline drops four times daily. The unconscious patient cannot blink periodically to cleanse and lubricate the eyes. Corneal drying or injury to the eye can lead to corneal ulceration and blindness. Many physicians order taping of the eyelids to reduce corneal abrasions. Application of an eye patch or eye shield may be helpful to protect the eye from injury.

Scalp and Hair Care.   The scalp and hair require attention:

- Examine the scalp for abrasions, pressure ulcers (especially in the occiput region), and edema. Treat any bruised or broken area.
- Patients with head trauma may have hair that is matted with blood, dirt, or glass; remove by combing and washing the hair, if not contraindicated, according to hospital procedure.
- Comb the hair; long hair can be braided or pulled to the side with an elastic band.

Fingernails and Toenails.   An unconscious patient may clench the fists, thereby digging the nails into the hands and causing injury. File and clip fingernails and toenails to protect the patient from injury.

Musculoskeletal Function

Immobility has a profound effect on the musculoskeletal system, including decreased muscle strength, shortening of muscles, increased muscle weakness and atrophy, contractures, and osteoporosis. At the cellular level, intracellular adenosine triphosphate (ATP) and glycogen concentrations decrease, rates of protein degradation increase, and contractility declines.[30]

- **Decreased muscle strength:** The degree of loss varies with the particular muscle groups and the degree of immobility. The antigravitational muscles of the legs lose strength twice as fast as the arm muscles, and recovery takes longer.
- **Decreased muscle mass and muscle atrophy:** Dramatic changes in muscle mass occur within 4 to 6 weeks of bed rest, accompanied by a decrease of 6% to 40% in muscle strength.[38] Muscle atrophy means loss of muscle mass. When a muscle is relaxed, it atrophies about twice as fast as one held in a stretched position. Because increased muscle tone prevents complete atrophy, patients with upper motor neuron disease and spastic paralysis lose less muscle mass. In contrast, with lower motor neuron disease and flaccid paralysis, muscle bulk lost is much more rapid. Muscle fibers are replaced by connective tissue with disuse.
- **Contractures:** A contracture is a loss of full range of motion, usually of a joint. When a muscle is maintained in a relaxed, shortened position for even 5 to 7 days, the mus-

cle shortens. Prolonged immobility results in loss of muscle mass. Joints change to dense connective tissue characteristic of a contracture.

- **Bone demineralization and osteoporosis:** Weight bearing and movement are critical to maintain bone formation and calcium balance. Immobilization results in significant bone loss. Significant loss of bone mineral density of the lumbar spine, femoral neck, and calcaneus observed in healthy men after bed rest are not full reversed after 6 months of normal weight-bearing activity. Further, the lost bone mass is not regained for some weeks or months after the muscle mass and strength have returned to normal, which increases the risk of fracture.[38] An osteoporosis state predisposes the patient to vertebral compression, long bone, and hip fractures. Hypercalcemia and hypercalciuria, which reflect loss of total body calcium, occur with bed rest. The high level of calcium in the urinary tract contributes to urinary calculus formation. When these physiologic changes are superimposed on elderly patients with decreased muscle and bone mass, the effects of bed rest are further enhanced.

Assessment

The muscles of the upper and lower extremities, neck, and shoulders should be assessed for tone, bulk, and range of motion, and both sides of the body should be assessed and findings compared.[39]

Musculoskeletal Problems

Abnormal findings commonly found in neuroscience patients include decreased muscle tone (e.g., flaccidity, paresis, paralysis), increased muscle tone (rigidity, decortication, decerebration, tremors), muscle atrophy, contractures, ankylosis, and joint dislocation. Common related patient problems include *impaired physical mobility and risk for trauma (e.g., contractures, stress fractures, and joint dislocation)*.

Nursing Interventions

The following nursing interventions are useful for preserving musculoskeletal function in the patient with a depressed state of consciousness:

- Position the patient in a neutral side-lying position in proper body alignment using pillows, rolls, and other equipment (e.g., positioning boots, splints, and trochanter rolls) as needed (see Chap. 11).
- Although the side-lying position is most often used, the dorsal position with the patient lying on his or her back is also useful. The same principles apply for alignment.
  - The head is in neutral position aligned with the spine.
  - The arms are slightly flexed at the elbows with the hands resting at the sides on pillows with the fingers extended over the pillows.
  - The hips are aligned with the head. Place a pillow between the legs to prevent internal rotation, adduction, and inversion of the upper leg.
  - The knees are positioned in slight flexion, often supported by a pillow for each leg. Care must be taken to prevent pressure on the peroneal nerve at the fibula head.

- The feet should be flexed at the ankles with the feet close to parallel with the wall. The heels should be elevated to prevent pressure and potential decubitus ulcer formation on the heels. Athletic shoes or positioning boots are useful to maintain the position of the feet.

CLINICAL PEARLS: Improper alignment/positioning may be a source of pain/distress. Assess position and/or foreign objects under the patient.

- Variations in positioning are required for *flaccid paralysis* and *flexor* or *extensor posturing, also known as decortication or decerebration.*
  - **Flaccid paralysis:** Position with boots or splints to prevent a contracture and trochanter towel rolls to prevent entrapment neuropathy of the peroneal nerve. Avoid compression at the elbows to prevent injury to the ulnar nerve.[40]
  - **Flexor or extensor posturing:** These patients are difficult to position because of the rigidity, and splints are usually not useful. Application of high-top athletic shoes assists in proper positioning of the feet.
- Points of positioning vary for *hemiplegia*. Whether on the back or in the side-lying position, align the head, neck, and spine in neutral position.
- In the side-lying position, position the patient on the unaffected side. The affected arm is slightly flexed, on a pillow that extends just below the axillary region. The pillow placement counteracts arm and shoulder adduction and internal rotation.
  - To prevent dependent edema, position each joint higher than the preceding joint, moving from the proximal to the terminal joints.
  - Flex the lower leg and place a pillow between the legs to align the legs properly.
  - For patients with a hemi-neglect syndrome, positioning the patient facing toward the affected side is useful.
  - Use a trochanter roll to prevent external rotation of the hip.
- In the dorsal position, lying on the back, use the pillow, as already described, to position the arms, hips, and legs.
- Reposition in proper body alignment every 1 to 2 hours or more frequently if reddened areas are present. Do not position the patient on reddened areas.
- If splints are used, take them off periodically and monitor skin for redness or breakdown.
- Administer passive range-of-motion exercises every 4 hours.
- Involve physical therapy/occupational therapy in the plan of care immediately and collaborate with them on the care. (An order is usually written for a physical therapy/occupational therapy consultation with admission orders.)

Genitourinary Function

Assuming the supine position while immobilized results in urinary stasis in the renal pelvis and urinary bladder, which provides a medium for bacterial growth. In addition, urinary retention and bladder distention may be present due to neurological pathology. The unconscious patient is at risk for two major problems: urinary tract infections and kidney and bladder stones (calculi). The causes of infection are the use of an indwelling catheter and urinary stasis. The stasis of urine in the bladder promotes bladder infections and ascending infections, which can involve the kidneys. The stasis of urine in the renal pelvis and bladder encourages formation of calculi. The increased levels of calcium being excreted from demineralized bones, another effect of immobilization, result in hypercalciuria and contribute to the formation of urinary calculi. In addition, acute renal failure can develop.

Assessment

- Monitor 24-hour intake and output record.
- Identify the characteristics of the urine (e.g., color, cloudiness).
- Monitor urinalysis, urine cultures, creatinine, and blood urea nitrogen.

Common related patient problems include *altered urinary elimination, incontinence, and risk for infection.*

Nursing Interventions

Methods of managing urine must be considered in patients with depressed states of consciousness. On admission, an indwelling catheter is usually inserted. This may be necessary to monitor fractional urinary output for patients receiving diuretic therapy (e.g., mannitol), those with diabetes insipidus, or other patients in whom careful and frequent monitoring of output is necessary. Another reason for catheter insertion is to keep the patient dry to prevent skin breakdown. The catheter itself is a foreign body and thus an irritant to the urinary tract. The literature supports a direct relationship between urinary catheters and urinary tract infection. There are some special considerations when weighing the benefits and risks of inserting and maintaining an indwelling catheter.

- If an indwelling catheter is necessary temporarily, remove it as soon as possible.
- For the male patient, a condom catheter may be a possible choice.
- An alternative to continuous urinary drainage is an intermittent catheterization program, useful in both genders.
- For some patients, absorbent incontinence pads that are changed frequently may be chosen to avoid the risk of infection from a catheter.
- Consider the condition of the skin. If areas of skin breakdown already exist, being wet for even a short time could increase that breakdown. (See Chap. 11 for further discussion.)
- The indwelling catheter should be removed as early as possible.

Gastrointestinal Function

Gastric ulcers, gastrointestinal bleeding, constipation, and fecal impaction are common in immobilized and unconscious patients. Gastric irritation can develop from drug therapy or hypersympathetic activity related to the primary neurological problems. Normal stimulation to peristalsis, such as physical activity or a high-fiber diet, is absent. Nutrition is commonly provided by enteral tube feeding, which does not generally stimulate peristalsis adequately. Some components of the therapeutic plan, such as drugs, contribute to constipation. Loose stools or diarrhea are also common in the unconscious immobilized patient, most often in response to poorly tolerated enteral feeding or drugs, especially antibiotics. In cases of severe diarrhea, pseudomembranous colitis due to *Clostridium difficile* should be suspected. A stool specimen for culture may be ordered.

Assessment

- Auscultate the abdomen for presence and strength (e.g., faint, sluggish, hyperactive) of bowel sounds.
- Note and record the consistency, color, amount, and frequency of stools.
- Review the intake and output record and 24-hour balance for the last several days to determine the hydration status of the patient.
- Review the medication record to identify drugs that may affect peristalsis and bowel evacuation.
- Ascertain the amount of fiber in the tube feeding the patient is receiving; seek consultation with the clinical dietician.
- Monitor stool for occult blood.
- If possible, monitor gastric aspiration for occult blood.
- Initiate a bowel program early.

Gastrointestinal Problems

Abnormal findings may include a distended abdomen with decreased or absent bowel sounds, paralytic ileus, hyperactive bowel sounds, or positive hemo-occult gastric aspirant or stools. Common related patient problems include *bowel incontinence, diarrhea (related to intolerance of tube feeding, effects of drugs, or infection), and colonic constipation.*

Nursing Interventions

A hospital-approved bowel program (e.g., stool softeners, bulk former, mild laxatives) should be instituted and followed. These drugs can be given through a feeding tube, gastrostomy, or jejunostomy tube. (See Chap. 11 for a sample protocol.) If constipation or diarrhea is a problem, a few points should be kept in mind.

- Constipation increases intra-abdominal pressure, which in turn can increase intracranial pressure.
- A drug to stimulate peristalsis may be added, such as metoclopramide (Reglan).
- In the case of diarrhea, the following should be kept in mind:
  - Review the type and rate of enteral feeding ordered; feeding intolerance, especially to lactose, may be present.
  - Consult with the clinical dietitian to determine dietary options (e.g., change the feeding to one of increased bulk or slow the rate of administration).
  - Consider an infectious process such as from pseudomembranous colitis if diarrhea is severe and ongoing.

- Concurrent drug therapy, especially antibiotics, can cause diarrhea. Discuss discontinuing a highly suspected drug or changing it to another drug.
- Consider adjusting the dosage and frequency of the drug.
- Add drug therapy to decrease peristalsis and control diarrhea.

Gastric aspirations and stool should be monitored for occult blood. This is necessary because gastrointestinal bleeding in the neurological patient is common, especially if a traumatic brain injury or intracranial insult has occurred. Another risk factor for gastrointestinal bleeding is concurrent drug therapy, such as dexamethasone, which is irritating to the gastrointestinal tract.

A gastric ulcer associated with neurological problems is called a Cushing's ulcer. All patients should be on a gastrointestinal prophylaxis drug regimen to prevent gastric ulcers. Proton pump inhibitors and histamine-2-receptor antagonists are the usual drug groups used for prophylaxis. It is unclear which drug group is superior.[41] Follow the unit protocol ordered by the physician.

> **CLINICAL VIGNETTE:** Mr. B is a 78-year-old man transferred to the medical floor after a long stay in the intensive care unit (ICU). During his ICU stay, he suffered a cardiac arrest, which resulted in hypoxic brain injury. For several weeks his Glasgow Coma Scale score has been stable at 8 (eye opening = 2, verbal = 1, motor = 5). He withdraws from painful stimuli and has 2/5 weakness on the right side. Vitals signs are stable. Mr. B expectorates copious amounts of secretions from his tracheostomy tube and requires frequent suctioning. He is obese and at risk of developing pressure ulcers. He has an indwelling urinary catheter and was treated for a urinary tract infection while in the ICU. Enteral nutrition is provided via a gastrostomy tube. The nurse creates a care plan for Mr. B.

Nosocomial Infections

Unconsciousness is related to high risk for infection for several reasons. Serious illnesses, often involving multiple body systems, challenge the body's immune system. Invasive procedures (e.g., surgery) and invasive equipment (e.g., central lines and urinary catheters) can lead to infection. Moreover, the use of antibiotics may result in opportunistic infections. Follow the Centers for Disease Control and Prevention (CDC) standards for body substance isolation. Body substance isolation means that gloves should be worn for anticipated contact with blood, secretions, and any moist body substances. Gloves are removed and properly disposed of between procedures and patients. When it is anticipated that contact with a patient could result in splashing of clothing, the skin, or face of the caregiver with secretions, blood, or body fluids, protective gear that includes gloves, a plastic apron, a mask, and goggles is worn. Proper disposal of contaminated material will isolate infectious material. The most effective method to prevent spread of infectious agents continues to be hand washing.

TABLE 15–1   CAUSES AND PREVENTION OF COMMON NOSOCOMIAL INFECTIONS

TYPE OF INFECTIONS	PREDISPOSING FACTORS	COMMON CAUSATIVE ORGANISMS*	PREVENTIVE MEASURES
Urinary tract infections	Indwelling catheters Straight catheterization	Gram-negative bacilli such as *Escherichia coli, Proteus mirabili, Enterococci faecali,* and *yeast;* in patients who had received an earlier course of antibiotic therapy *Pseudomonas aeruginosa, Serratia marcescens,* or *Enterobacter species* may be the causative organism.[†]	• Maintain a sterile closed urinary drainage system; no breaks in system when collecting urine samples. • Maintain dependent drainage. • Remove indwelling catheter as soon as possible. • Provide perineal care. • Prevent cross-contamination by strict adherence to handwashing protocol and wearing of gloves.
Respiratory infections (pneumonia)	Ventilatory assistance devices Dehydration Presence of tracheostomy or endotracheal tube Microaspiration	*Pseudomonas aeruginosa, Acinetobacter, Staphylococcus aureus, Haemophilus influenzae, Pneumococcus, Aspergillus* (chronic obstructive pulmonary disease patients with steroid use), multidrugresistant *S. aureus, Legionella,* anaerobes (aspiration)	• Change ventilation equipment according to hospital policy. • Follow aseptic suctioning procedure. • Administer tracheostomy care every 4 h. • Adhere to strict handwashing technique and principles of aseptic technique.
Vascular infections	Intravenous, arterial, and central catheters (phlebitis is the most common catheter-related infection) Hyperalimentation	Coagulase-negative *Staphylococci (Staphylococcus epidermidis* most common followed by *S. aureus, Enterococci, P. aeruginosa, Candida* organisms, *Enterobacter* organisms, *Acinetobacter* organisms, and *Serratia* organisms)[†]	• Change tubing according to hospital policy. • Inspect wound site for evidence of redness or infection. • Follow strict aseptic technique on insertion. • Change dressings according to hospital policy, using strict aseptic technique.
Intracranial; ventriculitis, other central nervous system infections	Intracranial monitors or catheters Contamination of craniotomy or spinal surgery incision Leakage of cerebrospinal fluid due to basal skull fractures	Ventriculitis: *S. epidermidis, S. aureus* Other infections: *S. aureus, Streptococcus, Neisseria meningitidis, H. influenzae, E. coli*	• Maintain a closed system. • Use strict aseptic technique for insertion and dressing change according to hospital policy. • Monitor insertion site and incision for evidence of infection.

*O'Grady, N. P., Barie, P. S., Bartlett, J., et al. (1998). Practice parameters for evaluating new fever in critically ill adult patients. *Critical Care Medicine, 26*(2), 392–408.
[†]Wijdicks, F. F. M. (1997). *The clinical practice of critical care neurology* (pp. 386–398). Philadelphia: Lippincott-Raven.

Follow CDC guidelines for hand washing. Table 15-1 lists major causes of infections.

Pain Management

Ongoing assessment and treatment of pain and anxiety aid in the prevention of secondary brain injury. Pain or anxiety can elevate intracranial pressure, heart rate, and systolic blood pressure, resulting in further physiologic damage. Recognizing pain and anxiety behaviors is necessary when caring for nonverbal patients. These behaviors may include grimacing, rigidity, wincing, brow furrowing, moaning, and restlessness. Pain-induced reflex responses may alter respiratory mechanics, increase cardiac demands, and cause contraction of skeletal muscles, muscle spasms, and rigidity.[42] Reassessment of pain and intervention efficacy ensures that the patient is progressing as expected and the chosen interventions are effective.[43]

CLINICAL PEARLS: When assessing neurological status (i.e., Glasgow Coma Scale), apply the least the amount of pressure to elicit a response.

Psychosocial Considerations

Although unconscious patients appear to be completely unaware of their environment, it is impossible to determine whether they are aware of any stimulus in the immediate environment. Many patients have regained consciousness and given accurate accounts of what happened and what was said to them when they were supposedly unconscious; therefore, it is important to maintain a positive attitude in the presence of these patients and assume that some stimuli do penetrate the complexities of unconsciousness.[44,45] Stimuli can be provided by playing the radio, touching the patient, and talking. In providing care, patients should be told what you will be doing. In addition, orient the patient to person, place, time, and the environment (weather and so forth).

CLINICAL PEARLS: Be mindful of discussions around patients; their ability to hear may still be intact.

Caring for patients with depressed states of consciousness includes not only caring for the patient, but for the patient's family as well. Relatives of these patients have been reported to experience a range of emotional reactions including shock, grief, anxiety, guilt, depression, and hostility toward caregivers. Family members may experience unexpected role changes such as assuming the role of primary caregiver or becoming the sole wage earner of the family while concurrently having lost a main source of emotional support. Psychological distress in family members can be exacerbated when relatives of the same patient experience different reactions.[46] For example, an adult patient's partner may have different expectations for outcomes than the patient's parents. It is important for health care organizations to be aware of the potential psychological stressors of illness and have protocols in place for support such as social workers, psychologists, and counselors.

THE CARE ENVIRONMENT

A safe and therapeutic care environment contributes to healing and recovery. The care environment is important for all patients, but particularly for those with depressed states of consciousness who are completely dependent on others for survival. A restorative care environment provides for the physical, emotional, and spiritual needs of the patient. Providing physical space that is clean, safe from hazards, and pleasing aesthetically increases the comfort levels of both patients and their families. Patient safety is of paramount importance; utilizing National Patient Safety goals is a priority for all health care providers.[47] A culture of patient safety is one that encourages clinicians, patients, and others to be vigilant in identifying potential or actual errors.[48]

Creating an environment for re-establishment of sleep-wakefulness cycles and other circadian rhythms is often challenging. Hospital settings are often very noisy from use of technology with monitors and alarms as well as the sounds created by the care providers, family, and patients. Newer architectural designs provide for therapeutic environments with control of temperature, light, sound, and air quality. However, it is the vigilant staff that implements the common-sense measure of a controlled environment to support the balance for patient care and rest. Strategic timing of nursing interventions allows for adequate time for restful sleep. Promoting undisturbed sleep may facilitate recovery from illness. The sleep/rest periods should not be filled with nursing activity.[49]

THERAPEUTIC COMMUNICATIONS

Therapeutic communications encompass a wide range of competencies. Communication skills facilitate imparting information and obtaining information. Active listening is a difficult discipline to acquire and requires intense concentration, attention, and focus to appreciate the obvious and subtle cues the patient is conveying, both verbally and nonverbally.[50] In a patient with a decreased level of consciousness, nonverbal cues and clinical findings may be the only source of assessing the patient's needs. For a patient with impaired consciousness, therapeutic touch combined with kind and soothing words can be a valuable means of providing reassurance and comfort.[10] Although unconscious patients

appear to be completely unaware of their environment, it is impossible to determine whether they are aware of any stimulus in the immediate environment. Many patients have regained consciousness and given accurate accounts of what happened and what was said to them when they were supposedly unconscious; therefore, it is important to maintain a positive attitude in the presence of the patient and assume that stimuli do penetrate the complexities of unconsciousness.[14,15] In providing care, the patient should be oriented to person, place, time, and the environment and told what you will be doing.

REGAINING CONSCIOUSNESS

Awakening from unconsciousness is usually a gradual process that has some degree of variability among patients over seconds, minutes, hours, or days. With improvement in the level of consciousness, the patient will be assessed for rehabilitation needs. See Chapter 11 for discussion of rehabilitation of neurological patients.

SUMMARY

There are few things more challenging than caring for a patient with a decreased level of consciousness. It is the quality of the nursing care and the ability of the nurse to identify risk factors, prevent complications, and maintain the highest functional level possible that will directly influence recovery and survival of the patient.

REFERENCES

1. Stevens, R., & Anish, B. (2006). Approach to the comatose patient. *Critical Care Medicine, 34*(1), 31–41.
2. Olson, D. M., & Graffagnino, C. (2005). Consciousness, coma, and caring for the brain-injured patient. *AACN Clinical Issues, 16*(4), 441–455.
3. Stevens, R. D., & Bhardway, A. (2006). Approach to the comatose patient. *Critical Care Medicine, 34*(1), 31–41.
4. Wijdicks, E. F. M., & Cranford, R. E. (2005). Clinical diagnosis of prolonged states of impaired consciousness in adults. *Mayo Clinical Proceedings, 80*(8), 1037–1046.
5. Milazzo, V., & Resh, C. (1981). Kinetic nursing—a new approach to the problems of immobility. *Journal of Neurosurgical Nursing, 14*, 120–124.
6. Brand, C., Campbell, D., Jones, C., Russell, D., Andrew, L., & Tweddle, N. (2003). A randomized controlled trial of an exercise intervention to reduce functional decline and health service utilization in the elderly. Retrieved February 12, 2006, from http://www.mh.org.au/ClinicalEpidemology/New_files?ProtocolFMP.pdf.
7. Szaflarski, N. L. (1996). Immobility phenomena in critically ill adults. In J. M. Clochesy, C. Breu, S. Cardin, A. A. Whitaker, & E. B. Rudy (Eds.). *Critical care nursing* (2nd ed., pp. 1313–1334). Philadelphia: W. B. Saunders.
8. Allen, C., Glasziou, P., & Del Mar, C. (1999). Bed rest: A potentially harmful treatment needing more careful evaluation. *Lancet, 354*, 1229–1233.
9. Convertino, V. A. (1997). Cardiovascular consequences of bed rest: Effect on maximal oxygen uptake. *Medical Science and Sports Exercise, 29*(2), 191–196.

10. Geraghty, M. (2005). Nursing the unconscious patient. *Nursing Standard, 20*(1), 54–64.

11. Mobily, P., & Kelley, L. (1991). Iatrogenesis in the elderly: Factors of immobility. *Journal of Gerontological Nursing, 17*(9), 5–10.

12. Sharp, J. T., Goldberg, N. B., & Druz, W. S. (1975). Relative contributions of rib cage and abdomen to breathing in normal subjects. *Journal of Applied Physiology, 39*, 608.

13. Harper, C. M., & Lyles, Y. M. (1988). Physiology and complications of bed rest. *Journal of the American Geriatric Society, 36*, 1047–1054.

14. Ropper, A. H., Gress, D. R., Diringer, M. N., Green, D. M., Mayer, S. A., & Bleck, T. P. (2004). Pulmonary aspects of neurological intensive care. In A. H. Ropper, D. R. Gress, M. N. Diringer, D. M. Green, S. A. Mayer, & T. P. Bleck (Eds.). *Neurological and neurosurgical intensive care* (4th ed., pp. 52–91). Philadelphia: Lippincott Williams & Wilkins.

15. Aherns, T., Kollef, M., Stewart, J., & Shannon, W. (2004). Effect of kinetic therapy on pulmonary complication. *American Journal of Critical Care, 13*(5), 376–383.

16. Hanneman, S. K., & Gusick, G. M. (2005). Frequency of oral care and positioning of patient in critical care: A replication study. *American Journal of Critical Care, 14*(5), 378–387.

17. Schleder, B. J. (2003). Taking charge of ventilator-associated pneumonia. *Nursing Management, 34*, 27–33.

18. Centers for Disease Control and Prevention. (1997). Guidelines for prevention of nosocomial pneumonia. *MMWR Recommendation Report, 46*(RR-1), 1–79.

19. Centers for Disease Control and Prevention. (2004). Guidelines for preventing health-care associated pneumonia. 2003: Recommendations of the CDC and the Healthcare Infection Control Practices Advisory Committee. *MMWR Recommendation Report, 53*(RR-3), 1–36.

20. American Thoracic Society. (2005). Guidelines for the management of adults with hospital-acquired, ventilator-associated, and healthcare-associated pneumonia. *American Journal of Respiratory Critical Care Medicine, 171*, 388–416.

21. Cook, D. J., Meade, M. O., Hand, L. E., & McMullin, J. P. (2002). Toward understanding evidence uptake: Semirecumbency for pneumonia prevention. *Critical Care Medicine, 30*, 1472–1477.

22. Kollef, M. H. (1999). The prevention of ventilator-associated pneumonia. *New England Journal of Medicine, 340*, 627–634.

23. Grap, M. J., Munro, C. L., Ashtiani, B., & Bryant, S. (2003). Oral care interventions in critical care: Frequency and documentation. *American Journal of Critical Care, 12*(2), 113–119.

24. Cutler, C. J., & Davis, N. (2005). Improving oral care in patients receiving mechanical ventilation. *American Journal of Critical Care, 14*(5), 389–394.

25. Cohn, J. L., & Fulton, J. S. (2006). Nursing staff perspectives on oral care for neuroscience patients. *Journal of Neuroscience Nursing, 38*(1), 22–30.

26. Schleder, B., Stott, K., & Lloyd, R. (2002). The effect of a comprehensive oral care protocol on patients at risk for ventilator-associated pneumonia. *Journal of Advocate Health Care, 4*, 27–30.

27. Scannapieco, F. A. (1999). Role of oral bacteria in respiratory infection. *Journal of Periodontology, 70*(7), 792–802.

28. Campbell, D. L. (2002). Development of a research-based oral care procedure for patients with artificial airways. *NTI News*, May 7, 2002.

29. Convertino, V. A., Bloomfield, S. A., & Greenleaf, J. E. (1997). An overview of the issues: Physiological effects of bed rest and restricted physical activity. *Medical Science and Sports Exercise, 29*(2), 187–190.

30. Resnick, N. M., & Dosa, D. (2005). Geriatric medicine. In D. L. Kasper, E. Braunwald, A. S. Fauci, E., S. L. Hauser, D. L. Longo, & J. L. Jameson (Eds.). *Harrison's principles of internal medicine* (16th ed., pp. 43–52). New York: McGraw-Hill.

31. Rubin, M. (1988). The physiology of bedrest. *American Journal of Nursing, 88*, 50–56.

32. Gillis, A., & MacDonald, B. (2005). Prevention deconditioning in the hospitalized elderly. *Canadian Nurse, 101*(6), 16–20.

33. Cree, C. (2003). Acquired brain injury: Acute management. *Nursing Standard, 18*(11), 45–56.

34. Bates, S. M., & Ginsberg, J. S. (2004). Treatment of deep-vein thrombosis. *New England Journal of Medicine, 351*, 268–277.

35. Saleem, S., & Vallbona, C. (1995). Immobilization. In S. J. Garrison (Ed.). *Handbook of medicine and rehabilitation basics* (pp. 185–196). Philadelphia: J. B. Lippincott.

36. Geert, W. H., Pineo, G. F., Hett, J. A., et al. (2004). Prevention of venous thromboembolism. *Chest, 126*, 338S–400S.

37. Panel for the Prediction and Prevention of Pressure Adults. (1992). *Pressure ulcers in adults: Prediction and prevention for assessment and management of patients*. Clinical Practice Guidelines, No. 3. AHCPR Publication No 92-0047, Rockville, MD: Agency for Health Care Policy and Research, U. S. Department of Health and Human Services.

38. Bloomfield., S. A. (1997). Changes in musculoskeletal structure and function with prolonged bed rest. *Medical Science and Sports Exercise, 29*(2), 197–206.

39. Markey, D. W., & Brown, R. J. (2002). An interdisciplinary approach to addressing patient activity and mobility in the medical-surgical patient. *Journal of Nursing Care and Quality, 16*(4), 1–12.

40. Wijdicks, E. F. M. (1997). *The clinical practice of critical care neurology* (pp. 4–14). Philadelphia: Lippincott-Raven.

41. Cash, B. D. (2002). Evidence-based medicine as it applies to acid suppression in the hospitalized patient. *Critical Care Medicine, 30*(6), S373–S378.

42. Puntillo, K., Morris, A. B., Thompson, C. L., et al. (2004). Pain behaviors observed during six common procedures: Results from Thunder Project II. *Critical Care Medicine, 32*(1), 421–427.

43. D'Arcy, Y., & McCarberg, B. (2005). Field guide to pain: Part 2: Developing a plan of care. *Nurse Practitioner, 30*(10), 60–62.

44. Jacobson, A. F. (2000). Caring for unconscious patients: Do they really remember? *American Journal of Nursing, 100*(1), 69.

45. Stein-Parbury, J., & McKinley, S. (2000). Patients' experiences of being in an intensive care unit: A select literature review. *American Journal of Critical Care, 9*(1), 20–27.

46. Crawford, S., & Beaumont, G. (2005). Psychological needs of patients in low awareness states, their families, and health professionals. *Neuropsychological Rehabilitation, 15*(3–4), 548–555.

47. Joint Commission on Accreditation of Health-Care Organization. (2006). Facts about 2006 National Patient Safety Goals. Retrieved February 28, 2006 from www.jcaho.org/accredited+organizations/patient+safety/06_npsg/06_cah_hap. htm

48. Phillips, J. (2005). Neuroscience critical care: The role of the advanced practice nurse in patient safety. *AACN Clinical Issues, 16*(4), 581–592.

49. Gerber, C. (2005). Understanding and managing coma stimulation. *Critical Care Nurse Quarterly, 28*(2), 94–108.

50. Robertson, K. (2005). Active listening: More than just paying attention. *Australian Family Physician, 34*(12), 1053–1055.

Neuroscience Critical Care

Susan Chioffi

Patients who have sustained severe central nervous system (CNS) insult require critically timed interventions, ongoing monitoring of multiple physiologic parameters, and frequent astute assessments by appropriately trained personnel. This chapter is intended to provide an overview of the environment in which these needs are best met and features of an ideal neuroscience critical care unit. Management of the neuroscience patient is discussed, with emphasis on ways in which scientific evidence has both supported and changed practice. Special characteristics of patients with significant CNS insults as well as commonalities with other critical care populations are addressed, including use of existing and emerging technologies. The ethical and legal considerations related to end-of-life care in the critical care environment are considered, with a particular emphasis on the management of the potential organ donor.

Caring for the critically ill patient with serious CNS injuries allows the bedside nurse to see the extent to which excellent nursing care can be a major factor in reducing morbidity and mortality. The frequent neurological assessments performed by the nurse are key to early recognition of new neurological deficits or deterioration of existing conditions. The nurse rapidly institutes ordered therapies, evaluates their effectiveness, monitors for the development of complications, consults with appropriate personnel for additional interventions, and generally ensures that care is provided according to accepted practice guidelines and protocols. In the acute and subacute stages of illness, while most of the focus is on preventing or minimizing secondary brain injury, the nurse is also responsible for preventing complications such as infection or those arising from prolonged immobility and bed rest. As the neuroscience patient is at high risk for self-injury related to temporary disorientation and confusion associated with CNS insult, special safety interventions are required.

CRITICAL CARE PERSONNEL

While the physical environment of the neuroscience critical care unit is of utmost importance, the model of care and the competencies of the professional staff determine the quality of care and patient outcomes. Best practices in neuroscience critical care emphasize the collaborative interdisciplinary team model of health care delivery with a particular focus on neuroscience and critical care training. The multiple disciplines of the core intensive care unit (ICU) team include physician

intensivists, bedside and advanced practice neuroscience critical care nurses, clinical pharmacists, and respiratory therapists. Interdisciplinary care is based on a comprehensive approach that includes standards, protocols, and guidelines consistent with high-quality evidenced-based care.[1,2] In critical care environments, physician intensivists are the gatekeepers who determine what services will be involved in the care of the patient. They conduct independent assessments of needs; establish discipline-specific goals, which they then work to meet; and communicate their assessment, goals, and progress to the rest of the team. A characteristic of an interdisciplinary team is the process of discussion among the team members leading to a comprehensive plan of care. This process engenders shared responsibility for outcomes.[3,4]

Physician Intensivists

Much attention has been focused on the usefulness of critical care trained physicians leading the care team in the ICU. Hospitals that use physician intensivists can show improved outcomes with fewer complications and decreased length of stay in intensive care units when compared with nonintensivist models of practice.[5] Various studies have shown that ICU teams directed by critical care board-certified physicians are associated with decreased morbidity and mortality as well as decreases in cost and sometimes length of stay.[6,7] Moreover, other studies looking at neuroscience ICUs in particular have shown improved patient outcomes with the use of intensivists.[5,8,9]

Critical Care Advanced Practice Nurses

Some health care facilities are also employing midlevel providers such as acute care nurse practitioners (ACNPs) to provide care in the ICU.[10,11] Advanced practice nurses (APNs) can participate in the team either in the role of a clinical nurse specialist or as an ACNP. As a clinical nurse specialist (CNS), the APN supports and promotes evidence-based practice, supports research initiatives, provides education and mentoring of the nursing staff, and assumes a leadership role in the education of patients and family.[12] By comparison, in the ACNP role, the APN is instrumental in implementing research-based protocols[13] while developing, ordering, and following through with a plan of care in collaboration with the intensive care physician.[14] Both the CNS and the ACNP have a positive influence on team collaboration, promoting clinical expertise and improved patient outcomes. A number of studies have established the benefits of APNs in the care of acute and critically ill patients.[15,16]

Critical Care Nurses

The bedside nurse, who is present on a round-the-clock basis, is the mainstay of care for the hospitalized ICU patient. Nursing staffing levels and nursing experience have been shown to affect such critical patient variables as infection rates of central venous catheters, preventable adverse events, and rapidity of ventilator weaning.[17] Critical care nurses perform the majority of patient assessments, evaluation of outcomes, and care delivery in the ICU. They are responsible for assessing the accuracy of technological devices that collect physiologic data, recording the data, and synthesizing the information for the development of an appropriate nursing plan of care tailored to the individual patient. The nurse must be able to keep the ever-expanding array of information in perspective while collaborating on the medical plan of care with the physician or midlevel provider. The data collected may also be used for approved research studies conducted on the unit, thereby contributing to the body of evidence supporting current therapies, investigational devices, or protocols.

Nurses require specialized training including completion of a critical care nursing course and unit orientation.[18] Nurses in neuroscience critical care units require additional training in neuroscience nursing. Studies examining the value of a neuroscience ICU emphasize not only specialized physician training, but also specialized nursing training as factors in improved patient outcomes.[9] Specialty nursing certification is desirable as it demonstrates practice experience and knowledge in that specialty, commitment to extensive continuing education activities, and an interest in the pursuit of excellence. Research is ongoing to assess how nursing certification is linked to improved patient outcomes, but it is difficult to isolate certification as a variable from the myriad other nurse-related variables that have an impact on patient outcomes.[19]

Critical Care Clinical Pharmacists

Clinical pharmacists who focus on the medications ordered for the critically ill, as well as medications most frequently used in the neuroscience population, are integral to the proper care of the patient with a severe CNS insult.[1] Many errors in the ICU are related to medication choice, dose, or delivery method.[20-23] The involvement of a clinical pharmacist has a positive effect on error reduction. The clinical pharmacist rounds with the critical care team, provides medication-related education, evaluates all drug therapy orders, monitors dosing and administration regimens, evaluates adverse reactions and medication interactions, and provides education as well as recommendations on cost containment issues.[17,18,24]

Critical Care Respiratory Therapists

Respiratory therapists familiar with weaning protocols and other advanced respiratory interventions are necessary to manage the ventilatory needs of the critically ill.[1] The critical care respiratory therapist brings expertise in mechanical ventilation and weaning protocols and proficiency in the transport of critically ill patients.[18] Respiratory therapists have specialized knowledge in the judicious use of noninvasive ventilation to avoid intubation and in the employment of strategies to prevent ventilator-associated pneumonia (VAP). As a result, their involvement contributes to improved outcomes.

Other Team Members

While the preceding intensive care providers comprise the interdisciplinary care team that works collaboratively throughout the day making changes in each patient's plan of care, there are other health care providers whose consultative services are only required intermittently though they are integral to successful patient care outcomes. These team members include nutritional support, speech pathology, physical therapy, occupational therapy, social work, and case managers. The workload for each of these providers includes patients outside of the ICU, so their involvement with patients, while important, is sporadic.

Nutritional Support: Clinical Dietician

Many critically ill neuroscience patients have an impaired ability to swallow due to an altered level of consciousness or neurological injuries and require nutritional support by an other-than-oral route. When use of the oral route is contraindicated, the enteral route is preferred; thus, patients will require the placement of a nasogastric, orogastric, postpyloric, or implanted feeding tube for nutrition. A registered dietician has the requisite knowledge to determine the most appropriate nutritional formula based on each patient's current illness, comorbidities, and nutritional requirements (see Chap. 8). The dietician can recommend other nutritional supplements and timing of diagnostic tests to assess the adequacy of nutritional support.

Speech Pathology: Speech Pathologist

As the patient's condition stabilizes or improves, a speech pathologist may be consulted. The speech pathologist evaluates the patient and makes recommendations in three areas. First, the pathologist assesses the patient's swallowing abilities and makes recommendations as to whether oral nutrition is safe based on a swallowing evaluation and, if so, what consistencies of foods and liquids should be ordered. Second, the patient's ability to communicate is assessed and communication tools such as special spelling or picture boards can be recommended and provided. Additionally, the use of speaking valves for patients with tracheostomies can be assessed and a plan implemented. Third, cognitive evaluation of the patient may be conducted, although this is often postponed until consciousness is re-established and mental status evaluation is possible.

Physical and Occupational Therapies: Physical Therapist and Occupational Therapist

The motor and cognitive impairments many neuroscience ICU patients experience require the involvement of a physical therapist and an occupational therapist. The physical therapist's focus is to maintain a patient's range of motion and assist with advancing the patient's mobility as his or her condition warrants. The physical therapist may recommend use of splints or other supportive devices to assist with motor recovery and prevention of neuromuscular complications. The occupational therapist's focus is to assist the awake patient to re-establish self-care abilities or to recommend alternative ways of adapting self-care activities to the patient's neurological deficits. Because the occupational therapist works with conscious patients who can engage in relearning of self-care activities, the occupational therapist may not see many patients in the neuroscience ICU but is more often consulted when that patient is recovering in an intermediate care unit.

Social Work: Social Worker

Some patients have complicated family situations that may affect transition along the continuum of care and the ability of the family to assist the patient in the recovery process. A social worker is particularly suited to assess family dynamics and support and to work with the family and social service agencies to meet the needs of the patient and family. Examples of situations in which the involvement of a social worker can be key include the following: the patient is a single parent with minor children and no immediate family available to assist with care decisions for the patient or children; or the patient has important family members in the military and arrangements must be made so the service member can be present at the patient's bedside.

Case Management: Case Manager

The job title and responsibilities associated with this position vary among health care facilities, but this is the health professional who oversees the patient discharge process. The case manager initially meets with the patient and family to discuss activities such as completing health care–related paperwork, evaluating the patient's current living situation and residence, and determining who will likely be the primary caregiver, should one be required, when the patient returns home. As the patient progresses, the case manager works with the interdisciplinary team to determine what posthospital care is best suited to the needs of the patient. The case manager then arranges for home health services or admission to a long-term acute care facility, rehabilitation facility, skilled nursing facility, or hospice.

The Importance of Teamwork

Whether the team approach leads to the best possible outcomes is not an aspect of care that can be easily studied due to the multiplicity of factors affecting patient outcomes (e.g., initial and ongoing severity of illness; time elapsed before appropriate care could be provided; availability of standard, emerging, and investigational therapies; the patient's comorbidities; and institutional variables). The functionality of the team is also key to assessing the effectiveness of such a model. Well-developed communication skills among members are critical to the success of a team. Effective communications allow the team to take full advantage of the expertise

each member brings to the group and to patients. Although further study is needed, the limited number of studies on this aspect of patient care do suggest that the adoption of the team model leads to better patient survival with lower hospital costs.[1,17]

There are significant barriers related to the widespread implementation of interdisciplinary critical care teams, including an impending shortage of critical care personnel and a growth in the need for critical care services associated with the looming increase in the numbers of elderly Americans.[1,6] It is expected that shortages of critical care physicians, nurses, pharmacists, and respiratory therapists will continue and worsen over the next 20 years.[6] Critical care delivery itself is currently very heterogeneous in America.[1] Some facilities have general ICUs, while others offer specialized ICUs such as neuroscience ICUs. Variations are also apparent according to university versus nonuniversity affiliation, state or city versus privately operated facilities, small versus large facilities, and urban versus rural settings. Some ICUs are "closed" units and others "open," based on physician admitting privileges. A closed unit refers to an ICU in which only the physician intensivists may admit a patient to the unit and the ICU staff assume complete responsibility for the patient until discharge from the unit. At that time, the primary admitting physician once again assumes responsibility for the medical management of the patient. In an open unit, any physician can admit a patient to the unit; that physician continues to assume responsibility and authority for the care administered in the ICU. The ICU physicians and staff are collaborators, but do not have final authority about the plan of care. There are wide variations in the availabilities and types of physicians, nursing care providers, and other providers. Even with all these variations, all ICUs are still responsible for the provision of quality care with optimal outcomes to critically ill patients.

While interdisciplinary collaboration is a key to successful teamwork, difficulties remain in nurse–physician collaboration related to the power differential between the professions. Nursing focuses on a holistic conceptual model of care, while physicians have a disease-based focus. With recognition of these differences, efforts can be made to utilize the strengths of each profession to improve understanding and collaboration.[25] Difficulties in communication at all levels have been identified as an ongoing problem in health care. Miscommunication, whether spoken or written, can contribute significantly to medical errors and subsequent patient harm; it can also contribute to an unhealthy work environment for all members of the patient care team.[14] Some barriers to effective communication of medical information are different communication styles, inadequate flow of information between team members, and human problems such as lack of knowledge, fatigue, and stress. Nurses in their educational programs learn to communicate narratively and descriptively, while physicians, in their search for answers, focus more narrowly on the facts. The critical care team needs a communication strategy to optimize clinical communication. The ideal model provides concrete and precise data about a particular patient within a specific situation, which includes an assessment of the patient care issue and recommendations for resolution of the issue. Some remedies for the inadequate flow of information include comprehensive written documentation forms and computerized health records, easily available to all, that list such key information as patient allergies; a standardized approach to "hand-off" communications with the opportunity to ask questions; and mechanisms for immediate reporting of critical values or information directly to the licensed responsible caregivers.

THE INTENSIVE CARE UNIT PHYSICAL ENVIRONMENT

The physical environment of any ICU encompasses several key features. The overall unit should be designed with nursing efficiency in mind, including easy access from all patient rooms of crucial supplies, storage, equipment, and medications. Families need adequate space for comfortable and pleasant waiting areas and rooms with privacy for meetings with health care providers, for counseling, and for grieving. Staff need space for work, a lounge/break area, and room for educational offerings.[26,27] While it is important that a patient room be designed so that multiple members of the care team can easily gain access to the patient at all times including crisis, this requirement must be balanced with patient and family needs to have a quiet and private setting. An ICU is by its very nature a bustling and noisy environment; it is all too easy to forget that patients experience that noise continuously. The ideal neuroscience ICU should have a structured program in which "quiet time" is scheduled and upheld.[28] Patient assessments, medications, and therapies are arranged so that none is required during quiet time. Lights (except those required for safety), televisions, and radios are turned off and curtains are drawn to create a quiet, dim environment. Family members are encouraged to leave the hospital and rest themselves. Besides allowing a very specific stretch of time in which all the patients can rest, it can help the staff to become more aware of the ambient noise levels and to take steps to decrease the intrusiveness of the environment outside of quiet time.[28]

A crucial component of any intensive care unit is the technology and monitoring equipment. An individual monitoring system provides numeric and real-time digitalized waveform representation of heart rate, blood pressure, and respirations as well as numeric representation of noninvasive blood pressure monitoring. It should be configurable so that numeric and visual representations of other monitoring devices can easily be added. Alarms must be easily adjustable according to individual patient needs and clearly indicate visually when an alarm has been turned off. An important aspect of alarm design is the need to create alarms for various devices that are easily distinguishable from other alarms as well as conveying some information about the clinical significance of the alarm. The sound of the alarm from a mechanical ventilator should sound more compelling than the alarm on a sequential compression device (SCD); an out-of-bed alarm should sound more important than an empty feeding pump. As the number of devices in use for critically ill patients increases, the difficulty in creating reasonably distinguishable alarms increases as well. Another difficulty associated with alarms is that people have different tolerances for alarms. For some, alarms are much more of a "foreground" noise and they are more alert to one going off; this is a useful attribute of an ICU nurse. It is far better to seek out and eliminate unnecessary alarms than it is to become accustomed to them and miss a critical alarm because some alarms have become "background" noise.

CLINICAL PEARLS: Eliminating alarms should focus on altering the reason for the alarm (e.g., ensuring that blood pressure alarms are set to the parameters for which interventions are required, carefully adjusting the sensitivity for a respiratory waveform so a respiratory rate will be counted accurately, or moving a pulse oximeter to a location where it will register correctly). Turning alarms off is *rarely* the appropriate course of action in these circumstances.

The bedside nurse is responsible for assessing the accurate function of equipment being used for a particular patient. The nurse must be properly educated about the setup and ongoing use of various machines, including troubleshooting. Some equipment requires a single training session, while others, as determined by individual institutions and specific unit management, require annual competency checkoffs. It is the professional responsibility of the individual nurse to obtain and maintain competency about equipment used regularly in the work area. Proper use of some equipment requires the ability to accurately calibrate and level the device; others require the ability to astutely assess waveforms and take appropriate action. Interventions can range from tightening connections and flushing lines as needed to requesting an assessment by the physician intensivist or midlevel provider for a damped ventriculostomy waveform, which could mean that the ventriculostomy is no longer draining, or a change in the pulmonary artery (PA) catheter waveform, which could mean a spontaneous wedging or that the catheter is no longer in the PA. A significant amount of nursing time can be dedicated to assessing and maintaining critical mechanical devices and technology.

Computerized documentation systems, while not yet universally available, are becoming an important tool for managing patient information. Critically ill neuroscience patients generate large amounts of data. Multiple physiologic parameters are assessed continuously and must be recorded every 5 to 15 minutes, and more frequently during critical time frames. A pen-and-paper system requires immediate recording on official forms or various personnel scribbling numbers on any available surface. A computerized system, with an interface to the monitoring system, can store the information until the appropriate personnel, generally the nurses, can download it and check it for accuracy before saving it, thus enabling the care team to concentrate on necessary interventions, not the recording of important data. Many computerized documentation systems have the capability to compress data, thus making it much easier to view large amounts of information and spot or track trends. Most systems also allow integration of information in a single place so that, for example, laboratory data can easily be tracked against physiologic data when assessing response to therapeutic interventions.

CLINICAL PEARLS: The nurse should regularly utilize the time compression feature to monitor patient response to therapy and look for trends that might point to an overlooked problem.

Computerized documentation systems can provide visual reminders to nurses about interventions such as oral care, patient repositioning, restraint-related activities, dressing changes, and weighing of patients. Nurses are thus reminded to document these interventions and add more detailed notes where appropriate. Drop-down menu lists encourage the use of standard medical terminology, which can facilitate interdisciplinary communication. It is important as well that a computerized information system have interdisciplinary documentation and support for alerts about new communications between disciplines; features that link orders and related documentation are also desirable.[29]

Maintaining and improving patient safety is of paramount importance in the hospital, and never more so than in the ICU. Medication administration has been identified as an especially error-prone aspect of hospitalization.[14,30,31] Safe medication administration becomes especially important in the intensive care setting where multiple medications are given by continuous intravenous infusion or intravenous bolus. A proposed intervention to improve patient safety is a computerized order entry system, particularly one that requires computerized entry of patient medications. Such a system alerts the person entering the medication order to patient allergies or to critical drug–drug interactions as well as whether a patient's home medications are nonformulary. It also requires that the drug name, route, dose, and frequency be clearly entered, and only standardized abbreviations are allowed in such a system. Necessary adjuncts to a computerized order entry system are standardized infusion concentrations and drip rate calculation programs to decrease the risk of incorrectly calculating medication doses. Another advantage of a computerized order entry system is that it encompasses routine admission orders, which include reminders on such things as venous embolism prophylaxis so that the initial orders are complete and comprehensive. Failure to provide such prophylactic treatment is another kind of medical error reported by the Institute of Medicine.[20] The initial expense of purchasing and implementing a computerized order entry system has slowed its adoption.

CLINICAL MANAGEMENT ISSUES

Cerebral Ischemia

After a patient has sustained the primary injury from a CNS insult, whether it is a cerebral contusion from trauma, an infarction from an embolic stroke, or subarachnoid hemorrhage from a ruptured intracranial aneurysm, multiple interventions must be undertaken to avoid secondary brain injury. Secondary brain injury occurs when normal tissue surrounding the injured area of the brain becomes ischemic due to a hypoxic cascade that can result in infarction, an irreversible state of neuronal death. Multimodal monitoring aids the critical care team in the early detection of the ischemic cascade so that appropriate interventions can be initiated before irreversible injury occurs.[32] The original CNS insult very often results in cerebral edema leading to increased intracranial pressure (ICP), which is a significant contributor to patient morbidity and mortality.[33] As intracranial pressure rises, compensatory mechanisms become exhausted and compromised cerebral perfusion leads to the risk for secondary brain injury. Concern about the effects of elevations in intracranial pressure led to the development of devices for monitoring intracranial pressure and, in some instances, to managing it. Some studies have shown that ICP monitoring, in conjunction with accepted brain injury management guidelines, appears to be associated with decreases in both mortality and morbidity.[33] Cerebral perfusion pressure (CPP) is derived from the ICP value by subtracting the ICP from the mean arterial pressure (MAP). The ICP and CPP are used together to guide therapeutic interventions for the patient who has sustained a severe CNS insult (see Chap. 13 for discussion of ICP).

CPP is an estimate of global cerebral blood flow. When a CNS insult results in impaired autoregulation, blood flow becomes pressure dependent and cerebral ischemia and infarct can occur if the perfusion pressure is inadequate. The recommended minimum CPP is 60 mm Hg,[34] and interventions to increase CPP are directed at increasing arterial blood pressure or decreasing ICP. In the management of vasospasm after subarachnoid hemorrhage, for example, hypertension and hypervolemia may be used to improve CPP and thereby increase cerebral blood flow.

Once a patient has an ICP monitoring device in place, the bedside nurse becomes the person most responsible for its proper use. The nurse must ensure that the device in question is appropriately calibrated, leveled, and properly connected to monitoring equipment. Furthermore, the nurse must protect the device from accidental dislodgement and be proficient in troubleshooting the device. Most importantly, the bedside nurse is responsible for accurately recording ICP device-generated data, recognizing the meaning of data, integrating it into the plan of care, and communicating the data to appropriate personnel in a timely and effective manner. Once a nurse has received adequate initial training about the use of an ICP monitoring device, competency validation on an annual basis is necessary. The types, uses, validity, reliability, and limitations of various ICP monitoring devices and systems available are described in detail in Chapter 13.

The nurse caring for a patient with an ICP monitor should frequently evaluate the effects of nursing and medical care, family presence, and spontaneous patient behaviors on the intracranial pressure value. This information is used to initiate measures to limit negative effects of selected activities on ICP elevations. For example, repositioning of a patient to facilitate care requires that the ICP device must always be correctly positioned so that an elevation in ICP can be promptly recognized and managed. Astute nursing judgment comes into play when the nurse must balance maintaining the ICP in the desired range with the need for necessary care activities such as performing pulmonary toilet activities to improve oxygenation and reduce the risk of pulmonary infection.[35] Family behaviors and interactions can be encouraged or discouraged based on observed physiologic responses, including changes in ICP. Studies to evaluate the effect of various nursing interventions continue to be conducted. Controversy exists about how often it is necessary to perform detailed neurological assessments on patients with significant elevations of ICP that have been difficult to control. Such patients often receive continuous sedation to control ICP, and temporarily discontinuing sedation to awaken a patient to conduct a neurological assessment can be associated with a dangerous elevation in ICP along with difficulty in returning the patient to an adequately sedated state.

CLINICAL PEARLS: The experienced critical care nurse continuously monitors trends and current physiologic parameters and collaborates with the interdisciplinary team in deciding on the necessity of continuing to frequently lighten sedation for neurological assessments. It is sometimes better for a patient to have the neuroscience ICU team maintain a steady level of sedation until physiologic data suggest that the ICP has improved enough for reversal of sedation to be safe.

Monitoring of the ICP and using the calculated derived CPP value to guide therapy is not considered adequate information for optimal medical management in some subgroups of patients. Adjunctive methods to assess intracranial dynamics such as cerebral blood flow (CBF) monitoring or assessment of cerebral oxygenation can be utilized. Technologies to provide continuous bedside monitoring of cerebral blood flow are emerging but are not the current standard of practice. Transcranial Doppler (TCD) studies are a noninvasive intermittent measure of cranial blood flow that can be used to evaluate flow disturbances in the circle of Willis.[36] TCD is frequently used to assess for changes in blood flow velocity, which can be an early indicator of cerebral arterial vasospasm in patients with subarachnoid hemorrhage following aneurysmal rupture. Changes in TCD values may precede clinical signs of vasospasm and can be a factor in altering therapeutic interventions. The American Association of Neurology advocates for the performance of TCD studies by trained ultrasonographers.[37] Although angiography is the "gold standard" for the detection of vasospasm, it is invasive and carries risks, which limit its use. TCD is better suited for serial monitoring since it is noninvasive and can easily be done on a daily basis at the bedside.[38]

An emerging adjunctive monitoring device looks at cerebral oxygen delivery by assessing brain tissue oxygenation, also known as $PbtO_2$, $PtiO_2$, $BtiO_2$, or $PbrO_2$. The retrograde jugular bulb catheter has been used to measure *global* oxygen extraction since the 1980s. A special oximetric catheter is placed up into the jugular vein to the level of the jugular bulb, a place where venous blood is minimally contaminated from extracerebral sources. Venous saturation is continuously recorded and blood is drawn intermittently to assess brain glucose and lactate levels. Unfortunately, the patient may experience significant cerebral ischemia before oxygen desaturation is recognized. Because the jugular catheter is a global measure, it does not reflect focal ischemia until it is significant enough to produce a change in global measurements.[39] There are also technical challenges associated with this technology. Careful management of the catheter by the nurse is required if reliable data are to be collected.[40]

A potentially better method of assessing brain tissue oxygenation involves direct measurement of cortical oxygenation. This new technology is being refined and its use is expected to become more prevalent in neurocritical care. There are currently two types of these monitors using different technology and generating slightly different values that require interpretation. Both monitoring systems involve a catheter, which, after appropriate calibration, is inserted by a trained physician or midlevel provider into the brain tissue, and the generated values are then used to guide therapy.[41] The location of the catheter is determined by the patient's diagnosis and possible coexisting injuries such as skull fractures. The normal $PbtO_2$ value falls between 25 and 50 mm Hg; a value below 20 requires intervention to prevent or limit secondary brain injury. Specific interventions are adjusted or initiated based on changes in the $PbtO_2$. Early studies show improved detection of brain hypoxia and a direct correlation between duration and severity of hypoxia and outcome.[40]

Perfusion computerized tomography (CT) studies are a form of CBF assessment used in acute ischemic stroke to differentiate areas of reversible and nonreversible ischemia.[42,43] Perfusion CT can also be used to predict outcome and some neurological deficits following traumatic brain injury.[38] CT angiography (CTA) studies are also used to assess CBF; CTA can look for intracranial aneurysms, arterial blockage, or narrowing when vasospasm is suspected. Perfusion CT and CTA both require the intravenous injection of iodinated contrast material.

From a nursing perspective, bedside monitoring technologies have better value for critically ill neuroscience patients than those, such as angiography, CTA, and perfusion CT, that require travel off the unit to the radiology department. Critically ill neuroscience patients are often exquisitely sensitive to position changes and relatively minor changes in oxygenation or carbon dioxide levels and can develop significant and dangerous increases in ICP when transported. Moving the patient from bed to table carries the risk of dislodging vital equipment or catheters or interrupting continuous intravenous infusion of medications. Conventional angiography and CTA studies as well as perfusion CT also require the nurse and the care team to consider possible adverse effects of the contrast material used for the study including patient allergy, possible renal damage, and volume shifts related to the osmotic diuretic effects of the agents used.

CLINICAL PEARLS: It is often the bedside nurse who reminds the team to think about the possibility of consequences of contrast dye.

Increasing intravenous fluid rates to prevent dehydration and the use of sodium bicarbonate infusions or Mucomyst (*N*-acetylcysteine) to mitigate possible renal damage in at-risk patients should be instituted as preemptive measures to limit the possibility of complications.[44,45] Any procedure that requires a critically ill patient, particularly one with a significant CNS insult, to be transported requires a clear answer to the question of how therapy for that patient will be immediately impacted by the resulting data before the procedure is undertaken.

Monitoring of Temperature, Blood Glucose, and Electrolytes

Temperature Monitoring. The patient's body temperature is a key concern in the neuroscience ICU, so it is frequently monitored on a continuous basis. As discussed later in the chapter, controversy exists in the literature about the clinical value of both treating fever and inducing hypothermia to improve patient outcomes. Physicians and nurses alike are concerned that sustained fever is detrimental to individual patients, so significant nursing efforts, based on physician-ordered therapies, are directed toward measures designed to avoid or treat fevers. The ambient room temperature is adjusted and portable fans are used for patient comfort. Acetaminophen is commonly used to treat fevers; ibuprofen is used more sparingly because of concerns about gastrointestinal disturbances or bleeding as a side effect. Many mechanical devices exist for the purpose of cooling febrile patients. External surface cooling devices have been in use for the longest amount of time. The hypothermia blanket is the most common one seen, but its effectiveness is limited by its slow cooling rate. Its use is also associated with shivering, "overshoot" of the temperature goal, patient discomfort, and concerns about skin integrity related to sustained contact with a very cold surface.[46] Mechanically ventilated patients frequently require the use of anesthetic agents and muscle relaxants to facilitate the cooling process. Other external devices that have been tried cool only the patient's head or are wrapped around the patient; these generate the same sorts of problems associated with the hypothermia blanket. Internal cooling is another mode that has been attempted. Cooled intravenous solutions have been used but tend to require large fluid volumes to achieve decreases in patient temperatures. Iced gastric lavage has been used. It is an especially labor-intensive therapy for nursing but is not particularly effective. Endovascular cooling using a special central venous catheter that works with a temperature-adjusted closed loop system is coming into use for patient temperature management. It has proven to be effective in decreasing patient temperature with less patient discomfort than other methods.[47]

Blood Glucose. Critically ill patients are frequently hyperglycemic on admission to the hospital. Increasing evidence suggests that hyperglycemia is associated with increased morbidity and mortality and that improving glycemic control improves patient outcomes.[48] Some studies have specifically shown worse outcomes in neuroscience patients,[49,50] while others have been directed at demonstrating the safety and benefits of intensive glucose management in patients with serious CNS injury.[51] Studies have focused on the use of continuous insulin infusion to maintain the patient's blood sugar between 80 and 110 mg/dL. Achieving tight glucose control requires that the critical care nurse obtain frequent measurements of the patient's blood sugar and make appropriate adjustments to the insulin infusion. There is no universal insulin infusion protocol, but the use of a continuous insulin infusion requires the adoption of an infusion protocol to facilitate rapid adjustment in the infusion as needed. Work continues on the best way to balance glycemic control and optimal patient safety, as avoidance of symptomatic hypoglycemia is paramount. When enteral feeds are suspended for procedures, high gastric residuals, or patient removal of feeding tubes, the need to adjust the insulin infusion to compensate for the lack of glucose intake should not be overlooked. Nursing vigilance is required to prevent the cognitively impaired patient from removing feeding tubes and increasing the risk of hypoglycemia.

Electrolyte Abnormalities. Neuroscience ICU patients are at risk for electrolyte disturbances related to their disease process, as a side effect of therapy, or a combination of the two. Sodium, potassium, magnesium, and phosphorus are the serum electrolytes that are most likely to require monitoring and repletion. The neuroscience ICU nurse is responsible for obtaining blood chemistries at ordered intervals, reporting abnormal values to the physician or midlevel provider, and collaborating on management. Many facilities have nurse-managed protocols for the repletion of potassium, magnesium, and phosphorus in the ICU. Sodium repletion can be associated with serious adverse patient outcomes, so it is managed on an individual patient basis.[52]

CLINICAL PEARLS: A *focal* change in a patient's neurological response should prompt concern for a structural cause such as cerebral arterial vasospasm or a cerebral infarct. A *global* change in neurological response is often associated with metabolic causes and the patient's temperature, glucose, oxygenation, and serum sodium should be carefully assessed and, if abnormal, treated in collaboration with the ICU team.

Sedation in the Intensive Care Unit

Sedation of the critically ill neuroscience patient can be a significant nursing challenge. The need to easily obtain the best possible neurological response from a patient is paramount for assessment data, but it must be balanced against minimizing cerebral ischemia and maintaining patient comfort. Undersedation carries the risk of unnecessary patient discomfort and anxiety, while oversedation can mean inaccurate assessment data suggesting a worse neurological examination or putting the patient at risk for hypoxemia from a depressed respiratory drive or hypotension from side effects from the sedating agent used. Existing sedation scales are not always adequate for assessing sedation in the neuroscience population. Some patients, such as those with Guillain-Barré syndrome, have extreme impairment of motor abilities and autonomic instability, which confound standard sedation scales. Still other patients receive infusion of paralytic medications that preclude the use of a standard sedation scale. The bispectral index monitor (BIS), introduced into the operating room to measure sedation during anesthesia, is gaining popularity as an objective method of monitoring sedation in the neuroscience population. The BIS monitor is a digitalized spectral electroencephalogram (EEG) that uses a statistically derived score to represent level of consciousness on a linear scale of 1 to 100. A score of 100 represents the awake and conscious patient; 80, the patient able to respond to loud commands; less than 60, the patient who does not respond to verbal commands; and 40, a deep hypnotic state. It is used to maintain a set level of sedation and gives the nurse another parameter by which to assess response to care activities and possibly avoid increases in ICP or decreases in CPP, which could lead to cerebral ischemia.[40,53]

CLINICAL VIGNETTE: MK is a 16-year-old girl who was the unrestrained driver in a single car motor vehicle crash. She sustained a severe closed head injury with the diagnosis of diffuse axonal injury based on initial brain CT. Her initial Glasgow Coma Scale (GCS) score was 8; she was intubated and placed on mechanical ventilation and an ICP monitor was inserted. Her ICPs were initially approximately 20 mm Hg but rapidly climbed to the 30s with any stimulation. A BIS monitor was added and she was placed on a propofol infusion, which was titrated to maintain a BIS of 60 to 70. Mannitol was instituted for ICP control, but the ICPs started rising before another dose was due, so 23% NaCl IV bolus was added as well. Within the first 24 hours, the nurses realized that lightening sedation to perform a neurological examination was associated with increases of ICP to the 50s as well as tachycardia, extreme hypertension, and ventilator dyssynchrony. It often took 30 minutes or more to return MK to an adequately sedated state. Using the data compression feature on the computerized documentation system to provide visual evidence of the progression of this behavior, the nurse worked with the interdisciplinary team to redefine the necessary neurological examination to include ICP, heart rate, blood pressure, serum osmolarities, BIS scores, and pupillary changes. These parameters were followed closely for the next 2 weeks, at which point her ICPs stabilized below 20 mm Hg; she was weaned from osmotic therapies and was able to tolerate discontinuation of sedation. MK made rapid progress in a neurological rehabilitation facility and went on to finish high school. She started college this fall.

Cardiovascular Monitoring

Patients with serious CNS insults are at risk for significant physiologic instability. Increases in ICP can trigger an increase in blood pressure so that CPP is maintained; the blood pressure can be elevated enough to cause cardiac ischemia or raise concerns about hemorrhage into an infarct or extension of existing hemorrhage. Decreased level of consciousness can lead to hypoventilation, with the resultant hypoxemia and hypercarbia having a deleterious effect on intracranial pressure and increasing the risk of secondary injury. Medications, such as anticonvulsants or sedatives, administered for a therapeutic purpose can produce unintended severe hemodynamic compromise. Guillain-Barré syndrome (GBS), for example, is associated with autonomic instability, which requires judicious intervention. Such patients require more intense cardiovascular monitoring including invasive monitoring of arterial blood pressure and invasive and noninvasive monitoring of volume status and cardiac function.

All critical care patients are on continuous cardiac monitoring. Electrocardiography (ECG) provides ongoing real-time information about abnormal patterns and life-threatening arrhythmias. Autonomic instability can result from cerebral injury and precipitate cardiac instability. Additionally, many older patients have significant cardiac comorbidities, which may put them at increased risk for myocardial ischemia and infarction. For some stroke patients, the diagnosis of cerebrovascular disease raises suspicions that the patient may have undiagnosed cardiovascular or peripheral vascular disease as well.

Invasive arterial blood pressure monitoring (arterial line) is instituted for many neuroscience ICU patients. It provides continuous monitoring of blood pressure, which can be crucial in patients with elevated ICP because CPP can then be calculated continuously as well. Many neuroscience ICU patients can be either severely hypertensive or hypotensive and may require continuous infusion of vasoactive medications. Sometimes, medical interventions are aimed at increasing or decreasing an otherwise normal blood pressure and continuous invasive monitoring is required to monitor to targeted physical values. Institutional policies vary, but, generally, if a patient requires intubation and mechanical ventilation, an arterial line is placed to facilitate measurement of arterial blood gases. The radial artery is most commonly used, although some patients require femoral arterial catheters. The most common complication of arterial line placement is thrombosis; its occurrence can be minimized by the use of nontapered Teflon-coated catheters, limiting the number of attempts to cannulate the same artery and using a continuous flush device.[54] The arterial line represents another instance in which the neurocritical care nurse must be skilled in calibrating and leveling a device as well as accurately interpreting the waveform and communicating key information to appropriate personnel.[55] The restless, confused, or agitated neuroscience ICU patient who requires an arterial line represents a particular nursing challenge.

For some critically ill neuroscience patients, heart rate and blood pressure do not provide enough hemodynamic information to adequately manage their care. Unclear volume status, adult respiratory distress syndrome (ARDS), neurogenic pulmonary edema, the possible diagnosis of sepsis, and apparent cardiac dysfunction necessitate measurement of preload and afterload. The flotation pulmonary arterial catheter (PAC) was introduced in 1970. The PAC is a right heart catheter, inserted at the bedside by trained personnel, which allows for direct measurements of right atrial pressures and indirect measurements of left heart function. It has the capability of measuring cardiac output through thermodilution and allows the calculation of oxygen delivery and consumption.[54] Proper use of the PAC requires that all personnel be educated on the interpretation of the data generated as well as the benefits and risks associated with its use. The Pulmonary Artery Catheter Education Program (PACEP) was developed by several specialty organizations, including the American Association of Critical Care Nurses (AACN), in conjunction with the Food and Drug Administration (FDA) and National Heart, Lung, and Blood Institute (NHLBI). It is designed to provide education for critical care providers on the use of information derived from the PA catheter. It can be accessed at http//www.PACEP.org. The critical care nurse must be particularly vigilant in the management of the catheter and interpretation of the waveforms; the PAC's position can change and the nurse must be able to act quickly should the catheter either move back into the patient's right ventricle or too far into a branch of the pulmonary artery as indicated by a change in the waveform or development of a cardiac arrhythmia. A daily chest radiograph should be performed to confirm that the PAC remains correctly positioned in the pulmonary artery. The risks associated with insertion of an invasive device and the potential life-threatening complications associated with the use of the PAC[56] have led to a search for noninvasive or less invasive devices to measure cardiac function, but none of these has come into widespread use as of yet.

CLINICAL VIGNETTE: RC is a 62-year-old man with a history of atrial fibrillation, hypertension, and chronic obstructive pulmonary disease who was admitted to the hospital with an embolic stroke. Though he did not initially require admission to the ICU, on hospital day 3, he became febrile and short of breath; ECG revealed uncontrolled atrial fibrillation, and the fever workup revealed a possible urinary tract infection. He required transfer to the neuroscience ICU for management of sepsis and respiratory failure. He had a difficult medical course necessitating the use of a PAC and vasopressors and required a tracheostomy and a percutaneous endoscopic gastrostomy (PEG) tube. After some initial progress weaning from the ventilator, RC slowly lost clinical ground; depression was suspected and antidepressants begun. Repeat brain imaging studies failed to show any new structural lesions to explain his worsening weakness. One of the nurses who had cared for him frequently reviewed many days' worth of physiologic data arranged graphically on the computer. It showed a trend over approximately 2 weeks during which his heart rate, blood pressure, and temperature slowly decreased. The ventilator section showed increasing ventilatory support to compensate for hypoventilation. The nurse thought about how he now complained of feeling cold and tired all the time, how slow he was in performing self-care activities, and how dry his skin had become as his hospitalization progressed. This is when the nurse realized that these were all signs of clinical hypothyroidism. Discussion with the ICU team led to the diagnosis and treatment of a previously unrecognized hypothyroidism. RC was able to eventually wean from the ventilator, have the PEG removed, and return home.

Respiratory Care Interventions

Many neuroscience ICU patients require respiratory care interventions ranging from noninvasive monitoring of ventilatory adequacy to noninvasive and invasive mechanical ventilation. Patients may hypoventilate related to a decreased level of consciousness or neuromuscular weakness from a disease process (GBS, myasthenic crisis), or as an iatrogenic complication of therapy (e.g., high-dose benzodiazepines for seizure control, barbiturate coma for ICP management or seizure control). Hypoventilation can lead to hypercarbia; since carbon dioxide (CO_2) is a potent vasodilator, this can cause significant elevations in intracranial pressure in at-risk patients. Others are hypoxemic from pulmonary edema, an aspiration event, or a pulmonary infection. These patients will require endotracheal intubation and mechanical ventilation; some will eventually require surgical tracheostomy for prolonged respiratory failure. A critically trained respiratory therapist should manage the ventilator settings according to established adult ventilator protocols. The nurse is responsible for ongoing respiratory assessments, periodic pulmonary toileting activities including oral care, turning, chest physiotherapy (either manual or with a specialty bed that provides timed percussion and vibration), and suctioning after the patient has been preoxygenated. Arterial blood gases are

assessed in accordance with institutional protocols; patients should have daily chest radiographs to assess for infiltrates, atelectasis, effusions, and edema as well to verify accurate placement of the endotracheal tube.

Sometimes the neuroscience ICU patient arrives with the diagnosis of obstructive sleep apnea requiring noninvasive continuous positive pressure ventilation (CPAP) during nighttime hours. Other times, patients are very reluctant to be intubated because of prior personal experience or negative experiences of people close to them. There are also occasions when aggressive treatment of pneumonia combined with CPAP will be adequate to prevent hypoxemia. Astute nursing management is required to ensure that the therapy is working and that a clear plan is in place regarding when and if intubation will occur. Patients may require considerable reassurance that they will receive adequate medication for pain and anxiety and that methods for communication will be consistently employed before they are willing to agree to intubation. Family members should always be involved in the discussions regarding the use of this potentially life-saving therapy.

CLINICAL PEARLS: If a patient's ability to communicate while mechanically ventilated will be limited to blinking or eye movements in response to yes-or-no questions, the indicators for yes or no should be well differentiated and posted in an easily visible location to facilitate rapid and accurate communication.

Two noninvasive methods of continuously assessing ventilatory adequacy are pulse oximetry (SpO_2) and capnography or end-tidal carbon dioxide ($ETCO_2$) monitoring. The pulse oximeter is a device that can easily be used on both ventilated and nonventilated patients to estimate arterial oxygen saturation of hemoglobin. It uses a combination of spectrophotometry and plethysmography principles and senses specific wavelengths of light emitted by hemoglobin in blood through a probe most frequently placed on a finger or earlobe. Clinicians can use the information acquired to noninvasively assess adequacy of oxygenation and quickly monitor response to changes in oxygen concentration. SpO_2 accuracy can be negatively impacted by anemia, irregular cardiac arrhythmias, skin pigmentation, and low perfusion states; additionally, nail polish or artificial nails can interfere with accuracy as well.[57] Capnography or $ETCO_2$ monitoring is used to monitor ventilated patients for adequacy of ventilation. Infrared spectrophotometry is the most common method for determining CO_2 concentration from a continuous sample of airway gas.[58] The $ETCO_2$ detector is most often incorporated into the mechanical ventilator circuit as an "in-line" device. Changes in $ETCO_2$ can be used to determine both over- and underventilation and can be an early cue of partial airway obstruction from a mucous plug or bronchospasm.[57]

ANXIETY, AGITATION, AND DELIRIUM
Anxiety

Many patients in the neuroscience ICU will either be heavily sedated for their medical management or be at a low level of neurological function without sedation. Still others will be anxious, agitated, or delirious. Though a certain amount of anxiety can be expected of any ICU patient or their family and friends, it is often more pronounced with the neuroscience patient. The seriousness of the patient's medical condition; the noise, monitors, and alarms of the ICU environment; the loss of control experienced by both the patient and family; and the difficulty in obtaining definitive medical information all combine to create a baseline of uncertainty and anxiety. For the critically ill neuroscience patient, there is the added concern about possible permanent deficits in neurological function such as cognition and mobility. If the initial brain insult is severe enough, it may be uncertain for many days whether the patient will survive; the possibility of lasting problems cannot even be considered.

The critical care nurse is positioned to assist in decreasing patient and family anxiety in this critical time period. The etiology of the anxiety is often different in the patient, and the nurse has more options, including pharmacologic intervention. Family interventions include a narrower scope of possibilities, responsibilities, and accountability.

The nurse can demonstrate, to the patient when possible but more likely to the family, interest in the patient as an individual. Attempts at coping can be supported, a sense of control can be restored, and information can be provided and reinforced. The perception on the part of the patient that the nurse is caring and competent can aid in the reduction of anxiety. Prompt management of pain; arranging for rest periods; providing brief explanations of procedures, alarms, and equipment; and avoiding the use of jargon are some ways to demonstrate caring and competent behavior. If the patient has some cognitive impairment, nursing behaviors can be tailored to this (i.e., increasing the use of gestures and pictures to convey information to a patient with aphasia or providing written information for the patient with short-term memory deficits).

While some anxiety associated with hospitalization is to be expected, the neuroscience ICU nurse should become concerned when patients exhibit excessive anxiety. Many neurocritical care patients arrive in the hospital due to an unexpected crisis and will pass their first several days of hospitalization in the ICU. Acute alcohol and/or sedative-hypnotic withdrawal should be suspected in patients who develop *extreme* anxiety in that time period. Other causes of this extreme anxiety should also be investigated by the interdisciplinary critical care team, particularly hypoxia, hyperventilation caused by pulmonary embolus, and partial complex seizures.

Agitation and Delirium

Some patients will move beyond being merely anxious into extreme restlessness, disorientation, irritability, and agitation. Agitation often precedes delirium; the patient starts picking at lines and bed linens or tries to get out of bed without assistance. Their sleep-wake cycle often becomes reversed; a patient who begins to sleep all day and stay up all night should be considered high risk for the development of delirium. Should the patient progress to true delirium, he or she will begin to show increasing deficits in attention and concentration coupled with a fluctuating level of arousal; this may be interspersed with periods of lucidity. The patient

is likely to swing between hypo- and hyperactivity and demonstrate emotional lability, and may exhibit delusions and paranoia as well as motor problems such as dysphagia, myoclonus, asterixis, and muscle tone changes.[59] When a patient becomes delirious, a search for an underlying cause should be initiated as delirium can be provoked by a wide range of underlying medical problems including infection, toxic or metabolic encephalopathies, altered cerebral perfusion related to edema or hypoxia, drug or alcohol withdrawal, or new CNS pathology. Early clinical assessment and treatment of the underlying medical problem combined with appropriate pharmacologic therapies can protect the patient from complications associated with delirium. Elderly patients represent the highest risk category for delirium. Malnutrition, polypharmacy, physical restraints, indwelling catheters, and volume overload have all been implicated as precipitating factors for delirium in this patient population.[60] Delirium is one of the leading causes of preventable injury in patients over the age of 65. It is associated with increased time on mechanical ventilation, increased hospital stays, and an increased risk of dying, both in the ICU and in the hospital.[59]

Specific treatment is directed at the underlying cause, but the general management of delirium includes orienting and reassuring the patient, decreasing the levels of environmental stimulation, establishing more normal day/night sleep cycles, and keeping the patient in contact with family, friends, and familiar objects. While these patients seldom respond to verbal interventions alone, sometimes the presence of a trusted family member or friend can help calm and orient the patient. Avoid physical restraints, if possible, as these may increase agitation and the possibility of patient injury. A patient care aide who can stay with the patient and provide gentle reorientation and diversionary activities while preventing the patient from removing catheters and other devices or from exiting the bed inappropriately may be a viable option. There are times when the neuroscience ICU patient will require pharmacologic intervention to manage agitation and delirium. The Society of Critical Care Medicine (SCCM) has published guidelines to aid the intensive care clinician in managing sedation, pain, and delirium in the critical care patient.[61]

TRANSPORT OF THE CRITICAL CARE PATIENT

Critically ill patients who require transport, whether intra- or interhospital, are at heightened risk for adverse events and must always be accompanied by appropriately trained personnel. Hospitals should have policies and procedures specifying who accompanies a patient during transport and who remains with the patient at the destination site. A critical care registered nurse should always accompany the patient. While specific personnel may vary, a minimum of two people should always accompany the patient.[62] The nurse ensures that properly functioning monitoring devices are in use, there is an adequate supply of intravenous fluids and continuously infusing medications, appropriate sedatives or narcotics accompany the patient, and resuscitation drugs and a defibrillator are immediately available. Tube feedings should be suspended to decrease the risk of aspiration during transport. If the patient is on mechanical ventilation, a respiratory therapist should accompany the patient. Studies have shown an increased incidence in VAP in patients requiring transport.[63] In the past, it was customary to ventilate patients during transport with a bag/valve/mask device and only connect them to a ventilator on arrival. Many facilities now have special transport ventilators to maintain patients on their optimal ventilatory support throughout the transport process. Patients with tenuous airways or significant decreases in level of consciousness should not be transported until a secure airway has been established.[62] In most critically ill patients, concern centers on hemodynamic instability, respiratory insufficiency, and the possibility of equipment failure.[64] The neurocritical care patient is at additional risk for altered cerebral perfusion related to elevations in ICP. Hypoxemia and hypotension have both been associated with increased secondary brain injury; both are potential complications of transport. Some institutions have dedicated intrahospital as well as interhospital transport teams to ensure the immediate availability of appropriately trained personnel in urgent and emergency situations.[65]

When there is concern about the patient's ability to tolerate transport, it can be useful to simulate the transport and destination environments for several minutes at the bedside.

CLINICAL PEARLS: Trying out the transport environment prior to transport can prompt increased anticipatory management of potential complications. Anticipatory management may include administration of mannitol prior to transport or adjustment of sedative or opiate infusion.

The patient should be connected to the transport monitor and ventilator and placed in the position he or she will sustain at the destination (generally supine and completely flat in bed), and the response assessed. If the patient becomes unstable, then the transport should be cancelled or delayed. When at all possible, diagnostic testing should be performed at the bedside as a matter of routine for the critical care patient.

While the neurocritical care nurse will most often be involved in the process of intrahospital transport, he or she may also be the nurse preparing a patient for interhospital transport or the nurse receiving the patient posttransport. Interhospital transport is most often initiated when an unstable critically ill patient has medical needs exceeding the capabilities of his or her current institution and must be transported to another facility for a higher level of care. The need for appropriately trained and equipped personnel with well-defined protocols for management during transport is a requirement. Again, a minimum of two health care providers should accompany the patient.[62] The transfer requires both physician-to-physician as well as nurse-to-nurse report of the patient's situation. Medical records, including pertinent laboratory and radiographic studies, should accompany the patient, but their preparation should not delay transport.

The patient must be stabilized to the best of the transferring institution's ability. Key components of stabilization include a secure venous access, a secured airway, an orogastric or nasogastric tube for decompression, a Foley catheter for urinary drainage, and, when necessary, spine immobilization, chest tube insertion for management of pneumothorax, and other immediate trauma stabilization. Patients should also receive medications necessary to manage agitation or combativeness during transport. Once the patient has been transported, the receiving nurse is responsible for assessing the patient for any deterioration during transport and contacting appropriate personnel, ensuring that monitoring continues, and that continuously infusing medications are not interrupted while the patient is transferred from the transport equipment to that of the receiving institution.

EVIDENCE-BASED PRACTICE AND RESEARCH

A driving force in the current health care environment is the use of "best practices" to improve patient outcomes through standardizing care based on protocols generated from research findings. In neuroscience critical care, many areas of previously accepted treatment have come under scrutiny as medical and nursing practitioners attempt to investigate whether there is evidence to support or change current practice.

While research involving large heterogeneous samples in a randomized double-blind controlled study is considered the "gold standard" for evidence-based practice,[66] such research is not always feasible. It would not be ethical to withhold a treatment considered the standard of care in the management of a particular disease process from a control group of patients in order to establish its value. There are other ways in which the efficacy of standard therapies for which the evidence base is lacking can be better tested. In some instances, it may be possible to use new monitoring methods or technology to prove or disprove the effect the treatment is believed to achieve. The therapy can also be tested by comparing it in research trials to a new therapy to see if either patient group has better outcomes. The search for scientific evidence to support the theories that guide patient care challenges the expert critical care nurse to incorporate research findings with existing clinical knowledge and practice.[66] Expertise in a particular field of nursing is a necessary component to working collaboratively with the interdisciplinary team when assessing the utility of implementing changes in practice based on the available evidence. For neuroscience critical care nurses, there is scientific evidence related to their specific patient populations that has either led to changes in practice or supported current clinical practices. Other research is ongoing regarding the value of other practices.

Sustained hyperventilation is an example of a standard therapy for the management of elevated ICP for which the available evidence does not clearly support its continued use. Hyperventilation induces hypocarbia; the associated vasoconstriction is thought to aid in the reduction of elevated ICP through a reduction in intracranial volume. New technology that measures brain tissue oxygenation has demonstrated that while sustained hyperventilation can decrease ICP, it also results in decreased $PbtO_2$, a measure of cerebral ischemia, in surrounding tissue.[32] A recent review of multiple studies suggests that the ability of hyperventilation to reduce ICP must be balanced not only against the possibility of cerebral ischemia from the cerebral vasoconstriction, but also against possible systemic effects, particularly hemodynamic instability. Controversy continues regarding the continued role of hyperventilation in the neuroscience population.[67]

Because management of ICP and CPP are considered to be key to improving outcomes in the neuroscience patient population, other research has focused on therapies aimed at altering either of these measurements. Studies of treatment options to decrease increased ICP, such as the use of mannitol as an osmotic diuretic to decrease cerebral edema and therapeutic hypothermia in the management of acute stroke and severe traumatic brain injury, are under way.

Evidence to date cautiously supports the use of mannitol for the acute management of elevated ICP,[68] but research is also underway evaluating the effectiveness of hypertonic saline as an alternative hyperosmolar agent.[69] Because hypertonic saline is a new treatment option without standardized protocols for use, it can be studied in controlled trials to establish its effectiveness and to determine which protocol produces the best effect before its use will be widely encouraged or discouraged.

Temperature management is an area of significant interest in the neuroscience patient population. Fever has long been thought to be detrimental, and aggressive measures are generally employed to return the patient's temperature to normal. Some studies that have attempted to link fever control and improvements in patient outcomes have not clearly shown such an effect.[46,70] There are other studies that do show a link between fever in neuroscience patients and increases in morbidity and mortality.[71–73] Induced hypothermia to aid in control of elevated ICP by reducing metabolic demand and thereby promoting reduction in ICP is a therapy that has seemed promising based on anecdotal evidence and results in small, early, single-center trials. However, these early results have not been replicable in larger multicenter trials and hypothermia seemed to be associated with an increase in adverse events, particularly pneumonia, coagulation abnormalities, and possible cardiac ischemia.[74] Clinical experiences involving individual patients have led to further studies as to whether there are very specific subpopulations in neuroscience that may clearly benefit from artificial manipulation of body temperature.

Research on the effects of critical care nursing interventions on patient outcomes has included assessment of the effects of head-of-bed elevation on vasospasm in subarachnoid hemorrhage,[36] methods of detecting inadvertent airway placement of gastric tubes,[75] ways to reduce unnecessary blood work,[76] and implementation of evidence-based oral care in neuroscience patients.[77] Research on providing oral care to patients may seem mundane compared to medical research on interventions that have a more obvious impact on patient outcomes, but a review of the literature reveals the link that has been established between poor oral care and an increase in local and systemic infections, including nosocomial and ventilator-associated pneumonia.[78–80]

Blood pressure optimization in the neuroscience patient population is an area of considerable interest and research. Accepted practice has allowed the patient's blood pressure to remain somewhat elevated out of concern for causing hypotension and worsening ischemic damage or raising intracranial pressure. There is the competing concern that elevated blood pressure may be associated with increased risk of hemorrhage or edema. Many patients present with elevated blood pressure after acute ischemic stroke. Studies report inconsistent associations with both good and poor outcomes related to maintaining an initial high blood pressure.[81] Current ischemic stroke guidelines arbitrarily set blood pressure (BP) guidelines at greater than 220 mm Hg systolic and greater than 120 mm Hg diastolic unless there is planned thrombolysis or evidence of noncerebral hypertensive organ damage such as myocardial infarction, aortic dissection, pulmonary edema, or renal failure.[82] Acute ischemic stroke is not the only neurologic emergency for which there is no high-quality data regarding optimal BP management. Intracerebral hemorrhage, subarachnoid hemorrhage, traumatic brain injury, acute spinal cord injury or infarct, and hypertensive encephalopathy are other patient populations in the neuroscience ICU for whom BP control is a major issue. Because cerebral autoregulation may not be intact in the injured areas of the brain, blood pressure control must be undertaken cautiously since hypotension is believed to be more injurious than hypertension in these patients. If vasoactive medications are used early in the course of treatment, short-acting continuous infusion agents are preferred. Phenylephrine, norepinephrine, and dopamine are the agents most often used to raise BP. Labetalol, esmolol, and nicardipine are those used most often to lower BP.[83]

INSTITUTE FOR HEALTHCARE IMPROVEMENT INITIATIVES

The Institute for Healthcare Improvement (IHI) is an organization dedicated to transforming U.S. health care by improving patient safety and preventing avoidable deaths. It is disseminating multiple initiatives, some specifically in the area of critical care. Critical care initiatives are targeted at the infection-related issues of ventilator-associated pneumonia, catheter-related bloodstream infections, and severe sepsis. The IHI promulgates protocol-based strategies that have been shown to improve outcomes and reduce costs. It presents the strategies in "bundles," which are groups of interventions related to a disease process that result in a better outcome implemented as a group rather than individually. The ventilator bundle centers around elevation of the head of the bed, daily "sedation vacation," assessment of readiness to extubate, peptic ulcer disease prophylaxis, and deep venous thrombosis prophylaxis.[84] The central line bundle involves hand hygiene, maximal barrier precautions on insertion, chlorhexidine skin antisepsis, optimal catheter site selection, and daily reassessment of continued need for the catheter.[85] The severe sepsis bundle, which is actually a pair of bundles, is based on the recommendations in the 2004 practice guidelines for the Surviving Sepsis Campaign. The sepsis resuscitation bundle outlines seven activities that should be done in the first 6 hours after patient presentation, and the accompanying sepsis management bundle encompasses interventions that should occur in the first 24 hours.[86] Neurocritical care nurses should be familiar with the recommendations in all the IHI bundles and be involved in their implementation at the institutions where they practice.

INTERACTING WITH THE FAMILIES OF NEUROSCIENCE INTENSIVE CARE UNIT PATIENTS

Many of the factors that can lead to anxiety in neuroscience ICU patients have the same effect on their families. The ICU environment is unfamiliar, noisy, and confusing; their loved one is seriously ill; and information can be difficult to obtain and understand. Often, families are far from home and their usual support systems. Studies have shown that the families of ICU patients have multiple needs, which continue throughout the patient's ICU stay. Families particularly continue to require honest answers with information presented in a clear and understandable manner along with the need to believe the patient is receiving the best possible care.[87] It is best to provide brief descriptions of the functions of the various mechanical devices in the patient's room, explain the meaning of the numbers and waveforms on the monitor, and avoid the use of jargon or abbreviations. Families value the information nurses are able to provide. APNs as well as bedside nurses can reinforce information already provided, clarify areas of confusion, and take care that possible misinformation acquired from other families in the waiting area is not perpetuated. Assure the family that they can contact the patient's nurse or physician when they are away from the patient's bedside and that the neuroscience ICU has appropriate contact numbers so the family can easily be reached if there is a change in patient status.

CLINICAL PEARLS: Anxious and tired people do not retain information well, so expect that repetition and reinforcement will be necessary. Assure the family that it is normal to need information reviewed.

CLINICAL VIGNETTE: JD was a 40-year-old man with severe Guillain-Barré syndrome. He was quadriparetic and ventilator dependent but able to move his head and eyes to communicate. He was married with a 3½-year-old son named Jay, who missed his hospitalized father a great deal. The mother was willing to have her son visit if the medical team felt it was appropriate. The nursing staff made sure the physicians and hospital administration approved of allowing such a young child to visit in the adult neuroscience ICU. The hospital's child-life specialists were contacted; they evaluated Jay and worked to be sure he understood that his dad couldn't move or talk right now but would get better. They were there the first time he visited JD; both father and son did well with the visit. For the remainder of JD's stay, when neither father nor son had an infection, Jay could often be found snuggled next to his dad, chattering happily about his day or sometimes just having a nap with him.

NURSING MANAGEMENT IN ORGAN DONATION

The potential organ donor is an unfortunate but distinct subpopulation found in the neuroscience intensive care unit. Although these patients have sustained a variety of especially severe CNS insults, their commonality is a failure to respond positively to maximal therapeutic interventions and to meet strictly defined criteria for the diagnosis of brain death. The possibility that a patient might be brain dead and might become an organ donor means that, from a nursing perspective, the acuity will increase, as these patients are often clinically unstable. The psychosocial needs of the family increase as they go from watchful waiting and hoping for a positive outcome to mourning the loss of a loved one while struggling to reach a consensus on the immensely difficult question of organ donation. The bedside nurse may be so occupied with managing the minute-to-minute interventions that he or she is unable to spend adequate time with the family. However, facilitating family presence and support are essential to the process; the ICU team must work collaboratively to meet the needs of the family.

Initial management of the potentially brain-dead patient involves recognizing that maximal therapies are failing or have failed. The nurse continues to have frequent discussions with the responsible physician or midlevel practitioner to ensure that all possible appropriate avenues of therapy are exhausted. Once it is clear, based on physiologic parameters and the lack of external response to noxious stimulation, that a patient will likely meet criteria for a diagnosis of brain death, intensive management does not cease. For a declaration of brain death to be made, the patient must have vital signs (blood pressure, temperature) and laboratory values close to normal parameters so that a lack of response to testing for brain death cannot be attributed to inadequate cerebral blood flow or a severe metabolic encephalopathy. American states and institutions vary somewhat in the criteria that must be satisfied for the declaration of brain death to be made. The variations are generally in regard to such things as time that must elapse since the patient received sedatives or narcotics or requirements for confirmatory tests such as EEG or cerebral blood flow studies. Currently, there is a federal requirement that the local organ donor agency be notified about all cardiac deaths, as well as impending brain death.

Throughout the process of determining brain death and the potential for organ donation, the bedside nurse's primary responsibility is maintaining the patient's physiologic stability. Brain-dead patients are often hemodynamically unstable and require significant volume and electrolyte repletion and the judicious use of pressors. They frequently develop marked metabolic, endocrine, and pulmonary derangements, which require aggressive management.[88,89] Efforts must also be undertaken to maintain normal body temperature as the patient no longer has the ability to thermoregulate.

It is extremely important to maintain ongoing and open communication with the family so they are not taken unaware by this turn of events. The interdisciplinary team works collaboratively to ensure that the family understands the nonsurvivable nature of the patient's CNS injury. The bedside nurse is available to answer subsequent questions and reinforce information provided regarding the diagnosis of brain death. Once the diagnosis is confirmed, the nurse facilitates conversations between the family and representatives of the local organ procurement organization. Discussions about organ donation are conducted separately from discussions about brain death; this allows families time to process the information and has been found to increase the rate of consent for organ donation.[88] Once the family has made a decision either for or against donation, the nurse assists in attending to the needs of the family as they say goodbye to their loved one. Pastoral care can be vital in tending to the spiritual needs of the family throughout this process.[90]

ETHICAL AND LEGAL CONCERNS

There are some ethical and legal concerns unique to the neuroscience ICU. Neuroscience patients, more than most intensive care patients, do not have the capacity to make their own health care decisions. Many of them, because of the nature of their cerebral insult, will not recover the ability to do so. While the role of the nurse is to be the patient's advocate in these situations, the best way to accomplish this is not always clear. Sometimes discussions with the family will clearly establish the existence of a durable health care power of attorney or advance directives. In the absence of either of those, it is usually easy to establish which family member should most appropriately be responsible for decision making for a particular patient. Other times the situation is murkier, such as when the patient's marital status is unclear or the immediate family has opposing views as to what would be best for the person or what that person would have wanted. Many institutions have patient–visitor relations personnel who can be a significant help in resolving these issues; other times, involvement of the institution's risk management department is necessary.

An especially difficult situation occurs when there is disagreement regarding the best course of treatment. This can involve interteam disagreement over whether to continue treatment or the extent to which a patient should be treated, ICU team–family conflicts regarding treatment, family difficulties in agreeing on the best course of action in the absence of clear written preferences from the patient, or some combination of all of these. There is support in the literature for the involvement of an ethics consult in such situations. Having a service available where an individual, team, or committee can address the ethical issues in a specific clinical case has been shown to reduce the conflicts that were prolonging inappropriate care and enable a shift in focus to comfort care.[91] The consultation service strives to be inclusive, educational, and culturally respectful throughout the process. Once the service is consulted, the medical record is reviewed, ethical concerns are clarified through discussion with the involved parties, and recommendations are made including arranging for further meetings for the purpose of improving communication. Studies have pointed out the need for improved physician–nurse communication and collaboration around end-of-life care in the ICU.[25] See Chapter 3 for further discussion.

FUTURE TRENDS

New research and clinical experiences will continue to broaden knowledge regarding severe CNS insults and will result in changes in medical and nursing management, including new drug therapies. Ongoing research into the neuroprotective effects of statins is promising, and their use may become widespread in the next several years.[92,93] Basic research will yield improved understanding of various brain pathologies. Biochemical markers in the bloodstream have been identified that correlate with the brain's ischemic response and have the potential to assist in the early diagnosis of stroke, prediction of infarct size, and possibly prediction of outcome.[94,95] Cerebral microdialysis is a technique for measuring brain extracellular chemicals. It is currently used for research in patients with ischemic stroke, brain injury, and subarachnoid hemorrhage, but limitations in the technology will continue to keep its use restricted to research for now.[96,97]

Current technologies for monitoring brain tissue oxygenation will come into widespread use over the next several years. Methods of noninvasive assessment of various physiologic parameters will undergo refinements and become a useful adjunct in the management of unstable critically ill patients. Refinements in the size of technologies will allow for more bedside diagnostic testing including CT brain scans,[98] thereby eliminating the risks to the patient associated with transport.

Increases in the numbers of advanced practice nurses will lead to review and use of existing nursing research as well as more nursing research into nursing behaviors and interactions regarding neurocritical care patients and their families.[13] Advanced practice nurses can work collaboratively with the interdisciplinary intensive care team to promote creative nursing responses to difficult situations. Nurse specialists are positioned to provide cost-effective and high-quality care in the intensive care environment.[15]

The bedside critical care nurse will continue to be the important link in ensuring communication between the patient and family and various members of the interdisciplinary intensive care team. The clinically competent and clinically confident neuroscience ICU nurse is key to providing holistic care and maintaining a human connection to the patient and family in the impersonal and mechanical world of the neuroscience ICU.

REFERENCES

1. Brilli, R. J., Spevetz, A., Branson, R. D., et al. (2001). Critical care delivery in the intensive care unit: Defining clinical roles and the best practice model. *Critical Care Medicine, 29,* 2007–2019.
2. Pronovost, P., & Goeschel, C. (2005). Improving ICU care: It takes a team. *Healthcare Execute, 20,* 14–16, 18, 20.
3. Dyer, J. A. (2003). Multidisciplinary, interdisciplinary, and transdisciplinary educational models and nursing education. *Nursing Education Perspectives, 24,* 186–188.
4. Mitchell, P. H. (2005). What's in a name? Multidisciplinary, interdisciplinary, and transdisciplinary. *Journal of Profession Nursing, 21,* 332–334.
5. Suarez, J. I., Zaidat, O. O., Suri, M. F., et al. (2004). Length of stay and mortality in neurocritically ill patients: Impact of a specialized neurocritical care team. *Critical Care Medicine, 32,* 2311–2317.
6. Ewart, G. W., Marcus, L., Gaba, M. M., Bradner, R. H., Medina, J. L., & Chandler, E. B. (2004). The critical care medicine crisis: A call for federal action: A white paper from the critical care professional societies. *Chest, 125,* 1518–1521.
7. Pronovost, P. J., Angus, D. C., Dorman, T., Robinson, K. A., Dremsizov, T. T., & Young, T. L. (2002). Physician staffing

patterns and clinical outcomes in critically ill patients: A systematic review. *Journal of the American Medical Association, 288,* 2151–2162.

8. Varelas, P. N., Conti, M. M., Spanaki, M. V., et al. (2004). The impact of a neurointensivist-led team on a semiclosed neurosciences intensive care unit. *Critical Care Medicine, 32,* 2191–2198.

9. Diringer, M. N., & Edwards, D. F. (2001). Admission to a neurologic/neurosurgical intensive care unit is associated with reduced mortality rate after intracerebral hemorrhage. *Critical Care Medicine, 29,* 635–640.

10. Hoffman, L. A., Tasota, F. J., Zullo, T. G., Scharfenberg, C., & Donahoe, M. P. (2005). Outcomes of care managed by an acute care nurse practitioner/attending physician team in a subacute medical intensive care unit. *American Journal of Critical Care, 14,* 121–130; quiz 131–132.

11. Christmas, A. B., Reynolds, J., Hodges, S., et al. (2005). Physician extenders impact trauma systems. *Journal of Trauma, 58,* 917–920.

12. Brooten, D., Youngblut, J. M., Kutcher, J., & Bobo, C. (2004). Quality and the nursing workforce: APNs, patient outcomes and health care costs. *Nursing Outlook, 52,* 45–52.

13. DeBourgh, G. A. (2001). Champions for evidence-based practice: A critical role for advanced practice nurses. *AACN Clinical Issues, 12,* 491–508.

14. Phillips, J. (2005). Neuroscience critical care: The role of the advanced practice nurse in patient safety. *AACN Clinical Issues, 16,* 581–592.

15. Kleinpell, R., & Gawlinski, A. (2005). Assessing outcomes in advanced practice nursing practice: The use of quality indicators and evidence-based practice. *AACN Clinical Issues, 16,* 43–57.

16. Russell, D., VorderBruegge, M., & Burns, S. M. (2002). Effect of an outcomes-managed approach to care of neuroscience patients by acute care nurse practitioners. *American Journal of Critical Care, 11,* 353–362.

17. Durbin, C. G., Jr. (2006). Team model: Advocating for the optimal method of care delivery in the intensive care unit. *Critical Care Medicine, 34,* S12–17.

18. Haupt, M. T., Bekes, C. E., Brilli, R. J., et al. (2003). Guidelines on critical care services and personnel: Recommendations based on a system of categorization of three levels of care. *Critical Care Medicine, 31,* 2677–2683.

19. Woods, D. K. (2002). Realizing your marketing influence, part 3: Professional certification as a marketing tool. *Journal of Nursing Administration, 32,* 379–386.

20. Bleich, S. (2005). Medical errors: Five years after the IOM report. *Issue Brief (Commonwealth Fund),* 1–15.

21. Paparella, S. (2006). Automated medication dispensing systems: Not error free. *Journal of Emergency Nursing, 32,* 71–74.

22. Tuohy, N., & Paparella, S. (2005). Look-alike and sound-alike drugs: Errors just waiting to happen. *Journal of Emergency Nursing, 31,* 569–571.

23. Simmons, D. (2005). Sedation and patient safety. *Critical Care Nursing Clinics of North America, 17,* 279–285.

24. Rudis, M. I., & Brandl, K. M. (2000). Position paper on critical care pharmacy services. Society of Critical Care Medicine and American College of Clinical Pharmacy task force on critical care pharmacy services. *Critical Care Medicine, 28,* 3746–3750.

25. Baggs, J. G., Norton, S. A., Schmitt, M. H., & Sellers, C. R. (2004). The dying patient in the ICU: Role of the interdisciplinary team. *Critical Care Clinics, 20,* 525–540, xi.

26. Fontaine, D. K., Briggs, L. P., & Pope-Smith, B. (2001). Designing humanistic critical care environments. *Critical Care Nursing Quarterly, 24,* 21–34.

27. Williams, M. (2001). Critical care unit design: A nursing perspective. *Critical Care Nursing Quarterly, 24,* 35–42.

28. Olson, D. M., Borel, C. O., Laskowitz, D. T., Moore, D. T., & McConnell, E. S. (2001). Quiet time: A nursing intervention to promote sleep in neurocritical care units. *American Journal of Critical Care, 10,* 74–78.

29. Staggers, N. (2003). Human factors: Imperative concepts for information systems in critical care. *AACN Clinical Issues, 14,* 310–319; quiz 397–418.

30. ICU patients at risk for preventable errors. AHRQ study puts spotlight on adverse events. (2005). *Healthcare Benchmarks Quality Improvement, 12,* 127–128.

31. The IOM medical errors report: 5 years later, the journey continues. (2005). *Quality Letter for Healthcare Leaders, 17,* 2–10, 11.

32. Unterberg, A. W., Kiening, K. L., Hartl, R., Bardt, T., Sarrafzadeh, A. S., & Lanksch, W. R. (1997). Multimodal monitoring in patients with head injury: Evaluation of the effects of treatment on cerebral oxygenation. *Journal of Trauma, 42,* S32–37.

33. March, K. (2005). Intracranial pressure monitoring: Why monitor? *AACN Clinical Issues, 16,* 456–475.

34. The Brain Trauma Foundation. The American Association of Neurological Surgeons. The Joint Section on Neurotrauma and Critical Care. (2000). Guidelines for the management of severe traumatic brain injury. *Journal of Neurotrauma, 17,* 451–553.

35. Olson, D. M., & Graffagnino, C. (2005). Consciousness, coma, and caring for the brain-injured patient. *AACN Clinical Issues, 16,* 441–455.

36. Blissitt, P. A., Mitchell, P. H., Newell, D. W., Woods, S. L., & Belza, B. (2006). Cerebrovascular dynamics with head-of-bed elevation in patients with mild or moderate vasospasm after aneurysmal subarachnoid hemorrhage. *American Journal of Critical Care, 15,* 206–216.

37. Alberts, M. J., Latchaw, R. E., Selman, W. R., et al. (2005). Recommendations for comprehensive stroke centers: A consensus statement from the brain attack coalition. *Stroke, 36,* 1597–1616.

38. Kirkness, C. J. (2005). Cerebral blood flow monitoring in clinical practice. *AACN Clinical Issues, 16,* 476–487.

39. Latronico, N., Beindorf, A. E., Rasulo, F. A., et al. (2000). Limits of intermittent jugular bulb oxygen saturation monitoring in the management of severe head trauma patients. *Neurosurgery, 46,* 1131–1138; discussion 1138–1139.

40. Littlejohns, L., & Bader, M. K. (2005). Prevention of secondary brain injury: Targeting technology. *AACN Clinical Issues, 16,* 501–514.

41. Jaeger, M., Soehle, M., & Meixensberger, J. (2005). Brain tissue oxygen (ptio2): A clinical comparison of two monitoring devices. *Acta Neurochirurgica Supplement, 95,* 79–81.

42. Eastwood, J. D., Lev, M. H., Wintermark, M., et al. (2003). Correlation of early dynamic CT perfusion imaging with whole-brain MR diffusion and perfusion imaging in acute hemispheric stroke. *AJNR American Journal of Neuroradiology, 24,* 1869–1875.

43. Harrigan, M. R., Leonardo, J., Gibbons, K. J., Guterman, L. R., & Hopkins, L. N. (2005). CT perfusion cerebral blood flow imaging in neurological critical care. *Neurocritical Care, 2,* 352–366.

44. Josephson, S. A., Dillon, W. P., & Smith, W. S. (2005). Incidence of contrast nephropathy from cerebral CT angiography and CT perfusion imaging. *Neurology, 64,* 1805–1806.

45. McCullough, P. A., & Soman, S. S. (2005). Contrast-induced nephropathy. *Critical Care Clinics, 21,* 261–280.

46. Cairns, C. J., & Andrews, P. J. (2002). Management of hyperthermia in traumatic brain injury. *Current Opinion in Critical Care. 8,* 106–110.

47. Diringer, M. N. (2004). Treatment of fever in the neurologic intensive care unit with a catheter-based heat exchange system. *Critical Care Medicine, 32,* 559–564.

48. van den Berghe, G., Wouters, P., Weekers, F., et al. (2001). Intensive insulin therapy in the critically ill patients. *New England Journal of Medicine, 345,* 1359–1367.

49. Parsons, M. W., Barber, P. A., Desmond, P. M., et al. (2002). Acute hyperglycemia adversely affects stroke outcome: A magnetic resonance imaging and spectroscopy study. *Annals of Neurology, 52,* 20–28.

50. Zygun, D. A., Steiner, L. A., Johnston, A. J., et al. (2004). Hyperglycemia and brain tissue ph after traumatic brain injury. *Neurosurgery, 55,* 877–881; discussion 882.

51. Van den Berghe, G., Schoonheydt, K., Becx, P., Bruyninckx, F., & Wouters, P. J. (2005). Insulin therapy protects the central and peripheral nervous system of intensive care patients. *Neurology, 64,* 1348–1353.

52. Diringer, M. N. (2001). Sodium disturbances frequently encountered in a neurologic intensive care unit. *Neurology India, 49,* Suppl 1, S19–30.

53. Olson, D. M., Chioffi, S. M., Macy, G. E., Meek, L. G., & Cook, H. A. Potential benefits of bispectral index monitoring in critical care. A case study. *Critical Care Nurse, 23,* 45–52.

54. Irwin, R. S., Rippe, J. M., Curley, F. J., & Heard, S. O. (Eds.). (2003). *Procedures and techniques in intensive care medicine* (2nd ed.). Philadelphia: Lippincott Williams & Wilkins.

55. Shaffer, R. B. (2005). Arterial catheter insertion (assist), care and removal. In: Lynn-McHale Wiegand, D. J., & Carlson, K. K. (Eds.). *AACN procedure manual for critical care* (pp. 451–463). Philadelphia: Elsevier Saunders.

56. Harvey, S., Harrison, D. A., Singer, M., et al. (2005). Assessment of the clinical effectiveness of pulmonary artery catheters in management of patients in intensive care (pac-man): A randomised controlled trial. *Lancet, 366,* 472–477.

57. Curley, F. J., & Smyrnios, N. A. (2003). Routine monitoring of the critically ill patient. In: Irwin, R. S. (Ed.). *Procedures and techniques in intensive care medicine* (pp. 226–246). Philadelphia: Lippincott Williams & Wilkins.

58. Good, V. S. (2005). Continuous end-tidal carbon dioxide monitoring. In: Lynn-McHale Wiegand, D. J., & Carlson, K. K. (Eds.). *AACN procedure manual for critical care* (pp. 87–93). Philadelphia: Elsevier Saunders.

59. Pandharipande, P., & Ely, E. W. (2006). Sedative and analgesic medications: Risk factors for delirium and sleep disturbances in the critically ill. *Critical Care Clinics, 22,* 313–327.

60. Barber, J. M. (2003). Pharmacologic management of integrative brain failure. *Critical Care Nursing Quarterly, 26,* 192–207.

61. Jacobi, J., Fraser, G. L., Coursin, D. B., et al. (2002). Clinical practice guidelines for the sustained use of sedatives and analgesics in the critically ill adult. *Critical Care Medicine, 30,* 119–141.

62. Warren, J., Fromm, R. E., Jr., Orr, R. A., Rotello, L. C., & Horst, H. M. (2004). Guidelines for the inter- and intrahospital transport of critically ill patients. *Critical Care Medicine, 32,* 256–262.

63. Bercault, N., Wolf, M., Runge, I., Fleury, J. C., & Boulain, T. (2005). Intrahospital transport of critically ill ventilated patients: A risk factor for ventilator-associated pneumonia—a matched cohort study. *Critical Care Medicine, 33,* 2471–2478.

64. Shirley, P. J., & Stott, S. A. (2001). Intrahospital transport of critically ill patients. *Anaesthesia and Intensive Care, 29,* 669.

65. McLenon, M. (2004). Use of a specialized transport team for intrahospital transport of critically ill patients. *Dimensions of Critical Care Nursing, 23,* 225–229.

66. Youngblut, J. M., & Brooten, D. (2001). Evidence-based nursing practice: Why is it important? *AACN Clinical Issues, 12,* 468–476.

67. Stocchetti, N., Maas, A. I., Chieregato, A., & van der Plas, A. A. (2005). Hyperventilation in head injury: A review. *Chest, 127,* 1812–1827.

68. Wakai, A., Roberts, I., & Schierhout, G. (2005). Mannitol for acute traumatic brain injury. *Cochrane Database of Systematic Reviews,* CD001049.

69. Ogden, A. T., Mayer, S. A., & Connolly, E. S., Jr. (2005). Hyperosmolar agents in neurosurgical practice: The evolving role of hypertonic saline. *Neurosurgery, 57,* 207–215; discussion 207–215.

70. Diringer, M. (2001). Reducing neurologic injury from hyperthermia: A hot topic. *Neurology, 56,* 286–287.

71. Diringer, M. N., Reaven, N. L., Funk, S. E., & Uman, G. C. (2004). Elevated body temperature independently contributes to increased length of stay in neurologic intensive care unit patients. *Critical Care Medicine, 32,* 1489–1495.

72. Azzimondi, G., Bassein, L., Nonino, F., et al. (1995). Fever in acute stroke worsens prognosis. A prospective study. *Stroke, 26,* 2040–2043.

73. Kilpatrick, M. M., Lowry, D. W., Firlik, A. D., Yonas, H., & Marion, D. W. (2000). Hyperthermia in the neurosurgical intensive care unit. *Neurosurgery, 47,* 850–855; discussion 855–856.

74. Alderson, P., Gadkary, C., & Signorini, D. F. (2004). Therapeutic hypothermia for head injury. *Cochrane Database of Systematic Reviews,* CD001048.

75. Burns, S. M., Carpenter, R., Blevins, C., et al. (2006). Detection of inadvertent airway intubation during gastric tube insertion: Capnography versus a colorimetric carbon dioxide detector. *American Journal of Critical Care, 15,* 188–195.

76. Beland, D., D'Angelo, C., & Vinci, D. (2003). Reducing unnecessary blood work in the neurosurgical ICU. *Journal of Neuroscience Nursing, 35,* 149–152.

77. Cohn, J. L., & Fulton, J. S. (2006). Nursing staff perspectives on oral care for neuroscience patients. *Journal of Neuroscience Nursing, 38,* 22–30.

78. Hanneman, S. K., & Gusick, G. M. (2005). Frequency of oral care and positioning of patients in critical care: A replication study. *American Journal of Critical Care, 14,* 378–386; quiz 387.

79. Kollef, M. H. (1999). The prevention of ventilator-associated pneumonia. *New England Journal of Medicine, 340,* 627–634.

80. Grap, M. J., Munro, C. L., Bryant, S., & Ashtiani, B. (2003). Predictors of backrest elevation in critical care. *Intensive Critical Care Nursing, 19,* 68–74.

81. Johnston, K. C., & Mayer, S. A. (2003). Blood pressure reduction in ischemic stroke: A two-edged sword? *Neurology, 61,* 1030–1031.

82. Adams, H., Adams, R., Del Zoppo, G., & Goldstein, L. B. (2005). Guidelines for the early management of patients with ischemic stroke: 2005 guidelines update a scientific statement from the stroke council of the American Heart Association/American Stroke Association. *Stroke, 36,* 916–923.

83. Rose, J. C., & Mayer, S. A. (2004). Optimizing blood pressure in neurological emergencies. *Neurocritical Care, 1,* 287–299.

84. Institute for Healthcare Improvement (2006). Implementing the ventilator bundle. Retrieved May 11, 2006, from http://www.ihi.org/IHI/Topics/CriticalCare/IntensiveCare/Changes/ImplementtheVentilatorBundle.htm

85. Institute for Healthcare Improvement. (2006). Implement the central line bundle. Retrieved May 11, 2006, from http://www.ihi.org/IHI/Topics/CriticalCare/IntensiveCare/Changes/ImplementtheCentralLineBundle.htm

86. Institute for Healthcare Improvement. (2006). Sepsis. Retrieved May 11, 2006, from http://www.ihi.org/IHI/Topics/CriticalCare/Sepsis

87. Tracy, M. F., & Ceronsky, C. (2001). Creating a collaborative environment to care for complex patients and families. *AACN Clinical Issues, 12,* 383–400

88. Arbour, R. (2005). Clinical management of the organ donor. *AACN Clinical Issues, 16,* 551–580; quiz 600–651.

89. Salim, A., Velmahos, G. C., Brown, C., Belzberg, H., & Demetriades, D. (2005). Aggressive organ donor management significantly increases the number of organs available for transplantation. *Journal of Trauma, 58,* 991–994.

90. Johnson, T. D. (2005). Intensive spiritual care: A case study. *Critical Care Nurse, 25,* 20–26; quiz 27.

91. Gilmer, T., Schneiderman, L. J., Teetzel, H., et al. (2005). The costs of nonbeneficial treatment in the intensive care setting. *Health Affairs (Millwood), 24,* 961–971.

92. McGirt, M. J., Woodworth, G. F., Lynch, J. R., & Laskowitz, D. T. (2004). Synthes award for resident research in spinal cord & spinal column injury: Statins for the treatment of neurological injury: A role beyond cholesterol lowering. *Clinical Neurosurgery, 51,* 320–328.

93. Lynch, J. R., Wang, H., McGirt, M. J., et al. (2005). Simvastatin reduces vasospasm after aneurysmal subarachnoid hemorrhage: Results of a pilot randomized clinical trial. *Stroke, 36,* 2024–2026.

94. Laskowitz, D. T., Blessing, R., Floyd, J., White, W. D., & Lynch, J. R. (2005). Panel of biomarkers predicts stroke. *Annals of the New York Academy of Sciences, 1053,* 30.

95. Smith, C. J., Emsley, H. C., Gavin, C. M., et al. (2004). Peak plasma interleukin-6 and other peripheral markers of inflammation in the first week of ischaemic stroke correlate with brain infarct volume, stroke severity and long-term outcome. *BMC Neurology, 4,* 2.

96. Marion, D. W., Puccio, A., Wisniewski, S. R., et al. (2002). Effect of hyperventilation on extracellular concentrations of glutamate, lactate, pyruvate, and local cerebral blood flow in patients with severe traumatic brain injury. *Critical Care Medicine, 30,* 2619–2625.

97. Johnston, A. J., & Gupta, A. K. (2002). Advanced monitoring in the neurology intensive care unit: Microdialysis. *Current Opinion in Critical Care, 8,* 121–127.

98. Hillman, J., Sturnegk, P., Yonas, H., et al. (2005). Bedside monitoring of CBF with xenon-CT and a mobile scanner: A novel method in neurointensive care. *British Journal of Neurosurgery, 19,* 395–401.

Section 5

Nursing Management of Patients With Injury to the Neurological System

Craniocerebral Injuries

Joanne V. Hickey and Bettina C. Prator

SCOPE OF THE PROBLEM

It is estimated that there are 1.5 million new cases of traumatic brain injury (TBI) annually in the United States; 235,000 of these will require hospital admission for treatment, approximately 50,000 people will die, and about 80,000 to 90,000 will have long-term disabilities.[1] The incidence of TBI is highest in younger people (15 to 44 years), although peaks are noted in infants, children, and the elderly. Males are more likely to have head injury, although it is noted that females have a higher mortality rate. Motor vehicle collisions (50%), falls (21%), assaults and violence (12%), and sports and recreational activities (10%) are the major causes of TBI. Driving while under the influence of alcohol and/or drugs, lack of use of restraints among automobile occupants, and lack of use of helmets among motorcyclists are commonly associated with motor vehicular crashes. Fatalities differ based on the cause of TBI, with firearm-related head injuries having a mortality rate of 91%.[2]

Disability after craniocerebral trauma has significant impact not only for the brain-injured person, but also for the family and society. Conservative estimates for permanent disability based on severity of head injury on presentation are 10% in mild, 66% in moderate, and 100% in severe injuries. The loss of human potential and the physical, emotional, psychosocial, and vocational impacts on the patient and family function are immeasurable and devastating. These impacts create the need for many health-related and community services.

OVERVIEW OF CRANIOCEREBRAL TRAUMA

Definitions and Classification

Craniocerebral trauma and **traumatic brain injury** are general designations to denote injury to the skull, brain, or both that is of sufficient magnitude to interfere with normal function and to require treatment. Chart 17-1 provides a classification of scalp and craniocerebral injuries.

Clinically, TBI is often classified according to a severity injury index called the Glasgow Coma Scale (Fig. 17-1). Alternatively, craniocerebral trauma can be classified according to location:

I. Scalp injuries: this may include contusion, abrasion, laceration, and subgaleal hematoma
II. Skull fractures: further classified according to:
   a. Type: include linear skull fracture, comminuted skull fracture, and depressed skull fracture
   b. Location: based on the anatomic location of the fractures such as frontal bone fracture, temporal skull fracture, and basilar skull fracture
III. Brain injuries: classified as:
   a. Focal injuries: include contusion, laceration, and hemorrhage. The latter is further classified as epidural hematoma, subdural hematoma, subarachnoid hemorrhage, and intracerebral hematoma
   b. Diffuse injuries: include concussion and diffuse axonal injury (DAI)

Anatomic Correlations

The cranial vault can be envisioned as a solid container with only one major opening at the base of the skull, the foramen magnum. The cranial vault is separated by bony buttresses into three compartments called fossae (anterior fossa, middle fossa, and posterior fossa). The internal plate of the intracranial vault varies in that it is smooth in some areas such as the occipital bone and highly irregular in other areas such as the frontal area. Some blood vessels lie close to the bone, such as the middle meningeal artery, while other blood vessels go through bony openings to get into the skull. See Chapter 4 for neuroanatomy review.

PATHOPHYSIOLOGY

There are two main stages in the development of brain damage after TBI: primary injury and secondary injury (Fig. 17-2).[3] **Primary injury** comes through direct contact to the head and brain as an immediate result of the initial insult at the moment of injury. The cerebral injury may be focal (contusion or laceration) or diffuse (concussion or diffuse axonal injury). **Secondary injury** results from complicating processes initiated at the moment of injury, which present later in the clinical course. These processes include intracranial hemorrhage, cerebral edema, increased intracranial pressure (ICP), hypoxic (ischemic) brain damage, and infection.[4]

CHART **17–1**   **Classification of Scalp and Craniocerebral Trauma**

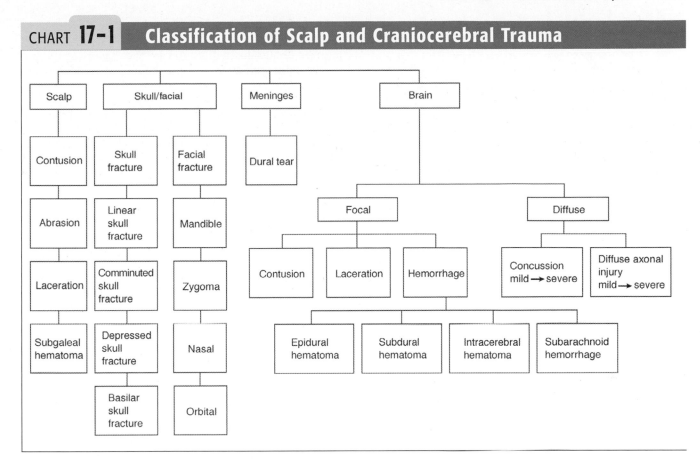

Flow–metabolism mismatch results in cerebral *ischemia*, unleashing the ischemic cascade and other biochemical changes on the cellular level that can lead to neuronal injury and cell death. Other later causes of *secondary injury* can result from a single event, series of events, or multisystem complications. For example, episodes of hypoxemia, systemic hypotension, sustained increased ICP, respiratory complications, electrolyte imbalance, or infections can precipitate additional insult to the injured brain.

PRIMARY BRAIN INJURY

TBI results from a mechanical force or load that sets the head in motion causing cellular damage.[5] Such mechanical forces are differentiated as impact, impulsive, and static. *Impact loading*

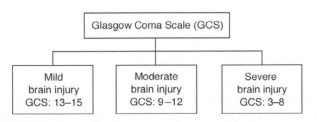

Figure 17-1 • Classification of brain injury according to the Glasgow Coma Scale.

involves direct contact of an object to the head, which results in skull deformation and/or fractures. *Impulse loading* results when another part of the body has direct contact to the object and the head moves as a consequence. This type of mechanical load does not cause skull fractures. *Static loading* is caused by a compressive force to the head, which may result in skull compression and fracture. Head motions caused by these mechanical forces result in contact phenomena injuries and head motions of accelerations and deceleration (Fig. 17-3).[6]

- **Contact phenomena injuries** are the direct result of an object striking the head and include local effects such as scalp laceration, skull fracture, extradural hematoma, contusions, lacerations, and intracerebral hemorrhage.[7] The velocity (low or high) of the impact determines whether the injury is restricted to the scalp or skull (low velocity) or includes the brain (high velocity) (Fig. 17-4).
- **Acceleration-deceleration** injuries are caused by abrupt changes in the velocity of the brain's principally rapid forward movement followed by an abrupt stop (inertia) within the cranial vault. It is produced by head motion at the instant after injury and causes strain on cerebral tissue.[8] These strains often operate simultaneously or in rapid succession to produce injury by compression (pushing together of tissue), tension (traction on tissue), or shearing (opposite but parallel sliding motion of the planes of an object).

A special type of acceleration-deceleration motion is **rotation** (sometimes called **angular acceleration**); it is common

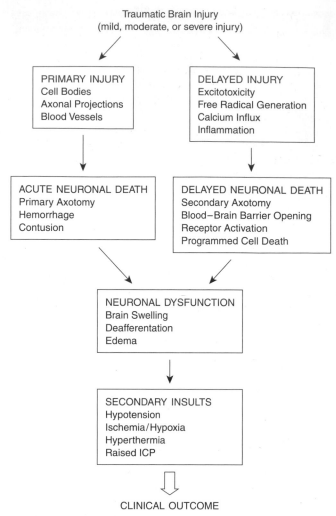

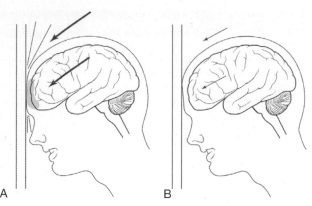

Figure 17-4 • (*A*) High-velocity contact impact on the brain and skull. (*B*) A low-velocity contact impact damages only the skull.

at sites where the brain tissue hits bony buttresses in the cranial vault. The effects of linear acceleration of the head are much less significant than those resulting from rotational forces. The acceleration-deceleration mechanism is responsible for two important types of injury encountered in blunt TBI, acute subdural hematoma and diffuse axonal injury.

Whether the head is fixed or free, a certain amount of acceleration-deceleration always occurs at the time of impact to the skull. The difference in density between the skull (a solid substance) and the brain (a semisolid substance) causes the skull to move faster than its intracranial contents. The brain, which is located within the rigid skull and compartmentalized by the dura and bony buttresses, responds to the force exerted on the skull by gliding forward and then rotating within the compartment. The rotational force produces distortion of the brain as well as tension, stretching, and shearing of involved tissue. Shearing may either result in coup (below the area of impact) and/or contrecoup (opposite of coup area) injuries.[9]

The maximal amount of injury is usually found at the frontal and temporal poles and on the inferior surfaces of the frontal and temporal lobes where brain tissue comes in contact with bony protuberances at the base of the skull. Shearing

Figure 17-2 • Key primary and secondary pathologic events with traumatic brain injury. ICP = intracranial pressure. (Dietrich, W. D. [2000]. Trauma of the nervous system A. Basic neuroscience of neurotrauma. In W. G. Bradley, R. B. Daroff, G. M. Fenichel, & C. D. Marsden [Eds.]. *Neurology in clinical practice* [3rd ed., pp. 1045–1054]. Boston: Butterworth & Heinemann.)

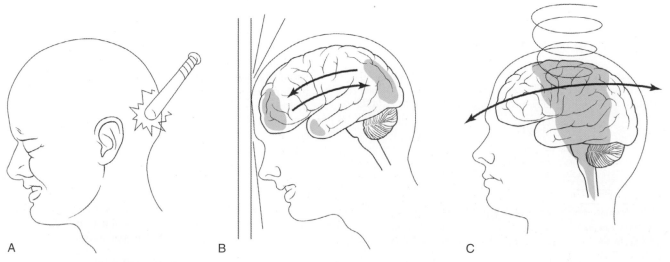

Figure 17-3 • Mechanisms of injury: (*A*) contact, (*B*) acceleration-deceleration, and (*C*) rotational acceleration-deceleration.

or sliding of cerebral tissue over another portion implies stresses on two different planes. With rotational acceleration, the stress of shearing is directed toward areas where tough, fibrous tissue and cerebral tissue meet. These high-risk areas include the crista galli, the sphenoid wing, the margins of the tentorium or falx, and the foramen magnum. The degree of injury will depend on the extent and direction of the angular acceleration. Rotational movement in the brain can cause damage to axons even without gross visible lesions.[10]

SECONDARY BRAIN INJURY

As discussed above, primary injury is the immediate response to the initial impact of mechanical force to the head, which results in cellular damage including neurons and glial cells, which further leads to axonal dysfunction. By comparison, secondary injury is a delayed, physiologic response to the primary injury. After the primary insult, neuropathological changes occur, which may include the activation of biochemical, metabolic, and inflammatory cascades, which may lead to ischemia, cerebral edema, inflammation, and neuronal death.[11] Cerebral pressure autoregulation is altered resulting in the brain's increased susceptibility to systemic blood pressure changes and other physiologic insults. Table 17-1 describes the intracranial and systemic insults that lead to secondary brain injury. The deleterious roles of these physiologic insults on TBI will be discussed later in this chapter in the management section.

Based on experimental models, several theories have been generated to explain the cause and mechanisms associated with secondary injury in TBI. Among the major theories that have been the focus of several clinical trials are neurotoxicity secondary to release of excitatory neurotransmitters that alters the cellular ionic homeostasis, membrane dysfunction due to the oxidative stress free radical cascade, and inflammation.[12]

Neurotoxicity. The release of excitatory amino acids such as glutamate and aspartate is widespread after trauma, resulting in cell swelling, vacuolization, and cell death.[13] Through activation of excitatory amino acid receptors (e.g., glutamate and aspartate), there is an abnormal intracellular calcium influx. In addition, extensive membrane depolarization, induced by trauma, allows for a nonselective opening of the voltage-sensitive calcium channels and an abnormal accumulation of calcium within neurons and glia. The calcium shifts are associated with activation of intracellular lipolytic and proteolytic enzymes, protein kinases (calpains), protein phosphatases, dissolution of microtubules, expression of neurotropic factors, altered gene expression, and activation of cell death genes.[14–17]

Axons first respond to injury by failure of aerobic glycolysis, phosphocreatine production, activation of high-energy cellular functions, and production of adenosine triphosphate (ATP). Failure of aerobic glycolysis increases lactate production and decreases intracellular pH, resulting in cellular acidosis. With failure of ATP production, the sodium-potassium pump can no longer maintain the homeostatic balance of intracellular ions (e.g., higher intracellular concentrations of potassium [K^+] and higher extracellular concentrations of sodium [Na^+]). The result is that extracellular K^+ increases as K^+ leaks out of the cell, and Na^+, calcium [Ca^{2+}], and water move into the cell from the extracellular space.[18]

A major final common pathway for cell death is loss of *calcium* homeostasis.[19] Loss of calcium homeostasis inhibits cellular metabolism. This, in turn, leads to increased breakdown of protein and lipids, increased breakdown of cell membrane from phospholipids hydrolysis, and the production of toxins (i.e., eicosanoid, platelet-activating factor, and free radicals). Concurrently, following trauma, there is immediate severe cellular energy failure causing a strikingly increased level of extracellular excitatory neurotransmitters (EENs). These EENs include the excitatory amino acids (EAAs) glutamate and aspartate and the amine acetylcholine. The source of EAAs is believed to be injured, energy-depleted, and depolarized neural cells (neurons and glia) that release their glutamate. Escalating levels of glutamate and aspartate stimulate specific EAA receptors that normally mediate excitatory synaptic transmission between neurons.

There are two subclasses of glutamate receptors: (1) metabotropic receptors that act by G protein and second messenger and (2) inotropic receptors that are ligand-gated ion channels. Three ion channels are known to be activated by glutamate and are named for the pharmacologic congeners of glutamate to which they respond maximally. These ion channels are kainate receptor ($\uparrow$ Na^+ influx and K^+ efflux), adenosine monophosphate (AMP) A receptor (α-amino-3-hydroxy-5-methyl-4-isoxazole propionic acid) ($\uparrow$ Na^+ influx and K^+ efflux), and N-methyl-D-aspartate (NMDA) receptor ($\uparrow$ Na^+, Ca^{2+}). Excessive stimulation of glutamate receptors opens ionic channels, which causes sodium-mediated cellular swelling and calcium-mediated neuronal disintegration from membrane lipid hydrolysis and protease activation.[20] Thus, overstimulated EAA receptors have been implicated as a final common pathway of neurotoxicity in numerous central nervous system problems, including traumatic injury.[21]

Oxidative stress free radical cascade. A metabolic cascade is activated after the primary injury that leads to oxygen radical superoxide anion formation, which includes superoxide, hydroxyl, hydrogen peroxide, singlet oxygen, and nitrous oxide. Their activity varies with tissue pH and the availability of superoxide dismutase (SOD). SOD converts superoxide to hydrogen peroxide, which in turn is converted to water by

TABLE 17-1   CAUSES OF SECONDARY BRAIN INJURIES

INTRACRANIAL CAUSES	SYSTEMIC CAUSES
• Intracranial hypertension	• Hypotension
• Cerebral edema/hematoma	• Hypoxemia
• Hydrocephalus	• Hypercarbia/hypocarbia
• Seizures	• Hyperthermia
• Cerebral vasospasm	• Hyponatremia
• Infection	• Hyperglycemia/hypoglycemia

catalase. Free radicals can damage proteins, the phospholipid components of cells, and organelle membranes, which results in membrane hydrolysis. The disruption of cellular membranes creates a vicious cycle of further generation of free radicals and ongoing cellular damage and neural injury.[22]

The blood and breakdown products within the brain following tissue injury become another source of oxygen free radicals. Free iron from hemoglobin breakdown can transfer an electron to oxygen-forming superoxide molecules or to hydrogen peroxide to form hydroxyl. These free radicals can overwhelm cytoplasm defenses and begin to oxidize cellular membrane by *lipid peroxidation*. Through lipid peroxidation, electrons are transferred to unsaturated fatty acids, which form free radicals called lipid peroxyl or alkoxyl moieties.[23] Ongoing lipid peroxidation causes breakdown of the cellular membrane and oxidation of membrane lipoproteins. The process also spreads to adjacent cells and perpetuates cell death and edema.[24]

Inflammation. An inflammatory cascade is activated within minutes of primary injury following TBI, which results in the release of several immune mediators known as cytokines. These cytokines are major players of a process that includes expression of adhesion molecules, cellular infiltration, and further release of more inflammatory cells and growth factors leading to either cell regeneration or cell death.[25] This dual role of cytokines in the pathophysiology of TBI has been widely studied and conflicting results have been found on whether or not cerebral inflammatory cascade following TBI is neuroprotective or contributory to neuronal and glial cell damage. Inflammatory mediators such tumor necrosis factor (TNF) and interleukins (ILs) that include IL-1, IL-6, IL-8, IL-10, and IL-12 have been noted in increased amounts in the cerebrospinal fluid (CSF) following TBI in several experimental studies.[26–30] Specifically, TNF has been associated with cerebral edema, blood–brain barrier (BBB) disruption, and neuronal cell death in the acute phase of TBI. Neutrophil and macrophage infiltration is also believed to exacerbate posttraumatic altered homeostasis of the brain and BBB disruption. On the other hand, IL-6 demonstrates neuroprotective function by preventing TNF synthesis, promoting nerve growth factor and neuronal regeneration, and neutralizing NMDA-mediated toxicity. Transforming growth factor-β (TGF-β) and IL-10 are believed to have beneficial roles in the inflammatory cascade following TBI by inhibiting the release of proinflammatory cytokines such as TNF and IL-1. Growth factors including nerve growth factor (NGF), basic fibroblast growth factor (bFGF), brain-derived and glial-derived neutrotrophic factor, and neurotrophin-3 (NT-3) are believed to have neuroprotective roles, specifically with neuronal repair and regeneration.

PRIMARY INJURY: DIAGNOSIS AND MANAGEMENT

Scalp Lacerations

The velocity and characteristics of the impacting contact object determine the extent of scalp injury. Injuries to the scalp can be classified as follows:

- **Abrasion**: the top layer of the scalp is scraped away; this is a minor injury that may cause slight bleeding. The area is cleaned and possibly dressed, and no other treatment is required.
- **Contusion**: the scalp is bruised with possible effusion of blood into the subcutaneous layer without a break in the integrity of the skin; there is no specific treatment.
- **Laceration**: the scalp is torn and may bleed profusely; suturing may be necessary.
- **Subgaleal hematoma**: a hematoma in the subgaleal layer of the scalp occurs and will usually absorb on its own.

A scalp contusion may benefit from the application of ice initially to prevent a hematoma from forming. Skull films may be ordered to rule out a skull fracture. Depending on other signs and symptoms, a computed tomography (CT) scan rather than a skull film may be ordered to rule out underlying skull or brain injury. Scalp lacerations often require suturing and aseptic management.

CLINICAL PEARLS: Scalp lacerations can be a source of acute blood loss; therefore, they should be evaluated immediately and sutured as indicated.

Skull Fracture

The mechanism of skull injury is direct contact. Factors that determine the degree of injury include the skull's thickness at the point of impact and the weight, velocity, and angle of impact of the intruding object. At impact, several actions are set in motion in split-second sequence. At the point of impact, there is a relative indentation that may be temporary or permanent, depending on velocity. Stress waves are set into motion, radiating throughout the entire skull. With *high-velocity impact*, a depressed skull fracture with or without a dual tear and cerebral laceration can occur. With *low-velocity impact*, the area of indentation rebounds outward and may result in no fracture, a linear fracture, or a comminuted fracture (see Fig. 17-4). The fracture line extends from the point of impact and is directed by bony buttresses toward the base of the skull.

Classification

Skull fractures are classified as follows:

- **Linear**: a singular fracture line occurring to the skull, which could be displaced or nondisplaced
- **Comminuted**: the skull is splintered or shattered into pieces
- **Depressed**: a fracture of the skull in which a fragment is depressed; the scalp and/or dura may or may not be torn
- **Open depressed fracture**: also known as compound skull fracture; is an opening of the skull as a result of comminuted depressed skull fractures and tearing of the dura mater and the scalp
- **Basal skull fracture**: often arises from extension of a linear fracture into the base of the skull. The frontal and temporal bones are usually affected so that the fracture involves the anterior or middle fossa. It is important to distinguish

between fractures of the cranial vault and those of the base of the skull. Although the mechanism by which the fractures arise is similar, the consequences of basilar fractures are more serious than those of cranial vault fractures. A feature of basal skull fractures is the frequency with which they traverse the paranasal air sinuses (frontal, maxillary, or ethmoid) of the frontal bone or the air sinuses located in the petrous portion of the temporal bone. The fragility of the bones in these areas and the intimate adherence of delicate dura account for the frequency of lesions in these areas and the consequent leakage of CSF through the dural tear manifested either by rhinorrhea (from the nose) or otorrhea (from the ear). Continued leakage of CSF can lead to serious infections. Such patients are at high risk for meningitis, abscess formation, and osteomyelitis from organisms gaining entry by way of the ear, nose, or paranasal sinuses through the dural tear.

Other complications associated with basal skull fracture include cerebrovascular injury such as internal carotid artery injury at the point of entry to the cranial vault through the foramen at the base of the skull. Fracture in or around the foramen can result in cerebral hemorrhage from laceration, thrombosis, development of a traumatic aneurysm, a carotid-cavernous sinus fistula, or carotid-cavernous sinus compression. A *carotid-cavernous sinus fistula* is characterized by chemosis, bruit, and pulsating exophthalmos. The oculomotor, trochlear, trigeminal, and abducens cranial nerves pass through the cavernous sinus. Compression of the sinus may be evident because of ophthalmoplegia or trigeminal dysfunction. Another potential complication is trapping portions of the frontal arachnoid and dura between the fracture edges, thus creating a permanent route for leakage of CSF. Radiographic and surgical identification of the exact area of the dural tear is extremely difficult, yet such identification is necessary to facilitate surgical repair.

A CT is used to diagnose a skull fracture. The ease with which a diagnosis of skull fracture is made depends on the site of the fracture. If a fracture is found on CT, there is always the question of associated brain injury, and magnetic resonance imaging (MRI) provides better resolution and clearer pictures at the fracture-cerebral site.

Most basal skull fractures are extensions of fractures of the cranial vault. A CT scan may not be sensitive enough to clearly show a basal skull fracture. A CT scan and clinical criteria are used to make a diagnosis. For example, a linear fracture of the parietal bone may be readily evident on a regular CT scan, whereas thin-slice CT may be necessary to find a basal skull fracture. If the paranasal sinuses are fractured, air may be evident in the frontal and maxillary sinuses on x-ray studies. With fracture of the temporal bone, the mastoid sinuses may be opaque. Common findings of **anterior fossa fractures** (fractures of the paranasal sinuses) include the following:

- Rhinorrhea (drainage of CSF, blood, or both from the nose)
- Subconjunctival hemorrhage of the eye
- Periorbital ecchymosis (raccoon's eyes)

With **middle fossa fractures** (fractures associated with fracture of the temporal petrous bone), common findings include:

- Otorrhea (drainage of CSF, blood, or both from the ear)
- Hemotympanum (blood behind the tympanic membrane)
- Battle's sign (ecchymosis over mastoid bone that develops 12 to 24 hours after injury)
- Conductive hearing loss (may be associated with signs of vestibular dysfunction, such as vertigo, nausea, and nystagmus)
- Possibly facial nerve palsy (Bell's palsy) that appears 5 to 7 days after injury

Treatment of skull fractures depends on the type of fracture. Generally, linear skull fractures do not require special medical management other than observation for underlying cerebral injury. A depressed skull fracture with an open scalp, skull, and dura mater requires surgery to débride, elevate, and remove bone fragments from the wound. If the fragments are extensive, a craniectomy may be necessary. Surgical elevation of depressed skull fractures may be necessary with greater than 8 to 10 mm depression, neurological deficit, CSF leak, and presence or absence of open depressed fracture.[31] For cosmetic and brain protective purposes, a cranioplasty with insertion of a bone or artificial graft may follow immediately or be postponed for a few months (approximately 3 to 6 months) if brain swelling is present.

Use of prophylactic antibiotics with basal skull fractures is controversial; many argue that prophylactic use allows for proliferation of other virulent organisms. Most CSF leaks resolve spontaneously within 7 to 10 days. To aid resolution of leakage lasting more than 4 to 5 days, a lumbar catheter for continual drainage of CSF may be inserted.[32] If leakage of CSF continues, a craniotomy may be necessary to repair the tear surgically or to repair the leakage with grafts.

Traumatic Brain Injuries

Injuries to the brain can be focal or diffuse. *Focal injuries* include contusions and hematomas. Concussions and diffuse axonal injuries are the major *diffuse injuries*. TBI could also be classified as penetrating or nonpenetrating. Common penetrating injuries are caused by gunshots and impalement and may result in contusions, hematoma, laceration, and cerebral edema. In all cases, the diagnosis of TBI is made with a noncontrast CT scan. In some instances, a contrast CT or MRI may be requested after a noncontrast CT scan, but neither a contrast CT scan nor MRI is required on an emergency basis. In severe TBI, a follow-up CT is often ordered 3 to 5 days postinjury or as necessary to follow progress and as needed for investigation of any neurological changes.

Focal Cerebral Injuries: Contusions, Lacerations, and Hematomas

Cerebral Contusions. The anterior and middle fossae at the base of the skull have irregular, bony buttresses that are capable of contusing or lacerating the brain on impact. The distribution of *contusions* in these particular areas is explained by the movement of the brain within the skull (Fig. 17-5). The frontal and temporal poles are vulnerable because of the relative restraint created by the sphenoidal ridges and other bony irregularities of the base of the skull. Less common sites of injury are the inferolateral angles of

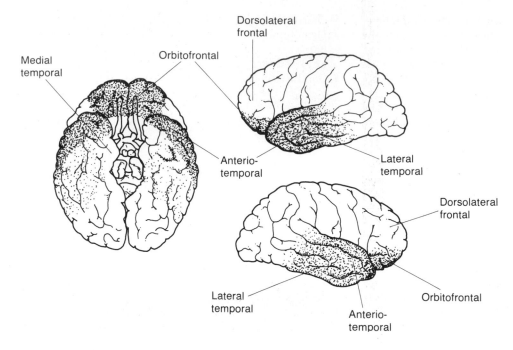

Figure 17-5 • Cerebral contusions. The most frequently involved areas of the brain in cerebral contusions are the orbitofrontal and anterior-temporal regions. These are the areas that come in direct contact with the irregular bony surfaces in the inside frontal skull area.

the occipital lobes, the medial surfaces of the hemispheres, and the corpus callosum. The firm falx cerebri and tentorium cerebelli not only restrict movement of the brain, but also contribute to contusion or laceration during impact as cerebral tissue impacts on these hard surfaces. This is particularly true when the rotational force of acceleration-deceleration is applied to the frontal-temporal area. Injury to the inferolateral angles of the occipital lobe and, less commonly, the inferior surface of the cerebellar and cerebral peduncles can result from impact by the tentorium. A blow to the vertex of the head may cause cerebellar, cerebellar-tonsillar, and brainstem contusions initiated by the downward thrust of the brain toward the foramen magnum.

A **cerebral contusion** is a bruising of the surface of the brain (cerebral parenchyma). Contusions may occur from blunt trauma (direct contact), a depressed skull fracture, a penetrating wound, or an acceleration-deceleration closed injury. With acceleration-deceleration, the sites of injury are generally predictable and are located where the brain has an impact on the bony protuberances within the skull (see Fig. 17-5). These areas include the frontal poles, frontal-orbital areas, frontal-temporal junction around the Sylvian fissure (where the brain is close to the lesser sphenoidal wings), and temporal poles (the inferior and lateral surfaces of the temporal lobes where there is a shelf-like separation between the anterior and middle fossae).

The clinical effect of a contusion depends on its size and related cerebral edema. Small, unilateral, frontal lesions may be asymptomatic, whereas larger lesions may result in neurological deficits. Contusions can cause secondary mass effect from edema resulting in increased ICP, and possible herniation syndromes. For patients with cerebral contusions, no surgical interventions are indicated and patients are managed medically with emphasis given toward prevention of secondary injuries such as intracranial pressure management.

Classification. Contusions are classified as gliding or surface contusions.[5] **Gliding contusions** result from rotational motion and are likely associated with DAI. Usual areas involved are the parasagittal regions of the brain with bilateral and symmetric focal hemorrhages of the cortex and surrounding white matter. **Surface contusions,** on the other hand, are injuries caused by contact forces and include[33]:

- **Fracture contusions** occur at the sites of fractures and are particularly severe in the frontal lobes when associated with fractures in the anterior fossa.
- **Coup contusions** are found directly under the areas of impact (contact).
- **Contrecoup contusions,** by contrast, are cerebral injuries at the *opposite pole* of direct contact. A contrecoup injury is most often a contusion, but occasionally it may be a laceration. Both coup and contrecoup injuries are caused by the rapid acceleration-deceleration of the semisolid brain within the rigid cranial vault.
- **Herniation contusions** occur at the time of injury at the point of contact where the medial part of the temporal lobe produces an impact at the edge of the tentorium or the cerebellar tonsils against the foramen magnum.

Cerebral Lacerations. A cerebral laceration refers to a traumatic tearing of the cerebral tissue. It is related to high-impact injuries and is treated in the same manner as a cerebral contusion is managed.

Intracranial Hemorrhage/Hematomas. Traumatic intracranial hemorrhage is a common complication of TBI. Although bleeding may begin immediately after injury, its presence may not be clinically apparent until sufficient blood accumulates to cause signs and symptoms of a space-occupying lesion and mass effect. The interval between bleeding and the appearance of clinical symptoms may be minutes or weeks, depending on the site and rate of bleeding. Intracranial hemorrhage may be an occult development in a patient who has sustained a seemingly minor TBI in which consciousness has been maintained or quickly restored. Other patients with hemorrhage may be unconscious from the moment of impact.

The major types of bleeding associated with head trauma are epidural hematoma (EDH), subdural hematoma (SDH), and intracerebral hematoma (ICH). Other focal bleeding includes traumatic subarachnoid hemorrhage (TSAH) and intraventricular hemorrhage (IVH). Each lesion is a distinct clinical entity, but two or more types of hemorrhagic lesions can coexist.

Epidural Hematoma. EDH, also known as an extradural hematoma, refers to bleeding into the potential space between the inner table of the skull (inner periosteum) and the dura mater. It accounts for about 0.5% to 6% of traumatic head lesions. Epidural hematomas are seen most often in children older than 2 years old and young adults because their dura is less firmly attached to the bony table than it is in older adults. Eighty-five percent of EDHs are arterial in origin, occurring from a tear of a branch of the middle meningeal artery in a patient who has sustained a skull fracture to the thin, squamous portion of the temporal bone, under which is located the middle meningeal artery. Therefore, common locations of the bleed are the temporal and temporoparietal regions, but may also occur in the frontal area. Occasionally an EDH may be venous, the result of torn dural venous sinuses particularly in the parieto-occipital region or posterior fossa. As the bleed expands, it gradually strips away the dura from the inner table of the skull, and a large, ovoid mass develops, creating pressure on the underlying brain and causing a mass effect.

Clinically, the "classic" description of an EDH was that of a momentary unconsciousness followed by a lucid period lasting for minutes to several hours. The lucid period was followed by rapid deterioration in the level of consciousness (LOC) from drowsiness to lethargy to coma as a mass effect and herniation developed. Only about 10% to 27% of patients with EDH present with the above classic manifestation. Other findings include ipsilateral pupillary dilation, contralateral hemiparesis, headache, vomiting, seizures, and hemi-hyperreflexia with a unilateral Babinski sign.[31]

In 60% of patients, a unilateral dilated ipsilateral pupil without loss of consciousness is found. Bradycardia and respiratory distress are late findings. If untreated, neurological deterioration may occur from drowsiness to lethargy and then to coma as mass effect and herniation developed.

EDHs are commonly identified through CT scan of the head (without contrast), which appears as a biconvex or lenticular high-density lesion adjacent to the skull (Fig. 17-6). Mass effect is frequently associated with this bleed, which can be seen radiographically. Lesions not noted on initial CT scan but on subsequent CT scans are known as delayed EDHs.

Immediate diagnosis and surgical evacuation of the hematoma are associated with lower mortality rate. Prognosis is associated with the severity and the duration of the brain compression caused by the EDH. Therefore, early diagnosis and management are important.[34] Surgical indication

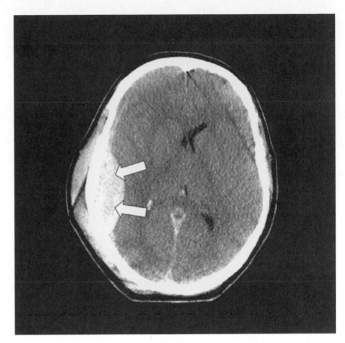

Figure 17-6 • Computed tomography scan: epidural hematoma.

includes symptomatic EDH and/or acute, greater than 1-cm bleed. Presence of coagulopathy associated with a hematoma should also be identified and optimally corrected to promote hemostasis and prevent rebleeding.

CLINICAL VIGNETTE: MJ, a 19-year-old white man, arrived at the emergency department (ED) via ambulance with altered mental status. Emergency medical service (EMS) personnel reported that the patient was an unrestrained driver in a motor vehicular accident. He was initially alert, oriented, and ambulatory on the scene, but apparently became confused and agitated. During transport to the emergency department (ED), the patient became obtunded. On arrival at the ED, the patient's Glasgow Coma Scale score was 5 and he subsequently required emergent intubation. Head CT scan revealed a right frontotemporal EDH with 0.7 cm right to left midline shift. The patient was taken to the operating suite for an urgent craniotomy for EDH evacuation.

CLINICAL PEARLS: Surgical indication for an EDH is symptomatic and/or acute bleed greater than 1 cm on CT scan.

Subdural Hematoma. An SDH refers to bleeding between the dura mater and arachnoid or pial layer. Approximately 30% of patients with posttraumatic intracranial lesions have SDHs. Most SDHs are caused by tearing of the bridging veins located over the convexity of the brain. Other causes include tearing of small cortical arteries, cerebral contusions, and acute bleeding into chronic SDHs. Bilateral SDHs are not uncommon. SDHs are categorized based on the interval between injury and the appearance of signs and symptoms.

Although there are no uniform definitions, three classes with approximate time intervals are recognized:

- *Acute:* up to 48 hours. This consists of clotted blood that is hyperdense on CT.
- *Subacute:* 2 days to about 2 weeks. The clot now lyses, and blood products and fluid are present. Clot will be seen isodense on CT scan.
- *Chronic:* longer than 2 weeks to several months. The clot is a fluid mass and is hypodense on CT.

Clinical presentations are usually due to brain compression and vary according to the location of the lesion and the interval between injury and presentation of symptoms. Common signs and symptoms associated with an *acute SDH* include gradual or rapid deterioration of the LOC from drowsiness, slow cerebration, and confusion to coma; pupillary changes; and hemiparesis or hemiplegia. *Subacute SDHs* are associated with less severe underlying compression. Signs and symptoms of subacute SDHs correspond closely to those of the acute SDH. *Chronic SDHs* can develop from seemingly minor TBIs. The time elapsed between injury and the development of symptoms may be months, so the initial injury itself may not be recalled. The lesion becomes encased within a membrane that is easily separated from the arachnoid and dura. The SDH slowly enlarges, probably because of repeated small bleeding, until a mass effect occurs. The most common symptoms of a chronic SDH include headache (progressing in severity), slow cerebration, confusion, drowsiness, and possibly seizure. Papilledema, sluggish ipsilateral pupillary response, and hemiparesis may later develop.

Elderly patients with cerebral atrophy associated with the normal aging process are prone to develop SDH because of traction on fragile bridging veins. This is particularly true with tear and rupture in the elderly with cerebral trauma. Atrophy also provides more free space into which bleeding can occur before symptoms are evident from a mass effect. With chronic SDH, the development of symptoms can be subtle because of gradual spatial compensation. Patients who have had long-term alcohol abuse with related cerebral atrophy and impaired blood clotting resulting from altered liver function and/or use of anticoagulants are also especially prone to SDH.

CT scan of the head will reveal a crescentic hyperdense lesion with edema/mass effect in acute SDH. Unlike EDH, CT scan findings of acute SDH appear concave over the brain surface and more diffuse (Fig. 17-7). The appearance of subacute and chronic SDH, as discussed earlier, varies according to density on CT scan.

Immediate surgical evacuation of the clot is recommended for symptomatic SDHs that are greater than 1 cm in thickness. Factors that affect outcome include initial Glasgow Coma Scale (GCS) score, pupillary status, time interval between trauma and treatment, clot size, mass effect, and presence of other traumatic lesions.[35] Low GCS score (<7), the presence of pupillary abnormalities, delay in treatment (>4 hours after injury), larger hematoma volume (>100 mL), midline shifts >1.5 cm, and associated cerebral contusions and/or traumatic subarachnoid hemorrhage are associated with poor functional survival and higher mortality rate.

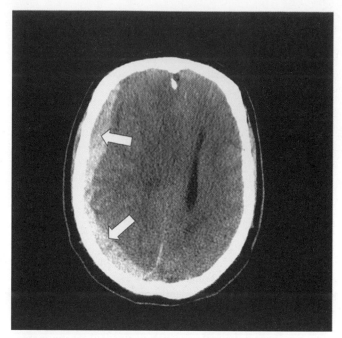

Figure 17-7 • Computed tomography: subdural hematoma.

CLINICAL VIGNETTE: JP is a 75-year-old Hispanic man who presented at the ED with a chief complaint of confusion. The family reports that the patient fell 3 weeks ago with no loss of consciousness noted at that time. Difficulty with balance and coordination was noted since the event, and the patient suffered from frequent falls. Confusion was noted 2 days ago, which appeared to be worsening. Past medical history includes coronary artery disease and hypertension for which patient is taking aspirin and metoprolol, respectively. The physical examination was unremarkable except for confusion and mild lethargy. Blood chemistry, complete blood count, and drug screen were unremarkable. Head CT scan revealed an acute and chronic left frontal, parietal, and temporal SDH with 1 cm left to right midline shift. The patient was then admitted to the neurotrauma intensive care unit (ICU) for monitoring with a planned craniotomy for SDH evacuation the following day, per neurosurgery. On arrival to the ICU, 6 units platelet transfusion was ordered for a suspected qualitative platelet dysfunction secondary to aspirin use.

CLINICAL PEARLS: Surgical indication for an SDH is symptomatic and greater than 1 cm thickness of bleed on CT scan.

Intracerebral Hematoma.   An ICH refers to bleeding into the brain parenchyma (Fig. 17-8) resulting from contusions or blood vessel injury. Approximately 16% of TBI cases are due to ICH.[36] Common locations are below the surface of the cortex in the basal ganglia or white matter. Manifestations include headache; altered mental status, which can vary from confusion to a reduced level of consciousness or coma;

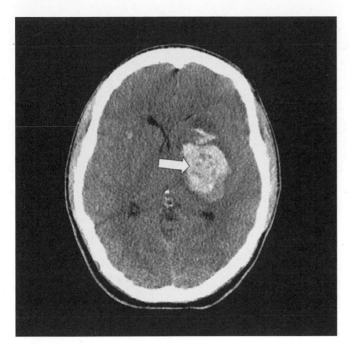

Figure 17-8 • Computed tomography scan: intracerebral hematoma.

contralateral hemiplegia; and ipsilateral pupil dilatation.[37] Clinically, ICHs behave as expanding, space-occupying lesions and consequently cause increased intracranial pressure, which could result in herniation. ICHs are seen on CT scan as high-density lesions in the brain parenchyma. They could be seen on the initial CT scan but could also be noted on later CT scans. **Delayed traumatic ICHs** may also occur a few hours to days after the head trauma.[38] They are noted in about 1% to 7% of TBI patients.

Similarly to EDH and SDH, the size of the ICH determines the best treatment approach. Considerable controversy exists regarding the indications for surgery in ICH. This is a complex decision based on the patient's neurological condition, size and location of the hematoma, patient's age, and patient/family wishes. Surgery rarely improves neurological outcome.[31] As a result, many patients are managed medically with supportive care and management of increased ICP.

CLINICAL VIGNETTE: ML is a 58-year-old white man who was found on the ground after a possible assault outside a bar. The patient was unresponsive with a GCS score of 4, requiring intubation for airway protection per EMS. No sedation and/or paralytic agent was given during the procedure. No change in GCS score was noted on arrival to the ED, with left pupil reactive to light at 2 mm and right pupil fixed and dilated at 5 mm. Emergent CT scan of the head revealed a large right basal ganglia hematoma with midline shift and effacement of the basal cisterns. Drug screen was unremarkable; however, a serum alcohol level of 130 mg/dL was noted. No neurosurgical intervention was planned, and the patient was transferred to the ICU for supportive care with an external ventricular drain (EVD) with ICP monitor placed.

Traumatic Subarachnoid Hemorrhage. TSAH is the accumulation of blood throughout the subarachnoid and is usually caused by surface contusions.[37] Onset of symptoms varies according to location and the rate of bleeding. Clinical presentation includes headache, reduced level of consciousness, nuchal rigidity, hemiplegia, and/or ipsilateral papillary abnormalities. Increased density spread thinly over convexity and causing fullness of the sulci and basal cisterns are usually noted on noncontrast CT scan of the head. Cerebral angiography is not indicated but may be done in cases when there is unclear history of trauma to exclude the presence of cerebral aneurysm.

There is no specific treatment indicated for TSAH. Management is usually supportive care. Some cases of cerebral vasospasm had been reported anecdotally as a consequence of TSAH, but its incidence is not well established; therefore, the use of calcium channel blockers (i.e., nimodipine) as prophylaxis is not a common practice. Cerebral angiogram to exclude vasospasm may be indicated in cases of delayed focal neurological deficits following TSAH.

Intraventricular Hematoma. IVH (Fig. 17-9) occurs secondary to traumatic subarachnoid hemorrhage or as an extension from an ICH and could be suggestive of severe head injury. It is reported in approximately 10% of severe head injuries.[39] Signs and symptoms include altered level of consciousness, hemiparesis, ipsilateral pupil dilation, and intracranial hypertension. Management consists of drainage of CSF with a ventriculostomy, intracranial pressure management, and prevention of secondary brain injuries.

Diffuse Cerebral Injuries: Concussions and Diffuse Axonal Injuries

Concussions. A cerebral concussion is defined as a transient, temporary, neurogenic dysfunction caused by mechanical

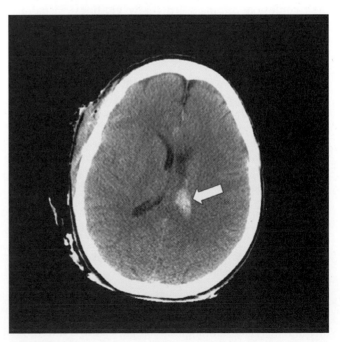

Figure 17-9 • Computed tomography scan: intraventricular hematoma.

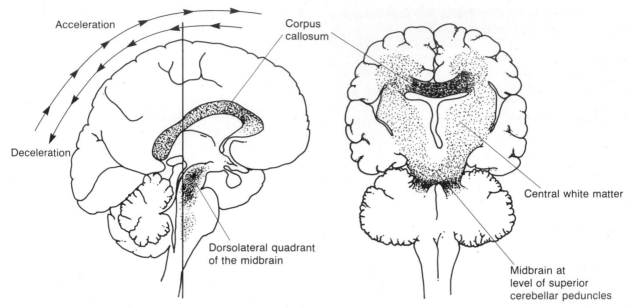

Figure 17-10 • Diffuse axonal injury. Diffuse axonal injury results from acceleration-deceleration and shearing force on the brain. Depending on the severity of the injury, the areas of the brain most often affected are the corpus callosum, the dorsolateral area of the midbrain, and the parasagittal white matter.

force to the brain. Acceleration-deceleration (with shearing stress on the reticular formation) is the mechanism of injury usually due to a nonpenetrating injury such as a sudden blow to the head. Signs and symptoms may include immediate unconsciousness lasting a few seconds, minutes, or hours; momentary loss of reflexes; and momentary (few seconds) and possible retrograde or antegrade amnesia (loss of memory for events immediately before and after the injury, respectively). Other presentations include headache, drowsiness, confusion, dizziness, irritability, giddiness, visual disturbances (seeing stars), and gait disturbances. Patients who have sustained other TBIs, such as contusions and hematomas, may have also sustained a concussion in most instances.

Concussions are classified as mild or classic, based on the degree of symptoms, particularly those of unconsciousness and memory loss. **Mild concussion** is defined as temporary neurological dysfunction without loss of consciousness or memory. By contrast, a **moderate** or **classic concussion** includes temporary neurological dysfunction, unconsciousness, and memory loss. Recovery of consciousness varies from minutes to hours. Some patients will develop a postconcussion syndrome (described later in this section).

CLINICAL PEARLS: Diagnosis of concussion is based on the patient's history and neurological examination.

The diagnosis of concussion is based on the patient's history and neurological examination. CT scan or MRI is usually unremarkable, although radiologic testing is still recommended in cases where concussion is suspected to exclude any other traumatic lesion and confirm absence of any focal lesion on a CT scan, if a CT scan is done. Depending on the severity of the concussion, a short-stay admission may be done to observe the patient's neurological status. In other cases, a patient may be discharged home under the supervision of a responsible adult. Specific verbal and written instructions about what signs and symptoms to look for and report immediately to the physician should be provided. The patient should also be cautioned in avoiding alcohol, illicit drugs, and/or other substances such as narcotic analgesics or sedatives that may mask any signs of neurological dysfunction.[40] For any persistent and/or worsening signs and symptoms, follow-up is imperative.

Diffuse Axonal Injury. DAI is a primary TBI associated with acceleration-deceleration during which shearing forces damage nerve fibers at the moment of injury (Fig. 17-10). Because of the difference in acceleration gradient on certain areas of the brain during primary impact, shearing forces at the white–gray junction, corpus callosum, brainstem, and sometimes cerebellum produce diffuse tearing of axons and small blood vessels.[41,42] DAI accounts for approximately 50% of primary brain injuries and 35% of deaths from all TBIs.[33,43] It is characterized by distinct gross and microscopic findings including axonal swellings that are widely distributed in the cerebral hemispheric white matter, corpus callosum, and upper brainstem; gross hemorrhagic lesions of the corpus callosum; and gross hemorrhagic lesions involving one or both dorsolateral quadrants of the rostral brainstem.[44]

An acceleration mechanism produces diffuse axonal injury with axonal shearing (*primary axotomy*) alone or together with tearing of blood vessels that cause microscopic petechial hemorrhage. In animal models, primary axotomy, in which axons are sheared, severed, or disconnected, is uncommon.[45,46] In transected axons, axoplasmic transport from the cell body to the axon terminal continues. However, the transported material cannot pass the damaged area, where it accumulates, causing the axon to swell.[47] Most axons undergo a series of changes that result in *secondary axotomy*. Although the timeline for neuronal death varies, primary axotomy usual occurs in approximately 1 hour, whereas secondary axotomy is more protracted.

The postulated sequence of axotomy is summarized as follows:

- **Primary axotomy** (<1 hour)
  - Axolemma permeability increases.
  - An influx of calcium occurs.
  - Microtubules are lost.
  - Mitochondria swell.
  - Focal loss of axonal transport occurs.

} Axotomy

Axonal injury is a dynamic, established, sequential pathophysiologic cascade of events that result in secondary axotomy.[48]

- **Secondary axotomy** (>4 hours)
  - Activation of intracellular leukocytic and proteolytic enzymes, including protein kinase, occurs.
  - Changes occur in phosphorylation.
  - Change occurs in the structure of neurofilament.
  - Loss of axonal transport occurs.
  - Axonal swelling occurs in 2 to 4 hours.
  - Neurofilament proteolysis occurs.

} Axotomy

A grading system based on the distribution of *pathologic findings* includes[32]:

- **DAI grade 1:** there is histologic evidence of axonal damage in the white matter of the cerebral hemispheres, corpus callosum, brainstem, and less commonly cerebellum.
- **DAI grade 2:** in addition to evidence of axonal injury, there are also focal lesions of the corpus callosum.
- **DAI grade 3:** in addition to findings of grades 1 and 2, there are lesions of the dorsolateral quadrant of the rostral brainstem.

Substantial recent research has increased our understanding of DAI. Diffuse injury to axons, which are apparent microscopically throughout the white matter of the cerebral hemispheres, the cerebellum, and the brainstem, has three presentation forms related to the length of the patient's survival.[33] In short-term survival (days), there are a large number of *axonal bulbs* throughout the white matter. It takes about 15 to 18 hours for the axonal bulbs to appear in humans.[49] In intermediate survival (weeks), there are large numbers of microglia clusters throughout the white matter. In long-term survival (e.g., vegetative state), there is *long tract degeneration* of the Wallerian type in these areas. In these survivors, the degenerative effects are finally replaced by *diffuse white matter gliosis*. Gliosis is the chief finding in long-term survivors and is related to severe and permanent disabilities.[50,51]

DAI is characterized clinically by functional cerebral failure, which may range from confusion to coma and death. It is also classified *clinically* as mild, moderate, or severe based on coma duration and brainstem signs.[52,53]

- **Mild DAI:** coma lasting 6 to 24 hours with the patient beginning to follow commands by 24 hours. *Outcome:* death is uncommon, but cognitive and neurological deficits are common.
- **Moderate DAI:** coma lasting longer than 24 hours, but without prominent brainstem signs. This is a common presentation (about 45% of all patients). *Outcome:* incomplete recovery in those who survive.
- **Severe DAI:** coma is prolonged and associated with prominent brainstem signs (e.g., decortication, decerebration). This presentation is seen in about 36% of all DAI patients. *Outcome:* death or severe disability.

CLINICAL PEARLS: Definite diagnosis of DAI can only be made microscopically; therefore, diagnosis is usually based on loss of consciousness with significant cerebral trauma but with unremarkable head CT scan; MRI of the head may occasionally demonstrate small lesions.

The clinical diagnosis of DAI is based on immediate onset of unconsciousness in a patient who has significant cerebral trauma and no intracranial lesion noted on CT scan. In some cases, an MRI may demonstrate small lesions not evident on a CT. Definitive diagnosis of DAI could only be made based on microscopic findings. The treatment is supportive care, specifically to the unconscious patient, which will be further discussed in this chapter. DAI is associated with significant disability or death whether or not there is a coexisting traumatic lesion such as contusion or hematoma.

Brain Injuries Caused by Gunshots and Impalement

Gunshot wounds to the head are responsible for most penetrating brain injuries, and they account for approximately 35% of deaths from brain injury in people younger than 45 years of age.[54] The wound created by the bullet depends on ballistics (i.e., the size, shape, velocity, and direction of the bullet). As the bullet propels forward and penetrates the skull, it compresses the air in front of it, thereby increasing the destruction of brain tissue locally and remotely.[55] The major effects of missile injuries are cerebral contusions and lacerations, focal tissue necrosis, hemorrhage from tearing of blood vessels, and focal or generalized cerebral edema. Hemorrhage and edema may produce increased ICP and possible herniation associated with rapid expansion during impact and in response to a space-occupying lesion. The severity of injury sustained depends on the structures involved and herniation. Cerebral abscesses are postinjury concerns because of the microorganisms that have been carried into the brain from surface debris of skin, hair, and bone fragments. Other late complications include traumatic aneurysms, seizures, and fragment migration.

Missile injuries are classified as follows:

- **Tangential injuries,** in which the missile does not enter the cranial cavity but produces a scalp laceration, facial injury, comminuted skull fracture, meningeal tear, or cerebral contusion-laceration.

- **Penetrating injuries,** in which the missile enters the cranial cavity but does not pass through it, resulting in the presence of metal, bone fragments, hair, and skin within the brain. There is direct injury to cerebral tissue in the path of the bullet as well as injury to tissue from the high-pressure waves created by the high-velocity bullet. This high pressure can cause coup and contrecoup injuries, spikes in ICP, and herniation.
- **Through-and-through injuries,** in which the missile perforates the cranial contents and leaves through an exit wound. Possible cerebral injuries are the same as for penetrating injuries. There is one tract created from a missile entering the brain, although several tracts are possible if the bullet ricochets off bony structures within the cranial vault.

The history and evidence of entrance and possible exit gunshot wounds indicate probable injury. A CT scan determines the amount of injury and identifies bone fragments and the location of bullets, if retained. Emergency surgical intervention is common for salvageable patients through evacuation of hematomas, such as EDH or SDH; to debride the wound and remove the bullet and necrotic tissue; and to treat other system injuries caused by bullets or trauma. Survivors usually require ICU management for intracranial hypertension and systems complications associated with severe TBI as well of injuries to other body systems.

OTHER INJURIES RELATED TO TRAUMATIC BRAIN INJURY

Facial Fractures

Facial fractures commonly coexist with TBI. Injuries may involve the soft tissue (contusions, lacerations), the facial bones (fractures), or both. The facial bones include most of the paranasal sinuses and the primary receptor organs for the senses of vision, hearing, taste, and smell. Facial injuries can result in disfigurement, motor and sensory dysfunction, and deficits in communication. Table 17-2 summarizes common facial fractures. A CT scan is used to diagnose a facial fracture that can lead to injury of the eye. Orbital fractures are often undiagnosed or are confused with cranial nerve injury.

Some facial fractures require surgical repair and reconstruction for cosmetic effects; therefore, appropriate consultation with oral-maxillofacial or plastic surgery is necessary. A series of surgical procedures may be necessary to achieve the desired outcome. Timing of surgery depends on stabilization and management of other higher-priority needs in a multitrauma patient. Some studies have shown that early craniofacial repair can be performed safely with appropriate general surgical and neurosurgical support in selected patients, thus avoiding costly delays and complications.[56]

Cranial Nerve Injuries Associated With Skull Fractures

Specific cranial nerves tend to be compressed or injured because of anatomic location, transection, and attachments.

Frontal bone fractures are associated with olfactory nerve (most vulnerable) and sometimes optic nerve injury. Cribriform plate fractures often produce anosmia because of injury of the olfactory nerve. Orbital plate fractures may affect the optic and oculomotor nerves, resulting in loss of vision and impaired eye movement. The orbits are created by the fusion of many bones. Any of these bones may become fractured in a TBI. Isolated lesions of the trochlear or abducens nerves are rare. *Temporal bone fractures* often result in facial nerve paralysis, the most commonly injured motor cranial nerve. Auditory nerve dysfunction of the cochlear or vestibular branches is seen with less frequency. Rare cases of palsies to the lower cranial nerve (glossopharyngeal, vagus, spinal accessory, and hypoglossal nerves) had also been reported with basal skull fractures, specifically those with occipital condyle fractures.[57] Treatment varies according to the cranial nerve affected but may include surgical decompression, steroid therapy, and supportive measures, such as the use of eye lubricant or patch in patients with facial nerve palsy and placement of a nasogastric tube to prevent aspiration for patients with dysphagia.

MANAGEMENT OF THE TRAUMATIC BRAIN INJURY PATIENT: THE CONTINUUM OF CARE

Minor and Moderate Traumatic Brain Injuries

The incidence of mild and moderate TBI is difficult to determine for several reasons, including the fact that many of these patients have no continuing contact with the health care system. First, there are varying definitions and classifications of mild and moderate TBI. Second, accessible data sets that follow patients do not exist. Third, TBI often coexists with other medical problems.

Although practitioners may intuitively distinguish among gradations of TBI, definitions of mild and moderate TBI are imprecise. Moreover, there are no good instruments to discriminate reliably among injury types. Additionally, victims are often seen at a doctor's office or ED, or not seen at all; consequently, they are often excluded from epidemiologic databases. The TBI may be concurrent with other injuries that are more prominent and serious and thereby receive primary attention. The GCS is one widely used classification method. However, it may not be sensitive enough to capture the deficits common to these injuries. It is unclear what influence a managed care environment has on the diagnostic and treatment options available to persons with mild TBI.

Mild TBI (GCS = 13 to 15) is a transient event in which there may be a dazed appearance, unsteady gait, and short-term confusion after a blow to the head. The patient feels well after a few minutes; most patients have full recovery without problems. Some will have posttraumatic amnesia and postconcussion syndrome. A subgroup of patients, who seem perfectly fine when seen, develop secondary brain injury and die.

No clear criteria exist for diagnosis or management of these patients. Whether all or only certain patients receive CT scans continues to be a clinical judgment of the caregiver. That all patients with a mild TBI need to be observed and monitored for evidence of deterioration is clear. Admission is

TABLE 17–2 COMMON FACIAL FRACTURES

BONE	FRACTURE	SIGNS AND SYMPTOMS
Mandible		
• Only movable bone of the face • Composed of lower jaw and ramus • Lower jaw or chin, portion that contains the teeth • Ramus portion vertical with condyloid processes that fit into the temporomandibular joint	• Most frequently fractured facial bone • Because of its arched shape, fractures common in two places	• Malalignment of the teeth • Pain • Bruising and laceration over the fracture site • Ecchymosis in floor of the mouth • Palpation of a "shelf" defect in the inferior border • Inability to palpate condylar movement when the little finger is placed in the external ear canal and the jaw is opened
Maxilla	**Midface Fractures**	**Midface Fractures**
• Holds upper teeth • Includes the palate • Forms a portion of the floor of the orbits • Forms part of floor and outer wall of the nasal fossa • Meets temporal and zygoma bones laterally • Contains maxillary sinus	• Involved in midface fractures (involves the maxillae, naso-orbital bones, and zygomatic bones) • Midface fractures classified using the system devised by René Le Fort: **Le Fort I fracture:** horizontal detachment of the maxilla at the nasal floor; leaves maxillary alveolar ridge of the hard palate mobile **Le Fort II fracture:** pyramid-shaped fracture of the central part of the face; includes transverse fractures across the medial maxillae and nasal bones, medial half of the infraorbital rim, and medial part of the orbit and orbital floor **Le Fort III fracture:** separates the cranial and facial bones; includes a Le Fort II fracture along with fractures of both zygomatic bones so that the fracture line cuts through both orbits transversely	• Distortion of facial symmetry (elongated face, flattened naso-orbital area) • Possible pushing of the upper and lower molar teeth together • Inability to close jaw • Pain • Edema • Ecchymosis of buccal mucosa in the lateral portions • Abnormal movement (free-floating maxillary segment) • Possible respiratory obstruction • Hemorrhage
Zygoma		
• Forms the prominence of cheekbone • Forms part of outer wall and floor of orbit • Part of temporal and zygomatic fossa	• Often involved in midface fractures • Fractures of the zygoma often called tripod fractures because of their shape • Fracture of the zygoma always involves the orbits	• Flatness of the cheek • Loss of sensation on the side of the face of the fracture • Diplopia • Ophthalmoplegia
Nasal		
• Forms bridge of nose • Forms part of upper inner orbit	• May occur alone or in conjunction with orbital or Le Fort fractures	• Ecchymosis and edema of the dorsum of the nose • Nosebleed • Laceration
Orbital	**Blow-out Fractures**	
• Seven facial and cranial bones that form the orbits (frontal, maxillary, zygomatic, lacrimal, sphenoid, ethmoid, and palatine)	• Fracture as Le Fort fractures or, less frequently, as orbital blow-out fracture • Blow-out fractures result from spike in intraorbital pressure caused by a blunt object (fist, baseball) directed at the globe; spike in pressure, fracture at the weakest point—the orbital floor or medial wall; the orbital contents may protrude into the maxillary sinus	• Sinking of globe • Diplopia (secondary to injury of the extraocular muscles) • Ophthalmoplegia • Possible blindness (secondary to detached retina) • Edema • Ecchymosis of the eyelid • Conjunctival hemorrhage • Paresthesia

Data from Bertz, J. (1981). Maxillofacial injuries. *Clinical Symposia 33*(4), 1–32; Black, J., & Arnold, P. G. (1982). Facial fractures. *American Journal of Nursing, 82*(7), 1086; and Lower, J. (1986). Maxillofacial trauma. *Nursing Clinics of North America, 21*(4), 611–628.

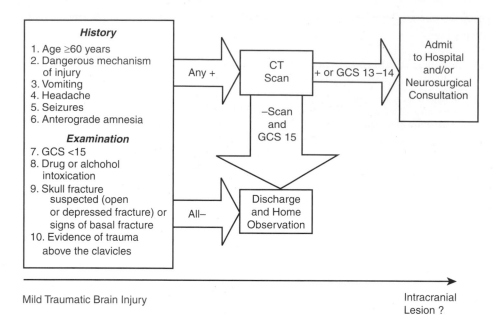

Figure 17-11 • Acute management of mild traumatic brain injury. CT = computed tomography; GCS = Glasgow Coma Scale. (Reproduced with permission from Cassidy, J. D., Carroll, L. J., Peloso, P. M., et al. [2004]. Incidence, risk factors and prevention of mild traumatic brain injury: Results of WHO Collaborating Centre Task Force on Mild Traumatic Brain Injury. *Journal of Rehabilitation Medicine, 36*[Suppl. 43], 28–60.)

warranted for patients in the following situations: loss of consciousness; neurological deficits; CSF leak or drainage from the nose or ear; alcohol consumption or other medical condition that makes assessment difficult; and absence of a support person to monitor them for 24 to 48 hours. People exhibiting no significant signs and symptoms may be sent home with a responsible person. Written instructions should outline what signs and symptoms may develop and what should be done if they appear. Figure 17-11 describes an evidence-based approach of mild TBI as recommended by the World Health Organization Collaborating Center for Neurotrauma Task Force on Mild Traumatic Brain Injury.[58]

The term **moderate TBI** (GCS = 9 to 12) indicates that more significant brain damage has occurred than with mild TBI. As this degree of brain injury is often concurrent with other organ system problems, the patient is often initially managed as a multisystem trauma patient with all the precautions (e.g., cervical neck injury immobilization) outlined for severe TBI. After the patient has been stabilized, a CT scan should be done as soon as possible. Because the moderate TBI patient is often admitted to an ICU that may not be a neurological ICU, the neurological injuries may be underestimated and thus not treated appropriately. An appropriate level of care for patients with moderate TBI requires frequent neurological monitoring and involves the same complement of management considerations outlined for severe TBI. Serious postinjury deficits may develop that can affect the person's ability to work and function effectively in changing roles, such as parent, spouse, or community member. Personality disorders are common. The moderate TBI patient needs to be monitored after discharge and provided with appropriate rehabilitation services and counseling, as needed.

Complaints of irritability, fatigue, headache, difficulty concentrating, dizziness, and memory problems, called **postconcussion syndrome,** often arise after moderate TBI. Anxiety and depression are also frequently noted, especially later in the course of the disorder. These symptoms were previously believed to be psychological in origin. However, current evidence supports the existence of a physiologic basis for these complaints. Targeted education is helpful in assisting the patient and family to cope with postconcussion syndrome. Supportive counseling may be necessary in dealing with emerging problems at work or at home. Symptoms usually subside with time but may last for months before resolution is complete.

Severe Traumatic Brain Injuries

Severe TBI refers to a brain injury that results in a GCS of 8 or less. This patient population is associated with high morbidity and mortality risks and requires intensive care. Laboratory and clinical research has remarkably increased our understanding of the pathophysiology of neurological damage that occurs not only at the moment of impact, but also over the following hours and days. An understanding of these processes has led to data on which traditional management strategies were scrutinized and novel strategies were developed and are being studied. With the goal of reducing if not reversing the devastating consequences of primary brain injury, evidence-based guidelines were developed with the ultimate goal of maximizing positive patient outcomes. In 2000, *Guidelines for the Management of Severe Traumatic Brain Injury* was published by the Brain Trauma Foundation, the American Association of Neurological Surgeons (AANS), and the Joint Section on Neurotrauma and Critical Care.[59] These guidelines are constantly in review and updated accordingly. In 2003, the cerebral perfusion pressure (CPP) guideline was updated by the AANS.

The above guidelines define evidence-based care and best practices for severe TBI and are the foundation for the care discussed in this chapter. The methodology used to develop the guidelines began with a thorough review of the evidence, followed by a classification into one of three categories:

- **Class I evidence:** prospective randomized controlled trials
- **Class II evidence:** prospective clinical studies (e.g., observational, cohort, or prevalence studies)

- **Class III evidence:** studies based on retrospectively collected data (e.g., registries, case review)

The overall degree of certainty of the evidence was further evaluated. As a result, the following three categories of recommendations were developed:

- **Standards:** represent principles of patient management that reflect a *high* degree of clinical certainty (strong class I evidence)
- **Guidelines:** represent a particular strategy or range of management strategies that reflect a *moderate* clinical certainty (mostly class II evidence)
- **Options:** include the remaining strategies for patient management based on *unclear* clinical certainty (class III evidence)

Guidelines for the Management of Severe Traumatic Brain Injury is an important resource and should be consulted for a more thorough discussion of the methodology, grading of evidence, degree of certainty, and literature reviewed.

The continuum of care begins at the trauma scene and continues throughout the various levels and settings of care. Continuity and smooth transition between settings are critical for obtaining optimal, cost-effective patient outcomes. This section addresses the essential components along the continuum and the evidence-based care needed to support optimal outcomes along the continuum.

PREHOSPITAL MANAGEMENT

All regions of the country should have an organized trauma care system in place. The *American College of Surgeons Committee on Trauma Resources for Optimal Care of the Injured Patient* has determined that neurosurgeons should have an organized and responsive system of care for patients with neurotrauma.[60] This system should include planning of care, prehospital management and triage, direct trauma center transport, maintaining appropriate call schedules, reviewing trauma care records for quality improvement, and participating in trauma education programs. Based on case reports and before-and-after comparison studies, mortality is reduced after major trauma in patients treated in an organized trauma system.[59]

CLINICAL PEARLS: Initial management of TBI includes:
  A: Airway
  B: Breathing
  C: Circulation
  D: Disability or neurological evaluation and stabilization

Prehospital management refers to the initial resuscitation and interventions to stabilize the patient at the injury scene and en route to the hospital. This care has a profound impact on the subsequent course of events and outcomes. Timely and effective brain resuscitation is critical because the brain has minimal reserves to meet ongoing metabolic needs. When insufficient substrates are available to the brain because of reduced cerebral blood flow (CBF) and cerebral oxygen delivery, ischemia and hypoxia develop, precipitat-

ing the pathophysiologic processes described earlier in this chapter. This inevitably leads to secondary brain injury and negatively affects patients' outcomes. Thus, hypoxemia and hypotension are indicators of poor outcome.

The American College of Surgeons has set national standards and developed Advanced Trauma Life Support (ATLS) training programs to prepare health care professionals to manage trauma victims effectively. Emergency medical services systems are designed to provide timely resuscitation and stabilization by well-trained personnel who can rapidly triage and transport victims to the appropriate health care facility. The emergency medical system includes telecommunication linkages with personnel at the health care facility where collaborative data analysis and clinical decision making occur through consultation that guides patient management at the trauma site and during transport. In collaboration with the Department of Transportation National Highway Traffic Administration, the Brain Trauma Foundation published the evidence-based *Guidelines for the Management of Severe Traumatic Brain Injury*.[61] Figure 17-12 summarizes these guidelines. In addition, because many TBI patients sustain multisystem trauma, primary and secondary trauma survey (see following section) is instituted to assess patients for evidence of these injuries systematically.

The first priority for the **initial management** for TBI patients is complete and rapid physiologic resuscitation, which includes airway, breathing, circulation, and disability. The latter was added to emphasize the significance of early recognition and stabilization of any neurological injury.

Airway

Patent airway should be assessed and secured. Patients with severe head injury with a Glasgow Coma Scale score of 8 or less, those with facial fractures, and/or those with other injuries that may compromise adequate oxygenation and ventilation should be intubated and assisted ventilation should be instituted. Intubation can be done with or without sedation and chemical paralysis. The use of sedative and paralytic agents should be done judiciously. Short-acting agents should be used so as not to interfere with the initial assessment of the neurotrauma patients. Chemical paralysis should also only be used by the emergency personnel who are skilled in endotracheal intubation and who are capable of performing surgical airway if the need arises. Cervical spine stabilization should always be done during field intubation due to the increased risk of cervical spinal injury among any TBI and/or multitrauma patients.

Breathing

Hypoxia, which is PO_2 less than 60 mm Hg on arterial blood gas or oxygen saturation of less than 90% measured via pulse oximeter, is associated with higher mortality.[62–64] Therefore, 100% oxygen should be administered and oxygen saturation should be continuously monitored and maintained at greater than 90%. Assisted ventilation, once initiated, should be done with the goal of maintaining $PaCO_2$ of approximately 35 mm Hg, which is the lower end of normocapnia.[61] Hyperventilation to a $PaCO_2$ of less than 35 mm Hg is only recommended when intracranial hypertension is suspected and herniation is imminent.

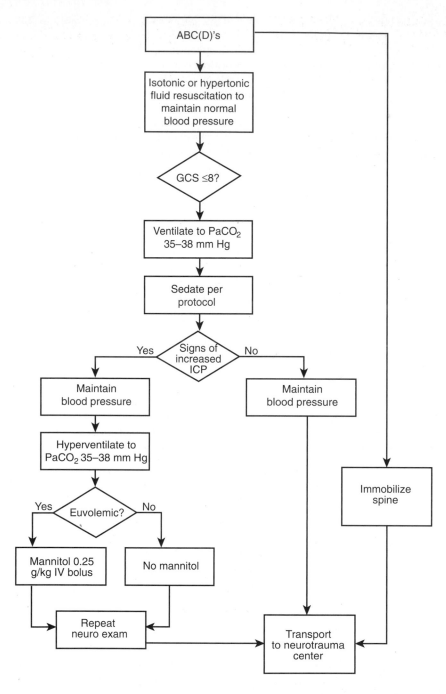

Figure 17-12 • Prehospital management of patients with traumatic brain injury. ICP = intracranial pressure. (Reproduced with permission from Gabriel, E. J., Ghajar, J., Jagoda, A., et al. [2002]. Guidelines for prehospital management of traumatic brain injury. *Journal of Neurotrauma, 19,* 81.)

Circulation

According to one study, raising blood pressure in hypotensive, severe TBI patients improves outcomes in proportion to the efficacy of the resuscitation.[65] Early hypotension, defined as a single episode of systolic blood pressure of 90 mm Hg or less, could significantly worsen the TBI patient's outcome.[62–64] Hence, the guideline emphasized the avoidance of hypotension as described above. In addition, the guideline recommended as a treatment option a mean arterial pressure (MAP) goal of 90 mm Hg based on the CPP goal of greater than 70 mm Hg using ICP of 20 mm Hg as a threshold. But recently, this guideline, specifically with regard to the CPP goal, was updated and rec-

ommended the maintenance of CPP at a minimum of 60 mm Hg based on findings that increasing blood pressure using artificial means to maintain CPP greater than 70 mm Hg could increase the risk of acute respiratory distress syndrome.[66]

Volume resuscitation is the primary method of attaining such blood pressure goal. In cases where hypotension is refractory to fluid resuscitation, the use of vasopressors may be initiated. Intravenous access should be established for fluid and/or drug administration. Isotonic fluids such as 0.9% normal saline (NS) are highly recommended, although there is growing evidence that the use of hypertonic saline for fluid resuscitation is more beneficial because it also reduces intracranial pressure. The use of hypotonic intravenous fluid in TBI patients is not recommended because it may cause and/or exacerbate cerebral edema.

Disability

Maneuvers to maintain airway patency must be modified to prevent cervical injuries. One cannot overemphasize the importance of treating all TBI patients for possible cervical fractures or spinal injury by immediately immobilizing the head and neck. All emergency medical personnel must be mindful of the disastrous consequences associated with neck manipulation, which include cord transection, quadriplegia, and death.

GCS scoring should be calculated by trained emergency personnel prior to administration of any sedative and paralytic agents. Pupils should also be assessed for any abnormalities. No specific treatment should be directed at intracranial hypertension without clinical evidence of transtentorial herniation or progressive neurological deterioration that is *not* attributable to extracranial causes. When there is clinical evidence of transtentorial herniation or progressive neurological deterioration not attributable to extracranial causes, the patient must be aggressively treated for intracranial hypertension. These interventions include[59,61]:

- Hyperventilation with goal PaCO$_2$ 30 to 35 mm Hg.
- Mannitol, but *only* if adequate volume resuscitation has been ensured.
- Hypertonic saline using small-volume resuscitation is being used more and more.
- Sedation and neuromuscular blockade are useful to optimize transport, but both interfere with the neurological examination. Sedation should be tried first, and short-acting neuromuscular blockade is provided only if sedation is inadequate.

Immediate transport to the nearest ED or trauma center for further evaluation and management of the TBI is very important. Depending on the circumstances, the above initial resuscitation strategies can be conducted during the transport. The guideline emphasized the significance of an established trauma system that will direct the emergency personnel or first responders where to transport patients with TBI. Specifically, severe TBI patients should be transported to a trauma center or hospital with 24-hour CT scanning, 24-hour neurosurgery service, and a capability for monitoring and managing intracranial hypertension.[61]

EMERGENCY DEPARTMENT OR TRAUMA CENTER MANAGEMENT

On arrival at the ED, multiple and concurrent activities are initiated by a well-trained team of health care professionals. Activity includes inserting arterial and central lines, inserting an indwelling urinary catheter, attaching monitoring equipment such as continuous electrocardiography, and conducting primary and secondary trauma surveys. The history and circumstances of injury and previous treatment are verified and clarified. The following are examples of important information to consider:

TABLE 17–3	COMMON DIAGNOSTIC TESTS FOR PATIENTS WITH TRAUMATIC BRAIN INJURY UPON ARRIVAL AT THE HOSPITAL

- Complete blood count; arterial blood gas; serum electrolytes, glucose, creatinine, and blood urea nitrogen
- Drug screen
- Serum alcohol level
- Chest radiograph
- Spine films usually cervical but may include thoracic and lumbar, as indicated
- Computed tomography (CT) scan without contrast of the head to exclude any traumatic lesion
- Pelvis radiograph to exclude fracture
- Focused abdominal sonography in trauma (FAST) examination to evaluate for abdominal trauma
- Abdominal and pelvis CT scan, as indicated for further evaluation of abdominal injury
- Urinalysis

- Circumstances of injury (e.g., direct blow to head, thrown from car, fell off bar stool)
- Seat belt or helmet worn (e.g., type of seat belt: lap or shoulder)
- How patient was found (e.g., lying face down)
- Unconsciousness (immediate; lucid period)
- Documented apnea or cyanosis and length of time
- Significant blood loss at the scene of accident

Resuscitation and stabilization treatment continue as discussed earlier; diagnostic testing is conducted (Table 17-3). A CT scan is the "gold standard" for diagnosis of TBI. It is a recommended diagnostic test for patients with a history of trauma and those at high risk for intracranial injury, which include patients with the following profile: a GCS score of 15 and a history of loss of consciousness or amnesia; a GCS score less than 15; and any patient with neurological deficits or signs of basilar or depressed skull fracture. The CT scan is ordered and completed immediately on admission, or it may be postponed until the patient's condition has stabilized in cases where there is hemodynamic instability. CT scan without contrast will provide visualization of most major intracranial injuries such as depressed skull fracture, EDH, SDH, ICH, and contusion. Cerebral angiograms or MRI may be ordered to exclude any vascular injury secondary to trauma such as arterial dissection, traumatic aneurysms, arteriovenous fistula, or venous occlusions. ICP monitoring, either by placement of an intraventricular catheter or subarachnoid screw (bolt), can be completed in the ED.

In summary, the management of the TBI patient in the ED is directed at resuscitation, stabilization, and establishment of a diagnosis. After these steps have been completed, a decision is made regarding immediate surgical intervention for life-threatening injuries or transfer to the intensive care unit (ICU) for medical management. These interventions are further outlined on Figure 17-13.[59]

INITIAL MANAGEMENT OF SEVERE BRAIN INJURY

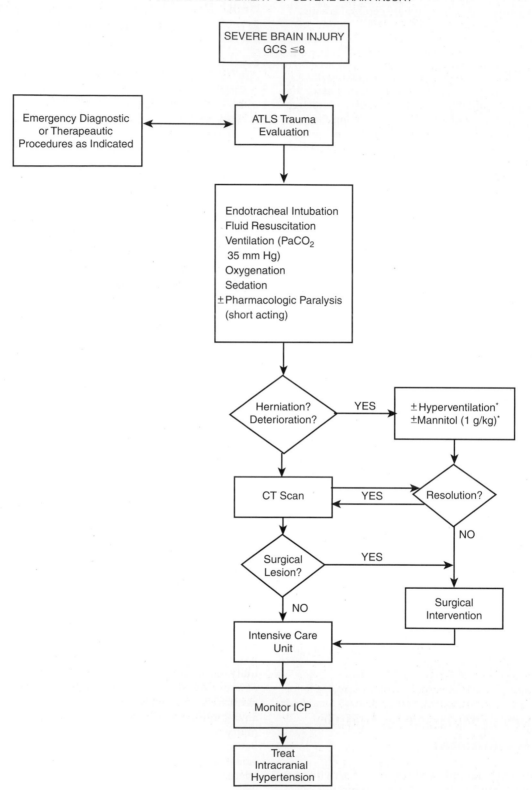

*Only in the presence of signs of herniation or progressive neurologic deterioration not attributable to extracranial factors.

Figure 17-13 • Initial resuscitation of severely head-injured patients. ATLS = Advanced Trauma and Life Support; ICP = intracranial pressure. (Reproduced with permission from Bullock, R., Chestnut, R., Clifton, G., et al. [2000]. Guidelines for the management of severe traumatic brain injury. *Journal of Neurotrauma, 17*[16/17], 465.)

INTENSIVE CARE UNIT MANAGEMENT OF SEVERE TRAUMATIC BRAIN INJURY

Severe TBI patients are admitted directly to the ICU from the ED or after emergency neurosurgery for close monitoring and technology interface. The goals of ICU care are to manage intracranial hypertension, maintain adequate cerebral oxygen delivery to meet cerebral metabolic needs, prevent secondary brain injury, and prevent or manage potential or actual systemic problems that can contribute to morbidity and mortality. Care maps for severe TBI are useful to guide care and address interdisciplinary care needs. The physician, nurse, respiratory therapist, case manager, physical therapist, speech therapist, occupational therapist, pharmacist, clinical nutritionist, and other health care professionals must work closely together to move the patient along in the continuum of care with the major goal of maximizing neurological recovery.

Monitoring

Systemic Monitoring

Included are cardiac rhythm monitoring via telemetry, pulse oximetry for oxygen saturation, invasive arterial blood pressure monitoring via arterial line, temperature monitoring, and end-tidal CO_2 monitoring.[67] Central venous pressure monitoring is also important to monitor the patient's fluid volume status; alternatively, a pulmonary artery flotation catheter may be placed in hemodynamically unstable patients for further monitoring and direction in management. Strict intake and output recording is also important to monitor the patient's hydration status and detect any complications such as polyuria secondary to central diabetes insipidus. Regular monitoring of blood glucose, serum electrolytes, and arterial blood gases are necessary to meet the optimum physiologic parameters (Table 17-4) to prevent and/or treat secondary brain injuries.

Cerebral Monitoring

ICP monitoring is recommended in all salvageable TBI patients with the following: abnormal head CT scan or a GCS score of 8 or less after resuscitation. It is also indicated in those with a normal head CT scan, if two or more of the following are noted at admission: age older than 40 years old, unilateral or bilateral motor posturing, or hypotension with systolic blood pressure of less than 90 mm Hg.[59] An abnormal CT scan of the head is one that reveals a hematoma, contusion, swelling, herniation, or compressed basal cisterns. Patients with mild to moderate TBI usually do not require an ICP monitor, but may be candidates depending on the physician's judgment or preference.

Intraventricular catheter placement connected to an external strain gauge is the most accurate, low-cost, and reliable method of monitoring ICP. It also can be recalibrated in situ. It not only provides ICP readings, but also allows EVD of CSF as treatment for intracranial hypertension. An intraparenchymal catheter with a fiberoptic or micro-strain gauge

---

TABLE 17-4 PHYSIOLOGIC PARAMETERS FOR THE MANAGEMENT OF SEVERE HEAD INJURY

- Intracranial pressure <20 mm Hg
- PaO_2: 90–100 mm Hg
- $PaCO_2$: 35–40 mm Hg (mild to moderate hyperventilation with $PaCO_2$ 30–35 mm Hg may be instituted for intracranial hypertension)
- SaO_2: 92%–100%
- Mean arterial pressure: 90 mm Hg or greater to support cerebral perfusion pressure >60–70 mm Hg
- Maintain systolic blood pressure 140–160 mm Hg
- Cerebral perfusion pressure: >60–70 mm Hg
- Cardiac output: 4–6 L/min; cardiac index: >3.0 L/min
- Systemic vascular resistance: 900–1400 dynes
- Central venous pressure: 8–10 mm Hg
- Pulmonary capillary wedge pressure: 14–16
- Serum osmolality: <320 mOsm
- Hematocrit: <32%; hemoglobin: >10 g
- Normal glucose (<150 mg/dL)
- Normal electrolytes
- Normothermia
- Normal range urine specific gravity (1.005–1.015)
- Urine output >30 mL/hr but <200 mL/hr

---

catheter tip transducer can also be used to monitor ICP, but unlike EVD, it does not allow for CSF drainage. Fiberoptic catheters are also used for ICP monitoring, but are more expensive and cannot be recalibrated. Other alternative methods that are known to be less reliable and more subject to artifacts are epidural devices and subarachnoid bolts. These are less frequently used.

Normal ICP is less than 15 mm Hg; the Brain Trauma Foundation guideline recommends treatment to be initiated for ICP above 20 mm Hg.[59] ICP reading allows the estimation of CPP (targeted CPP level is 50 to 70 mm Hg) by calculating the difference between MAP and ICP. See Chapter 13 for further discussion.

CLINICAL PEARLS: ICP monitoring indications: (1) abnormal head CT scan; (2) GCS score of less than 8; (3) normal head CT scan but age older than 40 years old with unilateral or bilateral posturing and/or hypotension with systolic blood pressure less than 90 mm Hg.

Jugular venous bulb oximetry may also be placed by insertion of a catheter into the jugular bulb to measure jugular venous oxygen saturation (SjO_2) and provide information on cerebral oxygen and supply. Normal SjO_2 is around 65%, with values of less than 60% indicative of compromised cerebral blood flow in association with the oxygen requirement of the brain.[68] As an option, the Brain Trauma Foundation recommends the use of this device in cases when hyperventilation therapy ($PaCO_2$ of 35 mm Hg or less) is necessary for intracranial hypertension refractory to sedation/analgesia, chemical paralysis, CSF drainage, and mannitol because hyperventilation can result in reduced cerebral perfusion.[59] Jugular venous saturation (<50%) or brain tissue oxygen tension (<15 mm Hg) are treatment thresholds.[59]

Management of Intracranial Hypertension

An important concept to understand in the management of intracranial hypertension is the Monro-Kellie principle, which states that the volume inside the rigid skull is equal to the sum of noncompressible contents, which include the brain, CSF, and blood. Any pathologic changes that may increase the quantities of these components or any addition of a new component (e.g., tumor or clot) will increase the volume without a corresponding change with the rigid skull. Compensatory mechanisms such as displacement/ decreased production of CSF or vasoconstriction to decrease cerebral blood flow may occur but are limited. When decompensation occurs, it results in an increase in intracranial pressure (>15 mm Hg), with an increase greater than 20 mm Hg requiring interventions. Intracranial pressure has an inverse relationship with cerebral perfusion pressure, which means the higher the ICP, the lower the CPP, which can result in cerebral ischemia. Low CPP can cause more neurological damage and cerebral edema, which result in a further increase in ICP. Moreover, intracranial hypertension can cause displacement and herniation of the brain resulting in death. Therefore, intracranial hypertension management is an integral part of the care of the TBI patient.

Applying the Monro-Kellie principle, intracranial hypertension can be therefore achieved by any of the following components:

- Decrease brain size: mannitol or hypertonic saline
- Decrease CSF: drainage
- Decrease blood: inducing vasoconstriction with hyperventilation
- Removal of the pathologic process (e.g., tumor or clot)
- Removal of a bone flap to allow expansion of the brain (craniectomy)

CLINICAL PEARLS: ICP threshold for treatment is 20 to 25 mm Hg with treatment in a stepwise approach, which may include CSF drainage, analgesia, sedation, hyperosmolar therapy with mannitol, hyperventilation, chemical paralysis, and pentobarbital coma.

Although no absolute ICP threshold exists above which treatment to lower ICP should begin, current data support a threshold of 20 to 25 mm Hg.[59,69] Figure 17-14 provides an algorithm for the treatment of intracranial hypertension.

Management of intracranial hypertension is usually done in a stepwise approach, moving from one therapy to another only if ICP remains uncontrolled with the present treatment. Conventional or first-tier therapies include CSF drainage, sedation/analgesia, chemical paralysis, hyperventilation (PCO2 35 to 40 mm Hg), and hyperosmolar therapy with mannitol. When intracranial hypertension is refractory to the conventional management as outlined above, second-tier therapies can be instituted, which include barbiturate coma, optimized hyperventilation (PCO2 <30 mm Hg), and craniectomy.

Cerebrospinal Fluid Drainage

As discussed earlier, intracranial hypertension can be reduced by reduction of the circulating CSF. This can be achieved by drainage of CSF via an external ventricular device or ventriculostomy. The physician will determine the threshold at which CSF will be drained. The order to drain CSF is set to a mean ICP. The threshold of greater than 20 mm Hg is recommended in the *Guidelines*.[59] Unit protocol for draining, if available, should be followed. The protocol should identify the duration of drainage (e.g., 5 minutes) and the characteristics of the CSF to be documented. The color or character of the drainage should be monitored (e.g., very bloody, pinkish), along with the amount of drainage.

Sedation, Analgesics, and Neuromuscular Blockade

The following must be taken into account when considering the use of potential drugs: effect of the drug on the cerebral metabolic rate of oxygen consumption (CMRO2), CBF, ICP, cardiovascular function, and respiratory function; toxicity; side effects; time to awakening after discontinuation of any sedating drugs; incidence of prolonged weakness after discontinuation; drug efficacy; effect on patient outcome; and cost.[70]

Sedation and Analgesics. Sedatives and analgesics are important management strategies in severe TBI patients. Both can be used to prevent and/or treat spikes in ICP related to agitation; restlessness; abnormal posturing; asynchrony with the mechanical ventilator; and painful interventions that increase CMRO2 and oxygen needs.

Benzodiazepines are the most commonly used sedatives and do not affect CMRO2, CBF, or ICP. Lorazepam (Ativan) and midazolam (Versed) are frequently used but have active metabolites that may cause prolonged sedation resulting in difficulty in conducting neurological assessment. Propofol (Diprivan), on the other hand, a sedative-hypnotic agent that is supplied in an intralipid emulsion for intravenous use, is the sedative of choice. It decreases CMRO2, CBF, ICP, and CPP. An ultra-short-acting, rapid-onset drug with elimination half-life of less than an hour, it has a major advantage of being titratable to its desired clinical effect but still provides opportunity for accurate neurological assessment.[71] The disadvantages are cost, its ability to cause dose-dependent hypotension, and muscle weakness with prolonged use. Because propofol is a lipid emulsion, serum triglyceride, liver, and pancreatic functions must be monitored and daily caloric requirement adjusted accordingly.

Sedatives do not possess analgesic properties. TBI patients may have other traumatic injuries aside from the cerebral injury such as fractures, wounds, and blunt injuries that cause pain. Without administration of analgesia, sedation of patients with pain may lead to increased agitation and combativeness. Therefore, the need for analgesics must be considered.[70] Parenteral narcotics, such as fentanyl or morphine sulfate, are frequently used for analgesia. These drugs do not increase CMRO2, CBF, or ICP in conventional doses. A low-dose continuous infusion of morphine is a frequently used method of administration. Respiratory depression is the major side effect of morphine and is a concern only if the

CRITICAL PATHWAY FOR TREATMENT OF INTRACRANIAL HYPERTENSION

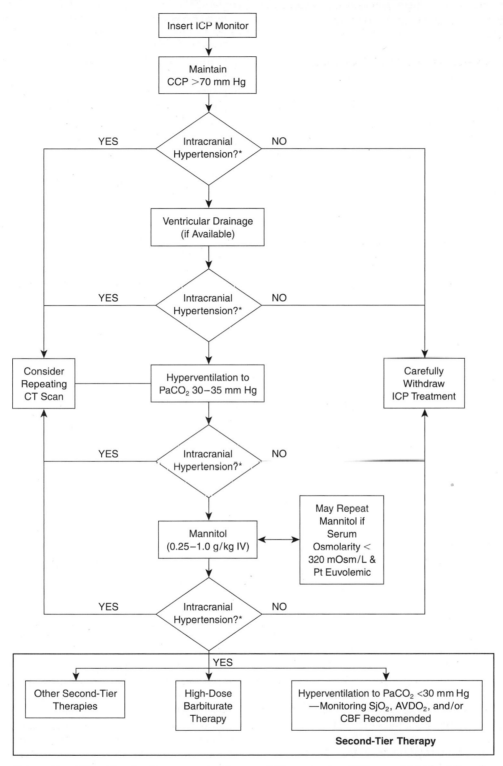

Figure 17-14 • Algorithm for the treatment of intracranial hypertension. CBF = cerebral blood flow; CCP = capillary closing pressure; CT = computed tomography; ICP = intracranial pressure. (Reproduced with permission from Bullock, K. H., Chestnut, R. H., & Clifton, G. L. [2000]. Guidelines for the treatment of severe TBI. *Journal of Neurotrauma, 17*[6/7], 538.)

patient is not intubated, which is unlikely in a severe TBI patient.

Neuromuscular Blockade. Between 1% and 10% of ICU patients now receive continuous administration of neuro-muscular blockade (NMB) drugs for more than 24 hours.[72]

NMB agents are usually used when sedation and analgesia are not enough to control intracranial hypertension. They are effective in reducing ICP spikes related to bedside activities such as turning and suctioning and in cases of patient–ventilator asynchrony. Drugs commonly used include rocuronium, pancuronium, vecuronium, pipecuronium, and atracurium. There use results in chemically induced paralysis, which limits neurological assessment to pupillary reaction; therefore, these drugs have the major disadvantage of masking any neurological changes or any seizure activity. The depth of paralysis is routinely monitored at the bedside using a peripheral nerve stimulator and an assessment method known as the "train-of-four."[73,74] A series of four low-voltage electrical stimulation devices (i.e., train-of-four) are applied to a peripheral nerve, such as the ulnar nerve or facial nerve, and the twitch response is noted. A complete blockade (0 of 4) response is related to deep paralysis. The major complication of chemical paralysis in patients is prolonged weakness or myopathy after extended use (i.e., longer than 24 hours). NMB use is also associated with longer intensive care unit stays and higher incidence of infection such as pneumonia.[71] TBI patients should be intubated, on assisted ventilation, and adequately sedated before administration of any NMB agent.

CLINICAL PEARLS: Patients on chemically induced paralysis should be routinely monitored at the bedside with a peripheral nerve stimulator and using the train-of-four (TOF) assessment method.

Mannitol

Osmotic diuretics are recommended based on level II evidence in the *Guidelines* for control of acute increased ICP caused by cerebral edema.[59] The osmotic diuretic of choice is mannitol, 0.25 to 1.0 g/kg through IV bolus (usual adult dose is 25 to 50 g) every 3 to 6 hours. It is indicated for intracranial hypertension and/or in patients exhibiting signs of transtentorial herniation or progressive neurological deterioration not attributable to extracranial causes. Mannitol acts by drawing edematous brain tissue water into the intravascular area resulting in reduced volume of the brain in a fixed skull, reducing the intracranial pressure. Aside from its osmotic effect, mannitol also has neuroprotective properties. It decreases blood viscosity by diluting the blood and deformability of the erythrocytes resulting in increased cerebral blood flow. Onset of action is within 15 to 30 minutes with peak in 60 minutes and duration of action for 6 to 8 hours.[59] With mannitol administration, euvolemia must always be maintained through adequate fluid replacement of urine losses. An indwelling urinary catheter is necessary to monitor urinary output. Serum osmolarity should be maintained at less than 320 mOsm/L to prevent renal failure. Blood pressure and electrolytes should be monitored carefully, because one danger associated with mannitol-induced diuresis is hypotension, which results in cerebral hypoperfusion and ischemia. Electrolyte imbalances (hypokalemia and hyponatremia) are common; therefore, serum electrolytes must be monitored and treated as necessary.

CLINICAL PEARLS: Serum osmolality should be maintained less than 320 mOsm/L to prevent renal failure with mannitol treatment.

Hypertonic Saline

The use of hypertonic solutions is gaining use in clinical practice. The principal effect of hypertonic saline on ICP is possibly due to osmotic mobilization of water across the intact blood–brain barrier, which reduces cerebral water content.[74a] A number of studies have been conducted to evaluate the use of hypertonic saline solutions from normal saline to 23.4% sodium chloride solutions to reduce intracranial pressure.[74b–74d] According to the 2007 *Guidelines*, there is not strong enough evidence to make recommendations for the use, concentration, and method of administration of hypertonic saline for the treatment of traumatic intracranial hypertension.[74e] See further discussion in this chapter.

Hyperventilation

Cerebral physiology and CBF after TBI are well understood, and this information forms the basis for the use of hyperventilation as a recommended standard and the *Guidelines* for management of TBI.[59] It is well established that CBF is lowest in the 24-hour period after TBI and remains low for approximately 3 additional days except in patients who do not survive because of uncontrolled intracranial hypertension.[75–79] The average CBF is about 30 mL/100 g/min during the first 8 hours after injury, and may be as low as 20 mL/100 g/min in the first 4 hours for the most critically ill patients.[59] Although the CBF threshold for irreversible ischemia or infarction is not clearly delineated, it is thought to be around the less than 15 mL/100 g/min level. Normal CBF is about 55 mL/100 g/min. Interestingly, in severe TBI patients, CBF is lowest in patients with SDH, diffuse injuries, and hypotension; it is highest in patients with an epidural hematoma with normal CT scans.[80–83]

Hyperventilation involves serious risks and its use should closely conform to the established *Guidelines*. The *purported* therapeutic effect of hyperventilation is that hypocapnia (lowered PaCO$_2$) causes vasoconstriction and decreases ICP. However, what happens is that hyperventilation reduces CBF, does not consistently reduce ICP, and may cause loss of autoregulation to cerebral blood vessels. Additionally, there is wide local variability of perfusion and vasoconstriction of cerebral tissue.[59,84] Accordingly, the *Guidelines*[59] note that prophylactic hyperventilation (PaCO$_2$ of 25 mm Hg or less) is not recommended. Hyperventilation is recommended as a temporizing measure for the reduction of elevated ICP. Hyperventilation should be avoided during the first 24 hours after injury when CBF is often critically reduced. If hyperventilation is used, jugular venous oxygen saturation or brain tissue oxygen tension (PbrO$_2$) measurements are recommended to monitor oxygen delivery.

So, when is hyperventilation a useful option? As an emergency measure, it can be helpful for *brief* periods when there is acute neurological deterioration. For *longer* periods, it may be useful when intracranial hypertension is refractory to the usual treatment strategies of sedation, chemical paralysis, drainage of CSF through a ventriculostomy, and use of osmotic diuretics. In these circumstances, hyperventilation becomes a second-tier strategy for a gravely ill patient. A final reminder is that abrupt cessation of hyperventilation can cause a rebound effect on ICP with spikes. The effect of hyperventilation on cerebral tissue and CSF acidosis is short lived.

The following is recommended for monitoring PaCO$_2$ values for evidence of cerebral ischemia during hyperventilation (PaCO$_2$ <30 mm Hg): jugular venous oxygen saturation (SjO$_2$); arterial-jugular venous oxygen (AVDO$_2$) content differences; brain tissue oxygen monitoring; and cerebral blood extraction (CBE) monitoring. Currently, there is no direct way to monitor for focal ischemia in the brain. Kept in mind that, although SjO₂ monitoring is helpful, it provides a *global* value of cerebral oxygenation and does not provide information on only the injured area.

Barbiturate Therapy

Barbiturates assist with intractable ICP by protecting the cerebrum and lowering ICP through the mechanisms of alterations in vascular tone, suppression of metabolism, and inhibition of free radical–mediated lipid peroxidation.[79,80] As a result, CBF is better matched to regional metabolic demands, and metabolic needs are lowered. The effect of these physiologic alterations is that ICP decreases and global cerebral perfusion improves.

The *Guidelines* make the following recommendation: "High-dose barbiturate therapy may be considered in hemodynamically stable salvageable severe head injured patients with intracranial hypertension refractory to maximal medical and surgical intracranial ICP lowering therapy."[59] See Chapter 13 for further discussion of barbiturate therapy.

Other Therapeutic Measures

Other available alternative management strategies for intracranial hypertension include decompressive craniectomy, use of hypertonic saline solution, and hypothermia. These methods are still less well studied and their efficacies are still not well established. Therefore, consensus on their use has not been reached within the evidence-based guideline efforts. Steroid therapy, once a standard of care for TBI patients, has been well studied and its effectiveness has not been proven. It is not a recommended treatment.

Decompressive Craniectomy. A craniectomy, whether unilateral or bilateral, has been used for intractable intracranial hypertension. It involves removal of the bone flap to allow expansion of the edematous brain. The indications for decompressive craniectomy are not well established. Anecdotal reports about its positive outcome when provided early for patients with no significant secondary brain injuries such as elevated and prolonged increased ICP, cerebral hypoperfusion, and herniation have been published.[85–87] However, no randomized controlled trials have been conducted regarding this therapy.

Hypertonic Saline. There has been increasing reports of the use of hypertonic saline (HTS) in TBI patients as an alternative osmotic agent for treatment of increased intracranial hypertension. Although there have been no large, randomized clinical trials conducted to date, several human prospective studies, anecdotal reports, and uncontrolled case studies have reported the use of hypertonic saline solution and its efficacy in the treatment of cerebral edema and intracranial hypertension.[88] Moreover, aside from its ability to reduce brain water content, laboratory-based studies demonstrate the extraosmotic action with its anti-inflammatory effects on excitatory neurotransmitters and on the immune system.[68] Administered intravenously either bolus or continuous at a set rate per hour, hypertonic saline can be delivered in a variety of strengths from 3% to 23.4%. With this therapy, close monitoring of serum sodium and serum osmolality is mandatory with targeted goals for severe TBI patients to a serum sodium concentration of 145 to 155 mEq/L and osmolality of 300 to 320 mOsm/L. Other serum electrolytes, specifically potassium, calcium, and magnesium, also must be monitored. Potential complications with HTS therapy include central pontine myelinolysis, encephalopathy, SDH, transient hypotension, pulmonary edema, heart failure, hypokalemia, hypochloremic academia, coagulopathy, intravascular hemolysis, and phlebitis if given via peripheral intravenous route.[89] There is a risk of rebound hyponatremia and rebound cerebral edema with withdrawal of treatment so that close monitoring is advised.

> **CLINICAL PEARLS:** Hypotonic and glucose-containing fluids should be avoided in TBI patients as they may cause an increase in cerebral edema and neurotoxic acidosis, respectively.

Hypothermia. Experimental and clinical studies demonstrate the effectiveness of hypothermia (32°C to 34°C) in reducing intracranial hypertension, but trials on its effect on patient outcome have conflicting reports. It is postulated that hypothermia has neuroprotective effects by reducing the biochemical cascade that leads to secondary brain injuries, which includes promoting antioxidant activity and reducing inflammatory markers and excitatory amino acids.[89,90] Based on this neuroprotective model, several clinical studies had been conducted to further develop this theory. Small clinical studies have demonstrated the beneficial effect of hypothermia in severe TBI patients. A large multicenter trial was not able to support that positive effect. Preliminary findings suggest that a greater decrease in mortality risk is observed when target temperatures are maintained for more than 48 hours.[59] Prophylactic hypothermia is associated with significantly higher Glasgow Outcome Scale scores when compared to scores for normothermia patients. It is clear that more well-designed studies need to be conducted to clarify the use and value of induced hypothermia.

Hypothermia can be induced with surface-cooling device such as cooling blankets or intravascular cooling devices with a specific target body temperature. Intubation with adequate sedation and chemical paralysis are usually required with this therapy for the patient's comfort. Close monitoring is very important. Potential complications of hypothermia include increased risk of infection, coagulopathy, cardiac arrhythmias, and electrolyte abnormalities. The presence of any of the above complications may warrant the need to cautiously rewarm the hypothermic TBI patient.

Steroids. Based on several prospective randomized controlled studies, steroids *do not* reduce ICP or improve neurological outcome, and are associated with increased mortality. Therefore, use of steroids for traumatic brain injury is contraindicated.[59]

> **CLINICAL VIGNETTE:** RF is a 20-year-old white man admitted to the neurotrauma ICU with multiple cerebral contusions sustained from a motor vehicular accident. His GCS score is 6; he is intubated and mechanically ventilated. An external ventricular drainage

device and an ICP monitor were placed on admission to the ICU. Initial opening intracranial pressure was noted to be 12 mm Hg. On ICU day 2, the ICP spiked to 25 to 30 mm Hg; it improved with sedation, analgesia, and mannitol. On ICU day 3, the patient's serum osmolality peaked at 325 mOsm/L with serum sodium of 151 mEq/L; mannitol was withheld. Elevated ICP readings to greater than 20 mm Hg persisted despite CSF drainage, sedation, and analgesia. Arterial blood gases were drawn, and showed a PCO_2 of 34 mm Hg. Repeat head CT scan revealed a slight increase to the cerebral edema with no change in character of the cerebral contusions. Chemical paralysis with pancuronium was initiated as well as continuing deep sedation, but intracranial hypertension persisted. After discussing treatment options, risks, and benefits to the family, the neurosurgery team gave orders to initiate pentobarbital coma for refractory intracranial hypertension.

Seizure Management

Posttraumatic seizures (PTSs) are classified according to the time of occurrence. Early PTSs occur within 7 days following injury, whereas late PTSs occur after 7 days after injury.[91,92]

Studies have shown that prophylactic anticonvulsants are effective in preventing early PTSs.[93] But they are not useful for prevention of delayed PTSs.[94,95] Based on class I evidence, a seizure management standard is recommendations in the *Guidelines for Management of Severe Traumatic Brain Injury*. Prophylactic use of phenytoin, carbamazepine, phenobarbital, or valproate is *not* recommended for prevention of *late PTSs*.[59,96]

CLINICAL PEARLS: Prophylactic anticonvulsants are only effective in preventing posttraumatic seizure that occurs within 7 days following injury.

Seizures must be controlled because they greatly increase $CMRO_2$ and ICP. Patients receiving neuromuscular blockade may have seizure activity or status epilepticus, but may not exhibit the usual motor activity typical of a seizure. Tachycardia, blood pressure instability, and intracranial hypertension may be the only evidence of seizure activity.[42] The rationale for seizure prophylaxis is based on the high risk of secondary injury from clinically undetected seizures. Patients who do not "wake up" inconsistent with other clinical data suggesting improved neurological status may have subclinical seizures. Use of compressed spectral array electroencephalography (EEG) bedside monitoring is becoming common in intensive care units to evaluate for seizures.

If seizures do occur, aggressive treatment is necessary to control the seizure and the concurrent cerebral hypoxia. Phenytoin is the most common drug used for acute seizure management. A loading dose of 15 to 20 mg/kg intravenous phenytoin with subsequent maintenance doses (usually 100 mg every 8 hours) is given to maintain a therapeutic level. Intravenous phenytoin should not be given any faster than 50 mg/min because of the possibility of hypotension and cardiac arrhythmias. Fosphenytoin is less likely to cause

hypotension and is usually administered in hemodynamically unstable patients. For maintenance, long-term anticonvulsant therapy phenytoin can be administered enterally. The usual dose of phenytoin is 300 to 400 mg daily. It is necessary to monitor blood levels of phenytoin to maintain a therapeutic range (10 to 20 mg/mL). Adjustment in dosage may be necessary when the patient is concurrently receiving tube feedings because phenytoin binds to the protein of the enteral formula. Holding the tube feeding 1 hour before and after phenytoin administration may be necessary.

In the ICU environment, seizure precautions are integrated into care. The patient's airway is maintained with an endotracheal tube or other airway, and suctioning equipment is readily available. Padded side rails are usually left up when the nurse is not at the bedside. Padding can easily be added to the side rails. Protection from injury is a consideration for an awake and ambulatory patient.

Multisystem Management

As discussed earlier in this chapter, extracranial factors such as hypotension, hypoxemia, hypercapnia, hypocapnia, hyperthermia, hyponatremia, hyperglycemia, and hypoglycemia can cause secondary brain injuries. Therefore, they should be prevented to further optimize the severe TBI patient's neurological outcome. The following addresses these common or potential problems in TBI according to each body system (Table 17-5).

Cardiovascular Management

Optimal volume resuscitation and cardiac function with maximum tissue perfusion should be a priority in TBI. Hypotension should be avoided with CPP goal of greater than 60 mm Hg. Adequate fluid resuscitation should be done with ongoing fluid replacement to maintain an acceptable MAP with CVP goal of 5 to 10 mm Hg or pulmonary artery wedge pressure of 10 to 14 mm Hg. There is still controversy regarding the choice of fluid between crystalloids and colloids, but avoidance of hypotonic and glucose-containing solutions is recommended. Hypotonic fluids will increase cerebral edema formation while glucose, an essential component of cerebral metabolism, could be converted to lactate in anaerobic states such as TBI and cause neurotoxic acidosis.[97] In cases where hypotension is refractory for fluid resuscitation, initiation of vasoactive drugs may be necessary. Many drug options are available to maintain higher blood pressure for patients with intracranial pathology. α- and β-adrenergic blockers do not directly affect CBF and have no effect on ICP in patients with intracranial hypertension; therefore, they may be preferred for control of blood pressure in brain-injured people.[98] Adequate MAP is facilitated with vasopressor drugs such as dopamine, phenylephrine, or norepinephrine, which are usually titrated according to a specific MAP or cardiac index parameter.

Cardiac arrhythmias are often reported in conjunction with TBI. Some are associated with acute coronary syndrome (ACS) and can be life threatening, while others could be caused by the hyperdynamic state due to stimulation of the sympathetic nervous system related to TBI. Dysrhythmias may include premature atrial contractions, atrial fibrillation

TABLE 17-5 MAJOR COLLABORATIVE PROBLEMS IN THE MANAGEMENT OF ACUTE, SEVERE TRAUMATIC BRAIN INJURY

SYSTEM	COLLABORATIVE PROBLEMS	ASSESS AND MONITOR	INTERVENTIONS/MANAGEMENT
Neurological	Increased ICP Herniation syndromes Seizures Cerebral ischemia	Monitor frequent neurological assessments Assess frequently for signs and symptoms of ↑ ICP Monitor anticonvulsant blood level (if anticonvulsants ordered) Monitor mean ICP with ICP monitor Monitor jugular venous oxygen saturation	Institute severe TBI protocol based on published *Guidelines for the Management of Severe Traumatic Brain Injury* Maintain seizure precautions
Respiratory	Atelectasis Pneumonia (aspiration and bacterial) Hypoxemia Ventilator dependency Neurogenic pulmonary edema ARDS Pulmonary embolus	Auscultate chest for breath sounds Monitor rate, rhythm, and pattern of respirations Monitor periodic arterial blood gases Monitor pulse oximetry Review periodic chest x-rays Monitor sputum cultures Monitor vital signs Monitor CBC	Administer oxygen Provide ventilatory support Oxygenate before suctioning Limit suctioning to no longer than 10 sec Turn patient periodically Provide chest physical therapy
Cardiovascular	Hypotension Hypertension Dysrhythmias Cardiogenic shock Deep vein thrombosis (DVT) Anemia DIC	Assess frequently vital signs Observe legs for DVTs Monitor CPP Monitor for dysrhythmias Monitor cardiac dynamics with arterial line and central line on ongoing basis Monitor ongoing ECG patterns Monitor hemodynamic data Monitor CBC, Hgb, Hct, electrolytes, and coagulation studies	Maintain systolic >90 mm Hg Maintain CPP >60–70 mm Hg Insert of arterial and central line for hemodynamic monitoring Maintain thigh-high elastic hose and sequential compression boots Use appropriate drug therapy to maintain blood pressure to targeted range
Gastrointestinal (GI)	GI hemorrhage Curling's ulcer Constipation Paralytic ileus Small bowel obstruction	Auscultate abdomen for bowel sounds and distension Monitor for GI bleeding Monitor for occult blood in stools Monitor serial Hgb and Hct	Administer prophylactic H₂ blockers Institute bowel program to prevent constipation
Genitourinary	Urinary tract infection (UTI) Acute renal failure Acute urinary retention	Monitor for evidence of UTI Monitor periodic urinalysis Monitor prn urine culture Monitor intake and output record Monitor periodic BUN and creatinine	Remove indwelling catheter as soon as possible Institute bladder retraining as soon as possible Maintain adequate fluid volume Treat UTI and acute renal failure
Skin/mucous membranes	Decubitus ulcer Laryngeal ulceration Oral thrush Corneal ulceration	Frequently inspect skin for redness/breakdown Inspect mouth for evidence of oral infection Inspect eyes for evidence of corneal ulceration Monitor oral-tracheal secretions for evidence of bleeding	Consider use of a special bed Turn and reposition patient frequently Insert artificial tears to each eye qid Maintain eye shields Secure endotracheal tube to prevent unnecessary movement Treat oral infection as needed Institute special skin treatment protocol for evidence of redness or decubitus
Metabolic	Electrolyte imbalance SIADH Cerebral salt wasting Diabetes insipidus Hyperglycemia Sepsis	Monitor frequent electrolytes, glucose, calcium, phosphorus, and magnesium Monitor serum and urine osmolality Monitor urine specific gravity Monitor ongoing core temperature Monitor for evidence of sepsis	Determine underlying fluid or electrolyte problem and treat Replace depleted electrolytes Maintain euvolemia Maintain tight control of glucose with regular insulin as necessary Administer mannitol as needed Maintain normothermia Treat sepsis as needed
Musculoskeletal	Contracture Spasticity	Monitor range of motion of joints Observe for spasticity	Request physical therapy consult and therapy Provide range-of-motion exercises qid Apply splints, casting, etc, as ordered

(continued)

TABLE 17–5 MAJOR COLLABORATIVE PROBLEMS IN THE MANAGEMENT OF ACUTE, SEVERE TRAUMATIC BRAIN INJURY (Continued)

SYSTEM	COLLABORATIVE PROBLEMS	ASSESS AND MONITOR	INTERVENTIONS/MANAGEMENT
Nutrition	Weight loss Dehydration Negative nitrogen balance	Monitor daily weight Monitor intake and output record Monitor daily caloric intake Monitor for need to adjust daily caloric goals Monitor blood chemistries	Consult with clinical dietician to calculate caloric/dietary needs, nutrition source, and frequency of feeding Insert enteral feeding tube Request metabolic cart, as needed Provide information at a scheduled time
Psychosocial	Agitation Family stress/dysfunction	Assess family function Assess family's understanding of patient status and prognosis Assess for any special needs of family	Provide compassionate support Offer counseling services Identify family spokesperson and contact

ICP, intracranial pressure; TBI, traumatic brain injury; ARDS, acute respiratory distress syndrome; CBC, complete blood count; CPP, cerebral perfusion pressure; ECG, electrocardiogram; Hgb, hemoglobin; Hct, hematocrit; BUN, blood urea nitrogen; SIADH, syndrome of inappropriate secretion of antidiuretic hormone.

or flutter, supraventricular tachycardia, ventricular tachycardia or fibrillation, intraventricular conduction defects, and atrioventricular block. To assess cardiovascular function, the patient's vital signs should be monitored frequently, and the continuous pattern on a cardiac monitor should be observed for arrhythmias. In addition, the following may be ordered: electrolytes; coagulation studies; CBC; cardiac enzymes to exclude ACS; perhaps an echocardiogram if cardiac mechanics are questioned; and a 12-lead electrocardiogram (ECG). Any abnormality should be analyzed promptly for its underlying cause, and the appropriate treatment promptly instituted.

Patients with TBI are at risk for deep vein thrombosis (DVT). The *Guidelines* recommend graduated compression stockings or intermittent pneumatic compression (IPC) stockings unless lower extremity injuries prevent their use. If in use, compression stockings should be continued until the patient is ambulatory. Low-molecular-weight heparin (LMWH) or low doses of unfractionated heparin should be used in combination with compression stockings. However, there is an increased risk for expanding intracranial hemorrhage.[59]

Respiratory Management

Patients with severe TBI usually have reduced mental status and require intubation and mechanical ventilation. Patent and secure airway should be maintained. The SaO_2 saturation, arterial blood gases, and the quality of respirations are major clinical parameters for assessment. Hypoxemia should be avoided. A PaO_2 greater than 60 and/or SpO_2 greater than 92 mm Hg are targeted therapy to be maintained at all times. Oxygen therapy is titrated according to these parameters. The use of positive end-expiratory pressure (PEEP) with mechanical ventilation is common, but caution is recommended with its use as it may cause ICP elevation.[99]

Ventilator setting should be adjusted with a goal $PaCO_2$ of 35 to 40 mm Hg. Chronic hyperventilation for ICP management was commonly used in the past. Recent research findings revealed that hypocapnia secondary to hyperventilation can lead to cerebral vasoconstriction and, consequently, impaired CBF to the ischemic threshold. Therefore, hyperventilation is only recommended acutely and transiently in cases of intracranial hypertension and/or neurological deterioration. As discussed earlier in this chapter, any use of therapeutic, optimized hyperventilation ($PaCO_2$ <30 mm Hg) requires real-time $PbtO_2$ monitoring.[59] Hypoventilation with its resulting hypercapnia ($PaCO_2$ > 45 mm Hg) should also be avoided. Carbon dioxide is a potent vasodilator and can cause cerebral vasodilatation, which increases cerebral blood volume and ICP.

Pulmonary problems are one of the major causes of complications in TBI patients. Common problems include pneumonia, neurogenic pulmonary edema, acute respiratory distress syndrome (ARDS), and pulmonary embolism.

Neurogenic pulmonary edema (NPE) is a complication seen commonly in severe TBI patients with increased ICP; it is also sometimes seen in patients after a major generalized seizure. This acute pulmonary edema is noncardiogenic in nature, is not related to injured alveolar epithelium or capillary endothelium, and occurs minutes to days after injury. Although poorly understood, the pathophysiology had been associated with a combination of hydrostatic forces and permeability changes caused by massive α-adrenergic discharge. At the time of impact, an abrupt rise in ICP and sympathetic discharge results in a release of catecholamines, which causes vasoconstriction, hypertension, and pulmonary edema. Clinical findings are nonspecific (dyspnea, tachypnea, tachycardia, hypoxemia, and mild elevation in leukocytes). On a chest x-ray, "fluffy" infiltrates are noted. Neurogenic pulmonary edema can progress to respiratory failure and a condition similar to ARDS, or it can be self-limiting, resolving in hours to days. Treatment consists of normalizing the underlying increased ICP with medical and nursing strategies and providing ventilatory support with adequate supplemental oxygen and PEEP; diuretics, specifically furosemide, are also useful.

ARDS may also occur. The specific mechanism is unknown, but it has been suggested that head trauma results in the release of thromboplastin, causing a pathophysiologic cascade that results in an increase in pulmonary vascular resistance and right to left pulmonary shunting.[100] Treatment includes mechanical ventilation and the use of PEEP.

Hematologic Management

Many TBI patients develop a problem with clotting in the absence of evidence of excessive bleeding. Some patients develop disseminated intravascular coagulation (DIC), a catastrophic insult in brain injury. This condition results from a combination of the release of large amounts of thromboplastin and the presence of tissue emboli. The tissue emboli are produced by circulating factor XII from the vascular endothelial lining.[100]

Abnormal findings on the activated partial thromboplastin time (PTT), prothrombin time (PT), platelet count, and plasma fibrinogen level do not present a complete picture. Therefore, careful and accurate diagnostic reasoning is important. High titer of fibrin degradation products (FDPs) and prolonged PT and PTT are highly suggestive of DIC. The double-D-dimer degradation product is used to confirm the diagnosis. Other useful analyses include PT, ethanol gelatin tests, and fibrinopeptide-A level. If the patient survives, DIC corrects within hours. The mainstay of treatment is replacement of clotting factors, platelets, and maintenance of adequate blood volume. Fresh frozen plasma is used to replace the fibrinogen and clotting factor VIII. Cryoprecipitate is used to replace clotting factor V. Activated factor VIIa (FVIIa) has also been used for correction of traumatic coagulopathy.[101] Although anecdotal reports and retrospective studies had described the efficacy of FVIIa in the treatment of coagulopathy among trauma patients, its use specifically on the indication, dose, and timing of treatment has not been established yet with a large, randomized, and prospective study.

Severe TBI patients, in the absence of coagulopathy, are high risk to develop DVT due to immobility, recent surgery, or trauma. About 40% of patients with TBI develop DVT.[102] For neurosurgical patients in general, the incidence of DVT in the calves is 29% to 43%. Therefore, DVT prophylaxis is an important therapy in the TBI population. Antithrombotic stockings and sequential compression devices are commonly used. Low-dose anticoagulants such as conventional heparin or LMWH are usually contraindicated in patients with any type of bleeding such as ICH, EDH, or SDH; during early course of trauma; and/or when extensive surgery is planned. A retrospective study revealed no difference in bleeding events between patients with severe TBI who received heparin within 3 days of injury and those who received it 3 days after surgery.[73] However, further studies need to be conducted to determine the safety of the timing of initiation of prophylactic anticoagulant use in TBI.

If DVT and/or pulmonary embolism (PE) are suspected clinically, diagnostic tests are indicated. Venography is the "gold standard" for the evaluation of DVT and pulmonary angiography for PE. However, both are invasive; therefore, Doppler ultrasound of the affected extremity is commonly done to exclude DVT and a radionucleotide ventilation/perfusion (V/Q) scan or CT angiogram of the chest is done to determine the presence of PE. Full anticoagulation is often contraindicated in patients with severe TBI, so alternative management strategy such as inferior vena cava filter placement is indicated once the diagnosis of thromboembolism is made.

Infection Control

Patients with TBI can develop sepsis from infection of initial injury sites (i.e., gunshot and other open head wounds), from infections associated with invasive procedures (i.e., ICP monitor, indwelling urinary catheter, pulmonary catheter, surgery), or from nosocomial infections. Universal precautions, strict aseptic technique, and adherence to culture and dressing protocols are critical for prevention.

> **CLINICAL PEARLS:** Prophylactic antibiotic use in patients with an EVD/ICP monitor is not common due to the lack of studies that establish the effectiveness of such practice, although a dose of a broad-spectrum antibiotic may be given prior to placement of the device.

In the ICU environment, the risk of nosocomial infections is high. Common sites of infection are the lungs, blood, and urinary tract. Pneumonia is common especially in patients on mechanical ventilation. *Aspiration pneumonia* from aspiration at the time of injury or thereafter, *bacterial pneumonia* from bacterial invasion, and *hypostatic pneumonia* from stasis of fluid in the lungs are common types of lung infections. *Nosocomial pneumonias* are also common and are usually caused by gram-positive organisms (*Staphylococcus aureus, Streptococcus pneumonia,* and *Haemophilus influenzae*) and sometimes gram-negative organisms (enteric bacteria or *Pseudomonas*). Surveillance, prompt identification, and treatment of pneumonia with appropriate antibiotics are important, although prevention takes precedence. Nursing measures to prevent pneumonia in severe TBI patients will be further discussed later in this chapter.

The following recommendations are made in the *Guidelines*: periprocedural antibiotics for intubation should be administered to reduce the incidence of pneumonia (however, it does not change the length of stay or mortality); and early tracheostomy should be performed to reduce mechanical ventilation days (however, it does not alter mortality or the rate of nosocomial pneumonia).[59]

Another common nosocomial infection is bacteremia. Sources may include the urinary tract, intravascular catheters, lungs, and surgical or traumatic wounds. Like any other infections, early identification of the source and initiation of appropriate antibiotics are important. Other treatment strategy includes removal of the source, if possible. This might include removal or replacement of intravascular catheters.

One of the complications of ICP monitors is infection, although colonization is more common than clinically significant infection such as ventriculitis.[31] The *Guidelines* state (level III) that routine ventricular catheter exchange or prophylactic antibiotic use for ventricular catheter placement is not recommended to reduce infection.[59]

If infection is suspected, a CSF sample should be sent to the laboratory for analysis and culture. Treatment includes removal of the ICP monitor or site change and antibiotics.

Temperature Control

Hyperthermia can result from local or systemic infections, central injury to the hypothalamus, cerebral irritation from hemorrhage, or drug response, particularly to anticonvulsants. With hyperthermia, cerebral metabolic rate increases 5% to 7% per degree centigrade.[103] This places the patient at high risk for inadequate oxygen supply at the cellular level and secondary injury. Therefore, frequent monitoring and aggressive management of an elevated temperature are critical. It is important to identify the cause of the elevated temperature and treat the primary cause. The patient should be pancultured (screening for the sites of infection) to determine the cause of the elevation. Treatment includes acetaminophen (650 mg every 4 to 6 hours, as needed) and other cooling measures (i.e., cooling blanket, removal of excess bed covers, environmental control). The goal is to maintain normothermia while preventing shivering. Chlorpromazine (Thorazine) is used to control shivering.

Electrolyte Management

Electrolyte imbalances are common in TBI patients. The most common electrolyte imbalance is hyponatremia often associated with either syndrome of inappropriate secretion of antidiuretic hormone (SIADH) or cerebral salt wasting. Hyponatremia can exacerbate cerebral edema or cause seizures. See Chapter 9 for further discussion. Therefore, early recognition of hyponatremia is important so that timely corrective measures can be instituted. Intravenous solutions with higher concentrations of saline, extra salt added to the enteral feeding, and drug therapy, such as fludrocortisone acetate (Florinef), are used. Fludrocortisone, a mineralocorticoid, increases sodium reabsorption in renal tubules and increases excretion of potassium and hydrogen. Dosage is 0.1 to 0.2 mg/day. Hypernatremia can also occur and is usually associated with diabetes insipidus or as a result of mannitol administration. Urine electrolytes and osmolality are important parameters in evaluating the cause of hyponatremia and hypernatremia. Distinction between causes should be made promptly to be able to institute the appropriate therapy.

CLINICAL PEARLS: Typical clinical presentation of central diabetes insipidus includes polyuria, acute hypernatremia, and hypoosmolar urine.

Diabetes insipidus can result in volume depletion, which is associated with poor outcomes in TBI patients. Therefore, volume depletion must be corrected promptly with appropriate fluid replacement. Serum magnesium is also monitored. Hypomagnesemia, if present, must be corrected because it can lower seizure threshold and cause secondary brain injury.

Endocrine Management

In patients with TBI, hyperglycemia may be due to a stress response to cerebral trauma or may be related to borderline or documented diabetes mellitus. As discussed previously in this chapter, an elevated serum glucose may aggravate ischemic insult to the brain in TBI patients and worsen neurological outcome. Therefore, intravenous solutions containing glucose should be avoided.[104] If serum glucose is elevated, a normal glucose range can be established and maintained by starting an intravenous drip with regular insulin. Fingerstick blood glucose testing should be moni-

tored and tight glucose control should be followed.[105,106] To date, there are no prospective studies conducted designed to determine an optimum blood glucose level to prevent secondary brain injury; however, a level of less than 150 mg/dL is currently considered acceptable. Hypoglycemia with blood glucose level of less than 60 mg/dL should also be avoided because it can cause seizures in TBI patients.

As discussed previously, central diabetes insipidus is common and should be identified and treatment initiated promptly. Clinical presentation includes polyuria (urine output >250 mL/hr), sudden increase in serum sodium, urine osmolarity of 50 to 150 mOsm/L, or urine specific gravity less than 1.005. Treatment includes volume replacement and vasopressin administration.

CLINICAL PEARLS: Blood glucose levels should be maintained between 60 and 150 mg/dL to prevent secondary brain injury.

Approximately 40% of TBI patients develop posttraumatic hypopituitarism (PTHP), which includes gonadotropin, somatotropin, corticotrophin, and thyrotropin deficiencies.[107] Hyperprolactinemia or hypoprolactinemia may also be manifested. Pituitary dysfunction is usually noted in the postacute phase of TBI, although some degree of hypopituitarism may be noted while the patient is still in the intensive care unit. Accurate diagnosis is important and adequate hormone replacement therapy is usually indicated. Consultation with the endocrine specialist may also be necessary for long-term management and follow-up.

Autonomic Management

Although alterations in autonomic function are common in the acute recovery phase of TBI, a syndrome of prolonged episodes of autonomic dysfunction has been noted to follow a wide variety of neurological conditions that include TBI, hydrocephalus, brain tumor, subarachnoid hemorrhage, and intracerebral hemorrhage. In TBI, the incidence is between 15% and 33% of patients most often associated with diffuse axonal injury and brainstem injury.[108] This syndrome has been described by a variety of terms including autonomic dysfunction syndrome (ADS), autonomic or sympathetic storming, and dysautonomic dysfunction.[109–113] Nurses in clinical practice most often refer to this constellation of acute signs and symptoms as "storming." The term *ADS* will be used here for purposes of discussion. The constellation of signs and symptoms include hypertension, elevated temperature, severe tachycardia, tachypnea, pupillary dilation, decerebrate or decorticate posturing, altered consciousness, and profuse sweating, all attributable to alternations in autonomic function. The severity of the sympathetic response can also lead to cardiac arrhythmias, myocardial injury, neurogenic pulmonary edema, and increased intracranial pressure.

The pathophysiology of ADS is not well understood. It is known that as a result of initial trauma there is an immediate sympathetic surge that provides the compensatory response to sustain vital functions compromised by injury.[114–116] A recognized center of sympathetic autonomic function is located in the hypothalamus. Cortical areas of the brain that influence the activity of the hypothalamus include the orbitofrontal, anterior temporal, and insular regions. Important subcortical areas that modulate hypothalamic function include the amygdala (particularly the central nucleus), the periaqueductal gray, the nucleus of the tractus solitarius, the cerebellar uvula, and the cerebellar vermis. Damage to these areas results in dysregulation of overall autonomic balance.[108] Through a series of feedback loops, the hypothalamus and brainstem through a number of midbrain and other structures interact, resulting in elevated temperature, hypertension, tachycardia, and tachypnea. In addition, there is a major response of the sympatho-adreno-medullary axis resulting in significantly elevated catecholamines.[117] The level of elevation of the catecholamines is hypothesized to predict the outcome in TBI, with higher levels associated with poorer outcomes.[118]

The clinical presentation of ADS can vary with a combination of the typical physical findings. The signs and symptoms of ADS prominent during the critical/acute stages include hypertension, fever, tachycardia, tachypnea, pupillary dilation, decreased level of consciousness, abnormal posturing, and diaphoresis. When all signs and symptoms are not present, the most common combination is tachycardia, fever, and hypertension as the main presenting signs.

Temperature elevation is a perplexing problem. The temperature may vary from being low-grade to high fevers with a sustained elevation. A fever typically prompts a search for the underlying cause to determine if it is of infectious or noninfectious origin. A special consideration in patients with TBI is that the intracerebral temperature may significantly exceed measured body temperature because of impaired blood flow in the injured area. Because fever increases metabolic rate and causes cerebral hypoxia that leads secondary brain injury, fever must be controlled aggressively and a search made for the etiology, which may identify an infectious source that requires antibiotic therapy. In addition to sepsis, other possible causes of an elevated temperature that must be ruled out are meningitis, neuroleptic malignant syndrome, malignant hyperthermia, and thyroid storm.[108]

The diagnosis of ADS is based on the clinical presentation. It may be present in the ICU environment or may not be noted until the patient is transferred to an intermediate unit. The nurse may notice certain triggers that precipitate a storm such as suctioning or turning the patient. Identification of a trigger can lead to pretreatment of the patient to abate or decrease the intensity of the storm.[114] The consequences of a prolonged storming event are secondary brain injury as well as myocardial injury or neurogenic pulmonary edema, as previously mentioned. Therefore, early recognition and treatment of ADS is critical for prevention of secondary injury.

A number of laboratory investigations may be ordered to rule out other causes of the clinical presentation. Common studies include the following:

- Complete blood count (CBC) to note presence of an elevated white blood count—rule out infection
- Blood cultures in a patient with a fever—rule out sepsis
- Sputum culture and Gram stain—rule out respiratory infection
- Urinalysis and urine culture—rule out urinary tract infection
- Thyroid panel—rule out thyroid storm

- Chest x-ray—rule out pneumonia or atelectasis
- Duplex ultrasound—rule out deep vein thrombosis
- Electrocardiogram—rule out myocardial infarction
- CT scan or MRI of brain—rule out abscess
- Lumbar puncture—rule out meningitis

The large number of neurotransmitters and pathways associated with the sympathetic hyperactivity found in ADS is reflected in the variety of treatment options available for specific clinical presentations. In general, opioids, beta blockers, sedatives, and central nervous system (CNS) depressants have been used with varying results. Drug therapy often begins with intravenous morphine sulfate (10 mg IV in ventilated patients with titration to effect by prn dosage or continuous IV drip). Other drugs used include propranolol (Inderal), clonidine (Catapres), chlorpromazine (Thorazine), bromocriptine (Parlodel), dantrolene (Dantrium), atenolol (Tenormin), and labetalol (Normodyne).[108]

In summary, ADS is associated with poorer functional outcomes.[109] Therefore, early recognition and treatment are important in preventing secondary brain injury.

Gastrointestinal Management

TBI patients are usually in a hypermetabolic and catabolic state so that nutritional support should be started without delay. If not addressed promptly, the compromised nutritional state can result in malnutrition, which can cause immunosuppression, delayed wound healing, loss of body mass, and organ failure. It is recommended that patients be fed to attain full caloric replacement by day 7 postinjury.[59]

There is no superior recommended route of feeding. Gastric, jejunal, and parenteral routes are available. Some prefer the *jejunal* feeding route because it avoids gastric intolerance and is easy to administer. By day 7 postinjury, at least 15% of the calories in the feeding formula should be from protein. A nutrition consultation should be obtained with the clinical dietitian within 24 hours of admission. Feeding should begin as soon as possible (within 24 hours of admission, unless contraindicated). Enteral nutrition is the preferred route of feeding because of consciousness alterations due to TBI. Insertion of a Dobbhoff feeding tube into the jejunum of the small intestines is common because it avoids the problem of gastric intolerance, regurgitation, and aspiration common with a nasogastric or orogastric feeding tube. The clinical dietitian recommends the type of feeding and daily nutritional goals until the patient is at the desired nutritional level. Feeding rate should be started at a low rate (i.e., 10 to 20 mL/hr), then gradually increased to the goal rate, based on the patient's tolerance and response. If the TBI patient is unable to tolerate enteral nutrition such as in cases of pentobarbital-induced ileus, parenteral nutrition can be instituted.

Stress ulcers in TBI patients are related to hypothalamic dysfunction and hyperacidity secondary to vagal hyperactivity, although their specific mechanism is unknown.[71] A stress ulcer can occur within 96 hours of the initial injury; therefore, stress ulcer prophylaxis should be promptly initiated. These ulcers are likely to affect the esophagus, stomach, and duodenum with the potential to cause bleeding and perforation. To prevent ulcer formation, gastric acid should be buffered to a pH of greater than 7.0 using H_2 receptor antagonists, such as the following:

- Ranitidine (Zantac): the usual dose of 150 mg twice daily through a nasogastric (NG) tube, or 50 mg every 6 to 8 hours IV
- Famotidine (Pepcid): 20 mg twice daily through an NG tube or 20 mg every 12 hours IV
- Sucralfate: 1-g suspension via nasogastric or orogastric tube

Monitor the patient for occult bleeding. An acute drop in hemoglobin levels may suggest gastrointestinal bleeding (GIB) and, therefore, should be monitored. Stools should be checked for occult blood and/or gastric lavage via nasogastric/orogastric tube can be conducted to exclude GIB.

Drugs used in managing the patient such as continuous intravenous propofol can lead to constipation. In the case of use of propofol to control elevated ICP and agitation in the ICU, severe gastric immobility can occur. Care providers must be attuned to monitoring the patient for evidence of gastric immobility and constipation.

To prevent constipation and initiation of Valsalva's maneuver, a bowel program is instituted. See Chapter 11 for discussion of a bowel program. A stool softener, such as docusate (Colace), 100 mg twice a day through a feeding tube, is useful. Laxatives such as bisacodyl or any magnesium-based laxative can also be added to the regimen. The frequency and consistency of bowel movements should be monitored daily. Stool softeners and laxatives should be withheld if diarrhea occurs, and the cause of the diarrhea explored such as sending a stool sample for *Clostridium difficile* toxin evaluation before initiating treatment. The abdomen should also be assessed for any signs of abdominal distention or paralytic ileus.

MANAGEMENT OF SEVERE TRAUMATIC BRAIN INJURY DURING THE POSTACUTE PHASE

After the patient has been physiologically stabilized and no longer needs continuous monitoring, the interdisciplinary team, working closely with the case manager, makes the decision to transfer the patient to an intermediate unit. The interdisciplinary care map that guided care in the ICU environment now continues into the next phase of recovery. Although the goals of patient management remain much the same, the major focus now becomes rehabilitation and discharge planning.

REHABILITATION

The presence and persistence of behavioral problems in TBI patients are associated with the site and severity of injury, the nature of the premorbid personality, and environmental factors. Personality changes may include silly, childish, or poorly controlled behavior, as characterized by self-centeredness, an inability to show empathy, impatience, and impulsiveness. Injuries predominantly involving the frontal lobe are characterized by decreased drive and initiative, flat affect, disinhibition, disregard for social norms, apathy, lethargy, lack of goal-directed behavior, difficulty with impulse control, and an impaired sense of self-identity. Lesions of the temporal lobe are characterized by episodes of violent behavior and possibly seizure disorders. Early intervention is helpful in modifying behavioral patterns and in assisting the patient and family in managing such behaviors before they become established.

The patient's psychosocial and personality deficits, alterations in the patient's roles and responsibilities, and the tremendous burden placed on the family resulting from injury disrupt family function. If the family was dysfunctional before the injury, the added stress of a family member with severe TBI compounds that stress on dysfunction. The stress on a marriage is significant because the uninjured spouse must now become the caregiver for someone quite different from the person he or she married. The enormous stresses on the caregiver, especially those related to fatigue, are well documented in the literature.

Traumatic brain injury can bring with it a wide range of physical, cognitive, behavioral, and psychosocial problems.[12] Physical deficits may include sensory, motor, and/or autonomic abnormalities. Common cognitive problems include memory deficits; attention and concentration problems; language and visual perception deficits; and difficulties in learning and problem solving, insight, judgment, and information processing. Behavioral problems, as discussed earlier, involve aggression, agitation, and mood disorders. The above neuropsychological consequences of TBI result in social issues that may include economic difficulties, relationship problems, unemployment, and increased suicide risk. Based on an individual patient's needs, a plan of rehabilitative care is developed using a comprehensive interdisciplinary approach. The location for rehabilitation center depends, among other factors, on the patient's functional deficits, the managed care options offered, and financial and other available resources. Most discharge and transition planning is coordinated by a case manager. It is the nurse's responsibility to contribute to the database and work with the case manager as an advocate for the needs of the patient and family. Information on available community and national resources of support and information for TBI patients and their families should be provided. Cognitive retraining, vocational rehabilitation, behavior modification, and psychotherapy may also be required, depending on the deficits of the patient.

Rehabilitation of TBI was addressed in a 1998 report published by the Agency for Health Care Policy and Research.[119] This report makes it clear that there are limited scientific data to support evidence-based practice and that there is a need to conduct studies to determine rehabilitation guidelines and standards.

The consequences of TBI are multifaceted and can be devastating, especially with severe TBI. Many of these problems are confronted initially in the rehabilitation setting and then in the community as the patient transitions to the highest level of function possible. For further in-depth discussion of this phase of recovery, consult the extensive rehabilitation literature.

PREDICTING OUTCOME FROM TRAUMATIC BRAIN INJURY

Clinical prediction of outcome following TBI is a widely discussed issue in neuroscience practice. Although prognostic indicators are many, no individual variable or cluster of variables is sufficiently reliable to predict outcomes accurately. Because of the interest in enhancing accuracy, many early clinical factors have been identified as possible predictors. A report about traumatic coma indicates that the clinical examination is unreliable, that electrophysiologic testing is much more useful, and that brainstem and sensory evoked potentials are helpful within the first week.[120] In an evidence-based methodologic approach to prognostic indicators for severe TBI,[121] a positive predictive value of at least 70% in key criteria was chosen as necessary for an indicator to be included.[122–131] The following indicators met these criteria and are considered reliable indicators for predicting poor outcome:

- Low score on GCS (≤8)
- Increased age
- Bilaterally absent pupillary light reflex
- Systolic blood pressure less than 90 mm Hg, further strengthened when combined with hypoxia
- Abnormalities on CT scan

The well-known **Glasgow Outcome Scale** places survivors of central nervous system trauma (Chart 17-2) into one of five categories, depending on the degree of their residual function and independence. The scale, which does not evaluate cognitive impairment, conveys only the examiner's general opinion of the patient's status.

Quality of life has become an important framework for describing outcome. However, this concept still has not been properly defined, and methods of measurement have not been well established. The most frequently mentioned proxy indicators for quality of life are independence in performing activities of daily living, ability to maintain social relationships, successful role implementation, gainful employment, and general ability to maintain control of one's life.

CHART 17-2   Glasgow Outcome Scale

- *Good outcome*—may have minimal disabling sequelae but returns to independent functioning and a full-time job comparable to preinjury level
- *Moderate disability*—capable of independent functioning but not returned to full-time employment
- *Severe disability*—dependent on others for some aspect of daily living
- *Persistent vegetative state*—no obvious cortical function
- *Dead*

Jennett, B., & Bond, M. (1975). Assessment of outcome after severe brain damage: A practical scale. *Journal of Neurosurgery, 4*, 673.

PREVENTION OF TRAUMATIC BRAIN INJURY

Prevention remains the primary management strategy in TBI. Programs with focus on the causes of TBI have been implemented. Direct public health initiatives with the goal to minimize incidence and/or injuries related to vehicular accidents, falls, violence, and sports and recreation are effective strategies in preventing TBI. Programs that discourage driving under the influence of alcohol or drugs, especially among young adults, have been implemented. The use of car restraint devices such as seat belts and airbags are highly mandated by most state laws. Although motorcycle helmet laws are still under debate, use of helmets is known to reduce fatalities and, therefore, is encouraged. Safety precautions to prevent falls, especially among the elderly, are also recommended. These include the use of handrails with stairs, grab bars in showers and tubs, ambulation assisted devices (i.e., walkers, canes, strollers), nonslip floor covers, adequate lighting, and avoidance of clutter. Programs to prevent violence both in the streets and schools have been established. Ongoing legislative laws to control the possession of firearms were established to further prevent firearm-related assaults. Moreover, safety precautions in sports training and coaching are highly recommended. The use of protective devices, such as helmets, in contact sports is also helpful in preventing injuries.

MANAGEMENT OF TRAUMATIC BRAIN INJURY: A DYNAMIC PROCESS THROUGH RESEARCH

Future advances in the care of TBI patients will be based on research focused on understanding the underlying mechanisms of injury. Both clinical and experimental research provide novel information that helps to develop new therapies and/or modify existing management strategies.

Advances in neuromonitoring technology are becoming available, although their efficacy still needs to be established with large clinical trials. Recently, continuous direct oxygen measurement in the brain became available. Neurotrend catheters or Licox catheters are introduced via a dedicated two-way or three-way bolt allowing for monitoring of ICP, brain tissue oxygen tension, and temperature.[119] As an alternative, these catheters can also be tunneled and placed locally in the affected brain tissue after intracranial surgery. The Licox catheter is marketed in the United States and has been studied extensively regarding its use, safety, and reliability. Several studies were focused on defining a critical value of brain tissue oxygen pressure ($PbrO_2$). Low values have been reported in TBI patients with $PbrO_2$ of 14 to 15 mm Hg, which is currently accepted as the ischemic threshold.[132,133] The localized nature of this brain tissue oxygen monitor is a limitation. To date, the site of $PbrO_2$ measurement within the brain has been addressed, with placement in the injured area or the undamaged area of the brain debated. Therefore, the use of $PbrO_2$ monitoring should be used as complementary to other established neuromonitoring devices such as the ICP monitor until further studies on its safety and reliability are conducted.

Another available device is cerebral microdialysis, which measures glucose, lactate, pyruvate, glutamate, and glycerol levels in the brain's extracellular fluid.[67] The lactate-to-pyruvate ratio provides information about the neuronal function; increased glutamate levels are indicative of ischemia; and increased glycerol levels are indicated of neuronal death. This device is currently being used as a research tool, but with its potential to predict and measure cerebral ischemia, there is much interest about its possible use as a monitor to support clinical decision making for patient management.

With the advent of the $PbrO_2$ monitoring device, oxygen-targeted therapy such as hyperoxia and packed red cell transfusion has been studied to improve cerebral oxygenation and prevent cerebral ischemia in severe TBI patients. To date, studies on hyperoxia or hyperbaric treatment in the TBI population are insufficient to establish efficacy, although a small decrease in mortality has been suggested.[134,135] Red blood cell transfusion to augment cerebral oxygenation by increasing $PbrO_2$ has been studied, but findings were not consistent.[136] Further studies are needed to establish the role of oxygen-targeted therapies in the management of severe TBI.

Potential neuroprotective agents have been studied and revealed promising results in animal studies, but failed to establish efficacy in human studies. These agents include glutamate antagonists,[137] free radical scavengers,[138] and calcium channel blockers. Dexanabinol, however, showed potential use as a neuroprotective agent. A synthetic, non-psychotropic cannabinoid, dexanabinol is a noncompetitive N-methyl-D-aspartate (NMDA) receptor antagonist found to scavenge free radicals, act as antioxidant, and inhibit cytokines in experimental studies. A phase II clinical trial conducted revealed an improvement in hypotension, ICP, and CPP in severe TBI patients with a promising benefit toward a positive neurological outcome.[139] This drug holds promise as a neuroprotective agent of choice for TBI patients, but further studies are needed.

ASSESSMENT AND CLINICAL REASONING: KEY ROLE OF THE NEUROSCIENCE NURSE IN PATIENT CARE

The following reviews key points of assessment and clinical reasoning as they apply to TBI patients.

Vital Signs

Chart 17-3 summarizes the significance of vital signs as they relate to neurological function and other body systems. The frequency for monitoring vital signs depends on the stability of the patient's condition. In the ICU setting, monitoring should occur at least every hour unless the patient is physiologically unstable.

Neurological Signs

After an initial baseline assessment is established, frequent subsequent assessments should be conducted to determine trends in neurological status (stability, deterioration, or improvement). For example, impending cerebral herniation and onset of new intracranial hemorrhage are major problems of acute deterioration that are life threatening; therefore, the importance of frequent serial assessments cannot be overstated. The frequency with which a serial neurological assessment is conducted depends on the patient's condition and degree of stability. In the unstable patient, neurological signs may be monitored as frequently as every 5 to 15 minutes. After the patient has been well stabilized, monitoring every 2 to 4 hours may be safe and appropriate. However, this time interval is the standard on regular care (postacute) units, but *not* in the ICU. The following are specific areas included in the neurological assessment:

- Level of consciousness and cognition (if responding verbally); if comatose, GCS is used
- Size, shape, and reaction of pupils to light (asymmetry seen with a focal lesion)
- Brainstem function, as evidenced by corneal and gag reflexes and extraocular movement (especially in an ICU environment)
- Motor function (focal mass indicated by asymmetry or lateralization)

Level of Consciousness

Level of consciousness is the most sensitive indicator of neurological change. If the patient is able to respond verbally, orientation to time, place, and person is assessed. Cognition is assessed by asking simple questions and making simple requests, such as "Show me two fingers," "Show me your left thumb," "Raise your left arm," and "Why are you here?" If comatose, the GCS is used.

Brainstem Reflexes

Assessing and monitoring brainstem function begin with the pupils. Pupils are normally equal in size and midposition, round, and briskly reactive to direct light. Any *new* change in the size or reaction of one or both of the pupils requires immediate evaluation. With lateral transtentorial herniation caused by localized cerebral edema (peaks about 72 hours after injury) or a focal lesion, one pupil will become dilated and progressively unresponsive to light. This is attributable to unilateral compression of the oculomotor nerve by the edematous herniating brain. An oval or ovoid pupil is also an early sign of transtentorial herniation. Immediate intervention may be necessary to prevent herniation and irreversible neurological deterioration. In addition, when looking into the eyes, observe their position in terms of spontaneous asynchronous movement (nystagmus) or extraocular movement (EOM) deviation.

The corneal and gag reflexes can be assessed easily at the bedside. The absence of either of these reflexes is a poor prognostic sign. Special protective eye care and lubrication should be applied if the corneal reflex is absent. Symmetry of the facial nerve can be checked by inserting a cotton-tipped applicator first in one nostril and then the other. By observing each side for grimacing, one can determine if a facial nerve deficit is present.

CHART 17-3   Vital Signs and Their Significance in a Head-Injured Patient

RESPIRATIONS

- Brain injuries can result in abnormal respiratory patterns that roughly correlate with the level of neurological dysfunction (see Chap. 7 for a discussion of abnormal patterns and level of injury).
- In general, an initial increase in intracranial pressure (ICP) results in slowing of respirations. If ICP continues to increase, the pattern becomes rapid and noisy until the terminal stage, when respirations cease.
- A few conditions can affect respirations:
  - Complications of metabolic disorders, such as diabetic acidosis, can change respiratory patterns (Kussmaul's respirations).
  - Injuries to the cervical spine below C-4 can cause respiratory difficulty, whereas injuries above C-4, the site of phrenic nerve innervation, can cause total arrest.

BLOOD PRESSURE

- Hypotension is rarely attributable to cerebral injury.
  - *Hypotension and tachycardia* are seen as terminal events in head injury.
  - *Hypotension and tachycardia* in a patient who is not terminal are usually related to occult bleeding, most likely in the abdominal, pelvic, or thoracic cavity.
  - *Note:* The inherent risk of hypotension involves its relationship to CBF, CPP, and subsequent hypoperfusion and ischemia CCP. Hypoperfusion is associated with CPP.
  - *Hypotension and bradycardia* may be a secondary response to cervical cord injury if the descending sympathetic pathways have been interrupted.
- Hypertension is commonly associated with ↑ ICP; it may also be associated with pain, fear, or anxiety.
  - *Hypertension and bradycardia* are associated with ↑ ICP; they are late signs that correlate with pressure on the brainstem.
    Cushing's response is an ischemic response of the body that maintains cerebral blood flow in the presence of rising ICP. Cushing's response includes hypertension, bradycardia, and a widening pulse pressure.

Cushing's triad includes hypertension, bradycardia, and an irregular respiratory pattern; it reflects a rising ICP in which there is direct pressure on the medullary center of the brainstem. It is often seen in the terminal stage and is associated with irreversible brainstem damage.

PULSE

- Pulse has been discussed in conjunction with blood pressure.
- *Bradycardia* is associated with increasing ICP or cervical injury.
- *Tachycardia* is associated with the following:
  - Occult (nonneurological) hemorrhage or hypovolemic shock
  - An autonomic response to injury of the hypothalamus or its connections
  - A terminal event in severe brain injury

TEMPERATURE

- *Hypothermia* can occur as a result of hypothalamic injury, because the hypothalamus is the heat regulatory center of the brain. The patient will assume the temperature of the ambient room air; if it is cold, body temperature will drop. Hypothermia (96°–97°F) is also seen early in cervical cord injuries.
- *Hyperthermia* in the brain-injured patient can be associated with direct injury to the hypothalamus or petechial bleeding into the hypothalamus or pons. Hyperthermia must be controlled because it *increases* the metabolic rate of all body cells, including those in the brain.
  - Oxygen consumption rises approximately 10% for every 1°C rise in temperature
    A rise from 37°C (98.6°F) to 40.5°C (105°F) results in a 35% increase in oxygen consumption.
    This can result in ischemia for the injured brain that was barely meeting metabolic needs when the temperature was within normal range.

CBF, cerebral blood flow; CPP, cerebral perfusion pressure; CCP, capillary closing pressure.

Without a gag reflex, the patient is at high risk for aspiration pneumonia. The ability to protect the airway and an intact gag reflex are criteria for consideration before removing an endotracheal tube. Provided there is no cervical fracture or dislocation, confirmed by cervical spine films, the eyes can be checked for doll's eye reflex (oculocephalic reflex) by the physician in the unconscious patient to provide information on severity of coma and prognosis.

Motor Function

Observe the patient for spontaneous movement. Asymmetry of movement or lateralization suggests a focal mass lesion on one side of the brain. Hemiparesis or hemiplegia, which involves only one side of the body, is a sign of lateralization, with the lesion located in the hemisphere opposite the side of motor weakness. Decortication (flexor) or decerebration (extensor) posturing is observed in comatose patients who have suffered severe TBI. Additionally, bilateral or unilateral flaccidity may be associated with spinal injuries.

Other Observations

The patient's face and scalp should be examined for signs of injury, such as abrasions or contusions that may have been missed during the initial assessment in the ED. Note the presence of ecchymosis on the mastoid bone (Battle's sign), periorbital ecchymosis (raccoon's eye), conjunctival hemorrhage, or clear or bloody drainage from the ear, from the nose, or postnasally. These signs indicate a basal skull fracture. Assuming that the patient has been cleared for presence of a cervical injury, assess the neck for evidence of nuchal rigidity, a sign of meningeal irritation. Nuchal rigidity can be caused by meningitis or blood in the CSF from subarachnoid hemorrhage.

If an ICP monitor is in place, observe for elevations in pressure and the shape of the P1, P2, and P3 components. Often, standing orders are in place for interventions to be implemented at a certain level of pressure elevation. The monitor also helps the nurse observe the effect of various nursing interventions on ICP. If the ICP is elevated, planned activities may be postponed until the pressure decreases. See Chapter 13 for further discussion of management of increased intracranial pressure.

NURSING MANAGEMENT OF TRAUMATIC BRAIN INJURY

A critical management and care focus for TBI patients is prevention of secondary brain injury by optimizing cerebral perfusion, early recognition of complications, and management of multisystem problems as previously discussed in this chapter. To achieve optimal outcomes for the patient, a collaborative interdisciplinary approach is needed. Some complications are more apt to occur in the first few days after injury; others are delayed. As a member of the collaborative interdisciplinary team, the nurse has both independent and interdependent roles. Evidence-based nursing practice, or best practice, should be provided.[140] A nurse with a strong knowledge of the neurological anatomy, physiology, and pathophysiology who can immediately identify complications and/or potential problems and provide prompt and appropriate interventions to prevent secondary brain injuries plays a very important role in the care of TBI patients.

Nursing measures to treat and/or prevent ICP elevation include proper positioning, elevation of the head of bed at 30 degrees, and prevention of jugular venous outflow obstruction by keeping the head in midline position. Cervical collar and endotracheal tubes must also be checked for tightness around the neck. Minimizing external stimulation is important. Use pharmacologic orders for sedation and analgesia as needed when providing potentially uncomfortable procedures such as wound care. Proper timing of the necessary procedures to allow for rest periods is also helpful. If the patient has an external ventricular drain, it may be necessary to open the drain to allow for CSF drainage to treat ICP elevations, according to unit protocol. The unit protocol for opening to draining of the ventriculostomy is based on an ICP reading (typically ≥20 mm Hg) and instructions about how long to keep the drain open (typically 5 minutes) and how fast to drain (very slowly, typically a few minidrops per minute). These specific parameters are given by the physician and provide the bedside nurse with clear instructions and guidance as to when to provide therapeutic intervention and when to notify the physician for further management instructions.

Hemodynamic stability is another important patient goal. The bedside nurse should be proficient with the use of available monitoring technology such as the cardiac monitor and the maintenance of the pulmonary catheter in critically ill patients. Knowledge about critical parameters is important, as is the ability to recognize any abnormalities to provide the appropriate interventions. Treatment is usually pharmacologic, and is guided by targeted physiologic values for hemodynamic variables, such as cardiac output and MAP. Drug administration is titrated to obtain the targeted range as ordered by the physician.

Maintaining a patent airway, the common pathway to the respiratory system, is another top priority in TBI management. In the acute phase of TBI, patients are neither able to manage their own secretions nor able to position themselves in the most expeditious way for adequate drainage of secretions. Meeting the patient's respiratory support needs is a nursing care objective of the highest priority. Suction is needed to prevent an increase in carbon dioxide and subsequent hypercapnia, which contributes to cerebral vasodilatation, cerebral edema, and increased ICP.

- Position the patient on the side to facilitate drainage of secretions and prevent aspiration, if not intubated.
- Preoxygenate with 100% oxygen before suctioning (with physician's approval).
- Limit the catheter insertion to 10 seconds or less to prevent an increase of CO_2.
- If a tracheostomy is present, provide tracheostomy care frequently, according to unit protocol, to prevent crusting and build-up of secretions that can obstruct the airway.
- Do not hyperextend or hyperflex the neck, because such maneuvers create a partial obstruction of the airway.

Atelectasis, a collapsed or airless state that may involve any part of the lung, is a respiratory problem that can develop rapidly. It is, therefore, important to be sure that all areas of the lungs are expanded. To assess the lungs for atelectasis, the nurse auscultates the chest for breath sounds, making sure to listen to the entire chest, especially the bases of the lungs. Nursing management directed at preventing atelectasis includes:

- **Adjust for sighs** on ventilator if this is an option.
- **Perform pulmonary percussion** if the patient is on a bed specially designed for this procedure.
- **Encourage deep breathing exercises and use the incentive spirometer** in the conscious patient to expand the lungs and loosen secretions.

The nurse should assess for the signs and symptoms of pneumonia by auscultating the chest for breath sounds and adventitious sounds and monitoring the character of the sputum for color and foul odor, as well as the temperature and white blood cell count for elevation. Nursing management to prevent pneumonia should incorporate the following:

- Maintain a patent airway.
- Turn from side to side every 2 hours to prevent stasis of fluid in the lungs.
- Do not position on the back, because this increases the possibility of aspiration.
- Administer chest physiotherapy to loosen and drain pulmonary secretions.

- Use meticulous aseptic technique when delivering care. The intubated or tracheotomized patient is at high risk for infection.
- Be sure to clear secretions from the back of the throat when suctioning.
- Elevate the head of the bed to 30 degrees.
- Maintain an inflated cuff on the tracheostomy tube to prevent aspiration.
- Confirm that the gag reflex is intact before feeding a patient.
- Provide meticulous oral hygiene care.

Nursing management should also be directed toward immediately addressing nutritional needs and beginning feeding expeditiously. Serum calcium, potassium, phosphorus, blood urea nitrogen, creatinine, and other laboratory values related to nutrition should be monitored. Interruptions in the feeding schedule should be avoided when possible as they can decrease the daily intake.[141] (See Chap. 8 for a discussion of nutritional needs.) Bowel movement should be monitored and abnormalities such as diarrhea and constipation should be noted. Unit protocols to address diarrhea or constipation should be implemented.

Another important nursing intervention is early initiation of rehabilitation therapies through referral to physical therapy, occupational therapy, and speech language pathology, as indicated. Patient positioning, range-of-motion exercises, and coma stimulation at the bedside may also be provided by the nurses.

NURSING MANAGEMENT FOR SPECIAL PROBLEMS

Basal Skull Fractures

The type of clinical evidence presented by a patient with a basal skull fracture depends on the particular basal skull fossa involved. Signs and symptoms may include ecchymosis of the mastoid process (Battle's sign), periorbital hemorrhage (raccoon's eyes) and ecchymosis, blood behind the eardrum (hemotympanum), decreased hearing, drainage from the nose (rhinorrhea) or ear (otorrhea), and postnasal drainage (postnasal drip). Nursing management addresses the risk of meningitis through the following strategies:

- Never suction through the nose if there is question of a basal skull fracture; the catheter could slip into the dural tear and become a source of contamination within the intracranial cavity.
- In a conscious patient, caution against blowing the nose; this act could introduce microorganisms into the meninges or brain through a dural tear.
- Do not introduce any foreign body into the orifice (nares or ear) or irrigate the area; sterile cotton or other absorbent material should be placed loosely around the orifice and changed frequently.

If there is any question whether the drainage is CSF, laboratory analysis of a test tube specimen for chloride concen-

tration is helpful. CSF's chloride concentration is greater than that of serum. Glucose testing for the presence of CSF is unreliable because nasal secretions can yield a positive reaction. The presence of drainage from the nose or ear is highly suggestive of CSF leakage. In clinical practice, drainage is often a combination of CSF and blood. A characteristic stain with a dark center and a lighter outer area (halo sign) is often seen. Most CSF leaks heal spontaneously within days. In rare instances, surgery is necessary to find and patch the tear. Use of prophylactic antibiotics for basal skull fractures is controversial.

A basal skull fracture can be very serious if rapidly developing local edema is close to vital brainstem structures. It can lead to life-threatening respiratory problems, including respiratory arrest. Nursing management includes monitoring for deterioration in vital or neurological signs as well as for signs of meningeal irritation.

Carotid-Cavernous Fistula

A carotid-cavernous fistula is a rare complication of TBI in which a laceration of the carotid artery results in direct communication between the high-pressure arterial blood of the internal carotid artery (ICA) and the low-pressure venous blood of the cavernous sinus. The cavernous sinuses are located at the basal skull on either side of the sphenoid body. The ICA, several of its branches, and the oculomotor, the trochlear, two divisions of the trigeminal, and the abducens nerves pass through the cavernous sinus. A patient with a carotid-cavernous fistula may present with one or more of the following signs: a bruit over the affected orbit; pulsating proptosis; conjunctival edema; orbital pain and chemosis; facial pain; limitation of extraocular movement; headache; diplopia; photophobia; and visual deficits (decreased visual acuity that can lead to blindness). The definitive diagnostic procedure is carotid angiography. Although spontaneous resolution may occur in a few patients, surgery is necessary for most. Surgical procedures include ligation of the ICA above and below the fistula or embolization. Nursing management includes neurological assessment, including all cranial nerves; auscultation of the bruit; assessment of pain; and monitoring for the presence of conjunctival edema. Special care is needed to prevent corneal ulceration and other injuries to the eyes.

Hygroma

A **hygroma,** an encapsulated collection of CSF, is caused by a tear in the arachnoid layer of the meninges, which allows fluid to escape into the subdural space. Concurrent cerebral edema locks the fluid into the space and creates pressure on the brain. The total accumulation of fluid may range from a few milliliters to, in rare cases, as much as 50 mL. A subdural hygroma is unilateral but may extend over the entire hemisphere or become encapsulated. The fluid's high protein content may account for its occasional coagulation. Symptoms corresponding to a slowly developing SDH occur, beginning with headache, which becomes severe and persistent. The only effective treatment is surgical removal.

SUMMARY AND FUTURE TRENDS

This chapter provides an overview of craniocerebral trauma, including diagnosis, treatment, and collaborative interdisciplinary management across the continuum of acute care. The evidence-based practice is discussed, particularly for the management of severe TBI. Research at both the physiologic and clinical levels will continue to develop the evidence base for management of TBI to achieve optimal patient outcomes.

Research continues on the pathophysiologic mechanisms of traumatic brain injury, with special interest in the cascade of neurotransmitters and potential neuroprotective drugs that could lead to prevention of secondary brain injury. A general trend toward use of noninvasive physiologic monitoring continues, although there has been little integration into practice. There is need to identify early indicators of neurological deterioration through more sensitive indicators such as spectral analysis of intracranial pressure waveforms, an area of promise that has yet to be realized. The continued revision of clinical practice guidelines based on evidence-based practice has been an outstanding contribution to standardization of practice protocols based on research. As evidence-based practice becomes the standard of care, better patient outcomes will be realized. Nurses need to conduct more research that contributes to the development of data-based nursing practice protocols.

REFERENCES

1. Thurman, D. J., Alverson, C., Dunn, K. A., et al. (1999). Traumatic brain injury in the United States: A public health perspective. *Journal of Head Trauma Rehabilitation, 14,* 602–615.
2. Jager, T. E., Weiss, H. B., Coben, J. H., & Pepe, P. E. (2000). Traumatic brain injuries evaluated in U.S. emergency departments, 1992–1994. *Academy of Emergency Medicine, 7,* 134–140.
3. Dietrich, W. D. (2000). Trauma of the nervous system A. Basic neuroscience of neurotrauma. In W. G. Bradley, R. B. Daroff, G. M. Fenichel, & C. D. Marsden. (Eds.). *Neurology in Clinical Practice* (3rd ed., pp. 1045–1054). Boston: Butterworth & Heinemann.
4. Graham, D. I., Adams, J. H., Nicoll, J. A. R., et al. (1995). The nature, distribution, and causes of traumatic brain injury. *Brain Pathology, 5,* 397–406.
5. Davis, A. E. (2000). Mechanisms of traumatic brain injury: biomechanical, structural, and cellular considerations. *Critical Care Nursing Quarterly, 23*(3), 1–13.
6. Gennarelli, T. A., & Thibault, L. E. (1985). Biological modes of TBI. In D. P. Becker & J. T. Povlishock (Eds.). *Central nervous system trauma status report: National Institute of Neurological and Communicative Disorders and Stroke* (pp. 91–404). Bethesda, MD: National Institute of Health.
7. Graham, D. I., & Gennarelli, T. A. (2000). Pathology of brain damage after TBI. In P. R. Cooper & J. G. Golfinos (Eds.). *Head injury* (4th ed., pp. 133–153). New York: McGraw-Hill.
8. Gennarelli, T. A. (1994). Animate models of TBI. *Journal of Neurotrauma, 11,* 357–368.
9. Nolan, S. (2005). Traumatic brain injury: A review. *Critical Care Nursing Quarterly, 28*(2), 188–194.
10. Valsamis, M. P. (1994). Pathology of trauma. *Neurosurgery Clinics of North America, 5*(1), 175–183.
11. Fritz, H. G., & Bauer, R. (2004). Secondary injuries in brain trauma: Effects of hypothermia. *Journal of Neurosurgical Anesthesiology, 16*(1), 43–52.
12. Lovasik, D., Kerr, M. E., & Alexander, S. (2001). Traumatic brain injury research: A review of clinical studies. *Critical Care Nursing Quarterly, 23*(4), 24–41.
13. Bullock, R., & Fujisawa, H. (1992). The role of glutamate antagonists for the treatment of CNS injury. *Journal of Neurotrauma, 9*(Suppl. 2), S443–S462.
14. Siejo, B. (1991). The role of calcium in cell death. In D. Price, A. Aguayo, & H. Thoenen (Eds.). *Neurodegenerative disorders: Mechanisms and prospects for therapy* (pp. 35–69). London: J. Wiley & Sons.
15. Mcintosh, T. K., Saatman, K. E., & Raghupathi, R. (1997). Calcium and the pathogenesis of traumatic CMS: Cellular and molecular mechanisms. *Neuroscientist, 3,* 169–175.
16. Mcintosh, T. K., Saatman, K. E., & Raghupathi, R. (1998). The molecular and cellular sequence of experimental traumatic brain injury: Pathogenic mechanisms. *Neuropathology Applied Neurobiology, 24,* 251–267.
17. Mcintosh, T. K., Saatman, K. E., & Raghupathi, R. (1996). Neuropathological sequelae of traumatic brain injury: Relationship to neurochemical and biomechanical mechanisms. *Laboratory Investigation, 74,* 315–342.
18. Graham, D. I., Adams, J. H., Nicoll, J. A. R., et al. (1995). The nature, distribution, and causes of traumatic brain injury. *Brain Pathology, 5,* 397–368.
19. Cruz, J., Minoja, G., Mattioli, C., et al. (1998). Severe acute brain trauma. In J. Cruz (Ed.). *Neurological and neurosurgical emergencies* (pp. 405–436). Philadelphia: W. B. Saunders.
20. Dietrich, W. D. (2000). Trauma of the nervous system A. Basic neuroscience of neurotrauma. In W. G. Bradley, R. B. Daroff, G. M. Fenichel, & C. D. Marsden (Eds.). *Neurology in clinical practice* (3rd ed., pp. 1045–1054). Boston: Butterworth & Heinemann.
21. Gennarelli, T. A., & Thibault, L. E. (1985). Biological modes of TBI. In D. P. Becker & J. T. Povlishock (Eds.). *Central nervous system trauma status report: National Institute of Neurological and Communicative Disorders and Stroke* (pp. 391–404). Bethesda, MD: National Institute of Health.
22. Graham, D. I., & Gennarellli, T. A. (2000). Pathology of brain damage after TBI. In P. R. Cooper & J. G. Golfinos (Eds.). *Head injury* (4th ed., pp. 133–153). New York: McGraw-Hill.
23. Valsamis, M. P. (1994). Pathology of trauma. *Neurosurgery Clinics of North America, 5*(1), 175–183.
24. Gennarelli, T. A., Thibault, L. E., Tipperman, R., et al. (1989). Axonal injury in the optic nerve: A model simulating diffuse axonal injury in the brain. *Journal of Neurosurgery, 71,* 244.
25. Morganti-Kossmann, M. C., Rancan, M., Stahel, P. F., & Kossmann, T. (2002). Inflammatory response in acute traumatic brain injury: A double-edged sword. *Current Opinion in Critical Care, 8,* 101–105.
26. Kossmann, T., Stahel, P. F., Lenzlinger, P. M., et al. (1997). Interleukin-8 released into the cerebrospinal fluid after brain injury is associated with blood brain barrier dysfunction and nerve growth factor production. *Journal of Cerebral Blood Flow Metabolism, 17,* 280–289.
27. Kossmann, T., Hans, V., Imbof, H. G., Trentz, O., & Morganti-Kossmann, M. C. (1996). Interleukin-6 released in human cerebrospinal fluid following traumatic brain injury may trigger nerve growth factor production in astrocytes. *Brain Research, 713,* 143–152.
28. Csuka, E., Morganti-Kossmann, M. C., Lenzlinger, P. M., Joller, H., Trentz, O., & Kossmann, T. (1999). IL-10 levels in cerebrospinal fluid and serum of patients with severe traumatic brain injury: Relationship to IL-6, TNF-alpha, TGF-beta1 and blood-brain barrier function. *Journal of Neuroimmunology, 101,* 211–221.
29. Morganti-Kossmann, M. C., Hans, V. H., Lenzlinger, P. M., et al. (1999). TGF-beta is elevated in the CSF of patients with severe traumatic brain injuries and parallels blood-brain barrier function. *Journal of Neurotrauma, 16,* 617–628.
30. Stahel, P. F., Kossmann, T., Joller, H., Trentz, O., & Morganti-Kossmann, M. C. (1998). Increased interleukin-12 levels in

human cerebrospinal fluid following severe head trauma. *Neuroscience Letters, 249*, 123–126.

31. Greenberg, M. S. (2006). *Handbook of neurosurgery* (6th ed., pp. 632–637). Lakeland, FL: Greenberg Graphics.

32. Chesnut, R. M., & Marshall, L. F. (1993). Management of severe TBI. In A. H. Ropper (Ed.). *Neurological and neurosurgical intensive care* (3rd ed., pp. 203–246). New York: Raven Press.

33. Graham, D. I., & Gennarelli, T. A. (2000). Pathology of brain damage after TBI. In P. R. Cooper & J. G. Golfinos (Eds.). *Head injury* (4th ed., pp. 133–153). New York: McGraw-Hill.

34. Servadei, F. (1997). Prognostic factors in severely head injured adult patients with epidural haematomas. *Acta Neurochirurgica, 139*, 273–278.

35. Servadei, F. (1997). Prognostic factors in severely head injured adult patients with adult subdural haematomas. *Acta Neurochirurgica, 139*, 279–285.

36. Roth, P., & Farls, K. (2000). Pathophysiology of traumatic brain injury. *Critical Care Nursing Quarterly, 23*(3), 14–25.

37. Soloniuk, D., Pitts, L. H., & Lovely, M. (1986). Traumatic intracerebral hematomas: Timing of appearance and indications for operative removal. *Journal of Trauma, 26*, 787–794.

38. Fukamachi, A., Kohno, K., Nagaseki, Y., et al. (1985). The incidence of delayed traumatic intracerebral hematoma with extradural hemorrhages. *Journal of Trauma, 25*, 145–149.

39. Le Roux, P. D., Haglund, M. M., Newell, D. W., et al. (1992). Intraventricular hemorrhage in blunt head trauma: An analysis of 43 cases. *Neurosurgery, 31*, 678–685.

40. Guskiewicz, K. M., Bruce, S. L., Cantu, R. C., et al. (2004). Recommendations on management of sport-related concussion: Summary of the National Athletic Trainer's Association position statement. *Journal of Athletic Training, 39*, 280–297.

41. Adams, J. H., Doyle, D., Ford, I., Gennerelli, T. A., Graham, D. I., & McLellan, D. R. (1989). Diffuse axonal injury in TBI: Definition, diagnosis, and grading. *Histopathology, 15*, 49–59.

42. Chedid, M. K., & Flannery, A. M. (1995). Head trauma. In J. E. Parillo & R. C. Bone (Eds.). *Critical care medicine: Principles of diagnosis and management* (pp. 1035–1058). St. Louis: C. V. Mosby.

43. Evans, R. W., & Wilberger, J. E. (1999). Traumatic disorders. In C. G. Goetz & E. J. Pappert (Eds.). *Textbook of clinical neurology* (pp. 1035–1958). Philadelphia: W. B. Saunders.

44. Jallo, J. I., & Narayan, R. K. (2000). Trauma of the nervous system: Craniocerebral trauma. In W. G. Bradley, R. B. Daroff, G. M. Fenichel, & C. D. Marsden (Eds.). *Neurology in clinical practice: The neurological disorders* (3rd ed., pp. 1055–1087). Boston: Butterworth-Heinemann.

45. Gennarelli, T. A., Thibault, L. E., Tipperman, R., et al. (1989). Axonal injury in the optic nerve: A model simulating diffuse axonal injury in the brain. *Journal of Neurosurgery, 71*, 244.

46. Povlishock, J. T., Becker, D. P., Cheng, C., et al. (1983). Axonal change in minor head injury. *Journal of Neuropathological Experimental Neurology, 42*, 225.

47. Le Roux, P. D., Choudhri, H., & Andrews, B. T. (2000). Cerebral concussion and diffuse brain injury. In P. R. Cooper & J. G. Golfinos (Eds.). *Head injury* (4th ed., pp. 175–199). New York: McGraw-Hill.

48. Maxwell, W. L., Povlishock, J. T., Graham, D. I., et al. (1997). A mechanistic analysis of non-disruptive axonal injury. *Journal of Neurotrauma, 14*, 419–440.

49. Graham, D. I., Lawrence, A. E., Adams, J. H., et al. (1994). βAPP is a marker of axonal injury. *Brain Pathology, 4*, P23–24.

50. Crooks, D. A. (1991). The pathological concept of diffuse axonal injury: Its pathogenesis and the assessment of severity. *Journal of Pathology, 165*, 5–10.

51. Slazinski, T., & Johnson, M. C. (1994). Severe diffuse axonal injury in adults and children. *Journal of Neuroscience Nursing, 26*(3), 151–154.

52. Gennarelli, T., Spielman, G., Langfitt, T., et al. (1982). The influence of the type of intracranial lesion on outcome from severe TBI: A multicenter study using a new classification system. *Journal of Neurosurgery, 56*, 26–32.

53. Gennarelli, T. A. (1993). Cerebral concussion and diffuse brain injuries. In P. R. Cooper (Ed.). *Head injury* (3rd ed., pp. 137–158). Baltimore: Williams & Wilkins.

54. Kaufman, H. H. (1993). Civilian gunshot wounds to the head. *Neurosurgery, 32*, 962–964.

55. Rosenberg, W. S., & Harsh IV, G. R. (1999). Penetrating cerebral trauma. In R. G. Grossman & C. M. Loftus (Eds.). *Principles of neurosurgery* (2nd ed., pp. 173–182). Philadelphia: Lippincott-Raven Publishers.

56. Brandt, K. E., Burruss, G. L., Hickerson, W. I., White, C. E., & McLellan, D. R. (1991). The management of mid-face fractures with intracranial injury. *The Journal of Trauma, 31*(1), 15–19.

57. Legros, B., Fournier, P., Chiaroni, P., Ritz, O., & Fusciardi, J. (2000). Basal fracture of the skull and lower (IX, X, XI, XII) cranial nerves palsy: Four case reports including two fractures of the occipital condyle—a literature review. *The Journal of Trauma: Injury, Infection, and Critical Care, 48*(2), 342–348.

58. Holm, L., Cassidy, J. D., Caroll, L. J., & Borg, J. (2005). Summary of the WHO collaborating center for neurotrauma task force on mild traumatic brain injury. *Journal of Rehabilitation Medicine, 37*, 137–141.

59. Brain Trauma Foundation, American Association of Neurological Surgeons, Congress of Neurological Surgeons, and AANS/CNS Joint Section on Neurotrauma and Critical Care. (2007). Guidelines for the management of severe traumatic brain injury, 3rd edition. *Journal of Neurotrauma, 24*(Suppl. 1), S7–S106.

60. American College of Surgeons Committee on Trauma Resources. (1998). *American College of Surgeons Committee on Trauma Resources for Optimal Care of the Injured Patient: 1999.* Chicago: American College of Surgeons.

61. Brain Trauma Foundation, American Association of Neurological Surgeons, Congress of Neurological Surgeons, and AANS/CNS Joint Section on Neurotrauma and Critical Care. (2007). Guidelines for the management of severe traumatic brain injury, 3rd edition. *Journal of Neurotrauma, 24*(Suppl. 1), S7–S13.

62. Chestnut, R. M., Marshall, L. F., Klauber, M. R., et al. (1993). The role of secondary brain injury in determining outcome from severe TBI. *Journal of Trauma, 34*, 216–222.

63. Fearnside, M. R., Cook, R. J., McDougall, P., et al. (1993). The Westmead TBI Project outcome in severe TBI: A comparative analysis of prehospital, clinical, and CT variables. *British Journal of Neurosurgery, 7*, 267–279.

64. Pigula, F. A., Wald, S. L., Shackford, S. R., et al. (1993). The effect of hypotension and hypoxia on children with severe TBI. *Journal of Pediatric Surgery, 28*, 310–316.

65. Vassar, M. J., Fisher, R. P., O'Brien, P. E., et al. (1993). A multicenter trial for resuscitation of injured patients with 7.5% sodium chloride. The effect of added dextran 70. The Multicenter Group for the Study of Hypertonic Saline in Trauma Patients. *Archives of Surgery, 128*, 1003–1011.

66. Brain Trauma Foundation. (2003). Guidelines for the management of severe traumatic brain injury: Cerebral perfusion pressure. Retrieved October 16, 2005, from http://www2.brain-trauma.org/guidelines/index.php

67. Martin, D., & Smith, M. (2004). Medical management of severe traumatic brain injury. *Hospital Medicine, 65*, 674–680.

68. Vincent, J., & Berre, J. (2005). Primer on medical management of severe brain injury. *Critical Care Medicine, 33*(6), 1392–1399.

69. Saul, T. G., & Ducker, T. B. (1982). Effects of intracranial pressure monitoring and aggressive treatment on mortality in severe TBI. *Journal of Neurosurgery, 56*, 498–503.

70. Prielipp, R. C., & Coursin, D. B. (1995). Sedative and neuromuscular blocking drug use in critically ill patients with TBI. *New Horizons, 3*(3), 456–468.

71. Yanko, J. R., & Mitcho, K. (2001). Acute care management of severe traumatic brain injuries. *Critical Care Nursing Quarterly, 23*(4), 1–23.

72. Murray, M. J., Strickland, R. A., & Weiler, C. (1993). The use of neuromuscular blocking drugs in the intensive care unit: A US perspective. *Intensive Care Medicine, 19*, S40–S44.

73. Ford, E. V. (1995). Monitoring neuromuscular blockade in the adult ICU. *American Journal of Critical Care, 4*(2), 122–130.

74. Kennedy, P. A., & Schalleri, G. (2001). Practical issues and concepts in vagus nerve stimulation: A nursing review. *Journal of Neuroscience Nursing, 33*(2), 105–112.

74a. Berger, D. P., Schurer, L., Hartl, R., et al. (1999). Reduction of post-traumatic intracranial hypertension by hypertonic/hyperoncotic saline/dextran and hypertonic mannitol. *Neurosurgery, 37*, 98–107.

74b. Bhardway, A., & Ulatowski, J. A. (2004). Hypertonic saline solutions in brain injury. *Current Opinions in Critical Care, 10*, 126–131.

74c. Qureshi, A. I., & Suarez, J. I. (2000). Use of hypertonic saline solutions in treatment of cerebral edema and intracranial hypertension. *Critical Care Medicine, 28*(9), 3301–3313.

74d. Ware, M. L., Nemani, V. M., Meeker, M., Lee, C., Morabito, D. J., & Manley, G. T. (2005). Effects of 23.4% sodium chloride solution in reducing intracranial pressue in patients with traumatic brain injury: A preliminary study. *Neurosurgery, 57*(4), 727–736.

74e. Bratton, S. L., Chestnut, R. M., Ghajar, J., et al. (2007). Guidelines for the management of severe traumatic brain injury, 3rd ed., II Hypersosmolar therapy. *Journal of Neurotrauma, 24*(Suppl. 1), S14–S20.

75. Bouma, G. J., Muizelaar, J. P., Choi, S. C., Newlon, P. G., & Young, H. F. (1991). Cerebral circulation and metabolism after severe traumatic brain injury: The elusive role of ischemia. *Journal of Neurosurgery, 75*, 685–693.

76. Jaggi, J. L., Obrist, W. D., Gennerelli, T. A., & Langfitt, T. W. (1990). Relationship of early cerebral blood flow and metabolism to outcome in acute head injury. *Journal of Neurosurgery, 72*, 176–182.

77. Marion, D. W., Darby, J., & Yonas, H. (1991). Acute regional cerebral blood flow changes caused by severe head injuries I. *Journal of Neurosurgery, 74*, 407–414.

78. Robertson, C. S., Clifton, G. L., Grossman, R. G., et al. (1988). Alterations in cerebral availability of metabolic substrates after severe head injury. *Journal of Trauma, 28*, 1523–1532.

79. Salvant, J. B., & Muizelaar, J. P. (1993). Changes in cerebral blood flow and metabolism related to the presence of subdural hematoma. *Neurosurgery, 33*, 387–393.

80. Bouma, G. J., Muizelaar, J. P., Stinger, W. A., et al. (1992). Ultra early evaluation of regional cerebral blood flow in severely head injured patients using xenon enhanced coupled tomography. *Journal of Neurosurgery, 77*, 360–368.

81. Obrist, W. D., Langfitt, T. W., Jaggi, J. L., Cruz, J., & Gennarelli, T. A. (1984). Cerebral blood flow and metabolism in comatose patients with acute head injury. *Journal of Neurosurgery, 61*, 241–253.

82. Obrist, W. D., Gennarelli, T. A., Segawa, H., & Dolinskas, C. A. (1979). Relation of cerebral blood flow to neurological status and outcome in head-injured patients. *Journal of Neurosurgery, 51*, 292–300.

83. Schroder, M. L., Muizellar, J. P., & Kuta, A. J. (1994). Documented reversal of global ischemia immediately after removal of an acute subdural hematoma. *Neurosurgery, 80*, 324–327.

84. Muizelaar, J. P., Marmarou, A., Ward, J. D., et al. (1991). Adverse effects of prolonged hyperventilation in patients with severe TBI: A randomized clinical trial. *Journal of Neurosurgery, 75*, 731–739.

85. Guerra, W. K., Gaab, M. R., Dietz, H., et al. (1999). Surgical decompression for traumatic brain swelling: Indications and results. *Journal of Neurosurgery, 90*, 187–196.

86. De Luca, G. P., Volpin, L., Fornezza, U., et al. (2000). The role of decompressive craniectomy in the treatment of uncontrollable of post-traumatic intracranial hypertension. *Acta Neurochirurgica Supplement, 76*, 401–404.

87. Albanese, J., Leone, M., Alliez, J. R., et al. (2003). Decompressive craniotomy for severe traumatic brain injury: Evaluation of the effects in one year. *Critical Care Medicine, 31*, 2535–2538.

88. Clifton, G. L. (2004). Is keeping cool still hot? An update on hypothermia in brain injury. *Current Opinion in Critical Care, 10*, 116–119.

89. Bhardwaj, A., & Ulatowski, J. A. (2004). Hypertonic saline solution in brain injury. *Current Opinion in Critical Care, 10*, 126–131.

90. Globus, M. Y., Alfonso, O., Dietrich, W. D., et al. (1995). Glutamate release and free radical production following brain injury: Effects of post-traumatic hypothermia. *Journal of Neurochemistry, 65*, 1704–1711.

91. Temkin, N. R., Dikmen, S. S., & Winn, H. R. (1991). Posttraumatic seizures. In H. M. Eisenberg & E. F. Aldrich (Eds.). *Management of head injury* (pp. 425– 435). Philadelphia: W. B. Saunders.

92. Yablon, S. A. (1993). Posttraumatic seizures. *Archives of Physical Medicine and Rehabilitation, 74*, 983–1001.

93. Temkin, N. R., Dikmen, S. S., Wilensky, A. J., et al. (1990). A randomized, double- blind study of phenytoin for the prevention of post-traumatic seizures. *New England Journal of Medicine, 323*(8), 497–502.

94. Manaka, S. (1992). Cooperative prospective study on posttraumatic epilepsy: Risk factors and the effect of prophylactic anticonvulsant. *Japanese Journal of Psychiatry and Neurology, 46*, 311–315.

95. McQueen, J. K., Blackwood, D. H. R., Harris, P., et al. (1983). Low risk of late post- traumatic seizures following severe head injury: Implications for clinical trails of prophylaxis. *Journal of Neurology, Neurosurgery, and Psychiatry, 46*, 899–904.

96. Chang, B. S., & Lowenstein, D. H. (2003). Practice parameter: Antiepileptic drug prophylaxis in severe traumatic brain injury—report of the quality standards subcommittee of the American Academy of Neurology. *Neurology, 60*, 10–16.

97. Gruen, P., & Liu, C. (1998). Current trends in the management of head injury. *Emergency Medicine Clinic of North America, 16*, 63–83.

98. Tietjen, C. S., Hurn, P. D., Ulatowski, J. A., & Kirsch, J. R. (1996). Treatment modalities for hypertensive patients with intracranial pathology: Options and risks. *Critical Care Medicine, 24*(2), 311–322.

99. Chesnut, R. M. (1997). The management of severe traumatic brain injury. *Emergency Medicine Clinic of North America, 15*, 581–604.

100. Pilitsis, J. G., & Rengachard, S. S. (2001). Complications of head injury. *Neurological Research, 23*, 227–236.

101. Dutton, R. P., McCunn, M., Hyder, M., et al. (2004). Factor VIIa for correction of traumatic coagulopathy. *Journal of Trauma, 57*(4), 709–718.

102. Nih, C. R. (1986). Prevention of venous thrombosis and pulmonary embolism. *Journal of the American Medical Association, 256*, 744–749.

103. Vandam, L. D., & Burnap, T. K. (1959). Hypothermia. *New England Journal of Medicine, 261*, 595–603.

104. Lam, A. M., Winn, H. R., Cullen, B. F., & Sundling, N. (1991). Hyperglycemia and neurological outcome in patients with TBI. *Journal of Neurosurgery, 75*, 5445–5551.

105. Zygun, D. A., Steiner, L. A., Johnston, A. J., et al. (2004). Hyperglycemia and brain tissue pH after traumatic brain injury. *Neurosurgery, 55*(4), 877–882.

106. Jeremitsky, E., Omert, L. A., Dunham, C. M., et al. (2005). The impact of hyperglycemia on patient with severe brain injury. *Journal of Trauma, 58*(1), 47–50.

107. Bondanelli, M., Ambrosio, M. R., Zatelli, M. C., et al. (2005). Hypopituitarism after traumatic brain injury. *European Journal of Endocrinology, 152*(5), 679–691.

108. Strum, S. (2002). Post head injury autonomic complications. Retrieved January 30, 2006, from http://www.emedicien.com/pmr/topic108.htm

109. Baguley, I. J., Nicholls, J. L., Felmingham, K. L., Crooks, J., Gurka, J. A., & Wade, L. D. (1999). Dysautonomia after traumatic brain injury: A forgotten syndrome? *Journal of Neurology, Neurosurgery, and Psychiatry, 67*, 39–43.

110. Rossitch Jr., E., & Bullard, D. E. (1988). The autonomic dysfunction syndrome: Aetiology and treatment. *British Journal of Neurosurgery, 2*, 471–478.

111. Ropper, A. H. (1993). Acute autonomic emergencies and autonomic storm. In P. A. Low (Ed.). *Clinical autonomic disorders* (pp. 747–756). Boston: Little, Brown.

112. Boeve, B. F., Wijdicks, E. F. M., Benarroch, E. E., & Schmidt, K. D. (1998). Paroxysmal sympathetic storms ("diencephalic seizures") after severe diffuse axonal head injury. *Mayo Clinic Proceedings, 73*(2), 148–152.

113. Fearnside, M. R., Cook, R. J., McDougall, P., & McNeil, R. J. (1993). The Westmead Head Injury Project outcome in severe head injury. A comparative analysis of pre-hospital, clinical and CT variables. *British Journal of Neurosurgery, 7*(3), 267–279.

114. Lemke, D. L. (2004). Riding out the storm: Sympathetic storming after traumatic brain injury. *Journal of Neuroscience Nursing, 36*(1), 4–9.

115. Keller, C., & Williams, A. (1993). Cardiac dysrhythmias associated with central nervous system dysfunction. *Journal of Neuroscience Nursing, 25*(6), 349–355.

116. Stanford, G. G. (1994). The stress response to trauma and critical illness. *Critical Care Nursing of North America, 6*(4), 693–702.

117. Rosner, M. J., Newsome, H. H., & Becker, D. P. (1984). Mechanical brain injury: The sympathoadrenal response, *Journal of Neurosurgery, 61*, 76–86.

118. Hamill, R. W., Woolf, P. D., McDonald, J. V., Lee, L. A., & Kelly, M. (1987). Catecholamines predict outcome in traumatic brain injury. *Annuals of Neurology, 21*(5), 438–443.

119. Agency for Health Care Policy and Research. (1998). *Rehabilitation for traumatic brain injury. Summary, evidence report/technology assessment, No 2.* Rockville, MD: Agency for Health Care Policy and Research. (http://www.ahcpr.gov/clinic/thisumm.htm)

120. Attia, J., & Cook, D. J. (1998). Prognosis in anoxic and traumatic coma. *Critical Care Clinics, 14*(3), 497–511.

121. Chesnut, R. M., Ghajar, J., Maas, A. I. R., et al. (2000). Early indicators of prognosis in severe traumatic brain injury. *Journal of Neurotrauma, 17*(6/7), 557–627.

122. Braakman, R., Gelpke, G. J., Habbema, J. D. F., et al. (1980). Systematic selection of prognostic features in patients with severe head injury. *Neurosurgery, 6*, 262–370.

123. Chang, R. W. S., Lee, B., & Jacobs, S. (1989). Accuracy of decisions to withdraw therapy in critically ill patients: Clinical judgment versus a computer model. *Critical Care Medicine, 17*, 1091–1097.

124. Foulkes, M. A., Eisenberg, H. M., Jane, J. A., et al. (1991). The Traumatic Coma Data Bank–Design, methods, and baseline characteristics. *Journal of Neurosurgery, 75*, S8–S13.

125. Jennett, B., & Bono, M. (1975). Assessment of outcome after severe brain damage. A practical scale. *Lancet, 1*, 480–485.

126. Jennett, B., Teasdale, G., Braakman, R., et al. (1979). Prognosis of patients with severe head injury. *Neurosurgery, 4*, 283–289.

127. Kaufmann, M. S., Buchmann, B., Scheidegger, D., Gratzl, O., & Radu, E. W. (1992). Severe head injury: Should expected outcome influence resuscitation and first day decisions? *Resuscitation, 23*, 199–206.

128. Langfitt, T. W. (1978). Measuring the outcome from head injuries. *Journal of Neurosurgery, 48*, 673–678.

129. Marshall, L. F., Becker, D. P., Bowers, S. A., et al. (1983). The National Traumatic Coma Data Bank. Part I. Design, purpose, goals and results. *Journal of Neurosurgery, 59*, 276–284.

130. Marshall, L. F., Gautille, T., Klauber, M., et al. (1991). The outcome of severe closed head injury. *Journal of Neurosurgery, 75*, S28–S36.

131. Teasdale, G., & Jennett, B. (1974). Assessment of coma and impaired consciousness. *Lancet, 2*, 81–84.

132. Haitsma, I. K., & Maas, A. I. R. (2002). Advanced monitoring in the intensive care unit: Brain tissue oxygen tension. *Current Opinion in Critical Care, 8*, 115–120.

133. Johnston, A. J., Steiner, L. A., & Coles, J. P. (2005). Effect of cerebral perfusion pressure augmentation on regional oxygen and metabolism after head injury. *Critical Care Medicine, 33*(1), 189–195.

134. McDonagh, M., Helfand, M., Carson, S., & Russman, B. S. (2004). Hyperbaric oxygen therapy for traumatic brain injury: A systematic review of the evidence. *Archives of Physical Medicine and Rehabilitation, 85*, 1198–1204.

135. Longhi, L., & Stocchett, N. (2004). Hyperoxia in head injury: Therapeutic tool? *Current Opinion in Critical Care, 10*, 105–109.

136. Smith, M. J., Stiefel, M. F., Magge, S., et al. (2005). Packed red blood cell transfusion increases local cerebral oxygenation. *Critical Care Medicine, 33*(5), 1104–1108.

137. Morris, G. F., Bullock, R., Marshall, S. B., et al. (1999). Failure of the competitive N-methyl-d-aspartate antagonist Selfotel (CGS 19755) in the treatment of severe head injury: Results of two phase III clinical trials. The selfotel investigators *Journal of Neurosurgery, 91*, 737–743.

138. Marshall, L. F., Maas, A. I., Marshall, S. B., et al. A multi center trial on efficacy of using tirilasad mesylate in cases of head injury. *Journal of Neurosurgery, 89*, 519–525.

139. Knoller, N., Levi, L., & Shoshan, I. (2002). Dexanabinol (HU-211) in the treatment of severe closed head injury: A randomized, placebo-controlled, phase II clinical trial. *Critical Care Medicine, 30*, 548–554.

140. Mcilvoy, L., Spain, D. A., Raque, G., Vitaz, T., Baoz, P., & Meyer, K. (2001). Successful incorporation of the severe head injury guidelines into a phased-outcome clinical pathway. *Journal of Neuroscience Nursing, 33*(2), 72–78.

141. Stechmiller, J., Treloar, D. M., Derrico, D., Yarandi, H., & Guin, P. (1994). Interruption of enteral feedings in head injured patients. *Journal of Neuroscience Nursing, 26*(4), 224–229.

RESOURCES

Websites for Providers, Patient, and Family

There are hundreds on the Internet; below are a few to begin a search for specific information.

Brain Injury Association USA: http://www.biausa.org/

Brain Injury Resource Center: http://www.headinjury.com/

Vertebral and Spinal Cord Injuries

Joanne V. Hickey

A PERSPECTIVE

The following statistical information describes spinal cord injuries (SCIs) In the United States in June of 2006.[1] There are an estimated 11,000 to 14,000 new SCIs per year.[2] Because no overall incidence studies of SCIs in the United States have been reported since the 1970s, it is not known whether the pattern of incidence has changed in recent years. The number of people living with SCIs is 253,000, with a range of 225,000 to 296,000 persons. The young are primarily affected by SCIs. From 1973 to 1979, the average age at injury was 28.7 years, with most injuries occurring between 16 and 30 years. Since 2000, the average age of injury is 38 years, and the number of people older than 60 years of age at time of injury has increased for 4.7% prior to 1980 to 11.5%. Seventy-seven percent of SCIs have occurred among males. Since 2000, the major categories of cause of injury include motor vehicle accidents (46.9%), falls (23.8%), acts of violence (primary gunshot injuries, 13.7%), and recreational sports (9.0%). At discharge, the most common diagnosis is incomplete tetraplegia (34.1%), followed by complete paraplegia (23.0%), complete tetraplegia (18.3%), and incomplete paraplegia (18.5%). Less than 1% of persons experienced complete neurological recovery by hospital discharge. Almost 65% of persons who sustain SCIs are employed at the time of injury. Generally, paraplegics have a higher employment rate than tetraplegics. Ten years postinjury 32.4% of paraplegics and 24.2% of tetraplegics are employed. At discharge from the hospital 88.1% of persons with SCIs return to noninstitutional settings such as their home. Only 5.4% are discharged to nursing homes. The length of stay in the hospital in 2004 was approximately 18 days and 39 days in acute rehabilitation. The average yearly expenses for SCIs are highest the first year, with higher costs for high-level (C-1 to C-4) tetraplegics. The estimated lifetime cost for a high-level tetraplegic who is 25 years old is $2,924,513, as compared to $1,721,677 for one who is 50 years old. For paraplegics, the cost for the same age categories is $977,142 versus $666,473, respectively. The major causes of death among persons with SCIs are pneumonia, pulmonary emboli, and septicemia.

In summary, the SCI statistics reported form the Spinal Cord Injury Information Network reflect some shifts in cause, length of hospitalization, and costs.[1]

Comprehensive Evidence-Based Practice

The model regional SCI care system program established in 1970 by the Rehabilitation Services Administration has helped to develop evidence-based and best-practice models that are cost effective for the care of SCI patients across the continuum of care, from accident scene through rehabilitation. The model SCI programs across the country provide a major research- and evidence-based practice focus. The American Spinal Injury Association (ASIA) and the International Medical Society of Paraplegia (IMSOP) published the *International Standards for Neurological and Functional Classification of Spinal Cord Injury*.[3] In addition, a number of professional organizations have published practice guidelines, such as the American Association of Neurological Surgeons and the Congress of Neurological Surgery, who published *Guidelines for Acute Cervical and Spinal Injuries* in 2002.[2]

UNDERSTANDING SPINAL CORD INJURIES

Anatomic Considerations

To appreciate the potential for injury to the spinal axis and its surrounding structures, one must understand the interrelated function of anatomic structures involved, namely, the vertebral column, the spinal cord, the supporting soft tissue, and the intervertebral disks. The vertebrae are irregularly shaped bones that support the muscles and protect the spinal cord. There are 33 vertebrae in the vertebral column: seven cervical, 12 thoracic or dorsal, five lumbar, five sacral (fused as one), and four coccygeal (fused as one). The vertebrae of each area have a distinctive shape. Stacked one on another to form the vertebral column, the vertebrae are laced into position by a series of supporting structures called *ligaments*. The ligaments, muscles, and other supporting structures are considered to be soft-tissue components (Figs. 18-1 and 18-2; see also Chap. 4).

There are two main parts to a vertebra: the body and the arch. The vertebral bodies are separated by intervertebral discs that serve as shock absorbers for the vertebral column during movement. The arch of the vertebra is created by a series of irregularly shaped projections. The fusion of the two pedicles and two laminae along with seven articular processes create a bony ring. The various projections of the vertebral

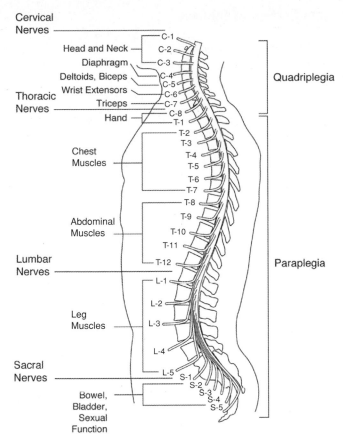

Figure 18-1 • Level of spinal cord injury and functional loss; the higher the spinal cord injury, the more motor, sensory, and autonomic functional losses are incurred.

arch allow for alignment, flexion, and movement of the vertebral column. The soft, vulnerable spinal cord passes through the bony arch of the vertebrae, which offer it protection.

The close anatomic relationship of the vertebrae, ligaments, and other soft-tissue structures; intervertebral discs; and spinal cord increases the probability that injury to any one of these structures can cause concurrent injury to any or all of the other structures. In other instances, injury to one structure, such as a vertebral fracture, can create the potential for injury to another structure, such as the spinal cord, if the primary injury is not treated promptly and effectively. Therefore, when discussing injury to the vertebral column and spinal cord, consider the interrelatedness of not only these two structures, but also the supporting soft-tissue structures and the intervertebral discs.

Vertebral, spinal cord, and soft-tissue injuries are discussed in this chapter, while intervertebral disc disease is the focus of Chapter 19.

Kinetics of Movement

The seven cervical vertebrae support the head, which weighs 8 to 10 lb. These vertebrae provide substantial movement of the neck and head in various directions, including flexion, extension, and rotation. The total amount of flexion and extension possible at the cervical spine is an 80-degree arc, 75% of which is extension. Rotation is made possible by the uniquely shaped atlas (C-1) and axis (C-2). Beneath the cervical vertebrae are the 12 thoracic vertebrae, which move very little owing to the anchoring of the ribs. Because the cervical spine is not fixed like the thoracic spine, it is extremely vulnerable to injury as a result of acceleration-deceleration forces.

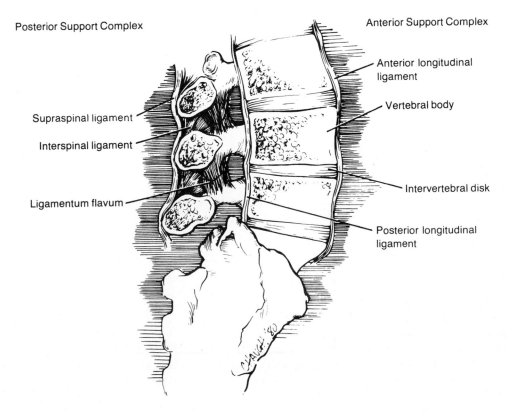

Figure 18-2 • Soft-tissue supporting structures of the spine. Two basic soft-tissue units constitute each spinal segment: the *anterior support complex*, formed by the anterior and posterior longitudinal ligaments, the disc, and the annulus, and the *posterior support complex*, formed by the supra-spinal ligament and inter-spinal ligament, the ligamentum flavum, and the facet capsules. When the posterior complex is disrupted, the spine is unstable, and surgical fusion is necessary. When the anterior complex is disrupted, the spine is usually more stable and can heal with use of a rigid brace. (From Weiner, W. J., & Goetz, C. G. [Eds.], [1989]. *Neurology for the non-neurologist* [2nd ed., p. 261]. Philadelphia: J. B. Lippincott.)

Mechanics of Injury

Vertebral injuries and SCIs result when excessive forces are exerted on the vertebral column. These forces are most often the result of acceleration-deceleration events that result in hyperflexion, hyperextension, deformation, axial loading, and excessive rotation.

Acceleration-Deceleration Events

Acceleration and deceleration are discussed together because they often occur in split-second sequence. At the moment of impact in a rear-end motor vehicle collision (i.e., external force applied from the rear), there is sudden **acceleration** of the portion of the body in contact with the seat. The head and upper back, which were not in contact with the seat or headrest, are violently thrust backward (hyperextension). After the head strikes the back of the seat or has hyperextended to its limit, it is then thrust forward. The head may strike the steering wheel or dashboard as it slows down (decelerates).

Deceleration is often the major mechanism of injury involved in a head-on motor vehicle collision. While the outside force, exerted from the front, abruptly arrests the vehicle's motion, the head and body continue moving forward until contact is made, usually with the dashboard. The person is forcibly hyperflexed while moving forward, hits the dashboard, and then snaps back into a forced hyperextension position.

Responses to Extreme Acceleration-Deceleration Events

Acceleration-deceleration can produce simultaneous and/or successive actions as detailed in the following descriptions:

- **Hyperflexion** tends to produce compression of the vertebral bodies with disruption of the posterior longitudinal ligaments and the intervertebral discs.
- **Hyperextension** usually causes fractures of the posterior elements of the spinal column and disruption of the anterior longitudinal ligaments.
- **Deformation** refers to the various alterations in the spinal column and supporting soft-tissue structures necessary to accommodate abnormal movements, such as hyperflexion, hyperextension, and excessive rotation. For example, in hyperextension of the cervical neck, the spinal canal shortens, the anterior longitudinal ligaments elongate, and the ligamenta flava are compressed and may bulge into the spinal canal, resulting in injury.
- **Axial loading**, also known as **vertical compression**, occurs when a vertical force is exerted on the spinal column. Axial loading is seen in injuries resulting from diving accidents, landing on the feet when jumping from a height, or landing on the buttocks when falling from a height.
- **Excessive rotation** refers to turning of the head beyond the normal range on the horizontal axis. This can result in compression fractures, tearing or rupture of the posterior ligament, dislocation at the facet joint, and fracture at the articular processes

Classification of Injuries

The velocity and angle of impact, as well as the type of exaggerated mechanical movement produced, influence the type of injury sustained. These factors are considered in the classification of injuries. Patients who have anatomic abnormalities or disease processes of the spinal column are much more vulnerable to SCI than those who do not. Chronic conditions, such as cervical spondylosis, spinal stenosis, arthritis, and scoliosis, are examples of conditions that increase the probability of injury.

A basic classification of the causes of injury to the vertebral column, spinal cord, and soft tissue includes the following categories and their characteristics.

Hyperflexion Injuries

Hyperflexion injuries (Figs. 18-3 and 18-4) caused by hyperflexion of the head and neck, as in sudden deceleration, are seen in head-on collisions and in diving accidents. If the pos-

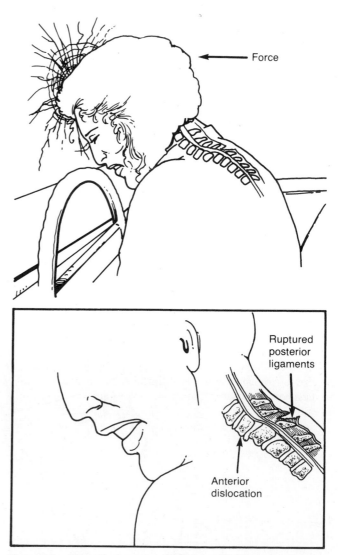

Figure 18-3 • Hyperflexion injury. With hyperflexion to the cervical spine, there may be tearing of the posterior ligamentous complex, resulting in anterior dislocation.

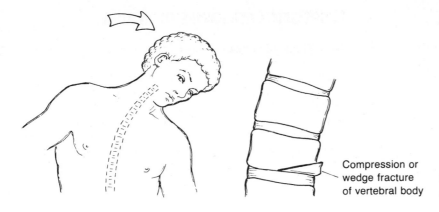

Compression or
wedge fracture
of vertebral body

Figure 18-4 • Lateral hyperflexion injury. Compression or wedge fracture of the vertebral body.

terior ligaments are intact, a **wedge** or **compression fracture** of the vertebral body is common. Because it is a relatively stable fracture, it does not usually require surgery. Flexion-extension imaging may be ordered to rule out a fracture not seen on plain x-rays. If the posterior ligaments are torn, the facets are usually disengaged and dislocated. Because this is an unstable fracture type, surgical stabilization will most likely required.

There is a high probability of cord damage with fracture dislocations or bilateral jumped locked facet fractures. These injuries occur most often in the cervical region and involve the greatest areas of stress, levels C-5 and C-6. A lateral hyperflexion injury can result from extreme lateral flexion or rotation of the head and neck.

Hyperextension Injuries

Injuries resulting from hyperextension (Fig. 18-5) of the head and neck, such as from a rear-end vehicular collision, tend to cause greater damage to structures than hyperflexion injuries because backward and downward movement involves a larger arc than flexion. If the head flexes forward, the chin strikes the chest and limits the arc. If the head flexes laterally, the head strikes the shoulder.

In a hyperextension injury, the spinal cord is stretched so that it lies against the ligamenta flava. Despite a negative result on radiographic examination, there may be contusion and ischemia to part of the spinal cord, and neurological deficits may appear. As a rule, ligaments remain intact and no fractures or dislocations occur. The greatest area of stress in a hyperextension injury is at the level of C-4 and C-5. Respiratory compromise, either from direct injury or ascending edema, is a concern.

Hyperextension injuries are commonly seen in elderly persons who have fallen and struck their chin. A less severe form of hyperextension injury is called a "whiplash" or acceleration injury, a stress and strain injury to the soft tissue (muscles and ligaments), but with no vertebral or SCI.

Compression Injuries

Compression injuries (Figs. 18-6 and 18-7) can result from axial loading, from vertical pressure (e.g., falling from a height and landing on the feet or buttocks), or from lateral flexion. The resulting fractures cause wedging, crushing, or bursting of the vertebral body. Compression fractures are sometimes categorized as **burst fracture, simple wedge fracture** (Fig. 18-8), and **teardrop fracture**, depending on the degree of compression or the fracture line noted on x-ray or imaging films.

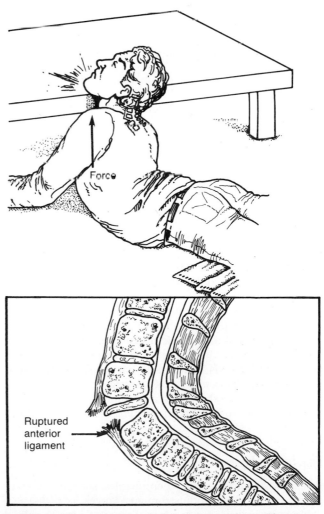

Force

Ruptured
anterior
ligament

Figure 18-5 • Hyperextension injury in the cervical area. The injury is related to a fall in which the chin is struck, forcing hyperextension of the neck and rupture of the anterior ligament.

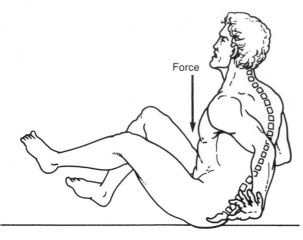

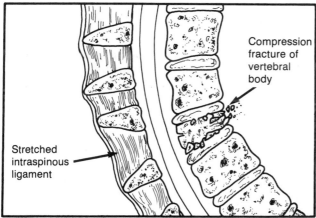

Figure 18-6 • Hyperflexion injury in the lumbar area. Injury can be caused by falling onto the buttocks. Note the compression fracture and the stretching of the intraspinous ligament.

Rotational Injuries

Rotational injuries (Fig. 18-9) are caused by extreme lateral flexion or twisting of the head and neck. Tearing and/or rupturing of the posterior ligaments may occur, allowing dislocation at the facet joint and fracture at the articular processes.

One or two facets may be involved. If one facet is dislocated or locked, usually no neurological deficits or temporary deficits result. In more than half the patients with two facets locked, neurological deficits can be expected. Reduction of the fracture is achieved by traction (cervical traction or halo with or without a jacket) or surgery to disengage the facets and stabilize the vertebral column (Cotrel-Dubousset [CD] rods; see surgical management section later in this chapter).

Penetrating Injuries

Penetrating injuries occur when missiles, such as bullets or shrapnel, or impalement instruments (knives, ice picks) penetrate the spinal column or supporting soft tissue. The object may shatter bone, create bone fragments, or transect a portion or complete plane of the spinal cord or soft tissue.

SPECIFIC CATEGORIES OF INJURIES

Soft-Tissue Injuries

Whiplash

Whiplash is a lay term for an acceleration injury involving hyperextension of the head during a rear-end vehicular collision. The ligaments and muscles of the neck sustain stress and strain injury. The usual signs and symptoms, which include stiff neck, pain in the neck and shoulder, limitation of movement, and muscle spasms, may not begin until 12 to 24 hours after injury. Other signs and symptoms may include headache, paresthesia, dizziness, vertigo, and tinnitus. The findings on physical examination are normal except for the previously listed signs and symptoms. The radiologic examination is negative. The diagnosis is based on the history of injury and the presence of the characteristic signs and symptoms. This is a common injury causing much pain and suffering to the patient, even though no abnormalities are noted on radiographic examination.

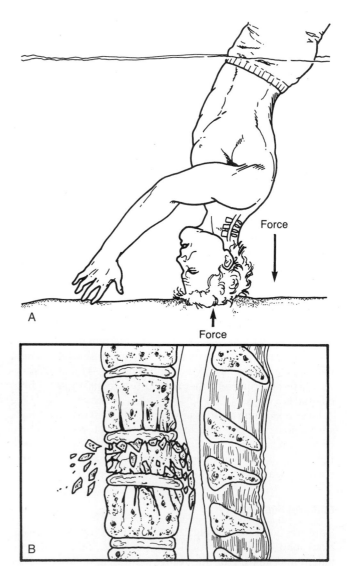

Figure 18-7 • Compression fracture secondary to axial loading.

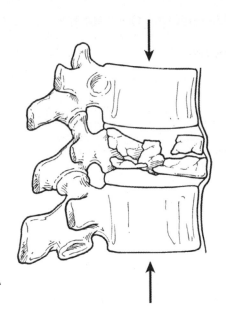

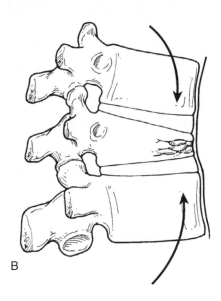

Figure 18-8 • Burst and compression fractures. (*A*) Burst fracture. Axial compressive forces may result in severe vertebral body fractures involving the anterior and middle columns with a collapse of the entire vertebral body, often with retropulsion into the spinal canal. This is a potentially unstable fracture, often with accompanying spinal cord injury. (*B*) Compression fracture. A compression fracture is a wedge-shaped fracture (also called wedge fracture) of the vertebral body involving the anterior column. It occurs in the thoracic and lumbar region, most often in the mid-thoracic and mid-lumbar region. Compression fractures can occur with minor trauma in older patients with osteoporosis and in younger people with significant trauma.

The pain caused by whiplash is thought to be attributable to the tearing, stretching, microhemorrhage, and edema incurred by the anterior neck muscles (sternocleidomastoid, scalenus, and longus colli muscles). The muscles, and possibly the ligaments, are strained. Patients with pre-existing cervical spondylosis and some with other conditions may have narrowing of the foramina and osteophytes and also increased rigidity of the spinal column. These conditions put them at greater risk of developing neurological problems if a whiplash injury occurs.

Treatment. Treatment of whiplash is directed toward making the patient comfortable. For less serious injuries, treatment involves mild analgesics (e.g., nonsteroidal anti-inflammatory drugs [NSAIDs], acetaminophen), local ice, and rest. More severe injuries are treated with short-term use of a soft collar, heat and cold application, analgesics, muscle relaxants, and anti-inflammatory agents.

Narcotic analgesics are reserved for severe pain and should be used sparingly to prevent dependency. NSAIDs are commonly ordered both for their anti-inflammatory effect and for their ability to inhibit prostaglandin synthesis, a substance known to be related to pain. Muscle relaxants such as cyclobenzaprine hydrochloride (Flexeril) and methocarbamol (Robaxin) are also used. Extended use of a cervical collar is controversial. Some physicians believe that collars hinder recovery of involved muscles if worn for more than a few days.

Other Soft-Tissue Injuries

The vertebral column depends on soft tissue for its stability. Therefore, any significant soft-tissue trauma (see Fig. 18-2) that occurs with vertebral injury can compromise the vertebral column. The other soft-tissue injuries with significance for vertebral stability are discussed in this chapter in conjunction with vertebral injuries and SCI.

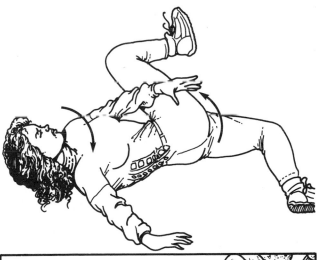

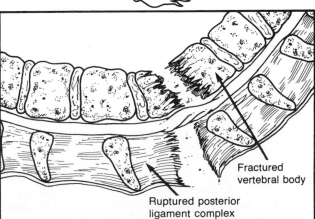

Fractured vertebral body

Ruptured posterior ligament complex

Figure 18-9 • Rotational injury. When rotational force occurs, there is concurrent fracture and tearing of the posterior ligamentous complex.

Vertebral Injuries

Classification

Although fractures can occur singularly in any part of the vertebral arch, most injuries occur in combination with vertebral body injuries. The "ends" of the vertebral column, the cervical and lumbar portions, have the greatest built-in mobility, which predisposes them to injury. The thoracic region is less prone to trauma because of the rigidity imparted to it by the rib cage. Vertebral injuries can be classified based on various perspectives of the injury:

- **Types of fractures**: simple or compression fractures
- **Fracture or dislocation**: pure fracture, pure dislocation, and fracture-dislocation
- **Stability or instability of injury**: according to a three-column framework
- **Segmental involvement**: upper cervical, subaxial cervical, thoracic, or lumbar and sacral

Each category offers a special practical perspective and is discussed in the following section.

Types of Fractures. For the purposes of this discussion, vertebral fractures are subdivided into simple and compression fractures (see Fig. 18-10 for a review of anatomic parts of a vertebra).

- **Simple fractures** appear as a singular break with the alignment of the vertebral parts remaining intact. These types of fractures usually occur to the spinous or transverse process, facets, pedicles, and vertebral body. There is usually no neural compression.
- **Compression fractures** are sometimes further subclassified as *simple wedge fractures, burst fractures,* and *teardrop fractures* (see Fig. 18-8). They are caused by axial loading and hyperflexion.
- **A simple (wedge) compression fracture** is caused by vertical compression when the cervical vertebral column is flexed. A burst fracture is caused by the same mechanical force, but the vertebral column is straight. Because the posterior ligaments are intact, the simple

(wedge) compression fracture is stable. No surgery is required. These fractures heal well with hard collar immobilization for about 2 months.[4] A halo jacket may also be used.

- **Burst fractures** are explosive fractures caused by severe axial loading on a straight cervical column. They shatter the vertebral body into several pieces. These fragments then can be driven into the spinal cord, resulting in serious injury. If there is no neurological damage and if the posterior ligaments are stable, wearing a hard collar for 2 months may be adequate therapy (Fig. 18-11). However, burst fractures often require a combined neurosurgical-orthopedic procedure for the removal of bone fragments, cord decompression, and vertebral column stabilization. Stabilization is accomplished by insertion of instrumentation, such as CD rods, a type of segmental rodding that can be accommodated to the individual's level of injury. See section on surgical management for further discussion.
- **Teardrop fractures** are caused by extreme flexion with axial loading. With this fracture a vertebral body is crushed by the vertebral body superior to it, causing the anterior portion of the compressed body to break away. These fractures, which are usually unstable (i.e., involving disruption of the posterior ligaments, resulting in forward dislocation), are managed with anterior decompression and fusion with halo immobilization.

Fracture or Dislocation. From another perspective, a vertebral injury can be a fracture without a dislocation, a dislocation without a fracture, or a fracture combined with a dislocation. **Dislocation** occurs when one vertebra overrides another, and there is unilateral or bilateral facet dislocation. Radiographic studies reveal a disruption in the established alignment of the vertebral column. Usually, the supporting ligaments are also injured, and the spinal cord may or may not be involved.

Subluxation is a partial or incomplete dislocation of one vertebra over another. Damage to the cord and supporting ligaments may or may not be present. With dislocation, re-establishment of alignment is necessary. This may be accomplished by traction followed by immobilization or by surgical stabilization (fusion or sometimes insertion of CD rods if the posterior ligaments are injured).

Fracture-dislocation, as the name implies, denotes a combined injury of a fracture and a dislocation that is usually accompanied by ligament and cord injury. As with simple dislocation, realignment is necessary. The fracture must be allowed to heal, and any bone fragments impinging on the cord must be removed. Therefore, surgery is indicated.

Stability or Instability of the Spinal Column. The concept of stability of the spinal column is addressed by White and Panjabi and modified by Greenberg.[5,6] *Clinical stability* is the ability of the spine under physiologic loads to limit displacement so as to prevent injury or irritation of the spinal cord and nerve roots (including cauda equina) and to prevent incapacitating deformity or pain due to structural changes. When the spinal column fails to respond appropriately, the spinal column becomes unstable, which results in injury and predisposes the spinal column, spinal cord, and soft tissue to further injury.

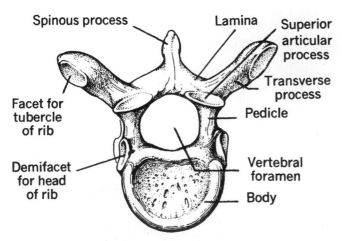

Figure 18-10 • The sixth thoracic vertebra with anatomic markings.

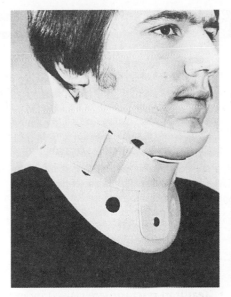

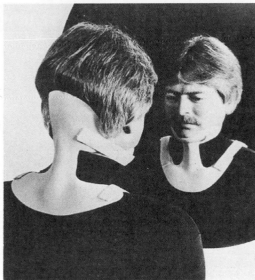

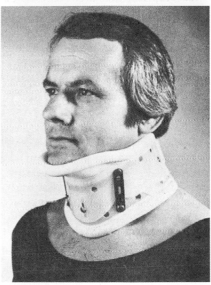

Figure 18-11 • Types of rigid cervical collars.

Therefore, nurses will hear much discussion about the clinical stability or clinical instability of the spinal column, which influences the medical and surgical management of the patient.

It is critical when considering vertebral fractures to distinguish between stable and unstable fractures and dislocations. This distinction is often based on the posterior ligaments. If the posterior ligaments are intact, the injury is considered stable. If they have been torn, usually by a rotational force, they are considered unstable. Stability of the vertebral-spinal elements is also addressed using a three-column theoretical framework. This approach is discussed in Chart 18-1. A stable fracture or dislocation is not apt to displace more than it was at the time of the injury, whereas an unstable fracture or dislocation is highly likely to displace further with extension of injury to the spinal cord. External immobilization or internal fixation may be unnecessary for stable injuries, whereas it is essential for unstable injuries. In addition, when ligaments heal, scar tissue forms. The scarred tissue, weaker than the preinjury tissue, may result in chronic instability and lead to SCI.

Vertebral Injuries According to Segmental Level

Vertebral injuries can be divided into four groups based on the involved segmental level: upper cervical, subaxial cervical, thoracic and lumbar, and sacral.[7]

Upper Cervical Segment

The four most commonly encountered upper cervical segment injuries are atlas fractures, atlantoaxial subluxation, odontoid fractures, and so-called hangman's fractures. Four less common injuries are occipital condyle fractures, atlanto-occipital dislocation, atlantoaxial rotary subluxation, and C-2 lateral mass fractures. A summary of upper cervical fractures and lower cervical fractures is presented in Table 18-1.

CHART 18-1   The Three-Column Framework: Spinal Stability and Instability*

Spinal stability refers to the ability of the vertebral support column to protect adequately the neural elements from injury during inactivity and activity. This determination is critical in managing patients because an unstable injury can result in extension of or new neurological deficits. Currently, criteria for determining spinal stability or instability are controversial.

Some physicians consider only the condition of the posterior ligaments when determining stability. Another approach is the three-column framework. The three-column approach provides an anatomic framework for considering stability. The cross-section of the spine is organized into three anatomic columns:

- The **anterior column** consists of the anterior longitudinal ligament, anterior half of the vertebral body, annulus fibrosis, and disc.
- The **middle column** consists of the posterior half of the vertebral body, annulus, disc, and posterior longitudinal ligament.
- The **posterior column** consists of the facet joints, ligamentum flavum, posterior elements, and interconnecting ligaments.

Applying this classification system to spinal injuries results in four classification categories, which are determined by the specific column(s) injured.

TYPE OF INJURY	COLUMNS INJURED		
	ANTERIOR	MIDDLE	POSTERIOR
Compression fractures	Yes	No	No
Burst fractures	Yes	Yes	No
Flexion-distraction fractures	Yes/no	Yes	Yes
Fracture-dislocations	Yes	Yes	Yes

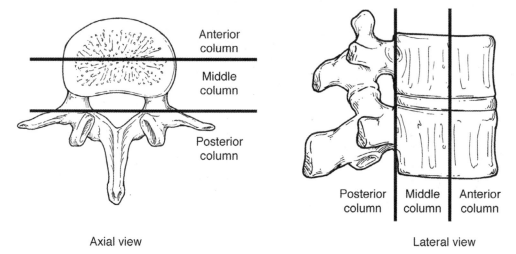

Axial view   Lateral view

*The rule of thumb is that when one column is injured, the spine is usually stable; when two or three columns are injured, the sustained injury is considered unstable.

Lenke, L. G., O'Brien, M. F., & Bridwell, K. H. (1995). Fractures and dislocations of the spine. In C. R. Perry, J. A. Elstrom, & A. M. Pankovich (Eds.). *The handbook of fractures* (pp. 157–189). New York: McGraw-Hill.

Subaxial Cervical Segments

Compared with the upper cervical segment, there is an increased risk of cervical cord damage in injuries to the lower cervical vertebrae (subaxial, i.e., below C-2). Two factors account for this: the size of the spinal canal is decreased in the lower spine, and there is an increased prevalence of injuries that narrow rather than expand the canal. Five types of subaxial cervical vertebrae injuries are discussed:

- **Isolated posterior element fractures** of the lamina, articular process, or spinous process occur when there is impact of the posterior elements on one another and compression-extension results.

- **Minor avulsion and compression fractures** of the subaxial cervical vertebrae include anterior compression or avulsion injuries of the vertebral body. Additionally, anterior and posterior concurrent bone injuries with minimal displacement and angulation can occur.
- **Vertebral body-burst fractures**, common in diving accidents, result from axial loading and flexion. The anterior and middle columns are involved, creating instability. Bone may protrude into the spinal canal.
- **With teardrop fractures** flexion and axial loading result in a teardrop fragment on the anteroinferior aspect of the affected body. SCI and three-column instability are usual.
- **Facet injuries causing spinal malalignment** result from a variety of biomechanical forces. Reduction may have to be

TABLE 18-1   CERVICAL VERTEBRAL INJURIES

TYPE	DESCRIPTION	TREATMENT

Lower Cervical Vertebral Injuries (Occiput to C-2)

Atlas (C-1) fractures 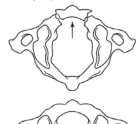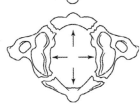	• Result from vertical compression of the occipital condyles on the arch of C-1; cause single or multiple fractures of the C-1 ring; bony pieces thrust away from the center, increasing the space for the spinal cord; thus, neurological injury is rare.
	• There are four types of atlas fractures:
	  1. **Isolated anterior arch fractures:** avulsion from anterior part of ring (usually stable)
	  2. **Isolated posterior arch fracture (fx):** hyperextension with compression of posterior arch of C-1 between occiput and C-2 (usually stable)
	  3. **Lateral mass fx:** fx anterior-posterior to articular surface of C-1 with unilateral displacement; stable fx
	  4. **Jefferson's fx:** burst fx into three or four pieces; can result in concurrent rupture of transverse ligament, resulting in instability
		• Isolated *anterior or posterior arch fx:* usually no neural injury; about 3 mo in cervical hard collar or halo vest
		• *Lateral mass fx:* hard collar or halo vest
		• *Jefferson's fx:* If transverse ligament strong, halo and vest; if weak, cervical traction followed by halo vest for 3–4 mo

Atlantoaxial subluxation
 	
Odontoid fractures
 	
Type I 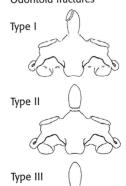
 	
Type II 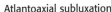
 	
Type III 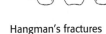
	• Caused by a weak or ruptured transverse ligament that stabilizes dens to anterior ring of atlas.
	• Produces atlantoaxial instability; high risk for spinal injury due to compression of upper cervical cord against the posterior arch of C-1
	• Need to rule out in all patients with neck pain following a motor vehicle accident (MVA) or in elderly with even minor injury to head or neck
	• Displacement, anterior or more often, posterior with rare (10%) neurological injury
	• Odontoid fractures classified into three types:
	  1. **Type I:** chip avulsion fx through the tip of the odontoid; stable fracture; heals well
	  2. **Type II:** fx through the base of the dens with separation, usually anteriorly, from the body of C-2; most common; poor blood supply to area; nonunion in 40%–50%; treatment depends on severity and response to treatment options
	  3. **Type III:** fx line extends into the body of C-2
		• Halo vest for 3 mo, only ligament injuries need a C-1 to C-2 posterior fusion
		• *Type I:* halo vest or hard collar.
		• *Type II:* difficult to treat; there are four options: traction to align then 3 mo in halo vest; halo vest; surgical fixation and fusion; or traction and surgery.
		• *Type III:* if reduced adequately, halo vest for 3 mo; if not, cervical traction first, then halo vest

Hangman's fractures
 	
Type I 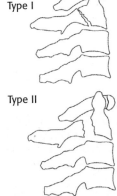
 	
Type II
	• Bipedicular fx with disruption of the disc and ligaments between C-2 and C-3 resulting from hyperextension and distraction
	• Named for injury seen in judicial hangings
	• Further classified according to amount of displacement and angulation of the C-2 body in relation to the posterior elements:
	  1. **Type I:** fx of neural arch without angulation and with up to 3 mm of anterior C-2 displacement on C-3; stable fx
	  2. **Type II:** <5 mm anterior displacement or angulation of C-2 on C-3
	  3. **Type IIA:** severe angulation of C-2 on C-3 with minimal displacement because anterior longitudinal ligament is hinge
	  4. **Type III:** bipedicle fx associated with unilateral or bilateral facet dislocations; unstable; often neurological deficits present
		• *Type I:* managed with a hard collar
		• *Type II:* <5 mm, halo vest if reduction maintained; if >5 mm, skeletal traction for 3–6 wk followed by halo vest
		• *Type IIA:* traction contraindicated; halo vest
		• *Type III:* open reduction when closed reduction not possible and posterior fusion of C-2–3; then halo vest for 3 mo

(continued)

TABLE 18–1 CERVICAL VERTEBRAL INJURIES (*Continued*)

TYPE	DESCRIPTION	TREATMENT
Type III	• Most types unstable; may or may not include neurological deficits depending on amount of displacement or angulation • Important to know type of fx to determine treatment	
Occipital condyle fractures	• Rare injury caused by concurrent axial loading and lateral flexion • Associated with severe head injury • Two types: avulsion or comminuted compression fx	• Cervical collar, such as Philadelphia type
Atlanto-occipital dislocations	• Rare injury caused by extension or flexion injury • Results in an avulsion of the atlas (C-1) body from the occipital bone and all ligaments • Almost always immediately fatal	• Traction contraindicated; halo vest
Atlantoaxial rotary sub-luxation	• Rare injury associated with MVAs • Diagnosis often missed	• Cervical traction for alignment, then a halo vest
Lateral mass fractures	• Rare injury associated with a combined axial loading and lateral flexion forces	• Usually hard collar

Lower Cervical Vertebral Injuries (C-3 to T-1)

Hyperflexion dislocation of C-3 to T-1	Most common cause of paralysis; only neck pain and no neurological deficits may be present	Reduction of the dislocation, then halo immobilization (for 3–6 mo) or a posterior fusion
Flexion-rotational injuries of C-3 to T-1	Usually, anterior subluxation with a unilateral subluxated facet	Reduction of the dislocation with traction; if unstable, posterior fusion
Hyperextension fractures	Usually involves only ligamental and muscle injury; often associated with central cord syndrome	Usually stable fractures; treated with a hard collar for 6–10 wk until the patient is pain-free
Compression fraction of C-3 to T-1	Results from flexion and significant axial loading; may be a simple wedge, burst, or teardrop fracture (see vertebral classification)	Treatment depends on the stability of the fracture; hard collar may be effective for stable fractures, whereas unstable ones may require surgical fusion

Based on Lenke, L. G., O'Brien, M. F., & Bridwell, K. H. (1995). Fractures and dislocations of the spine. In C. R. Perry, J. A. Elstrom, & A. M. Pankovich (Eds.). *The handbook of fractures* (pp. 166–189). New York: McGraw-Hill; and on Adams, J. C., & Hamblen, D. L. (1992). *Outline of fractures* (10th ed, pp. 79–108). Edinburgh: Churchill Livingstone.

done in stages to prevent additional injury. If traction is not possible, surgery is necessary. Traumatic disc herniation may also be present and usually requires an anterior discectomy and fusion.

The treatment options for subaxial cervical vertebral injuries include immobilization with sternal-occipital-mandibular orthonic device; halo vest; posterior fusion and stabilization with wires or instrumentation; anterior approaches for decompression; fusion with or without instrumentation; or a combination of these therapies. Treatment choices depend on the specifics of the fracture or malalignment and on the stability of the ligaments.

Thoracic and Lumbar Segments

Vertebral injuries in the thoracic and lumbar regions account for paralysis of the trunk and lower extremities. Compared with the lumbar region, there is normally little movement possible in the vertebrae of the thoracic region because of the inherent structural stability provided by the rib cage. The spinal cord ends at the upper border of the first lumbar ver-

tebra. The cord gradually tapers, beginning at the lower two thoracic vertebrae. As the cord tapers, it forms a cone called the *conus medullaris*, which continues at the filum terminale. The nerve roots coming off the lower segments of the spinal cord, termed the *cauda equina*, hang loosely and are susceptible to injury. However, injury to these nerves is less likely to be permanent than is injury to the spinal cord. In addition, the emergency procedures of decompression are less likely to be required because the nerve roots tolerate trauma far better than does the spinal cord itself.

There are four general categories of vertebral fractures of the thoracic, thoracolumbar, and lumbar spine:

• **Compression fractures,** caused by axial loading and hyperflexion, are common in the thoracic and upper lumbar regions of the vertebral column. Significant direct force must be applied to produce a fracture in the thoracic area. Injury is usually the result of a direct force applied to one vertebra, which is hyperflexed. The force is then transferred to the underlying cord, putting it at risk of injury. A compression fracture in the thoracic or lumbar region may be compressed anteriorly with or without subluxation of the vertebra. The other possibility is total compression of the vertebral body with anteroposterior protrusion.

- **Burst fractures,** which include injury to the anterior and middle columns and possibly the posterior column, are unstable. Axial loading with flexion creates the biomechanical force responsible for the injury. The vertebral body explodes or "bursts" as a result of the energy associated with injury, and often the vertebral body protrudes into the spinal canal.
- **Flexion-distraction injuries** (also called **Chance fractures)** involve three columns and are thus unstable. The fracture extends through the posterior elements, pedicle, and vertebral body. The mechanism of injury is acute flexion of the torso while restrained with only a lap belt. The flexion-distraction injuries (Chance fractures; Fig. 18-12) are classified according to the involvement of bone and soft-tissue components.
- **Fracture-dislocations** of the thoracic and lumbar areas are of three general categories: anterior or posterior dislocation of the whole vertebral body with fracture of the bony parts; comminuted fractures of the vertebral body with anterior or posterior displacement and rotation so that the rotational force usually tears the supporting ligaments; and lateral dislocation of the vertebra with fracture. All

three columns are involved so that the fracture is unstable, placing the patient at high risk for neurological injury.

Sacral Segments

Fractures of the sacrum and coccyx usually result from direct trauma, most frequently caused by falls. Any fall in the sitting position, such as falling on ice or being thrown from a horse and landing on the buttocks, can result in such a fracture. Nerve injury in this region can cause bladder, bowel, or sexual dysfunction and saddle anesthesia.

Lesions of the *conus medullaris* can occur with fractures in the lumbar region. These lesions can have confusing clinical presentations. Injury to the conus usually results in lower motor neuron symptoms (muscle flaccidity, muscle atrophy, hyporeflexia) because of the disruption of the anterior gray horn cells. A decompression laminectomy may be necessary if there is pressure on the neural elements. Lesions involving the *cauda equina* produce selected root syndromes. A decompression laminectomy may also be necessary for cauda equina injuries, but sacral roots are very delicate and sometimes do not recover even with early decompression.[8] An acute central disc herniation of L-4 to L-5 or L-5 to S-1 can result in major damage to the sacral roots that lie centrally within the dural

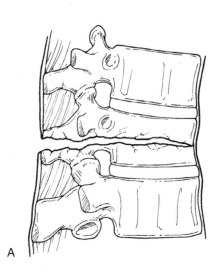

A

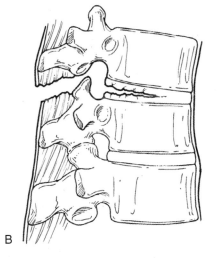

B

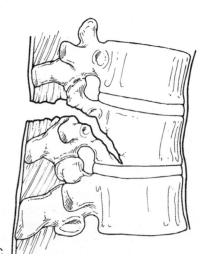

C

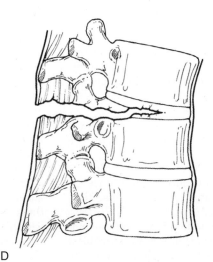

D

Figure 18-12 • Types of flexion-distraction (Chance) fractures. (*A*) Disruption through the entire bony elements. (*B*) Disruption through the entire ligamentous elements. (*C* and *D*) Disruption through bony and ligamentous elements.

sac. Another presentation is partial or complete sparing of the lumbar roots and often the S-1 roots. These patients may have total preservation of leg strength, but complete bowel and bladder paralysis and perineal anesthesia.

> **CLINICAL VIGNETTE:** A patient is admitted with sudden motor weakness to the lower extremities, inability to void, and absent reflexes. A Foley catheter is inserted and 1200 mL of urine is in the drainage bag in 5 minutes. Magnetic resonance imaging (MRI) reveals a large lumbar central herniation; emergent surgical decompression is undertaken. The surgeon describes the problem as a nerve root lesion. Eight hours after surgery, light touch and pinprick sensation are noted in the lower extremities. There is gradual recovery of sensory function; bladder function returns. With short-term physical therapy, the motor function to the lower extremity returns. The patient makes a full recovery in 3 months.

Spinal Cord Injuries

Injury to the spinal cord can be devastating because the resulting loss of body function also involves the loss of independence. The loss of function may be permanent or temporary, depending on the type of injury. The several syndromes related to SCI are summarized in Chart 18-2. Injuries to the spinal cord are classified by type of injury and by syndrome produced.

Classification by Cause

The spinal cord can be injured by concussion, contusion, compression, laceration, transection, hemorrhage, damage to the blood vessels that supply the cord, or damage to blood vessels within the cord.

- **Concussion:** a jarring (i.e., severe shaking) of the spinal cord can result in a temporary loss of function (i.e., spinal shock [see subsequent discussion]) lasting hours to weeks. No identifiable macro-neuropathological changes are noted on examination of the cord.
- **Compression:** as part of the distraction (i.e., distortion of the normal curvatures) of the spinal cord at the moment of injury, the neural element can be compressed and contused, lacerated, or transected.
- **Contusion:** contusion is bruising, which can lead to bleeding into the cord, subsequent edema, and possible necrosis from the compression caused by edema or direct damage to the tissue. The extent of the neurological deficits depends on the severity of the contusion and the amount of necrosis, if any. Fractures, dislocations, and direct trauma to the cord can cause a contusion.
- **Laceration:** an actual tear in the cord results in permanent injury to the cord. Contusion, edema, and cord compression accompany a laceration.
- **Transection:** a severing of the cord can be complete or incomplete. Actual complete transection is rare. However, clinical presentations, which mimic complete transection, are frequently seen.
- **Hemorrhage:** blood in or around the spinal cord is an irritant to the delicate tissue. Changes in the neurochemical environment, edema, and neurological deficits can result.

- **Injury to the blood vessels that supply the cord:** interference with or injury to the vessels that supply the spinal cord, the anterior spinal artery, or the two posterior spinal arteries results in ischemia and possible necrosis. Episodes of ischemia can cause temporary neurological deficits. Prolonged ischemia and necrosis causes permanent deficits.

The **syndrome of SCI without radiologic abnormality** (SCI-WORA) is more common in children than in adults. It is characterized by negative radiologic examination on plain films and tomography, either conventional or CT.[8,9] More common in adults is the syndrome of **SCI without radiologic evidence of trauma** (SCIWORET). In this syndrome the radiologic examinations are abnormal, but x-rays show no evidence of trauma. A review of SCIWORET patients reported evidence of compression on myelography or MRI and recommended early decompression surgery.[10] Use of MRI provides high sensitivity for detecting mild SCI and nonbony spinal column lesions, thus improving diagnosis.[8]

Pathophysiology

Spinal cord injury results from both the **primary injury,** which occurs at the time of the impact, and the **secondary injury,** which occurs after primary injury (i.e., minutes, hours, days) and is due to the complex systemic and biochemical processes on cellular function. The *primary injury* is the result of concussion, contusion, compression, laceration, transection, or disruption of the spinal cord or surrounding vascular components. The degree of injury depends on the magnitude of the force applied to the spinal cord and the angle of impact.

Collectively called *secondary injury*, several concurrent and overlapping vascular, chemical, inflammatory, and neuropathological changes occur following primary injury, which are interdependent cascades of systemic and cellular events initiated by the primary insult.[11] These intrinsically initiated destructive processes occur within minutes of injury and last for days to weeks.[12,13] Within minutes of injury, a cascade of concurrent events including alterations in blood flow, edema, hemorrhage, electrolyte abnormalities, membrane injury, and the release of vasoactive agents, cellular enzymes, cytotoxic mediators, excitotoxic neurotransmitters, and inflammatory mediators occurs and contributes to cellular membrane injury and posttraumatic ischemia.[14]

This interruption of the cord microcirculation results in *ischemic injury*; it is caused by direct vascular injury, hypotension related to neurogenic shock, loss of autoregulation, vasospasm, and vasospasm-induced thrombosis.[12,15] Ischemia, increased vascular permeability, and edema result. The microcirculatory changes are noted initially at the point of injury, but then encompass a wider area above and below the segment of injury. Injury site edema spreads from the primary core site to ascending and descending spinal cord levels, further decreasing neurological function. Ischemia also decreases adequate cellular oxygenation, which converts to anaerobic cellular function and the production of lactic acidosis. Hypoxia of the gray matter stimulates the release of catecholamines, which contribute to the hemorrhage and necrosis and cause further spinal cord dysfunction. The

(text continues on page 426)

CHART 18-2 Spinal Cord Injury Syndromes

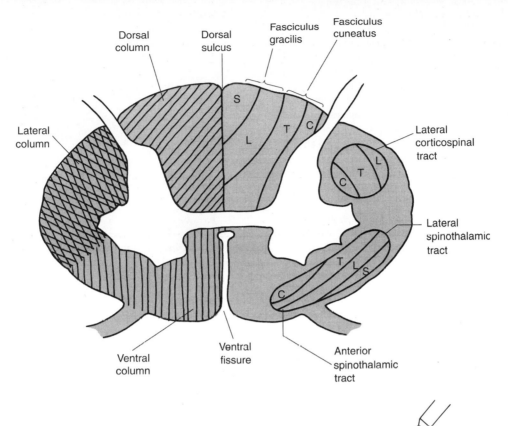

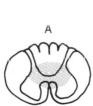

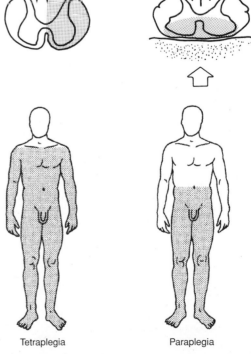

(A) Central cord syndrome. (B) Brown-Séquard syndrome. (C) Anterior cord syndrome.

Several terms related to spinal cord injury are defined.

- Tetraplegia refers to a lesion involving one of the cervical segments of the spinal cord that results in dysfunction of both arms, both legs, bowel, and bladder.
- Paraplegia refers to a lesion involving the thoracic lumbar or sacral regions of the spinal cord that results in dysfunction of the lower extremities, bowel, or bladder.
- A complete lesion (e.g., complete tetraplegia or complete tetraplegia) implies total loss of sensation and voluntary muscle control below the injury.
- An incomplete lesion implies preservation of the sensory or motor fibers, or both, below the lesion. Incomplete lesions are classified according to the area of damage: central, lateral, anterior, or peripheral.

Tetraplegia   Paraplegia

The shaded area shows the extent of motor and sensory loss.

(continued)

CHART **18-2**   Spinal Cord Injury Syndromes   (Continued)

CENTRAL CORD SYNDROME

- Presentation: There are more motor deficits in the upper extremities than the lower extremities; sensory loss varies but is more pronounced in the upper extremities; bowel/bladder dysfunction is variable, or function may be completely preserved.
- Cause: Injury or edema of the central cord, usually of the cervical area, is the underlying cause; hyperextension injuries, particularly if bony spurs are noted, can be causative.
- Result: Edema in the central cord exerts pressure on the anterior horn cells. The cervical fibers of the corticospinal tract are located in a more central position in the cord than the sacral fibers, which are located in the periphery. As a result, motor deficits are less severe in the lower extremities than in the upper extremities.
- Treatment: High-dose steroid (methylprednisolone) protocol for acute cord injury is controversial; immobilization or bed rest is the treatment of choice. Flexionextension radiographs are usually obtained. The prognosis varies.

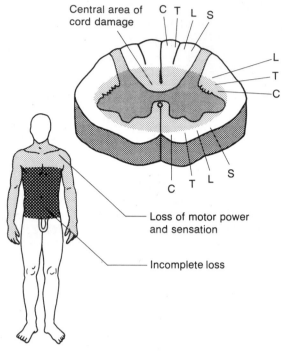

Central cord syndrome
A cross-section of the cord shows central damage and the associated motor and sensory loss (C, cervical; T, thoracic; L, lumbar; S, sacral).

ANTERIOR CORD SYNDROME

- Presentation: Loss of perception of pain, temperature, and motor function is noted below the level of the lesion; light touch, position, and vibration sensation remain intact.
- Cause: The syndrome may be caused by acute disc herniation or hyperflexion injuries associated with fracture- dislocation of a vertebra. It also may occur as a result of injury to the anterior spinal artery, which supplies the anterior two thirds of the spinal cord.
- Result: Injury to the anterior part of the spinal cord, which includes the spinothalamic tracts (pain), corticospinal tracts (temperature), and anterior gray horn motor neurons, is noted.
- Treatment: High-dose steroid (methylprednisolone) protocol for acute cord injury is controversial; surgical decompression is usually necessary to manage fracturedislocation. The prognosis varies.

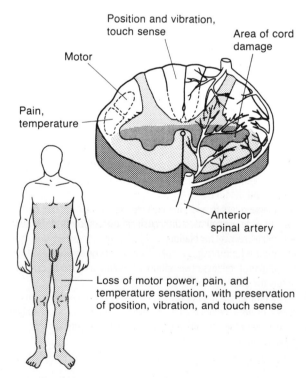

Anterior cord syndrome
Cord damage and associated motor and sensory loss are illustrated.

(continued)

CHART 18-2   Spinal Cord Injury Syndromes   (Continued)

BROWN-SÉQUARD SYNDROME (LATERAL CORD SYNDROME)

- Presentation: Ipsilateral paralysis or paresis is noted, together with ipsilateral loss of touch, pressure, and vibration and contralateral loss of pain and temperature.
- Cause: The syndrome may be caused by transverse hemisection of the cord (half the cord is transected from north to south), usually as a result of a knife or missile injury, fracture-dislocation of a unilateral articular process, or possibly an acute ruptured disc.
- Result: With right-sided cord transection, for example, the following would occur: paralysis of all voluntary muscles below the level of injury on the right side of the body (lateral corticospinal tract); loss of perception of touch, vibration, and position on the right side of the body below the level of injury (posterior columns, which include the fasciculus gracilis and fasciculus cuneatus); and loss of pain and temperature perception on the left side of the body below the injury (lateral spinothalamic tracts). Fibers that carry pain and temperature cross to the opposite side of the cord immediately after entering the cord and then ascend. The other tracts mentioned do not cross until they reach the brainstem.
- Treatment: High-dose steroid (methylprednisolone) protocol for acute cord injury is controversial; no specific treatment is undertaken except fracture-dislocation management.

CONUS MEDULLARIS SYNDROME

- Presentation: A lumbar enlargement of the spinal cord corresponds to the innervation for the lower extremities and extends from L-3 to S-2. Below the lumbar enlargement, the spinal cord narrows, ending as the conus medullaris. The *conus medullaris* is the cone-shaped lower end of the spinal cord. A fine pial thread called the *filum terminale* travels from the end of the conus medullaris to the first coccygeal segment.[*] The conus is located directly opposite vertebral bodies T-12 and L-1. The tip of the conus does not extend past the L-1–L-2 disc space. This anatomic area is a transition area of high stress from the rigid thoracic spine to the more mobile lumbar spine, which increases the risk of flexion-distraction and burst fractures.[*] *Lesions of the conus medullaris and cauda equina cause similar signs and symptoms and can be difficult to differentiate.* With conus medullaris, a range of lower extremity dysfunction, usually with lower extremity weakness or flaccid paralysis, loss of bladder and anal sphincter function early, male sexual dysfunction, and loss of Achilles reflex, is seen.[*] Sensory loss is variable, with saddle anesthesia possible and pain uncommon.
- Causes: Falls, vertebral trauma such as subluxation or dislocation, intervertebral disc herniation, and spinal epidural metastatic lesions are all possible causes.
- Result: Compression of the conus medullaris will result in the signs and symptoms outlined above.
- Treatment: A magnetic resonance imaging scan is useful to guide treatment decisions. Surgical decompression or radiation may be ordered depending on cause.[*] Use of steroids is controversial.

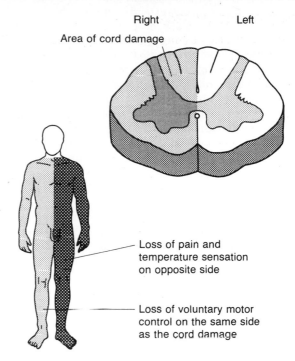

Right   Left

Area of cord damage

Loss of pain and temperature sensation on opposite side

Loss of voluntary motor control on the same side as the cord damage

Brown-Séquard syndrome
Cord damage and associated motor and sensory loss are illustrated.

CAUDA EQUINA SYNDROME

- Presentation: The spinal cord terminates at T-12 or L-1, and the cauda equina begins at lumbar disc space L-1 or L-2. The nerve roots from the lumbar, sacral, and coccygeal that extend distally from the conus medullaris are collectively called the *cauda equina*. Although the cauda equina is not a true spinal cord injury because it is outside the spinal cord, it is nonetheless a serious problem considered within the context of spinal cord injury. Patients present with weak or flaccid lower extremities with at least partial preservation of sensation. Pain is often severe, asymmetric, and radicular. The patellar and Achilles reflexes are absent. Sphincter disturbance is usually late and severe with urinary retention being most common.
- Causes: The most common cause is a large herniated disc. Other causes include epidural bony collapse, epidural tumor, epidural hematoma, trauma, and metastatic lesions.
- Result: The compression of the spinal nerves results in loss of neurological function that can be permanent if not relieved. Radiologic evaluation helps to determine treatment options.
- Treatment: Emergent surgery is indicated for cauda equina syndrome. The timing depends on the progression of motor deficits and pain, but is usually within 24 hours. The outcome of surgery varies, but is generally better than for spinal cord injury.

Cross-sections of spinal cord in this chart are from Kitt, S., & Kaiser, J. (1990). *Emergency nursing: A physiological and clinical perspective.* Philadelphia: W. B. Saunders.

[*]Barbeau, H., Ladouceur, M., Norman, K. E., Pepin, A., & Leroux, A. (1999). Walking after SCI: evaluation, treatment and functional recovery. *Archives of Physical Medicine Rehabilitation, 80,* 225–235.

release of catecholamines and vasoactive substances (norepinephrine, serotonin, dopamine, and histamine) from the injured tissue can cause vasospasm and impede microcirculation. These events further extend necrosis of blood vessels and neurons. The release of proteolytic and lipolytic enzymes from the injured cells causes vasospasm, delayed swelling, and necrosis in the spinal cord.

Calcium disruption in relation to spinal cord injury is important. A basic role of calcium is its role in regulation of the movement of sodium and potassium across the intracellular and extracellular space and also release of neurotransmitters at the synaptic junctions.[15] After initial injury, calcium balance changes from an increase of intracellular calcium to a decrease in extracellular calcium. The shift in intracellular calcium activates calcium-dependent proteases and impairs mitochondrial and other intracellular functions.

The exact triggers to the cascade are unclear, but within 8 hours of injury intracellular calcium elevation peaks and remains elevated for approximately 1 week postinjury.[16] Free fatty acids and free radicals are released from the cell membrane, thus stimulating the release of arachidonic acid and vasoactive eicosaoids.[11,12] The increased calcium levels stimulate protease and lipase activity, which stimulate lipid peroxidation of the cell membrane.[17,18]

Concurrently, the inflammatory process that was stimulated immediately after injury continues for several days as a complex multifactorial response, which includes endothelial damage; the release of inflammatory mediators such as catecholamines, prostaglandin, and endogenous opioids; changes in vascular permeability; development of edema; migration of peripheral inflammatory cells; and activation of microglia cells.[15]

The function of highly specialized central nervous system cells is disrupted by ischemia and hypoxia within minutes of injury. Micro-, petechial hemorrhage progresses to ischemia and possibly on to infarction and tissue necrosis. Irreversible nerve damage develops as a result of glial and neuronal tissue changes that replace normal neural elements with fibrotic scar tissue. As a result, neurological deficits become permanent.

ACUTE SPINAL CORD TRAUMA

Terminology

Incomplete Versus Complete Spinal Cord Lesions

A *complete spinal cord lesion* results in the absence of sensory and voluntary motor function below the level of injury including the lowest sacral segments (S-4 and S-5). An *incomplete spinal cord lesion* occurs when there is partial preservation of sensory (including position sense), motor (voluntary toe flexion), or a combination of sensory-motor function including the lowest sacral segments.[19,20] Sparing of the lowest sacral segments is called sacral sparing (sensation around the anus, voluntary rectal sphincter contraction). Types of incomplete spinal lesions include central cord syndrome, Brown-Séquard syndrome, anterior cord syndrome, and posterior cord syndrome (each discussed further in the chapter).

It is generally believed that there is virtually no chance of recovery when an SCI results in total loss of neurological function and no recovery has occurred within the first 24 hours after injury.[21]

Spinal Shock

Spinal shock refers to the clinical syndrome often seen in major SCI to the cervical and upper thoracic spinal cord. There is a temporary interruption of the sympathetic function leaving the parasympathetic function unopposed. Spinal shock is characterized by flaccid paralysis, loss of cutaneous and deep tendon reflexes, and anesthesia to all sensory modalities *below* the level of injury.[22] It includes the loss of urinary bladder tone, peristalsis (i.e., paralytic ileus), perspiration and piloerection, and vasomotor tone with the potential for dependent lower extremity edema. In addition, the autonomic dysfunction is characterized by systemic hypotension, warm skin, and bradycardia (50 to 70 beats/min). Concurrently, body temperature tends to be lower than normal (i.e., 96°F to 98°F [35.5°C to 36.5°C]) because of the break in the connection between the hypothalamus and the sympathetic nervous system. The body temperature responds to ambient room temperature.

Under normal conditions, the preganglionic axons of the sympathetic nervous system, which have origins in the thoracolumbar region of the spinal cord, receive impulses for reflex control of blood pressure and heart rate through the cardiac accelerator and vasoconstriction reflexes. In patients with cervical or upper thoracic spinal cord injuries, mild *hypotension* and *bradycardia* caused by sympathetic failure and peripheral vascular vasodilation accompany the state of "spinal shock."[23] The loss of sympathetic input to the systemic vasculature and the heart and subsequent decreased peripheral vascular resistance result in decreased peripheral vascular tone below the level of injury.[23] The bradycardia results from the suppression of the cardiac accelerator reflex. The unopposed vagal tone causes vasodilation and bradycardia. The mild hypotension, bradycardia, and loss of vasomotor tone are sometimes referred to as *neurogenic shock* to differentiate the hypotension from hypovolemic shock. Treatment with crystalloid solutions or plasma expanders, a mainstay of treatment of hypovolemic shock, may be helpful in some cases of neurogenic shock. By contrast, rarely is it necessary to use vasopressors to maintain adequate organ perfusion in neurogenic shock; it is usually necessary in hypovolemic shock.[23]

CLINICAL PEARLS: Note the difference between neurogenic shock and hypovolemic shock. In neurogenic shock, the nurse will see *mild* hypotension, bradycardia, warm skin, and areflexia. In hypovolemic shock, significant hypotension, tachycardia, cold and clammy skin, and normal reflexes are seen.

Clinically, it is difficult to ascertain a clear picture in the first few hours after SCI when there is a mixture of the temporary spinal shock with the permanent effects of SCI. In general, the loss of motor power and sensation that results from spinal shock resolves within *1 hour after injury*. Any weakness or sensory loss remaining after an hour is likely due to physical SCI rather than spinal shock. The loss of reflexes an autonomic tone may last days to months, depending on the spinal level and severity of the initial injury.[22] In most instances, it takes more than an hour to transport an injured patient from the site of injury to the hospital. Therefore, there may be differences in the motor and sensory examination at the injury site as compared with the examination conducted in the emergency room after there has been resolution of spinal shock.

Immediate Signs and Symptoms of Spinal Cord Trauma

When the spinal cord is suddenly injured, there is loss of motor and sensory function *below* the level of injury. See also the discussion of spinal shock above. If no motor or sensory function is present after spinal shock resolves, the injury is considered complete. The American Spinal Injury Association (ASIA) publishes the ASIA Impairment Scale often used by clinicians to determine the extent of SCI (Table 18-2). Specific functional losses, based on level of SCI, are also listed in Table 18-3.

The following losses are seen with *complete* SCI:

- Flaccid paralysis of all voluntary muscles *below* the level of injury
- Loss of all spinal reflexes *below* the level of injury
- Loss of pain perception, light touch, proprioception, temperature, and pressure *below* the level of injury (pain may be felt at the site of the injury because of a zone of heightened sensitivity [hyperesthesia] immediately *above* the level of the lesion)
- Absence of somatic and visceral sensations *below* the level of injury
- Loss of the ability to perspire *below* the level of injury (autonomic function)
- Bowel and bladder dysfunction.

Incomplete SCI syndromes and clinical presentation are found in Chart 18-2.

TABLE 18-2 ASIA IMPAIRMENT SCALE

A **Complete:** No motor or sensory function is preserved in the sacral segments S4–S5
B **Incomplete:** sensory but not motor function is preserved below the neurologic level and includes the sacral segments S4–S5
C **Incomplete:** motor function is preseved below the neurological level, and at least half of key muscles below the neurological level have a muscle grade less than 3
D **Incomplete:** motor function is preserved below the neurological level, and atleast half of key muscles below the neurological level have a muscle grade of 3 or more.
E **Normal:** motor and sensory function is normal

Clinical Syndromes

☐ Central cord
☐ Brown-Séquard
☐ Anterior cord
☐ Conus medullaris
☐ Cauda equina

Copyright, American Spinal Injury Association, from *International Standards for Neurological and Functional Classification of Spinal Cord Injury,* revised 2000.

EARLY MANAGEMENT OF PATIENTS WITH SPINAL CORD INJURY

Prehospital Management

The prehospital management of SCIs is critical to the patient's ultimate neurological outcome. Until proven otherwise, every trauma patient should be treated as if he or she has an SCI. This rule applies to any patient with a head injury and to the inebriated trauma victim whose mental status and cognitive functions are impaired (see Chap. 18).

Advance Trauma Life Support (ATLS) guidelines are followed.[12] The basic objectives of management at the injury site include (1) rapid assessment to determine the extent of vertebral injury or SCI; (2) immobilization and stabilization of the head and neck to prevent extension of injury; (3) extrication of the patient from the vehicle or injury site; (4) stabilization and control of any other life-threatening injuries; (5) triage to the appropriate facility; and (6) rapid and safe transport. The rescue personnel must be well trained because improper handling at the injury site can turn a minor vertebral injury into a major, irreversible SCI.

Emergency Department Management

On admission to the emergency department (ED), ATLS guidelines are followed. A report of the prehospital management and a history of the injury are collected rapidly. The focus is on rapid stabilization and assessment. After the primary survey and patient stabilization are completed, the secondary survey is conducted.

Transport of the patient with a hard collar and long spine board is critical; this keeps the patient immobilized in a neutral position to prevent further vertebral spinal injury.[24] The patient should be maintained with the hard collar and backboard until imaging is completed and the C-spine cleared. However, prolonged immobility on a backboard can lead to development of pressure ulcers within a few hours, especially if an SCI is present. Therefore, a backboard is used with full awareness of consequences and removed as quickly as possible. On arrival, the patient may be safely log-rolled off the backboard by well-trained ED personnel. If the patient is admitted to the ICU on a backboard, it should be removed with approval of the physician.

CLINICAL PEARLS: Note how long a patient has been on a backboard, recognizing the risk of the development of pressure ulcers on the sacrum, occipital region, shoulders, elbows, and heels. The nurse should alert the team to the time element and risk.

History of Accident

The history of the accident can be obtained from various sources, including the patient (if responsive), a family member, another accident victim, or first responders. Information about the circumstances of the injury, the neurological status of the patient immediately after injury, the treatment at the accident site, and the mode of transport is all vital. At the same time, a baseline assessment (primary survey) is conducted.

TABLE 18–3   FUNCTIONAL LOSS FROM SPINAL CORD INJURY

LEVEL OF SPINAL INJURY	MOTOR FUNCTION	DEEP TENDON REFLEXES	SENSORY FUNCTION	RESPIRATORY FUNCTION	VOLUNTARY BOWEL AND BLADDER FUNCTION	REHABILITATIVE POTENTIAL
C-1–4	• Tetraplegia: loss of all motor function from the neck down	All lost	• Loss of all sensory function in the neck and below (C-4 supplies the clavicles.)	• Loss of involuntary (phrenic) and voluntary (intercostals) respiratory function; ventilatory support and a tracheostomy needed	• No bowel or bladder control	• May be discharged home on a ventilator with home care
C-5	• Tetraplegia: loss of all function below the upper shoulders • **Intact:** sternomastoids, cervical paraspinal muscles, and the trapezius; can control head	C-5, C-6 biceps	• Loss of sensation below the clavicle and most portions of arms, hands, chest, abdomen, and lower extremities • **Intact:** head, shoulders, deltoid, clavicle, portion of forearms (C-5 supplies the lateral aspect of the arm.)	• Phrenic nerve intact, but not intercostal muscles	• No bowel or bladder control	• Use of extremity-powered devices to achieve some upper limb control • Head control facilitates wheelchair (W/C) balance • Adaptive tools, held in mouth, for typing and writing • Some adaptive tools and use of special computer technology
C-6	• Tetraplegia: loss of all function below the shoulders and upper arms; lacks elbow, forearm, and hand control • **Intact:** deltoid, biceps, and external rotator muscles of shoulders	C-5, C-6 brachioradials	• Loss of everything listed for a C-5 lesion, but greater arm and thumb sensation • **Intact:** head, shoulders, arms, palms of hands, and thumbs (C-6 supplies the forearm and thumb.)	• Phrenic nerve intact, but not intercostal muscles	• No bowel or bladder control	• Needs assistive devices to use arms (may be able to help feed, groom, and dress self) • Needs a motorized wheelchair • Dependent for all transfers
C-7	• Tetraplegia: loss of motor control to portions of the arms and hands • **Intact:** voluntary strength in shoulder depressors, shoulder abductors, internal rotators, and radial wrist extensors	C-7, C-8 triceps	• Loss of sensation below the clavicle and portions of arms and hands • **Intact:** head, shoulders, most of arms and hands (C-7 supplies the middle finger.)	• Phrenic nerve intact, but not intercostal muscles	• No bowel or bladder function	• Can perform some activities of daily living (ADLs) • Can use wrist extensor with a special splint to induce finger flexion • Can push a W/C with special hand-grasps • May be able to drive a specially equipped car
C-8	• Tetraplegia: loss of motor control to portions of arms and hands • **Intact:** some voluntary control of elbow extensors, wrist, finger extension, and finger flexors		• Loss of sensation below the chest and in portions of hands • **Intact:** sensation to face, shoulders, arms, hands, and part of chest (C-8 supplies the little finger.)	• Phrenic nerve intact, but not intercostal muscles	• No bowel or bladder function	• Able to push up in the W/C • Improved sitting tolerance • Can grasp and release hands voluntarily • Independent in most ADLs from W/C • Independent in use of W/C • Can use hands for catheterization and rectal stimulation for bowel movements

(continued)

TABLE 18–3   FUNCTIONAL LOSS FROM SPINAL CORD INJURY (*Continued*)

LEVEL OF SPINAL INJURY	MOTOR FUNCTION	DEEP TENDON REFLEXES	SENSORY FUNCTION	RESPIRATORY FUNCTION	VOLUNTARY BOWEL AND BLADDER FUNCTION	REHABILITATIVE POTENTIAL
T-1–6	• Paraplegia: loss of everything below the midchest region, including the trunk muscles • **Intact:** control of function to the shoulders, upper chest, arms, and hands		• Loss of sensation below the midchest area • **Intact:** everything to the midchest region, including the arms and hands (T-1 and T-2 supply the inner aspect of the arm; T-4 supplies the nipple area.)	• Phrenic nerve functions independently • Some impairment of intercostal muscles	• No bowel or bladder function	• Full control of upper extremities and completely independent in W/C • Full-time employment possible • Independent in managing urinary drainage and inserting suppositories • Able to live in a dwelling without major architectural changes
T-6–12	• Paraplegia: loss of motor control below the waist • **Intact:** shoulders, arms, hands, and long trunk muscles		• Loss of everything below the waist • **Intact:** shoulders, chest, arms, and hands (T-10 supplies the umbilicus; T-12 supplies the groin area.)	• No interference with respiratory function	• No bowel or bladder control	• In addition to the previously described capabilities, there is complete abdominal and upper back control. • Good sitting balance (allows for greater ease of W/C operation and athletics)
L-1–3	• Paraplegia: loss of most control of legs and pelvis • **Intact:** shoulders, arms, hands, torso, hip rotation and flexion, and some leg flexion	L-2–4 (knee jerk)	• Loss of sensation to the lower abdomen and legs • **Intact:** all of the above plus some sensation to the inner and anterior thigh (L-3 supplies the knee.)	• No interference with respiratory function	• No bowel or bladder control	• Independent for most activities from W/C
L-3–4	• Paraplegia: loss of control of portions of lower legs, ankles, and feet • **Intact:** all of the above, plus increased knee extension		• Loss of sensation to portions of the lower legs, feet, and ankles • **Intact:** all of the above, plus sensation to the upper legs	• No interference with respiratory function	• No bowel or bladder control	• Voluntary control of hip extensors; weak abductors • Walking with braces possible
L-4 to S-5	• Paraplegia: incomplete • Segmental motor control L-4 to S-1: abduction and internal rotation of hip, ankle dorsiflexion, and foot inversion L-5 to S-1: foot eversion L-4 to S-2: knee flexion S-1–2: plantar flexion S-1–2: (ankle jerk) S-2–5: bowel/bladder control	S-1–2 (ankle jerk)	• Lumbar sensory nerves innervate the upper legs and portions of the lower legs L-5: medial aspect of foot S-1: lateral aspect of foot S-2: posterior aspect of calf/thigh • Sacral sensory nerves innervate the lower legs, feet, and perineum	• No interference with respiratory function	• Bowel and bladder control possibly impaired • S-2–4 segments control urinary continence • S-3–5 segments control bowel continence (perianal muscles)	• Can walk with braces or may use W/C • Can be relatively independent

Assessment

For victims of trauma, a complete primary and secondary survey must be conducted, as outlined in ATLS. The **ABCs** (i.e., **a**irway, **b**reathing, **c**irculation) of life support are followed. The essential components of assessment include the medical history, physical examination, imaging studies, and other baseline tests. However, emphasis on these components varies depending on the circumstances of injury and patient acuity.[25] After the ABCs (see later discussion) have been stabilized, the clinical examination is conducted to assess the function of the spinal cord and approximate the level of injury.[22,26] By comparison, the purpose of imaging studies is to identify the extent of bone and ligament injury and to determine the best operative approach for decompression and stabilization, if surgery is indicated.

Treatment

Because hypoxia, hypotension, and hypertension can contribute to secondary SCI and other life-threatening complications, a few special considerations related to vertebral injury are noteworthy.[27] In addition, because trauma is involved, it is necessary to rule out the presence of other system injuries that could be life threatening.

Airway and Breathing. The airway is monitored for patency, and respirations are evaluated to determine whether the diaphragm and intercostal muscles are functional. Skin color, nail beds, and earlobes are also assessed for evidence of hypoperfusion. To prevent hypoxemia and secondary SCI, oxygen saturation should be maintained within normal range (94% to 100%) by administration of supplemental oxygen to all acute SCI patients. Patients with high cervical injuries may require intubation for ventilatory support with a mechanical ventilator. If a cervical injury is suspected and endotracheal intubation is necessary, a fiberoptic laryngoscopic insertion technique provided by a specially trained physician is necessary to prevent extension of the injury. Any injury compromising ventilation must be treated promptly.

> **CLINICAL PEARLS:**   The diaphragm is innervated by C-1 to C-4. If a high cervical injury is sustained, innervation to the diaphragm is affected, and the patient will have respiratory compromise. Intubation and mechanical ventilation are necessary. If the SCI is below the innervation to the phrenic nerve and above the innervation to the intercostal muscles, diaphragmatic breathing will be noted. These patients may also require varying degrees of respiratory support.

Monitor patients not requiring immediate intubation carefully for signs of ascending edema, which may rapidly compromise respirations and require emergent intubation. Continuous respiratory monitoring with pulse oximetry should be provided.

Circulation. Patients with SCIs (particularly within the cervical region) may show signs of hypotension, bradycardia, and lowered body temperature. These are symptoms of neurogenic shock, part of the spinal shock syndrome. The lowered blood pressure is attributable to vasodilation, which results from the loss of vasomotor tone

below the level of injury rather than blood volume. In most instances, treatment will not be necessary unless the hypotension is compounded by hemorrhagic shock (tachycardia will be present). However, if circulation is inadequate because of hemorrhage or cardiac compromise, treatment must be initiated immediately to hemodynamically stabilize the patient. The abdominal and thoracic cavities may be the sites of significant blood loss. A careful physical examination is necessary to rule out hemodynamic instability from occult bleeding. If the patient is cool to touch because of spinal shock, adding blankets will usually provide comfort.

Neurological Examination. The goals for the neurological examination include a neurological assessment, assessment of spinal cord function, and an approximation of the level of injury. In addition, the possibility of traumatic brain injury must be considered and excluded. Two scales for rating functional classification and impairment from SCI have been established by ASIA and are widely used in practice (Table 18-2 and Fig. 18-13).

Other Organ Systems. As already mentioned, trauma patients frequently have multiple injuries, including cardiac, intrathoracic, or abdominal injuries. The patient must be assessed for possible cardiac complications, especially cardiac contusion, with a 12-lead electrocardiogram (ECG). The presence of tachycardia with hypotension and cool and clammy skin should raise suspicion of visceral hemorrhage; a search should commence for signs of intra-abdominal or intrathoracic injury. Because pain perception is diminished or absent due to SCI, pain will not draw attention to a salient, life-threatening ruptured viscera. Neurogenic and hemorrhagic shock can be simultaneously present. Careful assessment and clinical reasoning must be used to recognize the problem and quickly institute appropriate treatment.

Methylprednisolone Protocol. Randomized controlled trials in the 1990s reported beneficial effects of high-dose methylprednisolone administered soon after SCI.[28–30] Soon after these study findings were published, the administration of high-dose methylprednisolone was considered the standard of practice. However, the validity of these studies has been questioned based on critical analysis of the original and additional data.[31,32] As a result, there is now a consensus that corticosteroids may offer only a slight benefit.[21] It is no longer considered the standard of care for acute SCI, although some centers continue to use the protocol.[33] If a methylprednisolone protocol is ordered, consult with the pharmacist for preparation of the drug in an intravenous solution. Note that there are contraindications for administration of the protocol.

The use of gangliosides for acute spinal cord injury has been proposed. However, according to a recent Cochrane review, the evidence available does not support the use of ganglioside treatment to reduce mortality in SCI patients. No evidence has supported improved recovery or quality of life in SCI patients who have received gangliosides.[34]

Other Considerations in the Emergency Department. The patient with an SCI has an atonic bladder that becomes rapidly overdistended. Urine may be retained and may overflow, and the bladder may feel distended on palpation. An indwelling urinary catheter is inserted to manage urinary output and prevent injury to the bladder from overdistention.

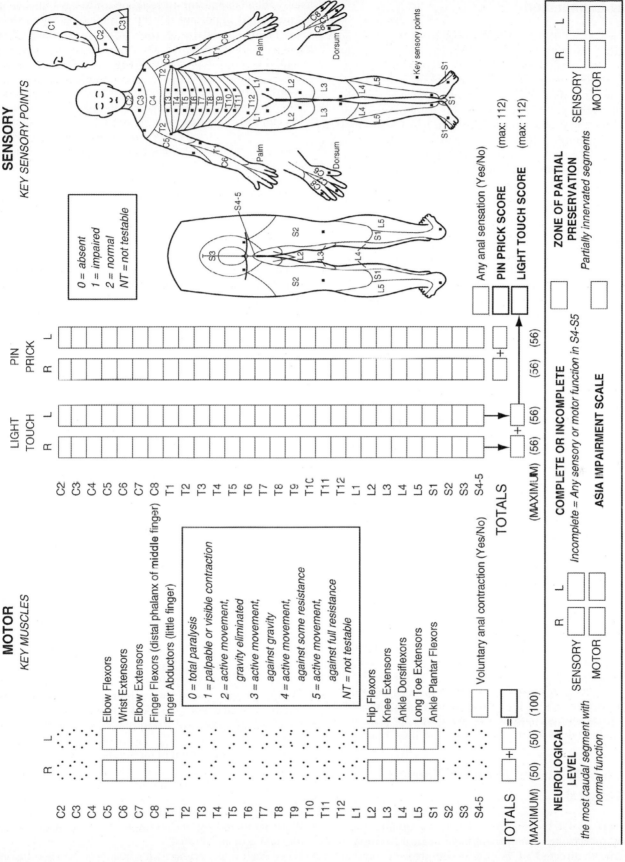

Figure 18-13 • ASIA motor and sensory scales. (Copyright, American Spinal Injury Association, from *International standards for neurological and functional classification of spinal cord injury*, revised 1996.)

431

Imaging Examination

Missing a cervical fracture or SCI can have devastating consequences. The following recommendations are made regarding radiographic cervical spine assessment in asymptomatic trauma patients: "Radiological assessment of the cervical spine is not recommended in trauma patients who are awake, alert, and not intoxicated, who are without neck pain or tenderness, and who do not have significant associated injuries that detract from their general evaluation."[2] In patients who are symptomatic, three cervical spine series (anteroposterior, lateral, and odontoid views) are recommended. Supplemental CT scan is further recommended in any suspicious or poorly visualized area.[2] Initial screening of the entire spinal anatomy (i.e., cervical to sacral) is conducted. Careful, expert management of the patient to prevent extension of injury is critical. The C-7 to T-1 vertebrae, normally difficult to visualize, may require special positioning techniques (i.e., swimmer's position) for visualization. The C-1 to C-2 level, especially the odontoid process, is also difficult to visualize. Films may be taken with the patient's mouth open to visualize the odontoid process. The physician must decide the specific type of x-ray studies necessary while considering patient cooperation and the risks of positioning.

CT imaging greatly enhances the detail with which bony, soft tissue, and spinal cord injuries can be identified. Both CT and MRI scans have their particular advantages and provide supplemental information for diagnosis and management decisions. CT scan is superior for detailed information about bony structures and fractures, whereas MRI provides better detail on soft tissues, including the spinal cord, ligaments, and discs.

Early Medical Management of Spinal Cord Injury

After initial stabilization and assessment in the ED, the SCI patient will most likely be admitted to the intensive care unit (ICU). In the ICU, a mechanical ventilator and supplemental oxygen, IV fluids, continuous cardiac monitoring, an indwelling urinary catheter, a nasogastric tube, elastic hose (i.e., TEDs), and sequential compression boots are provided. Depending on acuity, invasive monitoring with an arterial line and pulmonary artery catheter may be necessary. Other monitoring equipment is ordered as needed. After resuscitation measures are complete, further treatment decisions are made. The patient is continuously monitored for potential complications, which are treated promptly as they occur.

Selection of Treatment Approach: Surgical or Nonsurgical

The primary goal in treating spinal injury is to optimize outcomes by preserving or improving neurological function.[35] Treatment is directed at neural decompression, spinal realignment, and stabilization through either a nonsurgical or surgical approach. Decompression and stabilization may be done on an emergency basis, especially if neurological deterioration is apparent on serial neurological assessment. Stabilization is important to prevent new or further extension of neurological damage. The management of the patient depends on the type of SCI, the associated injuries, or the patient's other health problems, if any.

- **Neural decompression** of the spinal cord or spinal nerves is the first priority in preserving neurological function. Decompression is necessary to control and/or eliminate ischemia and necrosis in the involved spinal area. For treatment, either skeletal traction or immediate surgery is available. If surgery is chosen, a decompression laminectomy is the usual procedure.
- **Closed spinal realignment/reduction** of the vertebral column is necessary to re-establish normal spinal alignment and curvatures. Reduction is often associated with decompression management. Skeletal traction, a halo and vest application, and braces have been the mainstays of reduction. If the vertebral facets are locked, surgical intervention may be necessary to unlock the facets and align the vertebrae.
- **Stabilization** of the spinal column is accomplished with surgical instrumentation or by spontaneous fusion during the natural healing process. Skeletal traction and immobilization promote the natural healing process. These treatment options can be used alone or in combination with surgery to achieve the desired outcome. If surgery is indicated, stabilization is achieved either by fusing the spine using an analogous bone graft or by stabilizing the spine with the insertion of instrumentation (see later discussion).

SURGICAL MANAGEMENT OF SPINAL CORD INJURY

Neurological assessment data and imaging studies provide the foundation for determining the best approach to treatment. If surgery is indicated, selecting the best time for surgery is critical. Early surgery (within the first 12 to 24 hours) can preserve or improve spinal cord function. However, other clinicians prefer to have the patient well stabilized before proceeding to surgery. The following are reasons for early surgery:

- Evidence of cord compression
- Progressive neurological deficit
- Compound fracture of the vertebra (potential for bony fragments to dislodge and penetrate the cord)
- Penetrating wounds of the spinal cord or surrounding structures
- A bone fragment evident in the spinal canal

Early surgery is usually postponed in the following circumstances:

- When rapid and significant improvement in neurological function is demonstrated
- When staging is necessary, for instance, the need before surgery to first realign the vertebral column or to reduce dislocations or fracture-dislocations through traction or immobilization

• When a life-threatening injury or disease exists elsewhere in the body. With severe trauma, the patient may have other injuries such as a brain injury, contused kidney, cardiac contusion, intestinal rupture, or other problems in addition to SCI. Emergency surgery for life-threatening injuries, such as a ruptured spleen, may be necessary. The patient's condition may not be stable enough to tolerate prolonged anesthesia and spinal surgery.

Types of Procedures

For neural decompression, a posterior (most common), anterior, or lateral laminectomy is performed. For stabilization, the most common procedure is a posterior laminectomy. An open reduction and internal fixation with instrumentation is performed that utilizes plates, screws, wires, and rods. A fusion, using autologous iliac bone graft, may also be performed. It is beyond the scope of this text to summarize the selection criteria for surgical options or surgical instrumentation. Laminectomy and spinal fusion, along with nursing care, are discussed in Chapter 19.

All instrumentation systems have the same basic components that include a vertical device and a fixation or anchoring device.[14] The *vertical device* is a rod or a plate that is attached lengthwise to the vertebral column to provide stabilization. *Fixation or anchoring devices*, which attach the vertical rod or plate to the vertebra, are wires, screws, or hooks oriented at right angles to the vertical device. All systems pose potential complications because of system failure as well as postoperative wound infection.[36] There are a number of available systems include Harrington rods, Luque rods, and the CD system.

Harrington rods, developed in the early 1960s, were originally the cornerstone of spinal surgery instrumentation. The Harrington rod system consists of a rod or rods and wires affixed to the base of spinous processes and to the rod. This provides multiple fixation points for stabilization. In some cases, loss of reduction with progressive kyphotic deformity occurred in patients treated with Harrington instrumentation.[37] Current instrumentation systems are much more rigid and allow for segmental spinal fusion. **CD rods,** introduced in the early 1990s, are an example. These rods, used in conjunction with lamina hooks or pedicle screws, are the current approach for thoracic lumbar instrumentation.[38] This system provides for multiple points of fixation and greater stabilization. CD rod placement, although technically more difficult, does not usually require postoperative immobility. Ideally, use of CD instrumentation facilitates early mobility of the patient.

NONSURGICAL MANAGEMENT OF SPINAL CORD INJURIES

Nonsurgical management of the patient with an SCI commonly involves immobilization with a halo vest or brace and traction for reduction and realignment, singularly or more often in combination. Vertebral subluxation with or without cord involvement is often managed with immobilization with a halo vest and traction.

Approaches to Management Based on the Level of Injury

Cervical Injuries

Cervical Traction. Cervical traction is used much less frequently with the advent of earlier and better surgical stabilization. When cervical traction is used, its purpose is realignment or reduction of cervical vertebral dislocations. The most common type of cervical traction is the versatile halo traction system (described below). Skeletal traction greatly facilitates care and enhances patient comfort. After traction is in place, pain is greatly decreased or completely relieved. Traction ameliorates pain by separating and aligning the injured vertebrae and by reducing or eliminating spasms in the distracted muscles.

A regular, firm hospital bed is used with cervical traction. Some physicians prefer using one of the many special beds available. Depending on the type of injury and method of immobilization, special beds may be used to decrease the possibility of pressure areas. When in traction, a special technique is used to safely turn the patient for skin care and to change position to reduce pressure.

The Halo System. The halo is the most frequently ordered method for cervical and high thoracic vertebral injuries. The following are two uses for the halo

• Direct skeletal traction involving the application of hanging weights; the patient is maintained on complete bed rest and managed with special nursing care techniques (Fig. 18-14).

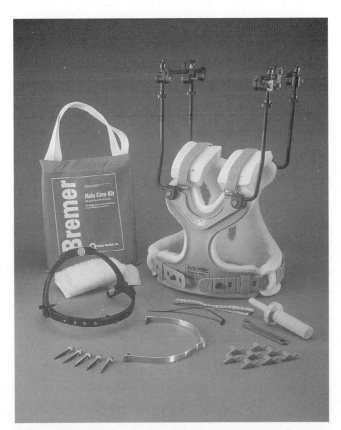

Figure 18-14 • Halo cervical skeletal traction. (Courtesy of Acromed Corp., Cleveland, OH.)

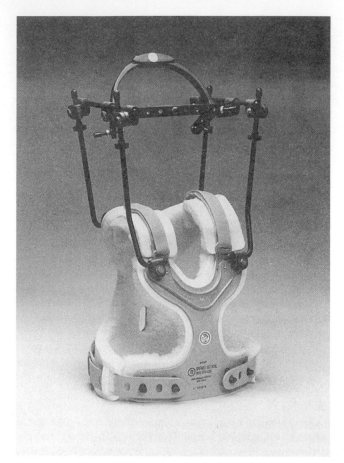

Figure 18-15 • Halo and vest. A lightweight, fleece-lined vest with a halo may be used to stabilize cervical vertebrae. Note that the vest comes in various sizes and does not need to be removed for magnetic resonance imaging studies. (Courtesy of Bremer Medical, Inc., Dawin Road, Jacksonville, FL 32207.)

• With a special body vest to stabilize the spine and allow healing. Ambulation is possible if the patient is neurologically intact (Fig. 18-15).

Using local anesthesia,[39] the halo (a metal ring) is inserted into the external bony table of the cranium and fixed with four pins, two posterior and two anterior. If direct traction is desired, a rope with hanging weights is applied. If immobilization and stabilization are desired, a vest with external metal rods is attached to the halo ring.[40] Small, dry, sterile dressings are placed around the pin sites.[41] Despite its appearance, the halo is comfortable, although some patients may develop a headache initially. In addition, any sound caused by bumping the halo can result in annoying vibrations. Rubber tips may be added to the pins to reduce this problem.

Using the halo for immobilization and fixation or stabilization allows for a shorter period of hospitalization, an outstanding cost advantage. If no paralysis exists, the patient is able to ambulate, thereby counteracting the multitude of potential problems associated with bed rest and immobility. The halo with vest is beneficial in cervical and very high thoracic fractures. Another feature of the halo is that surgery can be performed while the patient is in halo traction. This avoids the risk of malalignment of the injured area or extension of cord injury that could occur without the traction device.[42]

> **CLINICAL PEARLS:** The physician often applies skeletal traction before surgery to reduce the injury. When the best alignment possible is achieved, surgery (usually spinal fusion) is scheduled.

Thoracic and Lumbar Injuries

Depending on the specific type of injury, various treatment options are available for a patient with a thoracic or lumbar fracture or fracture-dislocation. If indicated, the surgical procedure most frequently performed is a laminectomy with instrumentation for stabilization, with or without a fusion. The following may be used to maintain thoracic or lumbar alignment either as an adjunct to surgery or as the only management protocol for the injury:

• A fiberglass or plastic vest (the vest, which is fitted to the patient, provides immobilization and support to the injured area)
• A Jewett brace, which extends the length of the spinal column (i.e., provides support to the lower thoracic and lumbar region)
• Other specially designed braces or orthotics

Sacral and Coccygeal Injuries

The usual treatment for sacral and coccygeal fractures is bed rest. The affected area is supported by a low support corset or special brace. A cushioning device (e.g., gel-filled cushion) can provide relief from pain and discomfort in the supine position. Pain is increased by sitting on a hard surface, so this should be avoided. The patient should be evaluated for bowel, bladder, and sexual dysfunction. Surgery is considered if there is evidence of compression.

FOCUS ON COLLABORATIVE MANAGEMENT IN THE ACUTE AND POSTACUTE PHASES

Acute Phase

Managing the patient with an acute SCI requires coordinated and collaborative interdisciplinary care that focuses on the patient. A clinical pathway provides a structure to map and integrate all components of care, in a timely manner, to achieve optimal measurable outcomes. The clinical pathway unites interdisciplinary team members and fosters collaboration around patient needs and outcomes. The pathway facilitates timely communications among the disciplines and assists the case manager in understanding the comprehensive needs of the patient. The core of the professional multidisciplinary team is composed of physicians, nurses, a physical therapist, an occupational therapist, a respiratory therapist, a case manager, a nutritionist, and a social worker. The major areas of focus for the collaborative team are included in Table 18-4.

(text continues on page 438)

TABLE 18-4   SUMMARY OF THE COLLABORATIVE MANAGEMENT OF MULTISYSTEM PROBLEMS IN THE ACUTE PHASE AFTER SPINAL CORD INJURY

SYSTEM-SPECIFIC CONSIDERATIONS	PATIENT PROBLEMS/ NURSING DIAGNOSES AND COLLABORATIVE PROBLEMS	ASSESSMENT AND MONITORING DATA	MANAGEMENT AND INTERVENTIONS
Neurological System			
• The level and pattern of neurological loss depend on the level of injury and need to be assessed and monitored for change; change can result from extension of injury or ascending edema. • As a result of spinal shock, many motor, sensory, and reflex functions are lost. Many specific deficits are listed under the body system that they primarily affect. • Hypothermia and orthostatic hypotension are commonly seen in the acute phase. • The patient who is tetraplegic is completely dependent on the care provider for self-care and mobility. • Often a cerebral concussion was also sustained at the time of injury; often memory is impaired for the circumstance of injury.	**Patient problems/Nursing diagnoses** • Risk for Altered Body Temperature • Hypothermia • Knowledge Deficit • Impaired Memory • Pain, acute • Impaired Physical Mobility • Self-Care Deficit, complete • Self-Care Deficit, instrumental • Sensory/Perceptual Alterations • Sexual Dysfunction • Sleep Pattern Disturbance • Impaired Swallowing • Risk for Injury **Collaborative problems** • Increased intracranial pressure if also sustained a brain injury	**Clinical data** • Assess baseline and monitor highest sensory level, motor function, and reflexes. • Monitor vital signs. • Assess baseline and monitor routine neurological signs for evidence of a concomitant brain injury. **Laboratory data** • Magnetic resonance imaging (MRI) or computed tomography (CT) scan • Plain x-rays of spine	• Provide for total care needs of patient. • Make sure that the patient is on the right type of bed based on the stability of the fracture and personal characteristics of the patient, such as weight. • Provide information to patient and family as requested; recognize that information will need to be repeated because of inability to comprehend fully the impact of the injury. • Be alert for decreased neurological function as a result of edema.
Respiratory System			
• Can develop varying degrees of respiratory difficulty depending on the level of injury: Injury at C-4 or above: Paralysis of diaphragm requires ventilator support. C-5 to T-6: Diaphragm is spared, but intercostals (T-1–6) are involved; patient is at high risk for respiratory problems and may need oxygen and special respiratory support. Even with lower injuries (T-6–12 innervating the abdominal muscles), there may be minor respiratory deficits. Also, immobilization and bed rest will decrease respiratory function (e.g., vital capacity), regardless of the level of injury. • The probability of certain respiratory complications decreases the lower the injury because the diaphragm and intercostals are spared. • Patients who cannot cough or manage their own secretions need a special respiratory management program. • Cervical surgery (both the procedure itself and the associated anesthesia) increases the risk of postoperative respiratory complications; thus, an optimal time for surgery (when the respiratory system is in the best condition possible) is recommended.	**Patient problems/Nursing diagnoses** • Ineffective Airway Clearance • Risk for Aspiration • Ineffective Breathing Pattern • Impaired Gas Exchange • Inability to Sustain Spontaneous Ventilation • Risk for Respiratory Infection • Risk for Altered Respiratory Function **Collaborative problems** • Hypoxemia • Atelectasis, pneumonia • Pneumothorax • Respiratory arrest	**Clinical data** • Determine baseline respiratory status. (Auscultate chest; note breathing pattern; assess the patient's ability to cough and deep breathe effectively.) **Laboratory data** • Chest x-ray studies • Blood gas levels • Complete blood count (CBC) • Sputum cultures • Pulmonary function studies (e.g., vital capacity)	• Intubate and provide ventilator support if the diaphragm is paralyzed or if respiratory function is ineffective. (The mode setting will depend on the needs of the patient.) • Provide supplementary oxygen as necessary. • Perform respiratory regimen (chest percussion; respiratory toilet; suctioning for patency; deep breathing if on a ventilator or sighing on ventilator setting). • Consult with a pulmonary physician as necessary. • Provide tracheostomy care every 4 h to maintain patency. • Provide chest physical therapy (PT) and deep breathing exercises every 2–4 h; if the patient is unable to cough effectively, assist with coughing by firmly depressing the abdomen when the patient coughs (place hands below the rib cage and above the umbilicus).

(continued)

TABLE 18–4   SUMMARY OF THE COLLABORATIVE MANAGEMENT OF MULTISYSTEM PROBLEMS IN THE ACUTE PHASE AFTER SPINAL CORD INJURY (*Continued*)

SYSTEM-SPECIFIC CONSIDERATIONS	PATIENT PROBLEMS/ NURSING DIAGNOSES AND COLLABORATIVE PROBLEMS	ASSESSMENT AND MONITORING DATA	MANAGEMENT AND INTERVENTIONS
• Other risk factors contributing to altered respiratory function include immobilization; bed rest; smoking; preexisting pulmonary disease (e.g., chronic obstructive pulmonary disease); concurrent chest trauma (e.g., fractured ribs, contused lungs); anemia; and gastric distention or paralytic ileus. Gastric distention may be associated with vomiting, aspiration, and compromised lung expansion. • Alert: Ascending edema can rapidly cause respiratory difficulty that requires immediate intervention; monitor rate and pattern frequently.	—	—	• Provide for intermittent positive-pressure breathing (IPPB) every 4 h. • Provide for use of incentive spirometer every 4 h.

Cardiovascular System

• Loss of sympathetic input from the higher brain centers results in bradycardia and vasomotor paralysis (vasodilation of blood vessels below the level of injury), so blood pressure is lowered. • Orthostatic hypotension results in pooling of blood below the level of injury because of vasodilation; this causes hypotension and decreased blood return to the heart. • Pooling of blood, coupled with immobility, greatly increases the risk of vascularstasis and orthostatic hypotension.	**Patient problems/Nursing diagnoses** • Impaired Gas Exchange • Decreased Cardiac Output • Altered Tissue Perfusion • Risk for Peripheral Neurovascular Dysfunction **Collaborative problems** • Decreased cardiac output • Dysrhythmias • Deep vein thrombosis (DVT) • Hypovolemia	**Clinical data** • Monitor vital signs. • Provide cardiac monitoring. • Monitor response to elevation of head (orthostatic hypotension). • Observe for signs and symptoms of thrombophlebitis, DVT, and pulmonary embolus. **Laboratory data** • Electrocardiogram • Electrolyte, coagulation studies	• Treat any life-threatening arrhythmias. • Apply elastic hose sequential compression boots. • Prophylactic use of heparin (5000 U every 12 h) helps prevent DVTs; this is *contraindicated* if any internal bleeding is present or if surgery has been performed. • Use vasopressors as necessary. • Cardiology consult may be necessary, especially if a cardiac contusion is suspected. • Assess for arrhythmias by observing the cardiac monitor. • Monitor patient's response to elevation of the head (orthostatic hypotension). • Observe for signs and symptoms of DVT and pulmonary embolus.

Integumentary System (Skin)

• Loss of vasomotor tone, paralysis, and bed rest contribute to the development of pressure areas and skin breakdown. • Once developed, broken areas of skin are very difficult to heal; therefore, use of a bed type to relieve continuous pressure while maintaining alignment should be considered.	**Patient problems/Nursing diagnoses** • Risk for Peripheral Neurovascular Dysfunction • Impaired Skin Integrity • Impaired Tissue Integrity • Altered Peripheral Tissue Perfusion **Collaborative problems** • Pressure ulcers	**Clinical data** • Monitor for signs and symptoms of redness or breakdown.	• Provide skin care and turn patient every 2–4 h. • When a special bed (e.g., a Roto Rest bed) is in use, adapt care measures appropriately.

(*continued*)

TABLE 18–4 SUMMARY OF THE COLLABORATIVE MANAGEMENT OF MULTISYSTEM PROBLEMS IN THE ACUTE PHASE AFTER SPINAL CORD INJURY (Continued)

SYSTEM-SPECIFIC CONSIDERATIONS	PATIENT PROBLEMS/ NURSING DIAGNOSES AND COLLABORATIVE PROBLEMS	ASSESSMENT AND MONITORING DATA	MANAGEMENT AND INTERVENTIONS
Musculoskeletal System			
• Prolonged immobility and paralysis have significant effects on bone, joints, and muscles (see Table 18–5).	**Patient problems/Nursing diagnoses** • Disuse Syndrome • Impaired Physical Mobility • Altered Protection **Collaborative problems** • Contractures • Ankylosis • Muscle atrophy • Osteoporosis	**Clinical data** • Monitor range of motion of joints for development of deformities, spasticity, or ankylosis.	• Consult with physical therapist to develop individualized PT program. • Provide range-of-motion exercises once daily. • Position the patient's extremities in proper body alignment.
Gastrointestinal (GI) System			
• Peristalsis is lost with spinal shock, resulting in paralytic ileus. • A distended abdomen interferes with adequate respirations. • Stress ulcers and gastric hemorrhage can also occur; because sensation is lost, the patient cannot feel the pain of ulceration. • Monitor for constipation.	**Patient problems/Nursing diagnoses** • Ineffective Breathing Pattern • Risk for Altered Respiratory Function • Risk for Injury • Bowel Incontinence • Constipation **Collaborative problems** • Paralytic ileus • GI bleeding • Constipation	**Clinical data** • Perform abdominal auscultation for bowel sounds. • Monitor stools for occult blood. • Monitor gastric pH. **Laboratory data** • CBC • Decreased hemoglobin	• Immediately insert a nasogastric tube to intermittent suction (low) for GI decompression. • Maintain patient's NPO status until bowel sounds return and the nasogastric tube is removed. • Initiate a bowel program as soon as possible. • Maintain a pH >5.0 by using Maalox, 30 mL every 3 h. • Administer drugs (e.g., cimetidine) for gastric prophylaxis. • Administer stool softeners/laxatives to facilitate a bowel program.
Genitourinary System			
• Bladder reflexes and control of micturition from higher brain centers are lost with cord injury; atonic bladder results. • An atonic bladder (loss of bladder tone) is distended and predisposes the patient to urinary tract infections (UTIs).	**Patient problems/Nursing diagnoses** • Reflex Incontinence • Altered Pattern of Urinary Elimination • Urinary Retention • Risk for Infection **Collaborative problems** • Acute urinary retention • Urinary tract infection	**Clinical data** • Palpate suprapubic area for bladder distention. • Review intake and output record. **Laboratory data** • Urine culture and sensitivity, urinalysis, blood urea nitrogen, and creatinine	• Insert an indwelling urinary catheter immediately. • Remove catheter and initiate intermittent catheterization program every 6–8 h once the patient is stable. • Aggressively treat UTI. • Maintain an intake and output record. • Use aseptic technique when managing the indwelling catheter.
Metabolic (Nutritional) System			
• The method of providing nutrition will depend on the associated injuries, level of consciousness, and presence or absence of peristalsis. • The body needs sufficient fluid, carbohydrates, and protein for energy and tissue repair.	**Patient problems/Nursing diagnoses** • Altered Nutrition: Less than body requirements • Fluid Volume Deficit • Fluid Volume Excess **Collaborative problems** • Negative nitrogen balance • Electrolyte imbalances • Acidosis • Alkalosis • Hypoglycemia, hyperglycemia	**Clinical data** • Assess skin turgor and mucous membranes for adequacy of hydration. • Monitor weight two times a week. • Monitor muscle mass of extremities. **Laboratory data** • Albumin, electrolytes, and other indications of nutritional levels	• Maintain NPO status until peristalsis returns. • Nutrition consult is necessary as soon as possible. • Total parenteral nutrition may need to be considered. • Use GI tract, if not contraindicated, as soon as peristalsis returns.

(continued)

TABLE 18–4   SUMMARY OF THE COLLABORATIVE MANAGEMENT OF MULTISYSTEM PROBLEMS IN THE ACUTE PHASE AFTER SPINAL CORD INJURY (*Continued*)

SYSTEM-SPECIFIC CONSIDERATIONS	PATIENT PROBLEMS/ NURSING DIAGNOSES AND COLLABORATIVE PROBLEMS	ASSESSMENT AND MONITORING DATA	MANAGEMENT AND INTERVENTIONS
Psychological or Emotional Response			
• If the patient is conscious, he or she is usually in a state of shock and denies what has happened and the impact on lifestyle. • Allow the patient to ask questions when ready. • The family may require the most support as they begin to comprehend what has happened and its impact on personal and family function.	**Patient problems/Nursing diagnoses** • Impaired Adjustment • Anxiety • Body Image Disturbance • Confusion • Decisional Conflict • Defensive Coping • Ineffective Denial • Diversional Activity Deficit • Grieving • Ineffective Individual Coping • Personal Identity Disturbance • Powerlessness • Impaired Social Interaction **Collaborative problems** • Depression • Anxiety	**Clinical data** • Assess the patient to determine what he or she is ready to hear. • Assess the family unit and its response to the injury and its impact.	• Be supportive of the patient and family. • Provide comprehensive information. • Make appropriate referrals for support.

After the patient has been physiologically stabilized and the vertebral column is also stable, rehabilitation efforts are begun. An increasingly precise picture of the extent of the overall deficits and how they will affect the patient's former lifestyle begins to emerge. Because level of consciousness (LOS) in acute care hospitalization is short, coordinated care is critical. In the current health care delivery system the continuum of care may also include subacute care, day hospitals, and community-based care. Careful coordination is necessary to move the patient along the continuum to provide seamless care. In conceptualizing the rehabilitation process, it must be recognized that rehabilitation is not complete until integration back into the community and into previous functional roles is achieved to the degree possible.

CLINICAL VIGNETTE: JC is a 24-year-old man who was traveling at high speed in his car when he skidded and hit a tree. He was wearing a seatbelt that was not on properly. He sustained a hyperflexion cervical neck injury. At the scene he was found unconscious, extricated from the vehicle, and then placed on a backboard. His vital signs were 94/64 with a pulse of 78 and respirations of 18. Upon arrival in the ED, he was conscious, but confused. He could not move his legs and had gross movement of his right arm and no movement of his left arm. Some light touch was intact on his arms and later on his right leg. His vital signs 2 hours after injury were 88/60 with a pulse of 70 and respirations of 18. On neurological exam his motor and sensory exam was the same except he had more light touch sensation on his right side. A diagnosis of anterior cord syndrome was made with fracture at C-6. He was placed in halo traction to align locked facets. Surgical fixation was planned later. His blood pressure increased gradually to 110/70 and pulse of 78. On further exam, the perineal area had intact sensation and the anal wink reflex was intact. He had a prognosis for a good recovery.

MAJOR PATIENT MANAGEMENT RESPONSIBILITIES OF THE NURSE

Selection of a Bed

Special beds are available that have been designed to provide support to the vertebral column, decrease the risk of multisystem complications associated with immobility, and facilitate administration of nursing care. Because of the additional cost associated with use of these beds, criteria should be established to determine appropriate bed use.

Signs and Symptoms of Acute Spinal Cord Trauma

The signs and symptoms of spinal cord trauma have been discussed in the previous section. The higher the level of injury, the greater will be the loss of motor, sensory, and reflex function. See Table 18-3 for a description of the functional loss that relates to specific levels of injury. The following section discusses several concurrent conditions associated with an acute SCI.

Spinal Shock and Related Neurogenic Shock

The temporary loss of autonomic function associated with neurogenic shock affects vital signs. Blood pressure is mildly decreased (especially with cervical injuries), and bradycardia is present. A cardiac monitor can monitor the patient for cardiac arrhythmias. The low blood pressure is related, in part, to orthostatic hypotension (see below). The ability to perspire is lost below the level of injury, so body temperature is responsive to the ambient room temperature. Most often, the temperature is low (possibly dropping to 95°F). In hot weather, the body temperature may be elevated, if temperature control is not available.

Orthostatic Hypotension

Orthostatic hypotension is defined as a rapid drop in blood pressure when the vertical position is assumed. Because the blood supply to the brain is inadequate, syncope results. Cerebral ischemia or stroke can result if the condition is not rectified. This condition is seen in patients who have been bedridden for a prolonged period, are postoperative from a lumbar sympathectomy, or have new SCI related to neurogenic shock.

With acute cervical and high thoracic SCI, the blood pressure tends to be unstable and lowered. After 1 to 2 weeks, it gradually rises until it is stabilized at a reading that corresponds to the preinjury norm for the patient. Orthostatic hypotension can impede the rehabilitative process if the patient cannot be raised in bed or assume the vertical position. Physiologically, orthostatic hypotension is caused by loss of arteriole vasomotor tone below the level of the lesion, which leads to a drop in arterial blood pressure when the patient assumes an upright position. Pooling of blood in the abdomen and lower extremities hampers adequate blood supply to the brain. Orthostatic hypotension is seen particularly in cord-injured patients with lesions above the T-7 level. Even slightly raising the head of the bed for a new tetraplegic patient can result in a drastic lowering of blood pressure.

Atonic Bladder

An atonic bladder is initially managed with an indwelling catheter for 24 to 48 hours. The nurse should follow meticulous aseptic technique in managing the catheter to prevent infections. As soon as possible, the catheter is removed and an intermittent catheterization program is initiated. There is urgency attached to early catheter removal because extended use of an indwelling catheter predisposes the patient to risk of urinary tract infection.

Ascending Spinal Cord Edema

With spinal cord trauma, edema develops soon after injury as a physiologic response. The swelling results in cord compression and compounds the functional loss. This is potentially life threatening, especially in association with cervical or high thoracic injury. Because edema can ascend the cord quickly and affect the C-4 level and above (the phrenic nerve innervates the diaphragm), a patient with previously adequate respirations may rapidly develop respiratory difficulty.

The spinal cord tolerates cord compression poorly. Permanent loss of function may result from frank damage to the cord itself, or temporary loss may occur related to exaggerated edema. With resolution of the edema, some functional return is possible, provided that irreversible damage has not been sustained. It is of critical importance for the nurse to observe the patient's status frequently for signs of deterioration from baseline function, especially in the early, acute phase of injury (during the first 72 hours or so).

CLINICAL PEARLS: Monitor the highest sensory and motor level frequently in the first 72 hours and document. Ascending edema can develop rapidly and result in respiratory difficulty in patients with cervical SCIs.

Respiratory Insufficiency

With C-1 to C-4 injuries, the intercostal muscles and often the diaphragm are paralyzed.[43] The patient depends on a ventilator for respiratory support. Although the diaphragm is spared in injuries at C-5 or below, a ventilator may be necessary in the acute phase owing to ascending cord edema. Evidence-based protocols are useful to guide rehabilitation and weaning of ventilator-dependent cervical SCI patients.[44] Related patient problems are listed in Table 18-4.

CLINICAL PEARLS: Carefully assess the respiratory rate, chest wall expansion, abdominal wall movement, cough, and chest wall for respiratory compromise. Arterial blood gases and pulse oximetry are useful at the bedside to monitor for hypoxia.

Paralytic Ileus

A nasogastric tube is often inserted and connected to suction to decompress the stomach and prevent vomiting and aspiration, and to facilitate free diaphragmatic movement. Acute paralytic ileus, characterized by abdominal distention, nausea, vomiting, and the absence of normal peristalsis, occurs with postacute SCIs. Paralytic ileus is not only a sign of spinal shock syndrome, but also can indicate intra-abdominal injury. Normally, the patient with an intra-abdominal injury will experience pain, but with an SCI, the sensation of pain may be lost.

CLINICAL VIGNETTE: Twenty-four hours after an SCI at level C-6, bowel sounds were absent. The cervical spine had been cleared. A nasogastric tube was inserted to decompress the gastrointestinal tract since it appeared that paralytic ileus had developed. The tube was necessary not only for decompression, but also to prevent vomiting and possible aspiration.

Deep Vein Thrombosis and Thromboembolism Prophylaxis

Patients with SCIs, and especially those with cervical SCIs, are at high risk for development of deep venous thrombosis (DVT) and thromboembolism (TE) that result in pulmonary embolism (PE). The contributing factors are immobility, flaccidity, and decreased vasomotor tone in the blood vessels below the level of injury. In addition to thigh-high elastic stockings, recommended prevention strategies include[45]:

- Use of low-molecular-weight heparins, rotating beds, adjusted-dose heparin, or a combination of modalities
- Low-dose heparin in combination with pneumatic compression stockings or electrical stimulation

Fatal PEs are reported in 1% to 2% of all patients with SCI within the first 3 months of injury. Focal pain, a common symptom of DVT, may not be noticed by SCI patients because of sensory deficits. Unilateral edema of the leg may be noted. Common laboratory studies include the D-dimer assay. Testing for those patients at higher risk of DVT includes impedance plethysmography, radiocontrast venography, Doppler ultrasound, and ventilation/perfusion lung scan.[46] For patients who have not achieved success with anticoagulation preventive therapy, a vena cava filter may be indicated. Prevention of thromboembolism continues into the rehabilitation phase and chronic phase of SCI.[47]

Pressure Ulcers

Patients with SCI are at high risk for the development of pressure ulcers. Clinical practice guidelines for prevention of pressure ulcers in spinal cord patients are available.[48] The high risk associated with use of backboards was discussed earlier in this chapter. Areas with sensory loss are at high risk for skin breakdown if relief from pressure is not provided. Special beds designed to relieve pressure are useful and cost effective for prevention.

After the patient is seated, relieve weight on the ischial tuberosities at frequent intervals (e.g., every 15 minutes initially), and gradually increase the time. Gel pads and other devices designed to relieve pressure are useful. A skin management and prevention program is an important responsibility, which is discussed in Chapter 11.

Nursing Assessment

The nursing database begins with the nursing history and assessment at the time of admission. Data collected in the history are part of the database for discharge planning, which is initiated during admission. Information about the family unit, work and leisure activities, and previous coping patterns is helpful in individualizing the plan of care. Assessment includes vital signs, neurological signs, spinal cord assessment, monitoring of laboratory data, and overall body systems assessment. Many physiologic assessment data are collected from instrument monitoring and a computer interface.

Vital Signs

Monitor vital signs frequently. A lower than expected blood pressure, bradycardia, and abnormal temperature may be noted, especially with cervical cord injuries. The basis for these changes in relationship to spinal cord trauma is discussed in the section of this chapter on neurogenic shock. However, SCI patients who have sustained concurrent trauma to other body systems may exhibit vital sign changes (hypovolemic shock) related to these other injuries. Because some injuries may not be noted immediately, a change in vital signs may be the first sign of occult internal hemorrhage or other potentially life-threatening problems. Therefore, frequent monitoring of vital signs for change and trends is important.

Neurological Signs

An abbreviated neurological assessment is conducted periodically, including evaluation of the level of consciousness and pupillary response. Patients with SCIs often have con-

current brain injuries of varying severity. A standard neurological assessment sheet may be used.

> **CLINICAL PEARLS:** Frequent (every 2 hours) neurological assessment and monitoring for trends is especially critical in the first 24 hours because of functional changes related to spinal shock changes, neurogenic shock, and the potential for occult injuries related to hypovolemic shock. After that time, assuming that the patient is physiologically stable, the time interval between assessments can be increased to every 4 hours and later to every 8 hours.

Spinal Cord Assessment Sheet

To determine exactly which functional levels remain intact, an extensive motor, sensory, and reflex assessment is necessary. A facility-created form, the ASIA Motor and Sensory Assessment form, or Chart 18-3 may be used for systematic assessment. Information collected in this database helps the nurse monitor the patient for neurological change and facilitates development of an individualized plan of care based on functional loss.

Body Systems Review

There are two reasons for conducting a systematic assessment of body systems in the patient with SCI. The first is to determine the location and extent of injuries to body systems other than the neurological system. The second is to determine the impact of the neurological injuries on other body systems (see Table 18-4).

Injuries to Other Body Systems. As discussed previously, patients with SCIs often sustain injury to other body systems as well. It is therefore important to consider the possibility of other injuries when assessing the patient. This assessment is complicated by the fact that all sensations are lost, including pain (often an indicator of a problem), below the level of injury. Because pain cannot be used as an objective indicator of dysfunction in affected patients, the nurse must rely on other indicators, such as laboratory data, to assess the patient. For example, gastric hemorrhage may be heralded by pain, decreased levels of hematocrit and hemoglobin, and a decline in central venous pressure. The nurse will need to concentrate on indications other than pain to monitor the patient for hemorrhage especially if the SCI is cervical or high thoracic.

> **CLINICAL PEARLS:** Monitor the blood pressure and pulse to differentiate between neurogenic and hypovolemic shock (related to occult injury). Maintain a high level of suspicion for occult internal bleeding in trauma patients.

Impact of Neurological Injury on Other Body Systems. Assessment data for problems arising in the acute phase of SCI are included in Table 18-4.

CHART 18-3   Nursing Assessment of Spinal Cord Function

Part I. Motor Function			Part II. Reflexes		
Left	**Muscle Action**	**Right**	**Left**	**Deep Tendon Reflexes**	**Right**
	Abduct upper arm			Ankle Jerk — S-1, S-2	
	Adduct upper arm			Knee Jerk — L-3, L-4	
	Extend upper arm			Biceps — C-5, C-6	
	Flex elbow			Triceps — C-7, C-8	
	Extend elbow			**Superficial Reflexes**	
	Flex wrist			Perineal — S-3–5	
	Extend wrist			Abdominals, upper — T-8–10	
	Flex fingers			Abdominals, lower — T-10–12	
	Extend fingers			Gag — cranial nerve IX and X	
	Thumb opposition				
	Upper abdominals				
	Lower abdominals				
	Flex upper leg				
	Extend upper leg				
	Flex knee				
	Extend knee				
	Dorsiflex foot				
	Plantarflex foot				
	Extend big toe				

A few selected reflexes are assessed.

The grading of deep tendon reflexes is assessed using the following scale:

- 4+ = very brisk; markedly hyperactive, often with associated clonus
- 3+ = more brisk than average
- 2+ = average or normal
- 1+ = diminished response
- 0 = no response

The grading of superficial reflexes is assessed using the following scale:

- 1 = present
- 0 = absent

Motor function is assessed using the following scale:

- 5 = normal strength
- 4 = slight weakness; can tolerate only a moderate amount of resistance
- 3 = moderate weakness; full range of movement against gravity only (no resistance)
- 2 = severe weakness; can move only when gravity is eliminated
- 1 = very severe weakness; a weak muscle contraction palpated but no visible movement noted
- 0 = complete paralysis

(continued)

CHART **18-3**   **Nursing Assessment of Spinal Cord Function**   (Continued)

Part III. Sensory Function

Left		Level	Right		Left		Level	Right	
Pain	POS/VIB	Cervical	Pain	POS/VIB	Pain	POS/VIB	Sacral	Pain	POS/VIB
		1					1		
		2					2		
		3					3		
		4					4		
		5					5		
		6							
		7							
		8							
		Thoracic							
		1							
		2							
		3							
		4							
		5							
		6							
		7							
		8							
		9							
		10							
		11							
		12							
		Lumbar							
		1							
		2							
		3							
		4							
		5							

Two sensory modalities are assessed: pain (pinprick), which is controlled by the lateral spinothalamic tract, and position (or vibration), which is controlled by the posterior columns. Pain perception is tested with pinprick. Position is tested by moving the thumbs and big toes up and down. If vibration is tested, a 256-Hz tuning fork is used. Using a dermatome, dermatomic areas are tested on each side of the body separately.

Sensory function is assessed using the following scale:

- 2 = normal
- 1 = present but abnormal
- 0 = absent

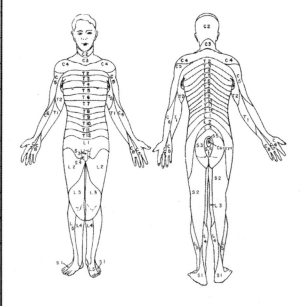

Dermatomes
Cutaneous distribution of the spinal nerves (See Figure 2-33, page 40. From Barr, M. L., and J. A. Kiernan [1988]. *The human nervous system* [5th ed]. Philadelphia: J. B. Lippincott.)

Laboratory Data

Laboratory data obtained during the acute phase of SCI include blood chemistry values (e.g., electrolyte studies, glucose and blood gas levels), microbiologic tests (e.g., cultures), and hematologic studies (e.g., complete blood count, hematocrit, hemoglobin). Also included among the diagnostic data are results from radiology (e.g., chest x-ray films, spinal films), imaging (e.g., CT scans, MRI), and other studies. Review of this database helps to correlate clinical observations of signs and symptoms with laboratory findings, to identify the need for special assessment and monitoring, and to determine specific nursing interventions.

Summary

Sources of data are numerous, and the needs of the patient can change dramatically, especially in the acute phase of SCI. Therefore, ongoing comprehensive assessment is required to provide a basis for analysis and to establish appropriate patient problems and nursing diagnoses.

Nursing Interventions

Given that patients admitted to the hospital with SCIs have self-care deficits, the nurse must determine to what degree the patient can perform such basic functions as bathing and hygiene, dressing and grooming, feeding, and toileting. The patient may be completely independent, in need of assistance, or completely dependent. An appropriate level of care is provided to meet basic needs. Other nursing interventions are included in Table 18-4. Based on the level of injury, the nurse can make some assumptions about patient needs (see Table 18-3).

Management of Cervical Skeletal Traction

Special protocols are used to manage patients who are being treated with halo cervical skeletal traction alone or combined with a vest used in association with the halo (Charts 18-4 and 18-5). Patients maintained in cervical traction are on complete bed rest and are at high risk for the multiple problems associated with immobility (see Table 11-2).

Spinal Cord Injury: Subacute Problems

In considering the comprehensive needs of patients along the continuum of care, several conditions can develop as the patient moves from the acute to the subacute phase. They include autonomic hyperreflexia, spasticity, bladder dysfunction, bowel dysfunction, sexual dysfunction, and psychosocial responses.

Autonomic Dysreflexia. Autonomic dysreflexia (AD), also known as autonomic hyperreflexia, is an acute syndrome of excessive, uncontrolled sympathetic output that can occur in patients who have sustained an SCI at or above the T-6 level. It is caused by spinal reflex mechanisms that remain intact after injury that results in hypertension.[49] The most common cause of AD is lower urinary tract stimulations. Noxious stimuli that can precipitate autonomic hyperreflexia include a distended bladder secondary to a plugged catheter, urinary calculus, or cystitis; constipation or fecal impaction; acute abdominal lesions; operative incisions; uterine labor contractions; pressure on the glans penis; and stimulation from skin lesions, such as inguinal rash, pressure ulcer, or ingrown toenail.

Clinically, the symptoms seen are severe pounding bilateral headache, nasal congestion, malaise, nausea, anxiety, and sometimes blurred vision, shortness of breath, and erythema of face, neck, and trunk. Common signs include profuse perspiration above the level of the spinal lesion, piloerection, and cool, pale skin below the spinal cord lesion. In addition to hypertension, bradycardia (secondary to vagal stimulation) or tachycardia may also occur.[49] The systolic blood pressure may rise as high as 240/120 or higher. The significance of the rise in blood pressure is judged based on the patient's usual baseline readings. If severe hypertension is left untreated, retinal hemorrhage, hemorrhagic stroke, subarachnoid hemorrhage, seizures (including status epilepticus), pulmonary edema, or myocardial infarction may result.

The pathophysiology of autonomic hyperreflexia is complex (Fig. 18-16). Afferent impulses ascend the spinal cord, but because of the spinal injury, upward ascension to higher centers is interrupted. A mass reflex stimulation of the sympathetic chain and nerves *below* the spinal injury occurs. This causes arteriolar spasms of the pelvic and abdominal viscera and of the skin, resulting in vasoconstriction *below* the lesion. The vasoconstriction produces cold skin and gooseflesh in the involved area and raises blood pressure. Baroreceptors in the aortic arch and carotid sinus are stimulated, and a message is sent through the vagus nerve to the vasomotor center (in the medulla), causing reflex slowing of the heart (bradycardia) and vasodilation *above* the lesion. The bradycardia represents an attempt by the body to cause vasodilation and lower the blood pressure.

Management. Nursing management is aimed at preventing conditions that are known to trigger AD. Treatment is directed toward rapid assessment for underlying cause and removal of the noxious stimuli and lowering of the blood pressure. AD represents a *medical emergency* and should be treated accordingly.

- Elevate the head of the bed.
- Loosen any constricting clothing.
- Assess for underlying cause.
  - Assess the bladder for distention. If a catheter is in place, check it for evidence of obstructed flow, such as a kink in the tubing. If the catheter is plugged, immediately irrigate it with a small amount (about 30 mL) of solution. If it still does not drain, replace the catheter immediately.
  - In patients who are being catheterized intermittently, catheterize the patient immediately, regardless of the time that has elapsed since the last catheterization.
  - AD may be triggered during bowel care or defecation. If symptoms develop, cease all activities until symptoms subside. Assess the lower bowel for impaction. If impaction present, attempt disimpaction.

CHART 18-4   Summary of the Nursing Management of a Patient in Cervical Skeletal Halo Traction

PATIENT PROBLEMS/ NURSING DIAGNOSES	NURSING INTERVENTIONS	EXPECTED OUTCOME(S)
ORTHOPEDIC TRACTION EQUIPMENT		
• Risk for Injury	• Check the orthopedic frame and traction daily to ensure that nuts and bolts are secure. • Check tongs daily to be sure that they are secure. • Be sure that traction weights are hanging freely and not resting on the floor or frame. (Releasing the traction is dangerous because cord injury could be extended.)	• The orthopedic frame will remain intact. • Tongs will not slip. • Traction weights will hang freely. • There will not be any extension of cord injury secondary to slippage of the traction apparatus.
SKIN INTEGRITY		
• Risk for Infection • Impaired Skin Integrity	• Inspect tong sites, and clean and dress daily as ordered (may be referred to as "pin care"). • Turn the patient every 2 hours from side to back to other side using a triple log roll technique as described below if a patient is on a regular hospital bed.	• The pin site will remain free of infection. • Skin integrity will be maintained. • The vertebral column will be maintained in a neutral position and in proper alignment.
	• Nurse # 1 stands behind the head of the bed and places hands firmly on the patient's head and neck, maintaining them in a neutral position; the head and neck are turned as a unit. • Nurse #2 stands at the patient's side and moves the patient's shoulders. • Nurse #3 stands at the patient's side and moves the patient's hips and legs. • Plan ahead, identifying desired position and pillow placement *before* moving the patient. When all three nurses are ready, turn the patient as a log on the count of three. Leave the patient positioned in the middle of the bed (if not, he or she will be uncomfortable); use pillows to support the patient's body in alignment. • Nurse #1 should hold the head and neck until the patient is supported adequately (if traction slips, manual traction can be supplied by Nurse #1).	
BASIC CARE		
• Self-Care Deficits	• Provide for basic care needs that the patient cannot do for self.	• Basic care needs will be met.
RESPIRATORY SYSTEM		
• Risk for Aspiration • Ineffective Airway Clearance • Risk for Infection • Impaired Gas Exchange • *Note:* The patient on a ventilator will need special care.	• Have suction available to maintain a patent airway. • Provide respiratory care. • Provide for deep-breathing, assistive coughing, and incentive spirometer exercises every 1–2 hours.	• Airway patency will be maintained. • The patient will not aspirate. • The patient will not develop a respiratory infection.
CARDIOVASCULAR SYSTEM		
• Impaired Tissue Integrity (venous stasis) • Altered Peripheral Tissue Perfusion • Decreased Cardiac Output	• Maintain thigh-high elastic (TED) stockings and sequential compression boots. • If the patient is receiving heparin, observe for signs and symptoms of bleeding. • Monitor for deep vein thrombosis (DVT) and pulmonary emboli (may be receiving minidoses of subcutaneous heparin q12h, if not contraindicated).	• Air boots and TEDs will be worn at all times. • Vital signs will be maintained within normal limits. • The patient will be observed for DVT and pulmonary emboli.

(continued)

CHART 18-4 Summary of the Nursing Management of a Patient in Cervical Skeletal Halo Traction (Continued)

PATIENT PROBLEMS/ NURSING DIAGNOSES	NURSING INTERVENTIONS	EXPECTED OUTCOME(S)
MUSCULOSKELETAL SYSTEM • Risk for Disuse Syndrome • Pain (related to muscle spasm) • Sensory Perceptual Alterations: visual and tactile	• Provide comfort measures. • Provide range-of-motion exercises qid • Position the patient in proper body alignment. • Reposition the patient frequently. • Stretch the patient's heel cord with exercises.	• The patient will be free from pain. • Contractures will not develop. • Strategies will be used to manage spasticity if it occurs.
GASTROINTESTINAL SYSTEM • Colonic Constipation	• Institute a bowel retraining program. • Auscultate the abdomen for bowel sounds. • Record the frequency and consistency of stool.	• Pattern of bowel evacuation every 1–2 day will be established.
GENITOURINARY SYSTEM • Altered Urinary Elimination • Risk for Infection • Sexual Dysfunction	• Monitor intake and output. • Force fluids. • If an intermittent catheterization protocol is initiated, use aseptic technique. • If the patient is voiding on his or her own, monitor postvoid residuals. • Provide information about sexual function.	• Intake will be 3000 mL unless contraindicated. • Postvoid residuals will be <100 mL. • Strict aseptic technique will be used for catheter protocols. • Sexual function and spinal cord injury are discussed with the patient when he or she is ready.
NUTRITION • Altered Nutrition: Less than body requirements • Fluid Volume Deficit	• Encourage an adequate diet. • Ask the dietician to see the patient. • Provide for adequate fluid intake up to 3000 mL daily. • Encourage the patient to take small portions of food into the mouth and chew well to prevent aspiration. • Keep suction equipment handy.	• A diet high in protein and carbohydrates, which includes a fluid intake of up to 3000 mL, will be provided. • Aspiration will be prevented.
EMOTIONAL AND PSYCHOLOGICAL SUPPORT • Powerlessness • Social Isolation • Ineffective Individual Coping • Diversional Activity Deficit • Body Image Disturbance • Knowledge Deficit	• Provide for social interaction and diversion based on the patient's functional level. • Reinforce a positive self-image. • Allow the patient to participate in decision making as much as possible. • Provide for patient teaching.	• The patient's mental health will be supported. • Social interaction and diversion will be provided based on the patient's ability to participate. • A positive body image will be supported. • Necessary information will be provided.

• Check skin and toenails for pressure ulceration or infection; spray with topical anesthetic.
• Monitor vital signs frequently (every 5 minutes).
• Antihypertensive drugs may be ordered to lower severe hypertension.

Prevention is the best approach. For patients discharged home or in community-based care, patients at risk need to be aware of the signs and symptoms of AD and know what can be done if they occur.

Neurogenic Heterotopic Ossification. Neurogenic heterotopic ossification (NHO) is characterized by the formation of new extraosseous (heterotopic) bone in soft tissue surrounding peripheral joints in patients with neurological disorders.[50] The cause is unclear. In SCI the incidence is in the range of

CHART **18-5**	**Summary of Nursing Management of the Patient in a Halo With Vest**

NURSING RESPONSIBILITIES

RATIONALE

MANAGEMENT OF THE HALO DEVICE AND THE BODY VEST

- Check the pins on the halo ring to be sure they are secure and tight.
- Check the edges of the fiberglass vest for comfort and fit by inserting the small finger or index finger between the vest and the patient's skin. If the vest is too tight, skin breakdown, edema, and possible nerve injury can occur.
- The vest should be supported while the patient is in bed.
- Place a rubber cork over the tips of the halo device to diminish magnification of sound if the pin is bumped.

- Ensures safety and integrity of the treatment
- Provides for comfort and prevents skin irritation

- Maintains proper body alignment
- Provides for comfort

METICULOUS SKIN CARE

- Inspect and cleanse the pin site once or twice daily, as prescribed, to prevent infection.
- Turn the patient in bed every 2 hour by means of the triple log roll technique to prevent the development of hypostatic pneumonia, atelectasis, and skin breakdown.
- Provide sponge pads to prevent pressure on prominent body areas, such as the forehead and shoulder, while the patient is in bed.
- Inspect under the vest, and keep all areas of skin dry.

- Maintains skin integrity and monitors the patient for infections

- Maintains proper body alignment and prevents injury

- Prevents injury and irritation to the skin

- Provides early identification of skin irritation or breakdown

ALTERED BODY IMAGE

- Help the patient adjust to the distorted body image that the halo device can create.

- Supports the patient's emotional well-being

CONTROL OF PAIN: COMFORT

- Administer mild analgesics to control headache and discomfort, which are common, around the pin site.
- Provide a soft diet, because many patients have jaw pain if they attempt to chew.

- Provides for comfort

- Provides for comfort

BASIC HYGIENIC CARE

- Encourage self-care as much as possible.

- Maintains the patient's independence and supports selfesteem

SUPPORT OF BODY SYSTEMS

- Maintain an intake and output record.

- Provide for a bowel program.

- Provide for range-of-motion exercises for all extremities.
- Provide for deep-breathing exercises at least four times daily.

- Apply thigh-high elastic hose (TED) to the legs to improve blood return to the heart.
- Observe the legs for development of thrombophlebitis or deep vein thrombosis.

- Provides information on urinary tract function and adequacy of fluid intake
- Prevents constipation and maintains a normal pattern of bowel evacuation
- Maintains muscle tone
- Encourages hyperinflation of the lungs and prevents infections and atelectasis
- Decreases the possibility of thrombus or embolus formation

- Allows early identification of potential problems so that treatment can be initiated

ASSESSMENT DATA

- Monitor neurological signs, vital signs, and vital capacity.

- Establishes a baseline and indicates change

(continued)

CHART 18-5   Summary of Nursing Management of the Patient in a Halo With Vest   (Continued)

NURSING RESPONSIBILITIES	RATIONALE

AMBULATION

If the patient's neurological function is intact, he or she will be able to ambulate in the halo ring and vest.

- Start to assess the patient's tolerance of the upright position by having him or her sit on the edge of the bed ("dangle"). Check vital signs. (Orthostatic hypotension may be a problem to overcome in the early stages.)
- Teach the patient to compensate for lost head and neck movement by making increased use of eye movement to scan the area.
- Accompany patients when ambulating because they are more accident prone owing to a displaced center of gravity, a tendency for loss of balance, and decreased peripheral vision.
- Consider the patient's use of a walker for ambulation as a means of support and greater safety.

- Prevents development of untoward side effects

- Provides for safety needs

- Same as above

- Same as above

PATIENT TEACHING

- If the patient is to go home with the halo and vest, begin a patient and family teaching plan using a booklet or other printed material. Review any written material prepared by the manufacturer for accuracy before giving it to the patient or family.

- Provides for safety and independence
- Meets the patient's and family's knowledge needs

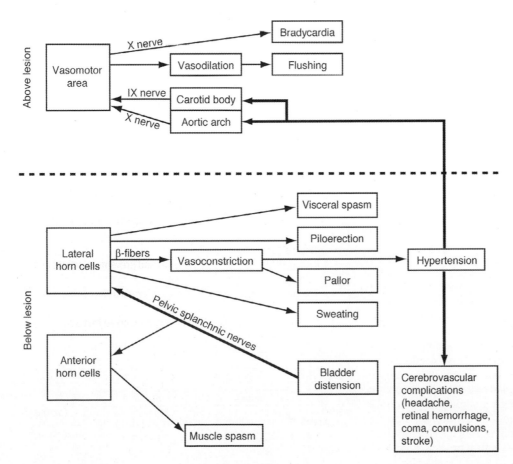

Figure 18-16 • Mechanism of autonomic hyperreflexia.

10% to 53%. The range of clinical presentation is wide from an incidental finding on x-ray to reduction in range-of-motion limitation (20% to 30%) to complete ankylosis (3% to 8%) of peripheral joints.

NHO always develops below the level of the SCI; it is most common in the hip. Other less affected joints in descending order include the knee, elbow, shoulder, hand, and spine. It is generally diagnosed between 1 and 6 months after injury, with 2 being months the mean. The signs and symptoms mimic those of acute arthritis with the exception that pain in SCI patients may be absent because of loss of sensation. Limitation in range of motion may be the first sign noted, followed by swelling of the affected limb.[50] Diagnosis of NHO is based on clinical signs. Periarticular erythema and warmth may also occur, sometimes with a low-grade fever.

The treatment for NHO includes sodium etidronate (20 mg/kg for the first 2 weeks followed by 10 mg/kg for 2.5 months for a total treatment period of 3 months), nonsteroidal anti-inflammatory drugs, and irradiation.[50–52] Surgical resection may be indicated to improve joint motion. Because NHO that exists at the time of diagnosis is not reversible, treatment is directed at prevention of further progression of the process. For patients with significant limitation of range of motion, surgery may be considered in 12 to 18 months. The time lapse allows for the maturation of the heterotopic bone, which minimizes the likelihood of recurrence. Surgery is directed at increasing the range of motion of the hip so that the patient can sit in a wheelchair without undue pressure. Because NHO can be the cause of significant pain and limitation of range of motion, its presence can significantly impede the rehabilitation phase and the achievement of an optimal outcome.

Spasticity.

Spasticity is a motor disorder characterized by an abnormal, velocity-dependent (i.e., how fast the joint is moved through its range of motion) increase in muscle tone resulting from interruption of the neural circuitry regulating the muscles.[53,54] There is an increase in tonic stretch reflexes (muscle tone) with exaggerated tendon reflexes, resulting from hyperexcitability of the stretch reflex, a component of the upper motor neuron syndrome.[53] The pathophysiology of spasticity is not completely understood, and it has been suggested that there are various types of spasticity.[55] The pathophysiology of spasticity involves interruption of the descending inhibitory pathways, causing increased tonic activity of gamma motor neurons through spindle afferent impulses, and centrally through reticulospinal and vestibulospinal pathways that act mainly on alpha motor neurons.

Spasticity is a common occurrence in both complete and incomplete SCI patients after resolution of spinal shock; it has a negative impact on rehabilitation potential and quality of life through restriction of activities of daily living and compromises patient safety. Recovery from spinal shock is a gradual process in which the spinal neurons slowly regain their excitability. The earliest indication heralding the end of spinal shock is the return of the perianal reflexes (bulbocavernous and anal-cutaneous reflexes). The bulbocavernous reflex is tested by squeezing the glans penis or pulling on the indwelling catheter and observing for slight muscle contraction and retraction of the scrotum. The anal reflex is present if there is a puckering of the anal sphincter ("anal wink") during digital examination of the rectum or scratching of the skin around the anal region. Muscle contraction may also be noted when inserting a rectal thermometer. Perianal reflexes return before deep tendon reflexes.

After a period of 1 to 3 days to a few weeks postinjury, the flaccid, hyporeflexic state is gradually replaced by spastic hyperreflexia and bilateral Babinski responses.[56,57] The flexors of the arms and the extensors of the legs are predominantly affected, and the predominant pattern is flexion or extension. The initial appearance of spasticity may be a false ray of hope for the patient. The "movement" noted is often misinterpreted by the patient or family as a return of normal voluntary function, rather than a heightened reflex response. Spasticity must be explained clearly and concisely to prevent any misinterpretation of its significance.

Management. The degree of spasticity can be assessed using a modified Ashworth scale.[58] The major day-to-day nursing problems encountered with spasticity are the difficulty of positioning the patient and the impact of spasticity on activities of daily living and mobility training. Spasticity is a difficult problem best managed collaboratively. No one treatment option is successful for all patients so that the most conservative options are used first and then ascend from there. The continuum begins with physical rehabilitation modalities, pharmacologic therapy, injection techniques, intrathecal baclofen, and finally surgery.[59] A spasticity management algorithm is found in Figure 18-17. Physical therapy options include a focus on specific muscle groups with proper positioning, exercises (e.g., passive range-of-motion exercises, stretching exercises), weight bearing, muscle strengthening, cold-heat application, and splinting. Pharmacologic management includes baclofen, dantrolene sodium, diazepam, clonidine, tizanidine, gabapentin, and cyproheptadine.[53,60,61] Newer forms of adjunctive therapy include oral and transdermal forms of clonidine and tizanidine. Injection with chemodenervation agents, phenol, or ethanol has also been used. Botulism toxin A (Botox) and intrathecal baclofen are also useful for spasticity management.[62] According to Cochrane systematic review of the literature, there is insufficient evidence to assist clinicians in a rational approach to spasticity

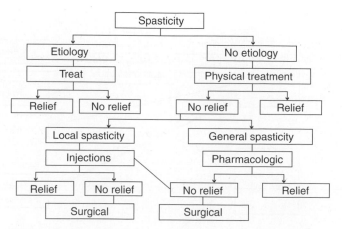

Figure 18-17 • Algorithm for spasticity management. (Adams, M. M., & Hicks, A. L. [2005]. Spasticity after spinal cord injury. *Spinal Cord, 43,* 577–586.)

management in SCI.[63] Surgical options include tendon lengthening, capsular release, rhizotomy, and dorsal root zone ablation.

> **CLINICAL PEARLS:** Factors that can increase spasticity include urinary tract infection, constipation, ingrown toe nails, pressure ulcers, and a poorly fitted brace or wheelchair.

The following are nursing interventions directed at preventing, controlling, or reducing spasticity:

- Provide passive range-of-motion exercises at least four times a day. Stiffness increases spasticity.
- Avoid circumstances that precipitate noxious stimuli known to increase spasticity (e.g., extremes in temperature, remaining in one position for an extended period, anxiety, pain, bladder or bowel distention, tight clothing or equipment, and decubitus ulcers).
- Turn and reposition the patient at least every 2 hours. Avoid rubbing or irritating the skin.
- Prevent the development of contractures. Flexor spasticity and contractures gravely limit the patient's ability to participate in activities of daily living (ADLs). Use proper positioning and consult with the physical therapist on the use of splints and for positioning options.
- Regard a sudden increase in spasticity as evidence of underlying noxious stimuli (e.g., a kink in the urinary drainage; fecal impaction; a skin abrasion or pressure ulcer; cold; and stiffness). The underlying cause should be treated or eliminated promptly.

Neurogenic Bladder and Retraining.

Urinary bladder control urination may be lost in SCI patients. Because prolonged use of a urinary catheter poses a major risk of urinary tract infections, earliest possible removal is indicated (24 to 48 hours)[64] and an intermittent catheterization protocol should be begun as soon as possible.[65] Aseptic technique, as well as careful handling of the catheter, drainage bag, and tubing, helps prevent urinary tract infections while the catheter is in place. As spinal shock resolves, a bladder retraining program can be instituted. Cystometric studies to evaluate bladder function may be scheduled. Various neurogenic bladder disorders are discussed in Chapter 11. A urinary antiseptic, such as methenamine mandelate, is often administered. Mandelamine is used for urinary tract infections. See Chapter 11 for a further discussion of bladder retraining.

Bowel Dysfunction and Bowel Retraining.

Most patients with SCIs are able to regain bowel control with an appropriate bowel training program.[66] An individualized bowel program is instituted and managed by the nurse (see Chap. 11). Prevention of constipation and fecal impaction is important for many reasons, including the risk of triggering autonomic hyperreflexia and of aggravating spasticity. The large bowel has its own neural center within the intestinal wall that responds to distention caused by feces. Dietary intake and digestive activities from the upper intestinal tract also influence bowel evacuation. The SCI affects bowel evacuation in the following way:

- Loss of the sensation of fullness in the lower abdomen or bowel
- Loss of awareness of bowel evacuation
- Loss of the ability to control the rectal sphincter
- Loss of the ability to contract the abdominal muscles and to expel the stool

In SCI patients, the abdominal muscles and diaphragm are used to facilitate bowel evacuation. If possible, position the patient comfortably with feet flat on the floor. If the abdominal muscles are impaired, the patient may be taught to exert pressure on the abdomen with the hands, or an abdominal belt may be recommended for someone who cannot strain at stool.

A well-balanced diet that is high in roughage, combined with an adequate fluid intake, produces softer stools and stimulates peristalsis. Medications, such as stool softeners, bulk producers, and lubricants, are also helpful. Mild cathartics and suppositories may be ordered. Digital dilation may be recommended. If these methods are not successful, a mild enema of limited fluid content can be administered.

A final important consideration is that selected body rhythms can be effectively used to help achieve bowel evacuation at predictable times. For example, the stimulus for defecation commonly occurs after meals because food is a stimulus for peristalsis, and peristalsis aids in moving the contents of the GI tract. The gastrocolic reflex responsible for strong contractions and peristalsis in the GI tract can be initiated by feeding the patient warm fluids and food at any time of the day. Therefore, planning for bowel evacuation and retraining should capitalize on normal body rhythms.

Bowel training must be a planned activity and must be individualized. Collaboration among the patient, nurse, and physician is necessary for successful outcomes. Patience and an optimistic attitude are necessary to provide a climate for success.

Sexual Dysfunction.

Sexuality and sexual adjustment should be an integral part of the overall rehabilitation for SCI patients. Sexual function is controlled by spinal levels S-2, S-3, and S-4. Therefore, several complete and incomplete SCI syndromes can affect sexual function. The initial step is referral to a physician who focuses on sexual dysfunction, such as a urologist, for diagnosis of specific problems and to provide information and options to a patient. Further counseling and education by a health care professional skilled in SCI and sexual function, both alone and with the patient's partner, are useful for successful adaptation.

Sexually active patients need counseling in birth control methods. Because the use of certain types of oral contraceptives may increase the risk of thrombophlebitis for women, careful determination of the best choice is important for the SCI patient.

Psychological Responses.

The impact of catastrophic illness, coupled with devastating functional loss, is overwhelming to the patient and family. Comprehensive patient and family education and support are required, as are sensitivity and compassion. The nurse should acknowledge the losses while being optimistic for the future with quality of life. The patient and family need accurate and comprehensive information to make appropriate decisions. Timing of information, that is, what information is provided at what point in the illness, is critical to prevent overwhelming the patient and family. In addition to the support provided by the individual practitioner, patient-centered conferences or family meetings incorporating an interdisciplinary team approach are useful in supporting the patient and family. A psychiatric consultation may be helpful for some patients.

The rapidity with which patients move from acute care settings to rehabilitation has been accelerated by managed care. Patients often do not have sufficient time to begin to process what has happened to them and what it means to their personhood. Psychological adaptation is a function of time.[67] A wide range of emotional responses are experienced by the patient with an SCI as he or she progresses from the acute to the rehabilitation phase. The sensory losses associated with SCI and the subsequent immobilization create sensory and perceptual alterations. Immobilization and confinement to bed by traction or paralysis limit and distort visual and auditory stimuli. For instance, vision may become distorted for the patient on bed rest, so that although fully aware of the ceiling, the upper half of the walls, and people from the waist up, he or she may not visualize most objects in their totality. A paralyzed patient may not even be able to scratch his or her nose. Confinement represents limited territoriality, with lack of control over access to one's surroundings. For those accustomed to using physical activity to relieve stress, immobility negates this stress reduction strategy. As a result, physical immobility can lead to psychological distress.

As the nurse assesses the patient and family, several of the following patient problems may be applicable: anxiety; fear; body image disturbance; ineffective coping; loneliness; dysfunctional grieving; personal identity disturbance; powerlessness; self-esteem disturbance; hopelessness; social isolation; and spiritual distress. In addition, the emotional and psychological responses of the family may require intervention. Family-focused nursing diagnoses include ineffective family coping and altered family processes.

Psychological Response: A Model for Intervention. Sudden catastrophic injury precipitates a crisis. Crisis theory and adjustment to long-term disability provide the nurse with a framework for viewing SCI and an approach to intervention.

Spinal trauma, a catastrophic event, is met with shock, disbelief, and denial. Initially, much of the activity in the hospital is directed toward life-saving measures and stabilization of the patient. The focus is on survival. If the patient is conscious, he or she is usually in a state of emotional shock. Shock and disbelief then evolve into denial. Patients who are experiencing denial do not believe that what they are being told has any bearing on their lives. They may acknowledge some of their injuries but may deny or downplay the seriousness of others. For example, a patient may recognize and acknowledge that his or her legs are dysfunctional but may believe that this is just a temporary state. Such patients may be convinced that next week or the week after, they will be back to normal. The nurse should listen but give no false hope. Focusing on the present helps to keep the patient firmly grounded in reality.[68]

The next stage is one of reaction, and it often lasts for a long time. There may be an acknowledgment that significant losses of body function have occurred that affect the patient's degree of independence and lifestyle. Reactions, which are varied, may include anger, rage, depression,[69] bargaining, verbal abuse of caregivers and family, ideation of suicide, and inappropriate sexual behavior. Listening, gentle reminders of intact functions, and support are helpful during this stage. Any suggestions of suicide should be taken seriously and the patient protected from self-harm. Next, the person begins to seek information about the injury, what can be expected in terms of outcome, and how care will be managed. At this stage, he or she becomes an active participant in care and rehabilitation. The nurse should allow the patient as much independence as possible and encourage the patient's efforts to maintain control of decision making. Finally, the person begins to cope effectively, provided adaptation has progressed. During this phase the patient develops a plan for a productive life, considering the limitations imposed by the injury. At this time, the patient can be integrated into the community.

The entire adjustment process just described can take many years to achieve. The nurse should be aware that because many patients are transferred almost immediately to specialized care centers from other hospitals, they may be only at the stage of denial or early reaction at the time of transfer.

The Nurse's Role. Caring for a patient who has sustained an SCI requires an awareness of the impact that the illness has had on the patient's emotional and psychological equilibrium. The following general suggestions provide guidance for patient care:

- Establish a therapeutic nurse–patient relationship.
- Cultivate a climate of trust.
- Allow the verbalization of feelings.
- Accept behavior without being judgmental.
- Let the patient know that it will take time to adjust to the disability.
- Encourage questions, referring those that you are unable to answer to the appropriate resource.
- Include written documentation of emotional and psychological reaction.
- Incorporate steps for meeting emotional and psychological needs into the care plan.
- Promote a good self-concept and body image by encouraging good grooming.
- Use team conferences to discuss the patient's emotional and psychological status.
- Encourage participation in the decision-making process related to care to foster a feeling of self-control.

Discharge Planning

In a managed-care environment, major decisions related to discharge planning are made almost immediately, that is, during initial evaluation of the patient.[70] The case manager who assumes facilitating and coordinating discharge planning and placement relies on assessments by the interdisciplinary team to provide a comprehensive database for matching patient needs with available resources. The assessments of health care team members should include specific recommendations for comprehensive patient management and long-term needs. Patient and family input and preferences must also be considered in planning. In addition to

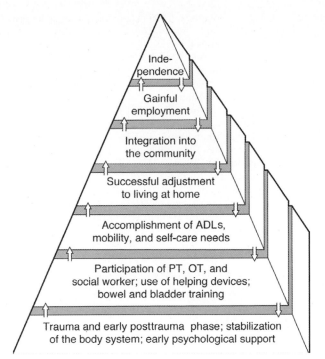

Figure 18-18 • The rehabilitation process following spinal cord injury. ADLs = activities of daily living; OT = occupational therapy; PT = physical therapy.

providing comprehensive assessment and recommendations, the nurse assumes an advocacy role for the patient and family.

Rehabilitation is a complex relearning process that addresses the holistic needs of the person. The continuum of care from critical care to rehabilitation is designed to help the patient achieve the highest level of independence and quality of life possible. The ultimate goal of the rehabilitation is the highest possible level of reintegration into the community and roles. The recovery of a patient with an SCI can be viewed in the context of Maslow's hierarchy of needs (Fig. 18-18).

If the patient is not already at an SCI center, transfer to a rehabilitation facility offers an opportunity for implementing a comprehensive and individualized program. The program may last from several weeks to several months. A multidisciplinary staff, including physicians, nurses, physical therapists,[71] occupational therapists, social workers, psychologists, vocational counselors, and other specialists, collaboratively provides a comprehensive rehabilitation program. Individual, group, and family counseling helps the patient and family accept and adjust to disabilities and changes in lifestyle resulting from the injury. Advice is also offered on necessary home environmental modifications that allow the patient to live at home. The social worker can help identify available resources to help meet the needs of the person with an SCI. For example, some states and private agencies provide funds to build ramps and purchase special equipment for the home.

The care within a rehabilitation facility is beyond the scope of this text. The reader is directed to other sources in the rehabilitation literature for this information.

Future Trends

According to the National Institute of Neurological Disorders and Stroke, spinal cord injury research has come of age.[72] Researchers have identified a wide variety of potential therapies for SCI, all of which need to be tested in well-designed studies. Equally exciting are the developments in medical engineering and robotics, which are changing rehabilitation programs for SCI patients. Enthusiasm and future potential must be tempered by the enormous work and strides that must occur to address the devastating effects of SCI.

SUMMARY

This chapter has provided an overview of SCI with an emphasis on stabilization and acute care management. Patients who sustain an SCI require a collaborative interdisciplinary approach to achieve optimal patient outcomes. Patients with paraplegia and tetraplegia require comprehensive rehabilitation and life-long management and care to reduce the risk of complications and to optimize independence. New options for delivering health care in the home and in subacute and long-term care facilities promise independence and improved quality of life. The most promising news for SCI victims, however, is new research, which is now under way. One day, new treatment protocols, including the actual regeneration of spinal cord tissue, may eliminate the devastating functional losses associated with SCI and restore mobility to those who, under current circumstances, have lost their ability to walk.[73]

REFERENCES

1. Spinal Cord Injury Information Network. Facts and figures at a glance, June 2006. Retrieved November 25, 2006, from http://spinalcord.uab.edu/shows.asp?durki=21446
2. Hadley, M. N., Walters, B. C., Grabb, P. A., et al. (2002). *American Association of Neurological Surgeons and the Congress of Neurological Surgery: Guidelines for acute cervical and spinal injuries.* New York: Thieme.
3. American Spinal Injury Association, International Medical Society of Paraplegia. (1992, revised). *International standards for neurological and functional classification of spinal cord injury.* Chicago, IL: Author.
4. Lenke, L. G., O'Brien, M. F., & Bridwell, K. H. (1995). Fractures and dislocations of the spine. In C. R. Perry, J. A. Elstrom, & A. M. Pankovich (Eds.). *The handbook of fractures* (pp. 166–189). New York: McGraw-Hill.
5. Greenberg, M. S. (2006). *Handbook of neurosurgery* (6th ed., pp. 698–699). New York: Thieme.
6. White, A. A., & Panjabi, M. M. (1990). *Clinical biomechanics of the spine* (2nd ed., pp. 277–278). Philadelphia: J. B. Lippincott.
7. Adams, J. C., & Hamblen, D. L. (1992). *Outline of fractures* (10th ed., pp. 81–85). Edinburgh: Churchill Livingstone.
8. Tator, C. H. (2000). Clinical manifestations of acute spinal cord injury. In C. H. Tator & E. C. Benzel (Eds.). *Contemporary management of spinal cord injury* (2nd ed., pp 21–32). New York: Thieme.
9. Schreiber, D. Spinal cord injuries. Retrieved November 21, 2006, from E-Medicine for WebMD, http:www.emedicine.com/emerg/topic553.htm

10. Saruhashi, Y., Huduka, S., Katsuura, A., et al. (1998). Clinical outcomes of cervical spinal cord injuries without radiographic evidence of trauma. *Spinal Cord, 36,* 567–573.

11. Dubendorf, P. (1999). Spinal cord injury pathophysiology. *Critical Care Nursing Quarterly, 22*(2), 31–35.

12. Tator, C. H. (1995). Update on the pathophysiology and pathology of acute spinal cord injury. *Brain Pathology, 5,* 407–413.

13. Chiles, B. W., & Cooper, P. R. (1996). Acute spinal injury. *New England Journal of Medicine, 334*(8), 514–520.

14. Marcotte, P. J., Shaver, E. G., & Weil, R. J. (1998). Acute spinal injury. In J. Cruz (Ed.). *Neurological and neurosurgical emergencies* (pp. 363–403). Philadelphia: W. B. Saunders.

15. Schwab, M. E., & Bartholdi, D. (1996). Degeneration and regeneration of axons in the lesioned spinal cord. *Physiological Review, 76,* 319–370.

16. Moriya, T., Hassan, A. Z., Young, W., et al. (1994). Dynamics of extracellular calcium activity following contusion of the rat spinal cord. *Journal of Neurotrauma, 11,* 255–263.

17. Buckley, D. A., & Gaunci, M. M. (1999). Spinal cord trauma. *Nursing Clinics of North America, 34*(1), 661–687.

18. Hall, E. D., & Springer, J. E. (2004). Neuroprotection and acute spinal cord injury: A reappraisal. *NeuroRx, 1*(1), 80–100.

19. Washington University School of Medicine. Physiology of spinal cord injury. Retrieved December 5, 2006, from http://www.neuro.wustl.edu/sci/physiolo.htm.

20. Waters, R. L., Adkins, R. H., Yakura, J., et al. (1991). Profiles of spinal cord injury and recovery after gunshot injury. *Clinical Orthopedics, 267,* 14–21.

21. Ropper, A. H., Gress, D. R., Diringer, M. N., Mayer, S. A., & Bleck, T. P. (2004). *Neurological and neurosurgical intensive care* (4th ed., p. 360). Philadelphia: Lippincott Williams & Wilkins.

22. Santago, P., & Fessler, R. G. (2004). Trauma of the nervous system. C. Spinal cord trauma. In W. G. Bradley, R. B. Daroff, G. M. Fenichel, & J. Jankovic (Eds.). *Neurology in clinical practice: The neurological disorders* (4th ed., pp. 1153–1154). Philadelphia: Butterworth Heinemann.

23. Ropper, A. H., Gress, D. R., Diringer, M. N., Mayer, S. A., & Bleck, T. P. (2004). *Neurological and neurosurgical intensive care* (4th ed., pp. 349–362). Philadelphia: Lippincott Williams & Wilkins.

24. Freeborn, K. (2005). The importance of maintaining spinal precautions. *Critical Care Nursing Quarterly, 28*(2), 195–199.

25. Marcotte, P. J., Shaver, E. G., & Weil, R. J. (1998). Acute spinal injury. In J. Cruz (Ed.). *Neurological and neurosurgical emergencies* (pp. 363–403). Philadelphia: W. B. Saunders.

26. Bondurant, F. J., Cotler, H. B., Kulkarni, M. V., et al. (1990). Acute SCI: A study using physical examination and magnetic resonance imaging. *Spine, 15,* 161–168.

27. Tator, C. H., & Fehlings, M. G. (1991). Review of the secondary injury theory of acute spinal cord trauma with emphasis on vascular mechanisms. *Journal of Neurosurgery, 75,* 15–26.

28. Bracken, D., Shepard, M., Collins, W., et al. (1990). Randomized controlled trial of methylprednisolone or naloxone in the treatment of acute SCI. *New England Journal of Medicine, 322,* 1405–1411.

29. Bracken, M. B. (1992). Pharmacological treatment of acute SCI: Current status and future prospects. *Paraplegia, 30,* 102–107.

30. Bracken, M. B., Shepard, M. J., Holford, T. R., et al. (1997). Administration of methylprednisolone for 24 or 48 hours or tirilazad mesylate for 48 hours in the treatment of acute spinal cord injury. *Journal of the American Medical Association, 227,* 1597–1604.

31. Hurlber, R. J. (2000). Methylprednisolone for acute spinal cord injury: An inappropriate standard of care. *Journal of Neurosurgery, 93,* 175–179.

32. Coleman, W. P., Benzel, D., Cahill, D. W., et al. (2000). A critical appraisal of the reporting of the National Acute Spinal Cord Injury Studies (I and II) of methylprednisolone in acute spinal cord injury. *Journal of Spinal Disorders, 13,* 185–189.

33. Hugenholtz, H. (2003). Methylprednisolone for acute spinal cord injury: Not a standard of care. *Canadian Medical Association Journal, 168*(9), 1145–1146.

34. Chinnock, P., & Roberts, I. (2005). Gangliosides for acute spinal cord injury (Cochrane review). *The Cochrane Database of Systematic Review, 2,* CD004444.

35. Wolf, A., Levi, L., Mirvis, S., et al. (1991). Operative management of bilateral facet dislocation. *Journal of Neurosurgery, 75,* 883–890.

36. Greenberg, M. S. (2006). *Handbook of neurosurgery* (6th ed., pp. 739–744). New York: Thieme

37. Gertzbein, S. D., Macmicheal, D., & Title, M. (1982). Harrington instrumentation as a method of fixation in fractures of the spine. *Journal of Bone & Joint Surgery, 64B,* 526–529.

38. Cotrel, Y., Dubousset, J., & Guillaumat, M. (1988). New universal instrumentation in spinal surgery. *Clinical Orthopaedics and Related Research, 277,* 10–23.

39. Hickey, J. V., & Namink, J. L. (2005). External fixation device insertion (assist). In D. J. Lynn-McHale Wiegand & K. K. Carlson (Eds.). *AACN procedure manual for critical care* (5th ed., pp. 806–810). Philadelphia: W. B. Saunders.

40. Hickey, J. V., & Monroig, J. L. (2005). Halo traction care. In D. J. Lynn-McHale Wiegand & K. K. Carlson (Eds.). *AACN procedure manual for critical care* (5th ed., pp. 811–817). Philadelphia: W. B. Saunders.

41. Hickey, J. V., & Davis, J. M. (2005). Tong and pin care. In D. J. Lynn-McHale Wiegand & K. K. Carlson (Eds.). *AACN procedure manual for critical care* (5th ed., pp. 818–820). Philadelphia: W. B. Saunders.

42. Hickey, J. V., & Hudgens, C. (2005). Traction maintenance. In D. J. Lynn-McHale Wiegand & K. K. Carlson (Eds.). *AACN procedure manual for critical care* (5th ed., pp. 821–826). Philadelphia: W. B. Saunders.

43. Winslow, C., & Rozovsky, J. (2003). Effect of spinal cord injury on the respiratory system. *American Journal of Physical Medicine and Rehabilitation, 82,* 803–814.

44. Gutierrez, C. J., Harrow, J., & Hanies, F. (2003). Using an evidence-based protocol to guide rehabilitation and weaning of ventilator-dependent cervical spinal cord injury patients. *Journal of Rehabilitation Research and Development, 40*(5, Suppl 2), 99–110.

45. Hadley, M. N., Walters, B. C., Grabb, P. A. et al. (2002). *American Association of Neurological Surgeons and the Congress of Neurological Surgery: Guidelines for acute cervical and spinal injuries* (pp. 203–204). New York: Thieme.

46. McKinney, D., & Garstang, S. V. Prevention of thromboembolism in spinal cord injury. Retrieved November 21, 2006, from http://www.emedicine.con/pmr/topic229.htm

47. Spinal Cord Injury Thromboprophylaxis Investigators. (2003). Prevention of venous thromboembolism in the rehabilitation phase after spinal cord injury: Prophylaxis with low-dose heparin or enoxaparin. *Journal of Trauma, 54,* 1111–1115.

48. Paralyzed Veterans of America. (2001). Pressure ulcer prevention and treatment following spinal cord injury: A clinical practice guideline for health-care professionals. *Journal of Spinal Cord Medicine, 24*(Suppl 1), S40–101.

49. Blackmer, J. (2003). Rehabilitation medicine: 1. Autonomic dysreflexia. *Canadian Medical Association Journal, 169*(9), 931–935.

50. Van Kuijk, A. A., Geurts, A. C. H., & van Kuppevelt, H. J. N. (2002). Neurogenic heterotopic ossification in spinal cord injury. *Spinal Cord, 40,* 313–326.

51. Spielman, G., Gennarelli, T., & Rogers, R. (1983). Disodium etidronate: Its role in preventing heterotopic ossification in traumatic brain injury. *Archives Physical Medicine Rehabilitation 64,* 539–542.

52. Garland, D. E. (1991). A clinical perspective of common forms of acquired heterotopic ossification. *Clinical Orthopedics Research, 263,* 13–29.

53. Adams, M. M., & Hicks, A. L. (2005). Spasticity after spinal cord injury. *Spinal Cord, 43,* 577–586.

54. Satkunam, L. E. (2003). Rehabilitation medicine: 3. Management of adult spasticity. *Canadian Medical Association Journal, 169*(11), 1173–1179.

55. Decq, P. (2003). Pathophysiology of spasticity. *Neurochirugie, 49,* 163–184.

56. Ditunno, J. F., Little, J. W., Tessler, A., & Burns, A. S. (2004). Spinal shock revisited: A four-phase model. *Spinal Cord, 42*, 383–395.

57. Peterson, P. L., O'Neil, B. J., Alcantra, A. L., & Michael, D. B. (1998). Initial evaluation and management of neuroemergencies. In J. Cruz (Ed.). *Neurological and neurosurgical emergencies* (pp. 1–20). Philadelphia: W. B. Saunders.

58. Bohannon, R. W., & Smith, M. B. (1987). Interrater reliability of a modified Ashworth scale of muscle spasticity. *Physical Therapy, 67*(2), 206–207.

59. Kirshblum, S. (1999). Treatment alternatives for spinal cord injury related spasticity. *Journal of Spinal Cord Medicine, 22*, 199–217.

60. Campbell, S. K., Almeida, G. L., Penn, R. D., & Corcos, D. M. (1995). The effects of intrathecally administered baclofen on function in patients with spasticity. *Physical Therapy, 75*(5), 352–362.

61. Saulino, M., & Jacobs, B. W. (2006). The pharmacological management of spasticity. *Journal of Neuroscience Nursing, 38*(6), 456–459.

62. Apple, D. F. (2000). Medical management and rehabilitation of the spinal cord injured patient. In J. M. Cotler, J. M. Simpson, H. S. Au, & C. P. Sliveri (Eds.). *Surgery of spinal trauma* (pp. 157–178). Philadelphia: Lippincott Williams & Wilkins.

63. Taricco, M., Pagliacci, M. C., Telaro, E., & Adone, R. (2006). Pharmacological interventions for spasticity following spinal cord injury: Results of a Cochrane systematic review. *European Medicophysiology, 42*(1), 5–15.

64. Cardenas, D. D., & Hooten, T. M. (1999). Urinary tract infections in persons with SCI. *Archives of Physical Medicine Rehabilitation, 76*, 272–280.

65. Giannantoni, A., Scivoletto, G., Di Stasi, S. M., et al. (1998). Clean intermittent catheterization and prevention of renal disease in spinal cord patients. *Spinal Cord, 36*, 29–32.

66. Kirshblum, S. C., Gulati, M., O'Connor, K., & Voorman, S. J. (1998). Bowel care practices in chronic SCI patients. *Archives of Physical Medicine Rehabilitation, 79*, 20–23.

67. Livneh, H., & Martz, E. (2003). Psychological adaptation to spinal cord injury as a function of time since injury. *International Journal of Rehabilitation Research, 26*(3), 191–200.

68. Dijkers, M. (1997). Quality of life after SCIs: A metaanalysis of the effects of disablement components. *Spinal Cord, 35*, 829–840.

69. Elliott, T. R., & Frank, R. G. (1996). Depression following SCI. *Archives of Physical Medicine Rehabilitation, 77*, 816–823.

70. DeVivo, M. J. (1999). Discharge disposition form model SCI care system rehabilitation programs. *Archives of Physical Medicine Rehabilitation, 80*, 785–790.

71. Fries, J. M. (2005). Critical rehabilitation of the patient with spinal cord injury. *Critical Care Nursing Quarterly, 28*(2), 179–187.

72. National Institute of Neurological Disorders and Stroke. Spinal cord injury concepts. Retrieved November 21, 2006, from http://www.ninds.nih.gov/news_and events/proceedings/sci_report.htm

73. Barbeau, H., Ladouceur, M., Norman, K. E., Pepin, A., & Leroux, A. (1999). Walking after SCI: evaluation, treatment and functional recovery. *Archives of Physical Medicine Rehabilitation, 80*, 225–235.

RESOURCES

Websites

American Spinal Injury Association: http://www.asia-spinalinjury.org/

University of Alabama: http://www.spinalcord.uab.edu

Back Pain and Spinal Disorders

Joanne V. Hickey and Andrea L. Strayer

This chapter focuses on selected spinal disorders common in neuroscience clinical practice, such as back pain and intervertebral disc disease. Other conditions such as osteoporosis and metastatic lesions are addressed only as risk factors rather than as primary conditions for a comprehensive discussion.

Back pain is a common and challenging health problem. Low back pain affects almost 90% of us at some time during our lifetime. It is second only to upper respiratory tract disease as a cause of temporary disability in all age groups. Because it ranks so high among the reasons for seeking health care, back pain has an enormous economic impact on providing health care. The economic toll to society is further increased by the lost productivity of sufferers and the income-associated disability costs. Likewise, neck pain is also a public health problem. Most patients with neck or low back pain suffer from musculoskeletal strain and will recover in 4 to 6 weeks. Others with more serious underlying causes require more aggressive treatment. Acute spine problems can become chronic conditions characterized by periods of exacerbation and temporary relief. Even after surgical intervention, some patients continue to experience symptoms of varying severity or have "failed back syndrome." Management of acute back or neck pain is challenging and controversial. Currently, scientific evidence in regards to many aspects of neck or low back pain is inconclusive.

CONDITIONS RELATED TO BACK OR NECK PAIN

Several conditions such as normal degenerative changes of aging increase the risk of back or neck pain. Other conditions are "red flags" for serious underlying problems and must be addressed rapidly (Table 19-1). Degenerative changes of aging are discussed later in this chapter. Other conditions mentioned elsewhere are summarized in Table 19-2 (see also Figs. 19-1, 19-2, 19-3, and 19-4).

Degenerative Changes Associated With Aging

The normal aging process decreases the fluid content in the nucleus pulposus, which at birth is about 90% and by age 70

is 70%.[1] Degeneration of the annulus fibrosus leads to tears in the rings of the annulus. Together these changes alter the absorption and redistribution of forces placed on the spine. These altered biomechanics may lead to disc bulging, herniation, and abnormal movement between vertebrae. This is commonly referred to as the degenerative cascade.[2]

As the degenerative cascade continues, further disc degeneration will eventually lead to changes in the endplates of the vertebral bodies. With motion, bone of one vertebra contacts the bone of the next, creating osteophytes in the area of the vertebral body and facet joints. Alternatively, disc bulging may ossify to form osteophytes. Ligament laxity and facet hypertrophy also develops. Disc degeneration, bony overgrowth, ligament laxity and buckling, and facet hypertrophy contribute to the creation of central canal and/or foraminal narrowing.[3,4] Spinal canal narrowing can lead to spinal cord compression in the cervical spine and cauda equina compression in the lumbar spine. Foraminal narrowing can lead to radiculopathy in the cervical and lumbar spine.

Osteoporosis

Osteoporosis is characterized by decreased bone mineral density (Fig. 19-4). Bone is normally in a continuous process of bone reabsorption (osteoclast activity) and bone formation (osteoblast activity). When there is more bone reabsorption than formation, osteoporosis occurs.[5] Peak bone mass occurs in the third decade of life, and decreases thereafter. Increasing age predisposes the person to net bone reabsorption, as does decreased estrogen (postmenopausal) and androgens, poor nutrition, alcohol and tobacco use, and corticosteroid use. According to the World Health Organization, when young healthy Caucasian women reach the age of 75 years, approximately 30% will have osteoporosis.[6]

Trabecular bone accounts for a large portion of the vertebral body and 90% of the load-bearing resistance. Because of the increased metabolic activity and more surface area of trabecular (also referred to as cancellous or spongiform) bone, it is especially affected by osteoporosis. Osteoporosis leads to a decreased density of horizontal trabeculae, which results in less tolerance to stress and biomechanical loads. This puts the patient at risk for fractures, which may lead to pain, alterations in daily activities, and disability.[7,8] Fractures often occur with minimal or no significant trauma. Low bone density also has

TABLE 19-1   "RED FLAGS" TO RECOGNIZE IN THE HISTORY AND PHYSICAL EXAMINATION OF PATIENTS WITH NECK OR BACK PAIN

- Possible tumor or infection
  - Tumor: pain in people under age 20 or age 50 or over; history of cancer
  - Infection: fever, chills, unexplained weight loss (note risk factors for spinal infection that include recent bacterial infection, e.g., urinary tract infection, IV drug abuse, immunosuppression)
  - Either tumor or infection: pain that worsens when lying down or the severity of which increases at nighttime

- Possible fracture
  - Major trauma (e.g., motor vehicle accident, fall from height)
  - Minor trauma or even strenuous lifting in older patients or those who potentially have osteoporosis

- Possible cauda equina syndrome
  - Lost or diminished sensation in the saddle area (e.g., perianal, perineal)
  - Recent onset of bladder dysfunction (e.g., retention, increased frequency, overflow)
  - Severe or progressive neurological deficit in the lower extremity
  - Poor rectal tone
  - Major motor weakness (quadriceps—weakness for knee extension; ankle plantar flexors, evertors, and dorsiflexors [foot drop])

- Possible spinal cord compression (myelopathy)
  - Gait disturbance; tripping, falling
  - Hand clumsiness; trouble buttoning, zipping, writing; hand weakness
  - Lhermitte's sign: shooting, electric shock sensations down back, usually noted with neck flexion
  - Hyperreflexia, spasticity, and clonus

implications for surgical or nonsurgical management options including surgical options and technique. The ultimate goal is for the patient to achieve an optimal outcome.

Low Back Pain

Health Care Guideline: Adult Low Back Pain, published by the Institute for Clinical Systems Improvement, sets a national standard for patient management.[9] The *Guideline's* recommendations, based on scientific evidence, are the consensus of expert practitioners. Acute low back problems are defined as activity intolerance resulting from lower back or back-related leg symptoms of shorter than 6 weeks' duration. Evidence and recommendations found in this guideline form the basis for the conservative care of the patient with acute low back pain outlined in this chapter.

About 90% of patients recover spontaneously from low back pain within 4 to 6 weeks.[10] A subsequent episode of low back pain is managed as a new acute episode. The focus of guidance has shifted from managing pain to helping patients improve activity tolerance and counseling patients to engage in lifestyle modifications to eliminate or reduce risk factors for future exacerbations of neck or back pain.[11]

Diagnosis of Back Problems

Because back pain is a symptom related to many conditions and disease processes, proper diagnosis is critical for treatment

and a satisfactory outcome.[12] During the initial encounter, usually at a clinic or primary care physician's office, the history and physical examination are directed at the following:

- Rule out signs or symptoms of potentially dangerous underlying conditions, that is, "red flags"; see Table 19-1.
- Collect a detail-focused history emphasizing limits to normal lifestyle, functional loss (including bladder and bowel dysfunction), and degree of pain.
- Perform a regional back examination (e.g., deformity, vertebral point tenderness, muscle spasm).
- Perform a neurological screening examination with particular attention to muscle strength, sensory dermatomes (pinprick and light touch), reflexes, evidence of muscle atrophy, flexibility (forward bending), and observation of the patient walking (e.g., posture, on toes, on heels, squat).
- Perform the straight leg raising test for low back pain (sometimes called Lasègue's sign); Figure 19-5 shows a way of testing for sciatic nerve root tension

In the absence of signs of serious problems, there is no need for special diagnostic studies because 90% of patients recover spontaneously within 4 to 6 weeks. These are patients who have a lumbosacral sprain. However, if a *serious underlying condition* is found or if there is *rapid progression of neurological deficits,* urgent diagnostic studies and definitive care should be sought.[13]

Initial Management

Patients with back problems are almost always treated on an outpatient basis. The cornerstones of early management are education and reassurance, patient comfort, and activity modification.

Education and Reassurance

In the absence of "red flags," patients need to be reassured that most people recover from back problems within 4 to 6 weeks. Education is a key element to recovery and prevention of future problems. The nurse often assumes the role of educator. Key elements of patient education during an acute episode of pain include:

- Gradually reintroduce activities as symptoms improve. Walking; gentle, gradual stretching; sitting for only short periods of time; and changing positions frequently are recommended.
- Ice alternating with heat, or whichever is preferred, may help decrease inflammation. Advise not to apply ice for more than 20 minutes of every hour and ensure heating pads are at a safe temperature.[14]
- Instruct on core strengthening and low back stabilization exercises.
- Stress will increase back pain. Take measures to decrease stress.
- Constipation will increase back pain; constipation prevention should not be overlooked.

A frank discussion on lifestyle modification that is advisable for the patient to reduce or eliminate risk factors of future

TABLE 19-2 CONDITIONS RELATED TO SPINAL PAIN

CONDITIONS	DESCRIPTION, SIGNS, AND SYMPTOMS	MANAGEMENT OR TREATMENT
Deformity		
Scoliosis • Abnormal sagittal, coronal, and axial curvature of the spine. May be idiopathic or degenerative • Predisposes the patient to disc and vertebral disease	Cause anatomic alterations; may result in: • Malalignment of one vertebra with the next • Disproportionate stress to selected areas of the vertebral column • A narrowed space within the spinal canal	Possible management approaches depend on exact etiology, degree of disability, and age of the patient: • Physical therapy • Braces • Fusion with extensive instrumentation
Osteoporotic compression fractures	• Decreased bone density leads to decreased tolerance to stress and increased risk of compression fractures. • One third of women over age 65 will develop a spinal fracture. Significant pain can accompany the fracture. Some are afflicted with multiple fractures.	• Treatment includes bracing, activity restrictions, and pain management. • Surgery may be indicated if there is uncontrolled pain, progressive deformity, neurological deficit, or spinal instability.
Neoplasms		
• Metastatic lesions involving the vertebrae or spinal cord • Primary tumors of the dura or spinal cord	• Metastasis is most often from prostate, lungs, breast, or gastrointestinal tract; deficits depend on the level of the lesion. – They cause pain and neurological deficits (e.g., bowel or bladder dysfunction, paresis, paresthesia). • With primary tumors, deficits depend on the spinal level involved; signs and symptoms are the same as for metastatic lesions.	Surgical decompression may be necessary; alternatively, irradiation with or without surgery (see Chap. 22) may be advised.
Infections		
• Abscess and/or osteomyelitis secondary to infections elsewhere in the body • Infections related to surgical procedures • Possible organisms include *Staphylococcus*, tubercle bacillus, *Aspergillus*, and *Streptococcus*	• Pain is the chief complaint; other deficits relate to the dermatomal level. If cervical spine epidural abscess is present, spinal cord compression can result.	Management may include: • Immobilization • IV antibiotics for 4–6 wk • Surgical drainage • Surgical decompression and possible reconstruction and spinal fusion, if necessary
Degenerative Diseases of the Vertebral Column		
• *Spondylosis:* degeneration of the intervertebral discs leads to disc collapse. There may be bulging of the annulus and buckling of the ligamentum flavum as well as decrease in neural foramen height. This leads to alterations in load transmission, which lead to osteophyte formation at the vertebral bodies and posterior facet joints. The degenerative process can lead to either stiffness between levels or instability from hypermobility. In the cervical spine, spondylosis can progress to cause central canal stenosis and spinal cord compression. If the patient has myelopathy on physical exam, it is called cervical spondylotic myelopathy.	• Pain can result from nerve root compression, fatigue, and additional stress on the vertebral column. • Disc protrusion can cause collapse of the disc space, resulting in narrowing of the intervertebral foramen and compression of the nerve roots.	Conservative management (effective in the majority of patients): • Activity modification • Stretching, strengthening, and aerobic exercise • Attaining appropriate weight Smoking cessation Psychosocial stressor management • Drug therapy (nonnarcotic analgesics; nonsteroidal anti-inflammatory agents [ibuprofen]; other types of anti-inflammatory drugs) Surgical approach: • If conservative treatment is ineffective, operative intervention may be warranted.
• *Spondylolisthesis:* slipping of one vertebra on an adjacent vertebra	• Most spondylolisthesis are degenerative. • The most frequently affected area is L-5, followed by L-4. • Symptoms are mild early in the course of the disease, then progress (lower back pain radiating to the thighs and legs; tenderness over L-4 and L-5; sensory and motor weakness). • Narrowing of the spinal canal and thecal sac are possible as a result of disc displacement. • There is also narrowing of the neural foramen, which can cause nerve root compression and radiculopathy.	• Management includes conservative pain control and physical therapy • Surgery for thecal sac or nerve root decompression is generally a decompressive laminectomy. A fusion may be indicated.

(continued)

TABLE 19-2   CONDITIONS RELATED TO SPINAL PAIN (*Continued*)

CONDITIONS	DESCRIPTION, SIGNS, AND SYMPTOMS	MANAGEMENT OR TREATMENT
Inflammatory Diseases		
• *Rheumatoid arthritis:* a generalized disease process affecting the connective tissue of the spine, hips, and hands – Cervical atlantoaxial area commonly affected – Cervical spine involvement is observed in 15%–70% of patients – Women ages 25–45 y affected three times more often than men	• As the disease progresses, occipitocervical instability can result from upper cervical spine ligament laxity, articular cartilage destruction, and bone abnormalities. • Cord compression can result from basilar invagination and instability. • Patients often present with neck pain.	Treatment of choice for upper cervical spine instability is surgical stabilization.
• Ankylosing spondylitis – Predominantly affects young men – Sacroiliac joints primary sites – Involves destruction of the joints and ankylosis – Slowly progressive disease; can result in complete calcification of the anterior longitudinal ligament with resulting immobilization of the spine – The spine is brittle and vulnerable to fracture because of the immobility of the spine.	• The chief symptom is pain in the center lower back. Morning stiffness is common, and decreased hip mobility may also occur. • Slow, progressive course lasts several years. • In early disease, symptoms precede roentgenographic changes; as the disease advances, the spine looks like a "bamboo spine" on x-ray studies. • Back pain, stiffness, and limitation of movement are the most common symptoms.	Management is symptomatic: • Pain control • Physical therapy • Other approaches, depending on the age of the patient and the degree of disability
Trauma		
• *Sprains and strains,* including whiplash • *Spondylolysis:* stress fracture of the pedicle	• Can be unilateral or bilateral • Often is a repetitive injury in young athletes, such as gymnasts. Spondylolysis can lead to a spondylolisthesis.	• Treatment is rest from the sport and physical therapy. • Surgery is only indicated if conservative treatment is not beneficial.
Referred Pain from Viscera		
• A patient may have back pain secondary to referral from viscera, such as the gallbladder and kidneys.	• A thorough physical examination will reveal underlying cause.	• Treatment depends on underlying cause.

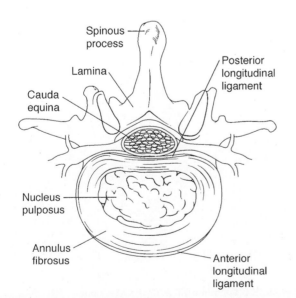

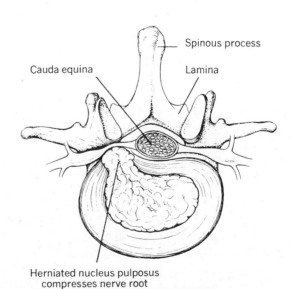

Figure 19-1 • Axial view of the lumbar spine, showing an intervertebral disc, the contents of the spinal canal, and the elements of the posterior bony arch.

Figure 19-2 • Ruptured vertebral disc. (From Chaffee, E. E., & Lytle, I. M. [1980]. *Basic physiology and anatomy.* Philadelphia: J. B. Lippincott.)

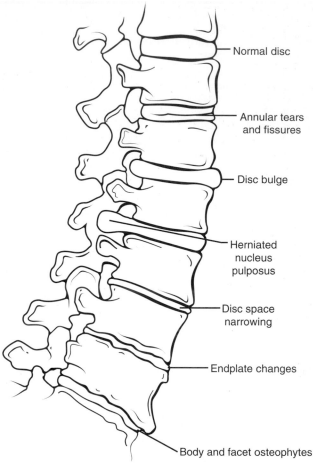

Normal disc

Annular tears and fissures

Disc bulge

Herniated nucleus pulposus

Disc space narrowing

Endplate changes

Body and facet osteophytes

Figure 19-3 • The degenerative cascade. (From Jeong, G. K. & Bendo, J. A. [2004]. Spinal disorders in the elderly. *Clinical Orthopaedics and Related Research 425,* 110–125.

episodes is often a difficult but important topic. Prevention of further episodes is the goal. To be successful, the patient needs to actively participate in good neck and back health. Education for the prevention of neck or back pain includes stretching exercise, aerobic activity, smoking cessation, and attaining the appropriate weight.[15]

Patient Comfort

Pain and discomfort are the usual reasons for seeking health care. The safest effective medication for acute low back problems is acetaminophen (no more than 4000 mg/d). Nonsteroidal anti-inflammatory drugs (NSAIDs), such as ibuprofen, are also recommended, but caution must be exercised because they may cause gastric irritation as well as renal and allergic side effects. Muscle relaxants may also be ordered. About 30% of patients experience drowsiness, which interferes with daytime activities. Narcotics are avoided if at all possible because of possible dependency. Application of heat or cold to the concentrated area of pain may provide some relief. While it is often recommended, evidence does not support the use of skin traction, massage, spinal manipulation, or acupuncture as effective treatment modalities.[16–18]

Activity Modification

Up to 6 Weeks. Activity is altered to avoid undue back irritation and debilitation from inactivity. Bed rest is not recommended. Prolonged bed rest (i.e., more than 4 days) has potentially debilitating effects, and its efficacy in the treatment of acute back problems is unproved.[19] For people with severe limitations resulting from leg pain, 2 days of bed rest may be necessary. It is important to continue routine activity, temporarily avoiding specific activities that increase stress on the spine and aggravate symptoms. Consideration should be given to the patient's specific circumstances.

To avoid undue stress to the back, patients need education on proper body mechanics (how to lift, sit, walk, and bend).

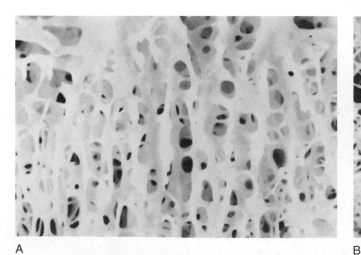

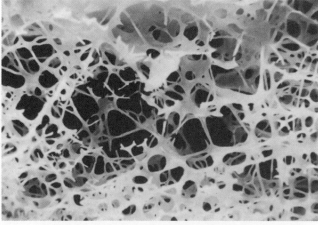

A   B

Figure 19-4 • Normal bone (*A*). Osteoporotic bone (*B*). (From Gill, S. S. & Einhorn, T. A. (2004). Metabolic bone disease of the adult and pediatric spine. In Frymoyer, J. W. & Wiesel, S. W. (eds in chief). *The Adult and Pediatric Spine.* (3rd ed, pp. 121–140). Philadelphia: Lippincott Williams & Wilkins.)

Clinical test for sciatic tension

The straight leg raising (SLR) test (A) can detect tension on the L-5 and/or S-1 nerve root. SLR may reproduce leg pain by stretching nerve roots irritated by a disc herniation.

A. Instructions for the Straight Leg Raising Test

(1) Ask the patient to lie as straight as possible on a table in the supine position.

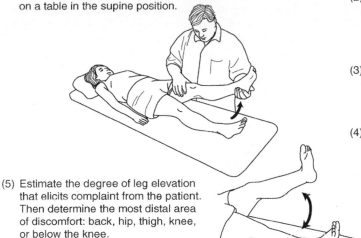

(5) Estimate the degree of leg elevation that elicits complaint from the patient. Then determine the most distal area of discomfort: back, hip, thigh, knee, or below the knee.

(6) While holding the leg at the limit of straight leg raising, dorsiflex the ankle. Note whether this aggravates the pain. Internal rotation of the limb can also increase the tension on the sciatic nerve roots.

Pain below the knee at less than 70 degrees of straight leg raising, aggravated by dorsiflexion of the ankle and relieved by ankle plantarflexion or external limb rotation, is most suggestive of tension on the L-5 or S-1 nerve root related to disc herniation. Reproducing back pain alone with SLR testing does not indicate significant nerve root tension.

(2) With one hand placed above the knee of the leg being examined, exert enough firm pressure to keep the knee fully extended. Ask the patient to relax.

(3) With the other hand cupped under the heel, slowly raise the straight limb. Tell the patient, "If this bothers you, let me know, and I will stop."

(4) Monitor for any movement of the pelvis before complaints are elicited. True sciatic tension should elicit complaints before the hamstrings are stretched enough to move the pelvis.

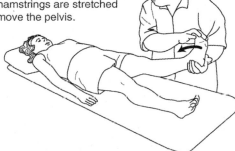

Crossover pain occurs when straight raising of the patient's well limb elicits pain in the leg with sciatica. Crossover pain is a stronger indication of nerve root compression than pain elicited from raising the straight painful limb.

Sitting knee extension (B) can also test sciatic tension. The patient with significant nerve root irritation tends to complain or lean backward to reduce tension on the nerve.

B. Instructions for sitting knee extension test

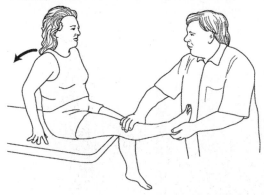

With the patient sitting on a table, both hips and knees flexed at 90 degrees, slowly extend the knee as if evaluating the patella or bottom of the foot. This maneuver stretches nerve roots as much as a moderate degree of supine SLR.

Figure 19-5 • Straight leg raising (SLR) test. (*A*) Instructions for SLR when the patient is lying down. (*B*) Instructions for SLR when the patient is sitting. (Bigos, S., Bowyer, O., Braen, G., et al. [1994]. *Acute low back problems in adults.* Clinical Practice Guideline, Quick Reference Guide Number. 14. Rockville, MD: U.S. Department of Health and Human Services, Public Health Service, Agency for Health Care Policy and Research, AHCPR Pub. No. 95–0643.)

Sitting, although generally a safe activity, may aggravate symptoms for some patients. Avoiding debilitation is accomplished by low-stress aerobic conditioning, such as walking, stationary biking, and swimming, with the time of exercise gradually increasing. Temporary activity restrictions for the workplace may be necessary, depending on the type of work an individual performs. Depending on gender and severity of symptoms, restrictions may need to be placed on the number of pounds that should be lifted without assistance. These recommendations range from 20 lb for patients with severe symptoms regardless of gender, to 60 lb and 35 lb, respectively, for men and women with mild symptoms.

After 6 Weeks. If after 6 weeks the patient has not recovered, and there is a question of an underlying problem or physiologic evidence of tissue insult or nerve impairment, imaging and possibly nerve conduction studies are ordered.

- Magnetic resonance imaging (MRI) is the "gold standard" for diagnosis of neural and soft-tissue problems (Fig. 19-6).
- Nerve conduction studies are ordered to evaluate for nerve compromise (radiculopathy) if the radiographic study, history, and clinical examination do not correlate and further diagnostic study is warranted.
- Other laboratory tests (e.g., erythrocyte sedimentation rate, complete blood count, and urinalysis) are helpful to screen for nonspecific medical problems; a bone scan is helpful if a spinal cord tumor, infection, or occult fracture is suspected. Generally, this would be completed with the initial evaluation if "red flags" are present.

More specific information is found in the *Health Care Guideline: Adult Low Back Pain*.[9]

Neck Pain

Neck pain is also a symptom in many conditions and disease processes; proper diagnosis is critical for treatment and a satisfactory outcome. Neck pain diagnosis and initial management generally follow the same algorithm as low back pain. Initially, the patient is seen and evaluated by the primary care physician. As with low back pain, "red flags" are ruled out. A detailed history is obtained, focusing on the neck and upper extremities. Neurological screening examination will focus on the strength, sensation, and reflexes of the upper extremities. Finger fine motor and dexterity as well as the Hoffmann's reflex and Babinski's reflex are also evaluated for any signs of myelopathy.[20,21]

As with low back pain, in the absence of signs of serious problems, there is no need for special diagnostic studies. The majority of patients have musculoskeletal strain and recover spontaneously within 4 to 6 weeks. However, if a *serious underlying condition* is found or if there is *rapid progression of neurological deficits*, urgent diagnostic studies and definitive care should be sought.

Initial management, education and reassurance, patient comfort, and activity alterations follow the same general guidelines as low back pain.

HERNIATED INTERVERTEBRAL DISCS

Herniation of cervical and lumbar intervertebral discs can cause significant pain and alterations in functional activity. The lumbar spine is most frequently affected by a herniated disc followed by the cervical spine. Thoracic herniation is uncommon. Patients may complain of arm or leg pain and be diagnosed with **radiculopathy** (pain and/or paresthesias in the distribution of a nerve root).

Men suffer from intervertebral disc herniation much more frequently than women. Most patients with disc disease are between 30 and 50 years old. About 90% to 95% of lumbar herniation occurs at the L-4 to L-5 or L-5 to S-1 levels.[22] When the cervical region is involved, the most common levels are C-6 to C-7 (C-7 radiculopathy) and then C-5 to C-6 (C-6 radiculopathy).[23] Multiple herniation sites occur in 10% of patients (Fig. 19-6).

Etiology

Trauma accounts for approximately 50% of all disc herniation. Examples of traumatic incidents include lifting heavy objects while in a flexed position (most common), slipping,

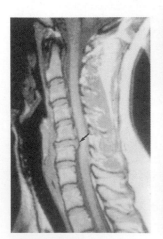 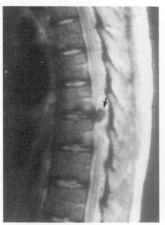 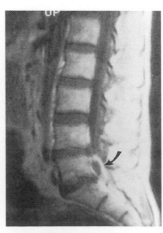

A (cervical)   B (thoracic)   C (lumbar)

Figure 19-6 • MRI views of herniated discs. *A* (cervical). Midsaggital T1-weighted MRI shows herniated disc (*arrow*) at C5–6 producing compression of the spinal cord. *B* (thoracic). Midsagittal T2-weighted MRI shows hypointense herniated disc (*arrow*) in mid-thoracic region resulting in compression of the spinal cord. *C* (lumbar). Midsagittal post-contrast T1-weighted MRI of the same patient shows that herniated disc (*arrow*) is not attached to any parent disc. There is peripheral disc enhancement. (Castillo, M. [1999]. *Neuroradiology companion* [2nd ed.]. Philadelphia: Lippincott-Raven.)

falling on the buttocks or back, and suppressing a sneeze in the lumbar area. In the cervical area flexion/extension injury of the neck can cause traumatic herniation. In some patients, no history of trauma can be identified. The cumulative result of repeated minor injuries is a chronic condition that places the patient at high risk for herniation.[24] The herniation syndrome also occurs in association with other degenerative processes, such as osteoarthritis or ankylosing spondylitis (Marie-Strümpell's spondylitis) and spinal stenosis. Patients with congenital anomalies, such as scoliosis, appear to be predisposed to disc injury because of malalignment of the vertebral column.

Pathophysiology

As previously mentioned, degenerative changes weaken the annulus fibrosus in middle and later life. Simultaneous degenerative changes occur in the nucleus pulposus, beginning after a peak level of development is reached in the early 30s. Fraying and tearing of the annulus fibrosus make the disc vulnerable to posterolateral displacement or bulging in response to biomechanical forces placed on the spine. This can occur with slight provocation, such as making an awkward movement, sneezing, or lurching forward. The nucleus pulposus can also protrude through the annulus fibrosus. A fragment may be laterally or centrally thrust into the spinal canal, where it encroaches on nerve roots (see Fig. 19-2). The presence or absence of symptoms is related to the degree of nerve root compression. In the lumbar spine, the majority of discs herniate in a posterolateral direction, just lateral to the posterior longitudinal ligament. In this position, the herniating disc may be in contact with the traversing nerve root at that level, causing symptoms. The cervical spine is more delicate, with a much smaller spinal canal. Disc herniation often causes radiculopathy; however, large central disc herniation can cause spinal cord compression.

Cervical and lumbar disc herniations are only problematic if spinal cord or nerve root compression results. Many people have bulging, protruding, or herniated discs and are *asymptomatic*.

Signs and Symptoms by Location

Lumbar Area

More than 90% of all clinically significant lower extremity radiculopathy is due to disc herniation at the L-4 to L-5 or L-5 to S-1 level. The signs and symptoms of herniated lumbar discs are grouped in the following general categories: pain, postural deformity, motor changes, sensory changes, alterations of reflexes, and nerve tension signs.[25]

Pain. Pain is the first and most characteristic symptom of a herniated disc. Pain varies in terms of quality, radiation, severity, and timing. Most describe the leg pain as sharp, shooting, burning, stabbing, or aching. The term **sciatica** is sometimes used to describe a syndrome of lumbar back pain that spreads down one leg to the ankle and is intensified by coughing and sneezing. The nerve roots L-4, L-5, S-1, S-2, and S-3 give rise to the sciatic nerve. The pain in the

buttock is described as deep, aching, or gnawing. The intensity of pain is influenced by leg position.

Pain from a herniated disc is aggravated and intensified by coughing, sneezing, straining, stooping, standing, sitting, blowing the nose, spasms of the paravertebral muscles, and any jarring movement while walking or riding. The character of pain ranges from mild discomfort to excruciating agony. Prolonged sitting is particularly painful. Pain may be alleviated by changing positions frequently, lying on the back with knees flexed and a small pillow at the head. Other patients prefer the lateral recumbent position, lying on the unaffected side with the knee flexed on the affected side.

Postural Deformity. The patient walks cautiously, bearing as little weight as possible on the affected side. The gait may be described as stiff or antalgic, and movement is deliberate to prevent jarring. Climbing stairs is particularly painful.

Motor Deficits. Slight motor weakness may be experienced, although major weakness does occur. Motor weakness can be difficult to evaluate because of the defensive reaction precipitated by pain. Weakness may be evident on plantarflexion or dorsiflexion of the foot (L-4) and dorsiflexion of the great toe (L-5, extensor hallucis longus [EHL]) and occasionally of the hamstring and quadriceps muscles. Weakness with plantarflexion correlates to the S-1 level. Foot drop occurs with significant dorsiflexion weakness. Atrophy of the affected muscles may develop, although it is not a common finding and can be minimal.

Cauda equina syndrome (CES) is caused by compression of the spinal nerves in the spinal canal at the level of the cauda equina. It can also be caused by any space-occupying lesion at the level from approximately L-2 to S-1. Symptoms include often bilateral progressive leg or foot weakness, urinary retention or incontinence, bowel incontinence, and saddle anesthesia. CES is rare; however, severe neurological compromise from a large herniated disc represents a surgical emergency

Sensory Deficits. The most common sensory impairments from root compression are paresthesias and numbness, particularly of the leg and foot. Note the specific areas of decreased sensation in the foot and leg using the pinprick method of sensory testing. Assess if the sensory deficit is dermatomal, that is, if it follows the distribution of a single nerve. Tenderness may be noted over the L-5 and S-1 vertebral spinous processes and along the tracking of the sciatic nerve.

Alterations of Reflexes. Depending on the level of the disc herniation, knee or ankle reflexes may be absent or diminished and there may be a negative Babinski's reflex because of the lower motor neuron component.

Nerve Root Tension Signs. Other signs found on the clinical examination commonly associated with evaluating patients with possible lumbar herniated disc disease include the straight leg raising test and crossed straight leg test. The **straight leg raising (SLR) test** (also called **Lasègue's sign**) is helpful in determining limitations of lower limb range of motion due to pain and the location of the pain during testing (see Fig. 19-5). Normally, it is possible when lying on the back to move the straightened leg about 90 degrees with only some slight discomfort in the hamstring muscles. The sciatic nerve becomes stretched with movement and creates traction on the proximal nerve roots. Traction and stretching of the nerve roots begin when the leg is at a 30- to 40-degree angle. In the patient with a herniated low back disc, the stretching of the sciatic nerve during passive, straight leg raising creates traction on the irritated nerve roots, thereby producing severe pain. Note the angle degree at which the patient experiences pain. This may be as little as 20 to 30 degrees. Repeating the Lasègue's maneuver on the unaffected leg produces pain of decreased severity on the contralateral side, also referred to as the crossed straight leg test.

Specific Lumbar Levels

The most common sites for lumbar disc herniation are the L-4 to L-5 and L-5 to S-1 levels, and in that order. Lesions at the L-3 to L-4 level are rare. Each level presents a characteristic syndrome of symptoms that is distinct from that of other levels (Figs. 19-7, 19-8, 19-9, and 19-10; Table 19-3). Note that multiple levels of disc herniation can exist.

L-3 to L-4 Level. Pain (L-4 radiculopathy) is located in the lower back, hip, posterolateral thigh, and anterior leg. Paresthesias are experienced in the middle section of the anterior thigh. Weakness may be noted in the quadriceps muscles, which may also demonstrate atrophic changes. The knee-jerk reflex is diminished.

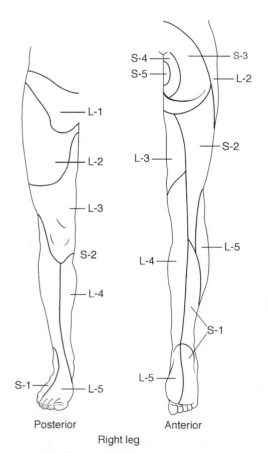

Figure 19-7 • Dermatomes of the leg.

TABLE 19–3	NEUROLOGICAL LEVELS OF THE LOWER EXTREMITIES		
ROOT	**REFLEX**	**MUSCLES**	**SENSATION**
L-2	–	Iliopsoas	Anterior thigh, groin
L-3	Patellar	Quadriceps	Anterior and lateral thigh
L-4	Patellar	Anterior tibialis	Medial leg and medial foot; medial malleolus
L-5	–	Extensor hallucis longus, hip abductors	Lateral leg and dorsum of foot; first web space
S-1	Achilles	Peroneus longus and brevis, gastrocsoleus	Lateral foot; little toe

From Scherping, S. C. (2004). History and physical examination. In J. W. Frymoyer & S. W. Wiesel (Eds.). *The adult and pediatric spine* (3rd ed., pp. 49–68). Philadelphia: Lippincott Williams & Wilkins.

L-4 to L-5 Level. Pain (L-5 radiculopathy) is perceived in the hip, groin, posterolateral thigh, lateral calf, dorsal surface of the foot, and first or second and third toes. Paresthesias may be experienced over the lateral leg and web of the great toe. There is tenderness at the femoral head and lateral gluteal region. There may be weakness with dorsiflexion of the great toe and foot. Foot drop can occur. Functionally, the foot cannot be picked up at the ankle, making walking difficult and putting the patient at risk for falls. The patient has difficulty walking on the heels. Atrophy, if present, is minor. Reflexes are usually not diminished.

L-5 to S-1 Level. Pain (S-1 radiculopathy) is perceived in the midgluteal, posterior thigh, and calf regions down to the heel and the outer surface of the foot on the side of the fourth and fifth toes. Paresthesias are found in the posterior calf and in the lateral heel, foot, and toe. Tenderness is especially apparent in the area about the sacroiliac joint. Weakness in plantarflexion of the foot may be evident. The patient has difficulty walking on the toes. The hamstring muscles may also show signs of weakness. If atrophy is present, the gastrocnemius and the soleus muscles are affected. The ankle-jerk reflex is often diminished or absent.

Remission of Pain. Pain associated with herniated disc disease can be recurrent. Patients may also present with a history of one or more similar episodes. Between acute exacerbations, pain may be completely absent or substantially diminished. The time between acute exacerbations is highly variable, with some having only weeks between episodes and some having complete relief with no recurrence.

Cervical Area

The cervical region of the spine is also prone to disc degeneration and spondylosis, as well as trauma, which predisposes the affected person to a wider range of pathologic conditions.

The most common cause of radiculopathy is decreased disc height and the associated degenerative changes (spondylosis) of the lower cervical region. Unlike the lumbar spine, disc herniation is only responsible for 20% to 25%

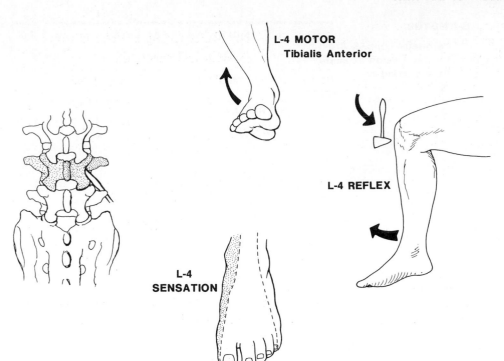

Figure 19-8 • L-4 neurologic level. (From Scherping, S.C. [2004]. History and physical examination. In Frymoyer, J. W. & Wiesel, S. W. [eds-in-chief]. *The adult and pediatric spine* [3rd ed., pp. 49–68]. Philadelphia: Lippincott Williams & Wilkins.)

of cases of radiculopathy, while degenerative changes account for 70% to 75% of cases.[23] Symptoms usually develop without any apparent precipitating event. However, symptoms may follow trauma, such as whiplash or hyperextension injuries. On radiographic investigation, there is disc degeneration and spondylosis, exhibited as

degenerative changes in the intervertebral and facet joints. These degenerative changes lead to neuroforaminal narrowing and subsequent nerve compression. The most common sites of cervical herniation are at the C-5 to C-6 and C-6 to C-7 levels, with pain along the affected sensory dermatomes. Anatomically, there is little free room within the

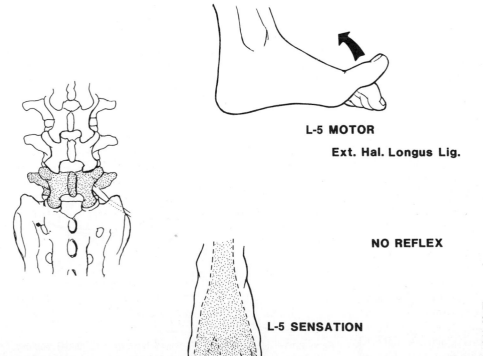

Figure 19-9 • L-5 neurologic level. (From Scherping, S.C. [2004]. History and physical examination. In Frymoyer, J. W. & Wiesel, S. W. [eds-in-chief]. *The adult and pediatric spine* [3rd ed., pp. 49–68]. Philadelphia: Lippincott Williams & Wilkins.)

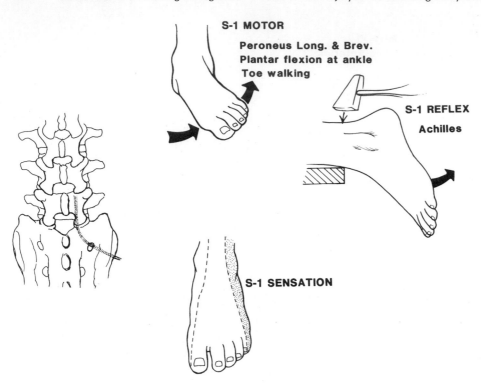

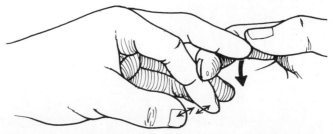

Figure 19-10 • S-1 neurologic level. (From Scherping, S.C. [2004]. History and physical examination. In Frymoyer, J.W. & Wiesel, S.W. [eds-in-chief]. *The adult and pediatric spine* [3rd ed., pp. 49–68]. Philadelphia: Lippincott Williams & Wilkins.)

spinal canal to accommodate any extraneous material. The cervical spinal cord is firmly positioned by the ligamenta denticulata. Disc protrusion in the cervical area can result not only in root compression, but also in cord compression because of the lack of free space. The particular presenting symptoms depend on the anatomic point and degree of disc protrusion.

Signs and Symptoms. The major signs and symptoms in the cervical area are discussed below.

Pain. Radicular pain in the shoulders, neck, and affected arm (Fig. 19-9) as well as paresthesias along the dermatome of the compressed nerve root is generally present. The pain is described as stabbing, burning, throbbing, and aching. It may be alleviated by raising the arm or holding the arm or head in certain positions, such as sitting with the head supported. The pain may be aggravated by driving, activities that require head flexion, and using the affected arm. Neck pain is often described as dull; pressure or aching is often also present. Paravertebral muscle spasms, which cause a stiff neck, often accompany the pain. Tenderness may be experienced when pressure is exerted over the involved cervical spine.

Motor Deficits. Radicular arm motor weakness or easy muscle fatigability may be present. Weakness may not be noted by patients if they have altered their activities due to pain. Neck movement is often restricted to some degree in all directions. Atrophy may also be detected on physical examination. A central disc herniation that is large enough to cause spinal cord compression can result in either insidious or acute spinal cord dysfunction. An acute herniation, as with trauma, will result in immediate extremity weakness, or if severe enough, paralysis. Spondylotic changes with a concomitant long-standing

disc protrusion or herniation will place the patient at risk for myelopathy. Myelopathy is clinically exhibited as decreased fine motor dexterity, gait difficulties, cramping in the extremities (often noted in the hands), and possible urinary difficulties. On examination, there is hyperreflexia, positive Hoffmann's sign (Fig. 19-11), upgoing toes (Fig. 19-12), and ankle clonus; there can be weakness, sensory changes, and poor tandem gait.

Sensory Deficits. As with lumbar radiculopathy, the most common sensory deficits are paresthesias and numbness in the distribution of the affected nerve root.

Alteration of Reflexes. Arm reflexes (biceps, triceps, and brachioradialis) may be absent or diminished in a radicular distribution, or increased if there is myelopathy.

Nerve Tension Test. "Spurling's sign," a nerve tension maneuver for the cervical spine, is conducted in neck extension. The

Figure 19-11 • Hoffman's sign. (From Scherping, S.C. [2004]. History and physical examination. In Frymoyer, J.W. & Wiesel, S.W. [eds-in-chief]. *The adult and pediatric spine* [3rd ed., pp. 49–68]. Philadelphia: Lippincott Williams & Wilkins.)

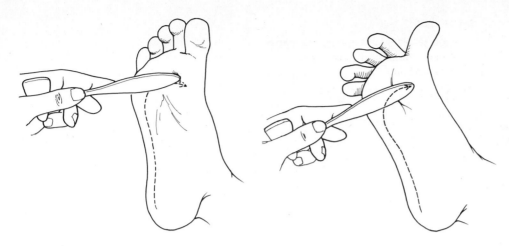

Figure 19-12 • Babinski reflex also referred to as "upgoing toes". (From Scherping, S.C. [2004]. History and physical examination. In Frymoyer, J.W. & Wiesel, S.W. [eds-in-chief]. *The adult and pediatric spine* [3rd ed., pp. 49–68]. Philadelphia: Lippincott Williams & Wilkins.)

neck is then bent laterally toward the symptomatic side. The Spurling's sign is positive if there is an exacerbation of the usual pain (Fig. 19-13).

Specific Cervical Levels

The most common affected cervical levels are at C-5 to C-6 and C-6 to C-7. Each level, and its associated spinal nerve, presents a characteristic syndrome of symptoms that is distinct from that of other levels (Figs. 19-14, 19-15, 19-16, 19-17, 19-18, and 19-19).

C-4 to C-5 Level (C-5 Radiculopathy). Pain is experienced in the neck and deltoid area. Paresthesias may also be pres-

ent. Weakness may be noted with arm abduction. Reflexes will be preserved.

C-5 to C-6 Level (C-6 Radiculopathy). Pain is experienced in the neck, shoulder, anterior portion of the upper part of the arm, radial forearm, and possibly the thumb and forefinger. Less frequently, pain extends to the scapular and clavicular regions. Paresthesias and sensory loss are found in the thumb, forefinger, radial and lateral forearm, and lateral aspects of the upper arm. Weakness is noted with flexion of the forearm (biceps). Tenderness is found in the supraspinal area of the scapula and the biceps region. The biceps and supinator reflexes are diminished or absent. The triceps reflex is either exaggerated or left intact.

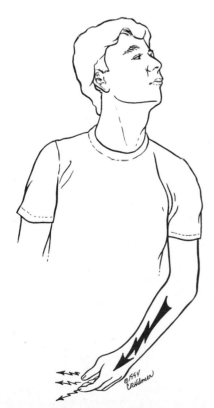

Figure 19-13 • New Spurling's sign. (From Scherping, S.C. [2004]. History and physical examination. In Frymoyer, J.W. & Wiesel, S.W. [eds-in-chief]. *The adult and pediatric spine* [3rd ed., pp. 49–68]. Philadelphia: Lippincott Williams & Wilkins.)

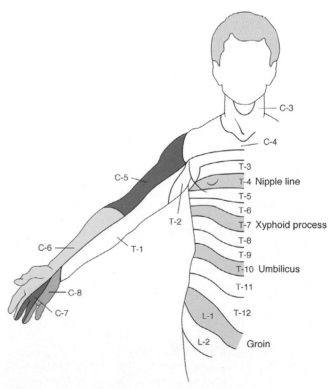

Figure 19-14 • Dermatomes of the cervical, thoracic, and upper lumbar regions.

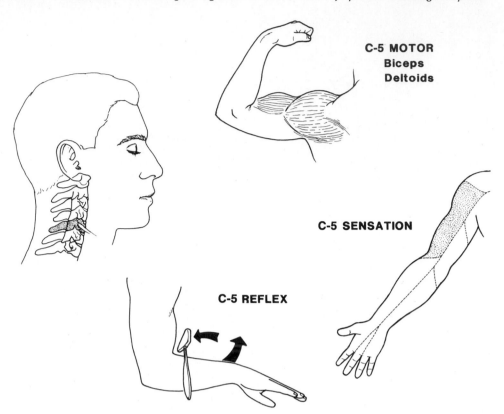

Figure 19-15 • The C-5 neurologic level. (From Scherping, S.C. [2004]. History and physical examination. In Frymoyer, J.W. & Wiesel, S.W. [eds-in-chief]. *The adult and pediatric spine* [3rd ed., pp. 49-68]. Philadelphia: Lippincott Williams & Wilkins.)

C-6 to C-7 Level (C-7 Radiculopathy). Pain is experienced in the neck, shoulder blade, and lateral surfaces of the upper arm and forearm. The index finger, the little finger, and sometimes the ring finger are plagued by pain, although all fingers may be involved. Paresthesias and sensory loss are most prominent in the second and third fingers and lat-eral forearm. Weakness is found in the triceps and extensor carpi radialis (extensors for forearm and hand grips). Occasionally, wrist drop may result. Tenderness is most apparent in the area over the medial shoulder blade. The biceps and supinator reflexes are preserved, whereas the triceps reflex is diminished or absent.

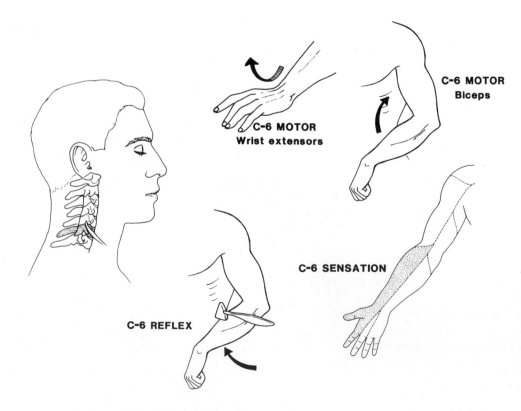

Figure 19-16 • The C-6 neurologic level. (From Scherping, S.C. [2004]. History and physical examination. In Frymoyer, J.W. & Wiesel, S.W. [eds-in-chief]. *The adult and pediatric spine* [3rd ed., pp. 49-68]. Philadelphia: Lippincott Williams & Wilkins.)

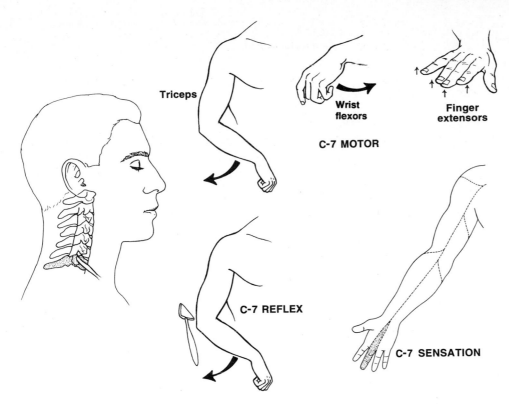

Figure 19-17 • The C-7 neurologic level. (From Scherping, S.C. [2004]. History and physical examination. In Frymoyer, J.W. & Wiesel, S.W. [eds-in-chief]. *The adult and pediatric spine* [3rd ed., pp. 49-68]. Philadelphia: Lippincott Williams & Wilkins.)

Diagnosis

Intervertebral disc herniation must be differentiated from other diseases causing neck or back pain, such as primary metastatic neoplasms. Diagnosis based on clinical examination alone is difficult, if not impossible. Additional information needed includes location, quality, and severity of pain; precipitating event (if any); alleviating and aggravating factors; history of trauma, and an abnormal MRI or computed tomography (CT) scan. MRI is preferred because it provides better visualization of the soft tissue. X-ray films, although not specific, can indicate a narrowing of the intervertebral disc space, osteophytes (spurs), or hypertrophic osteoarthritis. In special cases, an electromyogram with nerve conduction study may be performed to evaluate for a radiculopathy.

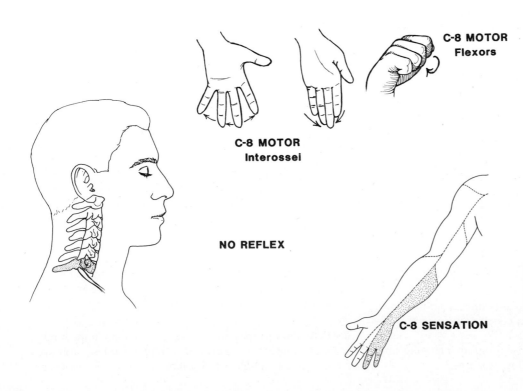

Figure 19-18 • The C-8 neurologic level. (From Scherping, S.C. [2004]. History and physical examination. In Frymoyer, J.W. & Wiesel, S.W. [eds-in-chief]. *The adult and pediatric spine* [3rd ed., pp. 49-68]. Philadelphia: Lippincott Williams & Wilkins.)

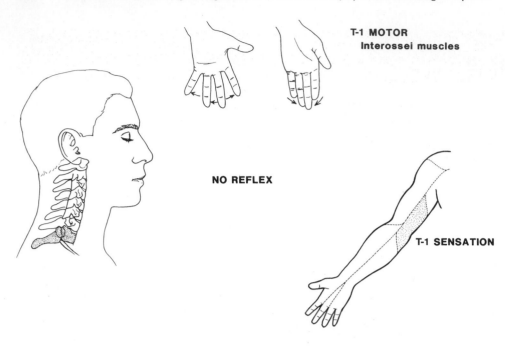

Figure 19-19 • The T-1 neurologic level. (From Scherping, S.C. [2004]. History and physical examination. In Frymoyer, J.W. & Wiesel, S.W. [eds-in-chief]. *The adult and pediatric spine* [3rd ed., pp. 49–68]. Philadelphia: Lippincott Williams & Wilkins.)

Treatment

There are two possible paths for treatments of herniated disc disease: *conservative treatment* or *surgery*. The belief that disc disease is caused by repeated biomechanical stress with degenerative changes is generally accepted. Most physicians, therefore, propose a course of treatment that will protect the involved area from added stress and provide an environment that will allow for healing of the injured degenerative discs by fibrosis. This two-pronged approach, together with pain control, constitutes conservative treatment.

Conservative Treatment

Conservative treatment for low back pain and neck pain follows the same general guidelines. Conservative treatment may be tried for at least 4 to 6 weeks. The three cornerstones of management are education and reassurance, patient comfort, and readjusting activity level to aid in recovery. The degree of activity alteration depends on the severity of symptoms. A patient with mild or moderate symptoms is generally advised to do the following:

• Modify general activity for a short time.
• Take nonnarcotic analgesics, anti-inflammatory drugs, and possibly muscle relaxants.
• Self-apply heat alternating with cold therapy, during an initial episode. Usually, apply each temperature for 20 minutes. Ice should not be applied for longer than 20 minutes at a time. During an exercise program, it may be helpful to use heat prior to exercise and ice after.
• For low back pain, avoid excessive lifting, bending, or twisting.
• For neck pain, ensure good posture and avoid neck flexion, such as desk work. Also check computer monitor height.
• Initiate a patient-specific exercise program including aerobic, stretching, and strengthening exercises.

• Set realistic, achievable goals; this enables the patient to quantify progress and increase self-control and confidence.
• Initiate patient-specific general health and well-being:
  • Smoking cessation
  • Weight appropriate for height
  • Reduction of psychological stressors
• Injections such as epidural or selective nerve root block may be prescribed.

The patient with *severe* symptoms is treated with bed rest for a short time. Resumption of light activity is advised to avoid undue back irritation and debilitation. Acupuncture and spinal manipulation as well as the use of traction or of physical modalities such as massage, diathermy, ultrasound, cutaneous laser treatment, biofeedback, and transcutaneous electrical nerve stimulation (TENS) have no proven efficacy in the treatment of low back pain.

Nursing Management During Conservative Treatment. The focus of care for this population, as with all patients, is education and reassurance, patient comfort, and activity modification. Goals of care are progressive mobilization; initiation of stretching, strengthening, and aerobic exercise program; education; patient-centered plan for general well-being; administering medications as appropriate; and preventing complications.[26] Chart 19-1 provides a summary of nursing management during conservative treatment (Figs. 19-20 and 19-21).

CLINICAL PEARLS: If a patient has experienced radicular pain without neurological deficit, 4 to 6 weeks of conservative treatment is warranted prior to operative intervention.

Bed Rest.   Bed rest for patients with severe pain in the lumbar region is limited to a short course (2 days or less), followed by resumption of light activity. If bed rest is necessary, proper

CHART 19-1 Summary of Nursing Management During Conservative Treatment of the Patient With a Herniated Intervertebral Disc*

PATIENT PROBLEM	NURSING INTERVENTIONS

Acute or Chronic Pain related to (R/T) inflammation or rupture of an intervertebral disc	• Advise alterations in activity.
	• Instruct family to apply ice packs to upper buttocks area on affected side.
	  —Apply no more than 20 minutes every hour to protect skin.
	  —Often sensation is decreased to involved area.
	• Use pain-relieving strategies, such as imagery and relaxation technique. Administer analgesics and muscle relaxants as necessary; assess the patient's severity of pain to decide which pain medication to give if more than one is prescribed.
	• Monitor the patient's response to pain-reducing treatments; use the visual analogue scale (scale of 1–10) for the patient to rate pain before and after interventions.

Risk for Trauma: extension of back injury R/T environmental factors and improper body mechanics	• Provide firm mattress. • Maintain shoulders and hips in alignment when turning the patient. • Teach proper body mechanics; caution the patient against twisting, stretching, pulling, or bending. • Maintain the patient in proper body alignment to decrease stress and strain. • For those with a herniated *cervical* disc, provide a small pillow in the nape of the neck. • For those with a herniated *lumbar* disc, provide a small pillow under the knees to relieve pressure; a small pillow can also be placed under the head (avoid pressure on the popliteal areas).
Risk for Constipation R/T decreased activity, bed rest, and drugs that decrease peristalsis	• Provide high-bulk diet. • Increase fluid intake. • Monitor the frequency of bowel movements and their consistency. • Institute a bowel program according to the physician's preference (e.g., stool softeners, laxatives.)
Impaired Physical Mobility R/T pain, numbness/tingling, fatigue, and muscle weakness	• Monitor degree of intact motor function. • Teach the patient to perform range-of-motion exercises at least four times daily. • Provide for progressive mobilization. • Assist the patient with ambulation as necessary. • Monitor the patient for use of proper body mechanics. • Provide assistive devices (e.g., brace, walker) as necessary.
Sensory/Perceptual Alterations: tactile, R/T diminished interpretation of tactile sensation secondary to inflammation or injury of the spinal nerves.	• Monitor degree of intact tactile perception in the affected areas. In patients with *cervical* disc, monitor sensation to arms, upper back, shoulders, and neck; in those with *lumbar* disc, monitor sensation to the lower back, buttocks, and legs. • Teach the patient to compensate for diminished function, such as by visually checking the position of an extremity.
Knowledge Deficit R/T body mechanics, modification of lifestyle, treatment plan, or use of braces, traction, or drugs	• Develop a teaching program tailored to the patient's needs; include proper body mechanics, a discussion of lifestyle adjustments, use of equipment, the prescribed treatment plan, use of drugs, and exercises, such as semi-sit-ups, pelvic tilt, knee–chest bends, and gluteal setting (Fig. 19–22) when patient is ready.
Risk for Disuse Syndrome R/T bed rest and immobility	• Provide for basic maintenance interventions. • Monitor vital signs and neurological signs periodically. • Apply elastic stockings to prevent deep vein thrombosis. • Encourage deep breathing exercises at least four times a day. • Monitor urinary output for urinary retention or urinary stasis. • Monitor for musculoskeletal changes, such as atrophy, contracture, and foot drop.
Anxiety R/T pain, immobility, hospitalization, uncertainty of outcome, and interference with previous lifestyle	• Explore areas of concern with the patient. • Help the patient develop strategies to reduce stress and anxiety. • Teach relaxation techniques and imagery techniques to control anxiety. • Help the patient set realistic goals. • Contact appropriate resources, such as a social worker, to assist in special problem solving.

* Differences in the management of a patient with a cervical or lumbar disc are noted when there is a variation.

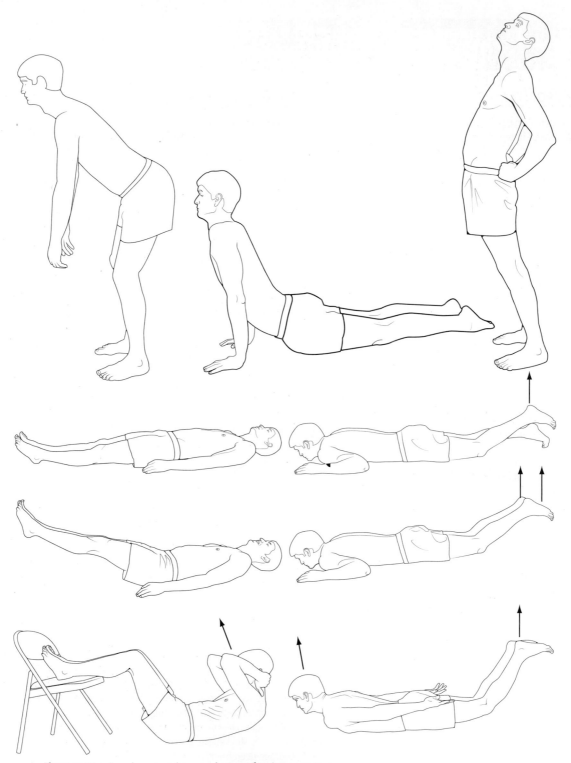

Figure 19-20 • Lumbar stretching and strengthening exercises.

positioning on the back with knees flexed is recommended. A pillow may be placed under the knees to prevent excess tension on the nerve roots. In addition, pressure must not be allowed to build up on the popliteal nerve. A small pillow may be placed under the head for comfort. For a patient with cervical pain, a small pillow may be placed in the nape of the neck. Because the purpose of bed rest is to reduce strain and pulling on the nerves, any items the patient may need should be within easy reach to avoid any undue stretching or moving. The nurse should discuss the overall purpose and goals of the bed rest regimen, as well as the duration, with the patient. Most physicians want the patient to resume walking as soon as possible; proper body mechanics should be reviewed and stressed during ambulation.

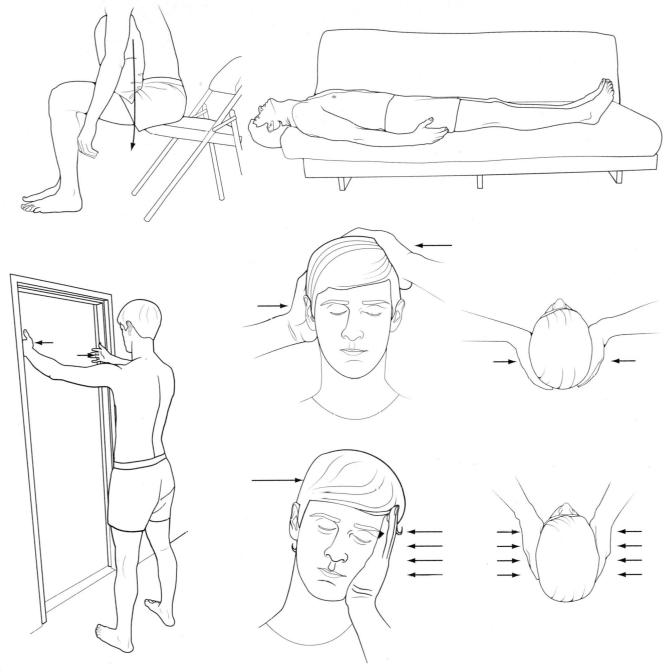

Figure 19-21 • Cervical stretching and strengthening exercises.

Activity Modification. Mobilization, staying as active as possible, is recommended. The patient may begin by walking short distances within the home, being careful to use good body mechanics. Bending, stooping, pushing, and pulling should be avoided. When symptoms and pain subside, activity is progressed and a stretching/strengthening/aerobic exercise program is initiated. Set specific, realistic goals for patients so that their progress can be quantified and goals achieved. This will increase their participation and commitment to the program.

General Health and Well-Being. When compared with nonsmokers, smokers reported more severe symptoms and had symptoms present for more time per day. Additionally, smokers had decreased psychological and physical health scores.[27,28] Of note is that smoking has a negative effect on bone healing, especially those in whom surgery is considered. Obese patients also report more severe symptoms and have increased risk of lumbar disc degeneration.[29,30] Obesity compounds the risk of surgery and prolongs recovery.[31] Psychosocial stress impacts disability and chronicity of low back

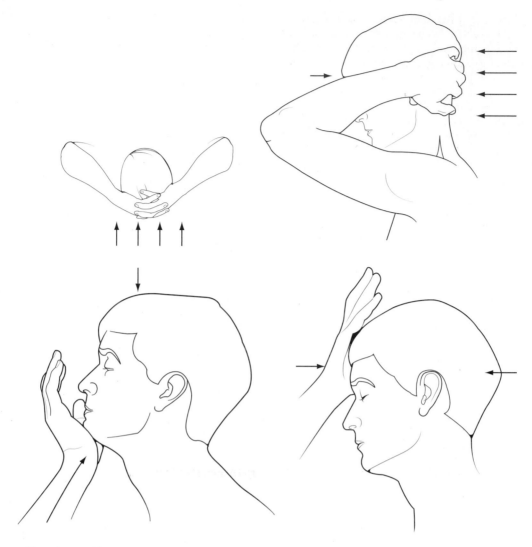

Figure 19-21 • (Continued)

pain in patients.[32,33] Patients who have psychosocial stressors and risk factors require reinforcement of education and reassurance so that they will actively participate in beneficial treatment activities.[34] If psychosocial issues are interfering with their participation, consideration is given for referral to psychological counseling.[35]

Drug Therapy. Analgesics, anti-inflammatory drugs, muscle relaxants, and sedative-tranquilizers are the major categories of drugs ordered to control the symptoms associated with back pain and intervertebral disc disease. All these drugs have side effects for which the patient should be monitored.

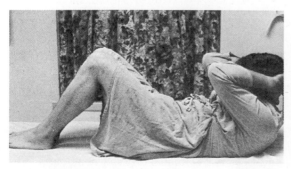
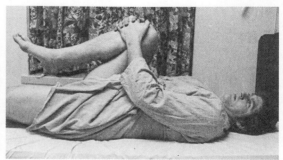

Figure 19-22 • An exercise program for patients with a herniated disc may include semi-sit-ups (*left*) and knee-chest exercises (*right*).

Analgesics. Analgesics are often necessary to manage mild to severe pain. Analgesics are classified as nonnarcotics or narcotics. For mild to moderate pain, nonnarcotic drugs are usually ordered. The following drugs are commonly used:

- NSAIDs
- Narcotic analgesics are reserved for severe pain (e.g., acetaminophen with codeine 30 mg or acetaminophen with hydrocodone 5 mg hydrocodone/500 mg acetaminophen or propoxyphene hydrochloride [Darvon] are common choices)

Pain is best controlled with a multifaceted treatment approach. Pain-relieving protocols include positioning, anxiety reduction, relaxation therapy, imagery, heat or cold local application, and analgesics. Analgesics are most effective when given before the pain becomes severe. Pain should be treated appropriately according to the guidelines for acute pain management. When chronic pain cannot be controlled adequately and interferes with a person's quality of life, referral to a multidisciplinary pain clinic may be helpful. If narcotics are considered, ensure that a bowel protocol to reduce constipation is used (e.g., Senna, laxatives) because constipation and straining at stool can exacerbate pain.

Anti-Inflammatory Drugs. Inflammation is triggered as part of a normal response to tissue injury. In the last decade or so, complex chemical substances, known as prostaglandins, have been identified as important mediators in the inflammatory process. Prostaglandins are synthesized and released in the presence of cellular injury. Drugs that treat inflammation are subclassified as steroidal or nonsteroidal drugs.

Steroidal agents are chemically related to cortisone (a hormone excreted by the adrenal cortex). Nonsteroidal agents are synthetic compounds that are *not* chemically related to substances produced by the body. NSAIDs are now the most important class of drugs used to treat inflammatory processes. These drugs have varying degrees of analgesic and antipyretic effects. They act by inhibiting the synthesis of prostaglandins.

NSAIDs are classified into salicylates and nonsalicylates. Aspirin is the most common and most prescribed of the salicylate group. In the nonsalicylate group, the following drugs are commonly used:

- Ibuprofen (Motrin, Advil)
- Naproxen (Anaprox, Naprosyn)

Keep in mind that these drugs can be irritating to the gastrointestinal lining, especially if there has been a history of gastric ulcers.

Muscle Relaxants. Several muscle relaxants are used. A few of the more frequently ordered drugs include:

- Cyclobenzaprine (Flexeril)
- Methocarbamol (Robaxin)
- Carisoprodol (Soma)
- Metaxalone (Skelaxin)

Most drugs are given orally, although in the hospitalized patient, rapid intravenous (IV) administration of certain muscle relaxants, such as diazepam (Valium) and methocarbamol, is possible. For example, IV methocarbamol 500 mg in 5% dextrose in water may be given because its dilution in solution decreases the highly irritative quality of the drug. The nurse who administers any drugs should be familiar with the many side effects and precautions for each.

Sedative-Tranquilizers. Sedative-tranquilizers are administered to decrease anxiety, which in turn decreases muscle tension and pain. One of the drugs frequently used is diazepam.

Summary of Nursing Management. The expected outcomes for the patient who is being managed conservatively for intervertebral disc disease include the following:

- Control of pain
- Improved mobility
- Tolerance of a progressive exercise program to strengthen muscles and improve posture
- Patient teaching and education related to good back health (e.g., going to a "back school" program)
- Active participation in plan to eliminate risk factors for future episodes of pain
- Resumption of previous lifestyle

Most patients treated conservatively will have a good recovery (see Chart 19-1). Unfortunately, some continue to have unresolved pain and may be considered as candidates for surgery.

Surgical Intervention

Herniated Intervertebral Disc. Within the first 4 to 6 weeks of acute symptoms, surgery is considered only when serious spinal pathology or nerve root dysfunction due to herniated disc is determined. These are patients who do not respond to conservative treatment or who, by the nature of the herniation or symptoms, require immediate surgical intervention to preserve neurological function. This latter group includes patients with:

- Cervical herniation that causes significant spinal cord compression
- Massive lumbar central herniation that compresses the cauda equina and results in sensory loss, paresis, and loss of sphincter control
- Compression, resulting in quadriceps weakness or foot drop
- Severe and unrelenting pain
- Slow-to-resolve or recurrent radiculopathy that interferes with normal lifestyle and employment

The surgical procedure selected depends on the location of the herniation (cervical, thoracic, or lumbar) and the findings on diagnostic work-up. The surgical options and the reasonably expected outcome of each option must be discussed with the patient. Possible surgical procedures for a ruptured intervertebral disc include:

Lumbar

- **Microdiscectomy**: removal of the nuclear disc material compressing the nerve and a small amount of nonherniated nucleus to help prevent reherniation; it may be completed with minimal access technology or with a laminectomy or partial laminectomy.

- **Hemilaminectomy**: part of the lamina and part of the posterior arch of the vertebra are excised.
- **Laminectomy**: the lamina, a part of the posterior arch of the vertebra, is removed. This procedure may be necessary for a large, central disc herniation.

Cervical

Anterior Approach

- **Anterior cervical discectomy with and without fusion** (most often with fusion): the intervertebral disc is removed and replaced with either an iliac crest autograft, a bone bank bone, or a synthetic spacer. A titanium plate is generally placed over the disc space. The patient may note some decrease in range of motion; however, because of prior degenerative disc disease, many have no noticeable change in range of motion.

Posterior Approach

- **Foraminotomy**: the intervertebral foramen is surgically enlarged to increase the space for exit of a spinal nerve. By enlarging the foramen, pressure on the spinal nerve that may be entrapped will be reduced, resulting in decreased pain, compression, and edema. This procedure is performed most often in the cervical region, because anatomically the cervical foramina are smaller than the lumbar foramina.

ADDITIONAL COMMON DIAGNOSES

In addition to herniated intervertebral discs, spinal stenosis, spondylolisthesis, and degenerative disc disease without herniation are common spinal diagnoses encountered. A brief description of these common spine disorders follows.

Spinal Stenosis. Spinal stenosis is any narrowing of the spinal canal or lateral recess. Often the diagnosis is made on imaging studies. Stenosis can be congenital, developmental, or acquired. A congenitally narrow cervical spinal canal with concomitant disc herniation or spondylosis can lead to cord compression more readily than with normal canal diameter.[36] Lumbar spinal stenosis is often an acquired degenerative condition as a result of spondylosis or spondylolisthesis.[37,38] Spondylosis is caused by facet hypertrophy, thickening and bulging of the ligamentum flavum, outward bulging of the disc, and disc degeneration.

Cervical stenosis, if severe enough, can lead to spinal cord compression. This can be an insidious process, cervical spondylotic myelopathy, or acute cord compression resulting in spinal cord injury. Lumbar stenosis leads to cauda equina compression, which can result in neurogenic claudication. In the symptomatic patient, it is theorized that either compression of the spinal nerve roots or insufficient blood flow to the nerve roots during walking leads to claudication symptoms.

Cervical spondylotic myelopathy is often insidious, and can present with a variety of signs and symptoms including poor fine motor dexterity, gait difficulties, neck pain in varying degrees, bladder dysfunction, hyperreflexia, positive Hoffmann's sign, upgoing toes, ankle clonus, motor weakness, sensory changes, and poor balance.[39,40]

Lumbar stenosis is also insidious. Typically patients seek medical care for leg pain with ambulation or a gradual decrease in walking distance; leg symptoms are decreased using a grocery cart or other device for support of forward flexion, there are usually hyperreflexic or absent leg reflexes, strength is generally intact, the patient may have decreased sensation, and the stance is often flexed forward.

Spondylolisthesis. Spondylolisthesis, the slippage of one vertebra on another, is most often seen at L-4 to L-5. While there are five types of spondylolisthesis, the most common is type III, degenerative. This is caused by chronic instability between two vertebrae leading to facet joint hypertrophy and laxity.

As previously mentioned, degenerative changes lead to disc dehydration and eventual osteophyte formation, facet joint hypertrophy, and ligament laxity. The biomechanical forces placed on the spine may lead to slippage of one vertebra on the adjacent one. This can be static or mobile, and can cause symptoms of stenosis.

Degenerative Disc Disease Without Herniation. The outer portion of the annulus fibrosus is innervated; however, the nucleus pulposus and the inner two thirds of the annulus fibrosus have no nerve endings. With aging, the disc dehydrates and tears develop in the annulus fibrosus. It is theorized that pain may occur if the outer third of the annulus is exposed to painful stimuli.[41]

The disc is secured to the vertebral cartilaginous endplates by Sharpey's fibers. With aging and disc desiccation, fissures occur in the endplates. Gas can accumulate in the disc. Annular bulging and further desiccation occur. There is adjacent level bone contacting bone, which leads to osteophyte formation.

Surgical Intervention

Stenosis

Decompressive laminectomy is the "gold standard" for decompressing the spinal canal in the cervical, thoracic, and lumbar spine. The number of levels surgically decompressed is dependant on the degree of stenosis and physician. Several factors are assessed in the physician's decision making as to whether or not a fusion is indicated following the decompression. These factors include spinal curvature, stability, and concomitant degenerative changes in the spine. In the cervical spine, a technique called laminoplasty is also an option for cervical canal decompression.[42]

Cervical, Thoracic, or Lumbar Procedures

Decompressive Laminectomy. The spinous process is removed first. Then the laminae are thinned with a high-speed drill. The lamina, once thinned, is then carefully removed to decompress the thecal sac. The extent of the decompression—the number of levels involved—depends on the degree of stenosis. The lateral recesses are checked for patency. During the preoperative planning, the physician will discuss with the patient if a fusion is necessary after the decompression is completed.

Cervical Laminoplasty. There are several different versions of the laminoplasty techniques performed. In general, the technique involves drilling a "hinge" through one lamina and drilling a "door" through the other lamina so that the lamina and spinous process are "opened" like a door to expand the spinal canal space. This is done at several levels in the cervical spine. Bone graft is often placed at the opening side. Mini-plates may be placed over the open side, and some physicians also place mini-plates over the hinged side.

Bone Basics and Healing

Bone provides support to the body and acts as a reservoir for chemicals necessary for bodily function as well as the stem cells of the hematopoietic system. Bone is composed of cortical (compact) bone and cancellous (trabecular) bone. Cortical bone is the compact, hard, outer layer bone, whereas cancellous bone is located between the cortical bone surfaces.

A living tissue, bone is constantly being reabsorbed and formed. Osteoclasts reabsorb bone components through enzymatic processes. Osteoblasts form new bone. The process of osteogenesis is bone forming only by living cells, while osteoconduction is the ability of a graft to allow growth into it, similar to a scaffold.[43]

Spinal arthrodesis is bone healing, or "fusing" together. The surgeon can employ a number of different techniques to create an environment conducive for the bone to heal. A fusion may be accomplished by utilizing autograft, allograft, synthetic materials, titanium or other metal spacers, and rod/screw systems.[44] A posterior rod and screw systems create internal stabilization.

- Specific vertebrae are stabilized by insertion of autograft bone or bone chips, allograft such as femoral ring, titanium cages, or synthetic spacers between the vertebrae. Autograft bone graft is usually obtained from the iliac crest (donor site). Allograft is purchased and comes in a wide variety of different types, shapes, and sizes. The purpose of spinal fusion is to internally immobilize and stabilize the vertebral column. With a spinal fusion, the patient must become accustomed to a permanent area of stiffness.
- External immobilization (collar or brace) may be indicated after surgery. This varies greatly depending on the type of procedure and the physician's preference. The goal of braces and collars is to externally immobilize the spine and prevent contraindicated movements, theoretically added to an environment to promote bony healing. In reality, most external immobilization devices allow for considerable movement.

Minimal Access Spinal Surgery

Tubular retractor systems are becoming more available to surgeons to perform minimal access discectomy. Proponents of this method report utilizing a smaller incision and, more importantly, limited soft-tissue retraction, which decreases the amount of pain the patient experiences after surgery. Techniques are also available to perform laminectomy for stenosis and lumbar fusions, thoracoscopic approaches, and cervical procedures such as microforaminotomy.[45] When possible, minimally invasive procedures are chosen.[46]

Nursing Management of the Patient Undergoing Lumbar Spine Surgery

Care of the patient who has undergone a microdiscectomy for an uncomplicated herniated disc; laminectomy for long-standing lumbar stenosis; or spinal fusion will require some similar and some very different types of nursing management (Chart 19-2).

> **CLINICAL PEARLS:** If a patient had left leg pain prior to a lumbar microdiscectomy and 6 hours postoperatively has right leg pain or weakness, this warrants immediate evaluation.

General Considerations. By the time a patient with a lumbar spine disorder is admitted for surgery, severe and debilitating symptoms have usually been present for some time. The decision to undergo surgery is often made because conservative treatment has failed, pain control is inadequate, and the quality of life is unacceptable. Other patients may have already undergone a surgical procedure but have experienced continued or renewed pain. For others, rapid onset of neurological deterioration has precipitated the need for urgent surgical decompression.

The length of hospitalization for a microdiscotomy is 23 hours or less. In many settings, it is an outpatient procedure. For a laminectomy, depending on the number of levels decompressed and the patient's comorbidities, the length of stay is 23 hours to 2 days. A spinal fusion length of stay varies depending on the actual procedure and patient comorbidities.[47-49]

Preoperative Teaching. Preoperative teaching may be provided in the physician's office before admission to the hospital or within the hospital setting if the surgery is related to other primary problems. Generally, if radiculopathy was present preoperatively, patients must understand that they are likely to experience some pain because of nerve root irritation and edema, which will gradually subside. The possibility of muscle spasms should also be discussed. All spinal surgery patients will experience varying degrees of postoperative back pain. The microdiscectomy patient, to a small extent, and the extensive lumbar fusion patient, to a large extent, can expect pain. Tactful handling and sympathetic understanding by the nurse creates a feeling of trust. Many patients experience uncomfortable muscle spasms in the low back, thighs, and abdomen during the early postoperative period. The nurse might say, "You may experience muscle spasms after surgery. It is a temporary occurrence that passes in a few days. It does not indicate that your surgery was not successful. You will be receiving your pain medication after surgery to keep you comfortable." Included in patient teaching are the need to turn the patient as a unit, keeping shoulders and hips aligned, and removing any undue stress on the back with the use of good body mechanics.

The preoperative patient teaching plan should include a discussion of the following:

- Basic preoperative routines, such as nothing by mouth (NPO) status before surgery and where the patient will go after the surgery (e.g., vital sign monitoring, frequent checking of dressing, deep breathing exercises)

CHART **19-2**   **Summary of the Nursing Management of Patients Following Lumbar Spine Surgery**

PATIENT PROBLEMS

Pain related to (R/T) tissue trauma, muscle spasms, and nerve root compression associated with surgical trauma and inflammation
- *Microdiscectomy:* pain and spasms in lower back, buttocks, and distribution of preoperative radiculopathy
- *Lumbar laminectomy:* pain and spasms in lower back, buttocks, or thighs
- *Lumbar fusion:* pain and spasms in lower back and buttocks radiating into legs

Urinary Retention R/T difficulty voiding in a horizontal position, the depressant effects of perioperative drugs, or sympathetic fiber stimulation during lumbar laminectomy

Constipation R/T decreased activity, bed rest, and drugs that decrease peristalsis

Sensory/Perceptual Alterations: tactile R/T nerve root compression associated with surgical trauma and inflammation

Impaired Physical Mobility R/T pain, numbness, tingling, and muscle weakness

NURSING INTERVENTIONS

A firm mattress is more supportive and easier to get in/out of bed.
- Position bed to reduce stress to the operative site.
  - *Microdiscectomy lumbar laminectomy:* head of bed at a comfortable position
  - *Lumbar fusion:* may have head of bed restrictions.
- Provide pillow for comfort.
  - *Microdiscectomy, laminectomy, fusion:* a small pillow may be placed under the head and one may be placed under the knees periodically (Fig. 19-23) to reduce strain.
- Keep shoulders and hips aligned when turning the patient.
- Maintain the patient in proper body alignment at all times so that spine remains in neutral position.
- Reposition the patient every 2 hour.
- Reinforce patient preoperative teaching to refrain from twisting, flexing, bending, hyperextending, or pulling on the side rails.
- Use pain-relieving strategies, such as imagery and relaxation techniques.
- Administer analgesics as necessary; assess severity of the patient's pain to decide which pain medication to give if more than one is prescribed.
- Monitor the patient's response to pain-reducing treatments; use the visual analogue scale (scale of 1–10) to allow the patient to rate pain before and after interventions.
- Provide for privacy and comfort. Assist the patient to the bathroom, if possible.
- Provide male patients with an opportunity to stand for urination if the physician permits.
- Palpate the bladder for distention. Utilize bladder scanner if available.
- Monitor the intake and output (I&O) record for adequate intake.
- Intermittent catheterization may be ordered if the patient is unable to void during the early postoperative period.
- Provide a high-bulk diet.
- Increase fluid intake.
- Monitor the frequency of bowel movements and their consistency.
- Auscultate the abdomen in all four quadrants for bowel sounds.
- Institute a bowel program according to the physician's preference (e.g., stool softeners, laxatives, etc.).
- Monitor the patient's perception of light touch and pain.
  - *Microdiscectomy, laminectomy, fusion:* monitor sensation to the lower back, buttocks, and legs. Compare with preoperative assessment. Preoperative numbness is slow and gradual to resolve, generally taking many weeks to reach maximum improvement.
- Protect the involved area from injury.
- Teach the patient to compensate for diminished function, such as by visually checking the position of the extremity.
- Monitor the patient's ability to move legs freely in bed; compare with preoperative baseline data.
- Perform range-of-motion exercises at least four times daily; the patient may be taught to do this independently.
- Provide assistive devices (e.g., brace, walker, etc.) as necessary.
- Provide for progressive mobilization as ordered.*
  - Microdiscectomy: stand at side of bed after return from postanesthesia care unit. Ambulate soon thereafter.
  - *Lumbar laminectomy:* begin mobilizing the afternoon/evening of surgery; follow the physician's protocol for mobilization.†

(continued)

CHART 19-2   Summary of the Nursing Management of Patients Following Lumbar Spine Surgery   (Continued)

PATIENT PROBLEMS	NURSING INTERVENTIONS
	– *Lumbar fusion:* usual is to begin mobilization the first postoperative day; follow the physician's protocol for mobilization. Highly variable dependent on procedure performed and physician preference.
Risk for Infection R/T surgical incision	• Observe the dressing for evidence of drainage (blood or cerebrospinal fluid).
	• Monitor the incision for swelling, redness, drainage, irritation, or pain.
	• Maintain strict aseptic technique when changing the dressing.
	• With a lumbar laminectomy, check the dry, sterile dressing to ensure that it has not become wet; if this occurs, change the dressing immediately.
Risk for Disuse Syndrome R/T surgery, perioperative drugs, bed rest, and immobility	• Provide for basic maintenance interventions.
	• Monitor vital signs and neurological signs periodically.
	• Apply compression boots to prevent deep vein thrombosis.
	• Encourage deep breathing exercises at least every 2 hours.
	• Auscultate the chest for breath sounds every 4 hours.
	• Monitor the patient for musculoskeletal changes, such as atrophy, contracture, and foot drop.
Knowledge Deficit R/T body mechanics, modification of lifestyle, treatment plan, or uses of braces, traction, or drugs	• Develop a discharge teaching program to decrease the risk of recurrent disc herniation by reducing stress on the back; include the following information:
	– Proper body mechanics
	– Use of adequate support when on a mattress and in a chair
	– Maintenance of optimal weight (a weight reduction program may be necessary)
	– Proper technique for any exercises prescribed by the physician, or reinforcement of exercises taught by the physical therapist, such as semi-sit-ups, pelvic tilt, knee–chest bends, and gluteal setting (see Fig. 19-22).
	– Any modifications in activity (e.g., for climbing stairs, lifting)
	• Explore areas of concern with the patient.
	• Help the patient develop strategies to reduce stress and anxiety.
	• Teach relaxation techniques and imagery techniques to control anxiety.
	• Help the patient set realistic goals.
	• If possible, provide written discharge instructions.

* The procedure for ambulation of patients varies from physician to physician. Some surgeons may ask that their patients dangle their feet from the edge of the bed on the evening of the day of surgery or the first postoperative day. Other surgeons do *not* allow their patients to dangle their feet at all, believing that excessive stress would be placed on the suture line. The individual protocols of the surgeon must be followed.

† *Technique for getting the lumbar spine surgery patient out of bed:* if possible, the head of the bed is raised with the patient comfortably positioned on the bed close to the edge of the side where he or she will be getting out of the bed. If the bed must remain flat, the patient is positioned on his or her side with knees and hips slightly flexed near the side of the bed from which he or she will rise. In either case, two nurses are necessary. One nurse grasps the patient under the arm and around the upper back and neck. The patient is instructed to place his or her arm around the nurse's shoulders. The other nurse grasps the patient's hips and legs. At the count of three, the nurses assist the patient to the upright position. If the patient is to walk, the support of two nurses is advisable, because weakness, dizziness, and light-headedness are common. A few steps to the door and back are sufficient for the first venture out of bed. Gradually, the patient will be able to tolerate ambulation for greater distances. As the patient becomes more mobile, he or she will require only assistance of one care provider and then be independent. Mobility is gradually increased. After a microdiscectomy, the patient is quickly ready to walk in the halls; after a multilevel laminectomy, the patient should be ready for the halls by early in the morning the first day after surgery. If the patient has had a fusion, the same technique is used; however, the patient may require a brace (per physician order), and he or she may not be walking in the halls until the afternoon or evening of the first postoperative day.

- Turning technique, keeping shoulders and hips aligned
- The correct technique for getting out of bed after surgery, pushing the torso up with the arms while swinging the legs over the side of the bed to eliminate twisting
- Rationale for maintaining proper body alignment at all times and ways in which alignment can be maintained
- Physical and/or occupational therapy, as indicated, may be ordered by the physician for gait retraining, mobilization, activities of daily living assessment, etc.

- The risks of twisting, pulling, stretching, or straining after surgery
  - Plan for general house/lawn care needs.
  - Be cautious of walking dogs that might unexpectedly pull.
- General hints to prepare for going home after surgery
  - Sit for only short periods of time; change positions frequently.
  - Take frequent short walks, gradually increasing endurance/distance.

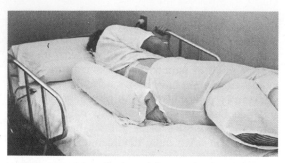

Figure 19-23 • Position of patient following lumbar laminectomy.

- Reminder about likely presurgery deconditioning
- Don't lift more than 10 lb (roughly 1 gallon of milk).
- Don't drive while on narcotic pain medications and it is until comfortable to do so.
- Monitor for potential voiding problems postoperatively, especially if receiving narcotics.
- Be aware that if a fusion was done and a graft from the hip used, the donor site may be more painful than the spine site.
- Surgery-specific hints
  - Microdiscectomy patients
    - Activity is decreased for the 2 to 6 weeks to allow for the annulus fibrosis to heal and prevent reherniation.
    - These patients can often return to a sedentary job 1 to 4 weeks after surgery.
    - After 4 to 6 weeks, there will be a gradual resumption of normal activities and core strengthening exercises.
  - Decompressive laminectomy patients
    - These patients are often deconditioned with a low walking tolerance.
    - In general, they are older individuals.
    - There will be a slow, consistent, gradual increase in activity.
  - Lumbar fusion
    - Very procedure- and surgeon-specific postoperative activity recommendations will be given.
    - Variables include instrumentation, bone quality, procedure and number of levels, and external bracing.

Preoperative Nursing Management. In addition to the routine preoperative preparation of the patient, thigh-high elastic stockings (TEDs) or lower extremity compression devices will be applied. This is done to facilitate blood return to the heart and to decrease venous stasis, which would place the patient at high risk for deep vein thrombosis. Vasomotor changes in the lower extremities secondary to autonomic stimulation can also contribute to stasis of blood.

Postoperative Nursing Management

General Care. Basic postoperative nursing management, such as frequent monitoring of vital signs, care of dressings, administration of IV fluids, and monitoring of intake and output, should be instituted. Follow your unit protocol for a lumbar surgery.

Special Assessment. In the postoperative period, the nurse should frequently assess sensory and motor function in the extremities. With lumbar surgery, the legs should be the focus of attention. When assessing motor and sensory function, the nurse compares present motor and sensory function with preoperative function. The patient is asked to move the extremities, wiggle the fingers or toes, and identify the part of the extremity that has been touched or squeezed. If there is apparent motor weakness, paralysis, or lack of awareness of touch or temperature in the postoperative period, nerve root compression should be suspected. Such deficits should be reported to the physician immediately.

> **CLINICAL PEARLS:** If after a lumbar laminectomy the patient is experiencing decreased motor function in his or her legs, this warrants immediate evaluation.

Several problems may arise following lumbar surgery including urinary retention, paralytic ileus, and muscle spasms. Urinary output should be monitored to be sure that the patient is voiding in sufficient amounts. Monitor for presence of bowel sounds and the girth of the abdomen for development of paralytic ileus. Muscle spasms in the operative region are often more painful than the incision site. Assess the character and location of pain.

The common patient needs associated with the postoperative lumbar surgery patient are discussed in Chart 19-2. In addition, many patients who have had more extensive surgery have an elevated temperature (up to 102.2°F [39°C]) for a day or two after surgery. Use acetaminophen (Tylenol) not to exceed 4000 mg in 24 hours (assuming no contraindications) orally to lower the temperature. Fluid intake should also be increased.

> **CLINICAL PEARLS:** Following lumbar surgery, in particular lumbar laminectomy, the patient may experience initial voiding difficulties. Pay close attention to avoid overextension of the bladder.

Table 19-4 presents special nursing considerations for the patient who has undergone spinal fusion or an anterior cervical fusion or discectomy.

> **CLINICAL VIGNETTE:** LR is a 42-year-old woman with 2 months of right leg pain. She describes the pain as radiating through her right buttock down the posterolateral right leg and the right calf to the bottom of her foot (as if there is "an arrow shooting down my leg"). Currently, she is participating in chiropractic treatment and massage therapy as well as taking muscle relaxants. She is not taking any nonsteroidal anti-inflammatory medications. On examination, her leg strength and sensation are intact, with an absent right Achilles reflex. Straight leg testing is negative. MRI reveals an L-5 to S-1 herniated nucleus pulposus, eccentric to the right. Her history and clinical and radiographic examination are concordant, exhibiting an S-1 radiculopathy. At this point she feels she is 50% better than at the onset of symptoms; nonsteroidal anti-inflammatory medications and physical therapy in addition to her current regimen were advised. One month later, she experienced an acute exacerbation of her symptoms. She underwent an L-5 to S-1 microdiscectomy for right S-1 radiculopathy with complete resolution of her symptoms.

TABLE 19-4   SPECIAL NURSING CONSIDERATIONS IN SPINAL FUSION*

PROBLEM OR PROCEDURE	SPECIAL CONSIDERATIONS	POSTOPERATIVE NURSING CONSIDERATIONS
Spinal fusion (in general) • Bone graft	A bone graft will be obtained from the patient (autograft), a bone bank (allograft), or a synthetic spacer. • If from the patient, the donor site is the iliac crest. • If from a bone bank, or if a synthetic device is used, there will not be a donor site.	If a donor site is present: • Monitor the incision for bleeding or drainage. • Assess the incision daily; change the dry sterile dressing as ordered. • Position the patient so that no undue pressure is placed on the donor site. • Instrumentation: a variety of options are available for spinal fusion instrumentation. Internal instrumentation is utilized by the surgeon to provide internal fixation and immobilization. It can be placed anterior, posterior, or both.
• Immobilization of the operative site	Some form of immobilization may be ordered. • *Cervical:* soft or rigid collar may be ordered; alternatively, a halo apparatus with jacket may be applied. • *Thoracic or lumbar:* a brace or body jacket may be ordered.	• Maintain the collar or brace as ordered. • Monitor the patient's skin for irritation. • Teach proper body mechanics. • Teach the patient the proper application of collar or brace. • If a halo apparatus has been applied, provide for patient teaching.
Posterior thoracic fusion	Autograft may be taken from a rib or the posterior iliac crest. Often these are lengthy incisions with significant postoperative pain.	
Posterior lumbar fusion	Autograft is generally taken from the posterior iliac crest, if enough is not available during the decompression. Usually, another incision is not necessary.	
Anterior cervical discectomy with fusion	Postoperatively, patients are mobilized as soon as they return from the PACU. Patients with allograft are generally discharged the same day or the next morning. Patients with autograft may require an additional night for donor site pain management and mobilization. • Collar if ordered. • Relatively pain free • Bothered by a sore throat or experiencing difficulty swallowing as a result of esophagus and trachea manipulation	• Provide comfort measures such as throat lozenges (viscous lidocaine [Xylocaine] may be ordered by the physician). • Additional complications are related to soft-tissue manipulation and swelling. The esophagus and trachea are retracted during surgery, and irritation of the recurrent laryngeal nerve and tracheal edema can result in hoarseness and difficulty coughing. • In addition, assess the quality of the patient's voice and the ability to cough; do not initiate oral intake if the patient cannot protect the airway adequately.

PACU, postanesthesia care unit.
* See Chart 19-2 for general principles of postoperative care.

Nursing Management of the Patient Undergoing Cervical Spine Surgery

There are some special considerations for the nursing management of the cervical spine surgery patient that vary from the above outlined lumbar spine surgery patient nursing management. In particular, anterior and posterior cervical spine surgery patients have very different postoperative expected courses and thus different nursing management (Chart 19-3).

General Considerations. The length of hospitalization for an anterior cervical discectomy and fusion is 23 hours or less. In some settings, it is becoming an outpatient procedure. For more extensive, multilevel anterior surgery, patient length of stay is 23 to 48 hours. Posterior cervical decompression with or without fusion generally requires 48 to 72 hours in the hospital. Pain control and mobilization tend to prolong length of stay.

Preoperative Teaching. Anterior cervical spine patients often experience intrascapular pain from intraoperative distraction of the vertebral bodies and some degree of sore throat. These patients usually have only minimal postoperative discomfort.

Posterior cervical spine patients will have significant posterior neck pain and muscle spasm. A multilevel cervical decompressive laminectomy with or without a fusion requires a long incision and soft-tissue disruption. Tactful handling by the nurse creates a feeling of trust. Reassuring the patient is important with statements such as, "Postoperative pain is a temporary occurrence that passes in a few days. It does not indicate that your surgery was not successful. You will be receiving your pain medication after surgery to keep you comfortable." Included in patient teaching is the need to turn the patient, keeping head and shoulders aligned, and removing any undue stress on the neck with the use of good body mechanics.

CHART 19-3 **Summary of Patient Problems With Cervical Spine Surgery**

PATIENT PROBLEMS	NURSING INTERVENTIONS
Pain related to (R/T) tissue trauma, muscle spasms, and nerve root manipulation associated with surgical trauma and inflammation • *Anterior cervical discectomy with or without fusion:* pain and spasms in upper back, shoulder, neck, or arms; may have sore throat and difficulty swallowing postoperatively as a result of manipulation of the esophagus during the procedure • *Posterior laminectomy with or without fusion:* pain and spasms in upper back, shoulder, neck, or arms	• Position bed to reduce stress to the operative site. 　– *Anterior-posterior cervical:* head of bed is usually elevated to a comfortable position. • Provide very flat, if any, pillow for comfort. 　– *Anterior or posterior:* Pillows need to be used cautiously to avoid forward flexion of the neck by forcing the head forward with a pillow. Good alignment of the spine is to be maintained. • Maintain the patient in proper body alignment at all times so that spine remains in neutral position. • Reposition the patient at least every 2 hours. • Reinforce patient preoperative teaching to refrain from twisting, flexing, hyperextending, or pulling on the side rails. • Use pain-relieving strategies, such as imagery and relaxation techniques. • Administer analgesics as necessary; assess severity of the patient's pain to decide which pain medication to give if more than one is prescribed. • Monitor the patient's response to pain-reducing treatments; use the visual analogue scale (scale of 1–10) to allow the patient to rate pain before and after interventions.
Urinary Retention R/T difficulty voiding in a horizontal position or the depressant effects of perioperative drugs	• Provide for privacy and comfort. Assist the patient to the bathroom, if possible. • Provide male patients with an opportunity to stand for urination if the physician permits. • Palpate the bladder for distention. Use bladder scanner if available. • Monitor the intake and output (I&O) record for adequate intake. • Intermittent catheterization may be ordered if the patient is unable to void during the early postoperative period.
Constipation R/T decreased activity, bed rest, and drugs that decrease peristalsis	• Provide a high-bulk diet. • Increase fluid intake. • Monitor the frequency of bowel movements and their consistency. • Auscultate the abdomen in all four quadrants for bowel sounds. • Institute a bowel program according to the physician's preference (e.g., stool softeners, laxatives, etc.).
Sensory/Perceptual Alterations: tactile R/T nerve root compression associated with surgical trauma and inflammation	• Monitor the patient's perception of light touch and pain. • Monitor sensation to the arms, upper back, shoulders, and neck. Compare with preoperative assessment. • Protect the involved area from injury. • Teach the patient to compensate for diminished function, such as by visually checking the position of the extremity.
Impaired Physical Mobility R/T pain, numbness, tingling, and muscle weakness	• Monitor the patient's ability to move legs and arms freely in bed; compare with preoperative baseline data. • Perform range-of-motion exercises at least four times daily; the patient may be taught to do this independently. • Provide assistive devices (e.g., brace, walker, reacher/grabber, etc.) as necessary. • Provide for progressive mobilization as ordered. 　– Roll the head of the bed up, align the patient at the edge of the bed, and gently assist the patient to a standing position by placing your arras across the patient's upper back and under the knees. The patient should *not* place his or her arm on the nurse's shoulder.

(continued)

CHART **19-3**   **Summary of Patient Problems With Cervical Spine Surgery** (Continued)

PATIENT PROBLEMS	NURSING INTERVENTIONS
Risk for Infection R/T surgical incision	• Observe the dressing for evidence of drainage (blood or cerebrospinal fluid). • Monitor the incision for swelling, redness, drainage, irritation, or pain. • Maintain strict aseptic technique when changing the dressing. • With a posterior cervical procedure, check the dry, sterile dressing to ensure that it has not become wet; if this occurs, change the dressing immediately.
Risk for Disuse Syndrome R/T surgery, perioperative drugs, bed rest, and immobility	• Provide for basic maintenance interventions. • Monitor vital signs and neurological signs periodically. • Apply compression boots to prevent deep vein thrombosis. • Encourage deep breathing exercises at least every 2 hours patients with a *cervical laminectomy* tend to have shallow respirations because of pain; such patients are at high risk for development of atelectasis and pneumonia. • Auscultate the chest for breath sounds every 4 hours. • Monitor the patient for musculoskeletal changes, such as atrophy, contracture, and foot drop.
Knowledge Deficit R/T body mechanics, modification of lifestyle, treatment plan, or use of braces, traction, or drugs	• Develop a discharge teaching program to decrease the risk of recurrent disc herniation by reducing stress on the back or neck; include the following information: – Proper body mechanics – Use of adequate support when on a mattress and in a chair – Maintenance of optimal weight (a weight reduction program may be necessary) – Proper technique for any exercises prescribed by the physician, or reinforcement of exercises taught by the physical therapist – Any modifications in activity (e.g., for climbing stairs, lifting) • Explore areas of concern with the patient. • Help the patient develop strategies to reduce stress and anxiety. • Teach relaxation techniques and imagery techniques to control anxiety. • Help the patient set realistic goals. • If possible, provide written discharge instructions.

The preoperative patient teaching plan should include a discussion of the following:

• Basic preoperative routines, such as NPO status before surgery and where the patient will go after the surgery
• Basic postoperative routines (e.g., vital sign monitoring, frequent checking of dressing, deep breathing exercises)
• Turning technique, keeping head and shoulders aligned
• If a cervical collar is used, using rails and being cautious of stairs and curbs
  • Cervical collar use and amount of time in a collar is variable, depending on surgeon preference and the specific procedure.
• Rationale for maintaining proper body alignment at all times and ways in which alignment can be maintained
  • Planning for general house/lawn care needs

• Being cautious of walking dogs that might unexpectedly pull
• General hints to prepare for going home after surgery
  • Taking frequent short walks, gradually increasing endurance/distance
  • Reminder about likely presurgery deconditioning
  • No lifting more than 10 lb (roughly 1 gallon of milk)
  • No driving while on narcotic pain medications, or if cervical collar is used

Surgery: Specific Hints

Anterior Cervical. Anterior cervical surgery patients often have some degree of sore throat. For those with multilevel surgeries, swallowing because of soreness can be difficult. The patient may also describe a "lump" feeling when swallowing, particularly for a C-3 to C-4 fusion. Instruct the patient to stay well hydrated, to start with soft food and gradually add food with more consistency as tolerated, and to chew well. If the patient has a lot of phlegm, dairy products may make it more tenacious. Clearing the throat may increase phlegm production.

CLINICAL PEARLS: Following an anterior cervical surgery, it is common to experience difficulties swallowing.

The intraoperative distraction of the vertebral bodies may cause postoperative pain at the base of the neck or between the shoulder blades. Heat or ice, massage, acetaminophen, muscle relaxants, or a short course of narcotic analgesics may be warranted.

Anti-inflammatory medications are contraindicated after a spinal fusion, because they interfere with bone healing. Ultimately the physician's preference is considered; these medications are often held for 6 to 12 weeks after surgery.

Posterior Cervical. The posterior cervical spine patient who has undergone multilevel surgery will require astute pain control postoperatively. Initially, patient-controlled analgesia and scheduled muscle relaxants are indicated. The patient will require maximal assistance immediately after surgery and the first postoperative day. Physical and occupational therapy are helpful postoperatively for most patients after spinal surgeries to encourage early and safe mobilization. However, the challenge is the short length of stay for most of these patients.

In the postoperative period, the nurse should frequently assess sensory and motor function in the upper extremities (Table 19-5). With anterior cervical surgery, swallow and voice quality should be assessed. Patients are likely to be monitored with a continuous pulse oximeter to ensure no respiratory difficulty. When assessing motor and sensory function, the nurse compares present motor and sensory

TABLE 19–5   THE NEUROLOGICAL LEVELS OF THE UPPER EXTREMITIES

ROOT	REFLEX	MUSCLES	SENSATION
C-5	Biceps	Deltoid Biceps	Lateral arm (Axillary nerve)
C-6	Brachioradialis	Wrist extensors Biceps	(Musculocutaneous nerve)
C-7	Triceps	Wrist flexors Finger extensors Triceps	Middle finger
C-8	—	Finger flexors Hand intrinsics	Medial forearm (Medial antebrachial cutaneous nerve)
T-1	—	Hand intrinsics	Medial arm (Medial brachial cutaneous nerve)

From Scherping, S. C. (2004). History and physical examination. In J. W. Frymoyer & S. W. Wiesel. (Eds.). *The adult and pediatric spine.* (3rd ed., pp. 49–68). Philadelphia: Lippincott Williams & Wilkins.

function with preoperative function. The patient is asked to move the extremities, wiggle the fingers or toes, and identify the part of the extremity that has been touched or squeezed. If there is apparent motor weakness, paralysis, or lack of awareness of touch or temperature in the postoperative period, spinal cord or nerve root compression should be suspected. Such deficits should be reported to the physician immediately.

CLINICAL PEARLS: Posterior cervical surgeries, such as cervical laminectomy, are quite painful with significant muscle spasm. These patients require astute attention and evaluation of effectiveness of pain control interventions.

The common patient problems associated with the postoperative spine surgery patient are discussed in Chart 19-3. In addition, many patients who have had more extensive surgery have an elevated temperature (up to 102.2°F [39°C]) for a day or two after surgery. Use acetaminophen not to exceed 4000 mg in 24 hours (assuming no contraindications) orally to lower the temperature. Fluid intake should also be increased.

Table 19-4 presents special nursing considerations for the patient who has undergone spinal fusion or an anterior cervical fusion or discectomy.

CLINICAL VIGNETTE: NP is a 41-year-old woman with a 4-week history of right arm pain. Awakening one morning with her arm sore (no precipitating event), her symptoms progressed to a pain intensity of 7 out of 10 at the best, and 10 out of 10 at the worst. She described her pain and paresthesias radiating into the anterolateral right arm, to the thumb and index finger. Additionally, she described sharp stabbing neck pain. Her symptoms were aggravated by head movement (she was having trouble finding any comfortable position) and alleviated only by narcotic pain medications; chiropractic treatment and nonsteroidal anti-inflammatory medications had not given her any symptom relief. Neurological examination revealed full strength and intact deep tendon reflexes; decreased sensation was noted in the anterolateral right arm, index finger, and thumb. NP's past medical history was significant for insulin-dependent diabetes, managed with an insulin pump. She was usually physical active, and had normal weight for height. NP was offered surgical intervention because of her 4 weeks' duration of increasingly severe pain despite conservative measures and an MRI demonstrating C-5 to C-6 herniated nucleus pulposus compressing the right C-6 nerve root. NP elected to undergo a C-5 to C-6 anterior cervical discectomy and fusion with allograft and plate. She did well postoperatively with complete resolution of her symptoms and return to her usual activities.

Potential Complications of Spine Surgery: Collaborative Nursing Problems

Although rare, complications can develop following a spinal surgery. Some are more apt to occur in the immediate postoperative period, whereas others usually arise later. Discharge teaching should include a discussion of signs and symptoms that should be reported to the physician immediately.

Complications after spinal surgery, when they arise, require medical assessment and intervention and are therefore collaborative problems. Early complications include hematoma at the operative site, cerebral spinal fluid (CSF) leak, and nerve injury. Later complications include infection, persistent CSF leak, arachnoiditis, and/or vertebral column instability. Following a fusion, potential complications include pseudoarthrosis (bone not healing, thus failing to fuse) and instrumentation failure.

Hematoma at the Operative Site. In rare instances, a hematoma can develop postoperatively as a result of bleeding at the operative site. The most prominent symptom is pain at the operative area that may or may not be described as throbbing. The pain is often out of proportion to what is expected after that specific surgery type. On assessment, there may be swelling around the incision, a decrease in motor function, and a decrease in sensation to the involved area. In the case of an anterior cervical surgery, respiratory difficulties such as stridor related to soft-tissue swelling or tracheal irritation/edema may develop. These findings warrant immediate notification of the physician. If a hematoma is present and is causing neurological deficits (decreased or lost motor and sensory function) or if there are concerns about respiratory compromise (for anterior cervical surgeries), the physician may reoperate to evacuate the hematoma. A hematoma, if left untreated, can result in irreversible motor and sensory deficits, including paraplegia and bowel or bladder dysfunction.

> **CLINICAL PEARLS:**   Following anterior cervical surgery, respiratory compromise warrants immediate evaluation.

CSF Leak. An intraoperative dural tear will be closed during surgery. However, occasionally, the closure will not suffice, and CSF will leak through the tear. The dressing should be assessed for drainage. Symptomatically, the patient will develop a headache. The physician will order flat bed rest, giving the dura time to heal. If the leak does not resolve, a lumbar drain may be placed or the patient may require re-exploration for surgical repair of the leak.[50]

> **CLINICAL PEARLS:**   If after a lumbar laminectomy the patient complains of a headache when standing that is alleviated by lying down, he or she may have a CSF leak; this warrants immediate evaluation.

Nerve Root Injury. Leg or arm weakness can occur as a result of nerve root injury. An aggressive program of physiotherapy is needed, along with slings, braces, or splints, depending on the involved extremity and the extent of injury. A short course of steroids (e.g., dexamethasone or methylprednisolone) may decrease the surrounding edema and improve function. Range-of-motion exercises should be incorporated into the nursing care plan, and careful attention must be directed toward preventing contractures, musculoskeletal deformities, and injury to the involved limb. The patient may sustain permanent disability even with an aggressive treatment program.[51]

Occasionally, a C-5 radiculitis can develop after extensive anterior or posterior cervical decompression. Clinically, the patient may exhibit pain in the C-5 distribution and deltoid weakness. This often resolves within 6 months after surgery.[52]

Iatrogenic Deformity. A laminectomy at more than one level of the vertebral column can cause spinal column instability and deformity. When the surgeon performs a laminectomy on two or more vertebral levels, or with other underlying degenerative disease such as spondylolisthesis, a spinal fusion may be necessary to ensure stability of the spinal column and prevent disability. This is often a delayed complication.

Infection. Caregivers require specific instruction on assessment and care of the incision. Changes in the wound (e.g., purulent drainage, odor) that indicate signs and symptoms of infection cannot be overemphasized. Early intervention for wound problems is imperative. If left untreated, local or systemic problems including discitis, abscess formation, or sepsis can develop.

CSF Fistula. A **CSF fistula** is an abnormal connection between the subarachnoid space and the incision, which causes CSF drainage; this will be evident on the dressing, either alone or in combination with serosanguineous drainage. The dressing is usually wet, and increased drainage occurs when the patient is lying on the back or standing. Of major concern is infection at the fistula site and meningitis, because microorganisms can ascend the fistula and flourish in the ideal environment of the cerebrospinal space.

Formation of a fistula is not an early postoperative complication. It often takes a week or more for evidence of a fistula to appear. Because CSF drainage on the dressing is the major sign of a fistula, it is important to monitor the dressing for continuous drainage that could be clear or yellowish in color. Patients and their caregivers should be advised to monitor the dressing and report abnormal drainage to the physician's office. If the fistula does not spontaneously seal itself, surgical closure will be necessary. Prophylactic antibiotics may be ordered, although this has not proven to be effective in the prevention of infection. If leakage of CSF is suspected, maintaining the patient on flat bed rest, thereby decreasing pressure on the meningeal defect, may help the leak to seal spontaneously.

Arachnoiditis. Arachnoiditis, an inflammation of the arachnoid layer of the spinal meninges, can result from infection, but more often the exact cause is unknown. It is theorized that it may be as a result of intraoperative nerve root manipulation. Arachnoiditis is a particularly worrisome complication because the scar tissue and adhesions that can form cause severe and chronic pain.

RECURRENT SYMPTOMS AFTER SURGERY

Surgery is not always synonymous with relief of pain and other symptoms. For example, a patient who has experienced long-term pain radiating down the leg before surgery will probably continue to have some pain after surgery. It may persist for several weeks postoperatively. If there has been considerable sensory loss because of nerve root compression preoperatively, pain perception may actually increase because of improvement of the sensory deficit. Such patients may experience paresthesias for several months after surgery.

Surgery for a herniated disc does not negate the possibility of recurrence of a disc herniation at the same level on the same or opposite side or at other levels. Repeated laminectomies in the same patient are not unusual. This possibility does underscore the need for patient teaching related to body mechanics, posture, and protection from injury. However, degenerative changes may already be present that predispose the patient to future problems, even if a teaching program is judiciously followed.

SUMMARY

Spine disorders that a patient may be afflicted with are numerous. Fortunately, most do not require surgery and the majority of patients with neck or back pain will have resolution of their symptoms within 4 to 6 weeks. Prevention of pain exacerbations is accomplished through education and collaborative goal setting with the patient. Included are realistic, attainable goals for stretching, strengthening, and aerobic exercise; stress management; weight appropriate for height; and smoking cessation. The evidenced-based and comprehensive *Clinical Practice Guideline* helps enormously in determining the most clinically effective and cost-effective approach to management.

When spine surgery is indicated, education is very important for the patient to guide him or her through the surgery and postoperative recovery. Postoperative expectations and recovery are as varied as the specific surgical interventions available. Nurses can reinforce necessary education and provide the framework for successful patient outcomes.

REFERENCES

1. Benzel, E. C. (2001). *Biomechanics of spine stabilization* (pp. 1–15). Rolling Meadows, IL: American Association of Neurological Surgeons.
2. Jeong, G. K., & Bendo, J. A. (2004). Spinal disorders in the elderly. *Clinical Orthopaedics and Related Research, 425,* 110–125.
3. Videman, T., Battié, M., Ripatti, S, Gill, K., Manninen, H., & Kaprio, J. (2006). Determinants of the progression in lumbar degeneration. *Spine, 31*(6), 671–678.
4. Hart, R. A., D'Alise, M. D., & Benzel, E. C. (2005). The geriatric patient. In E. C. Benzel (Ed.). *Spine surgery: Techniques, complication avoidance, and management* (2nd ed., pp. 1345–1355). Philadelphia: Elsevier.
5. Gill, S. S., & Einhorn, T. A. (2004). Metabolic bone disease of the adult and pediatric spine. In J. W. Frymoyer & S. W. Wiesel (Eds.). *The adult and pediatric spine* (3rd ed., pp. 121–140). Philadelphia: Lippincott Williams & Wilkins.
6. World Health Organization. Prevention and management of osteoporosis. WHO Technical Report Series 921. Geneva, Switzerland: Author. Retrieved May 11, 2006, from www.who.int. Online access.
7. Kis, J. E., & Kuko, T. R. (2005). Fracture risk, bone densitometry, and the medical management of osteoporosis. *Seminars in Spine Surgery, 17*(3), 137–143.
8. Lane, N. E. (2006). Epidemiology, etiology, and diagnosis of osteoporosis. *American Journal of Obstetrics & Gynecology, 194*(2 Suppl), 3–11.
9. Thorson, D. C., Vaneck, J., Campbell, R., et al. (2005). *Health care guidelines: Adult low back pain.* Institute for Clinical System Improvement. Retrieved May 11, 2006, from www.guideline.gov.
10. Atlas, S. J., & Nardin, R. A. (2003). Evaluation and treatment of low back pain: An evidence-based approach to clinical care. *Muscle and Nerve, 27,* 265–284.
11. Henwood, A. M., Adams, M. S., Sypert, G. W., & Benzel, E. C. (2005). Nonoperative management of neck and back pain. In E. C. Benzel (Ed.). *Spine surgery: Techniques, complication avoidance, and management* (2nd ed., pp. 1954–1963). Philadelphia: Elsevier.
12. Deyo, R. A., & Weinstein, J. N. (2001). Low back pain. *New England Journal of Medicine, 344*(5), 363–370.
13. Winters, M. E., Kluetz, P., & Zilberstein, J. (2006). Back pain emergencies. *Medical Clinics of North America, 90,* 505–523.
14. French, S. D., Cameron, M., Walker, B. F., Reggars, J. W., & Esterman, A. J. (2006). A Cochrane review of superficial heat or cold for low back pain. *Spine, 31*(9), 998–1006.
15. Grotle, M., Brox, J. I., Veierod, M. B., Glomsrod, B., Lonn, J. H., & Vollestad, N. K. (2005). Clinical course and prognostic factors in acute low back pain: Patients consulting primary care for the first time. *Spine, 30*(8), 976–982.
16. Heymans, M. W., van Tulder, M. W., Esmail, R., Bombardier, C., & Koes, B. W. (2005). Back schools for nonspecific low back pain. *Spine, 30*(19), 2153–2163.
17. Hurwitz, E. L., Morgenstern, H., Kominski, G. F., Yu, F., & Chiang, L. (2006). A randomized trial of chiropractic and medical care for patients with low back pain: Eighteen month follow up outcomes from the UCLA low back pain study. *Spine, 31*(6), 611–621.
18. Steele, E. J., Dawson, A. P., & Hiller, J. E. (2006). School-based interventions for spinal pain: A systematic review. *Spine, 31*(2), 226–233.
19. Hagen, K. B., Jamtvedt, G., Hilde, G., & Winnem, M. F. (2005). The updated Cochrane review of bed rest for low back pain and sciatica. *Spine, 30*(5), 542–546.
20. Côté, P., Cassidy, J. D., & Carroll, L. (2003). The epidemiology of neck pain: What we have learned from our population-based studies. *Journal of the Canadian Chiropractic Association, 47*(4), 284–290.
21. Rhee, J. M., & Riew, K. D. (2005). Evaluation and management of neck pain, radiculopathy, and myelopathy. *Seminars in Spine Surgery, 17*(3), 174–185.
22. Weidenbaum, M. (2004). Lumbar disc disease: Lumbar disc herniation and radiculopathy. In J. W. Frymoyer & S. W. Wiesel (Eds.). *The adult and pediatric spine* (3rd ed., pp. 913–926). Philadelphia: Lippincott Williams & Wilkins.
23. Carette, S., & Fehlings, M. G. (2005). Cervical radiculopathy. *New England Journal of Medicine, 353*(4), 392–399.
24. Jenis, L. G., Kim, D. H., & An, H. S. (2004). Cervical disc disease: Cervical radiculopathy. In J. W. Frymoyer & S. W. Wiesel (Eds.). *The adult and pediatric spine* (3rd ed., pp. 689–699). Philadelphia: Lippincott Williams & Wilkins.
25. Scherping, S. C. (2004). History and physical examination. In J. W. Frymoyer & S. W. Wiesel (Eds.). *The adult and pediatric spine* (3rd ed., pp. 49–68). Philadelphia: Lippincott Williams & Wilkins.
26. Prendergast, V., Jones, R., Kenny, K., Henwood, A., Strayer, A., & Sullivan, C. (2004). Spine disorders. In M. K. Bader & L. R. Littlejohns (Eds.). *AANN core curriculum for neuroscience nurses* (4th ed., pp. 403–488). St. Louis, MO: Elsevier Health Sciences.
27. Vogt, M. T., Hanscom, B., Lauerman, W. C., & Kang, J. D. (2002). Influence of smoking on the health status of spinal patients: The national spine network database. *Spine, 27*(3), 313–319.
28. Hadley, M. N., & Reddy, S. V. (1998). Smoking and the human vertebral column: A review of the impact of cigarette use on vertebral bone metabolism and spinal fusion. *Neurosurgery, 41*(1), 116–124.

29. Fanuele, J. C., Abdu, W. A., Hanscom, B., & Weinstein, J. N. (2002). Association between obesity and functional status in patients with spine disease. *Spine, 27*(3), 306–312.

30. Luike, M., Solovieva, S., Lamminen, A., et al. (2005). Disc degeneration of the lumbar spine in relation to overweight. *International Journal of Obesity, 29*, 903–908.

31. Cheng, J. S., Schmidt, M. H., Mueller, W. M., & Benzel, E. C. (2005). The obese patient. In E. C. Benzel (Ed.). *Spine surgery: Techniques, complication avoidance, and management* (2nd ed., pp. 1320–1332). Philadelphia: Elsevier.

32. Carragee, E. J. (2005). Persistent low back pain. *New England Journal of Medicine, 352*(18), 1891–1899.

33. Oleske, D. M., Lavender, S. A., Andersson, G. B., et al. (2006). Risk factors for recurrent episodes of work-related low back disorders in an industrial population. *Spine, 31*(6), 789–797.

34. Turner, J. A., Franklin, G., Fulton-Kehoe, D., et al. (2006). Worker recovery expectations and fear-avoidance predict work disability in a population-based workers' compensation back pain sample. *Spine, 31*(6), 682–689.

35. Walsh, T. L., Hanscom, B., Homa, K., & Abdu, W. A. (2005). The rate and variation of referrals to behavioral medicine services for patients reporting poor mental health in the national spine network. *Spine, 30*(6), 154–160.

36. Atlas, S., & Delitto, A. (2006). Spinal stenosis: Surgical versus nonsurgical treatment. *Clinical Orthopaedics and Related Research, 443*, 198–207.

37. Kim, S., & Lim, R. D. (2005). Spinal stenosis. *Disease-A-Month, 51*(1), 1–7.

38. Truumees, E. (2005). Spinal stenosis: Pathophysiology, clinical and radiographic classification. *Instructional Course Lectures, 54*, 287–302.

39. Rhee, J. M., & Riew, K. D. (2005). Evaluation and management of neck pain, radiculopathy, and myelopathy. *Seminars in Spine Surgery, 17*(3), 174–185.

40. Rumi, M. N., & Yoon, S. T. (2004). Cervical myelopathy history and physical examination. *Seminars in Spine Surgery, 16*(4), 234–240.

41. Baldwin, N. G. (2002). Lumbar disc disease: The natural history. *Neurosurgery Focus, 13*(2), 1–4.

42. Atlas, S., Keller, R., Wu, Y., Deyo, R., & Singer, D. (2005). Long term outcomes of surgical and nonsurgical management of lumbar spinal stenosis: 8 to 10 year results from the Maine lumbar spine study. *Spine, 30*(8), 936–943.

43. Kalfas, I. H. (2001). Principles of bone healing. *Neurosurgery Focus, 10*(4), 1–4.

44. Pilitsis, J. G., Lucas, D. R., & Rengachary, S. R. (2002). Bone healing and spinal fusion. *Neurosurgery Focus, 13*(6), 1–6.

45. Jaikumar, S., Kim, D. H., & Kam, A. C. (2002). History of minimally invasive spine surgery. *Neurosurgery, 51*(Suppl 2), 1–14.

46. Adamson, T. E. (2004). The impact of minimally invasive spine surgery. *Journal of Neurosurgery (Spine 1), 1*, 43–46.

47. Harvey, C. V. (2005). Spinal surgery patient care. *Orthopaedic Nursing, 24*(6), 426–440.

48. Starkweather, A. (2006). Posterior lumbar interbody fusion: An old concept with new techniques. *Journal of Neuroscience Nursing, 38*(1), 13–21.

49. Strayer, A. (2005). Lumbar spine: Common pathology and interventions. *Journal of Neuroscience Nursing, 37*(4), 181–193.

50. Bosacco, S. J., Gardner, M. J., & Guille, J. T. (2001). Evaluation and treatment of dural tears in the lumbar spine surgery: A review. *Clinical Orthopaedics and Related Research, 389*, 238–247.

51. Antonacci, M. D., & Eismont, F. J. (2001). Neurologic complications after lumbar spine surgery. *Journal of the American Academy of Orthopaedic Surgeons, 9*(2), 137–145.

52. Ikenaga, M., Shikata, J., & Tanaka, C. (2005). Radiculopathy of C5 after anterior decompression for cervical myelopathy. *Journal of Neurosurgery: Spine, 3*, 210–217.

RESOURCES

Websites

American Association of Neuroscience Nurses: http://www.aann.org

Lumbar Spine Surgery: A Guide to Preoperative and Postoperative Patient Care

Cervical Spine Surgery: A Guide to Preoperative and Postoperative Patient Care

Back Pain Resource Center: http://www.backpainreliefonline.com

Comprehensive information on neck and back problems: http://www.sofamordanek.com; http://www.spineuniverse.com

Information on neck and back pain: http://www.neckreference.com

Peripheral Nerve Injuries

Joanne V. Hickey

Injury to peripheral nerves can occur in the following three ways: *acute trauma* associated with vehicular accidents, mechanized industry, falls, and sports; *chronic entrapment syndromes* such as carpal tunnel syndrome; through exposure to toxins (e.g., alcohol), as well as some kinds of drug therapy; and through chronic disease (e.g., diabetes mellitus). In this chapter, peripheral injuries resulting from acute trauma are discussed. Chronic entrapment syndromes and other neuropathies are discussed in Chapter 33.

MECHANISMS OF INJURY

Acute traumatic events by which peripheral nerves are injured include partial or complete nerve transection, contusion, stretching, and electrical or thermal injury.

- A **partial or complete transection** of a nerve is a structural loss of integrity of some or all of the fascicles of a nerve, usually the result of a severe traumatic laceration nerve injury, such as from a chain saw or impact from a sharp instrument or bullet.
- With a **contusion**, the nerve remains structurally intact, but with undetermined axonal injury. The injury occurs from a direct blow to a nerve located close to the body surface, such as when an elbow is bumped, causing injury to the superficial ulnar nerve. It can also occur from a missile, such as a bullet or shrapnel, careening close to the nerve.
- **Stretch injuries** result from traction exerted on the nerve related to trauma (i.e., vehicular accidents) or improper use of orthopedic traction. In traumatic injuries, an unrestrained driver or passenger may be thrown into an abnormal position that stretches a peripheral nerve. Shoulder injuries are common and can result in a brachial injury. Excessive application of weight in orthopedic traction can also cause traction on a nerve. For example, the peroneal nerve may be injured by excessive traction.
- **Avulsion** is a tearing away from a structure or part of a structure by traction. This is a particular consideration in brachial plexus injuries. Root avulsions may be complete or incomplete; most avulsions are irreparable.
- **Electrical or thermal injuries** of peripheral nerves are often related to acute trauma. Electrical nerve injury results from a current passing through the peripheral

nerve when contact is made with electrical wires. The resulting injuries produce severe muscle and nerve coagulation, in addition to burns of the skin and destruction of bone. Prognosis for muscle reinnervation in these instances is generally poor. Thermal nerve injury causes similar types of local responses, with major damage resulting from burning and necrosis of tissue.

PATHOPHYSIOLOGY

Peripheral nerves are composed of nerves and connective tissue. The anatomy of a peripheral nerve includes the **endoneurium**, which is the connective tissue that surrounds both myelinated and unmyelinated axons. Each unit is grouped with many other axons into bundles of *fascicles* by the **perineurium**. Groups of fascicles are bound together by an outer covering of connective tissue called the **epineurium** (Fig. 20-1). Nerves are composed of afferent and efferent fibers. These axons can be differentiated on the basis of their size and presence or absence of myelin (i.e., myelinated or unmyelinated fibers). Each nerve fiber is composed of an axon encased in a series of *Schwann cells* that cover the length of the axon. The junctional points between Schwann cells are called the *nodes of Ranvier*. As nerves develop, one of two events can occur. Many unmyelinated axons become embedded in the Schwann cell, or the Schwann cell wraps around one axon in concentric circles to fuse together to form the myelin of the myelinated nerve fiber. The electrical activity of each nerve fiber is independent of the activity in all the other fibers in the nerve even though the fibers are close to each other. The endoneurium and the myelin isolate the action potentials of each fiber from other adjacent fibers.[1]

Axonal transport is the continuous and regulated flow of material from the cell body to the axons and synaptic terminals as well as in the reverse direction (antegrade and retrograde transport). This action is critical for neuronal function through the transport of material synthesized in the cell body and dendrites to reach the axon terminals, and for the material in the axon terminals to reach the cell body of the nerve. Without an operational axonal transport system, the nerve dies.[1] The resting and action potentials of axons are discussed in Chapter 4.

Axons may be affected by acute disorders of the axoplasm (i.e., cytoplasm of an axon). This may occur with a complete

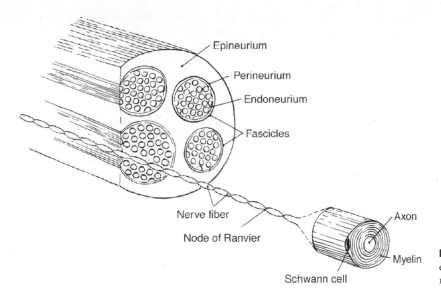

Epineurium

Perineurium

Endoneurium

Fascicles

Nerve fiber

Node of Ranvier

Axon

Myelin

Schwann cell

Figure 20-1 • Anatomic components of the periph-eral nerve. (Benanoch, C., et al. [1998]. *Medical neu-rosciences* [4th ed.]. Philadelphia: Lippincott-Raven.)

or partial laceration of the nerve or with severe local crush-ing, traction, or ischemia. In laceration the connective tissue framework is destroyed, whereas in the other lesions cited it remains intact. Common to all injuries mentioned are the loss of axonal continuity and the loss of the axonal transport sys-tem. Three degenerative reactions occur in response to this: changes in the cell body (chromatolysis), changes in the nerve fiber segment between the cell and body and the point of transection (primary degeneration), and changes in the distal nerve fiber or amputated stump distal to the injury (secondary or wallerian degeneration; Fig. 20-2). Chromatol-ysis appears within 24 hours after the axon is cut and pro-gresses until a maximum is reached between the second and third weeks. Concurrently, most degenerated debris at the distal stump undergoes wallerian degeneration and is

removed. Peripheral muscle atrophy accompanies wallerian degeneration. In lesions with a partial transection, not all axons are destroyed and some function may remain intact. If a nerve is completely severed, reinnervation is poor because the axonal buds or sprouts have no pathway to follow. They may grow haphazardly, form large abnormal tips, or form a painful neuroma.[1]

CLASSIFICATION OF PERIPHERAL NERVE INJURIES

Nerve injuries are classified using the Seddon[2] or Sunder-land[3] classification systems.[4] For purposes of this chapter,

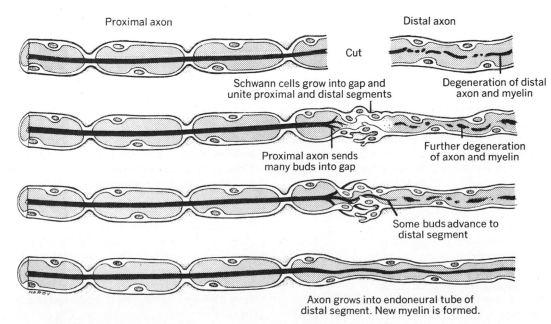

Proximal axon

Distal axon

Cut

Schwann cells grow into gap and unite proximal and distal segments

Degeneration of distal axon and myelin

Proximal axon sends many buds into gap

Further degeneration of axon and myelin

Some buds advance to distal segment

Axon grows into endoneural tube of distal segment. New myelin is formed.

Figure 20-2 • Wallerian degeneration: diagram of changes that occur in a nerve fiber that has been cut and then regenerates.

peripheral nerve injury is based on the simpler Seddon system, which classifies injury according to whether nerve or connective tissue is disrupted. Classification of injury is important to facilitate interpretation of clinical findings, provide guidance for treatment decisions, and suggest prognosis. If neither the nerve nor its connective tissue covering is disrupted, the injury is called a **neuropraxia**. It is a physiologic rather than an actual transection, but the axonal transport is impaired. Additionally, no wallerian degeneration occurs. Recovery may occur in hours to months, with an average of 6 to 8 weeks. If the neuronal components are disrupted but the connective tissue through which the nerve travels remains intact, the injury is called an **axonotmesis**. This type of injury is associated with wallerian degeneration of the involved neurons (see Fig. 20-2). Because the connective tissue components remain intact, the neurons are able to regenerate, albeit at a very slow rate. If the neuronal and connective tissue elements are disrupted, the injury is called a **neurotmesis**, and recovery depends on prompt and effective surgical intervention.

If a peripheral nerve has been completely severed, however, there is still a possibility for regeneration after surgical reapproximation of the severed nerve ends (see Fig. 20-1). Changes occur in the cell body of the injured peripheral nerve, for instance, swelling, chromatolysis, and side displacement of the nucleus. Chromatolysis usually indicates increased RNA and protein synthesis, an example of metabolic activity necessary for the regeneration of severed axonal fibers. In the isolated axonal segment, secondary degeneration occurs (wallerian degeneration). The axis cylinder and myelin sheath degenerate and are removed by the phagocytic cells. The only remaining evidence of the severed axonal segment is the Schwann (neurolemma) cells.

After surgical repair, the regeneration process begins with the proliferation of Schwann cells in the proximal stump near the transection and in the distal stump. These cells divide by mitosis to form continuous cords of Schwann cells, covering an area that encompasses the proximal stump, the gap across the transected area, the distal stump, and the area up to the sites of the sensory receptors and motor endings. The neurolemma cords act as guidelines for the regenerating axon.

Meanwhile, the cell body is directing synthesized protein and metabolites distally to provide the nutritional machinery for axonal regeneration. The axis cylinder of the proximal axon at the transection begins to generate tiny, unmyelinated sprouts that grow longitudinally. There may be as many as 50 sprouts. The random growth of buds or sprouts, which is accompanied by connective tissue proliferation, forms an enlargement called a *neuroma*; this can often be a source of intractable pain. Some sprouts will be misdirected and stray, but some will be successful in crossing the transected gap through the guidance of the neurolemma, finding their way to the distal stump. The rate of growth of a regenerating sprout is 1 to 4 mm per day. If the union is well aligned so that the axon will grow back into its former channel, functional return will be good.[1]

Successfully realigned nerves remyelinate, grow to their former size, and eventually claim a conduction velocity equivalent to about 80% of their former capacity. If the nerve realignments are mismatched, functional weakness, unintentional movements of muscles, and poor sensory discrimination and localization of stimuli may result. Sprouts unsuccessful in

making connections degenerate. Nerves proximal to the injured neurons are stimulated to produce collateral innervation to denervated areas. This process provides innervation long before the axon has regenerated to provide innervation. Therefore, some sensory return may occur before regeneration can realistically occur. This process is possible in the central and peripheral nervous systems.

DIAGNOSIS OF PERIPHERAL NERVE INJURIES

Diagnosis of plexus and peripheral nerve injury is based on a history of injury or presence of an irritative or injurious lesion and a complete neurological examination. The clinical examination is a very important step in establishing the type, degree, and site of injury. A motor and sensory examination is conducted, and pain characteristics evaluated. For upper extremity nerve injuries, Tinel's sign and evidence of Horner's sign are important. Plain x-rays of the chest (for upper extremity problems), computed tomography (CT) or magnetic resonance imaging (MRI), electromyography (EMG), and nerve conduction velocity (NCV) studies are conducted. The EMG and NCV studies are two diagnostic tests most useful to assess function nerve and muscle function. Newer MRI techniques have improved their value in diagnosis.

General Signs and Symptoms of Peripheral Nerve Trauma

Motor, sensory, and autonomic deficits and trophic signs and symptoms are the usual changes noted with peripheral nerve injuries. The degree of deficit in any area depends on the type and extent of injury. The general signs and symptoms include:

- Flaccid paralysis of the muscle or muscle groups supplied by the nerve. A paresis results if some, but not all, of the lower motor neurons innervating the muscle are functional.
- Absence of deep tendon reflexes (DTRs) in the affected area if all neurons are affected. If some neurons are functional, DTRs are weak.
- Atonic or hypotonic muscles.
- Progressive muscle atrophy that begins early (reaches peak in several weeks).
- Fibrillations and fasciculations that peak 2 to 3 weeks after the muscle is denervated. (**Fibrillations** are transitory muscle contractions caused by spontaneous stimulation of a single muscle fiber and can only be detected during EMG studies. **Fasciculations** are spontaneous contractions of several muscle fibers innervated by a single motor nerve filament and can be observed during the physical examination.)
- Diminished or complete sensory loss.
- Warm or dry skin (anhidrosis; does not perspire) caused by transection of the postganglionic sympathetic fibers.
- Trophic skin changes, which can be separated into a warm phase followed by a cold phase. The *warm phase* lasts about 3 weeks, during which time the skin in the affected areas is dry, warm, and flushed. The *cold phase* is characterized by cold, cyanotic skin; brittle fingernails; loss of hair; dryness and ulceration of skin; and lysis of bones and

joints. The digits are affected most. In some incomplete lesions of the median, ulnar, or sciatic nerve with causalgia (see below), the warm phase may persist and may be accompanied by sweating.

Types of Peripheral Nerve Trauma

Common Traumatic Syndromes

The **peripheral nerves** are the major nerve trunks in the extremities and are derived from the plexuses. Each nerve has a well-defined anatomic course in an extremity and innervates specific areas of the skin and muscles. A **plexus** is a complex network of axons that come together to form new combinations. The three major plexuses are the brachial, lumbar, and sacral plexuses. Specific traumatic syndromes commonly seen include brachial plexus injuries, upper extremity injuries (medial, ulnar, and radial nerves), and lower extremity injuries (femoral, sciatic, and common peroneal nerves).[5]

Brachial Plexus Injuries

Anatomic Considerations. The brachial plexus (Fig. 20-3) is created from spinal nerves C-5, C-6, C-7, C-8, and T-1. By a series of division and recombination, three major trunks result: the upper trunk (C-5 and C-6), the middle trunk (C-7), and the lower trunk (C-8 and T-1). Again, these trunks divide and recombine to create three cords that give rise to the following nerves:

- Lateral cord (chiefly derived from C-5 and C-6): musculocutaneous and the lateral half of the median nerve
- Median cord (chiefly derived from C-8 and T-1): ulnar nerve and the medial half of the median nerve
- Posterior cord (C-5, C-6, and C-7): axillary and radial nerves

Patterns of Injury. There are two common patterns of brachial plexus injury: an *upper plexus injury* that usually results from direct downward pressure on the shoulder; and a *lower plexus injury* from hyperabduction on the arm with traction and stretching.[6] The upper brachial injury produces a weak arm and shoulder with a functioning hand, whereas a lower brachial injury results in a strong arm but a hand held in flexion.

A severe traction injury usually involves avulsion of two or more spinal roots from the spinal cord. Simultaneously, other roots have probably experienced severe stretching. The result is total and permanent functional loss to both the avulsed and stretched nerves. The presence of Horner's syndrome strongly suggests C-8 and T-1 avulsion. (**Horner's syndrome** includes the sinking of the eyeball, ptosis of the upper eyelid, slight elevation of the lower eyelid, constriction of the pupil, and anhidrosis caused by paralysis of the cervical sympathetic nerve supply.) Table 20-1 lists specific injuries.

Upper Extremity Injuries. The radial, median, and ulnar nerves are the major peripheral nerves of the arm (Fig. 20-4).

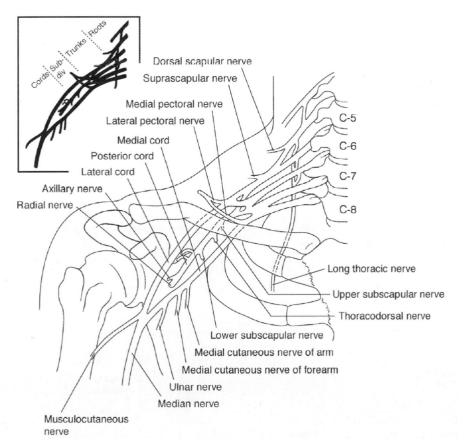

Dorsal scapular nerve
Suprascapular nerve
Medial pectoral nerve
Lateral pectoral nerve
Medial cord
Posterior cord
Lateral cord
Axillary nerve
Radial nerve

Cords Sub-div Trunks Roots

C-5
C-6
C-7
C-8

Long thoracic nerve
Upper subscapular nerve
Thoracodorsal nerve
Lower subscapular nerve
Medial cutaneous nerve of arm
Medial cutaneous nerve of forearm
Ulnar nerve
Median nerve
Musculocutaneous nerve

Figure 20-3 • Brachial plexus showing its various constituents and their relationship to structures in the region of the upper chest, axilla, and shoulder.

TABLE 20–1   BRACHIAL PLEXUS INJURIES: NERVE ROOTS, TRUNKS, MOTOR LOSS, AND SENSORY LOSS

NERVE ROOTS	TRUNK	MOTOR LOSS	SENSORY LOSS
C-5 and C-6	Upper	Most shoulder muscles are involved, except the pectoralis major	Deficit in the deltoid region and radial surface of the forearm
Also called Duchenne-Erb palsy		Loss or difficulty in abduction and external rotation of the arm and weak supination and flexion of the forearm	
C-7	Middle	Incomplete triceps loss and some involvement of the forearm flexors and extensors	Deficits in the middle fingers
		Difficulty in extending the forearm	
C-8 and T-1	Lower	Forearm muscle flexors and the hand muscles are chiefly involved	Deficit is in the medial side of the arm, forearm, and small finger
Also called Klumpke's palsy or Duchenne-Aran palsy		Paralysis and atrophy of the small hand muscles and wrist flexors, giving the appearance of a "claw hand"	

The radial nerve is most frequently injured at the point where the nerve winds around the humerus. A fracture of the humerus is the usual cause of injury, although a radius fracture may be the underlying cause. The median nerve may be injured in the upper arm by a shoulder dislocation or in the forearm or wrist by a laceration or a gunshot wound (Fig. 20-5). The ulnar nerve is most often injured at the elbow because of a fracture or dislocation of the elbow joint. Injury may also occur from a blow to the elbow that results in a contusion to the ulnar nerve. **Volkmann's contracture** refers to a muscle contraction of the arm and hand resulting from ischemic injuries at the elbow (Fig. 20-6). Table 20-2 shows specific motor and sensory deficits associated with each injury.

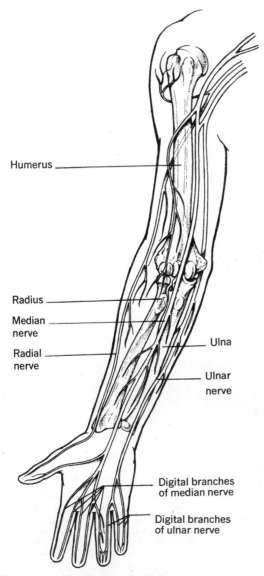

Figure 20-4 • Distribution of peripheral nerves of the arm.

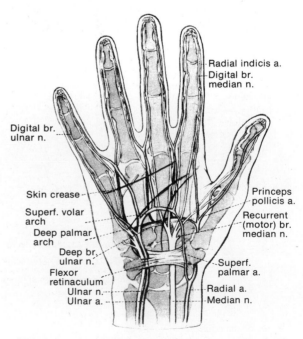

Figure 20-5 • Distribution of peripheral nerves of the hand.

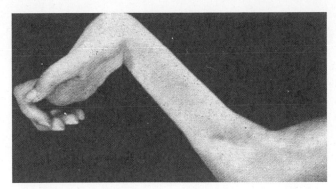

Figure 20-6 • Volkmann's contracture. (From Boyes, J. H. [1970]. *Bunnell's surgery of the hand* [5th ed.]. Philadelphia: J.B. Lippincott.)

Lower Extremity Injuries. The lumbar plexus gives rise to the femoral, sciatic, and common peroneal nerves (Fig. 20-7). The femoral nerve may be injured from compression of a pelvic tumor or a laceration during pelvic surgery. The sciatic nerve may be injured by pelvic or femoral fractures or gunshot wounds. Pelvic tumors and herniated intervertebral discs are other possible causes of sciatic compression. The common peroneal nerve can be injured from prolonged traction, prolonged application of a tourniquet, or compression at the lateral aspect of the knee during surgery. Table 20-3 provides specific motor and sensory losses with major peripheral nerve injuries of the leg.

PERIPHERAL NERVE INJURIES: TREATMENT

Treatment options are individualized to the particular injury incurred. If nerve injury is secondary to a primary problem, such as a tumor, attention is first directed to treatment of the primary problem. Fresh lacerations or transactions are explored and repaired with tension-free end-to-end anastomosis within 72 hours of injury.[7] Ideally, any associated injuries should be clean and healed. Selecting the optimal time for surgery, however, is most important. To determine the extent of nerve injury, surgical exploration may be planned immediately after injury. Primary nerve repair is usually scheduled for 3 weeks to 2 months after injury. Severed nerves may require resection and suturing to reapproximate the ends. Nerve grafts and transplantation are other options for treating injury.[4]

During surgical anastomosis of the severed nerve, the two nerve segments will have contracted, with each having formed scar tissue at the stump.[8] Dissection of the stumps further decreases the lengths of the ends to be joined. To compensate for this, the extremity is positioned in exaggerated flexion with a cast or splint applied to maintain the position after surgery. However, healing at the suture site takes 3 or 4 weeks. After healing has been ensured, the cast or splint is revised several times, with the degree of extension gradually increased by approximately 10 degrees each time. Cable grafting with autologous nerve tissue is a newer surgical technique that allows for anastomosis of nerves over large gaps, without the need for the exaggerated flexion position. Because denervated muscle begins to atrophy almost immediately after injury, it is important to use all available means to retard the process. As previously noted, axonal growth occurs at the rate of 1 to 4 mm per day. Some muscle atrophy will be evident before the slow process of nerve regeneration is completed.[9]

As soon as satisfactory healing has occurred, a physiotherapy program should be implemented to deal with the problems of immobility (stiffness, atrophy, and joint ankylosis). Special spring braces may be used to prevent foot drop or

TABLE 20–2   INJURIES TO THE RADIAL, MEDIAN, AND ULNAR NERVES

	RADIAL NERVE (FROM C-5 TO C-8 NERVE ROOTS)	MEDIAN NERVE (FROM C-6 TO T-1 NERVE ROOTS)	ULNAR NERVE (FROM C-7 AND T-1 NERVE ROOTS)
Motor paresis or paralysis	Loss of extension and abduction of the wrist, fingers, and thumb Wrist drop Inability to grasp an object or make a fist Forearm is pronated and flexed	Weakness of pronation of the forearm Weakness of wrist flexion Difficulty in abducting and opposing the thumb Inability to flex the distal phalanges of the index finger and thumb	Weakness of flexion of the wrist Flexion of the fourth and fifth fingers Inability to abduct and adduct the thumb See Volkmann's contracture (Fig. 20-6)
Sensory impairment or loss	Loss over the posterior aspect of the forearm and the radial aspect of the dorsum of the thumb or dorsum of hand	Loss of radial half of the palm; the palmar surface of the thumb, index, and middle fingers; and the radial half of ring finger	Loss of the fifth finger, the ulnar aspect of the fourth finger, and the ulnar border of palm With a nerve contusion, the chief symptom may be pain with little, if any, motor deficit
Atrophy	Extensor carpi ulnaris, extensor digitorum, extensor digiti minimi, abductor pollicis longus and brevis, and extensor indicis	Thenar muscles of hand and the flexor-pronator group of the forearm	"Claw hand" deformity (from wasting of the small hand muscles with hyperextension of the fingers at the metacarpophalangeal joints)
Other	Trophic changes at minimum	Loss of ability to sweat in affected areas	

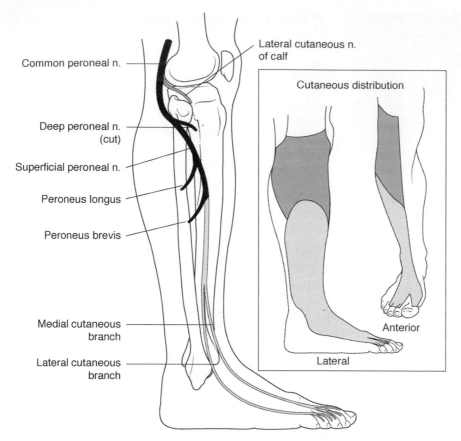

Figure 20-7 • Distribution of peripheral nerves of the leg.

wrist drop. Daily regimens of galvanic stimulation to minimize the atrophic change of muscle to fibrotic tissue may be instituted until the affected muscle demonstrates, on electromyography, that it has been reinnervated. Massage, whirlpool treatments, and an exercise program to re-educate the muscles are important components of an aggressive physiotherapy program.

The rehabilitation program is long and arduous. The prognosis varies depending on the type and location of the injury. It may be necessary to offer a total rehabilitation program at a center that provides vocational rehabilitation if permanent disability will prevent the patient from assuming his or her former place in society and returning to previous employment. The patient should be kept comfortable with appropriate analgesics, as necessary. The pain that sometimes accompanies peripheral nerve injury may seriously limit the functional rehabilitation of these patients and should be dealt with aggressively.

TABLE 20-3   INJURIES TO THE FEMORAL, SCIATIC, AND COMMON PERONEAL NERVES

	FEMORAL NERVE (FROM THE L-2, L-3, AND L-4 NERVE ROOTS)	SCIATIC NERVE (FROM L-4 TO S-3 NERVE ROOTS)	COMMON PERONEAL NERVE (FROM L-4 TO S-1 NERVE ROOTS)
Motor paresis or paralysis	Weakness of extension of the knee Weakness of hip flexion (if injury is near the psoas muscle)	Inability to flex the knee Weakened gluteal muscles Foot drop	Paralysis of dorsiflexion of foot and toes (foot drop) Difficulty with eversion of the foot (with involvement of the superficial peroneal nerve)
Sensory impairment or loss	Anterolateral thigh	Outer aspect of the leg and dorsum of the foot and sole and inner aspect of foot	Medial part of the dorsum of the foot and outer side of the leg
Atrophy	Wasting of the quadriceps muscles	Hamstrings and all muscles below the knee	Extensor digitorum brevis, perionei (foot eversion)
Other	Absence of the knee-jerk reflex	Loss of hair, changes in toenails, and changes in skin texture in distal leg below knee	—

COLLABORATIVE AND NURSING MANAGEMENT OF THE PATIENT WITH PERIPHERAL NERVE TRAUMA

The major collaborative problems associated with peripheral nerve injuries are **peripheral nerve impairment**, **paresis/paralysis**, **paresthesia**, and **pain management**. The medical or surgical plan will address the primary peripheral nerve problem. The loss of motor and sensory function in the involved area requires a multidisciplinary approach to care. In addition, pain management through a variety of strategies may be necessary.

Specific nursing care depends on the particular problem, type, and degree of injury. The patient with a peripheral injury may be hospitalized for surgery and discharged to recuperate at home. In other instances, a peripheral injury may be only one of several injuries seen as a result of multiple trauma. Management of the peripheral injury is incorporated into the total nursing management of the patient. However, general principles can be identified and followed when caring for patients with a peripheral nerve injury. These principles can be categorized into the following areas: assessment of function, maintenance of function, and rehabilitation.

Assessment of Function

A neurological assessment of the limb is made to determine which neurological functions remain intact. The assessment is initially conducted by the nurse to establish a baseline with which subsequent assessments can be compared. After the baseline has been established, subsequent assessments are conducted every 4 hours or at less frequent intervals, depending on the patient's condition.

Motor Function. Motor function is assessed by asking the patient to engage the limb through the normal range of motion, provided there is no contraindication to movement. In an acute traumatic injury, the injury is evaluated by the physician initially to determine whether movement is contraindicated, as would be the case if there were danger of a broken bone severing a nerve. If movement of the involved extremity is not contraindicated, range of motion is assessed. Any evidence of abnormal movements, such as tremors, fibrillation, or fasciculations, should be documented. Atrophy, contractions, paresis, and paralysis are abnormal findings. DTRs should also be assessed.

Sensory Function. Light touch, pain, position, and temperature are assessed. The patient should be questioned about whether he or she has experienced any abnormal sensations, such as tingling, a crawling sensation, or pain. All are examples of reportable findings.

Other Assessment Parameters. The involved limb should also be assessed for color, warmth, and texture. If the skin is cool to the touch or appears cyanotic, circulatory impairment or vasomotor tone may be indicated. Warm, dry, reddish skin indicates possible early trophic changes associated with autonomic alterations. Any evidence of scaling, brittle nails, or loss of body hair should be recorded.

Planning and Implementation

Following an assessment of the involved area, the nurse plans and implements the nursing care plan with consideration of the goals of medical management. If the physician has ordered immobilization of the involved area, the immobilization may be accomplished by a splint, a cast, or traction. The purpose of immobilization is to allow for the healing of a surgical incision in which there has been a reanastomosis or other surgical intervention for a severed nerve.

The following outlines major points of nursing management.

Splint and Cast Care. The splint is usually held secure with an Ace-bandage wrap or Velcro. The splint and wrap can become tight because of edema. The skin around the splint or cast should be checked for tightness, warmth, and color. If the splint or cast is too tight, as evidenced by tingling, blanched color, or coolness, steps can be taken to provide a better fit. In the case of a tight cast, the physician will need to decide which adjustments need to be made to ensure a better fit. It is best to refer the need for adjustments to the department that made the splint or brace originally, because all braces and most splints are custom-made to fit the contour of the wearer. A blanched appearance of the skin and coolness to the touch indicate interference with autonomic function and adequate blood supply. Any indications of drainage under the cast or splint should be addressed immediately.

Positioning of Extremity. If a cast or splint has been applied to the arm, a sling may be used to prevent dependence. In the case of a leg cast, the physician usually wants the leg to be supported and elevated on pillows to reduce the likelihood of edema.

Skin Care. Trophic changes of the skin are common signs and symptoms associated with peripheral nerve injury that make the skin susceptible to breakdown and injury. The skin should be examined for evidence of irritation or injury. Washing and careful drying are important, especially between the toes or fingers. If the skin is dry and scaly, lubricate with a lanolin preparation or other prescribed treatment. The nails should be filed and cut straight across to prevent skin injury.

Temperature. The involved extremity should be carefully protected from extremes in temperature. Because of lost or compromised sensory function, the area can be easily injured by extreme heat or cold without the patient being alerted to this through pain or discomfort.

Ambulation. Depending on the extent of injury of the involved extremity, the physician may limit ambulation and other activities of daily living (ADLs). The nurse should adjust the plan of care based on the limitations imposed by the injury and the medical treatment.

Rehabilitation

The length and complexity of the rehabilitative process can vary greatly. Patient education and support are important components of care. Patient education is directed at regaining the greatest possible level of independence. Help may be needed in developing alternative methods of performing ADLs. For example, if the dominant arm and hand are encircled by a splint, the patient will need to be helped to learn to eat with the other hand. If food is adequately prepared for the patient (beverage poured, food cut, and so forth), he or she will be able to manage with practice. In addition, anxiety is decreased, and the patient is better able to cope with the limitations imposed by the injury.

When an exercise program is initiated for the involved extremity, the patient will have to learn the active and passive (prescribed) exercises. Protect the involved limb from injury. The process of regaining motor and sensory function can be slow and thus lead to discouragement. Encourage the patient to commit to the outlined physiotherapy program to prevent skeletal deformities and slowly regain as much function as possible.

A decreased level of independence precipitates various emotional and psychological reactions. The patient experiences changes in body image, self-esteem, and lifestyle. Sensory deprivation, social isolation, and powerlessness result from the limitations imposed by the disability. Common behavioral manifestations from the various physical, emotional, and social disabilities include frustration, hostility, anger, and depression. Many patients go through a process of loss, grief, and bereavement over the lost function. The process of recovery is very slow (approximately 1 year with nerve transections). Physiotherapy is the major approach after surgical intervention has been completed. It is a slow process characterized by ups and downs, so it is easy for patients to become discouraged with the lack of apparent improvement. If the disability is permanent, the emotional impact imposes increased demands on the person's coping skills and adjustment patterns; therefore, it is extremely important that the nurse provide appropriate psychological and emotional support.

REFERENCES

1. Benarroch, E. E., Westmoreland, B. F., Daube, J. R., Reagan, T. J., & Sandok, B. A. (1999). *Medical neurosciences: An approach to anatomy, pathology, and physiology by systems and levels* (4th ed., pp. 382–384). Philadelphia: Lippincott Williams & Wilkins.
2. Seddon, H. J. (1942). A classification of nerve injuries. *British Medical Journal, 1,* 237–288.
3. Sunderland, S. (1968). *Nerves and nerve injuries.* Baltimore: Williams & Wilkins.
4. Murray, B. (2004). Trauma of the nervous system: Peripheral nerve trauma. In W. G. Bradley, R. B. Daroff, G. M. Fenichel, & J. Jankovic (Eds.). *Neurology in clinical practice* (4th ed., pp. 1179–1195). Philadelphia: Butterworth Heinemann.
5. Black, P., & Rossitch, E., Jr. (1995). *Neurosurgery: An introduction text.* New York: Oxford University Press.
6. Rankine, J. J. (2004). Adult traumatic brachial plexus injury. *Clinical Radiology, 59,* 767–774.
7. Greenberg, M. S. (2006). *Handbook of neurosurgery* (6th ed., pp. 560–563). Lakeland, FL: Greenberg Graphics.
8. Samii, M., & Penkert, G. (1998). Traumatic disorders of the peripheral nervous system. In J. Cruz (Ed.). *Neurological and neurosurgical emergencies* (pp. 349–362). Philadelphia: W. B. Saunders.
9. Chuang, D. C. (1999). Management of traumatic brachial plexus injuries in adults. *Hand Clinics, 15*(4), 737–755.

Nursing Management of Patients With Neoplasms of the Neurological System

Brain Tumors

Joanne V. Hickey and Terri S. Armstrong

OVERVIEW OF BRAIN TUMORS

The diagnosis of a brain tumor begins a journey of uncertainty, fear, and hope for the patient and family. The human saga is laden with confounding issues, including loss of neurological function ranging from subtle to significant, often including cognitive function; treatment options; quality of life; and often, end-of-life decisions. To care for the patient and family in a sensitive, compassionate, hopeful, and humanistic manner, the health care professional needs a broad knowledge base and particular skills. Within this framework of fundamental principles, concepts related to brain tumors and related management are explored in this chapter.

The Central Brain Tumor Registry of the United States (CBTRUS) estimates that in 2007, 51,410 new cases of primary malignant and nonmalignant brain and central nervous system tumors will be diagnosed.[1] This number is higher than incidence predicted by the American Cancer Society or the Surveillance, Epidemiology, and End Results (SEER) program, which collects primary malignant tumor data only. Overall, primary tumors are more common in females then males. In 2007, an estimated 12,750 deaths were expected to be attributed to primary malignant brain and central nervous system tumors in the United States.[2] In men 20 to 39 years of age, brain tumor malignancies were the second leading cause of cancer death in 1998, 1999, and 2001 and the leading cause of cancer death in 2000. Among women 20 to 39 years of age, brain tumors were the fifth leading cause of cancer death in 1998, 1999, 2000, and 2002.[1] Most adult brain tumors (30%) are located in the frontal, temporal, parietal, and occipital lobes of the brain (supratentorial region). Gliomas, particularly those of astrocytic origin, are the most common type of primary brain tumors and account for more than 40% of all neoplasms of the central nervous system (CNS) in adults.[3] The median age of diagnosis of all primary brain tumors is 57 years. The incidence of pilocytic astrocytomas, germ cell tumors, and medulloblastomas decreases with age. For all other tumors, the incidence increases with age.[1] Metastasis to the brain is found in 10% to 15% of cancer patients, with an estimated incidence of 80,000 annually.

The cause of most nervous system tumors remains unknown. Some inherited genetic syndromes predispose patients to the development of a brain tumor (e.g., neurofibromatosis types 1 and 2, tuberous sclerosis, von Hippel-Lindau disease). Specific chromosomal locations are related to specific types of tumors. For example, neurofibromatosis type 1 is located on chromosome 17q11 and is associated with astrocytomas or peripheral neurofibromas. In contrast, neurofibromatosis type 2, located on chromosome 22q12, is associated with acoustic and other neuromas, meningiomas, astrocytomas, ependymomas, and central neurofibromas.[4] Other tumors have a congenital basis (e.g., epidermoid, dermoid, and teratoid tumors and craniopharyngiomas). Some environmental agents, ionizing radiation in particular, clearly are implicated as causes of brain tumors, but they also appear to account for few cases.[4]

CLINICAL PEARLS: The cause of most nervous system tumors is unknown.

Classification of Brain Tumors

Classification of brain tumors is based primarily on histopathologic characteristics, which are important considerations for determining treatment options. For clinical purposes, other conventional classifications are also helpful in understanding the nature of brain tumors and will also be reviewed.

Histopathologic Basis of Classification

Although a tumor-node-metastases (TNM) staging system exists for primary brain tumors, the fact that most tumors do not spread outside of the central nervous system makes this system not useful clinically. Primary brain tumors are broadly classified by the presumed tissue of origin, with the degree of malignancy based on the degree of anaplasia. In specific tumors, location within the brain may also be considered. Several histologic[5] classification schemas exist, with the most widely used being the World Health Organization (WHO) system.[5,6]

The WHO system was initially developed in the 1970s and was subsequently revised. This system grades tumors on a continuum, utilizing the degree of anaplasia and survival into nine categories (Chart 21-1).[7] Tumors originating from neuroepithelial tissue account for the most prevalent glial tumors. The neuroepithelial category is further subclassified in Chart 21-2, with tumors of astrocytic origin being the most common subclassification.[8]

CHART 21-1   World Health Organization Classification of Central Nervous System Tumors

1. Tumors of neuroepithelial tissue
2. Tumors of cranial and spinal nerves
3. Tumors of the meninges
4. Hematopoietic neoplasms
5. Germ cell tumors
6. Cysts and tumor-like lesions
7. Tumors of the anterior pituitary
8. Local extensions from regional tumors
9. Metastatic tumors

Conventional Classifications

Other conventional classification systems are based on several distinguishing clinical considerations including primary versus secondary, neuroembryonic origins, anatomic location, and malignant versus benign.

CHART 21-2   Classification of Major Brain Tumors

Gliomas
    Astrocytic tumors
        Pilocytic astrocytomas (grade 1)
        Astrocytoma (grade 2)
        Anaplastic astrocytoma (grade 3)
        Glioblastoma multiforme (grade 4)
    Ependymomal tumors
        Ependymoma (variants)
        Anaplastic (malignant) ependymoma
        Myxopapillary ependymoma
        Subependymoma
    Oligodendroglial tumors
        Oligodendroglioma
        Anaplastic (malignant) oligodendroglioma
        Mixed oligodendroglioma
    Medulloblastoma
    Unclassified (mostly gliomas)
Meningiomas
    Menigiomas (multiple histologic types)
    Atypical types
    Anaplastic (malignant) meningioma
Pituitary adenoma
Neurinoma (schwannoma, acoustic neuroma)
Craniopharyngioma, dermoid, epidermoid, teratoma
Angiomas
Sarcomas
Miscellaneous (pinealoma, chordoma, granuloma, lymphoma)

Adapted from the WHO classification.

- **Primary versus metastatic brain tumors:** *primary brain tumors* originate from the various cells and structures that constitute the brain. *Metastatic brain tumors* originate from sites outside the brain, most often from primary tumors of the lung, breast, and melanomas. Primary brain tumors rarely metastasize outside of the central nervous system. *Carcinomatosis* is a condition in which carcinoma is widespread throughout the body and is sometimes used to describe multiple lesions in the brain or spread to the spinal fluid and meninges.

- **Neuroembryonic origins:** nervous system tumors originate from the ectodermal (outer) layer of the embryo. Chapter 4 briefly describes early embryonic development. At 16 days the *neural plate* appears, changing to the *neural groove* and *neural tube* by the third week. Those neuroectodermal cells not incorporated into the neural tube form *neural crests*. The neural tube and neural crests contain two types of undifferentiated cells called neuroblasts and glioblasts (spongioblasts). The *neuroblasts* become the basic unit of structure in the nervous system and are then called *neurons*. The *glioblasts* form a variety of cells that support, insulate, and metabolically assist the neurons. They are collectively called *glial cells*. Glial cells are subclassified into *astrocytes* (star-shaped cells), *oligodendrocytes* (glial cells with few processes), and *ependymal cells* (line the ventricles). This is the basis for the broad category of brain tumors called *gliomas*. Gliomas are further subdivided into *astrocytomas, oligodendrogliomas,* and *ependymomas*.

- **Anatomic location:** the anatomic location of the lesion affects signs and symptoms as well as presentation. Tumors can be extra-axial (located outside of the brain parenchyma) or intra-axial. Intra-axial tumors can be further defined by location by the specific site of the lesion such as the frontal or temporal lobe, pons, or cerebellum. Location may be noted by using the tentorium cerebelli as a reference point to differentiate between *supratentorial,* located above the tentorium (i.e., cerebral hemispheres), and *infratentorial,* located below the tentorium (i.e., brainstem or cerebellum). Knowing the location of the lesion helps to predict probable deficits based on an understanding of the normal function of that anatomic area. In addition, location is an important variable in selecting treatment options and prognosis.

- **Malignant versus benign:** using the word "benign" in the classification of brain tumors can be somewhat misleading. When a neoplasm is designated as benign, one suggests that a complete cure is possible; conversely, a malignant tumor would suggest a poor prognosis. The benign versus malignant distinction is made on the basis of histologic properties. Cells that are well differentiated are related to a better prognosis than poorly differentiated cells. However, when a tumor is located within the brain, other factors are equally important. A tumor that is considered to be histologically benign may be surgically inaccessible, as with a deep tumor requiring extensive dissection of tissue or one located in a vital area, such as the pons or medulla. A benign tumor that is partially or completely surgically inaccessible may continue to grow, and cause neurological deficits, if the tumor does not respond to other treatment options such as chemotherapy or radiation. These deficits can result in loss of significant neurological function and life. Tumors can be classified in regard to rate of growth or mitotic activity. Those tumors with slow growth are referred to as low-grade tumors. Those with a high growth rate are referred to as high-grade tumors.

> **CLINICAL PEARLS:**   The term *benign brain tumor* is misleading in that it only refers to a lower level of cell abnormality; it does not address or suggest a complete cure. Many other factors must be considered in patient outcomes.

Pathophysiology of Brain Tumors

The pathophysiology of brain tumors can be viewed from the perspective of molecular considerations and the effects of the tumor, both directly on cerebral tissue and indirectly through the development of increased intracranial pressure (ICP).

> **CLINICAL PEARLS:**   Most primary brain tumors do not spread outside of the central nervous system.

Molecular Considerations

Transformation of glial or neuronal cells into brain tumors is a complex process that is still incompletely understood. Brain tumors arise in association with multiple, specific structural molecular genetic alternations (i.e., mutations) within cells. These mutations can cause the cell to proliferate inappropriately as well as result in other malignancy attributes, such as the loss of differentiated characteristics of the tissue of origin, acquisition of the ability to invade surrounding normal tissues and metastasize, and the ability to resist antineoplastic therapies.[9] Two types of genetic molecular alterations trigger these changes in cellular behavior. The first change results in the complete cessation or partial decrease in cellular activities that physiologically restrain growth. These genes are known as *tumor suppressor genes.* The second change inappropriately activates genes that typically enhance cellular proliferation. Known as *proto-oncogenes*, these genes encode proteins that act as growth factors or growth factor receptors, mediators of signaling pathways, or regulators of gene expression. Mutations convert proto-oncogenes to oncogenes, which function in various ways to promote neoplastic changes, such as alterations in cell cycle progression, abnormalities in signal transduction pathways, glial cell invasion, and angiogenesis.[9]

The Effects of a Space-Occupying Lesion Within the Brain

Tumors directly affect the brain through *compression of cerebral tissue, through invasion or infiltration of cerebral tissue,* and sometimes through *erosion of bone.* A brain tumor usually grows as a spherical mass until it encounters a more rigid structure, such as bone or the falx cerebri. The encounter with an aplastic substance necessitates a change in the contour of the neoplasm. Neoplastic cells can also grow diffusely, with multiple cells infiltrating tissue spaces without forming a definite mass. The tumor enlarges because of cell proliferation, necrosis, fluid accumulation, hemorrhage, or the accumulation of degenerative by-products within the mass.

The clinical effects of a tumor within the brain and cranial vault depend on the location of the tumor, rate of growth, and consequences of increased ICP. A slow-growing tumor may become large before clinical signs and symptoms of increased ICP are noted. This happens because the tumor's volume is accommodated in the intracranial space over a long period of time, often years. A meningioma is a slow-growing tumor that can become large before signs and symptoms of increased ICP are noted. Conversely, depending on its location, evidence of a meningioma may be noted early because of focal deficits. With a fast-growing tumor, such as a glioblastoma multiforme, there is little time for the intracranial compartment to accommodate the lesion, and signs of increased ICP may be noted in a shorter time frame. In summary, an understanding of the pathophysiologic effects of brain tumors requires an understanding of the Monro-Kellie hypothesis and increased ICP along with the specific tumor type, location, and related focal deficits. See Chapter 13 for a discussion of increased ICP and its management.

In most patients with brain tumors, vasogenic edema develops in the surrounding tissue as a result of compression. At the cellular level, an increase in permeability of capillary endothelial cells of the cerebral white matter results in seepage of plasma into the extracellular space and between the layers of the myelin sheath. This alters the electrical potential of cells, impairing cellular activity. Cerebral edema may also develop rapidly from alterations in the blood–brain barrier caused by substances released from tumor cells.[3] As cerebral edema increases, a mass effect develops, and signs and symptoms of increased ICP become apparent. These signs and symptoms continue to develop as a tumor grows. The resulting increase in cerebral edema can result in cerebral herniation syndromes and death (see Chap. 13).

SIGNS AND SYMPTOMS OF BRAIN TUMOR

Given that brain tumors present in widely variable clinical patterns, there are no classic signs and symptoms. The particular clinical presentation depends on the size, location, compression or infiltration of specific cerebral tissue, related cerebral edema, and the development of increased ICP. Brain tumors are sometimes discovered as asymptomatic masses. Initially, neurological symptoms are subtle. Some symptoms found in association with brain tumors are also those found in less serious conditions, so patients need to be carefully evaluated. Patients often present with two categories of signs and symptoms, general or focal:

- General: headaches, nausea and vomiting, changes in the level of consciousness, and seizures
- Focal: specific *focal deficits,* such as hemiparesis, or *syndromes related to specific cerebral areas,* such as expressive aphasia or acromegaly (Fig. 21-1)

General Signs and Symptoms

The most common initial signs and symptoms of brain tumors are headache, nausea and vomiting, changes in the level of consciousness, and seizures.

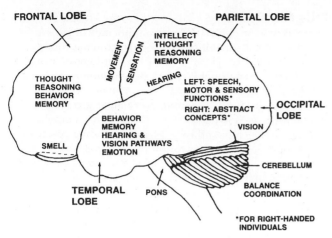

Figure 21-1 • Cerebral function and associated anatomic areas. (Reproduced with permission from the American Brain Tumor Association.)

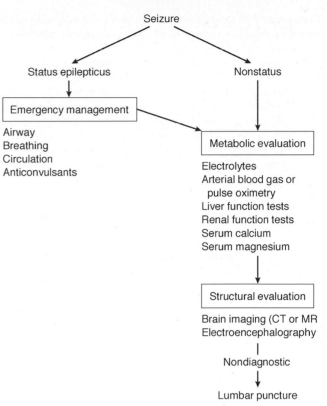

Figure 21-2 • Algorithm for initial evaluation of patients with suspected brain tumor based on type of seizure in presenting symptoms.

Headache. Headache is an early symptom in approximately one third of patients with brain tumors. The location and characteristics of the headache cover a wide range of possibilities. Headache is often described as intermittent and moderately severe; is usually worse in the morning because of irritation, compression, or traction of the blood vessels; and may be aggravated by acts known to increase ICP such as coughing or straining at stool. Onset of a new headache pattern, especially if it is worse in the morning or awakens the patient at night, deserves investigation. The area affected by the headache may be generalized or localized to the site of the tumor. As ICP rises, headache is generally bifrontal or bioccipital, regardless of the tumor location.

> **CLINICAL PEARLS:**   Headaches are the most common presenting symptom of a brain tumor.

Nausea and Vomiting. Vomiting may indicate increased ICP or a posterior fossa tumor, and it may or may not be accompanied by headache. Nausea or abdominal discomfort may accompany vomiting, although in most instances vomiting occurs without these symptoms. Vomiting associated with brain tumor is usually unrelated to meals, occurs most commonly in the morning, and can be projectile. The cause may be direct stimulation of the vomiting center (located in the medulla), especially with a posterior fossa tumor.

Change in the Level of Consciousness. Initially, alterations in consciousness may be very subtle, progressing from slight confusion, irritability, and somnolence to stupor and finally to coma. Blatant changes in consciousness, such as stupor and coma, are related to increased ICP.

Seizures. A new onset of seizures in an adult should prompt an immediate investigation for the underlying cause. Many patients experience seizures in the course of their illness. Seizures are either the initial symptom or occur during the illness in about 30% of patients. About 70% of patients with slower-growing tumors are likely to have seizure activity, whereas those with more rapidly growing tumors have a seizure rate of 30% to 40%.[10]

With brain tumors, hyperactive cells caused by cerebral edema and alterations in normal electrical potential produce abnormal paroxysmal discharges or seizure activity that may be generalized or focal. Focal seizures can aid in the localization of the tumor. Seizure activity is seen primarily with supratentorial tumors. Please refer to Chapter 29 for a more detailed review of seizure management and nursing implications.

The recommended work-up for a patient who presents with new onset of seizures is included in Figure 21-2. The work-up is divided into toxic/metabolic and structural factors. Possible metabolic factors include electrolyte imbalance, liver or renal failure, or side effects from radiation or chemotherapeutic agents. Structural causes include parenchymal metastases, dural metastases, or leptomeningeal disease. Additionally, hemorrhage, thrombosis, or meningitis can cause seizures in the patient with known brain tumor.

Focal Signs and Symptoms

Regardless of the histologic structure, location of a tumor will often give rise to focal signs and symptoms. Focal findings are often present and assist the health care provider in localizing the tumor. The possible manifestations of a brain tumor are many and include a new onset of seizures; gradual neurological deficits such as weakness or numbness on one side of the body; headache; new onset of vomiting; visual loss or field cuts; papilledema; loss of the gag reflex; ataxia; confusion; listlessness, somnolence or irritability; change in behavior or personality; memory deficits; and speech deficits. In addition, deficits may be noted in specific cranial nerves, including unilateral hearing loss or tinnitus; loss of smell; numbness on one side of the face; swallowing difficulty; and diplopia or blurred vision.[11] The next section reviews focal signs and symptoms as they relate to specific anatomic cerebral locations.

Frontal Lobe

Multiple higher cognitive, executive, behavioral, speech, and motor functions are controlled by the frontal lobe. Focal deficits can be traced to either anterior frontal or posterior frontal findings.

Anterior Frontal Lobe. Patients with tumors in the *anterior frontal lobe* present with a wide range of higher-level cognitive function and personality changes such as short- and long-term memory deficits, difficulty in concentration and vigilance, slowing of mental processes and reaction time, abulia, and difficulty with calculations, problem solving, insight, abstraction, and synthesis of ideas. Collectively, anterior frontal lobe symptoms are called the *frontal lobe syndrome.* Personality and behavioral changes may include emotional lability, flat affect, lack of initiative and spontaneity, loss of self-restraint, and loss of social behavior.

Posterior Frontal Lobe. Broca's area is located in the posterior-inferior frontal lobe. If a tumor is located in or around Broca's area in the dominant hemisphere, fluent speech deficits such as word finding may be noted. The primary motor strip is located in the posterior frontal lobe. Tumors in this area can cause focal findings of motor weakness such as monoparesis or focal seizure activity.

Parietal Lobe

The parietal lobe contains the sensory discrimination and association areas for body orientation, vision, and language. Parietal lobe tumors cause deficits in sensation, inability to recognize common objects, and neglect syndromes such as the lack of awareness of the opposite side of the body. If the lesion is in the dominant hemisphere and is located in the left angular gyrus of the parietal lobe, Gerstmann's syndrome may be present (i.e., finger agnosia, loss of right–left discrimination, acalculia, and agraphia). Seizure activity and homonymous hemianopsia are also possible with a parietal lobe tumor. A collection of symptoms associated with parietal lobe dysfunction is called the *parietal lobe syndrome.* Common symptoms include the following:

Sensory Changes
- Hypo- or hyperesthesia (impaired sensation with increased or decreased tactile sensitivity)
- Paresthesia (abnormal sensation involving tingling, crawling, or burning feeling on the skin)
- Loss of two-point discrimination (unable to determine by feeling if the skin is touched by one or two points simultaneously)

Recognition Deficits
- Inability to recognize letters or numbers
- Astereognosis (inability to recognize an object by feeling its size and shape)
- Autotopagnosia (inability to locate or recognize parts of the body)
- Anosognosia (loss of awareness or denial of specific motor or sensory deficits)
- Finger agnosia (inability to identify or select specific fingers of the hand such as thumb)

Orientation Deficits and Neglect Syndromes
- Loss of right–left discrimination
- Difficulty in going through doorways without knocking self on one side
- Neglect syndrome (a tendency to ignore the part of the environment or body opposite to the tumor)
- Construction apraxia (if asked to draw a face of a clock, ignoring the side of the clock opposite to the tumor)

Temporal Lobe

Neoplasms of the temporal lobe may cause psychomotor (complex partial) seizures, weakness, visual field deficits (often loss in the upper quadrant opposite the lesion), and memory deficits, most often for recent events. When the dominant side is involved, speech and language deficits are frequent because Wernicke's area is located in the dominant temporal lobe. Psychomotor seizures with visual, auditory, or olfactory hallucinations; automatism; and amnesia for events of the attack can occur. They may begin with an aura of peculiar sensations of the abdomen, epigastrium, or thorax.

Occipital Lobe

Tumors of the occipital lobe are infrequent compared with lesions involving the other cerebral lobes. When neoplasms do occur, the symptoms tend to be associated with vision. Symptoms include homonymous quadrantanopia (loss of vision in one fourth of the visual field), visual hallucinations, and failure to recognize familiar objects.

Pituitary and Hypothalamus Region

The pituitary gland and hypothalamus are closely related by location and endocrine production. Common symptoms resulting from tumors in these areas are visual deficit caused by optic atrophy and paralysis of one or more of the extraocular muscles; headache; and endocrine dysfunction of the pituitary gland with the subsequent precipitation of various syndromes, such as Cushing's syndrome, giantism, acromegaly, and hypopituitarism. In addition, tumors of the hypothalamus can affect fat and carbohydrate metabolism, water balance, sleep patterns, appetite, and sexual drive.

Lateral and Third Ventricles

If the tumor remains small, the patient may be asymptomatic. If the tumor grows into the cerebral hemispheres, deficits will depend on the particular function of the area involved. Tumors that grow within the ventricle may become of sufficient size to obstruct the flow of cerebrospinal fluid (CSF) resulting in noncommunicating hydrocephalus. If this occurs, headache, vomiting, and other symptoms of rapidly increased ICP will be noted. The patient may experience relief of symptoms by changing the position of the head. In this case, the position of the obstructing tumor is altered, thereby allowing the normal CSF flow pattern to be re-established.

Brainstem

Tumors of the brainstem may produce multiple symptoms such as lower cranial nerve deficits (swallowing, articulation, and gag reflex), motor and sensory deficits, vertigo, hiccups, ataxia, incoordination, nystagmus, dysphagia, nausea, and vomiting throughout the illness. Sudden death can occur from encroachment on vital centers (respiratory or cardiac arrest). Obstructive hydrocephalus may develop from encroachment on the ventricular system.

Midbrain

Neoplasms of the midbrain are rare. If present, they may result in occlusion of the cerebral aqueducts, cerebellar symptoms if the red nucleus is involved, Parinaud's syndrome (i.e., conjugate paralysis of upward gaze) if the quadrigeminal plate is involved, abnormal posturing, and ptosis and diminished light reflex as the tumor enlarges.

Fourth Ventricle

Tumors of the fourth ventricle obstruct the flow of CSF (noncommunicating hydrocephalus) and infiltrate and compress the brainstem or cerebellum. See Chapter 13 for a discussion of hydrocephalus. Headache, vomiting, and nuchal rigidity are common symptoms. Sudden death caused by compression of the cardiorespiratory center is possible. The lower cranial nerves, which control the gag and swallowing reflexes, become impaired, making aspiration a constant concern.

Cerebellum

Growth of a tumor in the cerebellar area is accompanied by cerebellar signs (ataxia, incoordination, nystagmus, vertigo, nausea), obstruction of flow of CSF, and potential for brainstem compression. The usual signs of increased ICP (headache, vomiting, and classic changes in vital signs) are common, particularly with CSF obstruction.

ASSOCIATED INCREASED INTRACRANIAL PRESSURE SIGNS

Many tumors are associated with increased ICP and present with or without localizing signs. They include medulloblastoma, ependymoma of the fourth ventricle, hemangioblastoma

of the cerebellum, pinealoma, colloid cyst of the third ventricle, and craniopharyngioma. These tumors are listed in Table 21-1.

The signs and symptoms associated with increased ICP are discussed in Chapter 13. Only papilledema and obstruction of CSF flow, as they relate to brain tumors, are discussed in this section.

Papilledema

Papilledema, seen in about 70% of patients with brain tumors, is associated with visual changes, such as decreased visual acuity, diplopia, and deficits in the visual fields. The visual pathways extend through the four lobes of the cerebral hemispheres. Therefore, it is reasonable to expect a high incidence of visual disturbances with supratentorial lesions. Dysfunction of the abducens nerve (cranial nerve VI), a symptom commonly seen in brain tumor lesions, results in an inability to move the eye outward on the horizontal plane. It is common that deterioration in vision is the main reason for referral to a neurologist by an optometrist or ophthalmologist, provided that the first examiner recognized the visual deficits as possibly being related to an intracranial lesion.

Obstruction to Flow of Cerebrospinal Fluid

Tumor encroachment from within or outside the ventricles or subarachnoid space interferes with the normal flow of CSF. This obstruction of CSF results in obstructive hydrocephalus. If the tumor encroachment occurs slowly, the development of hydrocephalus will be gradual. However, rapid tumor growth produces acute precipitation of signs and symptoms, such as a massive spike in ICP with rapid deterioration in neurological status.

APPROACH TO THE PATIENT WITH A BRAIN TUMOR

Patients and families going through the process of diagnosis and treatment of a brain tumor have multiple needs that can only be met by a collaborative interdisciplinary team of health care professionals who are knowledgeable about the disease. A partnership must be formed among the patient, family, and team to work together to create the best plan for the individual patient. There is an ongoing need for patient and family education as the patient progresses through the various stages of illness. Education provided in a supportive, honest environment empowers the patient and family to take control of the illness by making informed decisions. Through this process, good communication among the interdisciplinary team provides the support structure to assist the patient with the holistic impact of the illness.

Several potential collaborative problems should be addressed by the interdisciplinary team. Among potential neurological complications related to a brain tumor are increased ICP, seizures, hydrocephalus, cranial nerve impairment, paresis/paralysis, and peripheral nerve impairment. Other body systems are at risk for complications related to
(text continues on page 507)

TABLE 21-1   BRAIN TUMORS

TYPE OF TUMOR	DESCRIPTION	LOCATION OR DEMOGRAPHIC DATA	SIGNS AND SYMPTOMS	TREATMENT	PROGNOSIS
Common Brain Tumors					
Astrocytoma (grades I and II) Constitutes 25%–30% of all cerebral gliomas	Grade I: well-defined cells Grade II: cell differentiation less defined ↑ Cellularity	Usually found in cerebrum, cerebellum, hypothalamus, optic nerve and chiasma, and pons Cerebral hemisphere tumors most often found in adults 20–40 y	Neurological deficits depend on specific location of tumor and if it is supra- or infratentorial Onset of a focal or generalized seizure in previously seizure-free person is most common first sign	*Surgery:* gross total removal is treatment of choice, but complete removal rarely possible; partial removal may prolong life; tumor recurrence often associated with malignant progression *Radiation and Chemotherapy:* controversial; not done for grade 1	5–6 y survival on average Range, 2–20 y
Anaplastic astrocytoma (grade III)	Cellularity anaplastic: cellular atypia, ↑ mitosis				15–28 mo average survival
Glioblastoma (GBM) (also known as astrocytoma, grade IV) Constitutes 20% of all intracranial tumors and 55% of all gliomas	Malignant, rapidly growing Composed of heterogeneous cells Necrotic and hemorrhagic areas within tumor common	Usually found in a frontal lobe 40–60 y most common and with increasing age Male predilection	Memory loss, neurobehavioral changes, seizures, speech deficits, hearing/auditory (H/A), visual deficits Diffuse cerebral symptoms	*Surgery:* resection and debulking to relieve compression and ICP *Radiation* with *concurrent temozolomide followed by adjuvant temozolomide*	14–16 mo average survival
Astrocytoma of optic nerves and chiasma (spongioblastoma) Most common in children; sometimes seen in young adults	As the tumor grows, it enlarges the optic foramen with little distortion of surrounding structures Slow-growing tumor	Found along the optic nerves Girls > boys, with 2:1 predilection	Early symptoms include Dim vision Hemianopsia Optic atrophy Blindness Proptosis Hypothalamic imbalance	*Surgery:* removal possible but tumor often inaccessible *Radiation:* usually poor response	10 y or more
Ependymoma (low grade and anaplastic) Tumor of childhood and young adults	Arises from lining of ventricles Slow-growing	In ventricles, particularly fourth; can attach itself to roof or floor of ventricle, or grow directly into cerebral hemisphere Seen in children and adults up to 30 y, most often in men Supratentorial more common in adults; infratentorial in children	Rapid elevation in ICP secondary to CSF obstruction S&S vary by location If forth ventricle, ↓ level of consciousness, severe H/A, VS changes with ↑ ICP, N/V, pupillary changes, hemiplegia, hemiparesthesia, seizures If in cerebellar area, ataxia	*Surgery:* removal if surgically accessible; depends on location *Radiation:* for most *Chemotherapy:* usually not helpful *Shunting procedure:* prn to reduce ↑ ICP from obstructive hydrocephalus	About 5–10 y, depending on location

(continued)

TABLE 21–1   BRAIN TUMORS (*Continued*)

TYPE OF TUMOR	DESCRIPTION	LOCATION OR DEMOGRAPHIC DATA	SIGNS AND SYMPTOMS	TREATMENT	PROGNOSIS
Oligodendroglioma (low grade and anaplastic)	Calcification noted on radiologic examination in about 50% of patients	Cerebral hemispheres, particularly frontal and temporal lobes Found in patients 20–40 y	Depends on location Seizures are first symptoms in 50% of patients	*Surgery, chemotherapy* for those with loss of heterozygosity of the 1p and 19q chromosomes and radiation for those who are intact	5–10 y, depending on grade
Mixed gliomas Named for predominant tumor cell present	Composed histologically of two or more cell types of astrocytoma/ glioblastoma, oligodendroglioma, or ependymoma in any combination	Any place where various glioma types can be found	Depend on location of tumor	Depends on type of tumor *Surgery, radiation, chemotherapy*	≥5 y or more
Meningioma	Extra-axial tumor arising from dural elements Firm, encapsulated; can erode into bone Have estrogen and progesterone receptors; grow rapidly during pregnancy Slow-growing; can become large before symptoms appear Recur if not completely removed; can become malignant with reoccurrence Compresses brain	Predilection for areas proximal to venous sinuses Most common in women; average age, 50 y Parasagittal sinus Lateral convexities Sphenoid ridge Suprasellar Olfactory groove	Neurological deficits caused by compression and depending on area involved Progressive H/A, memory loss, or cognitive changes; paraparesis; seizures; urinary incontinence Gradual development of hemiparesis, speech abnormalities; other related to area of compression Extraocular nerve palsy, proptosis, seizures Bitemporal hemianopsia, optic atrophy, pituitary-related hormonal imbalance Anosmia, visual deficits, dementia, pupillary abnormalities	*Surgery:* complete removal, if possible, or partial dissection *Radiation:* after subtotal resection and at tumor recurrence Immunotherapy for atypical meningiomas	"Cure" with total removal Many years with partial excision with radiation
Metastatic brain tumors	20%–40% of cancer patients have metastasis to brain from other parts of the body (lungs, breast, lower GI most common) Spread to brain by blood Usually well differentiated from other brain tissue; lesion may be single or multiple	Can occur anywhere Seen as individual tumor or multiple tumors	Depend on location H/A, paresis, and cognitive deficits most common	*Surgery:* resection if possible, for singular lesion *Radiation:* with multiple lesions Gamma knife radiosurgery (for <3 lesions) Chemotherapy: similar as for primary tumor; methotrexate with oral leucovorin rescue common	Prognosis usually based on primary cancer 1–3+ y average
Malignant melanomas	Rare	Cerebral hemispheres from a primary lesion in skin	Depend on location	Surgery, radiation, chemotherapy	Few months to few years

(continued)

TABLE 21–1   BRAIN TUMORS (*Continued*)

TYPE OF TUMOR	DESCRIPTION	LOCATION OR DEMOGRAPHIC DATA	SIGNS AND SYMPTOMS	TREATMENT	PROGNOSIS
Primary cerebral lymphoma	Cellular tumor Behaves much like a glioblastoma Occurs in adults 40–50 y; more common in immunocompromised patients (immunosuppressive therapy for organ transplant or people with AIDS)	May arise in any part of brain May be either monofocal or multifocal	Neurocognitive and personality changes Focal signs or ↑ ICP signs	Biopsy followed by Decadron Chemotherapy Both radiation and chemotherapy are effective	After initial response, relapse common Average survival, 1–4 y

Cerebellopontine Angle Tumors (*includes several categories of tumors located in this anatomic area*)

TYPE OF TUMOR	DESCRIPTION	LOCATION OR DEMOGRAPHIC DATA	SIGNS AND SYMPTOMS	TREATMENT	PROGNOSIS
Miscellaneous astrocytomas and meningiomas	Can be confused with an acoustic neuroma without visualization Definitive diagnosis made by surgical exposure, biopsy, and histologic examination	Cerebellopontine angle	Variation of those seen with acoustic neuroma (see below)	*Surgery:* if possible; difficult surgical access (near vital centers) *Radiation:* may be selected over surgery	Depends on the type of tumor
Acoustic neuroma (schwannoma)	Arises from sheath of Schwann cells Usual size: pea to walnut Considered a benign tumor but located in an often inaccessible area Slow-growing Bilateral tumors are possible; when they occur, they result from a hereditary problem of chromosome 22; the tumors are part of central neurofibromatosis	Seen most often in patients 30–49 y Involves vestibular branch of CN VIII *Small tumors* are confined to internal auditory canal and involve CN VIII *Large tumors* extend outside internal auditory meatus *Large tumors* displace CN VII and compress CN V along with CN VIII; they may also encroach on CN IX and CN X, and possibly cerebellum	Depend on size; deficits noted on affected side *Small tumor (confined to internal auditory canal and involving CN VIII)* and include: Tinnitus/vertigo Hearing loss; most notable when using telephone or when source of sound is close to affected ear Dizziness *Large tumor (outside auditory meatus):* S&S listed above and *Facial:* loss of taste on anterior tongue, difficulty closing lower eyelid, facial weakness *Trigeminal:* facial paresthesia/anesthesia, difficulty chewing *Glossopharyngeal and vagus* (difficulty swallowing, hoarseness) *Cerebellar involvement* (ataxia/incoordination, possibly hydrocephalus, ↑ ICP from obstruction of CSF flow secondary to displacement of pons and medulla)	*Surgery:* microsurgical complete removal or debulking of larger tumors (debulking to preserve CNs involved in the tumors) Suboccipital retrosigmoid approach for smaller tumors Translabyrinthine approach for larger tumors With large tumors, the tumor may entwine other cranial nerves that would cause *severe* deficits if tumor were completely excised *Radiation:* focused radiation (proton beam, gamma knife) alternative in older patients; scar tissue a possible problem if later surgery needed. Also used in younger patients	Cure with small tumor and total resection; generally good outcome Tumor regrowth possible if subtotal resection Possible permanent hearing loss, loss of facial sensation on affected side, or facial droop Decreased or absent corneal reflex

(continued)

TABLE 21-1 BRAIN TUMORS (*Continued*)

TYPE OF TUMOR	DESCRIPTION	LOCATION OR DEMOGRAPHIC DATA	SIGNS AND SYMPTOMS	TREATMENT	PROGNOSIS
Chordoma	Arises from embryonic remnants May appear as a cerebellopontine angle tumor	Predilection M > F Occurs in patients 30–49 y Found in clivus (35%) dorsum of sellae to foramen magnum and (50% in sacrococcygeal area)	Loss of vision Extraocular muscle paralysis Paralyzed muscles of swallowing Noted on MRI or CT scan	*Surgery:* excision (approach varies depending on tumor location) *Radiation:* conventional or proton beam	Tumors tend to recur Poor prognosis with aggressive and metastatic tumors

Pituitary Tumors

Pituitary adenomas*
Classified by type of:
  Hormones secreted
  Effects (functioning or nonfunctioning)
  Grade of sella turcica enlargement or erosion
  Suprasellar extension
	Hormone(s) secreted
	  Prolactin (most common)
	  Growth hormone
	  ACTH
	  Nonfunctioning: produce S&S from compression of adjacent structures (e.g., optic nerves, bitemporal hemianopsia)
	Functioning (hormone-secreting): cause endocrine syndromes (e.g., acromegaly)
	Enclosed adenomas:
	  I—sella normal; floor may be indented
	  II—sella enlarged, floor intact
	  III—invasive adenomas; localized erosion of the floor
	  IV—entire floor diffusely eroded
	Classified A–D by suprasellar extension
	  A: No suprasellar extension
	  B: Suprasellar bulge does not reach floor of third ventricle
	  C: Tumor reaches third ventricle, distorting chiasmatic recess
	  D: Tumor fills third ventricle almost to foramen of Munro
		Most pituitary tumors in anterior lobe
		Both lobes can be damaged from compression of parasellar tumors
			In general:
			  Visual disorders (diminished vision with a scotoma; bitemporal hemianopsia)
			  Paresis of extraocular muscles
			  H/A
			  Various endocrine disorders (see below)
			  Abnormal sella turcica region on CT scan
			Endocrine disorders:
			Prolactin-secreting adenoma
			  Galactorrhea
			  Amenorrhea
			  Infertility
			  Loss of pubic hair
			  Impotence
			  ↑ Serum prolactin
			ACTH-secreting adenoma
			  Adrenal hyperplasia
			  Cushing's syndrome*
			Growth hormone–secreting adenoma
			  Giantism before puberty or closure of epiphyses
			  Acromegaly after puberty or closure of epiphyses (enlarged jaw, nose, tongue, hands, feet)
			  Thickening of soft tissue of face
			  Enlarged heart and pulmonary disease
			  Diabetes mellitus
			  Serum growth hormone levels >10 ng/mL
			Serious complications:
			Pituitary apoplexy syndrome: acute onset of ophthalmoplegia, blindness, drowsiness, and coma; death possible
				Depends on the size and type of the tumor, patient's age, and endocrine and visual deficits; surgery, radiation, or drug therapy separately or in combination
				Surgery: for smaller tumors, transsphenoidal microsurgery to remove total tumor and preseve or normalize pituitary
				Radiation: conventional radiation therapy or proton beam, if available
				Hormonal replacement: postsurgery, hormonal replacement possible
				Other drug treatment: bromocriptine may be used to inhibit prolactin; for some patients, this is only treatment necessary for prolactin-secreting tumors
					Curable with complete resection
					In others, very good outcome

(continued)

TABLE 21–1   BRAIN TUMORS (*Continued*)

TYPE OF TUMOR	DESCRIPTION	LOCATION OR DEMOGRAPHIC DATA	SIGNS AND SYMPTOMS	TREATMENT	PROGNOSIS
Developmental Tumors (seen sometimes in adults)					
Craniopharyngioma	Thought to arise from Rathke's pouch Solid or cystic tumors Can compress the pituitary and may even amputate the pituitary stalk About 75% with calcified areas Tumor growth is directed upward, resulting in invagination of the third ventricle and possible blockage of CSF flow Optic chiasm elevated by tumor, resulting in traction on optic nerves	In or about the sella pituitary area Usually affects children	Signs and symptoms of grossly ↑ ICP because of CSF flow blockage Pituitary or hypothalamic dysfunction Visual disturbance	*Surgery:* resection by intracranial or transsphenoidal approach *Radiation:* after *surgery;* tumor radiosensitive	Excellent if tumor is excised with microsurgery, cure rate, 80% Recurrence if only subtotal resection performed, even with radiation
Epidermoid and dermoid cysts	Cysts of congenital origin arising from the ectodermal layer; cysts lined with stratified squamous epithelium Epidermoid cysts contain keratin, cellular debris, and cholesterol; dermoid cysts contain hair and sebaceous glands	On bones of skull or within brain	Depends on location	*Surgery:* complete removal is usually possible	Very good
Genetically Related Autosomal Dominant Diseases					
Von Recklinghausen's disease (neurofibromatosis)	Genetic origin because of autosomal dominant mendelian trait Skin, nervous system, bones, endocrine glands, and other organs are sites of congenital anomalies, in addition to the multiple tumors of skin Firm, encapsulated lesions attach to the nerve	Benign, multiple, circumscribed dermal and neural tumors with increased skin pigmentation (cosmetically offensive) Tumors late in childhood or in early adolescence	Spots of hyperpigmentation (café au lait) and cutaneous and subcutaneous tumors	*Surgery:* possible, depending on the location of the tumor *Radiation:* tumor is radioresistant	Depends on involved area
Hemangioblastoma (with von Hippel-Lindau disease)	Vascular tumor Slow-growing	Cerebellum (as a single or multiple lesion); less common in the medulla and cerebral hemispheres; tumor in adults	Dizziness Unilateral ataxia Signs and symptoms of ↑ ICP Possible spinal cord involvement	*Surgery:* complete removal, if possible *Radiation:* with recurrence	Usually curable

ACTH, adrenocorticotropic hormone; AIDS, acquired immunodeficiency syndrome; CN, cranial nerve; CSF, cerebrospinal fluid; CT, computed tomography; GI, gastrointestinal; H/A, headache; ICP, intracranial pressure; MRI, magnetic resonance imaging; N&V, nausea and vomiting; S&S, signs and symptoms; VS, vital signs;

*Cushing's syndrome comprises moon facies, "buffalo hump," abdominal striae, pendulous abdomen; ecchymosis, hypertension, muscle weakness, osteoporosis, and high cortisol levels.

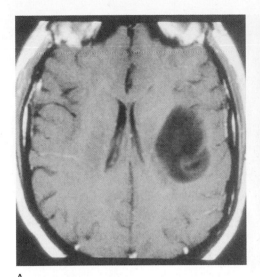

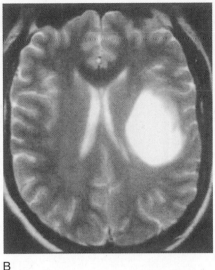

Figure 21-3 • Low-grade astrocytoma. (*A*) Axial postcontrast T1-weighted magnetic resonance image shows low-grade nonenhancing astrocytoma in the left temporal region. (*B*) Corresponding T2-weighted image shows well-defined margins and absence of surrounding edema. There is little mass effect.

A   B

treatment options such as sepsis, myelosuppression, gastric ulcer, and electrolyte imbalance. These more common problems seen in patients along the continuum of illness, as well as less common problems, require interdisciplinary effort for successful management.

Diagnosis

The clinical manifestations of brain tumors span a wide range of signs and symptoms, depending on the type, size, and location of the tumor. After a neurological examination, neuroimaging with magnetic resonance imaging (MRI) or computed tomography (CT) with and without contrast is performed. MRI with gadolinium is the preferred diagnostic test because it has high sensitivity; it can identify small tumors located near bone, especially in the posterior fossa, pituitary

fossa, internal auditory canal, and floor of the middle cranial fossa; it can identify cerebral edema accurately; and it provides improved anatomic detail allowing for better visualization of the extent of tumor and characteristics associated with degree of malignancy.[12] It is relatively easy to acquire multiplanar images that provide accurate localization and identification of the tumor without loss of detail (Figs. 21-3 through 21-10).[13] A CT scan provides satisfactory imaging in patients who have contraindications for an MRI, such as those with a pacemaker, who are claustrophobic, or who need rapid screening. The CT scan is done with and without contrast medium. If characteristics associated with metastatic lesions are seen (such as multiple lesions, spherical lesions with extensive surrounding cerebral edema), systemic work-up looking for a primary cancer is undertaken. If findings are consistent with a primary tumor, neuroimaging is often the only diagnostic test performed prior to a surgical procedure to obtain tissue diagnosis.

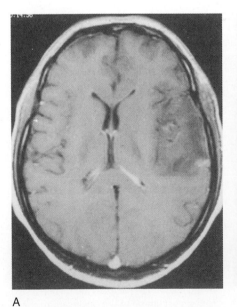

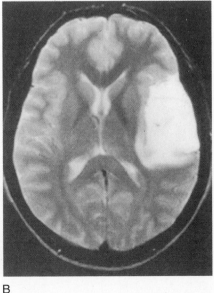

Figure 21-4 • Anaplastic astrocytoma. (*A*) Axial postcontrast T1-weighted magnetic resonance image shows left insular anaplastic astrocytoma with ill-defined margins and patchy enhancement. There is no obvious necrosis. (*B*) Corresponding T2-weighted image shows the tumor to have ill-defined margins.

A   B

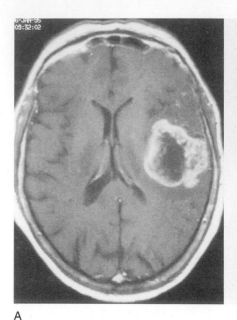

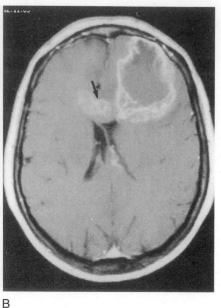

A   B

Figure 21-5 • Glioblastoma multiforme. (*A*) Axial postcontrast T1-weighted magnetic resonance (MR) image shows glioblastoma multiforme (GBM) in the left temporal lobe. Note irregular and thick ring enhancement. There is central necrosis. (*B*) Axial postcontrast T1-weighted MR image shows large and irregular enhancing GBM in the left frontal lobe with extension across the genu of the corpus callosum (*arrow*).

For tumors around the optic chiasm, such as pituitary tumors or gliomas, careful mapping of the visual fields by an ophthalmologist is necessary to determine the degree of visual deficits. With cerebellopontine angle tumors, such as acoustic neuromas, audiometric studies are helpful in determining the degree of hearing loss.

Endocrine studies (blood and urine levels of hormones controlled by the pituitary gland) are helpful when a pituitary adenoma or a craniopharyngioma is suspected. Common tests and their normal values are found in Table 21-2.

Surgery

With few exceptions after a brain lesion has been identified, tissue is required to make an accurate histopathologic diagnosis

before appropriate treatment can be initiated. The primary exception is when significant morbidity or mortality may occur as a result of lesion location, such as tumor involving eloquent areas of the brain or an infiltrating brainstem lesion.

Several surgical options are available. In some cases, complete tumor removal is possible, achieving a surgical "cure" without additional therapy.[14] This is true for many benign tumors such as juvenile pilocytic astrocytomas and meningiomas. Some tumors, although histologically benign, cannot be completely removed; nonetheless, a partial resection may be performed to relieve symptoms. Finally, in more malignant tumor forms, there appears to be a relationship between the extent of tumor resection and length of survival. Currently, neurosurgical and imaging techniques provide a safe means of partial or complete resection with a complication rate of

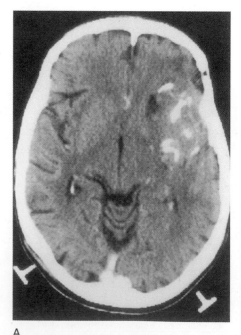

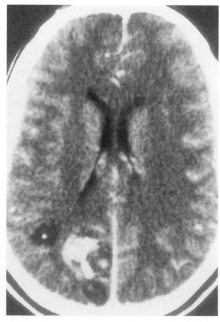

A   B

Figure 21-6 • Oligodendroglioma. (*A*) Axial postcontrast computed tomography (CT) scan shows an oligodendroglioma with multiple calcifications in the left frontotemporal region. (*B*) Postcontrast CT scan shows heavily calcified oligodendroglioma in the medial left occipital lobe. There is a tumor cyst lateral to the calcification.

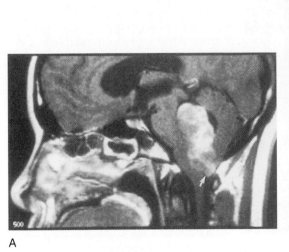

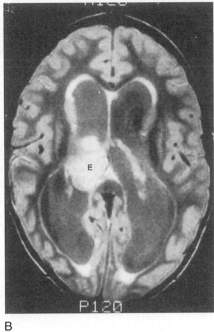

A

B

Figure 21-7 • Ependymoma. (*A*) Midsagittal postcontrast T1-weighted magnetic resonance image shows enhancing ependymoma in the fourth ventricle. The tumor extrudes (*arrow*) through the foramen of Magendie. (*B*) Proton density image shows ependymoma (*E*) inside the right lateral ventricle.

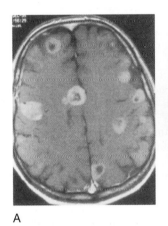

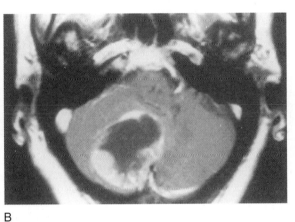

A

B

Figure 21-8 • Metastatic tumors. (*A*) Axial postcontrast T1-weighted magnetic resonance (MR) image shows multiple enhancing **metastases** (breast primary) at the gray–white junctions. (*B*) Axial postcontrast T1-weighted MR image of a different patient shows single necrotic metastasis from squamous cell carcinoma of the lung.

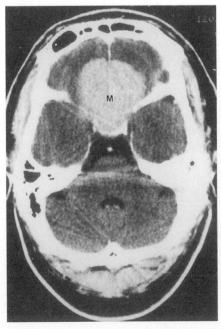

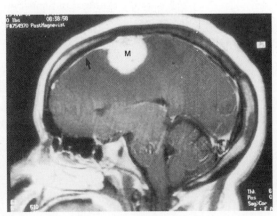

A

B

Figure 21-9 • Meningioma. (*A*) Contrast-enhanced computed tomography scan shows large frontobasal meningioma (*M*). (*B*) Parasagittal postcontrast T1-weighted magnetic resonance image shows parafalcine meningioma (*M*) with dural tail (*arrow*) of enhancement. There is surrounding edema.

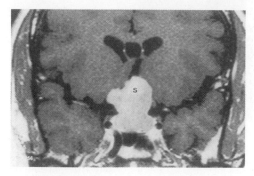

Figure 21-10 • Pituitary adenoma. Coronal postcontrast T1-weighted magnetic resonance image shows macroadenoma with typical figure-of-eight shape and suprasellar (*s*) extension.

less than 5% for most tumors. Preoperative embolization may be used to decrease bleeding during surgical resection with tumors that are very vascular such as a meningioma.

A craniotomy is the surgical procedure that most patients undergo. A bone flap is created by removing a portion of bone from the skull, allowing access to the dura, which can be opened. The tumor is either partially or completely resected and the bone flap replaced. Current technologies, such as stereotaxis and other image-guided systems, allow neurosurgeons to localize a tumor and other anatomic sites precisely. By identifying the margins of the tumor, surgery is minimally invasive and normal tissue preserved. Stereotaxis uses a computer to create a three-dimensional map of the tumor from CT or MRI information. Functional MRI allows identification of eloquent brain and assists with maximal resection with less morbidity. Intraoperative MRI also enables increased accuracy in resection. Stereotaxis is combined with microsurgical technology. Microsurgery enhances the neurosurgeon's visualization of the operative field through high-powered magnification. Ultrasonic aspirators combine two actions: high-frequency sound waves to break up the tumor and an aspirator to suction away the tumor fragments. Lasers, alone or in combination with conventional surgery, provide a beam of concentrated light energy capable of destroying tissue. A laser is useful for complete resection of a tumor, or it may be used in combination with partial surgical resection.

Other technologies allow treatment of tumors previously inaccessible to neurosurgeons such as those deep in the brain, those located on the motor strip or speech areas, or those at the base of the skull. Evoked potential electrophysiologic mapping of the brain's cortical surface is useful to measure electrical potential of nerves in response to stimulation with small electrodes.[14] Surgery can also be conducted under local anesthesia with brain-mapping techniques to allow for removal of tumors from the speech and motor areas. Finally, tumors at the base of the skull can now be successfully removed through the collaborative efforts of ear, nose, and throat (ENT) specialists, plastic surgeons, and neurosurgeons optimizing their skill and knowledge with available technology. See Chapter 14 for management of neurosurgical patients.

Whether biopsy or excision will be performed is based on several factors, including the location of tumor, the number of lesions, the presence of mass effect, and the patient's overall physical status. Biopsy, either open or stereotactic, to obtain tissue is associated with low morbidity and mortality but does not reduce tumor burden and may be associated with sampling error. Safely removing as much visible tumor without causing neurological deficit is the goal of surgery for most tumors, with few exceptions.

> **CLINICAL PEARLS:** Surgery is never curative for malignant primary brain tumors. Safely removing as much visible tumor is the goal of surgery for most tumors.

Medical Treatment

After the diagnosis of a brain tumor is established, the next major consideration is medical management. Methods for treatment of brain tumors in addition to surgery include the use of radiation and chemotherapy alone or in combination. In addition, supportive medications, such as anticonvulsants and corticosteroids, are often integral to patient management. The variables that are considered when selecting appropriate treatment include the type and grade of tumor, its location and size, surgical accessibility, presenting signs and symptoms, and the general condition of the patient. Informed consent for treatment must include the patient and/or his or her next of kin or designated significant other in the decision-making process.

General Drug Therapy

Most patients benefit from administration of corticosteroids (dexamethasone, prednisone, or methylprednisolone) to decrease cerebral edema. The reversal of symptoms can be remarkable. In the case of a CNS lymphoma, complete resolution of the enhancing tumor on scan can occur within weeks of initiating corticosteroids (although this is often a transient effect). As a consequence of this, if a CNS lymphoma is suspected, steroids will be held until after diagnostic biopsy. For other primary tumors, a corticosteroid is usually begun when the tumor is diagnosed and the presence of cerebral edema and increased ICP is confirmed. Dosing is based on the amount of edema and patient response. If surgery is recommended, dexamethasone is administered preoperatively, and tapered based on amount of resection and patient tolerance in the postoperative setting. Known side effects of steroid therapy include gastritis, peptic ulcer disease,

TABLE 21–2	COMMON TESTS FOR PATIENTS WITH SUSPECTED PITUITARY TUMORS	
HORMONE	**NORMS FOR WOMEN**	**NORMS FOR MEN**
Prolactin	Premenopausal women: 2.2–19.2 mEq/L Postmenopausal women: 1.0–12.8 mEq/L	Men: 1.9–11.7 mEq/L
Growth hormone	Women: 0–30 ng/mL	Men: 0–8 ng/mL
Cortisol	6:00 to 8:00 AM: 10–25 g/L	Same

alterations in healing, increased blood glucose levels, fluid retention, Cushing's syndrome (most commonly called "moon face" and "buffalo hump"), risk for infection, and corticosteroid-induced proximal myopathy. It should be taken with food, and an H_2 blocker (e.g., famotidine [Pepcid] or ranitidine [Zantac]) must be administered concurrently with corticosteroids to prevent gastric irritation.

Patients with supratentorial lesions who present with seizures will be placed on an anticonvulsant drug. The use of prophylactic anticonvulsants is controversial, with no study to date supporting their use. The agent used is based on potential toxicity and physician preference. Recently, anticonvulsants that utilize the P450 enzyme system for their metabolism, including phenytoin, phenobarbital, and carbamazepine, have been shown to enhance clearance of many chemotherapeutic agents.[15,16] As a consequence, agents that do not require this pathway for their metabolism are being used with increasing frequency. In some instances, a combination of two or three anticonvulsants is necessary to achieve seizure control. Appropriate management of seizures if they occur is an important teaching point. Chapter 29 discusses this in detail.

Radiation Therapy

Radiation therapy is the second major option in the treatment of most brain tumors, whether they are benign or malignant. In most cases, surgery is used for initial diagnosis and resection of as much tumor as possible. Radiation therapy is then employed to target the residual tumor with the goal of reducing or stabilizing its size. For malignant lesions, resection is never complete. Even if the entire visible tumor has been resected, there is usually microscopic seeding into normal adjacent tissue. Therefore, a course of postoperative radiation therapy is recommended to prevent or delay recurrent growth. Radiotherapy is usually recommended postoperatively for some benign tumors that have undergone subtotal resection and may be life threatening if growth continues. Other benign brain tumors may be treated with radiation to prevent recurrence.

Tumor cells are more radiosensitive than normal cells as a consequence of their increased mitotic activity. Damage to DNA is the mechanism by which radiation destroys tumor cells. Large numbers of hypoxic tumor cells are present in the core of malignant tumors. These cells are more resistant to the DNA-damaging effects of radiation, which may explain why radiation has a time-limited beneficial effect for malignant tumors.

Various options may be used to deliver radiation therapy. Standard external beam radiation therapy (EBRT) and, more recently, intensity-modulated radiation therapy (IMRT) are the cornerstones of radiation therapy. Additional methods of delivery include stereotactic radiosurgery, interstitial brachytherapy, and stereotactic radiotherapy. Each is briefly discussed.

External Beam Radiation Therapy. EBRT is the conventional form of radiation therapy used after a diagnostic surgical procedure, or in lieu of surgery for tumors that are either inoperable or extremely sensitive to radiotherapy. EBRT can be delivered to the area of tumor only (focal EBRT) or the entire brain (whole brain XRT). Total dose typically ranges between 40 and 60 Gy, delivered as once-daily treatments of a dosage of 1.8 to 2.0 Gy, five times per week.[17] Planning is typically based on the presurgical MRI for planning. For metastatic tumors, lower doses of EBRT are used with a commonly prescribed dosage of 30 Gy over 10 treatments. A CT scan is performed for planning and dose calculation, but an MRI is necessary to identify tumor margins. *Immobilization* devices such as the Aquaplast face mask are used to ensure that the patient remains in the same position each day during treatment.[17]

Proton Therapy. Proton therapy is similar to conventional EBRT, but proton particles are used instead of x-rays. Advantages to proton beam therapy is that a three-dimensional pattern can be constructed, thus limiting exposure to areas of normal brain and allowing for greater precision in delivery of therapy.[18] This treatment is currently only available at a few centers within the United States. Examples of CNS tumors treated with proton therapy include tumors such as chordomas, retinoblastomas, uveal melanomas, and meningiomas.[19]

Conformal radiation is that which uses high-dose external radiation beams that are shaped or "conformed" to match the shape of a tumor. This allows for a uniform high dose to be delivered to the tumor and minimizes radiation exposure to adjacent brain tissue. Radiosurgery is a form of conformal therapy that allows delivery of a highly focused dose of radiation in one fraction. This approach is beneficial for small (those <4 cm), well-circumscribed lesions.[17] For infiltrating lesions, undetectable tumor extension to surrounding brain tissue will not be targeted. There are two primary systems for delivery of radiosurgery: using a linear *accelerator (LINAC)* or using a *gamma knife*.

Intensity-Modulated Radiation Therapy. IMRT is a new approach to delivery of radiation therapy. IMRT uses computer programs to design the dose distribution, resulting in the radiation dose to the tumor differing from the radiation dose to the surrounding tissue. This advance benefits treatment planning for highly irregularly shaped tumors, limiting exposure to surrounding tissue, which should reduce associated toxicity.[20]

Interstitial Brachytherapy. Brachytherapy involves implantation of radioactive **seeds** directly into the tumor bed. These can be implanted on a temporary or permanent basis. This technique does require a neurosurgical procedure, and many patients require another surgical procedure to remove necrotic tissue.[17]

Responses to Radiation Therapy. Unfortunately, not all patients respond well to radiation therapy. Failure to completely annihilate malignant cells is the problem. This failure is attributed, in part, to the presence of hypoxic cells. Hypoxic cells are approximately three times more resistant to radiation than are well-oxygenated cells[21] and can remain viable after radiation therapy. As a consequence of the high failure rate of conventional radiation treatments for CNS tumors, methods to improve response are currently under investigation. Some are directed at making the treatment more specific, and others are aimed at making treatment more tumoricidal.[22] Examples include boron-neutron capture therapy and radioimmunotherapy. Another area of research is the use of radiosensitizers, including common chemotherapy agents and newer radiosensitizers such as motexafin gadolinium and RSR13, currently under investigation.

Side effects from radiation depend on location, total dose administered, and the technique used to provide radiation. The most common side effects of radiation in the acute phase are somnolence, hair loss, and skin disorders. Chronic side effects include loss of pituitary function, diminished intellectual function, hydrocephalus, and cerebral necrosis, especially with glioblastoma multiforme. In addition to follow-up for recurrence of the tumor, neuropsychological testing and endocrine evaluation may be helpful.

CLINICAL PEARLS: Radiation therapy is the standard treatment approach for most malignant tumors.

Chemotherapy

Chemotherapy is often used as an adjunct to surgery and radiation therapy, and is often the primary method of treatment at recurrence. Chemotherapy is most often used as part of a multimodal approach together with surgery and radiation. It may be given before, during, or after radiation therapy or at the time of tumor recurrence.

The most commonly used chemotherapeutic drugs are alkylating agents, particularly the nitrosoureas. Temozolomide (Temodar), carmustine (BCNU), lomustine (CCNU), Gliadel wafers (i.e., carmustine), procarbazine, or a combination of procarbazine, CCNU, and vincristine (PCV) is frequently used.

Most chemotherapeutic drugs are administered by the intravenous or oral route. In addition, the interstitial, intraarterial, and intrathecal routes have become options, depending on the particular drug and tumor site. These routes allow increased drug dosage, increasing the attack on malignant cells while limiting side effects. With *interstitial administration*, disc-shaped wafers impregnated with a biodegradable chemotherapeutic drug are placed directly into the surgical cavity after a tumor is removed to provide slow, direct drug to the tumor site without the drug spreading elsewhere in the body. The *intra-arterial* route helps to focus the chemotherapeutic agent as compared with an intravenous infusion in which the drug is mixed into the general circulation. *Intrathecal infusion* delivers a chemotherapeutic agent directly into the spinal fluid. This method has been used to treat some brain, spinal cord, and metastatic tumors.

Chemotherapeutic agents can be broadly classified into those that are cytotoxic (causing cell death) or cytostatic (those causing the cells to behave more like normal cells).[23] Cytotoxic chemotherapy can be further subdivided into classes based on the mechanism of action: cell cycle–specific agents (only active during certain phases of the cell's life cycle) and cell cycle–nonspecific agents (effective during all phases of the cell cycle). Some treatment protocols combine both categories of drugs to be effective against the maximum number of malignant cells.

Although chemotherapy has been the mainstay of treatment for various malignancies in other body systems, its use in brain tumor treatment has had limited success. Barriers to effectiveness include the presence of the blood-brain barrier, which is a network of blood vessels and cells that protect the brain and prevent certain molecules from passing through the cellular barrier. If chemotherapeutic drugs cannot be delivered to the focus of need, they will not be effective in killing the targeted tumor cells. A major challenge in brain tumor chemotherapy research has been to find drugs that will cross the blood–brain barrier without causing neurological injury to normal cells. In addition, tumor cells are able to block or become resistant to the agents prescribed.

The acute side effects of cytotoxic chemotherapy include anemia, leukopenia, thrombocytopenia, nausea, vomiting, and fatigue. The long-term effects are neurotoxic, hepatic, and pulmonary. The dosage of a drug is limited by potential toxicity to normal cells, called *dose-limiting toxicity*. Special concerns when treating a malignant lesion of the brain using chemotherapeutic agents include the following: cerebral edema affects drug entry into the tumor; drug resistance can occur; and the heterogeneity of tumor cells results in different chemosensitivity among cells within the same tumor.[24]

The major chemotherapeutic drugs are briefly discussed in the next section and also summarized in Table 21-3. The type and course of chemotherapy are dependent on tumor histology. Specific treatment approaches, incorporating information on surgical and radiation approaches in addition to standard chemotherapy for commonly occurring tumors, are also briefly discussed.

Glioblastoma. The current standard of care for patients with newly diagnosed glioblastoma multiforme (GBM) is a diagnostic surgical procedure, followed by combination therapy with temozolomide and EBRT followed by at least 6 months of adjuvant temozolomide.[25] Until recently, surgery and radiation therapy had been the standard treatment approach for GBM patients as a consequence of the modest benefit in terms of survival with the addition of adjuvant chemotherapy (or chemotherapy used in the postradiation setting).[26] Gliadel, a chemotherapy (BCNU)-impregnated polymer that is placed in the surgical bed after tumor removal, has also been shown to improve survival in patients with newly diagnosed malignant gliomas.[27] This approach has the benefit of minimal systemic toxicity and no limitation posed by the blood–brain barrier. Thus far, no studies have compared a systemic chemotherapy strategy with wafer treatment to determine the optimal treatment for patients with newly diagnosed glioblastoma, so definitive guidelines for the combined use have not been established.

The recurrent disease setting is where new agents or combinations are used in a clinical trial setting. In addition, additional surgery or various conventional chemotherapy treatments are used, including carmustine (BCNU) and lomustine (CCNU), irinotecan, carboplatin, or cisplatin and etoposide. As no standard therapy has been shown to have benefit over any other, patients with recurrent glioblastoma should be encouraged to participate in approved clinical trials in order to assess the development of more effective regimens.

Anaplastic Astrocytoma. For patients with anaplastic astrocytomas, surgical resection is the standard initial therapy, although some suggest that initially it should be radiation therapy.[28] The use of concurrent chemotherapy or chemotherapy in the adjuvant setting has not demonstrated a survival advantage for this patient population,

TABLE 21-3 CHEMOTHERAPEUTIC DRUGS COMMONLY USED TO TREAT BRAIN TUMORS

DRUG AND CLASSIFICATION	EARLY OR DELAYED TOXICITY	LABORATORY MONITORING	NURSING RESPONSIBILITIES
Carmustine (BCNU) Major drug used in treatment of malignant brain tumors Cell cycle nonspecific Nitrosoureas: cause breaks and cross-linking in DNA strands Crosses BBB	*Early* Nausea and vomiting Local phlebitis *Delayed* Bone marrow depression in 3–6 wk Pulmonary fibrosis (may be irreversible) with doses >200 mg/m² IV Renal and liver damage Veno-occlusive disease (hepatic or pulmonary) with high doses	Baseline data Weekly monitoring of CBC and BUN, creatinine, uric acid, SGOT, SGPT, and alkaline phosphatase levels Periodic chest x-ray studies	Administer antiemetics before and during drug administration. Apply ice to puncture site. Protect the patient from and monitor for infections. Monitor for respiratory, liver, and kidney dysfunction.
Lomustine (CCNU) Cell cycle nonspecific Nitrosourea Similar to BCNU	*Early* Nausea and vomiting *Delayed* Bone marrow depression (may be prolonged) Elevated AST level Pulmonary fibrosis Renal damage	Baseline data Same as for BCNU	Same as for BCNU
Cisplatin (Platinol) Heavy metal compound Exact mechanism of action unknown; appears to bind DNA Cell cycle nonspecific	*Early* Nausea and vomiting Anaphylactic reactions Fever Electrolyte imbalances *Delayed* Renal damage Ototoxicity Peripheral neuropathy Bone marrow depression Electrolyte imbalance Hypocalcemia	Baseline data Weekly monitoring of CBC and BUN, creatinine, electrolyte, and calcium levels	Administer antiemetics as necessary. Hydrate well. Monitor intake and output. Assess for hearing loss. Assess for numbness or tingling of fingers and toes. Monitor hearing. Monitor the patient for electrolyte imbalance.
Procarbazine hydrochloride Exact mechanism of action is unclear; probably inhibits protein, RNA, and DNA synthesis Given orally Rapidly absorbed Crosses BBB	*Early* Nausea and vomiting CNS depression *Delayed* Bone marrow depression Stomatitis Peripheral neuropathy Pneumonia Interaction with tyramine in food: hypertensive crisis	Baseline data CBC monitored weekly Chest x-ray studies	This is usually given as 28-d course (usually for first 72 h). Administer antiemetics as necessary. Monitor for signs of neurotoxicity. Monitor the patient for, and protect from, infection. Teach avoidance of foods high in tyramine (e.g., beer, ripe and aged cheeses). Teach avoidance of alcohol consumption (can cause severe GI toxicity because of Antabuse-like drug activity). Provide for special mouth care. Monitor peripheral nerve function. Monitor patient for respiratory problems.
Etoposide (VePesid) Also called VP16 Cell cycle nonspecific Appears to interfere with synthesis of DNA or RNA	*Early* Nausea and vomiting Red urine (not hematuria) Diarrhea Fever Hypotension *Delayed* Bone marrow depression Alopecia Peripheral neuropathy Mucositis Hepatic damage	Urinalysis CBC, AST, and ALT levels monitored weekly	Administer antiemetics as necessary. Monitor vital signs. Monitor the color of the urine. Monitor patient for, and protect from, infection. Prepare patient mentally for hair loss; support positive body image. Monitor peripheral nerve function.

(continued)

TABLE 21-3   CHEMOTHERAPEUTIC DRUGS COMMONLY USED TO TREAT BRAIN TUMORS (*Continued*)

DRUG AND CLASSIFICATION	EARLY OR DELAYED TOXICITY	LABORATORY MONITORING	NURSING RESPONSIBILITIES

Vincristine
  Plant alkaloid
  Inhibits mitosis
  Does not cross BBB
  Given IV
  Excreted by liver in bile
	Early
	  Leukopenia
	  Neuritic pain
	  Constipation
	Late
	  Hair loss
		CBC	Interacts with many drugs; consult pharmacists or other resources to determine possible interactions.
			Monitor blood levels of anticonvulsants (drug interaction with vincristine, which lowers blood level).

Temozolomide
  (Temodar/Temodal)
  First oral chemotherapeutic drug that crosses BBB
  Interferes with tumor growth
	Early
	  Nausea
	  Vomiting
	  Constipation
	  Headache
	Late
	  ↓ WBC
	  Fatigue
		CBC
		–
			Provide antiemetic and take at night.
			Monitor and treat headache.
			Monitor WBC.
			Protect from infection.
			Assist patient in developing strategies for fatigue.

ALT, alanine aminotransferase; AST, aspartate aminotransferase; BBB, blood–brain barrier; BUN, blood urea nitrogen; CBC, complete blood count; CNS, central nervous system; GI, gastrointestinal; IV, intravenous; WBC, white blood cell.

but is the focus of ongoing clinical evaluation. At recurrence, participation in evaluation of clinical trial therapies or the standard approaches as listed above are often administered.

Low-Grade Astrocytoma. The treatment of newly diagnosed low-grade astrocytomas is evolving.[28] Current guidelines recommend that younger patients (younger than 40 years) who have undergone extensive tumor resection be followed with serial imaging and treatment given at the time of recurrence. For those who are older or who have residual tumor after surgical resection, initial therapy often consists of radiation therapy.[29] Clinical trials are evaluating the role of early versus late therapy and the role of chemotherapy in this patient population.

Oligodendrogliomas. For patients with these tumors, a marker of response has been reported and is often used to define the treatment approach. Patients with anaplastic oligodendrogliomas with allelic loss of heterozygosity of the 1p and 19q chromosome arms have nearly a 100% response rate to chemotherapy and/or radiotherapy, while those without loss have a response in the range of 15% to 30%.[30] Often chemotherapy is used in initial therapy for those patients with tumors with demonstrated loss. Radiation therapy is still recommended for tumors that do not demonstrate 1p and 19q chromosomal changes but are felt to require treatment.

CNS Lymphoma. CNS lymphoma is an aggressive and rare form of non-Hodgkin's lymphoma. For this patient population steroids are often held until after a diagnostic surgical procedure, as their use may impact the ability to make a diagnosis. Biopsy is usually performed as a consequence of the infiltrative nature of these tumors. This patient population should undergo additional work-up, including evaluation for systemic lymphoma. The use of a methotrexate-based chemotherapy regimen is standard, and may be combined with radiation therapy.[28]

Brain Metastases. For patients with brain metastases, the treatment approach is dependent on the size and location of brain metastases and the status of the systemic disease. Radiation therapy is the most common form of treatment utilized. For those patients with a small number of lesions,

surgery and radiosurgery may also be used.[31] Chemotherapy has had a limited role in the treatment of brain metastasis, except in the use of intrathecal therapy with spinal fluid involvement. The roles of newer cytotoxic and cytostatic treatments are currently under investigation.

Future Directions

Despite ongoing efforts by many investigators, centers, consortia, and cooperative oncology groups, new treatments are clearly needed to impact the poor prognosis that persists for patients with high-grade primary brain tumors. Innovative approaches, including immunotherapies, gene therapies, and targeted therapies that block specific signal transduction pathways, are being actively investigated in clinical trials.

Various novel treatments are being investigated in an effort to increase the response rates to drugs and control tumor growth. Convection-enhanced delivery (CED) is a novel method of direct delivery of anticancer drugs to the brain tumor core and adjacent brain tissue surrounding the tumor core. CED uses positive pressure infusion to generate a pressure gradient to provide uniform distribution of anticancer drugs. Recent trials have shown that CED is an effective drug delivery approach to treat human nondiffused brain tumors with intratumoral injection of anticancer agents.[32] Although it appears to be effective, CED is highly invasive and is best used against small solid tumors since it has poor penetration of drug into diffused tumor tissue.[33]

For most tumors, cure is not possible. The development of new drugs and new methods of delivery begins with laboratory investigations and proceeds to clinical trials. Drug trials progress in four phases:

- Phase I establishes an optimal safe dose and defines toxicity.
- Phase II determines the action of the drug against specific tumors.
- Phase III compares the new drug with standard therapy for a specific tumor.
- Phase IV adopts the new treatment as part of standard treatment.

TABLE 21-4   NOVEL TREATMENTS IN CLINICAL TRIALS FOR MALIGNANT BRAIN TUMORS

CATEGORY	DESCRIPTION/ACTION OF DRUGS
BBB modifiers	Increase permeability of BBB to allow chemotherapeutic and radiation sensitizing agents access to the brain tumor
Angiogenesis inhibitors	Interfere with growth of tumor-associated blood vessels by preventing production of protein factors such as basic FGF and VEGF, thus cutting off tumors from critical nutrients and oxygen
Antimigration therapy	Interferes with ability of tumor cells to migrate by preventing breakdown of the extracellular matrix and preventing the production of cell surface proteins
Differentiation agents	Cause undifferentiated tumor cells to behave more like well-differentiated cells, encouraging tumor cell death through the normal process of programmed cell death (apoptosis)
Small-molecule growth inhibitors	Interfere with signal pathways, which tell cells to divide and replicate or cause signals to encourage apoptosis. These include agents that affect tyrosine kinase and epidermal growth factors.
Immunotherapy	Boosts immune system to fight tumors; tumor cells removed from patient are modified using a gene transfer technique, irradiated, and then injected back to the patient subcutaneously.
Gene therapy	The herpes simplex thymidine kinase gene (HSVtk) is the first gene to be used in humans with recurrent malignant tumors; p53 gene (transfer p53 gene into tumor cells using adenoviral vector) Injects modified viruses carrying toxic genes directly into tumor, making tumor vulnerable to drug therapy; HSVtk encodes for the viral enzyme thymidine kinase that phosphorylates ganciclovir. The phosphorylated metabolite is toxic to the tumor cells.

BBB, blood-brain barrier; FGF, fibroblast growth factor; VEGF, vascular endothelial growth factor.

Current therapies under investigation are summarized in Table 21-4.[23] Some of these novel drugs may eventually be used in combination with current standard drug protocols or in combination with other novel drugs currently under investigation.

Medical Management Along the Illness Continuum

For a patient with a brain tumor, great variability in outcome can occur depending on the type of tumor, the location, the treatment plan, and the multiple patient characteristics already discussed. The patient is at risk for developing complications from advancement of the disease process and treatment side effects. For example, a patient who has been seizure free may have a seizure. This suggests advancement of the disease process or failure to maintain a therapeutic blood level of an anticonvulsant drug.

Patients may also develop complications from treatment protocols such as myelosuppression or gastric bleeding. Both disease progression and treatment complications are opportunities for collaboration among the physician, the nurse, and other health care professionals to manage problems effectively across the continuum of the illness.

NURSING MANAGEMENT OF THE PATIENT WITH A BRAIN TUMOR

An Overview

The nurse is a member of a collaborative interdisciplinary team caring for the patient. The nurse's role comprises both independent and interdependent aspects. Many collabora-

tive problems confront the team caring for the patient. The specifics of nursing management for patients with brain tumors depend on the patient history, neurological deficits, diagnosis, and treatment plan. Role changes associated with the diagnosis and functional limitations often complicate the necessary care. Changes in patient status, as a consequence of tumor progression, toxicities of therapy, or neurological complications, often result in changes in the patient's needs and modification in the plan of care.

Factors impacting the patient's and the family's responses to a brain tumor include disease and treatment characteristics, individual and demographic factors, and comorbid conditions. Patients and families have an ongoing need for information and emotional support, which should be addressed by the nurse as part of the management plan.

The patient problem to address informational needs of the patient and family is *Knowledge Deficit*, and the nursing intervention for Knowledge Deficit is an individualized teaching plan for the patient and family. It includes information about the diagnosis and prognosis, medical plan of care, management of current deficits and disabilities, and future needs. Several organizations, including the American Brain Tumor Association, National Brain Tumor Foundation, and Brain Tumor Society, have written information concerning brain tumors in general, treatment of brain tumors, coping with brain tumors, and other related topics.

The emotional needs of the patient and family members are also within the province of nursing. Common patient problems related to emotional needs include:

- Fear
- Anxiety
- Personal Identity Disturbance
- Anticipatory Grieving
- Dysfunctional Grieving
- Altered Role Performance
- Social Isolation

- Impaired Social Interaction
- Altered Family Processes
- Impaired Adjustment
- Ineffective Individual and Family Coping
- Ineffective Denial

Nursing interventions are based on individual needs. In addition, referrals are made to appropriate and available resources. Patients and family members should be made aware of brain tumor support groups and counseling options.

In medical and nursing management of the patient with a brain tumor, quality of life and functional status for the patient is an ongoing concern. The *Karnofsky Performance Status Scale* (KPS) is widely used to quantify the functional status of cancer patients.[34] The KPS is an 11-point rating scale ranging from normal functioning (100) to dead (0). The increment from one category to another is 10 points (e.g., 10, 20, 30). Loss of function is viewed as being related to the cumulative physical, physiologic, and psychological effects of the illness. The KPS is helpful for monitoring the patient's functional status over time.

The importance of quality of life is apparent in discussing patients with primary brain tumors. Several instruments have been developed that allow the patient to report his or her quality of life or the severity of his or her symptoms.[35] Use of these standardized instruments can improve our understanding of the impact of the diagnosis and treatment on the patient's life. The patient's and family's perception of the quality of life is relative. The informed patient, who understands the diagnosis, prognosis, and potential impact on functional status, should guide decisions regarding treatment and supportive care.

Along with quality-of-life issues come decisions related to end-of-life care and intensity of care. (Chap. 3 discusses end-of-life decisions and palliative care.)

Nursing Management During Diagnosis

One of the nurse's main responsibilities during the diagnostic period is to provide information about the tests to be conducted. Since the possibility of a brain tumor can subject the patient to extreme emotional stress, the nurse must take the patient's deficits into account. The impact of such a diagnosis depends on the patient's ability to comprehend what the diagnosis means and how it will affect his or her life. Some patients have lost short-term memory. A patient who has an altered level of consciousness or impaired mental functions, such as memory loss, may not grasp the total impact of the situation but may react merely to the strangeness of the health care environment and interventions or loneliness. Memory loss has a major impact on patient teaching. The nurse must recognize if memory loss is present as well as the severity of loss. Depending on the severity of loss, teaching strategies may be modified to help the patient understand and remember. In severe memory loss, patient teaching is not possible and the focus of teaching is the family.

The patient who understands what is happening may initially deny the diagnosis. If this is the case, the patient will refuse to consider treatment, so informed consent is impossible. If the patient does accept the diagnosis, he or she may react with anger and hostility. Fear of death, mutilation, and loss of independence and mental functions are terrifying concerns. Mental images of other people with similar diagnoses may loom in the patient's mind and threaten body image and self-concept. A sense of powerlessness can overwhelm the patient.

A positive, supportive approach by the nurse can help the patient cope with the reality of the condition. Encourage questions and expression of feelings. The nurse should provide realistic reassurance about expected outcomes. At the same time, the patient should be included in the decision-making process as often as possible. Memory deficits have an impact on the process of providing support, because the patient may not recall previous information provided. Repetition of information is often necessary, and even repetition may not be sufficient to keep the patient informed.

Some organizations (and their telephone numbers) that provide information related to treatment options and support are listed below.

- National Brain Tumor Foundation, (800) 934-CURE, www.braintumor.org
- The Brain Tumor Society, (800) 770-8287
- American Brain Tumor Association, (800) 886-2282, www.abta.org
- American Cancer Society, (800) ACS-2345, www.acs.org
- Cancer Information Service, (800) 4-CANCER

CLINICAL VIGNETTE: Mrs. M was recently diagnosed with an anaplastic astrocytoma after undergoing a partial resection. She presents to the clinic to discuss treatment options. The patient is offered a choice of radiation, chemotherapy, or combination therapy. Assisting the patient to understand the treatment options is an important component of nursing care. Evaluating the patient's understanding of the information and providing written information that the patient can take home can assist the patient in making the decision regarding treatment options. If there is concern regarding the patient's ability to understand the information that is presented, a family member or designated significant other should be involved in the treatment choice.

Nursing Management Before and After Surgery

Nursing management for brain tumor surgery is the same as that outlined for other intracranial surgical procedures outlined in Chapter 14.

Nursing Management During Radiation Therapy

As the patient's advocate, the nurse facilitates collecting satisfactory answers to the patient's questions. If the patient's level of consciousness or mental functions have been impaired, the family will be afforded help so that informed consent can be ensured. The nurse's role during

CHART 21-3	Summary of Patient Problems During Radiation Therapy

PATIENT PROBLEMS	NURSING INTERVENTIONS	EXPECTED OUTCOME(S)
Knowledge Deficit related to (R/T) purpose, method, and goals of treatment protocol	• Ask the patient to tell you his or her understanding of the treatment protocol. • Clarify misconceptions. • Expand on areas of partial understanding. • Introduce new information as necessary. • Encourage the patient to ask questions. • Refer questions to another person, if necessary. • Develop a written teaching plan.	The patient will be able to verbalize and describe the purpose, goals, and method of administering the prescribed protocol.
Anxiety R/T approaching or current treatment	• Observe the patient for verbal and nonverbal cues indicating anxiety. • Provide emotional support. • Anticipate the needs of the patient.	The patient's anxiety will be reduced or controlled.
Altered comfort: acute nausea/vomiting R/T chemotherapy	• Assess the patient for nausea. • Provide small, frequent feedings that are easy to digest. • Administer antiemetic as ordered (give as prophylactic and as necessary). • Give nothing by mouth if vomiting occurs. • Offer mouth care frequently.	Nausea will be controlled or minimized; vomiting will be absent or controlled.
Altered Nutrition: Less than body requirements R/T nausea and vomiting	• Assess the patient's nutritional intake on a 24-hour basis. • Assess the patient's dietary preferences. • Request dietary consult as necessary • Offer small meals frequently (choose easy-to-digest foods).	The patient will maintain adequate nutritional intake.
Altered Oral Mucous Membrane R/T stomatitis	• Provide frequent mouth care. • Administer a soothing oral rinse or topical solution for oral comfort, such as glycerin swabs or viscous lidocaine suspension, as directed. • Avoid potentially irritating foods, such as citrus fruits. • Provide a soft, bland diet.	Discomfort from stomatitis will be eliminated or controlled.
Body Image Disturbance R/T hair loss	• Discuss the cause of alopecia, as well as the regrowth process. • Provide for meticulous personal hygiene. • Encourage female patients to use makeup and wear attractive head coverings. • Suggest the use of wigs when the patient is able to wear one. • Correct any misconceptions. • Allow the patient to verbalize feelings.	The patient will accept altered body image.
Fatigue R/T chemotherapy or radiation	• Allow the patient to express his or her feelings about general malaise. • Encourage and plan a schedule that allows for frequent rest periods. • Assess the patient's ability to perform activities of daily living (ADLs). • Provide for frequent rest periods. • Adjust the patient's schedule as necessary to conserve energy.	The feeling of fatigue will be minimized by frequent rest periods.
Altered Cerebral Perfusion R/T cerebral edema	• Assess the patient's neurological signs periodically. • Identify any signs of neurological deterioration; report any such changes to the physician and record findings. • Elevate the head of the bed 30 degrees. • Administer drugs and other protocols as ordered. • Continue to monitor the patient.	Neurological changes will be identified early and definitive action taken to control deterioration.

(continued)

CHART 21-3	Summary of Patient Problems During Radiation Therapy (Continued)	

PATIENT PROBLEMS	NURSING INTERVENTIONS	EXPECTED OUTCOME(S)
Risk for Infection R/T bone marrow depression	• Protect the patient from exposure to infections. • Monitor the patient for signs and symptoms of infection • Teach the patient and family the meaning of a decreased white blood cell (WBC) count and nadir (i.e., lowest point of WBC).	The patient and family will verbalize an understanding of preventive measures.
Risk for Injury R/T thrombocytopenia	• Monitor the complete blood count (WBC and platelet) and coagulation study results. • Be aware of and discuss with the patient delayed onset of bone marrow suppression (after 3 weeks). • Assess the patient for occult bleeding (stools, urine, gastric). • Assess the patient for easy bruising, petechial bleeding, nosebleeds, and bleeding from the gums.	The patient and family will verbalize an understanding of the precautions against and the risk factors for injury.
Risk for Impaired Skin Integrity R/T radiation-induced dermatitis (with radiation dermatitis, the skin becomes reddened, tanned, desquamatized, and sensitive)	• Institute special precautions for skin care at the site of radiation. • Protect the skin from rubbing, application of tape, and exposure to sunlight. • Do not use alcohol, powder, cream, or cosmetics on this area. • Do not wash off the skin markings used to localize the radiation exposure site.	Skin integrity will be maintained.
Knowledge Deficit R/T discharge and follow-up care	• Develop a written teaching plan for discharge. • Stress the importance of follow-up care. • Provide a written list of signs and symptoms that should be reported to the physician. • Caution against use of any drugs (e.g., aspirin) without prior approval of the physician. • Help the patient understand that some side effects of the treatment have a delayed onset. • Arrange for a follow-up appointment.	The patient will verbalize an understanding of the discharge plans and care.

Note: Some of the patient problems listed may not apply to all patients; however, those identified do include major nursing concerns.

radiation therapy is to provide emotional support to the patient and family, assess patient needs, manage side effects of treatment, and provide general comfort and hygienic needs.

The specific nursing responsibilities during radiation therapy include:

1. Before the start of treatment, inform the patient and family of the various activities that will occur in the radiation therapy department. As with most patient preparation of this kind, informing the patient of what to expect will help allay any fears caused by unfamiliarity with the procedure.
2. Provide proper skin care of the radiation site. Radiation dermatitis can be anticipated (the epidural layer is denuded in a 4- to 6-week period). The skin becomes reddened, tanned, and desquamated. Because the skin is sensitive, do not rub, apply tape, expose to sunlight, or apply alcohol, powder, cream, or cosmetics. The skin markings used to localize radiation exposure should not be washed off.

3. If the patient suffers from nausea, vomiting, or diarrhea, administer antiemetics and antidiarrheal agents as necessary.
4. To manage anorexia, offer small portions of foods that are easy to digest and liked by the patient.
5. For fatigue and general malaise, schedule activities to allow for rest periods. (Fatigue is a very common problem and needs to be vigorously addressed to customize treatment plans.)
6. Note the results of complete blood counts (CBCs), with special attention to white blood cell (WBC) and platelet counts. Bone marrow depression decreases platelets, which in turn increases the possibility of hemorrhage (petechiae, purpura, nosebleeds, or, most critical, intratumoral hemorrhage).
7. Monitor neurological signs for indications of increased ICP.
8. Provide emotional support by reassuring the patient that side effects will resolve after the treatment has been completed.

See Chart 21-3 for a summary of common patient problems.

CLINICAL VIGNETTE: Mrs. J is a 65-year-old woman scheduled to start radiation therapy today for a recurrent meningioma. She is concerned about side effects, particularly hair loss. The nurse provides emotional support and education regarding hair loss and care of the scalp including the following:

- Alopecia is expected in the area of the radiation field
- The skin may become reddened and sore and more sensitive to sunlight
- Appropriate scalp care, including the use of gentle shampoos for hair washing
- Avoidance of lotions with perfumes
- Use of a protective covering when outdoors
- Signs and symptoms to report, including excoriation of the scalp

Nursing Management During Chemotherapy

As previously discussed, the role of systemic therapy is increasingly at the forefront of treatment for patients with CNS tumors, especially malignant gliomas. The nurse should know which drugs the patient is receiving and the common side effects related to specific drugs. The patient and family should also be aware of this information. The most common side effects of intravenous chemotherapy include nausea, vomiting, diarrhea, stomatitis, anorexia, alopecia, and bone marrow depression (see Table 21-4).

Collaborative activities involving the nurse and physician include monitoring of vital signs and specific laboratory data and monitoring of the patient's response to the chemotherapy. The specific laboratory data to be collected depend on the toxicity of the drug, which may involve the kidney, liver, blood, or lungs. Clinical pathways, at the forefront of today's care, streamline care delivery and are helpful for drug protocols. With a clinical pathway, care and use of resources are standardized and streamlined, and expected outcomes are carefully monitored.

CLINICAL VIGNETTE: Mr. S is a 57-year-old man undergoing treatment with adjuvant temozolomide. He presents to the clinic for a follow-up visit. His primary complaint is constipation, which occurred at the end of the first week of temozolomide and is still continuing. Because constipation is a common side effect of temozolomide, the nurse asks about fatigue, nausea, and vomiting. The nurse provides education on the importance of diet, hydration, and exercise to help prevent constipation. Written information regarding over-the-counter options for stool softeners is also provided.

SUMMARY

Nursing management for the patient with a brain tumor spans a wide variety of circumstances, situations, and treatment modalities. Perhaps no role is more important than that of providing sensitive, supportive care of the patient and family.

REFERENCES

1. Central Brain Tumor Registry of the United States (2008). Statistical report: Primary brain tumors in the United States Statistical Report 2000-2004. Published by the Central Brain Tumor Registry of the United States, Hinsdale, IL.
2. Ries, L. A. G., Melbert, D., Krapcho, M., Mariotto, A., Miller, B. A., Feuer, E. J., Clegg, L., Horner, M. J., Howlader, N., Eisner, M. P., Reichman, M., Edwards, B. K. (eds). (2007). SEER Cancer Statistics Review, 1975-2004. National Cancer Institute, Bethesda, MD, http://seer.cancer.gove/csr/1975_2004/, based on November 2006 SEER data submission, posted to the SEER web site, 2007.
3. Kleihues, P., Soylemezoglu, F., Schauble, B., Scheithauer, B. W., & Burger, P. C. (1995). Histopathology, classification, and grading of gliomas. *Glia, 15*(3), 211–221.
4. Preston-Martin, S. (1996). Epidemiology of primary CNS neoplasms. *Neurology Clinics, 14*(2), 273–290.
5. Doolittle, N. D. (2004). State of the science in brain tumor classification. *Seminar Oncology Nursing, 20*(4), 224–230.
6. Gonzales, M. F. (2001). *Classification and pathogenesis of brain tumors* (2nd ed.). London: Harcourt.
7. Kleihues, P., Burger, P. C., & Scheithauer, B. W. (1993). The new WHO classification of brain tumours. *Brain Pathology, 3*(3), 255–268.
8. Wen, P. Y., & Kesari, S. (2008). Malignant gliomas in adults. *New England Journal of Medicine, 359*(5), 492-507.
9. Barker, F. G, & Israel, M. A. (1995). The molecular biology of brain tumors. *Neurology Clinics, 13*(4), 701–721.
10. Armstrong, T. S., Kanusky, J. T., & Gilbert, M. R. (2003). Seize the moment to learn about epilepsy in people with cancer. *Clinical Journal of Oncology Nursing, 7*(2), 163–169.
11. Lovely, M. P. (2004). Symptom management of brain tumor patients. *Seminar Oncology Nursing, 20*(4), 273–283.
12. Gilman, S. (1998). Imaging the brain. First of two parts. *New England Journal of Medicine, 338*(12), 812–820.
13. Castillo, M. (1999). *Neuroradiology companion: Methods, guidelines, and imaging fundamentals* (2nd ed.). Philadelphia: Lippincott-Raven.
14. Bohan, E., & Glass-Macenka, D. (2004). Surgical management of patients with primary brain tumors. *Seminar Oncology Nursing, 20*(4), 240–252.
15. Chang, S. M., Kuhn, J. G., Rizzo, J., Robins, H. I., Schold, S. C., Jr., Spence, A. M. et al. (1998). Phase I study of paclitaxel in patients with recurrent malignant glioma: a North American Brain Tumor Consortium report. *Journal of Clinical Oncology, 16*(6), 2188–2194.
16. Mathijssen, R. H., Sparreboom, A., Dumez, H., van Oosterom, A.,T., & de Bruijn, E. A. (2002). Altered irinotecan metabolism in a patient receiving phenytoin. *Anticancer Drugs, 13*(2), 139–140.
17. Hancock, C. M., & Burrow, M. A. (2004). The role of radiation therapy in the treatment of central nervous system tumors. *Seminar Oncology Nursing, 20*(4), 253–259.
18. Baumert, B. G., Norton, I. A., Lomax, A. J., & Davis, J. B. (2004). Dose conformation of intensity-modulated stereotactic photon beams, proton beams, and intensity-modulated proton beams for intracranial lesions. *International Journal of Radiation Oncology Biology and Physics, 60*(4), 1314–1324.
19. Lee, C. T., Bilton, S. D., Famiglietti, R. M., Riley, B. A., Mahajan, A., Chang, E. L. et al. (2005). Treatment planning with protons for pediatric retinoblastoma, medulloblastoma, and pelvic sarcoma: how do protons compare with other conformal techniques? *International Journal of Radiation Oncology Biology and Physics, 63*(2), 362–372.
20. Borgardus, C. R. (2003). IMRT: An overview. *Oncology Issues, 12*(2), 5–7.
21. Nelson, D. F., Urtasun, R. C., Saunders, W. M., Gutin, P. H., & Sheline, G. E. (1986). Recent and current investigations of radiation therapy of malignant gliomas. *Seminars in Oncology, 13*(1), 46–55.
22. Miyamoto, C. (2000). Radiation therapy principles for high grade gliomas. *Principles and Practice of Radiation Oncology Updates, 1*(3), 2–16.

23. Armstrong, T. S., & Gilbert, M. R. (2002). Glial tumors—new approaches in chemotherapy. *Journal of Neuroscience Nursing, 4*(6), 326–330.

24. Shapiro, W. R., & Shapiro, J. R. (1986). Principles of brain tumor chemotherapy. *Seminars in Oncology, 13*(1), 56–69.

25. Stupp, R., Mason, W. P., van den Bent, M., Weller, M., Fisher, B., Taphorn, M., et al. (2004). Concomitant and adjuvant temozolomide (TMZ) and radiotherapy (RT) for newly diagnosed glioblastoma multiforme (GBM). Conclusive results of a randomized phase III trial by the EORTC Brain & RT Groups and NCIC Clinical Trials Group. *Proceeding of ASCO, 23*, 1.

26. Stewart, L. A. (2002). Chemotherapy in adult high-grade glioma: A systematic review and meta-analysis of individual patient data from 12 randomised trials. *Lancet, 359*(9311), 1011–1018.

27. Westphal, M., Hilt, D. C., Bortey, E., Delavault, P., Olivares, R., Warnke, P. C., et al. (2003). A phase 3 trial of local chemotherapy with biodegradable carmustine (BCNU) wafers (Gliadel wafers) in patients with primary malignant glioma. *Neuro-oncology, 5*(2), 79–88.

28. Graham, C. A., & Cloughesy, T. F. (2004). Brain tumor treatment: Chemotherapy and other new developments. *Seminars in Oncology Nursing, 20*(4), 260–272.

29. Shaw, E. G., & Wisoff, J. H. (2003). Prospective clinical trials of intracranial low-grade glioma in adults and children. *Neuro-oncology, 5*(3), 153–160.

30. Ino, Y., Betensky, R. A., Zlatescu, M. C., Sasaki, H., Macdonald, D. R., Stemmer-Rachamimov, A. O., et al. (2001). Molecular subtypes of anaplastic oligodendroglioma: Implications for patient management at diagnosis. *Clinical Cancer Research, 7*(4), 839–845.

31. Armstrong, T. S., & Gilbert, M. R. (2001). Metastatic brain tumors: Diagnosis, treatment, and nursing interventions. *Clinical Journal of Oncology Nursing, 4*(5), 217–225.

32. Kunwar, S. (2003). Convection enhanced delivery of IL13-PE38QQR for treatment of recurrent malignant glioma: Presentation of interim findings from ongoing phase 1 studies. *Acta Neurochirurgica Supplement, 88*, 105–111.

33. Black, K. L., & Ningaraj, N. S. (2004). Modulation of brain tumor capillaries for enhanced delivery selectively to brain tumor. *Cancer Control, 11*(3), 166–173.

34. Mor, V., Laliberte, L., Morris, J. N., & Wiesmann, M. (1984). The Karnofsky performance status scale. *Cancer, 53*, 2002–2007.

35. Armstrong, T. S., Cohen, M. Z., Eriksen, L. R., & Hickey, J. V. (2004). Symptom clusters in oncology patients and implications for symptom research in people with primary brain tumors. *Journal of Nursing Scholarship, 36*(3), 197–206.

Spinal Cord Tumors

Joanne V. Hickey and Terri S. Armstrong

EPIDEMIOLOGY

Tumors can impact the spinal cord by causing external compression or by directly involving the cord or intradural space. Metastatic lesions causing external compression are by far the most common.[1] Primary tumors of the spinal cord constitute approximately 0.5% of newly diagnosed tumors and 7% of primary central nervous system neoplasms.[2] The exact incidence of metastatic disease affecting the spinal cord is not known, but is thought to impact up to 20% of all cancer patients. Their causes are unknown. The incidence and types of spinal cord tumors vary greatly between children and adults. Only tumors affecting adults are discussed in this chapter.

CLASSIFICATION

As with tumors involving the brain, spinal cord tumors have several classification schemas. The histology classification of spinal cord tumors includes primary tumors, which arise from the constituent elements of the central nervous system, or metastatic tumors, which spread from tumors originating in other organs. Table 22-1 provides the common histologic classification of tumors.[1] This system provides information on the histologic origin of the tumor as well as the grade, or degree of malignancy. From a histologic perspective, most primary spinal cord tumors are benign.

Spinal cord tumors are also classified according to their anatomic location with reference to the dural meningeal covering and the spinal cord, or to the vertebral column.

Location in Relation to Dura and Spinal Cord. Spinal cord tumors may be classified as extramedullary or intramedullary with respect to the dura and spinal cord.

Extramedullary tumors are located outside the spinal cord and are the most common location for primary spinal cord tumors, accounting for about 80% to 90% of cases.[3] Extramedullary tumors are subdivided into:

Extradural: outside the spinal dura; within the epidural space. The most common primary tumors are chordomas and sarcomas—20% of all primary spinal cord tumors. This is the most common location for metastatic cancer, with the most common primary sites being lung, breast, prostate, colon, kidney, and uterus.

Intradural: within the spinal dura, but not within the spinal cord. Primary intradural tumors include meningiomas and neurofibromas, which constitute 60% of all primary spinal cord tumors. Both primary and metastatic cancer can also involve the cerebrospinal fluid, often called leptomeningeal disease (LMD). Approximately 16,000 patients are diagnosed each year with LMD. The most common tumors to cause LMD are breast and lung cancer and lymphoma.

Intramedullary tumors are located within the substance of the spinal cord. Although metastatic cancer can cause intramedullary tumors, most of these lesions are primary spinal cord tumors, with ependymomas and gliomas occurring the most frequently. Ten to twenty percent of all primary spinal cord tumors are intramedullary. The locations of primary spinal cord tumors are shown on cross section in Figure 22-1.

CLINICAL PEARLS: Extradural tumors are the most common type of spinal cord tumor.

Location in Relationship to the Vertebral Column. Spinal cord tumors are roughly distributed as follows: cervical, 30%; thoracic, 50%; and lumbosacral, 20%. Locating a tumor more precisely helps to correlate the dermatome with specific functional assessment for that level (see Chaps. 4 and 19). Conversely, identifying deficits on examination can help to diagnose a spinal cord tumor and identify its location according to the involved dermatome.

Primary spinal cord tumors include neurofibromas and meningiomas usually found in the extramedullary area, and ependymomas and other gliomas usually found in the intramedullary area. Other types of primary spinal cord tumors include sarcomas, vascular tumors, chordomas, and epidermoids (Table 22-1). **Metastatic spinal cord tumors** are mostly extradural tumors. Although malignancies from almost any site can metastasize to the vertebral column, lesions from the lungs, breast, prostate, colon, kidney, and uterus, as well as lymphomas and multiple myelomas, are the most common.

Pathophysiology

Regardless of the type or location of a spinal cord tumor, the associated pathophysiologic changes can lead to cord

TABLE 22-1   COMMON SPINAL CORD TUMORS

TUMOR TYPE	HIGHEST INCIDENCE	GENDER	DESCRIPTION
Neurofibroma	30–50 y	Equally affected	60% above L-1, causing spastic paraparesis; 30% below L-1, causing a lateral cauda equina syndrome
Meningioma		M/F ratio 1:9	Most in midthoracic (T-3–6); a few in foramen magnum
Ependymomas	Average age 30 y	M/F ratio 2:1	Either intrinsic within the spinal cord at C-6–T-2 or on the filum terminate (central cauda equina syndrome). Very high incidence of associated syringomyelic cavitation, making the lesion seem much more extensive than its actual size
Gliomas	35–45 y	Equally affected	Almost all in cervical cord
Dermoids	15–20 y	No data	Located in sacrococcygeal area, usually associated with spina bifida
Chordoma	No data	Mostly males	Most in sacrococcygeal area; bone destruction and pain are major feature
Hemangioblastoma	Before the age of 40	No data	Well-circumscribed, encapsulated vascular tumor that can usually be completely removed; accounts for 3%–8% of intramedullary tumors

dysfunction and neurological deficits. These changes can result from direct cord compression, ischemia secondary to arterial or venous obstruction, or, in the case of intramedullary tumors, direct invasion (Figs. 22-2 and 22-3). Tumors causing cord compression can cause traction on or irritation of the spinal nerve roots, displacement of the spinal cord, interference with the spinal blood supply, or obstruction of cerebrospinal fluid (CSF) circulation. Cord compression alters the normal physiology involved in providing an adequate blood supply, maintaining stable cellular membranes, and facilitating afferent and efferent impulses for specific sensory, motor, and reflex functions of the spinal cord and related spinal nerves.

Invasive infiltration of the spinal cord is seen in association with intramedullary tumors. Edema associated with cord compression is seen in both extramedullary and intramedullary tumors. Edema can ascend the spinal cord, causing additional deficits to the sensitive cord. Control of edema is a major focus in management and will be discussed later. Focal (localizing) signs depend on the spinal level, the cross-section location, and the rate of growth and density of the spinal tumor.

CLINICAL PEARLS: Pathophysiologic changes can result from direct cord compression, ischemia secondary to arterial or venous obstruction, or, in the case of intramedullary tumors, direct invasion.

Spinal Level

Spinal level refers to the specific location of the tumor in the cervical, thoracic, or lumbosacral area. Sensory distribution from the spinal nerves at each level is mapped at dermatome levels (see Chaps. 4 and 19). Loss of sensation depends on the level of the tumor and correlates with the dermatome level. Motor deficits are also related to the tumor level, because motor components of various spinal nerves come together to innervate specific areas.

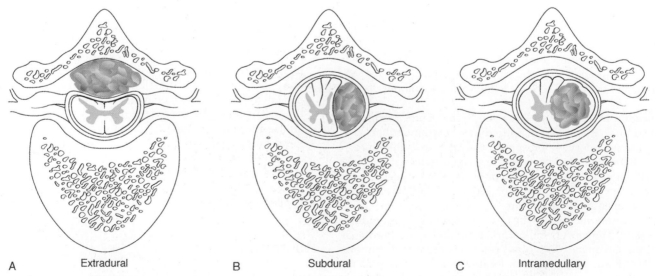

| A | Extradural | B | Subdural | C | Intramedullary |

Figure 22-1 • Location of intramedullary and extramedullary (subdural and extradural) tumors on cross section.

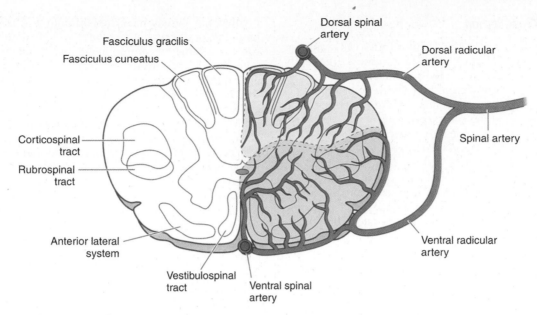

Figure 22-2 • Perfusion patterns of the spinal cord. (Kingley, R. E. [2000] *Concise text of neuroscience*. Philadelphia: Lippincott Williams & Wilkins.)

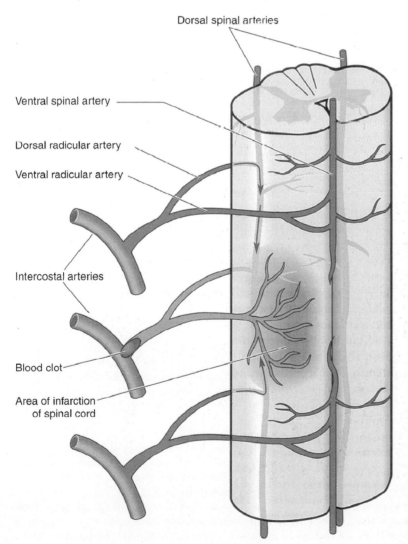

Figure 22-3 • Radicular arteries of the spinal cord. Not all of the 31 potential pairs of spinal arteries develop completely. Therefore, some parts of the spinal cord are perfused by only one or two radicular spinal arteries. Loss of a single artery at these sites can result in ischemic infarction of the spinal cord. The upper lumbar and thoracic spinal cord are particularly vulnerable. (Kingley, R. E. [2000]. *Concise text of neuroscience*. Philadelphia: Lippincott Williams & Wilkins.)

Location on Cross Section

Tumors involving the vertebral elements often cause anterior cord compression, because metastatic tumors frequently involve the vertebral body. In the anterior location, a pathologic fracture of the vertebral body with bone fragments driven back into the cord or tumor growth can encroach on the anterior aspect of the spinal cord. Isolated posterior element involvement is much less common.[4]

The major sensations conveyed by the spinal cord are light touch, pain and temperature, and position and vibration. A specific tract located in a designated anatomic area, noted on cross section (see Chap. 4), carries each sensation. The **posterior columns** (fasciculus gracilis and fasciculus cuneatus) convey *position and vibration sensations*. The **lateral spinothalamic tracts** convey *pain and temperature*. The **anterior spinothalamic tract** conveys *light touch*. On cross section, the spinothalamic tracts are located in the anterolateral area of the spinal cord (see Fig. 22-2). Therefore, the location of the tumor on cross section will help determine functional loss.

Rate of Growth and Density

The development of neurological deficits is directly related to the tumor's rate of growth and its density (i.e., soft or hard). A slow-growing tumor can accommodate itself to the limited space of the vertebral-spinal cord space within compensatory limits. Many primary spinal cord tumors grow very slowly over years, compressing the cord into a thin, ribbon-like structure with minimal neurological deficits. However, with a rapidly growing tumor, such as a primary malignant spinal cord tumor or a metastatic lesion, the cord fares poorly. Physiologically, the tumor produces major compression of the cord, resulting in substantial edema and, possibly, rapid paralysis (within hours).

A soft tumor can be of a consistency similar to that of the spinal cord. If it grows slowly, it causes gradual compression of the spinal cord. However, the cord's blood supply is able to respond to this alteration and adequately supply the vascular needs without interruption. The tumor adjusts to the available space for growth, becoming elongated, as necessary. Neither movement of the spinal column nor normal alterations in blood flow to the cord will produce injury by contusion or ischemia. By contrast, a hard tumor will respond to movement or vascular changes with spinal contusion, ischemia, and irreversible cord damage. Encroachment on neurological function is apparent earlier with hard tumors than with soft tumors because hard tumors do not conform to the available space.

Morphologically, spinal cord tumors are described as encapsulated or sharply outlined. Soft tumors are irregularly elongated and can extend for two or more segments, whereas hard tumors are more circumscribed. Some tumors have a fluid-filled cystic cavity called a *syrinx* that may require drainage.

Metastatic Spinal Cord Tumors

Compression of the spinal cord occurs in about 20% of all cancer patients. An epidural spinal tumor is the first sign of a malignancy in about 10% of patients.[5] Metastatic lesions can involve the vertebrae, grow through the intravertebral foramina, or directly impact the dura, spinal fluid, or spinal cord. The vertebral column is the most common site in the bony skeletal system for metastases. As mentioned previously, the most common primary sites of metastatic spinal cord tumors are the lungs, breast, prostate, colon, kidneys, and uterus. The malignant lesion tends to spread proximally from the primary organ affected to the adjacent vertebral body, spinous or transverse process, or pedicle. The lesion then causes epidural compression of the spinal cord or nerve roots. Tumors occur in the thoracic spine (70% of cases) followed by the lumbar spine (20%). Over 30% of patients have involvement at multiple spine levels.[1] Retroperitoneal neoplasms (especially lymphomas or sarcomas) may enter the spinal canal through the intervertebral foramina.

Typically extradural tumors produce radicular pain and signs of root involvement prior to cord compression. Metastatic lesions most commonly exert their effects on the spinal cord by direct compression, enlargement of a vertebral body or pedicle, collapse of an eroded vertebra, or direct extension of a paravertebral lesion through the intervertebral foramen. Edema of the cord, a consequence of compression, increases the degree of the deficit.

Signs and Symptoms Associated With Spinal Cord Tumors

Symptoms may develop insidiously and progress gradually, or they may progress rapidly as is common with metastatic lesions. The specific signs and symptoms depend on the anatomic location of the tumor (location on cross section), its location in relation to the level of the vertebral column (thoracic, lumbosacral), and the specific spinal nerves involved. Focal signs and symptoms aid in determining the level of the lesion; however, they can also be indistinct, misleading, and intermittently variable. Table 22-2 summarizes signs and symptoms according to the anatomic level of the tumor on or within the spinal cord.

Pain is the initial symptom in almost all patients. About 95% of patients with vertebral or spinal cord tumors have pain without neurological deficits as the *initial* symptom. At the time of diagnosis, 75% have pain and weakness, sensory disturbance, or sphincter dysfunction.[3] This highlights the importance of prompt diagnosis in order to preserve neurological function.

CLINICAL PEARLS: The specific signs and symptoms depend on the anatomic location of the tumor (location on cross section), its location in relation to the level of the vertebral column (thoracic, lumbosacral), and the specific spinal nerves involved.

Pain

The pain may be aching and localized or sharp and radiating (radicular pain). *Localized pain and point tenderness* are common over the involved vertebral area when pressure is applied to the spinous process. *Radicular pain* is defined as pain within the sensory distribution of a spinal nerve root. Pain, which can localize to the back or to an extremity, is caused by irritation, tension/traction, or compression of the

TABLE 22–2 SIGNS AND SYMPTOMS OF SPINAL CORD TUMORS BY VERTEBRAL LEVEL

LOCATION	SIGNS AND SYMPTOMS	COMMENTS
Cervical Levels		
C-4 and above • Especially dangerous because of innervation to the diaphragm (C-1–4) and the potential effect on respirations • High cervical tumors can affect the lower cranial nerves (VIII to XII).	• Possible respiratory difficulty • Quadriparesis or quadriplegia • Paresthesia • Occipital headache • Stiff neck • CN VIII: downbeat nystagmus • CNs IX and X: dysphagia; dysarthria • CN XI: difficulty shrugging shoulders; atrophy of shoulder and neck muscles • CN XII: deviation of tongue; difficulty speaking; unilateral tongue atrophy	Difficult surgical access; may consider proton beam therapy or another nonsurgical modality Downward gaze is controlled by pathways that extend from the brainstem to the upper cervical cord.
Below C-4	• Pain in shoulders and arms • Paresthesia • If the C-5–6 root is involved, there will be pain along the medial aspect of the arm. • If C-7–8 is involved, there will be pain along the outer side of the forearm and hand. • Weakness follows pain. • Atrophy of the shoulder, arm, and intrinsic hand muscles is often associated with fasciculation. • Horner's syndrome (ptosis, miosis, and anhidrosis on the affected side) • Hyperactive reflexes	Attributable to interference with sympathetic innervation
Thoracic Levels		

T-1–12
• Most metastatic lesions involve the thoracic region.
	• Pain in chest/back
	• Use of motor deficits to localize the lesion is difficult; spastic paresis may be evident.
	• Sensory deficits are more accurate in identifying the lesion's level:
	  —Know landmark areas, such as T-4 (nipple line) and T-10 (umbilicus).
	  —A band of hyperesthesia is often found above the level of the lesion.
	• A positive Babinski sign is noted.
	• Bowel and/or bladder dysfunction
	• Sexual dysfunction
		See Chapter 19 for an explanation and illustration of dermatomes.

Lumbosacral		
S-1–5	• Pain in lower back, which often radiates to legs; may also be felt in the perineal area • Paresis/spasticity of lower extremities, usually in one leg and later in the other • Sensory loss in legs and/or saddle area • Bowel and/or bladder dysfunction • Sexual dysfunction • Reflexes—ankle and knee-jerk reflexes are diminished or absent	Footdrop is common. Atrophy may affect certain muscle groups.

CN, cranial nerve

nerve root. The quality of pain can vary from mild to severe and from dull to piercing, but it is almost always present. Any activity that increases intraspinal pressure, such as the Valsalva maneuver (as occurs with coughing, sneezing, or straining) and movement, can cause pain to intensify and radiate. Pain can also be exaggerated by reclining, because this position stretches the spinal nerves. As a result, pain may awaken the patient at night.

Pain typically precedes signs of cord compression by weeks or even months, but after cord compression occurs, it is always progressive and may advance rapidly.[5] Pain can be focal or radiate in a known dermatomal pattern. Because the dermatomes supplying a particular area of the body overlap, pain can also be diffuse, mimicking such conditions as angina, an acute abdominal lesion, or intercostal neuralgia.

CLINICAL PEARLS: The most common presenting symptom of spinal cord tumor is pain.

Motor Deficits

The presenting motor signs and symptoms depend on the degree of involvement of the spinal nerve root and the spinal cord (Fig. 22-4). For example, involvement of the *anterior spinal nerve root* leads to a *lower motor neuron syndrome.* This is

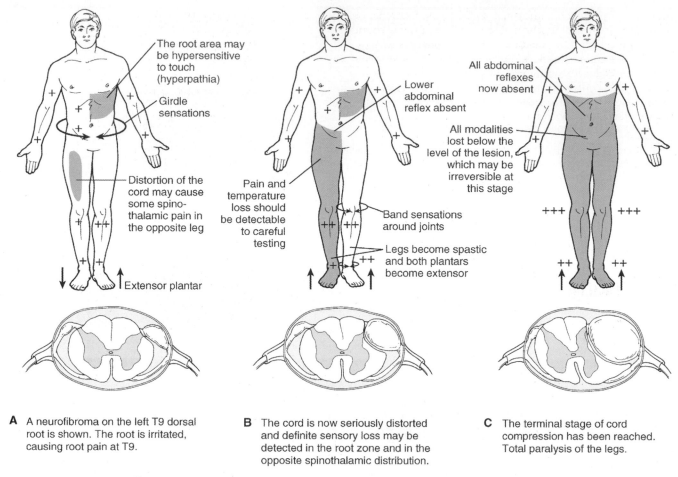

The root area may be hypersensitive to touch (hyperpathia)

Girdle sensations

Distortion of the cord may cause some spino-thalamic pain in the opposite leg

Extensor plantar

A A neurofibroma on the left T9 dorsal root is shown. The root is irritated, causing root pain at T9.

Lower abdominal reflex absent

Pain and temperature loss should be detectable to careful testing

Band sensations around joints

Legs become spastic and both plantars become extensor

B The cord is now seriously distorted and definite sensory loss may be detected in the root zone and in the opposite spinothalamic distribution.

All abdominal reflexes now absent

All modalities lost below the level of the lesion, which may be irreversible at this stage

C The terminal stage of cord compression has been reached. Total paralysis of the legs.

Figure 22-4 • Progression of deficits as the size of the mass and cord distention increase.

characterized by motor weakness; wasting and fasciculations of involved muscles; hypotonia (flaccidity); loss of tendon reflexes when neurons responsible for those reflexes are affected; and normal abdominal and plantar reflexes unless the neurons responsible for those reflexes are directly involved, in which case the reflex response is lost.

When the spinal cord becomes compressed, other motor deficits develop. Involvement of motor tracts results in an upper motor neuron deficit below the level of the lesion. An *upper motor neuron syndrome* includes weakness or paralysis, spasticity, increased tendon reflexes, a positive Babinski sign, loss of abdominal reflexes, and little or no muscle atrophy.[6]

The patient can have a *mixed presentation* of lower motor neuron disease and upper motor neuron disease, depending on the degree of compression present and the anatomic structures affected. Additionally, a combination of sensory and motor deficits may be noted as a Brown-Sequard syndrome (loss of motor function, light touch, vibration, and position sense on the side of the lesion, and contralateral loss of pain and temperature sense).

Sensory Deficits

Which specific sensory deficits develop depends on the presentation of the tumor on cross section. A lateral presentation affects pain and temperature sensation. Numbness or paresthesias, especially of the legs, appear as early symptoms.

Light touch sensation is preserved in the presence of a unilateral tumor resulting from the crossed and uncrossed components to the tract. Awareness of vibration and proprioception of body parts are affected if the posterior columns are involved. Compression from a tumor affects function below the lesion. Therefore, the highest intact sensory level should be determined. An intramedullary lesion may result in a "suspended sensory level" in which a band-like loss of sensation occurs at the level of the lesion.

Bowel, Bladder, and Sexual Dysfunction

Bowel, bladder, or sexual dysfunction is common. Constipation and, later, paralytic ileus are common bowel deficits. Early bladder deficits may present as urgency or difficulty in initiating urination gradually progressing to urinary retention. Decreased motor function and paresthesias of the perineum occur with some tumors, and impotence or other sexual dysfunction is possible. With a cervical intramedullary tumor (uncommon tumor location), *sacral sparing* may occur, with sensation to the perineum spared as a result of perineal sensation being controlled by the lateral spinothalamic tract.

Other Findings

As a tumor grows, it consumes all the space around the spinal cord, thus isolating the CSF below the tumor from normal CSF circulation, known as a CSF block. Examination of the CSF reveals xanthochromia, an increased protein count, few or no cells, and immediate clotting. Collectively, these findings are called **Froin's syndrome**. Some types of spinal cord tumor cause a syringomyelic syndrome from a syrinx found in the central intramedullary gray matter. This syndrome causes a chronic degenerative disorder of the spinal cord accompanied by motor weakness, spasticity, and pain.

DIAGNOSIS

Diagnosis begins with a complete medical history and physical examination, including a focused neurological examination. Diagnostic testing follows, with the urgency of some tests based on clinical findings.

Clinical Findings

In the early stages, subtle symptoms may not be evident. Collect a history of pain, including onset, location, and aggravating symptoms. Palpate the back and spine for localized point tenderness or spasms. Assess muscle strength and abnormal tone (flaccidity or spasticity) and look for signs of muscle wasting. Test deep tendon reflexes, superficial abdominal reflexes, and the Babinski sign.

Sensory assessment (i.e., pain, vibration, position, light touch) begins at the toes and moves upward to determine the highest intact functional level. The lesion level is often accompanied by a narrow band of hyperesthesia (abnormally increased sensitivity to stimuli) directly above its location. Assess for bladder dysfunction (urinary retention, urinary dribbling), bowel dysfunction (constipation), and sexual dysfunction (impotence).

As noted earlier, it is not uncommon for patients to initially experience pain without focal neurological deficits. The occurrence of focal deficits can assist in localization of the lesion, but their absence should not deter the clinician from further evaluation.

Diagnostics

The diagnostic test of choice for a patient with a suspected spinal cord lesion is magnetic resonance imaging (MRI) with contrast enhancement (gadolinium). In patients with systemic cancer, other diagnostic tests, including bone scan, positron emission tomography (PET) scan, and plan radiographs may also be performed. However, MRI with contrast exhibits superior sensitivity in detecting lesions in bony areas such as in the vertebral bodies. A noninvasive procedure, MRI allows multiple axial and midsagittal views demonstrating intramedullary pathology without radiologic exposure. Figure 22-5 shows an intradural-extramedullary meningioma. Optimal MRI requires that the patient remain motionless for a period of time during the procedure. This can be difficult if the patient is in pain. Imaging sequences that should be performed include axial and sagittal turbo-spin-echo T1-weighted images after gadolinium. These sequences are important for tumor detection, delineation, and tumor

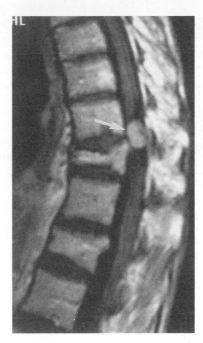

Figure 22-5 • Magnetic resonance image of an intradural-extramedullary thoracic meningioma. Note the incidental old compression fracture in the midthoracic region. (Castillo, M. [1999]. *Neuroradiology companion: Methods, guidelines, and imaging fundamentals* [2nd ed.]. Philadelphia: Lippincott-Raven.)

grading.[7] There are contraindications for MRI, such as previous surgery for placement of metal plates or rods. In these cases, alternative, less sensitive tests such as computed tomography (CT) may be used. However, in most circumstances, MRI has replaced myelography and CT as the standard of care.

With an intramedullary spinal cord tumor, the MRI demonstrates an enlarged or thickened cord. Often, the spinal cord is enlarged around the area of the slowly expanding tumor. The entire spinal axis should be examined to determine presence of areas of involvement. Although a specific type of tumor may be suggested by its location and pattern, the definitive histologic tumor type must be known before beginning treatment. Neurosurgical evaluation for possible biopsy or evacuation should be considered. Patients are at risk for sustaining significant neurological deficits both from the impact of the tumor on the spinal cord and from treatment modalities that may cause secondary cord injury.

For patients with intramedullary tumors or intradural tumors including LMD, evaluation of the CSF may be necessary to determine CSF involvement with tumor. This is obtained via lumbar puncture (LP). Brain imaging with either CT scan or MRI is necessary to rule out an intracranial abnormality that may lead to herniation as a result of the LP.[8] Analysis will include evaluation of glucose, protein, and cytology looking for tumor cells. Often, repeated lumbar punctures may be needed to make the diagnosis.

CLINICAL PEARLS: The diagnostic test of choice for a patient with a suspected spinal cord lesion is magnetic resonance imaging with contrast enhancement (gadolinium).

PRINCIPLES OF TREATMENT

For patients with suspected or diagnosed spinal cord tumors, the primary goals of treatment are preservation of neurological function, control of pain, and initiation of a treatment plan directed at tumor removal or control.[9] A combination of surgery, radiation therapy, and chemotherapy is often required. The degree of neurological dysfunction and the location of the lesion determine the urgency of treatment. For example, patients with sudden onset of focal neurological findings mandate an emergent work-up. For patients with signs of cervical cord dysfunction, immobilization of the neck is mandatory until stability has been obtained.

CLINICAL PEARLS: For patients with suspected or diagnosed spinal cord tumors, the primary goals of treatment are preservation of neurological function, control of pain, and initiation of a treatment plan directed at tumor removal or control.

Preservation of Neurological Function

Spinal cord tumors are often associated with localized edema. The spinal canal is narrow and provides little space for swelling without accompanying neurological dysfunction. Extensive pressure can compromise venous and arterial blood flow, resulting in ischemia and irreversible infarction of the spinal cord. The immediate administration of corticosteroids, most commonly dexamethasone (Decadron), can rapidly reverse this edema. The dosage and schedule of administration are controversial. Some recommend a bolus dose followed by a slow tapering dose over several days or until symptoms increase.[1] Corticosteroids are often given with chemotherapy and radiation protocols to control edema and preserve function. A patient receiving corticosteroids either PO or IV must also receive a gastric protection agent to prevent gastric irritation and bleeding.

Various supportive care measures may be necessary. If stability of the cervical spinal cord is in question, the patient should be immobilized with a cervical collar until the stability of the vertebral column can be assessed and surgical stabilization, if needed, can be undertaken. With a high cervical tumor, close monitoring of respiratory function is imperative and respiratory support may be necessary. These lesions can also be associated with difficulty with swallowing, and a feeding tube to prevent aspiration and support nutritional needs may be required. For the patient with tumors involving the lower spinal cord, urinary retention may occur. An indwelling catheter may be required or an intermittent catheterization program is started. Other supportive devices for ambulation or maintenance of independence of activities of daily living may be required dependent on lesion location and degree of deficit.

Improvement in function may occur after corticosteroid therapy is established and has become therapeutic. Physical and occupational therapy may also be necessary to assist with impaired ambulation related to paresis, muscle wasting, fatigue, and the concurrent high risk for falls.

With metastatic tumors, prompt diagnosis and treatment are the keys to preserving function. Most patients diagnosed with metastatic tumors have pain for an average of 3 months before the appearance of neurological deficits, which prompt a search for a cause.

Treatment Options

The treatment plan for a specific spinal cord tumor depends on the type of tumor, its location, and the rapidity with which signs and symptoms are developing. The overall medical condition of the patient is also an important consideration. Intradural-extramedullary tumors, such as neurofibromas, meningiomas, vascular tumors, chordomas, and epidermoid tumors, are usually treated with surgical excision alone. The management of intramedullary tumors, such as astrocytomas, ependymomas, and metastatic lesions, is much more difficult. These tumors often require a combination of surgery, radiotherapy, and possibly chemotherapy.

CLINICAL PEARLS: The prompt administration of corticosteroids is imperative to prevent irreversible infarction of the spinal cord.

Surgery

Surgical intervention is the primary treatment for most types of spinal cord tumors. Surgery is undertaken to establish a diagnosis through biopsy and to partially or completely resect the tumor. Rapid loss of motor, sensory, and bowel/bladder function indicates the need for *immediate surgery* to preserve or restore neurological function. Advances in surgical technique, such as intraoperative spinal cord evoked potential monitoring, intraoperative ultrasound localization, microneurosurgical approaches, and newer instrumentation (e.g., ultrasonic aspirators, lasers), are improving surgical outcomes. If a laminectomy is performed involving two or more levels, spinal fusion may be necessary.

For rapidly growing metastatic lesions, surgical decompression may be advised to maintain bowel, bladder, or motor function, thus preserving a reasonable quality of life even if the prognosis for the primary tumor is poor. Recently, decompressive surgery in combination with radiation therapy was shown to improve immediate ambulation, lengthen the time patients were able to walk, and lessen the use of narcotics and steroids compared to the use of radiation alone.[10] Therefore, surgery is often offered to patients with epidural disease in addition to radiation therapy. The outcome of surgery is better if extradural metastatic lesions are diagnosed early (for example, when only back pain is present without neurological deficits) then if the patient has significant neurological deficits. Plegia, once present, usually is irreversible.

Extramedullary intradural tumors, such as meningiomas or neurofibromas, can often be completely excised surgically. After complete resection, recurrence is rare for both tumor types. For neurofibromatosis patients with multiple spinal cord tumors, tumor removal is limited to symptomatic lesions. For intramedullary tumors, which are frequently malignant and often have microscopic infiltration of spinal cord parenchyma, attempts at complete surgical excision often pose substantial risk of loss of neurological function. Therefore, the goals of surgery are limited by the risk of neurological harm to the patient with the ultimate goal being to establish a diagnosis and decompress the spinal cord before embarking on additional treatment.

CLINICAL PEARLS: Decompressive circumferential resection of epidural tumor results in improved ability to walk for a longer period of time for patients with epidural tumors.

Procedures that are minimally invasive decrease recovery time because there is less surgical trauma to tissue. An example of a minimally invasive procedure is percutaneous vertebroplasty used for treatment of metastases to the vertebral body or compression fractures. A common problem in both conditions is varying degrees of pain. Although most patients are treated conservatively with analgesics, bed rest, and bracing, a small group of patients are left with severe persistent pain and limited mobility that is debilitating. Percutaneous vertebroplasty (PV) may be used as a treatment to provide pain relief from severe painful osteoporosis with loss of height and/or with compression fractures of the vertebral body. A compression fracture can occur from osteopenia that results from osteoporosis or chronic steroid therapy or from invasive vertebral body lesions such as a vertebral hemangioma, a myeloma, or metastasis. The PV procedure consists of injection of acrylic bone cement into the vertebral body to relieve pain and/or stabilize the fractured vertebrae. In some cases, the vertebral height will be restored to the vertebra as a result of the PV.[11]

Radiation

Most patients with primary spinal cord tumors do not require radiation therapy. However, radiation therapy is the mainstay of treatment for patients with spinal cord compression due to metastatic cancer. Some primary malignant spinal cord tumors (i.e., malignant gliomas, malignant ependymomas, and metastatic lesions) are also treated with radiation. Radiation therapy is also used for benign or low-grade spinal cord tumors that cannot be completely removed surgically.

Standard therapy includes the use of focal external beam radiation therapy to the affected area. The spinal cord is less tolerant of radiation therapy than the brain and other organs. The thoracic spinal cord, where half of all spinal tumors occur, is the most sensitive spinal tissue. Radiation oncologists work to minimize the risk of radiation-induced damage to normal spinal tissue by limiting the amount of radiation exposure to the spinal cord and surrounding structures. Studies suggest that the spinal cord can tolerate a maximum of 4500 cGy. Higher doses are associated with an increased risk of *radiation myelopathy*. Radiation myelopathy is a chronic, progressive condition initially seen as sensory impairment to the areas supplied by the affected cord. This irreversible complication of radiation exposure begins insidiously at least 6 months after completion of radiation therapy and, more frequently, 12 to 15 months after therapy. Motor deficits and changes in pain and temperature sensation develop, so that a Brown-Séquard syndrome is observed. This eventually converts to a transverse myelopathy with spastic paraplegia, loss of sensation in the affected areas, and loss of bowel and bladder control.

Current clinical trials are evaluating newer methods of delivery of radiation therapy, in an effort to maximize therapy and reduce toxicity. Current approaches currently under investigation include the use of intensity-modulated radiation therapy (IMRT) and proton beam therapy. In addition, the use of stereotactic radiation therapy for the treatment of spinal cord tumors is also being explored. These therapies are discussed in detail in Chapter 21. The impact on disease progression and neurological deterioration is yet to be determined.

CLINICAL PEARLS: Standard therapy includes the use of focal external beam radiation to the affected areas.

Chemotherapy

To date, the role of chemotherapy for spinal cord tumors is limited. Chemotherapy may be recommended in adults for spinal gliomas and other primary tumors as part of initial therapy or for tumors that progress after surgery and radiation. Chemotherapy may also be useful in a few chemosensitive cancers such as lymphomas and small-cell lung cancer as initial therapy. Its role is currently the focus of ongoing clinical trials evaluating therapy of metastatic disease to the brain and spinal cord.[9]

Adjunctive therapy such as hormonal manipulation may be useful for specific tumors. For example, tamoxifen (Megace) may be helpful for breast cancer, and androgen inhibition, either through chemical means (i.e., diethylstilbestrol) or orchiectomy, may be beneficial in prostate cancer.

For patients with LMD, intrathecal chemotherapy may be instituted. This involves direct administration of chemotherapy into the CSF either by lumbar puncture or a reservoir implanted in the lateral ventricle (i.e., Ommaya reservoir).[8] Several agents are available for treatment, including methotrexate, cytosine arabinoside, and DepoCyt (a liposomal formulation of cytosine arabinoside). Current clinical trials are evaluating the effects of other chemotherapeutic agents directly instilled into the CSF and the role of systemic therapy in treating this disease. For most patients, the prognosis remains poor despite treatment.

Prognosis and Discharge Planning

Prognosis will vary greatly, depending on the type of tumor and the neurological deficits present. With primary tumors, some resolution of neurological deficits may occur gradually, sometimes over months to years. Each patient should be evaluated to identify individual rehabilitation needs. Most patients with neurological deficits will benefit from a short-term, aggressive rehabilitation program. Patients with metastatic lesions often do not fare as well because of the advanced stage of the primary tumor. For these patients, further treatment of the primary cancer may be planned. For others, palliative care with hospice care or placement in a chronic care facility may be chosen.

NURSING MANAGEMENT OF THE PATIENT WITH A SPINAL CORD TUMOR

Some commonalties in nursing management exist in the care of patients with spinal cord injuries and those with spinal cord tumors (see Chap. 18). Specifics of care depend on the segmental level of the tumor and the presenting signs and symptoms. If the patient is treated surgically, nursing management follows that outlined for a laminectomy patient (see Chap. 19). Some patients develop metastatic lesions to the spinal cord as a complication of a primary cancer. The nurse will need to consult a text on oncologic nursing for specific management and treatment that should be integrated into the plan of care.

The objectives of care for the hospitalized patient with a spinal cord tumor include early recognition of neurological change through ongoing monitoring; control of pain; management of sensory and motor deficits and their impact on activities of daily living (ADLs); and management of bowel and bladder dysfunction. See Chart 22-1 for a summary of assessment parameters.

CLINICAL VIGNETTE: Mrs. H is a 58-year-old woman with a history of breast cancer. She presents to the oncologist's office after experiencing new onset back pain. Any new neurological symptom warrants investigation. The nurse explores the location of the pain, precipitating factors, and characteristics. The patient should undergo a complete neurological evaluation. The absence of neurological deficits should not preclude further investigations. This may include a bone scan, but the diagnostic test of choice to rule out spinal cord disease is MRI with gadolinium.

Assessment

The nurse should conduct a baseline assessment of vital and neurological signs. Neither the level of consciousness nor pupillary signs are apt to be affected unless the sympathetic innervation of the cervical spinal nerves is involved. In this instance, Horner's syndrome will be seen. The key areas of assessment include pain, motor, sensory, bowel, and bladder function.

Pain. Assess the quality (on a scale of 1 to 10), location, and type (e.g., dull, piercing) of pain present, using the visual analogue scale. Note whether and where the pain radiates and any circumstances that exacerbate the pain.

Motor Function. Assess motor strength and grade on a 0 to 5 scale as outlined in Chapter 6. Palpate the muscles for signs of atrophy. Note presence of abnormal motor tone, reflexes, involuntary movement, and limited range of motion. If the patient is able to walk, assess the gait, as well as the ability to sit and stand up without assistance. Note any functional deficits that impact on ADLs.

Sensory Function. All sensory modalities must be evaluated, including light touch, pain and temperature, vibration, and position sensations (see Chap. 6). With the patient's eyes closed, begin at the toes and work your way up the body, assessing each side of the body and distal to proximal function and comparing findings. Determine which modalities are absent or diminished. Patients often experience a "level" of sensory loss, in which they have

---

CHART 22-1   Assessment Parameters for a Patient With a Spinal Cord Tumor

SENSORY ASSESSMENT

- With the patient's eyes closed, assess the following sensory modalities:
  - Light touch
  - Pain (pinprick)
  - Position
- Beginning at the feet and working upward systematically, assess each side of the body and compare findings; often, sensory loss is asymmetrical. (See Chap. 6 for technique.)
- Note the highest level of sensation recorded in relation to an anatomic marking (e.g., umbilicus) or dermatome level. (See Chaps. 4, 6, and 20.)
- If pain is present, describe the characteristics of pain using standard pain assessment criteria.
- Assess progression/change in pain over time.
- Assess for cervical vertebral, thoracic vertebral, and lumbar vertebral pain for *tenderness* while palpating vertebrae.
- Identify highest level of intact sensory function on each side of body.
- Document highest level of function for pain so pain level can be monitored over time.

MOTOR ASSESSMENT

- Systematically assess each side of the body for muscle strength and muscle tone; compare findings. (See Chap. 6 for technique.)
- Observe the patient's gait pattern, if ambulatory.

- Note the presence of spasticity or other abnormal movement.
- Assess deep tendon reflexes and coordination.

BOWEL ASSESSMENT

- Assess the normal bowel evacuation pattern for the patient (frequency, consistency, time of day, etc.).
- Assess for any changes in bowel habits.
- Assess use of any home remedies for regularity (food, drugs).
- Auscultate the abdomen for bowel sounds and distention.

BLADDER ASSESSMENT

- Assess the patient's normal voiding pattern.
- Assess the patient for any changes or discomfort in voiding pattern.
- Palpate the suprapubic area for distention or pain.

RESPIRATORY ASSESSMENT (FOR CERVICAL TUMORS)

- Assess rate, depth, and rhythm of respirations.
- Observe chest movement for asymmetry, abdominal breathing, or abnormal chest movement.
- Auscultate the chest bilaterally for breath sounds.

OTHER NOTATIONS

- Assess the patient for orthostatic hypotension.
- Note any absence of perspiration (e.g., Horner's syndrome).

lack of sensation corresponding to lesion location and involving areas of the body below this level. A band of hyperesthesia often exists over the level of sensory loss. Note any abnormal sensations (paresthesias), such as burning or a pins and needles sensation.

Bowel Function. Auscultate the abdomen for bowel sounds. Determine the normal pattern of bowel function, and ascertain whether there has been a change in bowel patterns such as constipation, diarrhea, or incontinence of stool. A bowel program may need to be instituted.

Bladder Function. Note the urinary voiding pattern. Determine whether there is evidence of urinary retention (a common problem with spinal cord tumors) or incontinence. Urinary retention will place the patient at high risk for urinary tract infection. Monitor intake and output. A bladder retraining program may be necessary.

CLINICAL PEARLS: Urinary retention commonly occurs with spinal cord tumors.

Collaborative and Patient Problems

After assessment data have been collected, a list of collaborative and patient problems with interventions is developed (Chart 22-2). The major collaborative problems are:

- Spinal cord compression
- Paresis/paresthesia/paralysis
- Fecal impaction
- Urinary retention
- Infection
- Intractable pain

| CHART **22-2** | **Summary of Nursing Management of the Patient With a Spinal Cord Tumor** |

PATIENT PROBLEMS	NURSING INTERVENTIONS	EXPECTED OUTCOME(S)
Pain Related to (R/T) Spinal Cord and/or Spinal Nerve Compression and Muscle Spasms	• Monitor pain at least every 4 hours. —Monitor quality (dull, piercing), location, and other characteristics. —Monitor the severity of pain by asking the patient to use the visual analogue scale (VAS) to report pain severity on a scale of 1 to 10. —Monitor nonverbal signs of pain (e.g., facial expression, emotional control). —Monitor the effect of pain on activities of daily living (ADLs). • Identify activities/factors that aggravate pain.	• The patient will accurately describe pain phenomena. • The patient will identify changes in pain intensity using the VAS. • The patient will participate in controlling activities/factors that aggravate pain.
	• Administer analgesics and steroids as ordered, and before the pain intensity has escalated. • Provide physical comfort measures. —Reposition the patient every 1 to 2 hours. —Maintain proper body alignment. —Administer massage (e.g., a back rub). • Apply a special mattress based on any limitations (e.g., a water mattress, an alternating pressure mattress). • Teach stress-reducing techniques for pain control (e.g., relaxation, imagery, distraction activities). • Assist the patient to plan individual pain control strategies that are most effective.	• The patient will report the his or her response to analgesics using the VAS. • The patient will identify measures that facilitate comfort. • The patient will learn and use stress-reducing techniques to control pain. • The patient will participate in developing an overall pain control plan.
Impaired Physical Mobility R/T muscle weakness, paralysis, spasticity, and pain	• Monitor motor function every 8 hours (muscle strength, muscle tone, gait, ability to move in bed). • Teach the proper use of assistive devices. • Provide assistance, as necessary, in transfer and ambulation once spinal cord is stabilized. • Administer range-of-motion exercises every 4 hours. • Position the patient in proper body alignment every 2 hours; use supportive devices as necessary.	• The comparison of data to baseline data will identify any changes.

(continued)

CHART 22-2	Summary of Nursing Management of the Patient With a Spinal Cord Tumor (Continued)

PATIENT PROBLEMS	NURSING INTERVENTIONS	EXPECTED OUTCOME(S)
Related Patient Problems: • Self-Care Deficits • Risk for Impaired Skin Integrity • Risk for Disuse Syndrome	• Monitor the effect of impaired mobility on ADLs. • Develop specific interventions to compensate for deficits. • If spasticity is present, keep the involved extremity warm; reposition periodically; seek suggestions from the physical therapist. • Provide analgesics at least 30 minutes before a planned activity. • If bed rest is ordered, consider protocols to counter the effects of immobility (deep breathing exercises, skin care, turning schedule, etc.). • Request physical therapy (PT) and occupational therapy (OT) consults once patient's spinal cord is stabilized.	• Any ADLs that the patient cannot do independently will be provided by the nurse, or an alternative way of doing the activity with an adaptive device will be developed. • The patient will report a decrease in pain and an increase in activity tolerance. • Interventions will be in place to prevent the development of disuse syndrome.
Sensory/Perceptual Alterations: Tactile and Kinesthetic, R/T neurological sensory deficits (spinal cord compression, edema) Related Patient Problems: • High Risk for Injury	• Monitor sensory function; identify the highest level of intact sensory function. • Teach the patient to compensate for any deficits by checking the position of the involved area visually. • Protect the involved area from injury (e.g., burns, bruising). • Monitor ability to ambulate secondary to sensory deficits.	• Comparison of data to baseline data will identify any changes. • The patient will find ways to compensate for the lost sensory modality so that the effect on performance of ADLs will be minimized.
Urinary Retention R/T spinal cord compression and edema Related Patient Problems: • Risk for Urinary Tract Infection	• Monitor the patient's voiding pattern and amount per voiding. • Maintain an accurate intake and output record. • Monitor the patient for suprapubic distention or pain. • Explain the rationale for treatment and management. • Insert indwelling catheter or establish intermittent catheterization schedule. • Remove the indwelling catheter as soon as possible. • Develop a bladder retraining program: 　—Teach the Credé and stretch maneuvers. 　—Measure postvoid residuals after attempts to empty the bladder. 　—Teach intermittent catheterization. 　—Set a catheterization time schedule to obtain about 500 mL of urine each time.	• The patient will accurately report his or her former voiding pattern. • The patient will verbalize an understanding of the treatment regimen and the underlying rationale. • The patient will establish a regular pattern of urinary elimination. • The patient will learn self-catheterization technique.
Constipation R/T decreased peristalsis secondary to spinal cord compression/edema	• Establish the patient's previous bowel elimination pattern. • Auscultate the abdomen for bowel sounds. • Palpate the abdomen for distention. • Increase bulk in diet. • Encourage an adequate fluid intake. • Begin a bowel protocol that will provide for satisfactory bowel elimination.	• The patient will accurately report the previous bowel elimination pattern. • Presence of peristalsis will be monitored. • A diet high in bulk and fluids will be encouraged unless contraindicated by the medical plan. • A bowel protocol will be established that ensures bowel movements (with stools of soft consistency) every 1 to 2 days.
Risk for Injury R/T sensory/ perceptual alterations and impaired physical mobility	• Teach the patient to: 　—Check the position of the affected limbs visually. 　—Check the integrity of the skin daily, especially affected parts, for evidence of injury. 　—Check the temperature of the unaffected limb before applying heat to affected areas. 　—Use heating devices very cautiously.	• The patient and family will recognize the patient's highrisk status secondary to neurological deficits. • Strategies will be developed to prevent injury.

CHART 22-2 Summary of Nursing Management of the Patient With a Spinal Cord Tumor (Continued)

PATIENT PROBLEMS	NURSING INTERVENTIONS	EXPECTED OUTCOME(S)
Anxiety R/T pain, uncertainty about the disease process, and outcome	• Assist the patient with ambulation. • Allow the patient to express his or her feelings. • Correct misinformation and clarify information as necessary. • Refer the patient to appropriate resource people, as necessary. • Help the patient set realistic goals. • Be supportive. • Help the patient find ways to reduce anxiety (e.g., relaxation techniques, diversion).	• The patient will seek assistance in ambulation. • Anxiety will be reduced to a manageable level.

Other possible Patient Problems—general:
• Knowledge Deficit R/T
  —Disease process
  —Treatment modalities (surgery, irradiation, chemotherapy)
• Sexual Dysfunction
• Functional Incontinence
• Fatigue
• Fear
• Ineffective Individual Coping
• Ineffective Family Coping
• Powerlessness
For patients with cervical tumors:
• Ineffective Breathing Pattern
• Ineffective Airway Clearance
• Impaired Swallowing		

Management

For the hospitalized patient, in preparation for discharge, the nurse will make a complete assessment of the patient to determine the level of independence in performing ADLs, home activities, and activities within the community. Working collaboratively with other health team members, a discharge plan is developed. These patients need a case manager to assist with the planning of care that is often complex and long term. As mentioned previously, some patients will benefit from a short-term rehabilitation program through an in-house rehabilitation facility or through outpatient services. For the patient with a metastatic lesion, contacting the primary physician managing the cancer and any community resources previously involved in the patient's care will help ensure continuity of care. Hospice care in the home or nursing home is an option for patients in the terminal stages of illness.

CLINICAL VIGNETTE: Mr. L is 48-year-old man who recently underwent a resection of an ependymoma involving the lower thoracic cord. He is being discharged today. The nurse should assess the patient's current level of neurological dysfunction. Deficits in self-care, including wound care, lower extremity weakness, and bowel/bladder control, should be evaluated. Education regarding wound care, limitations placed on activities, symptoms to report, and follow-up should be reviewed.

Follow-Up in the Community

Patients with either primary or secondary spinal cord tumor may require long-term follow-up and management. From the nursing perspective, functional ability in ADLs, nutrition, comfort (pain control), and quality of life provide a framework for assessment and care. In addition to monitoring motor, sensory, bowel, and bladder function, other functional deficits may become apparent, such as impotence. Persistent problems may require further evaluation and possible referral for resolution.

REFERENCES

1. Van Goethem, J. W., van den Hauwe, L., Ozsarlak, O., De Schepper, A. M., & Parizel, P. M. (2004). Spinal tumors. *European Journal of Radiology, 50*(2), 159–176.
2. Goetz, C. G., & Pappert, E. J. (1999). *Textbook of clinical neurology.* Philadelphia: W.B. Saunders.
3. Maher de Leon, M. E., Schnell, S., & Rozental, J. M. (1998). Tumors of the spine and spinal cord. *Seminars in Oncology Nursing, 14*(1), 43–52.
4. Cruz, J. (1998). *Neurologic and neurosurgical emergencies.* Philadelphia: W.B. Saunders.
5. Gucalp, R., & Dutche, J. (2005). Oncologic emergencies. In: D. L. Kasper, E. Braunwald, A. S. Fauci, S. L. Hauser, D. L. Longo, & J. L. Jameson (Eds.). *Harrison's principles of internal medicine* (6th ed., pp. 575–583). New York: McGraw-Hill.

6. Aminoff, M. J., Greenberg, D. A., & Simon, R. P. (1996). *Clinical neurology* (3rd ed.). Stanford: Appleton and Lange.

7. Runge, V. M., Lee, C., Iten, A. L., & Williams, N. M. (1997). Contrast-enhanced magnetic resonance imaging in a spinal epidural tumor model. *Invest Radiology, 32*(10), 589–595.

8. Armstrong, T. S., & Gilbert, M. R. (2004). The treatment of neoplastic meningitis. *Expert Opinion in Pharmacotherapy, 5*(9), 1929–1935.

9. van den Bent, M. J. (2004). Management of metastatic (parenchymal, leptomeningeal, and epidural) lesions. *Current Opinion in Oncology, 16,* 309–313.

10. Patchell, R. A., Tibbs, P. A., Regine, W. F., Payne, R., Saris, S., Kryscio, R. J., et al. (2005). Direct decompressive surgical resection in the treatment of spinal cord compression caused by metastatic cancer: a randomised trial. *Lancet, 366*(9486), 643–648.

11. Patel, J., & Singh, M. K. (2006). Percutaneous vertebroplasty. Retrieved July 12, 2007, from http://www.emedicine.com/neuro/topic682.htm

RESOURCES

Published Material

General information about the effects of spinal cord disease can be assessed from the National Spinal Cord Injury Association at (800) 962-9629.

American Brain Tumor Association. *About metastatic tumors to the brain and spine.* Available by phone at (800) 886-2282.

Brain and Spinal Cord Tumors. *Hope through research* (NIH Publication No. 93-504). Available by phone at (800) 352-9424.

Murphy, R. F. (1990). *The body silent.* New York: W. W. Norton (written by an anthropologist coping with an inoperable ependymoma).

Price, R. (1994). *A whole new life: An illness and a healing.* New York: Atheneum Press (a prize-winning author who has survived more than 15 years with a malignant spinal cord astrocytoma).

Nursing Management of Patients With Cerebrovascular Problems

Cerebral Aneurysms

Deidre A. Buckley and Joanne V. Hickey

OVERVIEW

A **cerebral aneurysm** is a saccular outpouching of a cerebral artery. Intracranial saccular aneurysms or berry aneurysms account for approximately 80% to 90% of all intracranial aneurysms and are the most common cause of nontraumatic subarachnoid hemorrhage. These small, berry-like projections occur at arterial bifurcations in the circle of Willis, with other shapes such as pedunculated, sessile, and multilobulated aneurysms occasionally seen.[1] Rupture of a cerebral aneurysm usually results in a **subarachnoid hemorrhage (SAH)**, which is defined as bleeding into the subarachnoid space. The prevalence of unruptured intracranial aneurysms is variable based on current studies. Autopsy studies have shown that the overall frequency of unruptured intracranial aneurysms in the general population ranges from 0.2% to 9.9% (mean about 5%). It is estimated that approximately 10 to 15 million Americans have a cerebral aneurysm, most of which are small, are innocuous, and do not bleed throughout life. Most recent prospective autopsy and angiographic studies indicate an overall frequency of about 2% to 4%, suggesting that unruptured intracranial aneurysms will affect about 6 million individuals in the United States at some point in their lives.[2,3] An intracranial aneurysm is a common postmortem finding, with a prevalence ranging from 1% to 6% of adults in autopsy findings. The prevalence of aneurysms in adults undergoing angiography is between 0.5% and 1%. This suggests that between 1 million and 12 million Americans have intracranial aneurysms.[4]

The mean age of the U.S. population is increasing, and intracranial aneurysms seem to develop with increasing age. The incidence of SAH from aneurysms also increases with age. Most studies have found an increased occurrence of aneurysms in women compared with men, although in childhood and adolescence the ratio appears to be opposite, with a male-to-female ratio of 2:1.[1]

SAH is one of the most feared causes of acute headache upon presentation to the emergency department. Headache accounts for 1% to 2% of emergency room visits and up to 4% of visits to primary care offices. Among all the patients who present to the emergency room with headaches, approximately 1% has subarachnoid hemorrhage. One study put the figure at 4%. Two prospective studies found that if only patients with "the worst headache" of their lives and a normal neurological exam were considered, 12% of the patients had subarachnoid hemorrhage.[5-7]

The annual incidence of SAH in North America is about 15 cases per 100,000 or roughly one hemorrhage every 18 minutes. About 80% of patients with nontraumatic SAH have ruptured saccular aneurysms, which occur in 30,000 patients annually in the United States.[8]

Accurate early diagnosis is critical, as the initial hemorrhage may be fatal, may result in devastating neurological outcomes, or may produce minor symptoms. Despite widespread neuroimaging availability, misdiagnosis or delays in diagnosis occur in up to 25% of patients with SAH[9] when initially presenting for medical treatment. A list of common misdiagnoses is shown (Table 23-1).[10]

Variation in Presentation

Misdiagnosis often results from three repetitive patterns of error: failure to understand limitations of computed tomography (CT), failure to appreciate the spectrum of clinical symptoms, and failure to correctly interpret lumbar puncture (LP). There are between 20% and 50% of patients with documented SAH that report a distinct, severe headache (known as a "thunderclap headache") in the days to weeks before the index episode of bleeding, known as a "warning headache."[5] Thunderclap headaches develop in seconds, achieve maximal intensity in minutes, and can last hours to days. The differential diagnosis includes subarachnoid hemorrhage, acute expansion, dissections or thrombosis of unruptured aneurysms, cerebral venous thrombosis, brief headaches during exertion and sexual intercourse, and benign thunderclap headaches. All patients who present with thunderclap headaches should be evaluated immediately for SAH.[5]

Almost half the patients with SAH have episodes of minor bleeding. In one series of 500 patients with SAH, 34% had bleeding during nonstrenuous exercise and 12% during sleep. The headache may be in any location, may be localized or generalized, may be mild, may resolve spontaneously, or may be alleviated by analgesics. Patients with less severe headaches may be given the diagnosis of a more common condition such as sinusitis, tension headache, or migraine.[5,11] When vomiting is present, especially with a low-grade fever, some of the common misdiagnoses include viral syndrome, viral meningitis, flu, or gastroenteritis. Those patients with significant neck pain may be given the diagnosis of arthritis or cervical neck pain, and those with pain radiating down

TABLE 23-1 COMMON MISDIAGNOSES OF SUBARACHNOID HEMORRHAGE

No diagnosis made, or headache of unknown etiology	Transient ischemic attack/ischemic stroke
Headache (migraine, tension, or cluster headache)	Trauma
Meningitis or encephalitis	Hypertensive crisis
Neck problems (arthritis or cervical disc disease)	Sinusitis
Alcohol or drug intoxication	Psychiatric diagnoses

the leg may be given the diagnosis of sciatica. Patients who present with confusion or agitation may be diagnosed with a primary psychiatric disorder.

Most patients who present with SAH will have abrupt onset of severe, unique headache or neck pain. Some will have abnormal findings on neurological exam, such as subtle meningismus or ocular findings. An understanding of the wide presentation of symptoms along with careful history taking and physical examination is the best strategy for identifying patients who should be evaluated for SAH.

Evaluation Tools

The first diagnostic test should be a noncontrast CT scan. Very thin cuts (3 mm in thickness) through the base of the brain are suggested because the thicker cuts (10 mm) may miss small collections of blood. The sensitivity of CT decreases over time from the onset of symptoms. The dynamics of the cerebrospinal fluid (CSF) and spontaneous lysis can result in rapid clearing of old subarachnoid blood.[5,8,12] Four studies have evaluated modern, third-generation CT scanners.[5,7,13–15] In retrospective studies of patients admitted to the hospital with subarachnoid hemorrhage, 100% of patients who underwent scanning within the first 12 hours[14] and 93% of patients who had a CT scan within the first 24 hours[13] after onset of headache had positive findings on CT scanning. Prospective outpatient studies found a sensitivity of 98% (117 of 119) for scanning performed in the first 12 hours[15] and a sensitivity of 93% (14 of 15) for scanning performed in the first 12 hours.[7]

Although magnetic resonance imaging continues to advance and detects aneurysms, standard magnetic resonance imaging is inferior to CT for the detection of acute SAH. CT remains the imaging method of choice because of its wider availability, lower cost, and greater convenience for sick patients and because there is a greater experience with its interpretation.

Lumbar puncture should be performed in a patient whose clinical presentation suggests SAH and whose CT scan is negative. "Traumatic taps" occur in up to 20% of lumbar punctures and must be differentiated from true hemorrhages. Most experienced practitioners agree that the presence of xanthochromia is the primary criterion of subarachnoid hemorrhage in patients with negative CT scans.[12]

Some believe that the presence of erythrocytes, even in the absence of xanthochromia, is more accurate. This difference

can be explained by the various methods of detecting xanthochromia. Those who believed that xanthochromia is most important used spectrophotometry, and those who believed that erythrocytes are most important used visual inspection, which can miss discoloration in CSF in up to 50% of patients.[5]

Most warning headaches are indications of unrecognized subarachnoid hemorrhages that can be diagnosed by appropriate methods. Properly performed and interpreted CT scan and lumbar puncture in patients with acute severe headache will identify the majority of patients with SAH. Some patients whose diagnostic test results are ambiguous or who are at unusually high risk for aneurysm should undergo neurological or neurosurgical evaluation and vascular imaging by magnetic resonance, CT, computed tomography angiography (CTA), or conventional cerebral angiography.

Eighty-five percent of aneurysms in adults occur in the anterior circle of Willis in the proximal arterial bifurcations. The most common sites in the anterior circulation include the anterior communicating artery (A-comm) to anterior cerebral artery (ACA) junction, internal carotid artery (ICA) bifurcation in the posterior communicating artery (P-comm) origin, and proximal middle cerebral artery (MCA). In the posterior circulation, the most common locations include the basilar tip (BA), the superior cerebellar artery (SCA), and the anterior inferior cerebellar arteries (AICAs). In children and adolescents, the ICA bifurcation is noted by many investigators to be the most common location[16,17] and the frequency of posterior circulation aneurysms appears higher in children than adults, with some series reporting from 4% to 16% and others reporting a higher incidence in the range of 30% to 57%.[17] The incidence of posterior circulation aneurysms in people under 18 years of age was 24% as compared to 6% in the adult population. In the literature, the incidence of giant aneurysms in the younger population (under 18 years) ranges from 14% to 54%.[17]

Multiple aneurysms occur in 20% to 25% of patients with saccular aneurysms, with approximately 20% of patients with saccular aneurysms having a family history of intracranial aneurysms or subarachnoid hemorrhage.[18] A variety of other pathologic entities have been associated with intracranial aneurysms, such as polycystic kidney disease, arteriovenous malformations (AVMs), coarctation of the aorta, moyamoya disease, Marfan's syndrome, Ehlers-Danlos syndrome, pituitary tumors, and pseudoxanthoma.[3]

Each year in the United States there are approximately 30,000 new cases of SAH secondary to rupture of intracranial aneurysm.[8] Patients age 18 years or less account for 1% to 2% of aneurysmal SAH.[17,19] Despite considerable advances in diagnostic, surgical, anesthetic, and perioperative techniques, the outcome for patients with ruptured aneurysms remains poor; in fact, only one third of people who experience aneurysmal SAH recover without major disability. Cerebral aneurysm rupture is most prevalent in the 35- to 60-year-old age group, with 50 being the mean age of occurrence. Aneurysmal SAH occurs more often in women than men by a ratio of 3:2.[20]

FAMILIAL ANEURYSMS

There have been many families with documented intracranial aneurysms. *Familial intracranial aneurysms* are generally defined as the presence of two or more family members among first- and second-degree relatives with proven aneurysmal SAH or incidental aneurysms.[21–23] Incidence of familial aneurysms among SAH patients is 6% to 20%.[24,25] It has been estimated that the prevalence of familial intracranial aneurysms among patients with SAH is somewhere in the order of 7% to 10%. Ogilvy states that in his experience with patients with ruptured and unruptured aneurysms, approximately 22% will have family members with aneurysms. Familial intracranial aneurysm is defined as two or more blood relatives who harbor intracranial aneurysms.[26] Leblanc et al. reviewed 13 families with intracranial aneurysms and found the occurrence in the same decade in two affected siblings in 10 of 12 cases (83%). Although the usual incidence of morbidity and mortality from initial rupture of hemorrhage is about 40%, when familial patients are reviewed, the incidence of patients who suffered death or disability in the initial hemorrhage is 70%.[27]

The familial occurrence does suggest the possibility of a genetically determined defect of the arterial wall. Several studies suggest that individuals with familial intracranial aneurysms are more likely to have multiple aneurysms and that these aneurysms are more likely to rupture at a smaller size than those patients with an isolated aneurysm.[28] Therefore, treatment considerations are different than for patients with an unruptured isolated aneurysm. No genetic locus has yet been identified, nor has a biologic marker been found that can identify patients with familial intracranial aneurysms. The likelihood of finding such a genetic locus is highest in patients with multiple lesions and familial tendency, so blood samples can be obtained from many members of the same family possibly harboring the gene.

The Familial Intracranial Aneurysm (FIA) Study has recruited a number of families, and its goal is to identify genes that underlie the development and rupture of intracranial aneurysms. The National Institute of Neurological Disorders and Stroke (NINDS)-funded study is the largest genetic linkage study to date. The study includes 26 clinical centers that have broad experience in clinical management and imaging patients with intracranial aneurysms. The study will recruit 475 families with affected sib pairs or with multiple affected relatives through retrospective and prospective screening of potential subjects with an intracranial aneurysm.[29]

The *primary hypothesis* of this study is that there are specific human chromosomal regions that are associated with an increased risk of intracranial aneurysms (IAs). There is evidence that suggests that a genetic component plays an important role in the development of IAs, but specific loci affecting the risk of IAs have not been identified. The long-term *objective* is to identify susceptibility genes that are related to the formation of intracranial aneurysms.[29]

Population-based studies suggest that genetic factors play an important role in aneurysm formation and aneurysm rupture. The risk of unruptured aneurysms, as determined by noninvasive screening such as magnetic resonance angiography (MRA) in unaffected relatives of families with two or more members who have an intracranial aneurysm, is about four times greater than the risk among the general public.[30] These disorders account for less than 1% of all intracranial aneurysms in the population and hence cannot explain the familial aggregation of intracranial aneurysms.[29]

Another important aspect of the genetic study is the critical need to consider environmental factors in disease risk such as smoking. Nearly 80% of patients with an IA have a history of smoking at some time in their life.[31] Not all individuals who smoke develop IA. Smoking may increase the risk of IA in individuals with specific genotypes at IA susceptibility loci.

The FIA Study has excellent power to detect genes associated with the development of intracranial aneurysm rupture and may hopefully determine the complex relationships between genes and the environment that can lead to death.[29]

Various genetically determined conditions have been associated with intracranial aneurysm; a definite link has only been associated with autosomal dominant polycystic kidney disease. The percentage of these patients that have cerebral aneurysms varies from 10% to 40%. There is no identified definitive pattern of inheritance. Other diseases frequently mentioned such as Marfan's syndrome, Ehlers-Danlos syndrome type 4, neurofibromatosis, and pseudoxanthoma elasticum are more often associated with carotid cavernous fistulas than with aneurysms.[26] The current recommendation for screening is that each family member should undergo magnetic resonance imaging (MRI), MRA, or CTA. It is recommended that family members be screened in their 20s and every 5 to 10 years thereafter. It is thought that patients who have a family history of aneurysm may develop them at a younger age than those with spurious aneurysms, although there is no conclusive study.[26]

After an aneurysm is identified in a patient with a family history of aneurysms, treatment is often recommended. Endovascular, surgical, or combined options are considered, and the treatment with the lowest risk and highest efficacy of obliterating the aneurysm is recommended to the individual.[26]

ETIOLOGY

Although the precise etiology of cerebral aneurysms remains unclear, many extrinsic, congenital, and genetic factors have been implicated in the formation and rupture of intracerebral aneurysms. One theory suggests that a congenital/developmental defect exists in the medial and adventitial layers of the artery in the circle of Willis. There is little scientific basis for this theory, because these defects are commonly found postmortem in persons without aneurysms. The degenerative theory is strongly supported by current research and ascribes causation to hemodynamically induced degenerative vascular disease.[32] According to this theory, the intima, covered only by the adventitia, bulges from a local weakness. By late midlife, stress causes vessel ballooning and rupture. There may be a predisposition to aneurysm formation in individuals with hypertension and in those in whom connective tissue disease promotes fragility of the arterial wall.[32] Forbus suggested aneurysms were acquired lesions resulting from degeneration of the elastic membrane due to continued overstretching, combined with an underlying congenital defect in the muscularis portion of the arterial wall.[33] Glynn proposed that the degeneration of the internal elastic lamina, possibly caused by atherosclerosis, was the leading cause in the formation of a saccular aneurysm. He stated that both congenital medial defects and acquired internal elastic defects had to be present before aneurysm formation.[34]

Phillips et al. noted that the distribution of the defects was inconsistent with the frequency of distribution of berry aneurysms in humans.[35] He further rationalized that the thinning of the arterial wall occurred early and was associated with the degeneration of the cells in the elastica and of the muscle cells of the intracellular matrix. He also noted that the increased rate of aneurysmal SAHs with increasing age suggests that they are not congenital lesions. This does not preclude congenital predisposition.

More recently, research has demonstrated an association between the presence of specific human leukocyte antigen alleles and the genetic role they may play in aneurysm formation.[36] There are some families in which several members are found to have aneurysms. When this occurs, other close family members should be monitored for vascular lesions.

Although the etiology of most aneurysms is as yet unknown, there are types of intracerebral aneurysms in which the etiology has been well demonstrated. Head trauma can result in traumatic intracranial aneurysms resulting from localized arterial tear. Bacterial and fungal infections have also been known to cause infectious (mycotic) aneurysms. Infectious aneurysms form when bacteria, usually from septic emboli, break off and actually invade and destroy the vessel wall. Atherosclerotic aneurysms can form in vessel walls that have been damaged by deposits of atheromatous material, resulting in fusiform aneurysms. Fusiform aneurysms are rarely associated with SAH.

Intracranial Aneurysms in the Pediatric Population

Intracranial aneurysms in children (younger than 18 years old) are rare, with a reported prevalence ranging from 0.5% to 4.6%,[30] and their epidemiology is poorly understood. Pediatric intracranial aneurysms occur more often in male patients and have a predilection for the terminal ICA bifurcation.

There are 706 aneurysms occurring in the pediatric population that have been reported in the English literature since 1939. Male-to-female occurrence is 1.8:1, and subarachnoid hemorrhage was the mode of presentation in 80% of the children. The most common overall location was the ICA terminus, which was the location in 26% of the cases. Only 17% occurred in the posterior circulation, and one fifth were giant lesions. Surgical treatment was performed in 79% of the cases. There was an overall good outcome in 60% of the cases, with mortality in 28%.[16]

The sex predominance (male-to-female ratio 1.8:1) may suggest the existence of differences in pathogenesis of aneurysm formation in the pediatric patient. One interpretation is that congenital factors present in all aneurysm patients may be expressed more in boys, but environmental factors may contribute to the increased incidence in girls.[16]

Aneurysms in the pediatric population are four times as likely to present with SAH versus no SAH. Also, pediatric aneurysms are twice as likely to be of a better grade. Of the published series of pediatric aneurysms, almost all the earliest series before 1981 were composed of SAH patients. Unruptured aneurysms were detected more often thereafter, a reflection in the improvement of neuroimaging techniques.

The ICA terminus location, representing 26% of the 706 patients reviewed in the literature, was the most common location of intracranial aneurysms, followed by the next predominant location, which was the anterior communicating complex, accounting for 19% of the aneurysms. Posterior circulation aneurysms accounted for 17% of all pediatric aneurysms.[16]

Pathogenesis of Pediatric Aneurysms

Pediatric aneurysms are likely to be pathologically distinct from adult saccular aneurysms.[37] The characteristic abrupt termination of the internal elastic lamina and muscularis media at the entrance to adult saccular aneurysms at arterial bifurcations that is thought to be susceptible to sheer stress or to hypertensive and atherosclerotic deterioration was not found in autopsy series of pediatric aneurysm specimens.[16]

Other theories for aneurysm formation in children include a connective tissue abnormality, an infectious process, a congenital anomaly causing an internal or medial elastic membrane defect, or head injury including birth trauma.[17] More studies are necessary to better understand the differences in aneurysm formation in children versus adults. The male dominance and distinct anatomic location suggest the expression of a yet undetermined pathologic mechanism of aneurysm formation in children.[16]

ANEURYSM HEMODYNAMICS

The occurrence, growth, thrombosis, and rupture of intracranial saccular aneurysms can be directly related to the effect of hemodynamic forces. Strong evidence favors the idea that aneurysms of this nature occur because of hemodynamically induced degenerative vascular injury.[32] Despite in vitro studies over the last decade, the exact mechanisms of action of these stresses remain to be completely understood, and guidelines for determining the likelihood that a particular aneurysm will grow, rupture, regress, or thrombose do not exist.

Evolving imaging techniques that depict accurate vascular morphology as well as evaluate and in some instances quantify particular aspects of cerebral hemodynamics enable an opportunity to add to the natural history of saccular aneurysms.[38] An assessment of the chance of rupture of an asymptomatic saccular aneurysm is almost entirely based on a statistical analysis of the natural history of "similar lesions." Several factors combine to influence the magnitude of this risk (history of smoking, age, gender, number of aneurysms), and they all play a role in formulating techniques that would allow a more objective and individual estimation of risk. Research directed at the use of several evolving techniques in angiography, magnetic resonance, and ultrasound aimed at the improved imaging of hemodynamic stresses that affect aneurysms may better define the relationship between the stresses and the vascular remodeling seen in aneurysm wall degeneration and healing.[38] Aneurysm growth is a dynamic process that results from complex and incompletely understood interactions between hemodynamic forces and production of structural components that compose an aneurysm's wall. Due to physical limitations in the collagen present at the site where aneurysms form, it would be expected that a growth much larger than 8 mm in diameter would result in rupture. However, in most instances this does not occur. Changes in various hemodynamic factors (shear stress, pressure, and impingement force) as well as the presence of several humoral factors (inflammatory mediators and adhesion molecules) are potential signs of arterial injury. Sensing these signs, endothelium has the capacity to regulate the activity of substances that act to either promote or inhibit the repair of an aneurysm wall.[38] Combinations of CT, CTA, MRI, MRA, and ultrasound can in some instances measure both geometric relationships and physiologic parameters such as shear stress, pulse pressure, and compliance before and after a given intervention. As these techniques evolve, improve, and become more widely used, they will provide data that will be valuable in both the laboratory and in a clinical setting.[38]

CLASSIFICATION

Cerebral aneurysms present in a variety of sizes, shapes, and etiologies. When classified by size, the following categories are used:

- Small: to 10 mm
- Medium: 10 to 15 mm
- Large: 15 to 25 mm
- Giant: 25 to 50 mm
- Super-giant: larger than 50 mm

Classification by shape and etiology yields the following categories:

- **Berry aneurysm:** most common type; berry or saccular shaped with a neck or stem (Fig. 23-1)
- **Fusiform aneurysm:** an outpouching of an arterial wall, without a stem
- **Traumatic aneurysm:** any aneurysm resulting from a traumatic head injury (accounts for a small number)
- **Mycotic (infectious) aneurysm:** rare; caused by septic emboli from infections, such as bacterial endocarditis; may lead to aneurysmal formation
- **Charcot-Bouchard aneurysm:** microscopic aneurysmal formation associated with hypertension; involves the basal ganglia and brainstem

- **Dissecting aneurysm:** related to atherosclerosis, inflammation, or trauma; an aneurysm in which the intimal layer is pulled away from the medial layer and blood is forced between the layers

LOCATION

Cerebral aneurysms usually occur at the bifurcations and branches of the large arteries at the base of the brain (circle of Willis). Eighty-five percent of aneurysms develop in the anterior part of the circle of Willis. The remaining 15% are found in the posterior circulation, known as the vertebrobasilar system. (See Fig. 23-2 for distribution of aneurysms.)

The most common sites of saccular aneurysms are:

- 85% to 95% in the carotid system, with the following three most common locations:
  - A-comm is the single most common: 30%
  - ACA are more common in males
  - P-comm: 25%
  - MCA: 20%
- 5% to 15% in the posterior circulation (vertebrobasilar arteries)
  - About 10% on BA: basilar bifurcation, known as basilar tip, most common followed by basilar artery–superior cerebellar artery (BA-SCA), basilar artery–vertebral artery (BA-VA) junction, and AICA
  - About 5% on vertebral artery (VA) and posterior inferior cerebellar artery (PICA) junction is the most common
- Fusiform aneurysms are more common in the vertebrobasilar system
- 20% to 30% of patients who suffer an aneurysm will have multiple aneurysms

RUPTURED ANEURYSM

SAH is a type of intracranial hemorrhage in which bleeding occurs into the subarachnoid space. It accounts for 6% to 8% of all strokes and continues to be a significant cause of morbidity and mortality. Approximately 12% of patients die before receiving medical attention.[28] SAH is associated with mortality rates between 25% and 50% from the consequences

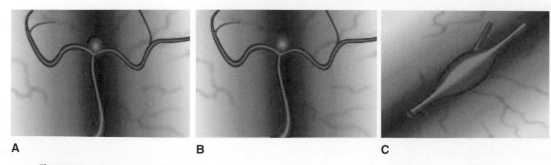

| A | B | C |

Figure 23-1 • Aneurysms. (*A*) Saccular (sac-like), with a well-defined neck. (*B*) Broad based with a wide neck. (*C*) Fusiform (spindle shaped) without a distinct neck. (Copyright 2005 University of California Regents.)

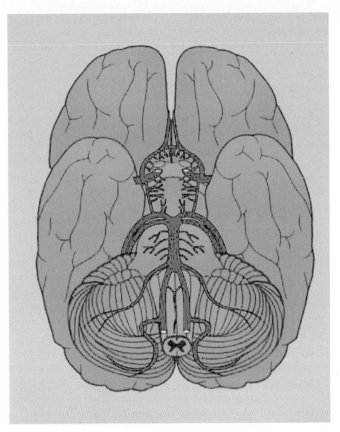

Figure 23-2 • Aneurysms located on arteries of the circle of Willis. (Netter Medical Images.)

The incidence of aneurysmal SAH is higher than most other neurological diseases such as brain tumor, multiple sclerosis, and bacterial meningitis. The incidence of other types of stroke (intracerebral hemorrhage and cerebral infarction) has declined over the years, while the incidence of aneurysmal subarachnoid hemorrhage remains the same.[4]

There is a possible reduced occurrence of SAH in some premenopausal women, especially those without a smoking history. In the same study, hormone replacement reduced the risk in postmenopausal women who had never smoked.[41] Racial differences have been infrequently studied, although there are data that indicate that the incidence rate in the African-American population is twice that of whites.[42] Age-related differences are detected, with increasing incidence of SAH with age.

Pathophysiology

At the time of aneurysmal rupture, blood under high pressure is forced into the subarachnoid space at the base of the brain (circle of Willis), spreading by way of the sylvian fissures into the basal cisterns. Less often the aneurysm ruptures into one of the following areas of the brain, resulting in formation of a hematoma: the brain parenchymal tissue (intracerebral hematoma); the ventricles (intraventricular hematoma); the subarachnoid space (subarachnoid hematoma); or the subdural space (subdural hematoma). When rupture occurs, it usually occurs at the thin-walled dome of the aneurysm, causing blood to enter into the subarachnoid space. Tissue pressure surrounding the aneurysm stops the bleeding, and fibrin, platelets, and fluid form a plug that seals off the site of bleeding. The resulting clot can occlude the area or interfere with CSF absorption. The blood released irritates the brain tissue, setting up an inflammatory response that enhances cerebral edema.

Concurrent with the time of rupture, significant SAH occurs, raising intracranial pressure (ICP) toward the mean arterial pressure and lowering cerebral perfusion pressure. These hemodynamic changes probably account for the transient loss of or altered level of consciousness. Clinically, a stroke syndrome with associated increased ICP develops. The specific signs and symptoms associated with the event depend on the location of the hemorrhage and the degree of ICP.

of the initial rupture. Approximately half of the untreated survivors will rebleed within the next 6 months, and among this group, morbidity and mortality are even higher.[39] Approximately 30% of people die within the first 2 weeks following the acute event, and many survivors have persistent long-term deficits. Although advanced imaging techniques have allowed the noninvasive detection of an aneurysm or AVM as the potential source of a bleed, most aneurysms are detected following rupture. After SAH has occurred, medical complications are aggressively treated, but morbidity from factors other than rebleeding is still common.

Natural History and Incidence of Subarachnoid Hemorrhage

Many questions regarding natural history of SAH can be answered from available data. SAH of any cause represents from 4.5% to 13% of all strokes. Age-adjusted incidence rates of SAH are available from numerous studies, with reported rates from 7.9 per 100,000 persons per year in Oxfordshire, England, to 15.1 per 100,000 in Helsinki, Finland. In Japan, there has been higher incident rates reported—21 to 25 per 100,000. Long-term trends are only available from Rochester, Minnesota, in population-based studies, which demonstrate that there is no change in the incidence rate of SAH through 1989. There are some gender-related differences, with female incidence higher than male in some population-based studies.[40]

SIGNS AND SYMPTOMS

Signs and symptoms arising from an aneurysm can be divided into two categories: those presenting before rupture or bleeding (**unruptured**), and those appearing after rupture or bleeding (**ruptured**).

Unruptured Aneurysms

Most patients are completely asymptomatic until the time of bleeding. A recent publication of the American Heart Association outlines the recommendations for management of patients with unruptured intracranial aneurysms.[43] In approximately 40% of cases, there are warning signs, often called *prodromal signs,* that are either ignored or attributed to other causes. Prodromal signs may suggest the location of the aneurysm or enlargement of the lesion. Localizing signs and symptoms include:

- Dilated pupil (loss of light reflex; oculomotor nerve [cranial nerve (CN) III] deficit)
- Extraocular movement deficits of the oculomotor (CN III), trochlear (CN IV) or abducens (CN VI) cranial nerves
- Possible ptosis (oculomotor nerve [CN III] deficit)
- Pain above and behind eye
- Localized headache
- Nuchal rigidity (neck pain on flexion)
- Possible photophobia

Small intermittent aneurysmal leakage of blood may result in generalized headache, neck pain, upper back pain, nausea, and vomiting. Management of unruptured intracranial aneurysms is controversial because of the lack of knowledge of the natural history of these lesions and the risks of repairing them.[18] A large multicenter study was conducted to determine the risk of rupture and the risks associated with the repair of unruptured intracranial aneurysms.

Whether all unruptured aneurysms should be treated has been debated for years. Clinical outcomes depend on various factors and require balancing early and delayed risks. There is minimal information available in the literature regarding the natural history of unruptured aneurysms. A published study of the natural history of aneurysm studies observed 130 patients for a follow-up that lasted 8.3 years. None of the aneurysms smaller than 1 cm in maximal diameter at discovery ruptured during follow-up, whereas 15 of 51 aneurysms 1 cm or larger ruptured during follow-up. In a review of 142 patients harboring 181 unruptured aneurysms (some had multiple aneurysms), 27 hemorrhages occurred during 1,944 patient-years of follow-up (mean 13.9 years) with an annual rupture rate of 1.4%. The size of the aneurysm was a predictor of hemorrhage. Other studies have suggested that there was not an insignificant risk of hemorrhage in small aneurysms and in others, selected locations, such as anterior communicating artery aneurysms, had been associated with increased rupture rate.[1]

International Study of Unruptured Intracranial Aneurysms

In 1998, the investigators of the Internation Study of Unruptured Intracranial Aneurysms (ISUIA) reported results from the initial aspects of the international collaborative study of unruptured intracranial aneurysms. The retrospective cohort study included patients with unruptured intracranial aneurysms diagnosed among 53 participating centers from 1970 to 1991. Patients with and without SAH were included, but analysis was performed based on the following categories:

- Group 1: patients without SAH
- Group 2: patients with an earlier SAH from an aneurysm, but with that ruptured aneurysm definitively treated, and having had another unruptured aneurysm

Patients with traumatic, mycotic, or fusiform aneurysms were not eligible. A prospective component including those

with and without surgical or endovascular treatment was also conducted, and the surgical results were reported in 1998. Hard copies of cerebral angiograms from all patients were reviewed at the Mayo Clinic. Long-term follow-up was conducted in both prospective and retrospective groups. In the retrospective cohort, 1449 patients with 1937 unruptured intracranial aneurysms (727 group 1 and 722 group 2) were observed during follow-up. There were 1085 (75%) who had a single unruptured intracranial aneurysm, and 364 had multiple unruptured intracranial aneurysms. Signs and symptoms leading to diagnosis of unruptured intracranial aneurysms included ischemic cerebrovascular disease, headaches, cranial nerve deficits, aneurysmal mass effect, ill-defined spells, and convulsive disorders.[1]

Several aneurysm characteristics were analyzed, including site, size, presence of daughter sac, and presence of multiple lobes. During the follow-up period, 32 of the 1449 patients had an aneurysm rupture, with 28 of 32 ruptures within the first 7.5 years of follow-up. Among group 1 patients with SAH, 1 of 12 was smaller than 10 mm in diameter, whereas 17 of 20 patients in group 2 with ruptures had aneurysms smaller than 10 mm in diameter.[1]

In group 1 patients, the only significant predictors of rupture were size and location of aneurysm. Aneurysms that were smaller than 10 mm were less likely to rupture than those 10 to 24 mm. There were other selected sites—basilar tip, vertebrobasilar and posterior communicating—that were at increased risk of rupture. In group 2, the relative risk of rupture was 5.1 ($p = 0.004$) for aneurysms at the basilar tip and 1.31 ($p = 0.04$) for older age. Size of aneurysm did not predict rupture in group 2 patients.

The cumulative rates of rupture for patients were:

- Group 1 patients (no previous SAH) with aneurysms smaller than 10 mm in diameter were 0.05% per year.
- Group 1 patients with aneurysms larger than 10 mm in diameter were 20 times higher—approaching 1% per year.
- Group 2 patients—smaller aneurysms (i.e., smaller than 10 mm) were 11 times more likely to rupture as aneurysms of the same size in group 1, at about 0.5% per year.
- The rupture rate of larger aneurysms (i.e., larger than 10 mm) was similar in group 2 patients compared with those in group 1, at about 1% per year.

Mortality for SAH was 66%. The paper also reported surgical intervention-related morbidity and mortality of the prospective cohort. At 1 month, group 1 patients' surgical mortality was 2.3%. Overall morbidity and mortality for all patients in group 1 were 17.5% at 1 month and 15.7% at 1 year.[1] A meta-analysis was performed in 1997 that reviewed 23 studies of prevalence and risk of rupture of intracranial saccular aneurysms. For adults without specific risk factors, the prevalence of intracranial saccular aneurysm was 2.3%, which increased with age. Nine studies were used to analyze risk of rupture, totaling 3907 patient-years. The highest risk per year was 1.9%. For aneurysms equal to 10 mm, the annual risk was 0.7% per year. The risk was slightly higher in women. The risk was also higher for those aneurysms larger than 10 mm in diameter, those that were symptomatic, and those in the posterior circulation.[44]

Since the publication of phase I of the ISUIA data in 1998, an expert panel concluded that "in consideration of the apparent low risk of hemorrhage from incidental small (<10 mm) aneurysms in patients without previous SAH, treatment rather than observation cannot be generally advocated."[43] The newest ISUIA information allows a more individualized and sophisticated assessment of the risks of natural history versus the risk of treatment (either surgical or endovascular) on the basis of much more than aneurysm size. With the group 1 patients with aneurysms smaller than 7 mm in size, it is unlikely that the natural history of these lesions can be improved, particularly with older patients and those with anterior circulation aneurysms. Current natural history studies including ISUIA include very few symptomatic patients with small unruptured intracranial aneurysms. An important element in decision making is age of the patient, as age has a major effect on operative morbidity and mortality and very little effect on natural history. It is also important to consider the long-term effects of the efficacy and durability of treatment of both surgical and endovascular procedures and to re-enforce the need for long-term follow-up in these patients.[3]

Asymptomatic Aneurysms

During the last two decades, detection of unruptured intracranial aneurysms has increased because of new and improved diagnostic tests (MRA, digital subtraction angiography, and three-dimensional CTA) and a more active treatment approach for patients with ruptured intracranial aneurysms. In addition, older patients are more likely to be treated than in the past.

The natural history of unruptured intracranial aneurysms is poorly understood, as are the risk factors. This is due to the lack of studies with sufficient patient numbers and follow-up years. The current knowledge of the natural history of unruptured aneurysm is based on only a few studies, with the risk factors being even more controversial because of the differing results published from these studies. Therefore, treatment decisions for unruptured aneurysms vary.[18,45-47]

In a long-term cohort study of 142 patients with unruptured aneurysms, Juvela et al.[47] conducted follow-up of 2575 person-years. They found an approximate rupture rate of 1.3% per year for an unruptured aneurysm. This overall rupture rate is similar to earlier observations of 1% to 2% per year[45] but somewhat lower than those reported in another study (2.3% per year),[46] and it is higher than that in the ISUIA study (0.3% per year).[18]

Aneurysms may be acquired degenerative lesions that develop as a result of hemodynamic stress, or they may be familial or associated with connective tissue diseases.[23] There may be unknown factors that increase the risk of aneurysm formation or SAH. Some of these factors include hypertension, cigarette smoking, use of oral contraceptives, female gender, atherosclerosis, aging, alcohol consumption, arterial deficiency in collagen type III, viral infections, arteriovenous malformations, asymmetry of the circle of Willis, pituitary tumors, and certain human leukocyte antigen–associated factors.[47,48]

The results of the studies conducted by Juvela et al. suggest that unruptured aneurysms should be treated regardless of size, at least in patients younger than 50 years old.[47,48] In older patients with small aneurysms, smoking cessation alone may be treatment enough. In North America and Europe, the prevalence of smoking in patients who suffer SAH ranges from 45% to 75%, whereas in the general adult population the range is 20% to 35%.[49] These studies concluded that unruptured intracranial aneurysms should be surgically treated, regardless of size, if technically possible, and that patient age and concurrent diseases do not increase surgical risk. Although cigarette smoking seems to increase the risk of aneurysm rupture, surgery should not be withheld in these cases because of the devastation that can result from aneurysmal rupture compared with the success rates attained in surgical treatment of unruptured aneurysms.[47]

Ruptured Aneurysm

The most frequent presentation of aneurysms is rupture, which most often produces SAH. Intracerebral hemorrhage occurs in 20% to 40% of cases (more common in those with aneurysms distal to the circle of Willis, e.g., MCA). Intraventricular bleeding occurs in 13% to 28% (most common in anterior communicating artery aneurysm; prognosis appears worse with about 64% mortality), whereas subdural blood is present in 2% to 5% of cases. At the time of rupture or bleeding, blood is forced into the subarachnoid space. The patient experiences a violent headache, often described as "explosive" or "the worst headache of my life." Immediate loss of consciousness may occur, or the level of consciousness may decrease. Vomiting is common. Other signs and symptoms include:

- Cranial nerve deficits (especially CNs III, IV, and VI); non–pupil-sparing CN III palsy produced by expanding posterior communicating artery aneurysm
- Those related to meningeal irritation, including nausea, vomiting, stiff neck, pain in the neck and back, and possible blurred vision or photophobia. Signs of meningeal irritation usually appear 4 to 8 hours after the SAH. Mild temperature elevation may accompany SAH.
- Those related to a stroke syndrome, including signs and symptoms related to the vascular territory involved and intracerebral hemorrhage (e.g., hemiparesis, hemiplegia, aphasia, cognitive deficits)
- Those related to cerebral edema and increased ICP (mass effect), including seizures, hypertension, bradycardia, and widening pulse pressure
- Those related to pituitary dysfunction secondary to irritation or edema resulting from the proximity of the gland to common locations of aneurysms and possibly causing diabetes insipidus and hyponatremia

Hunt-Hess Classification

Many different SAH grading systems have been proposed; the most widely used is the Hunt-Hess Classification. This system was initially designed for patients with SAH. It is a helpful tool to guide the physician in diagnosing the severity of SAH secondary to aneurysmal bleeding, as well as in timing surgical intervention if surgery is an option. The patient is assigned to a category on admission to the hospital (Table 23-2). Changes in the patient's condition are then monitored according to baseline. The original paper did not consider the patients' age, site of aneurysm, or time since hemorrhage; patients were graded on admission and preoperatively.

TABLE 23–2	HUNT-HESS CLASSIFICATION OF SUBARACHNOID HEMORRHAGES

GRADE	DESCRIPTION
I	Asymptomatic, or mild headache and slight nuchal rigidity
II	Cranial nerve (CN) palsy (e.g., oculomotor [CN III], abducens [CN VI]), moderate to severe headache, nuchal rigidity
III	Mild focal deficit, lethargy, or confusion
IV	Stupor, moderate to severe hemiparesis, early decerebrate rigidity
V	Deep coma, decerebrate rigidity, moribund appearance Add one grade for serious systemic disease (e.g., hypertension, chronic obstructive pulmonary disease) or severe vasospasm on angiography Modified classification adds the following:
0	Unruptured aneurysm
1a	No acute meningeal/brain reaction, but with fixed neurological deficit

TABLE 23–3	FISHER GRADING SCALE (AMOUNT OF BLOOD ON CT SCAN IS A PREDICTOR OF VASOSPASM)

FISHER GROUP	BLOOD ON CT
1	No subarachnoid blood detected
2	Diffuse or vertical layers <1 mm thick
3	Localized and/or vertical layers ≥1 mm
4	Intracerebral or intraventricular clot with diffuse or no subarachnoid hemorrhage

DIAGNOSIS

Diagnosis of a cerebral aneurysm is based on:

- History and results of neurological examination.
- CT scan, without contrast media; a good-quality fourth-generation CT will detect SAH in 95% or more of cases if scans are done within 48 hours of SAH. Blood appears as high density (i.e., appears white) within subarachnoid spaces.
- If the CT findings are negative, lumbar puncture is used in selective cases. Red blood cell (RBC) counts usually exceed 100,000 per mm.
- CTA is now being used in many institutions as the first radiographic tool. It is a more recent development than MRA, and its role is being refined, with a reported sensitivity of 95% and specificity of 83%. Unlike conventional angiography, CTA provides a three-dimensional image and demonstrates the relationship to nearby bony structures. With improved techniques in CT scanning, a scan can be completed in a matter of minutes to obtain data necessary to complete three-dimensional imaging of intracranial aneurysms.
- MRI is not sensitive within the first 24 to 48 hours, especially with thin layers of blood; it is more satisfactory after 4 to 7 days. MRA is also used.
- Cerebral angiography remains the "gold standard" for evaluation of cerebral aneurysms. It demonstrates a source of the aneurysm in about 80% to 85% of cases and radiologic vasospasm (i.e., a narrowing of the cerebral blood vessels as seen on radiographic films).

Imaging

Computed Tomography

CT remains the mainstay of initial detection of SAH, with 90% or better sensitivity in detecting a clinically significant SAH in the first 2 days after the event. It is important to realize that a negative CT scan never excludes SAH and that a clinical suggestion of an SAH, even in the face of a negative CT scan, still requires a lumbar puncture.[87]

A plain CT scan obtained within 48 hours of aneurysmal rupture is usually the initial diagnostic procedure ordered. If the scan is performed within 24 hours of the initial SAH, a high-density clot in the subarachnoid space can be demonstrated in 92% to 95% of cases; if done within 48 hours, the clot can be demonstrated in 75% to 85% of cases.[8,45] A CT scan also aids in establishing the extent and location of subarachnoid bleeding and is useful for identifying patients at high risk for the development of vasospasm and for pinpointing the potential vascular territory of the vasospasm.

The Fisher Grading Scale (Table 23-3) is used to assist in prediction of outcome. The amount of blood on CT scan correlates with the severity of cerebral vasospasm.

If an angiogram is ordered and multiple aneurysms are seen, the CT scan is helpful in identifying which aneurysm bled, based on the presence of a clot.

Spiral Computed Tomography Angiography

Spiral CTA using the slip ring technology allows visualization of arterial anatomy after IV administration of a timed bolus of contrast material and can acquire images in a very short time. This new technique is often used as a first step in evaluation of patients with a diagnosis of SAH who are being transferred into a tertiary care facility. The images can provide an immediate diagnosis for the physician managing the patient. Patients have been brought to the operating room or endovascular suite based on these images to reduce any further time from treatment of the lesion. Imaging time is generally 30 to 40 seconds. This is an extremely helpful technology in the primary evaluation of patients with diagnosis of SAH. One disadvantage of the technique is the load of contrast material that is administered, although the benefits often outweigh the risks.

- The examination is begun in the location of interest, either the circle of Willis or the carotid bifurcation, using contiguous unenhanced 5-mm-thick axial sections. After the area of interest is determined, nonionic contrast is injected IV via an automated power injector into an 18-gauge angiocatheter in the antecubital vein at a rate of 5 mL/sec for a total of 120-mL volume, with a 25-second delay between the injection and the onset of data acquisition.[50]

- Two-dimensional maximum intensity projection (MIP) views and three-dimensional surface-rendered and volume-rendered reconstructions are reformatted from the raw image data from the workstation by neuroradiologists, CTA technicians, and/or treating neurovascular specialists in a three-dimension lab. By using this new technology, the Massachusetts General Hospital (MGH) neurovascular group has been able to diagnose and manage approximately 80% of aneurysm patients using CTA alone. This is true for both ruptured and unruptured aneurysms.[50] CTA was able to detect 100% of symptomatic aneurysms (ruptured aneurysms plus presenting aneurysms) in this MGH study.

Another nice feature of CTA is its rapidity. For patients presenting in the emergency room with presumed diagnosis of subarachnoid hemorrhage, the data can be acquired and analyzed within 15 to 20 minutes. The films can be expeditiously reviewed by the clinicians, and a decision can be made to treat the aneurysm with either a surgical or an endovascular approach. This technology has greatly facilitated the care of some critically ill patients who can forgo angiography prior to aneurysm treatment. Patients can be studied as outpatients as well, and the study can be completed in 30 to 40 minutes.[50]

Overall, the advantages of CTA are that it is noninvasive; it is much quicker (the actual scanning time is 2 to 3 minutes); it requires fewer resources (equipment, staffing, and cost); it does not require sedation (in the majority of patients); it is not painful to the patient; and it is a suitable test for the critically ill patient. CTA can detail the anatomy of branch vessels in relation to the aneurysm (Fig. 23-3). It can also detail the bony anatomy in relationship to the aneurysm. These details give the treating physician an excellent idea of what

the surgery or endovascular treatment may involve prior to undergoing the procedure. This minimizes the risk to the patient, as the potential pitfalls of surgery can be anticipated prior to undergoing the treatment. Images can also be rotated in any direction to view the aneurysm from a variety of angles on the computer workstation. The view from the surgical approach can be chosen well in advance to the surgery. CTA has proven to be a useful tool in the diagnosis and management of aneuryms.[50]

CTA is a reliable alternative to MRA in evaluating the circle of Willis and carotid bifurcation. At some institutions, specific applications include triaging patients for possible superselective thrombolysis, following patients with carotid stents, and evaluating multiperspective approaches to intracranial aneurysms. Additionally, CTA may ultimately demonstrate advantages in the screening of aneurysms in the appropriate patient population.

Angiography

Cerebral angiography (Fig. 23-4) is still the mainstay of diagnosis for cerebral aneurysms in most centers, but with the advent of CTA, this appears to be changing. Angiography provides visualization of all four major cerebral vessels and their branches. Angiography is commonly scheduled immediately following diagnosis of SAH by CT scan or CTA in patients who are deemed clinically stable. If not clinically stable, the CTA often provides enough information to offer complete treatment of the aneurysm. Early angiography or CTA allows for definitive diagnosis and enables the cerebrovascular team of physicians (neurosurgeon, interventional neuroradiologist, and neurologist) to advocate a treatment plan for the patient. In addition to the specific location

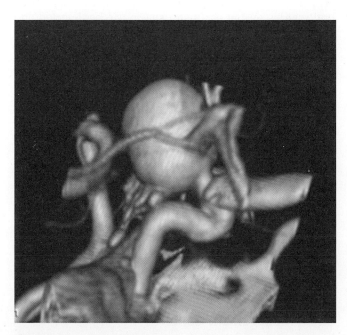

Figure 23-3 • Computed tomography angiogram demonstrating right paraclinoid. (Courtesy of Christopher S. Ogilvy, MD, Massachusetts General Hospital, Boston, MA.)

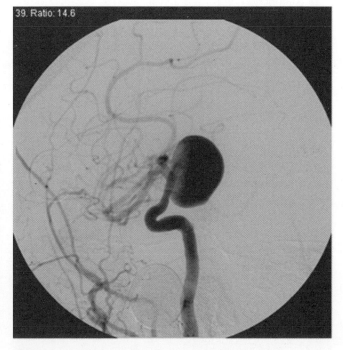

Figure 23-4 • Angiogram demonstrating right paraclinoid aneurysm. (Courtesy of Christopher S. Ogilvy, MD, Massachusetts General Hospital, Boston, MA.)

of the aneurysm, the following points can be identified using angiography:

- The particular characteristics of the aneurysm (shape, size, presence of daughter sac)
- Any anomalies of cerebral vasculature (e.g., involving the circle of Willis) that will affect treatment decision
- The presence of vasospasm, which may influence the urgency to obliterate the aneurysm either surgically or endovascularly, so that triple H (hypervolemic, hemodilution, and hypertensive) therapy or some combination, such as hypervolemic hypertensive management, can be initiated

Repeat Cerebral Angiography. Repeat angiography may be performed for the following reasons:

- Confirmation of diagnosis when no aneurysm is found on early angiography (small aneurysms can be missed, particularly in the posterior circulation). Angiogram is usually repeated 10 days to 2 weeks after the initial study.
- Identification of reversal of previously observed vasospasm
- Detection and treatment of vasospasm when there is deterioration of neurological function (change in level of consciousness is the most common situation)

Negative Angiogram and Subarachnoid Hemorrhage. It is generally believed that if an aneurysm is not found with a thorough cerebral angiogram in a patient with a documented SAH, in approximately 5% of the cases, this represents a false-negative result. Explanations range from transient thrombosis of the aneurysm to vasospasm, technical error, or ruptured pial vascular malformation. Repeat angiography, looking at both the cerebral anatomy as well as the spine to rule out spinal arteriovenous fistula or AVM in conjunction with head and neck CTA, is generally recommended in such patients 1 week to 10 days after the initial angiogram. Historically, many practitioners recommended a third angiogram, usually at 3 months after the initial angiogram, to ensure normal cerebral vasculature. Currently, some centers are comfortable with two negative angiograms and CTAs if the hemorrhage pattern on the CT scan is in fact perimesencephalic. Other centers are opting to have the patient undergo a CTA rather than conventional angiography at 3 months to further confirm normal vasculature of the brain and spine.

Perimesencephalic nonaneurysmal SAH is a distinct entity and considered a benign condition with a good outcome. This group has less risk of rebleeding and vasospasm than other patients with SAH of unknown etiology. The actual etiology is yet to be determined, but it may be secondary to rupture of a small perimesencephalic vein or artery. Small aneurysms may obliterate themselves after rupture, leaving no aneurysm to be found on angiography. This type of aneurysm may be referred to as a *cryptic aneurysm.*

Magnetic Resonance Imaging

MRI plays only a minor role in the diagnosis of acute SAH because of the unstable condition of many of these patients and the relatively high insensitivity of MRI to acute subarachnoid blood. The inherent contrast of MRI depends on clot retraction and deoxygenation of the hemoglobin. In the acute stages of a bleed, this clot retraction does not occur readily when blood is mixed with CSF. The hemoglobin molecule remains better oxygenated after an SAH than after bleeding into the parenchyma. Thus, CT scan remains the examination modality of choice in the evaluation of an acute SAH.

Magnetic Resonance Angiography

MRA evaluation of aneurysms yields the best results with aneurysms 0.5 to 1.5 cm. MRA can assist in the evaluation of aneurysms, particularly when they are larger than 3 mm in diameter. MRI and MRA should be reserved as tools to assist in the evaluation of patients with possible symptoms of aneurysm and not used in those who have had an acute hemorrhage. This procedure will also screen for possible causes that may elicit symptoms relative to headache or mass effect, such as an arteriovenous malformation or arterial fistula. Given these limitations, high-resolution angiography may still be necessary to exclude aneurysms smaller than 3 mm.[51]

Lumbar Puncture

LP is used only if a CT scan is unavailable, if there is no evidence of increased ICP (e.g., papilledema) and the CT scan results are negative or inconclusive, and if there is also the need to establish evidence of SAH. An LP is contraindicated in the presence of increased ICP because of the risk of brainstem herniation; it also increases the risk of rebleeding. CSF analysis reveals blood; xanthochromia (discoloration of CSF) is noted when the CSF is centrifuged.

Transcranial Doppler

Transcranial Doppler (TCD) series is a technology that is often used on a daily basis in most neurological intensive care units (NICUs) in patients who have suffered SAH. The purpose of TCD is to monitor flow velocities in major cerebral arteries so that early vasospasm can be detected and treated. Mean velocities of greater than 120 cm/sec are considered mild vasospasm, greater than 150 cm/sec moderate vasospasm, and greater than 200 cm/sec severe vasospasm.

▨ INITIAL APPROACH TO MEDICAL MANAGEMENT

The patient who survives the initial rupture of a cerebral aneurysm is beset by various potential problems and complications that can lead to additional morbidity and mortality. Consideration of whether to treat or how to treat a ruptured cerebral aneurysm depends on various factors: age of the patient, the neurological condition of the patient (Hunt-Hess grade), Fisher grade, or size of the aneurysm. The patient's current or previous medical condition may also factor into the decision-making process.

Initial Management Concerns

- Rebleeding—the major concern during the initial workup. Maximal frequency of rebleeding is in the first day

(4% on day 1, then 1.5% daily for 13 days). Between 15% and 20% rebleed within 14 days, and 50% will rebleed within 6 months; thereafter, the risk is 3%/year with a mortality of 2%/year.

- Acute hydrocephalus—usually obstructive because of obstruction of CSF by a blood clot
- Delayed ischemic neurological deficit most likely related to vasospasm
- Hyponatremia with hypovolemia
- Deep venous thrombosis (DVT) and pulmonary embolism
- Seizure
- Determining source of bleeding; a CTA or four-vessel cerebral angiography is required depending on the institution.

The **goals of initial medical management** include:

- Augmenting cerebral blood flow (CBF) by:
  - Increasing cerebral perfusion pressure (CPP)
  - Improving blood rheology
  - Maintaining euvolemia (the majority of patients become hypovolemic in the first 24 hours after SAH)
  - Maintaining normal ICP
- Neuroprotection

Patients are admitted to the NICU where the following can be provided:

- An arterial line is placed (for those patients who are hemodynamically unstable, stuporous, or comatose).
- Patient is intubated (comatose or unable to protect airway).
- Pulmonary artery catheter (PAC) line is placed for those with a Hunt-Hess grade of 3 or higher, those with syndrome of inappropriate antidiuretic hormone (SIADH), or those who are hemodynamically unstable.
- Cardiac monitor attached—SAH may be associated with cardiac arrhythmias and there are changes measurable on electrocardiogram in more than 50% of cases.
- Intraventricular catheter is placed in patients developing hydrocephalus and with a Hunt-Hess grade of 3 or higher.

Nursing responsibilities include:

- Vital signs with neurological checks every hour
- O_2 saturation monitoring
- Bed rest with head of bed (HOB) elevated by 30 degrees
- Low level of external stimulation; restricted visitation
- Strict intake and output (I&O) record
- Thigh-high antiembolic (TED) hose and pneumatic compression boots
- Indwelling urinary catheter if patient is lethargic, incontinent, or unable to void

Fluid Volume Control

One of the goals of medical management is to maintain fluid volume within a normal range (euvolia). The underlying reason for this is that dehydration increases hemoconcentration, which is thought to increase the incidence of cerebral vasospasm. If cerebral edema is present, a regimen of moderate fluid restriction and steroids may be ordered. Mannitol may be ordered to decrease cerebral edema. Early aggressive fluid therapy may prevent cerebral salt wasting.

- Normal saline IV solution with 20 mEq KCl/L at 2 mL/kg/hr
- 5% albumin, 500 mL over 6 hours, started immediately at admission

Blood Pressure Control

In the early hours after rupture, blood pressure is commonly elevated, probably reflecting a physiologic response to increased ICP. As ICP is decreased, the blood pressure also decreases. If the blood pressure continues to be elevated owing to increased ICP from mass effect of cerebral edema or a hematoma, mannitol may be administered. The drug is beneficial for two reasons: (1) it decreases cerebral edema and neurological deficits, and (2) it improves CBF. Decreased cerebral edema lowers the ICP and blood pressure.

Hypertension is controlled to prevent rebleeding. The goal of therapy is to maintain the systolic blood pressure between 120 and 150 mm Hg. Systolic pressures above this level are treated with drugs such as labetalol, nitroprusside, or nicardipine. Nitroprusside and nicardipine are used in conjunction with an arterial line. They are vasodilators and may increase the risk of rupture with an unsecured aneurysm. These drugs effectively lower the pressure without sudden drops in the systolic pressure and are easily titrated.

CLINICAL VIGNETTE: LW is a 46-year-old woman with a history of migraines. She had severe headaches with intermittent nausea 3 weeks prior to hospital admission. Twelve days prior to admission she experienced the worst headache of her life and presented to her local emergency room several times. She was treated with pain medication and sent home. One day prior to admission, she went to a different emergency room for her persistent headaches. A CT scan was performed, which demonstrated intraparenchymal hemorrhage (Fig. 23-5) and a subarachnoid hemorrhage with a Hunt Hess grade of 1 and Fisher grade of 4. She was transferred to a tertiary care facility where a CTA (Fig. 23-6) was performed demonstrating a 12-mm right distal M1 multilobulated saccular aneurysm with large right frontal intraparenchymal hemorrhage causing mass effect. There is also a 4-mm aneurysm on the left distal M1 segment pointing superiorly. She was neurologically intact with some intermittent nausea. She is a 20-pack-year smoker and currently smokes one pack per day.

The cerebrovascular team decided surgery was the best mode of treatment due to the hematoma and aneurysm location and proceeded the following morning with a right frontotemporal craniotomy for clot evacuation and right MCA aneurysm clipping. Since she presented several days with postsubarachnoid hemorrhage, she remained at some risk for vasospasm. She was on nimodipine 60 mg PO q4h and had daily TCD monitoring. She did very well postoperatively with no vasospasm. She was neurologically intact, had minimal pain, and was discharged home on postoperative day 6 with home health care nursing and physical therapy.

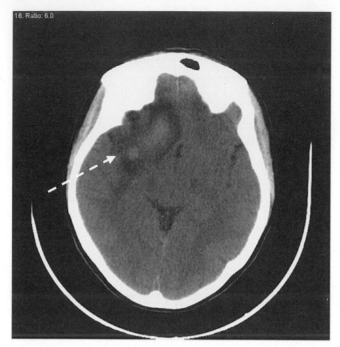

Figure 23-5 • Computed tomography scan demonstrating an intraparenchymal hemorrhage. (Courtesy of Christopher S. Ogilvy, MD, Massachusetts General Hospital, Boston, MA.)

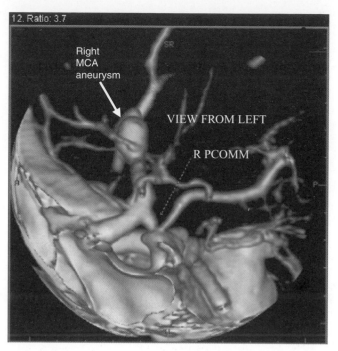

Figure 23-6 • Computed tomography angiogram demonstrating a 12-mm right distal M1 multilobulated saccular aneurysm with large right frontal intraparenchymal hemorrhage causing mass effect. MCA, middle cerebral artery; R PCOMM, right posterior communicating artery. (Courtesy of Christopher S. Ogilvy, MD, Massachusetts General Hospital, Boston, MA.)

> **CLINICAL PEARLS:** Patients who present to the emergency room with the "worst headache of their life" need a thorough neurological evaluation, which includes diagnostic testing such as a CT scan and/or lumbar puncture to evaluate for SAH.

Electrocardiographic Changes

The association between SAH and electrocardiography (ECG) has been known since 1954 when Burch et al. noted an ECG pattern of Q-T prolongation and T-wave inversion in patients with SAH.[52] Subsequent investigations have determined that ECG abnormalities occur in 25% to 75% of patients with SAH.[53]

The pathophysiology of cardiac injury in patients with SAH appears to result from an excess of catecholamines in the myocardium. The "catecholamine hypothesis" remains controversial, and other proposed mechanisms include coronary arterial spasm, coronary artery disease, and injury caused by elevated myocardial wall stress in the setting of tachycardia and hypertension.

The prognostic importance of ECG changes in association with SAH has been examined in small studies with varying results. It is unclear whether these ECG changes are predictive of cardiac mortality or are simply a reflection of the underlying central nervous system process.

Zaroff et al.[54] conducted a retrospective study of 439 patients with SAH with abnormal ECG changes and determined the incidence of cardiac and all-cause mortality. They found that 27% of the study population had ECG readings that met the criteria for myocardial ischemia or infarction. This study indicates that patients with SAH and ischemic ECG readings are at low risk for cardiac mortality, with or without aneurysm surgery.

One may conclude that surgery should not be withheld from patients with SAH on the basis of ischemic ECG changes alone. The patients with a higher Hunt-Hess grade may be at greater risk for poor neurological outcomes without aggressive therapy such as surgery or endovascular treatment.[54]

Drug Therapy

The following drugs are usually ordered for the patient with an aneurysmal rupture:

- The calcium channel blocker nimodipine (Nimotop) 60 mg q4h orally or through nasogastric tube, initiated within 96 hours of SAH, is given for 21 consecutive days. Nimodipine may also be given 30 mg q2h as it can decrease blood pressure significantly. Nimodipine has been shown to enhance collateral blood flow and improve long-term outcomes in patients with SAH from aneurysm rupture.
- Anticonvulsants may be given as prophylaxis against seizures. Phenytoin is the usual agent used; provide a load with 17 mg/kg, maintenance with 100 mg three times daily.
- Stool softeners prevent constipation and straining at stool, which results in initiation of Valsalva's maneuver, increased ICP, and increased blood pressure, which in turn can cause rebleeding of the aneurysm.
- Use of steroids is controversial; however, some believe it is beneficial for treatment of cerebral edema and the inflammatory effect of the meningeal irritation. A typical regimen is Decadron taper: 4 mg PO/IV/NG q6h × 1 day;

3 mg PO/IV/NG q6h × 2 days; 2 mg PO/IV/NG q6h × 2 days; 1 mg PO/IV/NG q6h × 1 day.

- Nexium 20 mg PO daily or ranitidine 150 mg PO bid to prevent gastric irritation from steroids and antacids such as Mylanta 30 mL PO/NG QID PRN
- Analgesics (acetaminophen or codeine/morphine/Dilaudid) are administered as necessary to control headache.
- Sedatives may be prescribed, because an agitated patient is at risk for elevated blood pressure.
- Heparin 5000 units SQ bid or Fragmin 2500 units SQ daily to help prevent emboli
- Insulin (regular human) drip sliding scale may be ordered. For blood sugar (BS) less than 200 units, give 0 units; for BS 201 to 250 units, give 4 units; for BS 251 to 300 units, give 6 units; for BS 301 to 350 units, give 8 units; for BS 351 to 400 units, give 10 units; for BS greater than 400 units, give 12 units and call house doctor; SQ q6h.
- Replacement of minerals such as potassium, magnesium, calcium, and phosphorus is necessary based on laboratory testing. Magnesium 1000 mg PO tid is a frequently seen order. Magnesium level should be greater than 1.8.

Monitoring for Complications

In the acute phase, most patients are managed in the NICU, where they can be observed frequently and monitored with invasive hemodynamic monitoring equipment by a well-trained and knowledgeable nursing staff. The rationale for monitoring of neurological signs and other parameters is early detection of complications. The major complications of aneurysmal rupture are *rebleeding, cerebral vasospasm,* and *hydrocephalus,* which are discussed in a later section of this chapter. Other problems associated with aneurysmal rupture/bleed are reflected in laboratory studies and the results of an electrocardiogram. The following are pertinent data.

Blood Studies

- White blood cell (WBC) count: often elevated (15,000 to 18,000) as a result of meningeal irritation
- Hematocrit, fibrinogen, and platelets; bleeding time and osmolality: indicators of development of cerebral vasospasm
- Electrolytes: hyponatremia often develops as a result of SIADH or salt wasting
- Blood gases: monitor adequacy of oxygenation
- Glucose: hyperglycemia can worsen outcome for subarachnoid hemorrhage patients, as it can increase free radical formation, promote inflammation, disrupt the blood–brain barrier, and increase calcium influx.[55]

Electrocardiogram

Changes related to hypothalamic dysfunction result in elevated serum catecholamine levels. Catecholamines stimulate alpha-adrenergic receptors in the myocardium, possibly causing ST changes, prolonged QRS, prolonged Q-T interval, and tall T waves. ECG changes may be consistent with endocardial damage and sometimes myocardial ischemia. Consultation with a cardiologist experienced in the care of patients with SAH is beneficial and can avoid delay in treatment with early intervention.

SURGICAL/INTERVENTIONAL TREATMENT

Surgery historically has been the treatment of choice for a ruptured or bleeding cerebral aneurysm. Currently, the endovascular approach for treating ruptured aneurysms has been gaining increasing worldwide acceptance as an alternative to neurosurgical clipping due to the recent publication of the International Subarachnoid Aneurysm Trial (ISAT) in *Lancet* on October 26, 2002. The ISAT produced exciting results with potential benefits for coiled patients, but the long-term efficacy of coils remains questionable.

With the advent of interventional procedures using such devices as the Guglielmi detachable coil (GDC), balloons, and stents, there are now options in the modality of treatment. Technical advances since the GDC development over 10 years ago include three-dimensional and complex shaped coils and ultrasoft coils, balloon-assisted embolization, and intravascular stent-assisted embolization. Placement of GDCs and other embolic devices into cerebral aneurysms is rapidly gaining acceptance as an alternative to surgical clipping and in many centers is the treatment of choice. Consideration of various factors, including age of the patient, size and shape of the aneurysm, location of the aneurysm, the neurological condition of the patient (Hunt-Hess grade), and previous medical conditions, is necessary when deciding the best treatment option. The goal of treatment, either surgical or interventional, is to prevent rebleeding by sealing off the aneurysm so that the aneurysm is totally obliterated with either a clip or coil. In situations in which the patient is gravely ill, the decision may be to coil the dome of the aneurysm (where rupture occurred) and after the patient's condition stabilizes, operate and clip the entire aneurysm.

Timing of Treatment

Timing of treatment is critical to patient outcome. As a result of studies demonstrating improved outcomes from earlier treatment, there has been a definite trend toward early (within 24 to 48 hours after hemorrhage) treatment for those patients who present with aneurysmal SAH. Even patients whose condition is assessed as poor (Hunt-Hess grades 4 and 5) are considered for early treatment, depending on the stability of their overall medical condition. The following are the benefits of early treatment:

- Results in superior management in overall care
- Eliminates the problem of rebleeding
- Allows for removal of basal cistern clots associated with vasospasm
- Permits institution of previously mentioned triple H (hypervolemic, hemodilution, and hypertensive) therapy for postoperative vasospasm without the risk of rebleeding

Surgical Approaches and Considerations

Microsurgical techniques and improved anesthesia allow for a precise surgical approach and clipping of aneurysms. The surgical approach and method of aneurysmal obliteration depends on the location and characteristics of the aneurysm. An aneurysm with a stem or neck is usually managed with a

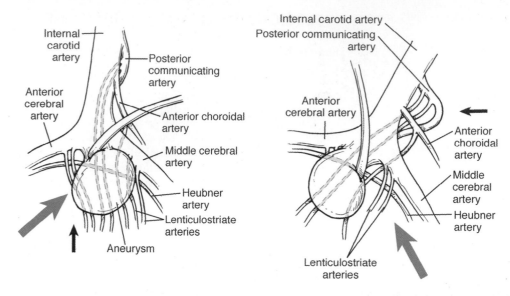

Figure 23-7 • Microexposure and visualization of the perforating vessels near the aneurysm. *Shaded arrows* indicate frontal and temporal surgical access. *Small black arrow* indicates lateral carotid accesses. *Small black arrow* points to sylvian accesses. (Courtesy of Christopher S. Ogilvy, MD, Massachusetts General Hospital, Boston, MA.)

surgical clip on the neck (Figs. 23-7, 23-8, and 23-9; see also Chap. 14). Depending on the location and size of the aneurysm, more than one clip may be necessary to obliterate it (Figs. 23-10 and 23-11). The surgeon may choose from a wide selection of commercial clips of different sizes, shapes, and angulations. For aneurysms that are difficult to reach, the surgeon may have to modify a clip to accommodate the

vessels and structures at the aneurysmal site. Before permanent clips are positioned, temporary clips are often applied medial or distal to the aneurysm to minimize blood flow to the aneurysm so as to improve the exposure to the aneurysm and to ensure proper placement of the permanent clip. The temporary clips, which are softer and gold tipped, are removed after the aneurysmal neck has been securely

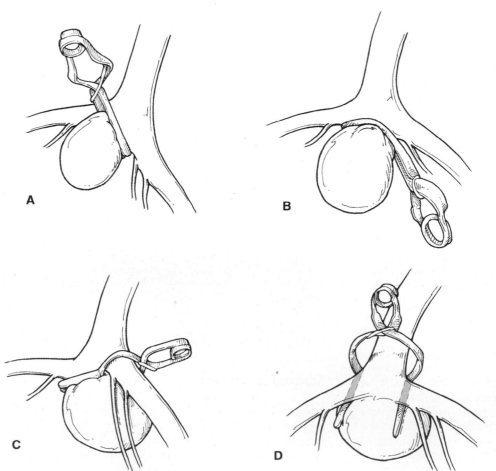

Figure 23-8 • Clipping techniques. (*A*) Straight clip for small aneurysms. (*B*) Curved clip to reconstruct the vessel. (*C*) Fenestrated clip encircles the middle cerebral artery to keep it open while clipping the aneurysm. (*D*) Fenestrated clip encircles the internal carotid artery to occlude the neck of an inferiorly directed aneurysm. (Courtesy of Christopher S. Ogilvy, MD, Massachusetts General Hospital, Boston, MA.)

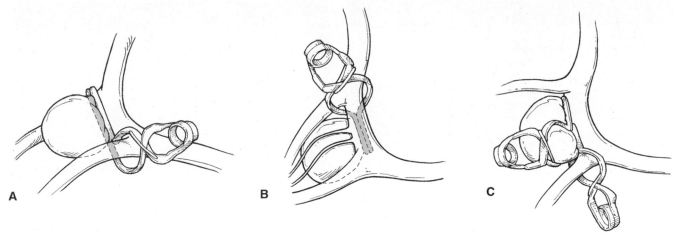

Figure 23-9 • Clipping strategies with fenestrated clips. (*A*) Here, a side-deflected fenestrated clip is used to occlude the aneurysm neck while reconstructing the neck of the A2 vessel. (*B*) An angled fenestrated clip reconstructs the anterior communicating artery, saving perforating branches. (*C*) Two fenestrated clips are used to clip a wide neck aneurysm. (Courtesy of Christopher S. Ogilvy, MD, Massachusetts General Hospital, Boston, MA.)

clipped. The adequacy of vascular territory circulation is verified before the permanent clips are applied (Figs. 23-12, 23-13, and 23-14).

Intraoperative angiography, CBF studies, or intraoperative Doppler studies may be conducted during surgery to verify the adequacy of circulation and the security of the clip. Some aneurysms, such as fusiform aneurysms, are not amenable to clipping because of their shape or location. In such situations, the aneurysm may be surgically wrapped in muslin, which provides support to the weakened arterial wall and also induces scarring. Newer techniques for obliterating fusiform aneurysms include a bypass and an end-to-end anastomosis of arteries once the fusiform section is dissected and removed.

If multiple aneurysms are present, it may not be possible to obliterate all lesions at one surgery. The priority site is the aneurysm that has bled, after it has been identified by

CT/CTA and angiography. A second surgical or endovascular procedure may be planned for a later date, if indicated. Alternatives to direct surgical clipping of an aneurysm include:

- Wrapping—although this is usually not the goal of surgery, situations may arise in which little else can be done (e.g., fusiform aneurysms).
- Trapping—effective treatment requires distal and proximal arterial interruption by direct surgical means (ligation or occlusion with clip), by placement of a detachable balloon, or a combination. It may also necessitate extracranial-intracranial (EC-IC) bypass to maintain flow distal to the trapped segment proximal ligation.

Certain situations require special considerations by the neurosurgeon. For example, with a large aneurysm involving the

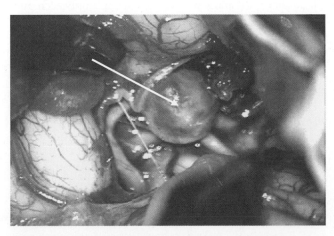

Figure 23-10 • Intraoperative photo of middle cerebral artery aneurysm. (Courtesy of Christopher S. Ogilvy, MD, Massachusetts General Hospital, Boston, MA.)

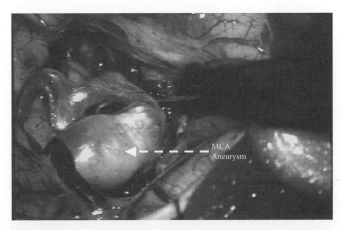

MCA Aneurysm

Figure 23-11 • Intraoperative photo of dissection of middle cerebral artery aneurysm prior to clipping. *Dashed arrow* points to middle cerebral aneurysm. (Courtesy of Christopher S. Ogilvy, MD, Massachusetts General Hospital, Boston, MA.)

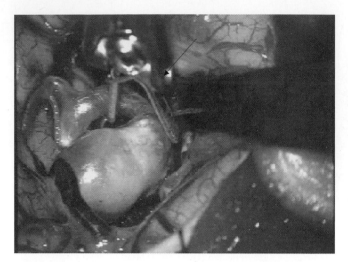

Figure 23-12 • Intraoperative photo of surgeon about to place clip on middle cerebral artery aneurysm. (Courtesy of Christopher S. Ogilvy, MD, Massachusetts General Hospital, Boston, MA.)

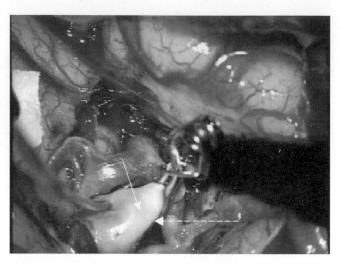

Figure 23-14 • Intraoperative photo demonstrating final clip placement. *Arrows* point to deflated aneurysm. (Courtesy of Christopher S. Ogilvy, MD, Massachusetts General Hospital, Boston, MA.)

basilar tip, special precautions must be taken to prevent injury to the small perforating branches emitted from this area. If these vessels are compromised, the patient may not awaken and may develop thalamic infarcts, depending on the extent of the injury. Some neurosurgeons consider using cardiac arrest bypass surgery to clip these large posterior circulation lesions. More often, these lesions are considered for endovascular coiling therapy. Prolonged cardiac arrest can be tolerated under deep hypothermia and artificial extracorporeal circulation. The techniques involved are very complicated, and a skilled surgeon who is confident in the use of this technique is necessary.

Special considerations are also warranted with a mycotic aneurysm. Mycotic aneurysms account for approximately 4% of intracranial aneurysms and occur in 3% to 15% of patients with subacute bacterial endocarditis. Usually located at the distal end of a vessel, the most common location is the distal

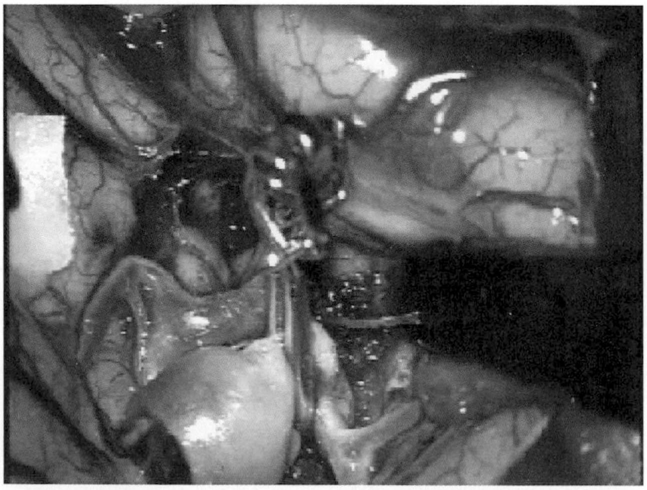

MCA branches (75% to 80%). Treatment with antibiotics for 4 to 6 weeks may result in disappearance of the lesion. However, if the aneurysm remains and enlarges, surgical or endovascular treatment may be necessary.

International Subarachnoid Aneurysm Trial

The ISAT is a multicenter randomized trial comparing neurosurgical clipping with endovascular coiling in patients with ruptured intracranial aneurysms.[56] The ISAT, funded by the United Kingdom's Medical Research Council, is the first multicenter randomized study in the world to compare the two modes of treating aneurysms.

The ISAT randomly assigned 2143 patients with a ruptured aneurysm to either clipping or coiling. Centers had to have expertise in both surgical and endovascular management of ruptured aneurysms. All participating centers were major neurosurgical sites treating between 60 and 200 cases annually. Endovascular physicians had to have performed a minimum of 30 aneurysm procedures, while only accredited neurosurgeons with experience in aneurysm surgery were able to participate in this trial. Patients were enrolled in 43 centers throughout Europe, North America, and Australia and one center in the United States. The ISAT started recruitment in 1997 and stopped enrollment in 2002 after an interim analysis showed a benefit of endovascular treatment on the primary endpoint—death or dependency at 1 year. It was discovered that at 1 year, 23.7% of coiled patients were dead and disabled compared to 30.6% of patients who underwent surgical clipping of their aneurysm. There was an absolute overall risk reduction of 6.9% in the coiled patients.[57]

The results of the study were statistically significant, but the biologic significance must be considered. The coiling treatment leaves the possibility for coil compaction or aneurysm growth over time. This may result in aneurysm rebleeding. Longer-term follow-up is important to assess the question of durability and efficacy. The ISAT found that the

Figure 23-13 • Intraoperative photo securing aneurysm clip at neck of middle cerebral artery aneurysm. (Courtesy of Christopher S. Ogilvy, MD, Massachusetts General Hospital, Boston, MA.)

risk of rebleeding after coiling was 26 out of 1048 with available follow-up at 1 year after treatment (2.4%). In their surgical group, there were 10 out of 994 patients who bled after treatment by 1 year (1%). Surgical clipping reduced the bleeding by over 50% compared to the endovascularly treated patients. If this rate continues, surgical treatment may be the optimal means to treat ruptured aneurysms.

These data highlight the need for short-term and long-term follow-up for ruptured aneurysms after treatment. The ISAT reveals exciting results for endovascularly treated patients, but the long-term efficacy and durability of coils remain a question. The study provides a framework for other future studies in the United States and other countries.

Endovascular Treatment of Aneurysms

Despite recent advances in neurological surgery and intensive care management, the morbidity and mortality rates of patients who survive an initial SAH remain high. A high percentage of patients may not be surgical candidates for various reasons. The management of intracranial aneurysms continues to evolve, particularly the endovascular management component. The use of electrically detachable platinum coils for the endovascular treatment of intracranial aneurysms was first described by Guglielmi et al.[58] GDCs were prospectively evaluated in selected North American medical centers to determine their use in treating intracranial aneurysms that were not amenable to direct surgical treatment. Electrothrombosis occurs when a positively charged electrode that has been placed in the bloodstream attracts negatively charged blood elements—RBCs and WBCs, platelets, and fibrinogen. Electrolysis occurs when two electrodes positioned in a solution are connected to a direct current. When direct current is applied to the coil system, the positively charged platinum coils promote electrothrombosis while at the same time electrolysis of the junctional stainless steel wire occurs, detaching the coil in the aneurysm without traction.

The platinum coils are soft and have their own preformed helix of 2 to 14 mm. Once released from the catheter tip, the coil forms loops to prevent unnecessary stress to the aneurysm wall. When the correct size coil is introduced into the aneurysm, it adopts the shape of the lumen, not deforming the aneurysm.

Endovascular Technique. Using proper angiographic technique, a 5-Fr to 7-Fr guiding catheter is introduced into the carotid artery or VA under systemic heparinization. The microcatheter, either Tracker 10 or 18, depending on the size of the aneurysm, is coaxially advanced into the aneurysm. It is necessary to use a soft-tipped guidewire when entering the aneurysm, not only to direct the catheter into the lumen, but also to minimize risk of rupture to the aneurysm wall.

Once the microcatheter is in the proper position, a detachable coil is introduced into the lumen. If the coil migrates, it can be repositioned. When the coil is in the proper position, the positive end of a direct current source is connected to the proximal end of the detachable wire and the negative end is connected to a needle inserted in the groin. Current of 0.5 or 1 mA is provided by a battery-operated generator. The detaching end must be beyond the catheter tip to promote electrolysis. This can be ensured by markers on the catheter (3 cm from the tip) and the wire (28 mm from the uninsulated segment).

The direct current induces thrombus formation around the platinum coil. More than one coil and often multiple coils (depending on aneurysm size) are used to sufficiently pack the aneurysm. These patients have follow-up angiograms 6 months to 1 year after the procedure to ensure complete obliteration of the aneurysm and to assess whether recanalization has occurred. If recanalization does happen, the patient will most likely require repeated embolization procedures to obliterate the remaining open portion. Endovascular treatment of intracranial aneurysms by using coils is proving to be a safe method of preventing aneurysm rupture.

The treatment of aneurysms by using electrically detachable electrothrombolytic coils was developed by Guglielmi in 1989, and the first patient was treated in 1990.[58,59] Since 1990, many centers have published their experience with the GDC modality, and these data show this procedure to be both safe and effective in preventing most intracranial aneurysms from rupture.[60,61]

The exception to this usually favorable outcome is seen in patients with giant intracranial aneurysms measuring 2.5 cm or larger. In the early GDC series, it was demonstrated that although post-GDC aneurysm rupture was exceedingly uncommon in all aneurysms smaller than 2.5 cm in diameter, a significant number of giant aneurysms bled after GDC treatment. It is important to stress that protection of the aneurysm from hemorrhage is the primary goal of any treatment. In September of 1995, the U.S. Food and Drug Administration approved the GDC, which is now widely used.[62]

In an attempt to improve outcome, endovascular embolization of aneurysms performed using GDCs and newer types of coils/stents has been evaluated as a viable treatment option and as an adjunct to the proven definitive treatment of surgical clipping in selected cases in which clipping is not desirable or feasible. Patients in poor medical condition and those who have aneurysms that are inaccessible may benefit from endovascular treatment because it may at least provide protection from early rebleeding during the acute period.

Coil embolization of ruptured basilar tip aneurysms not amenable to surgical clipping appears to decrease morbidity and mortality rates compared with available natural history data on ruptured aneurysms treated conservatively. Some patients with ruptured basilar tip aneurysms who are not surgical candidates should be offered embolization as a treatment option. The role of endovascular treatment in patients with unruptured basilar tip aneurysms remains unclear.[63]

In those patients in whom giant aneurysms can be surgically clipped with acceptable risks of morbidity and mortality, that approach remains the treatment of choice because the embolization option does not appear to offer the same durability of protection from rupture. Coil embolization does offer an alternative in those cases in which patients presenting with mass effect symptoms on CNs cannot be surgically treated with acceptable risks of morbidity and mortality.[59]

CLINICAL VIGNETTE: DG is a 44-year-old woman who presents to her primary care doctor with a chief complaint of "pulsations in the back of her neck," which resolved after taking blood pressure medication. As part of the work-up, an MRA and CTA (Fig. 23-15) were done, which demonstrated an 11-mm basilar tip aneurysm. After review at a cerebrovascular conference, the team decided that the aneurysm would be amenable to either surgery or endovascular treatment. The patient opted for the coil treatment (Figs. 23-16, 23-17, and 23-18). She was placed on aspirin 325 mg daily and Plavix (clopidogrel)75 mg PO daily 10 days preoperatively. She was admitted the morning of the procedure and discharged home neurologically intact 2 days later on aspirin 325 mg and Plavix 75 mg PO for a period of 3 weeks. She also had a skull film (Fig. 23-19) done prior to discharge to assess coil placement. She will be followed up with skull films again in 6 months and then an angiogram in 1 year, 3 years, and 5 years.

CLINICAL PEARLS: Many patients present with "incidental" aneurysms. As a clinician, it is important to sort out symptomatology as it relates to a particular lesion. It is necessary to educate patients about the current treatment modes, including observation if deemed appropriate. It is also important to reassure patients that the presenting symptoms may not be associated with the aneurysm, as in the previous Clinical Vignette. With endovascular treatment, follow-up is critical, and this should be stressed with the patient prior to treatment.

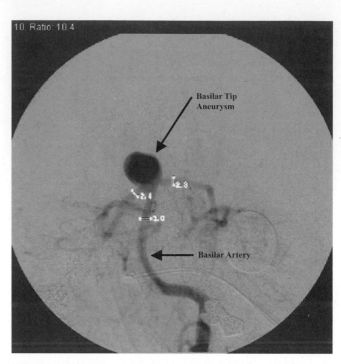

Figure 23-16 • Angiogram showing basilar tip aneurysm (*top arrow*) arising from the basilar artery (*bottom arrow*). (Courtesy of Christopher S. Ogilvy, MD, Massachusetts General Hospital, Boston, MA.)

Parent Vessel Occlusion

Another treatment approach that is utilized less often today due to technological advances involves occluding the parent vessel that supplies blood to the aneurysm. It is desirable to preserve the parent vessel whenever possible. The evolution

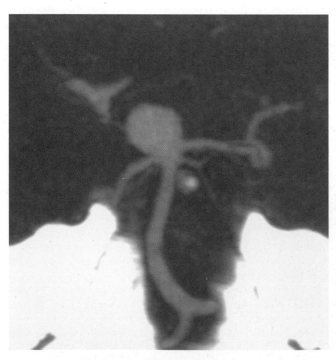

Figure 23-15 • Computed tomography angiogram maximum intensity projection image demonstrating basilar tip aneurysm. (Courtesy of Christopher S. Ogilvy, MD, Massachusetts General Hospital, Boston, MA.)

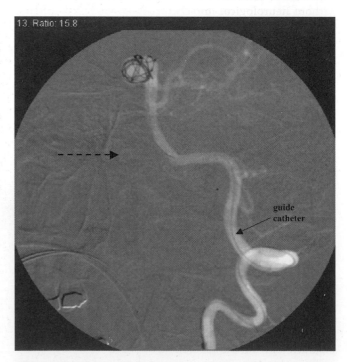

Figure 23-17 • Angiogram showing a 5-Fr guide catheter advancing into the left vertebral artery. Coils are detached within the basilar aneurysm (*dashed arrow*). (Courtesy of Christopher S. Ogilvy, MD, Massachusetts General Hospital, Boston, MA.)

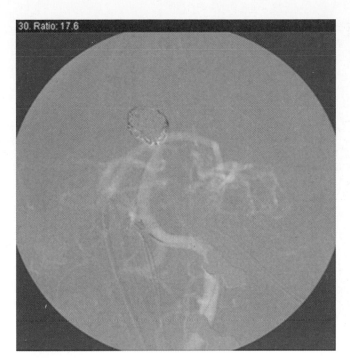

30. Ratio: 17.6

Figure 23-18 • Angiogram shows completion of coil embolization with coils tightly packed within aneurysm. (Courtesy of Christopher S. Ogilvy, MD, Massachusetts General Hospital, Boston, MA.)

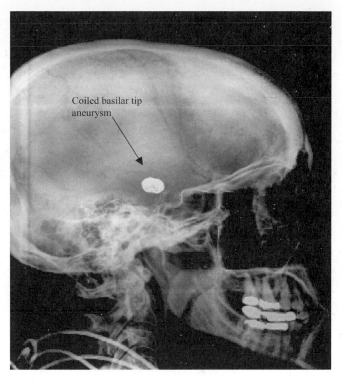

Coiled basilar tip aneurysm

Figure 23-19 • Skull film showing coiled basilar tip aneurysm. (Courtesy of Christopher S. Ogilvy, MD, Massachusetts General Hospital, Boston, MA.)

of stents and coils has allowed the preservation of the parent vessel while providing finite treatment of the aneurysm.

If parent vessel occlusion is deemed appropriate, it is important to establish whether the vessel can be sacrificed without neurological impairment. Various methods have been documented as effective, but not as absolute predictors of tolerance. A basic method is to constantly monitor motor, sensory, and cognitive functions in an awake patient during temporary occlusion (15 to 20 minutes). A patient's electroencephalogram (EEG) can be monitored to detect any ischemic focus that may lead to clinical symptoms.

Preparation for temporary occlusion testing is similar to routine angiography. The occlusion balloon is inflated with contrast material until internal carotid artery flow is completely stopped. An experienced neurologist monitors neurological functions continuously for 20 minutes. Some centers may be monitoring EEG changes or stump pressure measurements during this interim. A challenge test may be applied by reducing systolic blood pressure to approximately 80 mm Hg. If the patient tolerates this occlusion and has sufficient collateral circulation on high-volume angiogram, the patient is ready for permanent occlusion.

Indications for Permanent Occlusion.
Aneurysms treated by parent vessel occlusion are those of the cavernous or petrous extracranial internal carotid artery or extracranial VA that are generally not amenable to stent and/or coil treatment. Giant subarachnoid aneurysms inoperable because of their size or undefined neck and aneurysms that are unclippable and located below the level of the circle of Willis or carotid bifurcation are often considered for stent and/or coils before the option of parent vessel occlusion. Dissecting aneurysms of

the internal carotid or vertebral arteries and fusiform aneurysms without a well-defined neck may be eliminated by trapping or proximal occlusion.

Postocclusion Care.
Hemodynamic changes following carotid occlusion can persist for at least a week. Low-level heparinization (partial thromboplastin time [PTT] level 40 to 60) should be maintained for 24 to 48 hours postoperatively and the patient's activity regulated. For the first 24 hours, the patient is on complete bed rest. By the second or third day, the patient is out of bed and ambulating. If symptoms of cerebral ischemia are detected, the blood pressure is further elevated and blood volume expanded by increasing fluid intake. Gradual increase in activity helps the proper adjustment of cerebral circulation to postocclusion hemodynamic changes, thus minimizing the risk of cerebral ischemia.

Patients are usually discharged home on some type of anticoagulation therapy, often one aspirin daily. If proximal occlusion of the parent artery is achieved, aneurysms of the internal carotid artery below the ophthalmic artery or VA undergo complete obliteration. For those internal carotid artery aneurysms above or at the level of the ophthalmic artery and for basilar aneurysms, the rate of complete obliteration drops to the 50% range. This is as a result of persistent flow in the aneurysm lumen through collateral circulation.

Balloon Remodeling Technique

Aneurysms selected for endovascular treatment are usually spherical and have a dome-to-to-neck ratio greater than or equal to 2. The absolute diameter of the aneurysm neck should be less than 4 mm and less than one half the diameter of the parent vessel.[64,65] Many aneurysms do not fall within these guidelines and are not considered for coil placement. Recent reports in the literature discuss the feasibility, efficacy, and safety of the balloon-assisted technique first described by Jacques Moret as the "remodeling technique."[64,66,67,69]

In the treatment of wide neck aneurysms, one of the major risks is the possibility of the coil herniating into the parent vessel causing thromboembolic events, which is the most serious and frequent complication associated with endovascular treatment of aneurysms.

The technique involves temporary occlusion of the aneurysm neck with a detachable balloon while a coil is in place. The balloon prevents coil migration out of the aneurysm or protrusion into the parent vessel, allowing for an increased percentage of successful aneurysm treatment. There are several types of balloons that can be used, including over-the-wire occluded balloons and ones without end holes. Each type has distinct advantages and disadvantages.

Many aneurysms are amenable to coil treatment using the Moret balloon-assisted technique.[68] The balloon is placed across the neck of the aneurysm, which prevents coil protrusion and migration. The balloon stabilizes the microcatheter in the aneurysm during coil delivery and also allows the coil to assume the three-dimensional shape of the aneurysm without occluding the parent vessel. The remodeling technique is a practical extension of endovascular coil embolization of cerebral aneurysms and increases the number of aneurysms that can be treated. It may offer a second treatment approach in aneurysms in which surgical clipping has failed and may provide an alternative treatment in aneurysms that are surgically inaccessible or require a different surgical approach. It provides an alternative to second or third craniotomies in patients with multiple aneurysms and a less invasive treatment in patients with severe concomitant medical problems.[69]

Findings to date show that aneurysms completely occluded postprocedure remain occluded on follow-up examination. Aneurysms that are subtotally occluded (i.e., more than 95%) immediately after coil placement tend to remain stable (30%), have progressive thrombosis (14%), or progress to occlusion (22%). Neck remnant growth in aneurysm subtotally occluded is not unique to aneurysms treated with coils and can be found in the surgical literature. Some believe that growth of a neck remnant in aneurysms treated with coils is directly related to the density of the coil packing within the treated aneurysm and the relationship of the neck remnant to the parent artery. A 10% failure rate of this procedure has been reported in the literature. Embolic phenomena were the most noted risk.[70] Wide neck aneurysms continue to be a challenge to both neurosurgery and interventional neuroradiology. With the introduction of new technology and devices such as stents and bioactive coils, lesions may be treated more effectively and safely.

Future of Interventional Endovascular Treatment

Interventional endovascular technology has great potential for the future. Endovascular therapy over the past 10 years has revolutionized the treatment of aneurysms. The current combined morbidity and mortality rate related to the neurosurgical clipping of an incidental cerebral aneurysm is between 5% and 10%. The indication for surgical treatment of incidental surgical aneurysms is influenced by the location and size of the aneurysm and the patient's age and medical condition. The overall morbidity and mortality in patients treated in a series by Murayma et al. are comparable to the best neurosurgical series for the treatment of incidental aneurysms.[71] The combined clinical and procedural morbidity and mortality rate of the endovascular technology has dramatically decreased over the last couple of years because of the development of better delivery systems and softer and newer types of coils as well as the increased experience of the neurointerventional teams. The long-term anatomic results have also been improved by the combined use of three-dimensional coils, soft coils, and GDC balloon-assisted technology.[72]

The Newer Endovascular Techniques

In the last 10 years, there have been several technical advances since the advent of GDC coils in 1990s that have improved endovascular treatment of aneurysms. Although there has been remarkable progress with endovascular treatment of aneurysms, over 25% of cerebral aneurysms show some reopening of the lumen over time.[73,74] Coil compaction over time is the greatest contributing factor to the recanalization of the aneurysm. This phenomenon is thought to be caused by the water hammer effect of pulsatile blood flow. Previous studies have shown that coil compaction is directly related to the density of the packing, defined as the ratio of inserted coil volume to the volume of an aneurysm. Higher aneurysm packing can be achieved by higher volumes of coils.[75]

New coil designs including soft coils, three-dimensional coils, ultrasoft coils, and coils that are coated with polymers (hydrocoils) have contributed to the improved ability to obliterate aneurysms. There are new bioactive coils, which include Matrix® (Boston Scientific, Freemont, CA), Polyglycolic-Polylactic acid (PGLA) coated detachable coils (Fig. 23-20), which combine a pure platinum backbone with an added biodegradable copolymer. These promote organization of intra-aneurysmal thrombus and neointimal growth

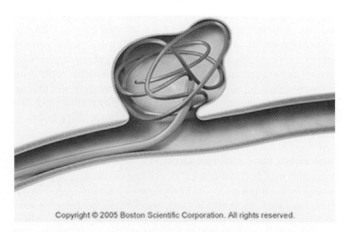

Figure 23-20 • Aneurysm with the insertion of Matrix detachable coils (Boston Scientific, Fremont, CA), which combines a pure platinum backbone with an added biodegradable copolymer. (Courtesy of Boston Scientific Corporation.)

at the neck of the aneurysm.[70] Cerecyte coils (Micrus Endovascular, San Jose, CA) have recently been developed and provide an induced tissue response. The Nexus coil (Micro Therapeutics, Inc., Irvine, CA) is a platinum alloy coil enlaced with absorbable polymer fibers and attached to a stainless steel guiding system with a radiopaque positioning coil.

Hydrophilic coils, such as the HydroCoil (MicroVention, Aliso Viejo, CA), are hydrogel-coated coils that, when deployed in the aneurysm, swell to three times their original size. They hydrate and expand once they are inserted in the aneurysm, facilitating a more complete occlusion in the aneurysm. These new coils may promote healing at the aneurysm neck, where recanalization and recurrence most commonly occur.[70] New devices and technologies continue to improve our ability to treat complex aneurysms endovascularly. The introduction of bioactive coils, hydrophilic coils, and intracranial stents allows a safe and effective means of treating difficult aneurysms with an endovascular technique.[70]

The Neuroform microstent (Fig. 23-21) provides the ability of neck reconstruction, facilitating more complete aneurysm obliteration by reducing the risk of coil prolapse into the parent vessel. The stent provides a matrix for endothelial growth.[72,76]

Stents and Treatment

A *stent* refers to a device used to hold a skin graft in position that was originally composed of a substance invented by British dentist Charles Thomas Stent (1807 to 1901), called Stent's mass, which he used to make impressions of teeth. The origin of the term stent is controversial. Another belief is that the word may have derived from the word "stint," which means to restrain within certain limits.

According to Palmaz, a stent is a coil or mesh tube that is introduced into the body through a catheter in a constrained form. The device is deployed by various mechanisms. The device's original role was thought to be to:

1. Prevent elastic recoil of a vessel after balloon angioplasty by holding a vessel open to a predetermined diameter
2. Prevent dissection after balloon angioplasty by pushing the dissected layers against one another and against the arterial wall
3. Provide a cylindrical vessel lumen wall by forcing asymmetric plaques eccentrically[77]

The application of stenting to ICA disease grew out of the success that such procedures had in both the coronary and peripheral arenas. In the mid-1990s, interest grew in the use of stents in the management of pseudoaneurysms and arterial dissections.[78] One of the limitations of coil embolization of wide neck aneurysms or fusiform aneurysms is permanent obliteration. Stents may provide a means of covering an aneurysmal neck to allow for coil deposition within the fundus without the fear of parent vessel occlusion or stenosis. In 1997 Higashida et al. successfully placed a Palmaz-Schatz PS 1540 articulated stent (Johnson & Johnson Interventional Systems, Warren, NJ) across the neck of a ruptured fusiform basilar aneurysm and used the stent to hold coils in the aneurysmal fundus and out of the basilar artery lumen.[79] In 1998, Lanzino et al. used an AVE (Arterial Vascular Engineering [Santa Rosa, CA]) coronary stent in the management of a paraclinoid aneurysm.[76]

Stent-assisted coil embolization (Fig. 23-22) prevents protrusion of the coils into the parent vessel. The introduction of intracranial stents has contributed positively to treatment options for coil occlusion of fusiform and wide neck

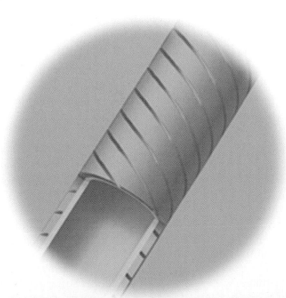

Figure 23-21 • Neuroform stent delivery system. (Courtesy of Boston Scientific Corporation.)

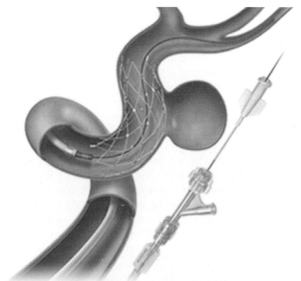

Figure 23-22 • The Neuroform microstent inserted via the parent vessel to treat aneurysm. The stent provides for neck reconstruction, facilitating more complete aneurysm obliteration by reducing the risk of coil prolapse into the parent vessel. (Courtesy of Boston Scientific Corporation.)

aneurysms. Stents may also help to prevent recanalization, which can occur despite the use of balloon remodeling and bioactive coils.

The Neuroform stent (Boston Scientific) is the first intracranial stent developed and on the market. It is made of nitinol (a nickel titanium alloy that assumes a predetermined shape in appropriate conditions). This flexible material allows the stent to be navigated within the tortuous intracranial vessels and to span the neck of a branch point effectively.[80]

The stent serves as a mechanical scaffold for placement of the coils into the aneurysm. The stent can allow for safe packing of the lesion, preventing herniation into the parent vessel. Some technical problems with the stent have been reported, such as stent displacement after delivery during microcatheter manipulation. Newer stents have been developed with increased radial force and are more easily positioned and deposited. A newer-generation Neuroform stent, the Neuroform 2, has additional cross-links allowing for increased radial force. This new self-expanding stent has an open-cell mesh design and is specifically designed for intracranial anatomy.

The newest generation of nitinol stents is the Enterprise stent (Cordis Neurovascular, Miami, FL). It has been designed specifically for the treatment of wide neck aneurysms. The benefits of this system are that it can be introduced into a standard microcatheter after access is achieved and can be partially deployed almost 70% within the parent artery and be recaptured and redeployed if necessary. The closed-cell design allows the coils to remain in the aneurysm and not protrude into the normal parent artery.[81]

The disadvantage of all these stents is that they are very thrombogenic. A stent stimulates platelet aggregation upon exposure to the patient's blood. It is recommended that patients receive dual antiplatelet treatment at least 3 days before stent treatment. In the study by Benitez et al., patients were given clopidogrel 75 mg and aspirin 325 mg by mouth 3 days prior to the stent procedure. After the procedure, intravenous heparin was continued for 24 hours with partial thromboplastin time in the range of 60 to 70 seconds. After the heparin was discontinued, dextran 40 was started for another 24 hours. Dextran is a volume expander and has an intrinsic antiplatelet effect. Femoral sheaths were removed on postoperative day 1, when partial thromboplastin time had normalized. The patients were maintained on aspirin and clopidogrel for 6 weeks. After 6 weeks, the clopidogrel was stopped and the aspirin maintained indefinitely.[82]

For ruptured aneurysms, Howington and Hopkins recommend clopidogrel 450 mg and aspirin 325 mg either the night before or morning of the procedure. At least 2 hours should pass before the stent is deployed. In the case of an acutely ruptured aneurysm, the use of antiplatelet therapy is anxiety producing, but the risks of thromboembolic complications without the use of antiplatelet therapy can have devastating consequences. The risks of utilizing a stent without proper antiplatelet therapy and the knowledge of possible thromboembolic complications are too high to proceed.[82] Antiplatelet therapy is most appropriate with unruptured aneurysms, as it would be contraindicated in ruptured aneurysms.[70] Practice varies regarding use of anticoagulation with ruptured aneurysms.

Others have used stents to assist with coil embolization of wide neck VA aneurysms. Stenting is an exciting new neurointerventional procedure that assists the practitioner with the management of some challenging and otherwise unmanageable neurovascular disease processes. As new devices are developed and as controlled trials are undertaken to assess their effectiveness, older surgical procedures may be replaced in favor of less costly and less debilitating endovascular procedures.[78]

COMPLICATIONS OF ANEURYSMAL RUPTURE/BLEEDING

The major complications of aneurysmal rupture/bleeding, which can lead to significant mortality and morbidity, include rebleeding, vasospasm, and hydrocephalus.

Aneurysmal Rebleeding

Of the 18,000 persons who survive the initial rupture of an aneurysm annually, 3000 either die or are disabled from rebleeding. Some believe the incidence of rebleeding is as high as 30%. The highest incidence occurs in the first 2 weeks after initial hemorrhage. Peaks in the incidence of rebleeding occur in the first 24 to 28 hours and at 7 to 10 days. Rebleeding within the first 24 to 48 hours is the leading cause of death in persons surviving the initial bleed. Peaking of rebleeding episodes at about 7 to 10 days appears to correlate with normal clot dissolution by natural fibrinolysis or from hypertension. Approximately 70% of patients who rebleed will die.[8]

Signs and Symptoms/Treatment

The onset of rebleeding is usually accompanied by sudden severe headache, often associated with severe nausea and vomiting; a decrease in or loss of consciousness; and new neurological deficits. Death may occur. Rebleeding can be confirmed by a CT scan or a sudden spike in ICP with new blood seen in the bag if a ventricular drain is in place. Early treatment, with either surgical or endovascular methods, of the aneurysm is the most effective means of preventing rebleeding.

Cerebral Vasospasm

Of the 18,000 persons annually who survive initial aneurysmal rupture, 3000 either die or are disabled from cerebral vasospasm. Vasospasm occurs in approximately 30% of patients. By definition, *cerebral vasospasm* is narrowing of a cerebral blood vessel and causes reduced blood flow distally, which may lead to delayed ischemic deficit and cerebral infarction if left untreated. Besides the damage done by the initial SAH, brain damage produced by vasospasm is an important cause of morbidity and mortality after hemorrhage, with 14% to 36% of patients suffering disability and death. Clinical signs of vasospasm are evident in about one third of patients after SAH, whereas angiographic and transcranial Doppler studies reveal spasm in 70% of cases.

Since improved treatment of aneurysmal subarachnoid hemorrhage has occurred with early and improved microsurgery, new endovascular techniques, and better postoperative care and monitoring, vasospasm has significantly decreased as the cause of death over the last 10 years (from 35% in the 1970s to <10% at this time). The present rescue therapies, which include triple H (hypertension, hypervolemia, and hemodilution), interventional procedures such as balloon angioplasty, and intra-arterial nicardipine and other vasodilators, are associated with significant morbidity and are labor intensive and expensive.[83] A drug that would prevent delayed ischemic effects and minimize the amount of rescue therapy and optimize late outcome is desirable.

Current medical management is centered on maintaining cerebral perfusion and blood pressure at high levels by using vasopressors and hypervolemia therapy. Patients are also maintained on the calcium channel blocker nimodipine orally for a period of 21 days. When nimodipine is orally administered in good-grade patients, a number of studies have shown a reduced morbidity and mortality. The nimodipine therapy may be limited due to hypotension, which may lead to decreased perfusion pressure and cerebral ischemia.[84]

When the patient's condition deteriorates 3 to 14 days after SAH, vasospasm should be considered as the possible cause. A CT scan should be performed immediately to rule out hydrocephalus, infarction, or rebleeding. Vasospasm can decrease cerebral perfusion to an area, causing ischemia and perhaps infarction, and can lead to further deterioration of neurological function. The etiology of vasospasm is unknown, although many hypotheses have been proposed. Current hypotheses range from the suggestion that spasmogenic agents are released as the clot breaks down to the more recent hypothesis that an endothelium relaxing factor, such as nitric oxide, is somehow inhibited from exerting its relaxing effect because of changes in the endothelial cells that produce nitric oxide. These cellular changes may be induced by the release of blood into the extravascular compartment.

Vasospasm may be differentiated as either angiographic or symptomatic. **Angiographic vasospasm** refers to narrowing of a cerebral arterial territory, as noted on angiography, without clinical symptoms. **Symptomatic vasospasm** is the clinical syndrome of delayed cerebral ischemia associated with angiographically documented narrowing of a major cerebral arterial territory and TCD elevation of a specific arterial territory. Vasospasm develops 3 to 14 days after SAH (peaking at 7 to 10 days), although the onset may be delayed up to 21 days.[1]

Etiology

The etiology of vasospasm is uncertain, but recent studies have demonstrated that nitric oxide (NO) prevents and reverses vasospasm after aneurysmal subarachnoid hemorrhage.[85]

Vasospasm is produced by extravasated blood and occurs maximally in arteries surrounded by the thickest clot. There are many sources of evidence incriminating ET-1 in the pathogenesis of cerebral vasospasm.[86] The etiology of vasospasm is related to the release of hemoglobin and oxyhemoglobin, which in turn stimulates the release of a host of vasoconstricting agents including ET-1. After a subarachnoid hemorrhage, oxyhemoglobin stimulates ET-1 production. Lysed red blood cells seem to be a source of ET-1, which is a

potent and long-lasting constrictor of cerebral arteries. In several animal models of aneurysmal subarachnoid hemorrhage, ET-1 receptor antagonists (ET-A or ET −A+B) were able to prevent or reverse cerebral vasospasm.[87–90] Hence, ET-1 seems to play a major causal role in the pathophysiology of delayed ischemic effects of subarachnoid hemorrhage. Endothelin receptor agonists block the effect of an important causative factor of cerebral vasospasm.

Signs and Symptoms

Vasospasm is characterized by a gradual neurological deterioration related to a vascular territory. The clinical manifestations of vasospasm are variable. At least 50% of patients remain asymptomatic, whereas some 20% to 30% will have some delayed neurological ischemia. These deficits may be focal, but a clinician may also see confusion, decreased level of consciousness, and coma. The neurological deficits may be specific to a particular vascular territory, such as ACA or MCA, or they may be multifocal and diffuse, as when the cortical areas and boundary zones are involved. Most patients will have impaired level of consciousness. Deficits may include paresis/paralysis of a limb or side of the body, cranial nerve deficits, and aphasia. As a consequence of the severity and location of the ischemia caused by the vasospasm, cerebral infarction may develop, thus contributing to increased permanent neurological deficits or death.

Prediction of Vasospasm and Vascular Territory

An initial CT/CTA scan taken at the time of the bleed has gained credibility as a predictor of the incidence, location, and severity of vasospasm (see Table 23-3). The extent and location of clots in the basal cisterns of the subarachnoid space and cerebral fissures are the specific determinants considered. Patients who have subarachnoid clots larger than 5 × 3 mm in the basal cisterns or who have layers of blood 1 mm thick or more in the cerebral fissures have a high incidence of vasospasm. Fisher has demonstrated that the amount of blood in the basal cisterns, as shown by the initial CT scan, can reliably predict which patients will develop symptomatic vasospasm, with the amount of blood directly related to the incidence and severity of vasospasm. Bleeding into the brain or ventricles does not result in vasospasm.

Information concerning the probability and location of vasospasm can be helpful to the physician and nurse. Correlation of the vascular territory supplied by the artery at risk with the specific neurological functions of that territory helps to focus attention on those specific functions during neurological assessments. A decreased level of consciousness, the presence of focal signs, or both, together with a CT scan correlated to the cerebral territory, along with elevated TCDs, are indicative of vasospasm *when no other changes can explain the neurological deterioration*. When subtle or significant deficits occur, the nurse can quickly alert the physician to these findings so that prompt interventions can prevent extension of the neurological deficits or even death.

Treatment

The result of vasospasm is decreased cerebral perfusion (blood flow) to the clinically affected arterial territory. Currently, treatment for symptomatic vasospasm is directed at the primary goal of increasing cerebral perfusion pressure, using hypervolemic, hypertensive, and hemodilution (triple H) therapy. With a craniotomy, there is usually a 300- to 400-mL blood loss that produces hemodilution with a hematocrit of 30% to 32%.[144] Hemodilution improves CBF. The balance of oxygen-carrying capacity and viscosity is optimized at a hematocrit level of 32% to 35%. To maintain the hematocrit in the desired range, albumin and packed RBCs may be used as volume expanders, or blood may be removed and mannitol may be administered (to decrease volume).

Central venous pressure is maintained at approximately 8 to 10 mm Hg, and the pulmonary capillary wedge pressure is 14 to 18 mm Hg. This is achieved by administration of colloid (5% albumin) on a regular basis (every 6 or 8 hours) to expand the intravascular volumes. Therapy is also aimed at maintaining a heart rate of greater than 70 beats per minute and a 30% rise in mean arterial blood pressure (160 to 170 mm Hg) for the duration of the vasospasm. If necessary, hypertension can be induced with vasopressors—dopamine (Intropin), phenylephrine (Neo-Synephrine), or dobutamine. The level of hypertension may be carefully controlled in the case of an unclipped aneurysm because of the concern for rebleeding. If vasospasm occurs after surgical clipping of the aneurysm, systolic blood pressure is often maintained between 180 and 200 mm Hg. Special care is warranted in patients with cardiac, pulmonary, or renal dysfunction. Central venous pressure monitoring is indicated in these cases, and some patients will need pulmonary artery catheters to guide therapy. One must watch for pulmonary edema, electrolyte imbalances, and cerebral edema in such complex patients.

Mannitol has been shown to increase CBF in the setting of vasospasm, with improvement in neurological function. A calcium channel blocker, nimodipine, has been standard treatment for nearly a decade and has been shown to have a beneficial effect on stroke after SAH, and a beneficial effect on blood flow as well. Nimodipine is begun at 60 mg PO or through nasogastric tube every 4 hours. Multiple studies demonstrate a modest effect in neurological outcome, although no clear angiographic demonstration of improved spasm was noted. It is believed that the site of effect is at the cellular level where it acts as a neuronal protector. Nimodipine therapy seems reasonable as long as the ability to treat with hypertension is not compromised. If it does lead to unmanageable drops in blood pressure, the dose is split or reduced or use of the drug is eliminated. TCD is an invaluable tool in the management of vasospasm. It is noninvasive, is rapidly interpretable, and can be done on a daily basis to guide therapy. TCD gives flow velocities in the basal segments of the cerebral vessels, and increases in velocities may be seen in increased perfusion states or with narrowing of the basal segments. It is difficult to precisely correlate ischemic symptoms with TCD velocities because of variability of collateral supply. Vasospasm of the ACA and MCA will be symptomatic at lower velocities than isolated MCA spasm. As TCD velocities increase, the intensity of medical management is also increased.

Medical therapy may be nearly exhausted by the time ischemic symptoms appear, and emergency and invasive alternatives are immediately begun. Angiography with the intention of angioplasty or intra-arterial drugs infused to open the narrowed arterial wall can be extremely useful. The major goal is to proceed with invasive therapy before prolonged clinical deficits to maximize neurological function.

Endovascular Therapy. Not all patients who develop anatomic spasm will develop clinical vasospasm. If a patient develops a new deficit that is suggestive of clinical vasospasm despite maximal medical prophylaxis, cross-sectional imaging is required (CT or CTA is preferable and easier than MRI). This will allow exclusion of other conditions that can produce such a deficit (such as rehemorrhage, hydrocephalus, or postoperative extra-axial hematoma) and permit identification of infarction or hemorrhagic transformation if already present in the ischemic territory. If infarction has already occurred in the zone of the vasospastic arteries, endovascular therapy is precluded.

Two forms of endovascular therapy are available: balloon angioplasty and intra-arterial transcatheter infusion of a potent vasodilating drug, such as papaverine (less commonly used); the more commonly used calcium channel blockers, nicardipine and verapamil; and the newer agent, milrinone, a phosphodiesterase enzyme inhibitor. Papaverine is a short-acting vasodilator that is infrequently used today for the treatment of spasm due to its short duration necessitating frequent angiographic procedures and since the discovery of newer more effective agents. Intra-arterial nicardipine and verapamil are given through superselective angiography in varying doses depending on the intensity of the spasm and the physician. Some physicians give between 3- and 10-mg doses per patient. Arterial dilation is the goal, and is generally achieved with these doses. Milrinone, a cardiac inotrope, is a phosphodiesterase inhibitor and has been used as an intra-arterial vasodilator, similar to papaverine. It also has a short half-life, but can be followed up with an intravenous infusion, and has the additional benefit of enhancing cardiac output. It also can induce hypotension.[91] Balloon angioplasty uses a low-pressure nondetachable microballoon to dilate the spastic segment mechanically. This is done under systemic anticoagulation. Once dilated, arteries generally do not experience spasm again unless a second hemorrhage occurs. Intra-arterial drugs are sometimes used in combination with the angioplasty, depending on the degree of vasospasm. Intra-arterial verapamil, nicardipine, or milrinone infusions can be efficacious in situations in which spasm is quite distal in the arterial bed or inaccessible by balloon.

Outcomes are clearly best when such intervention is early. The risks of either angioplasty or intra-arterial vasodilating drugs include reperfusion hemorrhage in an already infarcted territory, mechanical arterial rupture, arterial dissection, and thromboembolism. The risks are warranted in the hands of an experienced endovascular therapist at $2000 to $10,000 per procedure, which is a small price compared with the potential life-long cost of stroke in a patient in whom it could have been prevented.[92]

New Therapies for Vasospasm on the Horizon

There are hopeful therapies on the horizon for the prevention and/or treatment of vasospasm. Once such therapy is the use of an endothelin A receptor antagonist, clazosentan, which is being studied in patients with aneurysmal subarachnoid hemorrhage. The intention is that it will reduce the incidence and severity of vasospasm following rupture of an aneurysm. In the following study, clazosentan or placebo was given to patients following surgical clipping of the ruptured aneurysm: between October 2002 and April 2003, patients were recruited from five neurosurgical centers in Germany to participate in a phase IIa, multicenter study that had two parts: a randomized, double blind component (part A), where some patients were given either clazosentan (0.2 mg/kg/hr) or placebo, and an open label component (part B), where patients with established vasospasm were given clazosentan (0.4 mg/kg/hr for 12 hours followed by 0.2 mg/kg/hr) for exploratory purposes only. There were 40 patients screened. Thirty-four patients fulfilled the enrollment criteria and were subsequently enrolled.

This study was the first to demonstrate that clazosentan significantly decreases the incidence and severity of angiographic vasospasm after aneurysmal subarachnoid hemorrhage. Due to the limited number of patients in this study, the observed benefits cannot be generalized to the overall subarachnoid hemorrhage population. Further studies are being done to assess dosage as well as clinical outcome.

Clazosentan is a selective endothelin A receptor antagonist. It has been developed as an intravenous infusion as to treat patients with SAH to prevent vasospasm. Clazosentan shows high specificity for the endothelin receptor. In preclinical pharmacology studies, clazosentan appeared to be selective for the cerebral circulation, having cerebral vasodilating effects but little effects on the peripheral hemodynamic.[93] There will be more studies to determine the effectiveness of clazosentan for the treatment of vasospasm.

Hypomagnesia occurs in more than 50% of patients with subarachnoid hemorrhage and is related to poor outcome and delayed cerebral ischemia (DCI) in patients after 3 months.[94] DCI usually occurs 4 to 10 days after hemorrhage, so it is important that neuroprotective agents be started before the start of ischemia. In many stroke models, magnesium was shown to have a neuroprotective effect and reduced infarct volume in experimental SAH in rats.[95] Magnesium is a potent cerebral vasodilator and there has been interest in its use as a neuroprotectant and antivasospastic agent. There have been promising studies in the IV supplementation of magnesium in patients with vasospasm.[96,97] Magnesium may increase cerebral blood flow and reduce the contractions of cerebral arteries caused by various stimuli such as blood. Magnesium is inexpensive and readily available and has a well-established clinical profile in cardiovascular and obstetric practice. There is a lack of knowledge on the dosage for the extended use of magnesium and large randomized trials are needed.

Statins have many biologic properties independent of their cholesterol-lowering effects that make them an interest for prophylaxis against delayed cerebral ischemia after aneurysmal subarachnoid hemorrhage. The statins have the ability to down-regulate inflammation and up-regulate endothelial NO synthesis. In one study, the primary finding as a result of simvastatin treatment (80 mg/d for 14 days) was that patients had a lower incidence of clinical vasospasm (confirmed angiographically or by TCD criteria) and a significant reduction in MCA velocities. The hypothesis is that simvastatin exerts its therapeutic effects

by anti-inflammatory and endothelial protective properties. This suggests that the use of simvastatin is safe and well tolerated. More studies are needed to determine the optimal dosage, and whether the decreased incidence of vasospasm is reflected in the functional outcome of patients is yet to be determined.[98]

Another area of study is in regard to the molecular basis of delayed vasospasm, including endothelial disruption by NO depletion, free radical injury, and inflammation. Nitric oxide is a potent vasodilator and inhibitor of vascular smooth muscle proliferation and endothelial cell apoptosis. After a subarachnoid hemorrhage, decreased NO production by the endothelium and increased utilization of NO during inflammation are some of the mechanisms for the depletion of NO. Statins seem to increase the bioavailability of vascular NO and to lessen the inflammatory response and ameliorate free radical production. More studies are necessary to assess the potential benefits of statins in patients with aneurysmal subarachnoid hemorrhage.

There are ongoing studies to evaluate the effectiveness of NO donors or nitric oxide synthase (NOS) substrates to evaluate the effectiveness on ameliorating vasospasm in experimental and clinical settings.

High-Risk Factors: Hyponatremia and Fluid Restriction

Hyponatremia is the most common electrolyte abnormality following SAH, detected in 10% to 25% of the cases, whereas mild hyperkalemia occurs less frequently. This is an important clinical finding because hyponatremia and decreased fluid volume are recognized high-risk factors for development of vasospasm. In aneurysmal hemorrhage, hyponatremia can be caused by SIADH or salt wasting (see Chap. 9). If hyponatremia is caused by true SIADH, an expanded blood volume is present that requires fluid restriction. If hyponatremia is attributed to salt wasting (in which case there is also hyponatruria), blood volume is decreased. The treatment for salt wasting is fluid replacement. Widjicks et al. measured plasma volume, fluid and sodium balance, and serum vasopressin (i.e., antidiuretic hormone [ADH]) levels in patients with ruptured saccular aneurysms.[99] They found that vasopressin values were elevated at the time of the patient's admission but declined in the first week, regardless of the presence of hyponatremia. By definition, SIADH is associated with an increased serum ADH level. The conclusion drawn was that the natriuresis and hyponatremia were the result of primary salt wasting rather than SIADH. Further, they suggested that the natriuresis and hyponatremia should be corrected by fluid replacement rather than by fluid restriction, which is the treatment of SIADH.

The degree of hyponatremia is usually mild, occurring within 2 to 4 days of SAH, reaching a peak occurrence at about 7 days, and then becoming less frequent. Management should be with salt repletion, either orally or parenterally as needed to maintain sodium balance. Volume restriction is rarely necessary and often dangerous in the setting of vasospasm. Clinical manifestations may include a decreased level of consciousness or seizures, with delayed ischemic deficit and vasospasm reported as outcomes of previously used treatment with fluid restriction. The overall clinical outcome is worse for patients with hyponatremia.[100]

Seizures

The frequency of seizures following SAH is not known with certainty. In the early period, seizures occur between 16% and 90%.[1,76] Risk factors for seizures in the early period after SAH include previous history of hypertension, CT-documented presence of focal intraparenchymal blood, occurrence of a cerebral infarction, middle cerebral aneurysm location, and duration of coma after SAH.[1] Seizures generally occur within 18 months (if they do occur) and may be generalized, focal, or complex. On the basis of available data, many treat all aneurysmal SAH patients with anticonvulsants. If the hemorrhage is mild, anticonvulsants are tapered after 1 month. If the hemorrhage is more severe and if intraparenchymal brain injury has occurred, extended therapy and EEG monitoring are employed. Phenytoin 100 mg every 8 hours is given after an initial loading dose with 1 g (or 15 mg/kg) given slowly.

Communicating Hydrocephalus

Hydrocephalus is a condition in which there is an obstruction to the flow of CSF within the ventricular system or subarachnoid space (noncommunicating hydrocephalus) either due to intraventricular mass lesions or to external compression or a problem with reabsorption of CSF (communicating hydrocephalus). The type of hydrocephalus that occurs with SAH is communicating hydrocephalus. Hydrocephalus can be classified as acute, subacute, or delayed. The profiles for each are different and are briefly discussed here. With SAH, hydrocephalus develops as a result of blood in the CSF, which plugs the arachnoid villi, thus interfering with the reabsorption of CSF. Diagnosis is established on the basis of CT findings, which will reveal dilated ventricles with blood within the ventricles.

Signs and Symptoms/Treatment

The following summarizes the signs and symptoms of the three types of hydrocephalus, as well as the appropriate treatment for each.

Acute

- Occurs within the first 24 hours after hemorrhage
- Occurs in up to 20% to 67% of affected patients within 3 days following SAH
- Associated with intraventricular hemorrhage or excessive blood in the basal cisterns of posterior fossa
- Characterized by the abrupt onset of stupor or persistence of coma
- Management: immediate ventriculostomy to drain the CSF periodically, especially when ICP is elevated above a predetermined level such as 20 mm Hg

Subacute

- Occurs within the first few days to 7 days after hemorrhage
- Associated with blood in the CSF secondary to SAH
- Characterized by drowsiness, the onset of which is gradual, although an abrupt onset is possible
- Management: ventriculostomy, or serial lumbar puncture or lumbar drainage of CSF

Delayed

- Occurs 10 or more days after hemorrhage
- Associated with blood in the CSF secondary to SAH
- Characterized by a gradual onset of symptoms when the patient is recovering from surgery; symptoms include gait difficulty and behavioral changes (dull, quiet, and blunted animation)
- Management: surgical placement of a ventriculoperitoneal shunt

Because signs and symptoms of hydrocephalus are nonspecific, changes in responsiveness may be attributed to other problems, thus delaying appropriate treatment.

NURSING MANAGEMENT OF THE PATIENT WITH AN ANEURYSM

Nursing management of the patient with a cerebral aneurysm can be divided into three areas: management before treatment, management during complications, and management after treatment.

Nursing Management Before Treatment

The patient who has sustained aneurysmal rupture/bleeding requires ongoing neurological and systems assessment, supportive care, preventive strategies, implementation of specific protocols (e.g., drug therapy), and management of increased ICP.

Assessment/Monitoring

The initial and ongoing neurological and systems assessment and monitoring require not only a focus on neurological function, but also include other body systems such as the cardiovascular, respiratory, renal, and endocrine systems. These symptoms can be directly affected by cerebral aneurysm pathophysiology as well as by multiorgan dysfunction associated with severe illness. Cardiac monitoring for arrhythmias and ischemic events has already been discussed, along with respiratory and other system concerns. The initial assessment and ongoing monitoring of the neurological system includes:

- Level of consciousness*
- Pupillary size, shape, and reaction to light*
- Motor function (e.g., hand grasps, pronator drift, motor strength of extremities)*
- Other CN deficits (blurred vision or diplopia, extraocular movement deficits, ptosis, facial weakness)
- Aphasia
- Headache and facial pain (e.g., pain behind the eyeball).
- Nuchal rigidity (stiff neck, pain in neck, and back pain with flexion of neck), photophobia

Neurological assessments are conducted periodically. The frequency of assessments depends on the acuity and stability of the patient. Those assessment components marked with an asterisk (*) are the most sensitive to change in neurological function. The neurological assessment may be conducted every 15 minutes to 4 hours, depending on the stability of the patient and care setting. New assessment data are compared with previous findings to determine change and trends. Accurate documentation and intershift sharing and reporting of information are essential in identifying trends in neurological function.

On confirmation of diagnosis of cerebral aneurysm, the patient is assigned a grade category according to the Hunt-Hess Classification and the Fisher Grading Scale. Both classification systems alert the nurse to the acuity of the patient and give an indication of the probable treatment. Usually, patients who present with an SAH are admitted to an intensive care setting where the technology and proper monitoring devices are available to assist in neurological and other body systems monitoring. See Chapter 16 for a discussion on neurological critical care.

Altered consciousness diminishes the patient's ability to comprehend the significance and implications of the events happening around him or her. Because there may not be one clear cause to which altered consciousness can be attributed, determining the etiology of deterioration in the level of consciousness, restlessness, or agitation may be difficult. Such alterations may result from rebleeding, hydrocephalus, ischemia, vasospasm, hypoxia, increased ICP, or electrolyte imbalance. Alterations may also be caused by the psychological effects of immobility, sensory deprivation, powerlessness, or other responses to hospitalization.

Common Patient Problems and Collaborative Problems

The most common patient problems are found in Chart 23-1. The following are the major collaborative problems associated with aneurysmal SAH:

- Aneurysmal rebleeding
- Hydrocephalus
- Cerebral vasospasm
- Increased ICP (i.e., secondary brain injury)
- Seizures
- Stroke
- Cardiac ischemic injury, dysrhythmias
- DVT
- Electrolyte-endocrine imbalance (hyponatremia, SIADH, diabetes insipidus, cerebral salt wasting, hyperglycemia)
- Neurogenic pulmonary edema
- Infections, especially aspiration or bacterial pneumonias
- Meningitis, particularly in patients where an extraventricular drain is required

Most of these have been discussed briefly. Rebleeding, hydrocephalus, and vasospasm are the most critical complications in which astute nursing care and assessment can lead to early treatment and ultimate prevention of permanent neurological disability or death. The affected patient is also prone to DVT and related pulmonary emboli, for unknown reasons. The nurse needs to keep these potential problems in mind when caring for the patient.

Nursing Care: Additional Points of Care

Nurses are responsible for preventing complications. These responsibilities are singled out as being extremely important

because they are within the realm of the nurse to monitor and control. First, a bowel program is initiated to prevent straining at stool. Most patients receive a narcotic for headache control. A side effect is decreased peristalsis, which can result in constipation if action is not taken to counteract this trend. In addition, bed rest and immobility also contribute to constipation. A bowel management program must be instituted immediately on hospitalization. By the time constipation becomes a problem, the peak time for high incidence of rebleeding is reached. Straining at stool (initiating Valsalva's maneuver) is dangerous because it can cause rebleeding and increase ICP.

The second concern is that the patient who is maintained on bed rest is at high risk for DVT and pulmonary emboli. This risk factor can be controlled by the use of elastic hose (TEDs) and sequential compression boots. It is the nurse's responsibility to make sure TEDs and boots are worn at all times. The patient's legs should be monitored periodically for the development of DVT.

Third, *seizure precautions* are instituted. As a precaution in the event of seizure activity, aspiration, or deterioration, a standby suction setup is kept in readiness at the bedside along with an oral airway. Padded side rails are also in place to protect the patient from injury.

Drug Therapy. In addition to care, the nurse is responsible for administering prescribed medications and for being aware of the action, toxicity, and interactions of the various drugs used. In this way, pertinent observations can be made in assessing the patient's response to the drug therapy. Nimodipine is given for 21 days to all patients who have suffered an SAH. With discharge from the hospital occurring earlier, it is important to ensure that the patient's pharmacy has the medication available before the patient is sent home. It is also necessary that the patient and family comprehend the importance of completing the drug.

With the development of stents and coils, and because of their thrombogenic characteristics, there is a need for unruptured aneurysm patients to take Plavix and aspirin prior to the procedure. There may be some variation in amount and length of time a patient is on the antiplatelet regime. Generally, Plavix 75 mg PO daily and aspirin 325 mg PO daily is given to the patient 10 days before the coil and/or stent procedure. If just coils are placed, the patient will remain on aspirin 81 mg or 325 mg daily for a 6-week period. If stents are placed in addition to the coiling, the patient is discharged home on Plavix 75 mg PO daily and aspirin therapy for at least a 6-week period.

Psychological Support

Considering the sudden diagnosis, it is important to monitor the patient's and family members' psychological and emotional responses. If the patient presents with an unruptured aneurysm, they may want to talk to another patient who has already experienced treatment—either surgical or endovascular. This may alleviate fears and anxieties that only "survivors" can share. Providing written material is also helpful to explain treatment and recovery. Patients may want to contact organizations such as the Brain Aneurysm Foundation

CHART **23-1**   **Summary of Patient Problems Associated With Cerebral Aneurysms**

PATIENT PROBLEMS	NURSING INTERVENTIONS	EXPECTED OUTCOMES
Pain (headache, neck/back pain) related to (R/T) meningeal irritation	• Assess the type, location, and specific characteristics of the headache. • Assess the patient for pain and other signs and symptoms of meningeal irritation. • Reposition the patient gently, avoiding any unnecessary movement of the neck or head. • Administer analgesics as ordered. • Darken the patient's room. • Apply a cold, wet cloth or ice pack to the patient's head for comfort.	• The characteristics of the headache will be noted and recorded. • Analgesics and comfort measures will be administered. • The patient will provide objective evidence that the pain has been relieved.
Sensory/Perceptual Alterations, Visual, R/T photophobia secondary to meningeal irritation	• Note any evidence of discomfort when assessing direct light response of the pupils. • Maintain a darkened room by drawing the blinds or shades and avoiding direct light.	• Photophobia will be controlled by maintaining a darkened room.
High Risk for Injury R/T seizure activity secondary to cerebral irritation	• Maintain seizure precautions. • Monitor the patient for any signs of seizure activity and document in the patient's chart. • Administer anticonvulsant drugs prophylactically, as ordered.	• Seizure activity will be prevented. • If a seizure does occur, the patient will not be injured.
Anxiety (mild, moderate, or severe) R/T illness and/or restrictions of aneurysm precautions	• Assess the patient for objective and subjective evidence of anxiety. • If anxiety is present, try to identify the specific causes. • Attempt to clarify, control, or change the circumstances surrounding the anxiety. • Make appropriate referrals, as necessary. • Reassure the patient. • Depending on the patient's level of consciousness, use imagery, relaxation techniques, and other methods to control anxiety. • Administer sedatives, if ordered.	• Depending on the patient's level of consciousness, he or she will demonstrate an understanding of the purpose of the aneurysm precautions. • The patient will be informed of the plan of care and reassured. • The specific causes of anxiety will be identified. • Anxiety will be minimized or controlled.
High Risk for Secondary Brain Injury R/T rebleeding or cerebral vasospasms	• Assess neurological signs frequently for evidence of neurological deterioration. • Report immediately any significant changes in the patient's condition. • Recognize the peak times of occurrence of rebleeding and vasospasm. • If deterioration occurs, implement nursing protocols and standing orders so that ischemic response is treated.	• The patient will be carefully monitored so that any signs or symptoms of neurological deterioration will be identified quickly. • If there is evidence of deterioration, the physician will be notified immediately. • Nursing interventions and standing orders will be implemented quickly.

(see Resources section at end of chapter) for additional support and educational material.

When a patient has suffered an SAH, he or she will need reassurance and frequent orientation to the hospital environment. If the Hunt-Hess grade is high (associated with unconsciousness), it is often the family that will need education and guidance through a tenuous and often uncertain hospitalization course. A calm and reassuring approach to the patient and family is most therapeutic.

The following are general suggestions to prevent adverse behavioral or psychological responses in the patient who has suffered an SAH secondary to immobility, sensory deprivation, and powerlessness:

• Orient the patient frequently to time, place, and person.
• Familiarize the patient/family with the environment.
• Be alert for cues from the patient/family indicating areas of concern.
• Provide information in a clear and simple manner to clarify any concerns.
• Clarify any misconceptions and quickly reorient the patient.
• Report any severe responses to the patient's restrictions that may indicate the need for modification by the physician.
• Be supportive and available to the family throughout the hospitalization and follow-up.

Nursing Management After Surgery/Endovascular Therapy

Nursing management after a craniotomy for aneurysm clipping follows that outlined in Chapter 14. Because there is some incidence of vasospasm even after surgery, the nurse must monitor the patient for any neurological deterioration that may herald the onset of vasospasm. (Note that such onset may be gradual, as evidenced by a slight pronator drift or confusion.) A CT scan is often done when new neurological change occurs.

For the patient who has undergone endovascular therapy with either coils and/or stent, nursing management focuses on monitoring vital signs and neurological signs for evidence of vasospasm or ischemia. In addition, the femoral puncture site where the sheath is placed is monitored for evidence of bleeding, and the pedal pulses are assessed for evidence of occlusion. The patient is maintained on bed rest with the involved leg extended for a period of time until the sheath is removed. If the patient is receiving intra-arterial treatment for vasospasm, the sheath may be left in for a longer time. It is important to assess for potential signs and symptoms of a retroperitoneal bleed, such as decreased hematocrit, low systolic blood pressure, and abdominal pain and discomfort. Such symptoms need to be reported to the physician immediately.

Discharge Planning

Even with the technological advances that have been made in the management of patients with aneurysms, the outcome for patients includes significant neurological deficits. Throughout hospitalization, there needs to be interdisciplinary patient management to address the patient holistically and ensure early diagnosis and treatment of deficits. Many patients will need further rehabilitation after discharge from the acute care setting. Discharge planning should begin at admission or shortly thereafter and should address the individual needs of the patient. Much patient and family teaching is necessary to assist them in making decisions and coping with the multiple problems that may arise.

Cost Analysis and Predictors of Outcomes

There is a growing concern in our health care environment to minimize cost while maintaining quality care. It is a major challenge to all health care personnel and requires a collaborative effort of the managers of the health care delivery system and the providers of health care. Patient outcomes are such indicators and should be the focus in evaluating the achievement of quality, effectiveness, and appropriateness of patient care. Nurses should be active in collaborative decision making to optimize patient outcomes.

Although there are 30,000 reported cases of aneurysmal SAH in the United States annually, most aneurysms remain asymptomatic and undetected. In the past, unruptured aneurysms came to the attention of a neurosurgeon only after an SAH in a patient with multiple aneurysms. Since the development of microneurosurgical techniques and endovascular procedures, many neurosurgeons and neuroradiologists advocate elective treatment either surgically or endovascularly of an unruptured, asymptomatic, intracranial aneurysm. The superiority of elective aneurysm treatment has not been tested in any prospective clinical trials, although decision analysis models show more favorable outcomes with surgery. Economic implications of treatment decisions are in the forefront of the minds of physicians and society. Cost-effectiveness analysis is a technique designed to evaluate treatment options by using both economic and clinical outcome data. In this era of economic health care constraints, treatments that are not cost effective will be increasingly denied public and private insurance reimbursement.

Advances in treatment of patients who present with an unruptured intracranial aneurysm have changed the outlook for those who receive surgical or endovascular treatment. Substantial improvements in surgical morbidity and mortality do not seem to have had much of an impact on the clinical course of SAH when the total patient population is studied. The mortality rate from SAH is as high as 50%, and the many patients who do survive incur significant morbidity.[101]

The search for more accurate outcome predictors and the continued development of ever more precise outcome-based measures and their relationship to the management of cerebral aneurysms and SAH are critical.[102] Neurological deficits that occur after aneurysmal SAH may vary according to location of the lesion. Saccular intracranial aneurysms are the most common cause of SAH. The Hunt-Hess Classification (previously described) is based on a patient's clinical condition and correlates with surgical risk. A newer grading system, the MGH Scale, has been proposed to better predict outcome of aneurysm patients. It recognizes several predictive variables such as age, Fisher Grading Scale (amount of blood on CT scan), clinical presentation, and location of the aneurysm that the traditional Hunt-Hess Classification ignores. The Hunt-Hess Classification only looks at the clinical condition of the patient. The MGH Scale is designed to better predict cost and length of stay for aneurysm patients.[103]

Much of the literature states that clinical grade on admission is strongly associated with outcome and encompasses many of the reported outcome predictors, such as extent of the initial hemorrhage and age. Economic concerns require a concomitant improvement in methods for assessing and predicting management costs. Length of stay (LOS) provides a reasonable estimate of medical resource use.[102] Health care professionals realize that the risk of disability and death and the cost of medical care is particularly high, especially in those patients who have suffered an SAH and are 65 years or older. Increasing knowledge about predictors that can help determine patient outcome can only serve to enhance our care for these patients and families. Treatment options must be evaluated in terms of quality of life, functional outcome, and financial details.

The current and anticipated health care environment demands that nurses and other health care providers shift focus from planned care to a managed care system. The emphasis on "care planning" is moving toward ensuring the achievement of acceptable patient outcomes within an efficient time frame with the appropriate use of resources. The changing health environment requires health care professionals to explore alternative ways to deliver quality patient care, reduce length of stay, and manage resources.

Stachniak et al. looked at age as an influence on cost and effectiveness of treatment in patients with SAH.[104] The results from their study suggest that elderly patients, certainly those over 65 years, can benefit from aggressive treatment. Stachniak determined that cost was indeed higher in every area of care for those aged 65 years or older compared with younger patients. Interestingly, when evaluated by decade, there were no significant cost differences. The data analyzed indicates that aggressive treatment is appropriate unless and until the patient or family determines that for nonmedical reasons, nonsurgical treatment is preferred. Even though hospital costs may be higher for treating elderly patients with SAH, the decision of whether access to care should be based on the cost of care provision is a moral and ethical question that cannot be answered based on financial data.

To better understand the effect of severity of hemorrhage and the clinical course on resource use, researchers compared demographic and clinical information as well as hospital costs for the following four groups of patients: patients with unruptured aneurysms, those with acute aneurysmal SAH, those with SAH and vasospasm, and those with SAH and a negative angiographic result. The results of the study revealed three high-cost areas that accounted for almost 50% of the total costs in the care and treatment of patients with SAH: ICU stay, arteriography, and medical/surgical supplies. Strategies for cost containment include minimizing the ICU stay, limiting stays to those patients who need aggressive management (e.g., patients in vasospasm). A step-down unit may be a viable alternative for some of these patients. This is an area in which nurses could collaborate in critical decision making to determine which patients could be safely managed in a less acute setting. A major cost savings in this population could be reduced consumption of disposable supplies. Development of new treatment modes to manage vasospasm may also reduce the need for angiograms, thus reducing costs.

After reviewing 543 SAH patients over a 10-year period, Elliott et al. correlated clinical grade on admission (Hunt-Hess grade) with hospital LOS and cost.[102] As the Hunt-Hess grade increased, so did LOS. The patients with the worst clinical grade (i.e., grade 5) showed a reduction in both LOS and cost because of devastating bleeding followed by death soon after admission. More than 50% of the costs of patients with cerebral aneurysms, both ruptured and unruptured, are associated with LOS and surgery.[102] Surgical repair of aneurysms before rupture could represent tremendous savings in expense and use of neurosurgical and other hospital resources. This conclusion is supported by other reports of direct costs for patients with SAH to be 1.5 times greater than costs for the care of patients with unruptured aneurysms.[105] These studies emphasize a need for a more detailed evaluation of how preoperative and postoperative factors influence LOS, particularly in regard to nursing and medical interventions. Further research needs to be done to stratify radiographic, clinical, and treatment factors that will better predict cost and LOS for each grade of aneurysm patient. Such information could be useful in nursing research allocation. Therefore, there are several factors to consider when deciding to treat a patient with a ruptured intracranial aneurysm. Age, size of the lesion, neurological condition of the patient, and aneurysm location are important factors.

Advances in aneurysmal SAH management have been documented by a decrease in mortality after surgical management.

Ropper and Zervas highlighted that significant neurological morbidity and decreased rates of patients returning to work are common, even in patients presenting in the best neurological condition.[106] Recently, outcome analysis has assumed a prominent role for caregivers, patients, and payers who are interested in standardized assessments of the clinical sequelae of different treatment practices. With the advent of multiple-modality treatment of SAH, as well as advanced intensive care units and endovascular options for vasospasm treatment, there is little doubt that regional variations in the practice of SAH management will continue to evolve. To document the effect of these practice variations accurately, specific standardized assessments of outcomes are essential.

Most data about outcomes after SAH have relied on physician-oriented global assessments, such as the Glasgow Outcome Scale (GOS). This reliable tool is used to assess outcomes in various illnesses and has five categories: dead, persistent vegetative state, severe disability, moderate disability or fair recovery, and good recovery. Good recovery describes the patient's neurological and physical status and the assessor's perception of the patient's capacity to return to work and return to "normal" or "near normal" functioning. The nature of this scale has made it difficult to analyze specific factors that may contribute to global outcome. The assessment of "good recovery" is not usually based on a full evaluation of both the patient's cognitive and behavioral changes. Standardized neuropsychological tests provide objective measures of cognitive function, but if they are used alone, disabling behavioral changes and problems in everyday life may be underestimated.[107]

Buchanan et al.[107] assessed behavioral and personality changes, psychosocial function, and family burden in a mixed sample of 28 patients who underwent surgery for SAH and were viewed by their neurosurgeon as having a "good recovery" or "moderate disability." Despite good physical recovery 19 months after SAH, more than half the patients had not returned to their previous level of employment. Their daily lives were affected by mental and physical fatigability. Intolerance to being rushed, to groups of people, to small children, to lack of order or routine, and to normal sound levels were common complaints. It is difficult to measure these problems objectively, and they can compromise personal relationships and employment. Family relationships suffered, and intimate relationships were affected by lack of libido. Carter et al. examined the prevalence of physical disability and depression in a cohort of patients who had sustained aneurysmal SAH who presented initially in good neurological condition (Hunt-Hess grades I to III).[108] Other factors analyzed included patient age and initial neurological status; a standard global outcome assessment, the Reintegration to Normal Living Status Index; and the patient's self-report of work status.

Measures such as the GOS or Rankin Scale provide for a ready assessment of outcome, and the use of a standardized self-reported outcome assessment has the ability to further our understanding of deficits after SAH from a patient's perspective. By identifying and analyzing factors associated with quality of life, it may be possible to identify specific interventions (i.e., antidepressive therapy or cognitive rehabilitation programs) that may help quality-of-life perceptions.

SUMMARY

This chapter has provided a comprehensive discussion of the state of the science of cerebral aneurysm treatment and care. The future trends have been addressed within the context of discussing treatment. The trend toward more endovascular approaches rather than surgical intervention is clear. Determining the best approach for the individual patient lies in the availability of treatment options and sound clinical judgment.

REFERENCES

1. Brown, R. (1999). Natural history of intracranial aneurysms. *Neurovascular Update: Present Practices and Future Directions*
2. Rinkel, G. J., Djibuti, M., Algra, A., & van Gijn, J. (1998). Prevalence and risk of rupture of intracranial aneurysms: A systematic review. *Stroke, 29,* 251–256
3. Wiebers, D. O., Piepgras, D. G., Meyer, F. B., et al. (2004). Pathogenesis, natural history, and treatment of unruptured intracranial aneurysms. *Mayo Clinic Proceedings, 79,* 1572–1583
4. Schievink, W. I. (1997). Intracranial aneurysms. *New England Journal of Medicine, 336,* 28–40.
5. Edlow, J. A., & Caplan, L. R. (2000). Avoiding pitfalls in the diagnosis of subarachnoid hemorrhage. *New England Journal of Medicine, 342,* 29–36.
6. Linn, F. H., Wijdicks, E. F., van der Graaf, Y., Weerdesteyn-van Vliet, F. A., Bartelds, A. I., & van Gijn, J. (1994). Prospective study of sentinel headache in aneurysmal subarachnoid haemorrhage. *Lancet, 344,* 590–593.
7. Morgenstern, L. B., Luna-Gonzales, H., Huber, J. C., Jr., et al. (1998). Worst headache and subarachnoid hemorrhage: Prospective, modern computed tomography and spinal fluid analysis. *Annals of Emergency Medicine, 32,* 297–304.
8. Mayberg, M. R., Batjer, H. H., Dacey, R., et al. (1994). Guidelines for the management of aneurysmal subarachnoid hemorrhage. A statement for healthcare professionals from a special writing group of the Stroke Council, American Heart Association. *Stroke, 25,* 2315–2328.
9. Meyer, F. B., Sundt, T. M., Jr., Fode, N. C., Morgan, M. K., Forbes, G. S., & Mellinger, J. F. (1989). Cerebral aneurysms in childhood and adolescence. *Journal of Neurosurgery, 70,* 420–425.
10. Cheung, A. C. O. (2004). Subarachnoid hemorrhage diagnosis and management. *Neurovascular News, Massachusetts General Hospital, Winter/Spring 2004,* 1–2.
11. Mayer, P. L., Awad, I. A., Todor, R., et al. (1996). Misdiagnosis of symptomatic cerebral aneurysm. Prevalence and correlation with outcome at four institutions. *Stroke, 27,* 1558–1563.
12. Vermeulen, M. (1996). Subarachnoid haemorrhage: Diagnosis and treatment. *Journal of Neurology, 243,* 496–501.
13. Sames, T. A., Storrow, A. B., Finkelstein, J. A., & Magoon, M. R. (1996). Sensitivity of new-generation computed tomography in subarachnoid hemorrhage. *Academic Emergency Medicine, 3,* 16–20.
14. Sidman, R., Connolly, E., & Lemke, T. (1996). Subarachnoid hemorrhage diagnosis: Lumbar puncture is still needed when the computed tomography scan is normal. *Academic Emergency Medicine, 3,* 827–831.
15. van der Wee, N., Rinkel, G. J., Hasan, D., & van Gijn, J. (1995). Detection of subarachnoid haemorrhage on early CT: Is lumbar puncture still needed after a negative scan? *Journal of Neurology, Neurosurgery, & Psychiatry, 58,* 357–359.
16. Huang, J., McGirt, M. J., Gailloud, P., & Tamargo, R. J. (2005). Intracranial aneurysms in the pediatric population: Case series and literature review. *Surgical Neurology, 63,* 424–432; discussion 432–433.
17. Krishna, H., Wani, A. A., Behari, S., Banerji, D., Chhabra, D. K., & Jain, V. K. (2005). Intracranial aneurysms in patients 18 years of age or under, are they different from aneurysms in adult population? *Acta Neurochirurgica (Wien), 147,* 469–476; discussion 476.
18. Unruptured intracranial aneurysms—risk of rupture and risks of surgical intervention. International study of unruptured intracranial aneurysms investigators. (1998). *New England Journal of Medicine, 339,* 1725–1733.
19. Norris, J. S., & Wallace, M. C. (1998). Pediatric intracranial aneurysms. *Neurosurgery Clinics of North America, 9,* 557–563.
20. Heiserman, J. F., & Bird, C. R. (1994). Cerebral aneurysms. *Neuroimaging Clinics of North America, 4,* 799–822.
21. Kasuya, H., Onda, H., Takeshita, M., Hori, T., & Takakura, K. (2000). Clinical features of intracranial aneurysms in siblings. *Neurosurgery, 46,* 1301–1305; discussion 1305–1306.
22. Leblanc, R. (1997). Familial cerebral aneurysms. *Canadian Journal of Neurological Sciences, 24,* 191–199.
23. Ronkainen, A., Miettinen, H., Karkola, K., et al. (1998). Risk of harboring an unruptured intracranial aneurysm. *Stroke, 29,* 359–362.
24. Leblanc, R. (1996). Familial cerebral aneurysms. A bias for women. *Stroke, 27,* 1050–1054.
25. Raaymakers, T. W., Rinkel, G. J., Limburg, M., & Algra, A. (1998). Mortality and morbidity of surgery for unruptured intracranial aneurysms: A meta-analysis. *Stroke, 29,* 1531–1538.
26. Ogilvy, C. S. (2000). Familial intracranial aneurysms. *Circle of Friends Newsletter, Brain Aneurysm Foundation, 4,* 1–2.
27. Leblanc, R., Melanson, D., Tampieri, D., & Guttmann, R. D. (1995). Familial cerebral aneurysms: A study of 13 families. *Neurosurgery, 37,* 633–638; discussion 638–639.
28. Schievink, W. I., Wijdicks, E. F., Parisi, J. E., Piepgras, D. G., & Whisnant, J. P. (1995). Sudden death from aneurysmal subarachnoid hemorrhage. *Neurology, 45,* 871–874.
29. Broderick, J. P., Sauerbeck, L. R., Foroud, T., et al. (2005). The familial intracranial aneurysm (FIA) study protocol. *BMC Medical Genetics, 6,* 17.
30. Ronkainen, A., Hernesniemi, J., Puranen, M., et al. (1997). Familial intracranial aneurysms. *Lancet, 349,* 380–384.
31. Kissela, B. M., Sauerbeck, L., Woo, D., et al. (2002). Subarachnoid hemorrhage: A preventable disease with a heritable component. *Stroke, 33,* 1321–1326.
32. Stehbens, W. E. (1989). Etiology of intracranial berry aneurysms. *Journal of Neurosurgery, 70,* 823–831.
33. Forbus, W. D. (1930). On the origin of military aneurysms of the superficial cerebral arteries. *Bull John Hopkins Hospital, 47,* 239–284.
34. Glynn, L. E. (1940). Medial defects in the circle of willis and their relationship to aneurysm formation. *Journal of Pathological Bacteriology, 51,* 213–222.
35. Phillips, L. H., Whisnant, J. P., O'Fallon, W. M., & Sundt, T. M., Jr. (1980). The unchanging pattern of subarachnoid hemorrhage in the community. *Neurology, 30,* 1034–1040.
36. Ryba, M., Grieb, P., Podobinska, I., Iwanska, K., Pastuszko, M., & Gorski, A. (1992). Hla antigens and intracranial aneurysms. *Acta Neurochirurgica (Wien), 116,* 1–5.
37. Herman, J. M., Rekate, H. L., & Spetzler, R. F. (1991). Pediatric intracranial aneurysms: Simple and complex cases. *Pediatric Neurosurgery, 17,* 66–72; discussion 73.
38. Strother, C. (2000). Aneurysm hemodynamics. *Neurovascular Update: The New Millennium,* May 25, 2000.
39. Ellegala, D. B., & Day, A. L. (2005). Ruptured cerebral aneurysms. *New England Journal of Medicine, 352,* 121–124.
40. Brown, R. (2000). Ruptured intracranial aneurysms: Morbidity and mortality. *Neurovascular Update: The New Millennium,* May 25, 2000.
41. Longstreth, W. T., Nelson, L. M., Koepsell, T. D., & van Belle, G. (1994). Subarachnoid hemorrhage and hormonal factors in women. A population-based case-control study. *Annals of Internal Medicine, 121,* 168–173.
42. Broderick, J. P., Brott, T., Tomsick, T., Huster, G., & Miller, R. (1992). The risk of subarachnoid and intracerebral hemorrhages

in blacks as compared with whites. *New England Journal of Medicine, 326,* 733–736.

43. Bederson, J. B., Awad, I. A., Wiebers, D. O., et al. (2000). Recommendations for the management of patients with unruptured intracranial aneurysms: A statement for healthcare professionals from the Stroke Council of the American Heart Association. *Circulation, 102,* 2300–2308.

44. Raaymakers, T. W., Rinkel, G. J., & Ramos, L. M. (1998). Initial and follow-up screening for aneurysms in families with familial subarachnoid hemorrhage. *Neurology, 51,* 1125–1130.

45. Taylor, C. L., Yuan, Z., Selman, W. R., Ratcheson, R. A., & Rimm, A. A. (1995). Cerebral arterial aneurysm formation and rupture in 20,767 elderly patients: Hypertension and other risk factors. *Journal of Neurosurgery, 83,* 812–819.

46. Yasui, N., Suzuki, A., Nishimura, H., Suzuki, K., & Abe, T. (1997). Long-term follow-up study of unruptured intracranial aneurysms. *Neurosurgery, 40,* 1155–1159; discussion 1159–1160.

47. Juvela, S., Porras, M., & Poussa, K. (2000). Natural history of unruptured intracranial aneurysms: Probability of and risk factors for aneurysm rupture. *Journal of Neurosurgery, 93,* 379–387.

48. Juvela, S. (1996). Prevalence of risk factors in spontaneous intracerebral hemorrhage and aneurysmal subarachnoid hemorrhage. *Archives of Neurology, 53,* 734–740.

49. Weir, B. K., Kongable, G. L., Kassell, N. F., Schultz, J. R., Truskowski, L. L., & Sigrest, A. (1998). Cigarette smoking as a cause of aneurysmal subarachnoid hemorrhage and risk for vasospasm: A report of the cooperative aneurysm study. *Journal of Neurosurgery, 89,* 405–411.

50. Ogilvy, C. S. (2004). Improved neuroimaging streamlines care of aneurysm patients. *Neurovascular News, Winter/Spring,* 3–5.

51. Sevick, R. J., Tsuruda, J. S., & Schmalbrock, P. (1990). Three-dimensional time-of-flight MR angiography in the evaluation of cerebral aneurysms. *Journal of Computer Assisted Tomography, 14,* 874–881.

52. Burch, G. E., Meyers, R., & Abildskov, J. A. (1954). A new electrocardiographic pattern observed in cerebrovascular accidents. *Circulation, 9,* 719–723.

53. Davis, T. P., Alexander, J., & Lesch, M. (1993). Electrocardiographic changes associated with acute cerebrovascular disease: A clinical review. *Progress in Cardiovascular Diseases, 36,* 245–260.

54. Zaroff, J. G., Rordorf, G. A., Newell, J. B., Ogilvy, C. S., & Levinson, J. R. (1999). Cardiac outcome in patients with subarachnoid hemorrhage and electrocardiographic abnormalities. *Neurosurgery, 44,* 34–39; discussion 39–40.

55. Song, E. C., Chu, K., Jeong, S. W., et al. (2003). Hyperglycemia exacerbates brain edema and perihematomal cell death after intracerebral hemorrhage. *Stroke, 34,* 2215–2220.

56. Molyneux, A. J., Kerr, R. S., Yu, L. M., et al. (2005). International Subarachnoid Aneurysm Trial (ISAT) of neurosurgical clipping versus endovascular coiling in 2143 patients with ruptured intracranial aneurysms: A randomised comparison of effects on survival, dependency, seizures, rebleeding, subgroups, and aneurysm occlusion. *Lancet, 366,* 809–817.

57. Molyneux, A., Kerr, R., Stratton, I., et al. (2002). International Subarachnoid Aneurysm Trial (ISAT) of neurosurgical clipping versus endovascular coiling in 2143 patients with ruptured intracranial aneurysms: A randomised trial. *Lancet, 360,* 1267–1274.

58. Guglielmi, G., Vinuela, F., Sepetka, I., & Macellari, V. (1991). Electrothrombosis of saccular aneurysms via endovascular approach. Part 1: Electrochemical basis, technique, and experimental results. *Journal of Neurosurgery, 75,* 1–7.

59. Malisch, T. W., Guglielmi, G., Vinuela, F., et al. (1998). Unruptured aneurysms presenting with mass effect symptoms: Response to endosaccular treatment with guglielmi detachable coils. Part i. Symptoms of cranial nerve dysfunction. *Journal of Neurosurgery, 89,* 956–961.

60. Guglielmi, G., Vinuela, F., & Duckwiler, G. (1995). Coil induced thrombosis of intracranial aneurysms. In R. J. Marcunias (Ed.). *Endovascular neurological intervention* (pp. 179–188). Park Ridge, IL: AANS.

61. Malisch, T. W., Guglielmi, G., Vinuela, F., et al. (1997). Intracranial aneurysms treated with the Guglielmi detachable coil: Midterm clinical results in a consecutive series of 100 patients. *Journal of Neurosurgery, 87,* 176–183.

62. McDougall, C. G., Halbach, V. V., Dowd, C. F., Higashida, R. T., Larsen, D. W., & Hieshima, G. B. (1998). Causes and management of aneurysmal hemorrhage occurring during embolization with Guglielmi detachable coils. *Journal of Neurosurgery, 89,* 87–92.

63. Eskridge, J. M., & Song, J. K. (1998). Endovascular embolization of 150 basilar tip aneurysms with Guglielmi detachable coils: Results of the food and drug administration multicenter clinical trial. *Journal of Neurosurgery, 89,* 81–86.

64. Debrun, G. M., Aletich, V. A., Kehrli, P., Misra, M., Ausman, J. I., & Charbel, F. (1998). Selection of cerebral aneurysms for treatment using Guglielmi detachable coils: The preliminary University of Illinois at Chicago experience. *Neurosurgery, 43,* 1281–1295; discussion 1296–1297.

65. Fernandez Zubillaga, A., Guglielmi, G., Vinuela, F., & Duckwiler, G. R. (1994). Endovascular occlusion of intracranial aneurysms with electrically detachable coils: Correlation of aneurysm neck size and treatment results. *AJNR American Journal of Neuroradiology, 15,* 815–820.

66. Mericle, R. A., Wakhloo, A. K., Rodriguez, R., Guterman, L. R., & Hopkins, L. N. (1997). Temporary balloon protection as an adjunct to endosaccular coiling of wide-necked cerebral aneurysms: Technical note. *Neurosurgery, 41,* 975–978.

67. Takahashi, A., Ezura, M., & Yoshimoto, T. (1997). Broad neck basilar tip aneurysm treated by neck plastic intra aneurysmal GDC embolization with protective balloon. *Interventional Neuroradiology, 3,* 167–170.

68. Aletich, V. A., Debrun, G. M., Misra, M., Charbel, F., & Ausman, J. I. (2000). The remodeling technique of balloon-assisted Guglielmi detachable coil placement in wide-necked aneurysms: Experience at the University of Illinois at Chicago. *Journal of Neurosurgery, 93,* 388–396.

69. Moret, J., Pierot, L., Boulin, A., et al. (1994). "Remodeling" of the arterial wall of the parent vessels in the endovascular treatment of intracranial aneurysms (abstract). *Proceedings of the Society for Neuroradiology, 36,* (Suppl. 1), S83.

70. Wells-Roth, D., Biondi, A., Janardhan, V., Chapple, K., Gobin, Y. P., & Riina H. A. (2005). Endovascular procedures for treating wide-necked aneurysms. *Neurosurgical Focus, 18,* E7.

71. Murayma, Y., Vinuela, F., Duckwiler, G. R., Gobin, Y. P., & Guglielmi, G. (1999). Embolization of incidental cerebral aneurysms by using the Guglielmi detachable coil system. *Journal of Neurosurgery, 90,* 207–214.

72. Lanterna, L. A., Tredici, G., Dimitrov, B. D., & Biroli, F. (2004). Treatment of unruptured cerebral aneurysms by embolization with Guglielmi detachable coils: Case-fatality, morbidity, and effectiveness in preventing bleeding—a systematic review of the literature. *Neurosurgery, 55,* 767–775; discussion 775–778.

73. Raymond, J., Guilbert, F., Weill, A., et al. (2003). Long-term angiographic recurrences after selective endovascular treatment of aneurysms with detachable coils. *Stroke, 34,* 1398–1403.

74. Sluzewski, M., van Rooij, W. J., Rinkel, G. J., & Wijnalda, D. (2003). Endovascular treatment of ruptured intracranial aneurysms with detachable coils: Long-term clinical and serial angiographic results. *Radiology, 227,* 720–724.

75. Slob, M. J., van Rooij, W. J., & Sluzewski, M. (2005). Coil thickness and packing of cerebral aneurysms: A comparative study of two types of coils. *AJNR American Journal of Neuroradiology, 26,* 901–903.

76. Lanzino, G., Wakhloo, A. K., Fessler, R. D., Hartney, M. L., Guterman, L. R., & Hopkins, L. N. (1999). Efficacy and current limitations of intravascular stents for intracranial internal carotid, vertebral, and basilar artery aneurysms. *Journal of Neurosurgery, 91,* 538–546.

77. Palmaz, J. C. (1992). Intravascular stenting: From basic research to clinical application. *Cardiovascular and Interventional Radiology, 15*, 279–284.

78. Horowitz, M. B., & Purdy, P. D. (2000). The use of stents in the management of neurovascular disease: A review of historical and present status. *Neurosurgery, 46*, 1335–1342; discussion 1342–1343.

79. Higashida, R. T., Smith, W., Gress, D., et al. (1997). Intravascular stent and endovascular coil placement for a ruptured fusiform aneurysm of the basilar artery. Case report and review of the literature. *Journal of Neurosurgery, 87*, 944–949.

80. Howington, J. U., Hanel, R. A., Harrigan, M. R., Levy, E. I., Guterman, L. R., & Hopkins, L. N. (2004). The Neuroform stent, the first microcatheter-delivered stent for use in the intracranial circulation. *Neurosurgery, 54*, 2–5.

81. Higashida, R. T., Halbach, V. V., Dowd, C. F., Juravsky, L., & Meagher, S. (2005). Initial clinical experience with a new self-expanding nitinol stent for the treatment of intracranial cerebral aneurysms: The cordis enterprise stent. *AJNR American Journal of Neuroradiology, 26*, 1751–1756.

82. Benitez, R. P., Silva, M. T., Klem, J., Veznedaroglu, E., & Rosenwasser, R. H. (2004). Endovascular occlusion of wide-necked aneurysms with a new intracranial microstent (Neuroform) and detachable coils. *Neurosurgery, 54*, 1359–1368.

83. Kassell, N. F. (1993). The role of vasospasm in overall outcome from aneurysmal subarachnoid hemorrhage. In J. M. Findlay (Ed.). *Cerebral vasospasm* (pp. 27–28). Philadelphia: Elsevier Science Publication.

84. Robinson, M. J., & Teasdale, G. M. (1990). Calcium antagonists in the management of subarachnoid haemorrhage. *Cerebrovascular and Brain Metabolism Reviews, 2*, 205–226.

85. Gabikian, P., Clatterbuck, R. E., Eberhart, C. G., Tyler, B. M., Tierney, T. S., & Tamargo, R. J. (2002). Prevention of experimental cerebral vasospasm by intracranial delivery of a nitric oxide donor from a controlled-release polymer: Toxicity and efficacy studies in rabbits and rats. *Stroke, 33*, 2681–2686.

86. Cosentino, F., & Katusic, Z. S. (1994). Does endothelin-1 play a role in the pathogenesis of cerebral vasospasm? *Stroke, 25*, 904–908.

87. Foley, P. L., Caner, H. H., Kassell, N. F., & Lee, K. S. (1994). Reversal of subarachnoid hemorrhage-induced vasoconstriction with an endothelin receptor antagonist. *Neurosurgery, 34*, 108–112; discussion 112–113.

88. Roux, S., Loffler, B. M., Gray, G. A., Sprecher, U., Clozel, M., & Clozel, J. P. (1995). The role of endothelin in experimental cerebral vasospasm. *Neurosurgery, 37*, 78–85; discussion 85–86.

89. Zimmermann, M., Seifert, V., Loffler, B. M., Stolke, D., & Stenzel, W. (1996). Prevention of cerebral vasospasm after experimental subarachnoid hemorrhage by RO 47-0203, a newly developed orally active endothelin receptor antagonist. *Neurosurgery, 38*, 115–120.

90. Zuccarello, M., Soattin, G. B., Lewis, A. I., Breu, V., Hallak, H., & Rapoport, R. M. (1996). Prevention of subarachnoid hemorrhage-induced cerebral vasospasm by oral administration of endothelin receptor antagonists. *Journal of Neurosurgery, 84*, 503–507.

91. Kosty, T. (2005). Cerebral vasospasm after subarachnoid hemorrhage: An update. *Critical Care Nursing Quarterly, 28*, 122–134.

92. Dowd, C. (1999). Endovascular treatment of vasospasm. *Neurovascular Update: Present Practices and Future Directions*

93. Vajkoczy, P., Meyer, B., Weidauer, S., et al. (2005). Clazosentan (axv-034343), a selective endothelin a receptor antagonist, in the prevention of cerebral vasospasm following severe aneurysmal subarachnoid hemorrhage: Results of a randomized, double-blind, placebo-controlled, multicenter phase IIa study. *Journal of Neurosurgery, 103*, 9–17.

94. van den Bergh, W. M., Algra, A., van Kooten, F., et al. (2005). Magnesium sulfate in aneurysmal subarachnoid hemorrhage: A randomized controlled trial. *Stroke, 36*, 1011–1015.

95. van den Bergh, W. M., Algra, A., van der Sprenkel, J. W., Tulleken, C. A., & Rinkel, G. J. (2003). Hypomagnesemia after aneurysmal subarachnoid hemorrhage. *Neurosurgery, 52*, 276–281; discussion 281–282.

96. Chia, R. Y., Hughes, R. S., & Morgan, M. K. (2002). Magnesium: A useful adjunct in the prevention of cerebral vasospasm following aneurysmal subarachnoid haemorrhage. *Journal of Clinical Neurosciences, 9*, 279–281.

97. Macdonald, R. L., Curry, D. J., Aihara, Y., Zhang, Z. D., Jahromi, B. S., & Yassari, R. (2004). Magnesium and experimental vasospasm. *Journal of Neurosurgery, 100*, 106–110.

98. Lynch, J. R., Wang, H., McGirt, M. J., et al. (2005). Simvastatin reduces vasospasm after aneurysmal subarachnoid hemorrhage: Results of a pilot randomized clinical trial. *Stroke, 36*, 2024–2026.

99. Widjicks, E. F. M., Vermeulen, M., Hijdra, A., et al. (1985). Hyponatremia and cerebral infarction in patients with ruptured intracranial aneurysms: Is fluid restriction harmful? *Annals of Neurology, 17*, 137–140.

100. Hasan, D., Wijdicks, E. F., & Vermeulen, M. (1990). Hyponatremia is associated with cerebral ischemia in patients with aneurysmal subarachnoid hemorrhage. *Annals of Neurology, 27*, 106–108.

101. Taylor, C. L., Yuan, Z., Selman, W. R., Ratcheson, R. A., & Rimm, A. A. (1997). Mortality rates, hospital length of stay, and the cost of treating subarachnoid hemorrhage in older patients: Institutional and geographical differences. *Journal of Neurosurgery, 86*, 583–588.

102. Elliott, J. P., Le Roux, P. D., Ransom, G., Newell, D. W., Grady, M. S., Winn, H. R. (1996). Predicting length of hospital stay and cost by aneurysm grade on admission. *Journal of Neurosurgery, 85*, 388–391.

103. Ogilvy, C. S., & Carter, B. S. (1998). A proposed comprehensive grading system to predict outcome for surgical management of intracranial aneurysms. *Neurosurgery, 42*, 959–968; discussion 968–970.

104. Stachniak, J. B., Layon, A. J., Day, A. L., & Gallagher, T. J. (1996). Craniotomy for intracranial aneurysm and subarachnoid hemorrhage. Is course, cost, or outcome affected by age? *Stroke, 27*, 276–281.

105. Wiebers, D. O., Torner, J. C., & Meissner, I. (1992). Impact of unruptured intracranial aneurysms on public health in the united states. *Stroke, 23*, 1416–1419.

106. Ropper, A., & Zervas, N. (1984). Outcome 1 year after SAH from cerebral aneurysm: Management morbidity, mortality, and functional status in 112 good risk patients. *Journal of Neurosurgery, 60*, 909–915.

107. Buchanan, K. M., Elias, L. J., & Goplen, G. B. (2000). Differing perspectives on outcome after subarachnoid hemorrhage: The patient, the relative, the neurosurgeon. *Neurosurgery, 46*, 831–838; discussion 838–840.

108. Carter, B. S., Buckley, D. A., Ferraro, R., Rordorf, G., & Ogilvy, C. S. (2000). Factors associated with reintegration to normal living after subarachnoid hemorrhage. *Neurosurgery, 46(6)*, 1326–1334.

RESOURCES

Websites

The following websites provide information on cerebral aneurysms. The Brain Aneurysm Foundation: http://www.bafound.org
http://www.brain-surgery.com/aneurysm.html
http://brainavm.oci.utoronto.ca
http://www.bostonscientific.com/
http://www.mayoclinic.com/health/brain-aneurysm/DS00582
http://dpi.radiology.uiowa.edu/nlm/app/aneur/brain/aneur.html
http://www.cedars-sinai.edu/1146.html?wt.srch=1&cpid
http://www.mgh-interventional-neurorad.org/
http://www.snisonline.org

Patient and Family

Organizations

Brain Aneurysm Foundation, 612 East Broadway, South Boston, MA 02127, Tel: 617-269-3870.

Arteriovenous Malformations and Other Cerebrovascular Anomalies

Deidre A. Buckley and Joanne V. Hickey

Cerebrovascular malformations are believed to be developmental vascular anomalies that result from failure of the embryonic vascular network to develop properly.[1] The incidence of cerebrovascular malformations is unclear because many lesions are asymptomatic and are found only incidentally at autopsy. They are relatively common lesions that can cause a variety of symptoms. Some lesions present with serious symptoms such as hemorrhage, seizure, or headaches, whereas other lesions are quite benign with no symptoms at all. The presentation, location, and natural history of these lesions will determine whether management will be surgical, endovascular, radiosurgical, or observation.

CLASSIFICATIONS OF VASCULAR MALFORMATIONS

Cerebrovascular malformations are classified into five major categories: capillary telangiectases, venous malformations (VMs), arteriovenous malformations (AVMs), dural arteriovenous fistulas (DAVFs), and cavernous malformations (CMs).[2] The term *malformation* is preferable to the previously used *angioma*. Angioma has a connotation of neoplasia, a connotation that is inaccurate with these lesions. The incidence of vascular malformations varies from 0.1% to 4% in various autopsy studies. In a large autopsy series, the detection of AVMs was 1.4% (46 AVMs among 3200 brain tumor cases). Vascular malformations are about one seventh as common as intracranial saccular aneurysms. AVMS are the most common type of vascular lesion, followed by CMs and VMs. With improvement in cross-sectional imaging in both computed tomography (CT) and magnetic resonance imaging (MRI), higher detection rates are being reported and in patients with increasing age.[2] Because some of these lesions do not have direct arterial vessel input, they may not be visible on angiography.[1,3,4]

Telangiectases

Telangiectases are small (0.3 to 1.0 cm) capillary lesions that are composed of clusters of vessels that look something like dilated capillaries separated by normal-appearing parenchyma. These lesions have little clinical significance because they rarely cause any symptoms; they are not apparent on radiologic examination. Telangiectases are an incidental finding at autopsy and are most commonly located in the posterior fossa or spinal cord and have an overall frequency of 0.1%.[2]

Cavernous Malformations

CMs, also called cavernous hemangiomas, cavernous angiomas, and cavernomas, are congenital nodular lesions. They resemble a mulberry- or "popcorn-like"–appearing lesion in the brain, spinal cord, or nerve roots and are composed of sinusoidal-type vessels that are not separated by normal-appearing parenchyma (neural tissue). Microscopic examination often reveals small hemorrhages with numerous, hemosiderin-laden macrophages and gliotic tissue in the adjacent parenchyma. Elastic fibers are absent in the walls of these vascular caverns. Thrombosis may be present in some of the dilated venules.[2] Calcification within the lesion is common.

CMs are well-defined, purple lesions that may grow to an appreciable size and may be mistaken for a brain tumor on CT scan. Other cavernous malformations are found incidentally at autopsy. The overall frequency of CMs was approximately 0.4% in a large autopsy study. A retrospective review found a detection rate of 0.4% to 0.9% on MRI studies. CMs are rare in children and account for about 10% of all symptomatic vascular malformations.[2] The peak occurrence is in the third and fifth decades of life.[5] CMs occur in two forms, either *sporadic*, which is characterized by one lesion, or *familial*, which is characterized by multiple lesions with an autosomal dominant mode of inheritance.[6] Genetic linkage studies revealed a locus for CM on chromosome 7q. Two additional loci have also been identified mapping to chromosomes 7p and 3q. The CM gene was successfully identified as KRIT1.[5]

These low-flow lesions are not apparent on angiography but may be visualized on CT scan and MRI (Fig. 24-1) as a combination of high and low T1 and T2 signals with surrounding hemosiderin. Most often CMs present on MRI with no symptoms. Some cavernous malformations may cause

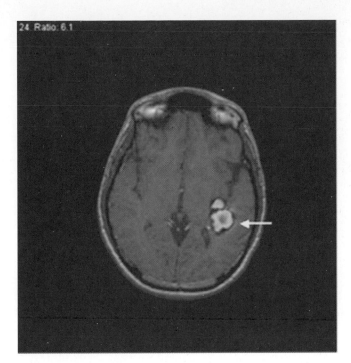

Figure 24-1 • Magnetic resonance image (T1 axial image) demonstrates a left temporal cavernous malformation with a peripheral rim of hemosiderin suggesting recent hemorrhage. (Courtesy of Christopher S. Ogilvy, MD, Massachusetts General Hospital, Boston, MA.)

seizures and intracerebral hemorrhage. Symptom presentation depends on location and lesion size. A CM of any size can present with hemorrhage. These hemorrhages tend to occur at lower pressures and with less severity than those bleeds associated with AVMs, although serious hemorrhages that are life threatening or with serious consequences can occur with CMs of the cerebellum or brainstem. The frequency of hemorrhage among those who present with either incidental diagnosis or seizures is approximately 0.4% to 2% per year. In those who present with hemorrhage, the annual recurrence rate would be higher, with a rate of about 4% to 5% in the next year. Location also plays an important role in hemorrhage risk such that patients with brainstem, thalamic, cerebellar, or basal ganglia lesions have an initial annual hemorrhage risk of 4.1% compared to 0.4% among those with superficial lesions.[2]

Treatment is considered in patients who present with multiple episodes of hemorrhage that are either clinically or radiographically significant or in patients suffering from uncontrolled seizures. The optimal treatment is stereotactic surgical assistance for the supratentorial lesions. Many surgeons choose to observe lesions in critical areas such as the brainstem, basal ganglia, central sulcus, and spinal cord. They may be pushed to treatment with repetitive hemorrhages. The hemorrhage can create a clot cavity, thus providing a route for surgical access and creating a plane for dissection of the lesion.

It is unclear whether radiosurgery has any effect on CMs compared with the natural history. Some groups have noted that radiosurgery may have a greater risk of morbidity compared with AVM radiosurgery. Surgical resection can be performed safely in some patients with deep CMs. Only a select group of patients are considered candidates for radiosurgery. This group would include patients with repetitive hemorrhages where surgery would have prohibitive risks.[2]

Venous Malformations

VMs, also referred to as venous anomalies, are composed of anomalous veins, separated by normal parenchyma, which drain into a dilated venous trunk. A VM is important to brain tissue because it provides normal venous drainage. VMs are the most common vascular anomaly of the brain and are detected in up to 2.6% of all performed autopsies.[2] These lesions have no recognizable direct arterial input. Calcification within the lesion is rare. The predominant location of venous malformations is in the cerebrum, although some are found in the cerebellum (3:1 ratio). Clinically, the patient may present with seizures. Venous malformations may be evident on CT scan, MRI (Fig. 24-2), or angiography. Those found in the cerebrum rarely cause hemorrhage and are treated conservatively. At times, venous anomalies may be adjacent to cavernous malformations. If the cavernous malformation is symptomatic so that the patient presents with hemorrhage, the cavernous malformation may need to be removed with care to avoid obstruction on the functional drainage represented by the venous anomaly. The VM is left untreated. Rarely, vascular malformations may be associated with seizures, motor symptoms, trigeminal neuralgia, or motor deficits. These lesions are simply an anomalous pattern of functionally normal venous drainage. An attempt to resect or

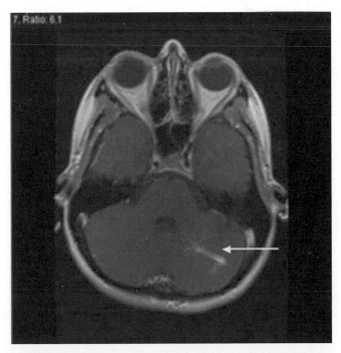

Figure 24-2 • T1 axial magnetic resonance image with gadolinium enhancement shows a developmental venous malformation within the left cerebellar hemisphere. (Courtesy of Christopher S. Ogilvy, MD, Massachusetts General Hospital, Boston, MA.)

treat may result in occlusion, which frequently causes a venous infarction. Therefore, resection of VMs is not recommended and conservative management is the goal.[1]

Dural Arteriovenous Malformations (Fistulas)

Dural AVMs, also called dural arteriovenous fistulas, are almost always acquired lesions, rather than developmental. Dural AVMs comprise 10% to 15% of all intracranial AVMs. They are defined by the following criteria: (1) the nidus of the arteriovenous shunting is within the cranial dural matter, (2) arterial supply arises exclusively from the extracranial circulation or from the meningeal branches of the intracranial branches, and (3) venous drainage is either directly into the dural venous sinus or into nearby leptomeningeal veins.[7]

Venous outflow obstruction, at times associated with sinus thrombosis, can precede development of dural AVMs. The clinical presentation of dural AVMs is primarily related to the pattern and location of venous drainage, rather than to the characteristics of the nidus of the malformation or the arterial feeders.[8] Clinical symptoms are manifested as *generalized* nervous system signs (e.g., papilledema, headache, visual disturbances, or hydrocephalus due to malabsorption of the cerebrospinal fluid) and *focal* signs (e.g., seizure, transient ischemic attack, intraparenchymal hemorrhage, and fixed cortical, brainstem, and cerebellar deficits). The general symptoms are related to generalized venous hypertension in the dural sinuses and the focal symptoms indicate direct or indirect retrograde cortical venous drainage. Leptomeningeal venous drainage is the most important risk factor for focal neurological deficits and hemorrhage.[7] Symptoms of lateral and sigmoid sinus dural AVMs include a pulse-synchronous tinnitus or bruit (70% of cases), papilledema, and headaches, while anterior cranial fossa and tentorial dural AVMs often present with intradural bleeding in 84% and 71% of cases, respectively.[7]

The natural history of dural arteriovenous malformations is highly variable, ranging from spontaneous regression of the lesion, to stable persistence with minor clinical manifestations, to gradual progression to major neurological disability, to acute intradural hemorrhage. Pulsatile tinnitus often occurs with lesions of the transverse or sigmoid sinus.[9] Cortical-based lesions may cause seizures or progressive deficits. With cavernous sinus lesions exophthalmos, diplopia or impaired vision may occur. A superior sagittal sinus lesion may cause papilledema, visual loss, and pseudotumor cerebri.

A head CT scan usually does not detect dural AVMs, but may detect blood, abnormal density in the white matter (due to venous congestion), mass effect, hydrocephalus, and dilatation of major venous sinuses while failing to reveal the lesion.[9] An MRI is more sensitive in detecting abnormal enhancement near the cranial vault, dilated pial veins, or thrombosed venous sinuses. A four-vessel angiogram with selective external carotid artery injection is still the "gold standard" for treatment planning.[2] Computed tomography angiography (CTA) is a newer diagnostic tool that is helpful in localizing a dural AVM.

Management of dural AVMs often requires a multiple modality approach. Treatment may be required urgently if the patient presents with aggressive symptoms such as hemorrhage (intraparenchymal or subarachnoid) or other acute symptoms such as progressive visual loss. Those patients with proptosis, intractable pulsatile tinnitus, or chemosis may be considered for curative or at least palliative treatment.[2] Treatment of DAVFs has evolved over the last three decades.

Transarterial embolization, transvenous embolization, and surgical resection of the lesion may be used alone or in combination depending on the anatomy of the lesion and clinical setting. Stereotactic radiosurgery may also be used, although a larger series is needed to define the role of this modality.[10]

Arteriovenous Malformations

An AVM is composed of a tightly tangled collection of abnormal-appearing, dilated blood vessels that directly shunt arterial blood into the venous system without the usual connecting capillary network. Blood vessels of the AVM are thin walled and tortuous and lack the normal characteristics of veins or arteries. The three morphologic components of an AVM are the nidus, the feeding arteries, and the draining veins. (The literature often refers to the nidus when discussing AVMs; a *nidus* is defined as the focus of the AVM, that is, the tangle of abnormal vessels.) The vessels of the AVM vary greatly in diameter, but the veins are generally larger than the arteries. The arterial vessels, also called *feeder arteries*, supply the AVM. Dilated veins without the usual intervening capillary network drain the lesion. As a result of the absence of the capillary network, blood flow is accelerated and the pressure is elevated within the fragile vessels of the AVM. These conditions predispose the lesion to hemorrhage.

AVMs may be small and focal, or they may be large, involving an entire hemisphere. Some are conical, with the apex pointing inward and the base positioned on the surface of the cerebral cortex. In rare instances, the lesion is so deep that the ventricles and choroid plexus are involved, thus predisposing the person to intraventricular hemorrhage. The parenchyma between the vessels of the AVM is usually abnormal, with nonfunctional gliotic tissue (proliferation of neuroglia [i.e., supporting tissue] in the brain). Frequently, there is evidence of old hemorrhage and hemosiderin deposits (iron-containing glycoprotein pigment found in tissue, excessive amounts of which occur in pathologic conditions). Patients may have a radiographic hemorrhage without clinical signs or symptoms of hemorrhage.

The AVM is the most common cerebrovascular lesion that causes symptoms and is, therefore, clinically significant. Over the last decade, there have been significant developments in the treatment of intracranial AVMs. There has been an evolution in microsurgical, endovascular, and radiosurgical techniques to treat these lesions. As the management options have evolved, combined modality treatment protocols have developed in various institutions. AVMs are found in both children and adults. AVMs in adults constitute the focus of most of this chapter.

ARTERIOVENOUS MALFORMATIONS IN THE ADULT: AN OVERVIEW

Several important points can be made to describe AVMs: they account for 8.6% of subarachnoid hemorrhages; this means that 1% of strokes are attributable to ruptured AVMs. The Harvard Cooperative Stroke Registry did a 3-year study documenting 9 AVM cases among 494 cases of stroke from all causes of stroke in a population of 100,000. This yields an incidence of about 3 per 100,000 annually.[3,23] The ratio of AVMs to intracranial aneurysms is 1:10.[3,23] Approximately 90% of AVMs are located in the supratentorial area and involve the cerebral hemispheres; only 10% of this group are located in the deep subcortical areas (e.g., basal ganglia, thalamus, corpus callosum). The location of 10% of AVMs is within the cerebellum and brainstem. Of those patients with AVMs, 80% develop symptoms between the ages of 20 and 40 years of age; the remaining 20% develop symptoms before the age of 20 years.

Pathophysiology and Pathologic Characteristics of Parenchymal Arteriovenous Malformations

There are two pathophysiologic characteristics related to AVMs. The first is the effect of shunting of blood from the arterial to the venous system without the intervening capillary network. Normally, the capillary network provides capillary resistance to blood flow, thus decreasing the intravascular pressure. However, when an AVM is present, blood is shunted from the high-resistance normal vascular bed to the low-resistance vessels within the AVM, thus exposing the draining venous channels to elevated intravascular pressure. These dynamics predispose the vessels to rupture and hemorrhage.

The second is the effect of impaired perfusion of the cerebral tissue adjacent to the AVM. Elevated intravascular and venous pressure impairs cerebral perfusion pressure. When the AVM is large and has a high flow, the diversion of blood to the AVM may cause ischemia to the adjacent normal tissue. Clinically, this is evidenced by slowly progressive neurological deficits. The diversion of blood to the AVM is called the *vascular steal phenomenon*.

Parenchymal AVMs result from abnormalities in the vasculature during fetal development from fetal age of 3 to 12 weeks. Failure of normal involution of embryonic vasculature networks is thought to occur as AVMs develop. Some AVMs may enlarge by recruitment of new blood vessels during childhood and early adulthood.[1]

AVMs are circumscribed vascular lesions that displace, rather than encompass, normally functioning brain tissue. They are separated from normal tissue by abnormal and nonfunctional gliotic parenchyma. Evidence of microscopic or gross hemorrhage is very common. This is true even in patients who have no clinical manifested hemorrhage. Partial thrombosis of an AVM is not uncommon and can occur spontaneously. This may explain why some AVMs appear smaller on repeat angiography than on a previous study. This may also explain why some AVMs that are classified as "occult" are not seen on angiography.

Clinical Presentation

The major clinical presentation of AVMs is hemorrhage, seizures, headache, and progressive neurological deficits.

The following section provides a brief discussion of each symptom.

Hemorrhage. Hemorrhage is the most common initial manifestation of AVMs. More than 50% of AVMs present with intracranial hemorrhage.[11] When an AVM ruptures, it usually causes intraparenchymal hemorrhage.[12,13] If the AVM is superficial, a subarachnoid hemorrhage can occur. In the rare instance of an AVM that involves the choroid plexus, rupture can result in intraventricular hemorrhage. The available natural history studies demonstrate an overall risk of initial hemorrhage of approximately 2% to 3% per year.[14] Mortality associated with initial AVM rupture is reported to be between 6% and 30% with an average of about 15%. Serious morbidity is between 15% and 80% with an average of about 30%. The combined morbidity and mortality rates from an AVM bleed may be as high as 15% to 80%.[15–18] The chance of rebleeding during the first year is approximately 6%.[19] After the first year, the incidence of recurrent hemorrhages decreases to 4% per year. This is the same as the rate of hemorrhage from AVMs that have never bled. In addition to annual risk of hemorrhage, the lifetime risk must be considered. With the assumption of a 2% to 4% annual hemorrhage risk, the lifetime risk of a bleed among people with previously unruptured AVMs is calculated by the following formula: lifetime risk (percentage) = 105 minus the patient's age in years.[20] The hemorrhage associated with rupture of an AVM is not as devastating as that associated with a ruptured cerebral aneurysm. In addition, the vasospasm and acute rebleeding (20% to 40% rebleed within 14 days) associated with aneurysms are not characteristic of AVMs.[4] Vasospasm does not occur within the AVM because there is no blood in the basilar subarachnoid cistern around the major intracranial arteries as is commonly found with aneurysmal rupture.

Seizures. Seizures are the second most common manifestation of AVMs.[12,14,19] Seizures occur in approximately 20% to 25% of patients.[14,21,22] It has been suggested that approximately 70% of patients with AVMs have seizures at some time.[13] Of those patients who have seizures, about 50% experience the focal type. The natural history of a patient with an AVM presenting with seizures is still not certain.

The etiology of seizures in patients with AVMs is also not clear, but two explanations have been suggested. First, cortical injury from hemorrhage into areas adjacent to the AVM may cause foci for seizure activity. Second, chronic ischemia from the vascular steal phenomenon may also cause abnormal cells that may become the foci for seizure activity.[23]

In patients who present with seizure, there is a 25% chance of hemorrhage within 15 years, or 4% per year.[24] It is thought that medical therapy is generally successful in the control of seizure activity. The prognosis for patients who have surgery or embolization in combination with surgery to resect the AVM is favorable in that the frequency of seizures lessens in most patients.[25] It is also thought that seizures improve after radiosurgery.[26]

Headache. Other presentations of AVMs include headaches in 15% of affected patients.[27] Recurrent headache that does not respond to usual drug therapy may be the only symptom of an AVM. Some patients experience migraine-like headaches. A headache work-up with an MRI scan may suggest the presence of an AVM. It is important to remember that some types of headaches are related to AVMs. Some AVMs in the occipital lobe cause migraine-like headaches. Often after the removal of the AVM, the patient's headaches resolve.[28] Because of the high frequency of headaches in the population, the relationship of AVM to headache is difficult to define. As technology improves and becomes more readily available, MRI scans are being ordered by physicians for headaches or other complaints, and an AVM or other lesion may be found incidentally. In certain circumstances headaches are clearly related to an underlying AVM, but in other situations there is a much less well-defined relationship. In cases in which differentiation of symptoms from lesions is less clear, it would be dangerous to assume the headaches are caused by the malformation and will be relieved by treatment, either partial or complete. The patient must understand that symptoms may be incidental to the lesion.

Progressive Neurological Deficits. The development of progressive neurological deficits is primarily attributed to cerebral ischemia resulting from vascular steal. The signs and symptoms will depend on the specific area of cerebral tissue deprived of adequate blood supply. Progressive deficits may also be related to repeated small hemorrhages that have not been clinically apparent.

Venous hypertension from arterialization of the venous system may account for neurological deterioration. Hydrocephalus is another mechanism that plays a role in progressive neurological deficits caused by ventricular compression from dilated veins.

Neuropsychiatric Manifestations

AVMs may cause neuropsychiatric manifestations. Approximately 10% of patients with an AVM manifest some sort of neuropsychiatric behavior. The vascular steal syndrome is thought to be responsible for such symptoms.[23]

Diagnosis

Diagnostic Procedures

CT Scan. The CT scan is one of the initial screening tools for AVMs. It is a diagnostic test in which cross sections of the brain are examined through the use of x-rays and a computer. The picture of the various layers produced by the scan accurately reflects anatomic structures inside the brain, such as the ventricles, basal ganglia, and thalamus. A CT scan without contrast has a low sensitivity and is often ordered to rule out the presence of an acute hematoma. Calcification and hypointensity may be noted on these films. If the AVM has hemorrhaged, serial CT scans are helpful in monitoring blood clot and observing for resolution of blood over time.

MRI/Magnetic Resonance Angiography (MRA). MRI is an initial diagnostic tool and is ordered more commonly than a CT scan for complaints such as headaches. The MRI is very sensitive, showing a homogeneous signal void on T1- and T2-weighted sequences, often with hemosiderin suggesting prior hemorrhage.[14] The MRI is critical in defining the treatment plan of the AVM to determine the site of its nidus (the central part of the AVM), as well as its relationship to other critical anatomic structures in the brain. It is also better than CT scanning in demonstrating subtle changes in tissue composition (e.g., edema and old hemorrhage).

MRA is the same procedure as MRI, but with the difference that blood vessels are examined instead of body tissue. The MRA can provide some data on the presence of intranidal or feeding artery aneurysms, some information on venous drainage patterns, and subtle AVM nidus qualities.[14] MRI and MRA are both noninvasive types of studies.

Computerized Tomography Angiography. CTA is an exam that uses x-ray to observe blood flow in arterial and venous vessels throughout the body. It is performed with a series of thin-slice axial images during a bolus of IV contrast. Data are accumulated and manipulated by technicians in a three-dimensional lab to show the blood vessels in the head or cervical region. This study may be done in addition to traditional cerebral angiography. CTA will unlikely ever replace digital subtraction angiography (DSA) because arteriovenous (A-V) shunting may only be defined by frames of the angiogram over time. CTA is a more static snapshot of the vasculature, which can help localize the lesion.

Angiography. Cerebral angiography is the definitive diagnostic procedure for AVMs. It demonstrates the feeding arteries, the nidus, and the draining veins. This information is important for making decisions about the advisability of surgery, endovascular therapy, or radiosurgery. Cerebral angiography is also useful for following the progress and development of the AVM over time. As mentioned earlier, some AVMs are angiographically occult lesions. These lesions are discovered in the diagnostic work-up of patients presenting with intracranial hemorrhage or in patients with seizures.

Treatment

Decisions regarding the best approach to management of AVMs are complex. Among the factors that influence patient outcomes, the two that are critical are the reputation of the hospital and, in particular, the experience and skill of the neurosurgeon and interventional neuroradiologist with AVMs. The natural history of the lesion for hemorrhaging, along with the specific characteristics of the particular lesion for an individual patient, must be carefully weighed. The physician must compare the long-term risk presented by an untreated AVM with the more immediate risk of surgery or other treatment options.

Natural History of Arteriovenous Malformations

Understanding the biologic behavior or natural history of AVMs is helpful in weighing treatment approaches. The following provides statistics about the natural history of AVMs.

Unruptured AVM. There is approximately a 3% risk of bleeding per year, with about a 1% risk of death per year.

Ruptured AVMs. *The peak age for hemorrhage is between 15 and 20 years.* The mortality rate for the first hemorrhage is about 10%; morbidity exists in the 30% to 50% range (neurological deficit from each bleed). Small AVMs tend to present more often as hemorrhages than larger ones.[29] It was postulated that larger AVMs presented as seizure simply because their size made them more likely to involve the cortex. The smaller AVMs are now thought to have a much higher pressure in the feeding arteries. Thus, smaller AVMs are assumed to be more lethal than larger ones.

The average risk from hemorrhage from an AVM is approximately 2% to 4% per year.[30] The risk of rebleeding is approximately 6% to 17 % during the first year; it then decreases to a baseline level by the third year. After a second bleed, the risk of another hemorrhage may be as high as 25% during the first year.[2]

The mortality associated with a second hemorrhage is approximately 13%; subsequent hemorrhages carry a mortality rate of about 20%. Prior hemorrhage is a strong predictor of future hemorrhage. Impaired venous drainage and a single draining vein has been a predictor of hemorrhage. The presence of distal aneurysms on small feeding arteries as well as nonnidal aneurysms may also increase hemorrhage risk.[2]

With wider use of MRI for screening of patients for various neurological signs and symptoms, asymptomatic AVMs are being detected more frequently. The risk of hemorrhage is about 4%.[30] Of all patients with AVMs who have no previous clinical history of hemorrhage, 25% to 33% demonstrate evidence of previous hemorrhage.[28]

The natural history of AVMs suggests a high probability for hemorrhage at some time. Statistics also suggest that the incidence of rebleeding is the same regardless of whether the AVM is unruptured or ruptured. Although the physician makes the decisions about medical management, it is important for the nurse to understand the basis for the decision. This information is helpful in teaching both the patient and family and in reinforcing the information provided to the patient and family by the physician.

Cerebral Aneurysms and Arteriovenous Malformations. Seven percent of patients with AVMs also have cerebral aneurysms. Approximately 75% of such aneurysms are located on a major feeding artery, most likely resulting from increased flow. Aneurysms may form within the nidus or on draining veins. When treating tandem lesions, the symptomatic aneurysm or AVM is usually the one treated first. When feasible, they both may be treated at the same time with either surgery or embolization. If it is not clear which had produced the bleeding, the odds are usually with the aneurysm.[31]

Grading of Arteriovenous Malformations

The most commonly used grading system for AVMs is that described by Spetzler and Martin, who developed their system according to their degrees of surgical difficulty.[32] The Spetzler-Martin AVM Grading Scale (Fig. 24-3) provides a simplified scheme based on size, location, and venous drainage:

SIZE	
0–3 cm	1
3.1–6.0 cm	2
>6 cm	3
LOCATION	
Noneloquent	0
Eloquent	1
DEEP VENOUS DRAINAGE	
Not present	0
Present	1

Eloquence refers to areas of the brain that have readily identifiable neurological function; if injury to any of these areas occurs, a disabling neurological deficit will be noted. According to this grading system, the eloquent areas are the sensorimotor, language, and visual cortex; the hypothalamus and thalamus; the internal capsule; the brainstem; the cerebellar peduncles; and the deep cerebellar nuclei.

Each of these three variables becomes a subscale that is assigned a numerical value. The scores of each subscale are added together, and the total score indicates an AVM grade from I to V. Angiographic findings are used to collect data for each subscale.

Within this system, grades I and II lesions have a low morbidity, whereas higher-grade lesions are associated with gradually increasing morbidity. Spetzler and Martin recommend surgery for all grade I and II lesions. Grade III lesions should be treated case by case; however, they usually recommend surgery for both symptomatic and asymptomatic lesions. Grade IV and V lesions necessitate a multidisciplinary approach. There are other grading systems that focus on anatomic, hemodynamic, and physiologic properties associated with AVMs; however, it was found that the three factors identified in the Spetzler-Martin systems were most accurate in predicting surgical outcomes.[27]

Treatment Options

The treatment options available for AVMs include surgery, embolization, radiosurgery, and conservative treatment. Comprehensive evaluation of a patient with an AVM includes a detailed clinical examination and radiologic clarification of the anatomy with MRI and arteriography. After the comprehensive evaluation, decisions can be made regarding the best management approach by comparing the natural history of the lesion with the intervention-related morbidity and mortality.

There is evidence suggesting that the radiologic parameters may be predictive of hemorrhage risk. There is a complex combination of variables that may predict the risk of hemorrhage from AVM. Some have noted that patients with seizures may be at slightly higher risk, but this has not been noted consistently.[15,19] There are also data to suggest that prior hemorrhage is a strong predictor of hemorrhage.[33] Small AVM size in maximal diameter[19] or volume may also be a predictor for higher hemorrhage risk.[34] AVMs in the intraventricular or periventricular location may also be at an increased risk to bleed,[35] although this is not found consistently.[36]

The angiographic characteristics of an AVM are complex. There are both arterial and venous factors that are predictive of an increased risk of hemorrhage, although studies are not *definitive*. Characteristics of the venous drainage system,

GRADE I   GRADE III   GRADE IV

GRADE II

GRADE V

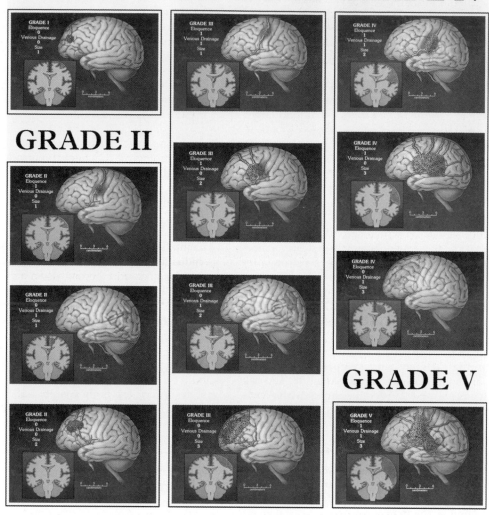

Figure 24-3 • Spetzler-Martin Grading System for arteriovenous malformations. (From Spetzler, R. F., & Martin, R. A. [1986]. A proposed grading system for arteriovenous malformations. *Journal of Neurosurgery, 65,* 476–483.)

including the presence of deep venous drainage, have been reported to be a predictor of presentation with hemorrhage.[37,38]

Surgery. With rare exceptions, surgery for an AVM is always elective. Only if there is an intracerebral hematoma or subdural hematoma is early surgery considered. Even when surgery is anticipated after hemorrhage, it is usually delayed for about 3 weeks. This timetable allows for the patient to be stabilized and for the brain to recover from the effects of hemorrhage.

Applying the grading system for AVMs discussed earlier, the experienced neurosurgeon is able to assess the degree of surgical difficulty. The physician considers the age of the patient along with the anatomic location of the lesion and other characteristics that influence the technical approach to the lesion. The goals of surgery are (1) complete excision of the AVM to prevent hemorrhage completely and (2) excision of the lesion without causing hemorrhage or injury to adjacent tissue during the surgery. Ligation of the feeder

vessels does not provide protection from hemorrhage.[39] Lesions are typically excised using standard microsurgical techniques with the microscope (Fig. 24-4). The arterial feeders are generally attacked first, followed by excision of the nidus of the lesion and then resection of the draining vein. To ensure complete obliteration of the lesion, intraoperative or postoperative angiogram is recommended. If there is residual lesion, immediate resection should be considered to avoid potential hemorrhage from the remaining vessels. If it is thought not to be safe to resect remaining vessels, alternative treatment should be considered, which may include stereotactic radiosurgery. There is a risk of hemorrhage during the interval period until the lesion has been obliterated.[27] The lesion may have to be treated in stages with a combination of embolization and surgery.

A special concern related to surgery for large AVMs (i.e., larger than 4 to 5 cm) is normal perfusion pressure breakthrough.[40] Normal perfusion pressure breakthrough is a rare occurrence and is described as severe, protracted, and

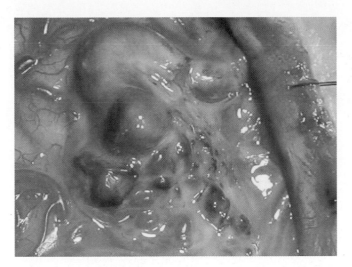

Figure 24-4 • Arteriovenous malformation as seen under the microscope at surgery.

unexplained brain edema accompanied by diffuse hemorrhage or focal deep hemorrhage in the parenchyma immediately adjacent to the area of resection. To prevent this occurrence, the interventional neuroradiologist plans one, two, or more stages of endovascular treatment to reduce the blood supply to the AVM.

Embolization. Embolization of brain AVMs is a subspecialty of interventional neuroradiology that has made tremendous strides over the past few years. Improvement in catheters—that is, flow-directed and flow-assisted microcatheters—have made navigation of intracranial vessels safer and have allowed more accurate delivery of embolic material. Improvement in imaging equipment has led to safer, more effective treatment. Depending on size, location, symptoms, hemodynamics, and anatomic vasculature of AVMs, embolization may be curative, palliative, or adjunctive to surgery or radiosurgery.[41]

The goal of preoperative embolization is to minimize blood loss and occlude vessels that may be a challenge surgically, such as intranidal arteriovenous fistulas and deep feeding arteries. Preoperative embolization is generally not indicated for small, noneloquent AVMs, as these lesions are generally respectable with a low morbidity and mortality. The decision to perform preoperative embolization is indicated when the anatomy or size of the lesion adds to the surgical risk, and the addition of embolization will favorably minimize surgical risk.[2,32]

As with surgery, the interventional neuroradiologist's experience with embolization procedures greatly influences outcomes for the patient. Improvements in microcatheter technology have allowed for superselective catheterization of distal vessels as well as intranidal aneurysms. Digital subtraction angiography and the development of "road mapping" techniques are essential to endovascular treatment. The use of heparin during the procedure has been proved to minimize thromboembolic complications and is a necessary adjunct to embolization and minimizes the risk of gluing the catheter to the vessel. With longer injections, more nidus can be occluded.

Current embolic materials are divided into solid and liquid agents. Solid agents consist of polyvinyl alcohol particles, microcoils, fibers, and microballoons.[42,43] Liquid agents consist of cyanoacrylate monomers, such as I-butyl cyanoacrylate (IBCA) and n-butyl-cyanoacrylate (NBCA), which is a short-acting liquid polymerizing agent. In its solidified form, it is relatively soft, making it easy for the surgeon to resect the lesion.[39] NBCA has been officially approved by the Food and Drug Administration (FDA) for use in cerebral AVMs. Polyvinyl alcohol (PVA) and Gelfoam particles are easier to use but are nonpermanent embolic agents. Microcoils and silk thread are highly thrombogenic, although not permanent. Another agent that is a polymer solution is ethylene vinyl alcohol (i.e., EVAL copolymer).[44] Other liquid agents include absolute ethanol, with and without the use of contrast agents for visualization under fluoroscopy.

PVA and NBCA have been the most commonly used embolic agents to date. The process of embolization and nidus occlusion is slower with particulates such as PVA as compared with liquid agents. NBCA is injected into the nidus to form an acrylic cast. Although revascularization has been noted to occur when acrylic agents are used, NBCA is one of the most permanent embolic agents. Since acrylics are adhesive, the neurointerventionalist must be aware of the risk of gluing the catheter to the blood vessel. To avoid such complication, rapid withdrawal of the catheter is necessary at the termination of the injection. The adhesive properties of NBCA prohibit prolonged injections, and only a limited amount of nidus can be occluded with a single injection.

The Onyx Liquid Embolic System (Microtherapeutics, Inc., Irvine, CA) is the newest embolic agent available and recently approved by the FDA. Onyx is a new nonadhesive liquid embolic agent and is a derivative of ethylene vinyl alcohol polymer dissolved in dimethyl sulfoxide (DMSO). Onyx is supplied in a ready-to-use vial, so no mixing of components is required before injection. The nonadhesive property of Onyx allows the physician greater latitude in varying the rate and amount of liquid agent delivered during a single injection.[45]

The advantage of Onyx is that it is a liquid, nonadhesive agent that is opaque and easily injected through a microcatheter. The disadvantage of Onyx is that it uses DMSO as a solvent. If Onyx is given in too high a concentration or volume, DMSO is potentially toxic to blood vessels and may lead to damage, vasospasm, or necrosis.[46]

The goal of embolization for definitive or palliative treatment is permanent occlusion of the nidus and feeding vessels and to attempt to occlude deep surgically inaccessible or deep arterial feeding vessels to facilitate surgical excision. Other goals of preoperative embolization are to occlude intranidal aneurysms and high-flow fistulas to promote thrombosis of the AVM's nidus. It is important that different embolization materials be evaluated and developed in order to improve the quality and care of patients with complex cerebrovascular disease.

Radiosurgery. The underlying goal of radiation therapy for AVMs is to induce an inflammatory response in the vessel walls of the lesion that will result in permanent thickening of pathologic vascular channels, with ultimate thrombosis and obliteration of the lesion.[23] The purpose of radiosurgery is to irradiate the blood vessels of the AVM to cause progressive luminal obliteration and hence prevent hemorrhage. With focused radiation, the dose of radiation to surrounding brain tissue around the AVM can be minimized. Radiosurgery can be an important management strategy in a selected group of patients for lesions in deep brain locations (brainstem, thalamus, internal capsule, basal ganglia) or for eloquent areas (sensorimotor or visual cortex).[2] The success in achieving this goal is determined, in part, by the ability to provide partial or total radiation to the lesion. If obliteration is incomplete, the patient is at risk for hemorrhage.

Preradiosurgical embolization for AVMs is also a consideration. Three potential goals when endovascular therapy is to be undertaken before radiosurgery are (1) to decrease target size to less than 3 cm in diameter, because it is known from the radiosurgical data that smaller volumes have a higher cure rate; (2) to eradicate angiographic predictors of hemorrhage, such as intranidal aneurysms or venous aneurysms; and (3) to attempt to reduce symptoms related to venous hypertension.[27] There has been no ideal embolic agent identified for preradiosurgical use.[47,48]

Various types of ionizing radiation have been used in the treatment of AVMs, including x-rays (produced by x-ray tubes or megavoltage linear accelerators); gamma rays (produced by cobalt); and Bragg peak therapy (proton beam and helium beam).[49] A delayed complication common to all types of radiation therapy is radionecrosis of healthy neural tissue. This can occur in a matter of months (3 to 11 months) or years (1 to 8 years) after radiation therapy. It is evidenced by development of new neurological deficits or worsening of previous deficits.

Conventional Radiation Therapy. Conventional radiation therapy is defined as orthovoltage or megavoltage external beam radiation or cobalt-60 gamma rays without stereotactic technique. Its use has generally not been considered effective in treating AVMs. However, recent publications recommend a re-examination of the use and patient selection criteria for conventional radiation therapy. The literature suggests that this type of radiosurgery induces desirable changes within the wall of lesions.

Gamma Knife Radiosurgery. Leksell pioneered stereotactically directed gamma radiation.[50] This so-called bloodless surgery is used to treat surgically inaccessible lesions that are 2 to 3 cm in diameter (see Chap. 14). For larger lesions, only partial radiosurgery can be offered. Current AVM stereotactic radiosurgery studies report obliteration rates of 64% to 95% for AVMs with average diameters smaller than 3 cm after radiosurgery. Factors that influence successful radiosurgical treatment include smaller AVM volume, fewer draining veins, hemispheric AVM location, and younger patient age.[51]

Bragg Peak Proton Beam Therapy. For surgically inaccessible AVMs, proton beam radiosurgery has been useful as an ablative approach to shrink the lesion.[17] This is a noninvasive procedure that uses the radiation emitted by protons that have been accelerated in a cyclotron. Stereotactic technique controls the focus of the beam to the target area.

The major advantage of proton beam radiosurgery over gamma and x-rays is that it makes use of the quantum wave properties of protons to reduce doses to surrounding tissue so that tissue beyond the target receives very little to no radiation. Protons deposit most of their radiation in what is known as the Bragg peak, which occurs at the point of greatest penetration of the protons in tissue. After the diagnostic work-up has been completed, radiation therapy is administered on an outpatient basis or during a brief hospitalization. There is no immediate risk to the patient from such irradiation. The major drawback is the possibility of hemorrhage before the effect of the therapy is realized. Radiosurgery effects develop gradually, requiring 12 to 24 months to reach a therapeutic level that provides protection against hemorrhage. As a result of radiosurgery, the walls of the lesion thicken, and there may be some obliteration of the lesion and reduction in its size. Complications related to proton beam therapy are uncommon, although radiation-induced necrosis has been reported. The physician attempts to keep the risk below 3% to 5%. The possibility of complications in a patient reflects the location of the AVM relative to brain structures.

Conservative Management. In some instances, the treatment of choice may be conservative management. A discussion of any restrictions on activities, such as contact sports, is necessary. For patients who present with seizures, seizure activity can be well controlled with anticonvulsant therapy.

Summary of Treatment

There are four treatment options for patients with a cerebral AVM, the first being observation. The AVM can be monitored with the understanding that the patient would have some risk of neurological symptoms or hemorrhage. Otherwise, intervention includes single or combined modalities of surgery, endovascular therapy, or radiosurgery. Each has associated risks and benefits. Regardless of the treatment approach recommended to a particular patient, it is necessary to monitor him or her over time. In addition to follow-up appointments, periodic cerebral angiography, MRI, or both are ordered to check the progress of the lesion.

PEDIATRIC ARTERIOVENOUS MALFORMATIONS

AVMs account for 30% to 50% of hemorrhagic stroke in children, and more often than adults have hemorrhage as their presenting symptom. Neonates and infants can present with cardiac failure from arteriovenous shunting due to the large amount of arteriovenous shunting relative to cardiac output. Other presenting symptoms are seizure, neurological deficit, headache, or incidental.[14]

Hemorrhagic episodes from an AVM have been associated with mortality as high as 25%.[54,63] Thus, the high risk of hemorrhage would tend to warrant treatment whenever possible. Pediatric lesions are more often found in eloquent locations such as the basal ganglia and thalamus.[55,56]

Treatment includes surgery, embolization, and radiosurgery, as well as a multimodality approach. If a lesion is considered too high risk for surgery due to eloquence of location or pattern of venous drainage, radiosurgery is often the treatment of choice. Surgery provides an immediate definitive obliteration, but radiation may be less risky in those considered high grade on the Spetzler-Martin Scale. The negative aspect of radiosurgery is the time to obliteration, which takes at least 2 to 3 years, where the patient remains at risk for hemorrhage. Embolization is generally an adjunctive treatment to surgery or radiosurgery with the goal to reduce the nidus size. Rarely embolization is a curative modality of treatment.[63]

Many of the large series of pediatric AVMs have been associated with higher rates of morbidity and mortality compared to adults regardless of treatment modality. One of the largest surgical series reported a series of 160 pediatric AVMs in which morbidity and mortality were 18% and 11%, respectively.[57]

Many authors have reported recurrence of AVM in their pediatric patients after total excision and radiographic evidence of total obliteration.[56–59] One study suggested that the recurrence of pediatric AVMs may express higher astrocytic vascular endothelial growth factor than adult AVMs, which may explain why they may reappear.[59] Such recurrence of pediatric AVMs may indicate a need for radiographic follow-up later in life.[14] An AVM in a pediatric patient will have a high risk of hemorrhage or rehemorrhage over a lifetime. If there is a 2% annual risk of hemorrhage over a 50-year horizon, there is a 65% chance of hemorrhage over a lifetime.[63]

Vein of Galen Malformations

A vein of Galen aneurysm is a rare high-flow vascular malformation of the brain in which there is marked dilatation of the venous system. It is a congenital malformation of blood vessels of the brain that occurs prior to birth. The vein of Galen is a large deep vein at the base of the brain. This malformation shunts blood from the arteries to the brain very quickly, increasing overall blood flow, thus increasing the work of the heart. This can result in cardiac failure, which is the most common presentation of the disease.[60]

Similar to other AVMs, the capillaries that normally slow blood flow and allow oxygen exchange to surrounding tissues are missing. Blood flows directly from arteries to veins without slowing down. The high blood flow can also interfere with the normal blood drainage of the brain, leading to hydrocephalus.

Diagnosis of this malformation is sometimes made in utero during the third trimester of pregnancy with prenatal ultrasound. MRI is the imaging tool of choice for evaluating these lesions. It can demonstrate the location of the fistula, the nidus, arterial components, and the venous sac and drainage. It is important to diagnose properly and not confuse the lesion with an AVM. An AVM is a very thin-walled lesion that may be more likely to hemorrhage than the vein of Galen malformation, which tends to have a thicker wall. The angiogram is also an important test and often will be done in conjunction with endovascular treatment.

Vein of Galen malformations have been subjected to a variety of classification schemes. Morris et al. described two disorders, the vein of Galen aneurysmal malformation (VGAM) and the vein of Galen aneurysmal dilatation (VGAD).[60] The VGAM is a lesion of early embryologic occurrence and the VGAD is a later lesion seen when the venous system of the brain is more developed. The VGAM is a pathologic varix of the embryologic median vein of the prosencephalon that drains the flow from the fistulous malformation. There may be single or multiple arterial feeders.

The clinical manifestation of VGAMs and VGADs is determined by the volume of flow to the fistulous connection, the severity of venous constraints, the stage of venous development at which the lesion became dominant, and anatomic configuration. The dominant clinical complications in neonates relate to cardiac effects of the high-flow lesion. Immediate neurological complications in neonates are thought to be related to brain ischemia due to venous hypertension, tissue edema, and ischemia compounded by decreased perfusion due to cardiac failure.[60]

VGAMs have lower rates of flow that tend to present later in childhood with hydrocephalus or macrocephaly, failure to thrive, and other focal neurological signs. Generally, the degree of arteriovenous shunting correlates with the exact age of the patient at presentation. The higher-flow lesion often presents at 1 year of age, and the lower-flow lesion presents later in childhood. Sometimes retardation may be a variable at the time of diagnosis. With early treatment some of the intellectual deficits are frequently reversed. Seizures and intracranial hemorrhage may also be present at the time of diagnosis. If these lesions are untreated, the prognosis is universally poor.

Endovascular occlusion of the arterial components of these malformations by either a transvenous or transarterial approach is the treatment of choice. The embolization materials include coils, particulate matter, suture material, and glue such as (NBCA). When surgery follows the embolization, it is targeted at the remaining fistula. It may be necessary to partially treat a neonate who presents with cardiac failure with a vein of Galen malformation with an endovascular approach in order to stabilize the cardiac condition. Definitive treatment can be performed when the child is older and more stable. Direct surgical treatment is associated with very high morbidity and mortality, with rates up to 70%. At times staged surgical obliteration of aneurysm feeders should be considered if endovascular methods are unsuccessful.[64]

Those neonates or infants presenting with hydrocephalus and a vein of Galen malformation need special care in treatment decisions; the hydrocephalus may be related to increased venous pressure that inhibits reabsorption of the cerebrospinal fluid. In this case, a shunt may only promote clinical deterioration in the infant since the reduction in intracranial pressure may worsen the venous hypertension. Generally, partial or complete obliteration of the vein of Galen lesion with embolization results in resolution or stabilization of the hydrocephalus. The exception would be the presence of obstructive hydrocephalus due to a large vein of Galen. This type may also respond to partial or complete embolization of the lesion. The management strategy tends to be avoidance of a shunt and endovascular treatment of the malformation to manage hydrocephalus.[60]

CLINICAL VIGNETTE: SB is a 14-year-old boy, previously healthy, who was found obtunded by his younger brother after inhaling a toxic agent. He arrived to the emergency department unresponsive with a Glasgow Coma Scale (GCS) score of 3. A CT scan demonstrated a large cerebellar hemorrhage (4 × 3 cm) and a CTA showed a 1.0 (anteroposterior) × 1.1 medial/lateral (ML) × 1.9 superior/inferior (SI) cm posterior fossa AVM involving the right cerebellar tonsil and vermis (Fig. 24-5). He was immediately taken from the scanner

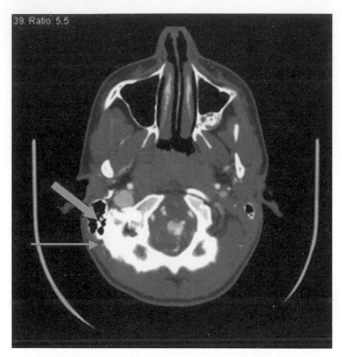

Figure 24-5 • Computed tomography angiogram shows a 4 × 3 cm cerebellar hemorrhage within the third and lateral ventricles (*thin arrow*) and a posterior fossa arteriovenous malformation with a nidus involving right cerebellar tonsil and vermis (*thick arrow*). (Courtesy of Christopher S. Ogilvy, MD, Massachusetts General Hospital, Boston, MA.)

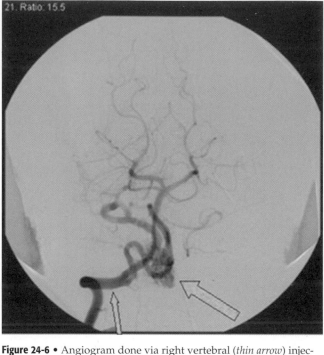

Figure 24-6 • Angiogram done via right vertebral (*thin arrow*) injection shows the arteriovenous malformation (*thick arrow*) within inferior posterior cranial fossa. (Courtesy of Christopher S. Ogilvy, MD, Massachusetts General Hospital, Boston, MA.)

to the operating room, where a suboccipital decompression for resection of cerebellar hematoma was performed along with a right frontal ventriculostomy. A CT scan was performed after the procedure demonstrating the tip of the ventricular catheter in the right lateral ventricle, diffuse intraventricular blood, and new suboccipital craniectomy. He was brought to the pediatric intensive care unit (PICU) where he was closely monitored with instructions to keep the drain at 12 mm and clamped and to open for intracranial pressure (ICP) measurements greater than 15 mm. His blood pressure targets remained tight with a systolic blood pressure goal between 80 and 120 mm Hg. He was also given mannitol 25 g q6h and Decadron. During his course in the PICU, he experienced a drop in his hematocrit from 28 to 19 over a period of 10 hours, which was the result of a stress ulcer causing a gastrointestinal bleed in the setting of steroid administration. He received frequent blood transfusions.

After 17 days in the PICU, he was ready for transfer to rehab. His neurological status had improved, with the following being noted: awake and following commands; at times disoriented upon awakening, but orients with command; face symmetric and strength full bilaterally; reports sensation intact throughout; attempting to pull out lines. After reviewing the patient and films at the cerebrovascular conference, it was decided to attempt embolization of the AVM with hope of cure. The AVM was predominantly fed by the right posterior inferior cerebellar artery (PICA) and with a single large draining vein going to basal vein of Rosenthal (Fig. 24-6). About 10 weeks later, the patient was brought to the

embolization suite for treatment. The interventional neuroradiologist injected NBCA three times into the nidus. After the third NBCA injection, there was no further opacification into the AVM nidus (Fig. 24-7). The impression at the conclusion of treatment was complete

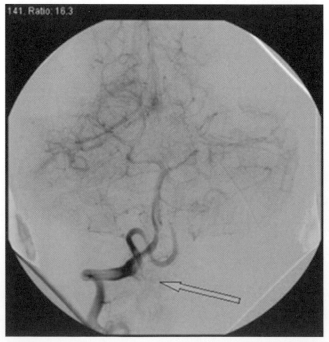

Figure 24-7 • n-Butyl-cyanoacrylate embolization of cerebellar arteriovenous malformation. (Courtesy of Christopher S. Ogilvy, MD, Massachusetts General Hospital, Boston, MA.)

obliteration of the AVM with no remaining nidus or early draining vein after the final NBCA deposition. His postprocedure course was uneventful and he was discharged back to rehab in good condition 3 days after embolization treatment, where he would continue physical therapy for his balance problems.

Four months later, he was brought back to the hospital for a diagnostic angiogram to ensure the AVM was totally obliterated. He had been doing well at home with some balance issues and diplopia. The angiogram demonstrated the following: "hypervascular blush apparently arising from a small C1 dural branch of the left vertebral artery. A small, slightly early draining cerebellar cortical vein drains to the right transverse sinus. Findings are consistent with a small residual AVM" (Fig. 24-8). An MRI was done during this admission that also documented the residual AVM: "A 1.4 cm AP × 1.0 cm TV enhancing nodule within the cerebellar resection cavity may represent a residual nidus." Three weeks later, he underwent a suboccipital craniotomy with microsurgical resection of the arteriovenous malformation. Postoperative angiogram immediately following the surgery demonstrated "no evidence of residual posterior fossa arteriovenous malformation" (Fig. 24-9). He was discharged home in excellent condition 2 days after surgery with some mild nystagmus. In a follow-up office visit almost 1 year after his initial admission, he was in excellent condition, in school full time, and doing most activities. He was encouraged to resume physical education and all activities as tolerated. The plan is a follow-up CTA in approximately 9 months to ensure the lesion is gone.

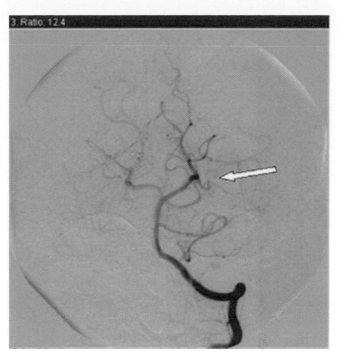

Figure 24-9 • Postoperative angiogram via left vertebral injection demonstrates no evidence of residual arteriovenous malformation. (Courtesy of Christopher S. Ogilvy, MD, Massachusetts General Hospital, Boston, MA.)

CLINICAL PEARLS: An AVM in a pediatric patient will have a high risk of hemorrhage or rehemorrhage over a lifetime. If there is a 2% annual risk of hemorrhage over a 50-year horizon, there is a 65% chance of hemorrhage over a lifetime.[63] AVMs can recur in the pediatric population. It is suggested that delayed imaging studies should be considered in children at least 1 year after their initial negative postoperative arteriogram, and perhaps even a longer-term study considered to exclude a **recurrent** AVM.[58]

CLINICAL VIGNETTE: JF is a 25-year-old white man who in April fell approximately 10 feet with loss of consciousness. A CT scan was performed, which demonstrated a lesion. An MRI was performed in further work-up of the lesion that demonstrated a 3-cm left cerebellar AVM. The patient had noticed episodes of aphasia lasting approximately 2 minutes occurring over the past 2 years that have become more frequent, up to a few times per month. His maternal grandmother died of a cerebellar hemorrhage at the age of 55 years and his mother was diagnosed with a left parietal lobe venous malformation.

In August, a diagnostic angiogram (Figs. 24-10 and 24-11) was performed, which demonstrated the left cerebellar AVM with arterial flow from the left PICA, superior cerebellar artery (SCA), and dural branches of the left posterior cerebellar artery (PCA). There was a left PICA aneurysm. The multidisciplinary cerebrovascular team recommended embolization and surgery. In November, a stage I embolization was performed using Onyx to the left SCA and left PICA supply. Two weeks later, stage II Onyx embolization was performed, again injecting glue into the left PICA supply. The angiogram

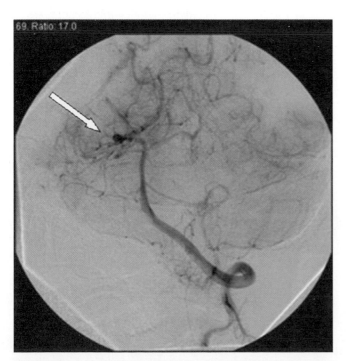

Figure 24-8 • Angiogram demonstrates hypervascular blush consistent with small residual arteriovenous malformation. (Courtesy of Christopher S. Ogilvy, MD, Massachusetts General Hospital, Boston, MA.)

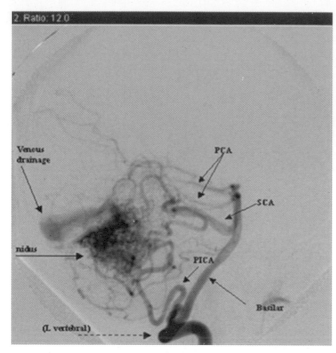

Figure 24-10 • Angiogram demonstrates lateral views of vertebral artery injection (*dashed arrow*), showing cerebellar arteriovenous malformation supplied by the left posterior inferior cerebellar artery (PICA) and left superior cerebellar artery (SCA). (Courtesy of Christopher S. Ogilvy, MD, Massachusetts General Hospital, Boston, MA.)

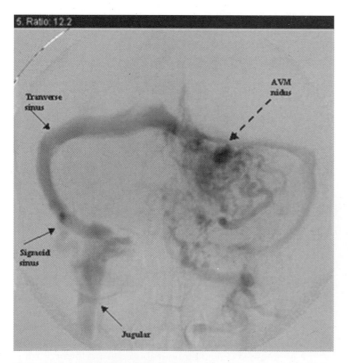

Figure 24-11 • Angiogram demonstrates anteroposterior view of left cerebellar arteriovenous malformation (AVM). *Dashed arrow* points to AVM nidus. (Courtesy of Christopher S. Ogilvy, MD, Massachusetts General Hospital, Boston, MA.)

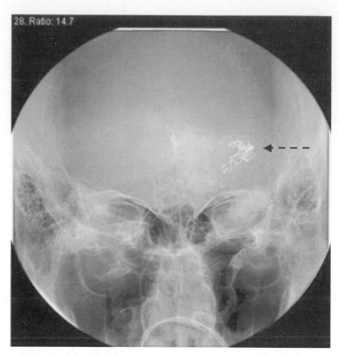

Figure 24-12 • Anteroposterior view of stage II embolization. *Arrow* points to glue cast using Onyx. (Courtesy of Christopher S. Ogilvy, MD, Massachusetts General Hospital, Boston, MA.)

demonstrated minimal to moderate supply to the AVM via the left PICA and minimal residual supply via the left SCA (Fig. 24-12). In December, 5 days after stage II embolization, the patient underwent a left posterior fossa craniotomy for resection of the left cerebellar AVM. After the successful surgery, he underwent an angiogram that demonstrated no residual AVM (Fig. 24-13). He spent the night in the neurological intensive care unit. Postoperatively he was neurologically stable, with the following noted: alert, oriented ×3, right third nerve palsy, speech fluent, following all commands, no drift, moving all extremities 5/5. He was transferred on postoperative day 1 to the neurological floor, and discharged home in good condition on postoperative day 3. He was instructed to wear a patch, alternating eyes, to minimize his diplopia. The 6-week postoperative visit demonstrated improvement in third nerve palsy, with resolution of diplopia on upgaze, but diplopia remaining on downgaze. Given the magnitude of the AVM, he is making excellent progress. He complains of some mild nausea and fatigue, but feels he is getting stronger each day. He hopes to return soon to his job as a disc jockey.

CLINICAL PEARLS: The occurrence in this Clinical Vignette was an incidental lesion. It is important to treat these dangerous lesions if treatment can be offered with a high efficacy and with minimal risk. The risk of JF's hemorrhage over his lifetime is 80%. This is based on the assumption of a 2% to 4% annual hemorrhage risk. The lifetime risk of a bleed among people with previously unruptured AVMs is calculated by the following formula: lifetime risk (percentage) = 105 minus the patient's age in years.[20] This calculation makes the assumption that the yearly risk of hemorrhage is constant and that the risk of hemorrhage in any given year is not influenced by events in other years.[61]

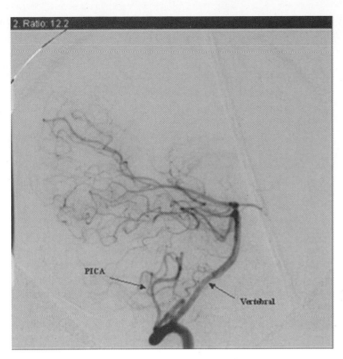

Figure 24-13 • Postoperative angiogram of the left vertebral artery showing no residual arteriovenous malformation. PICA = posterior inferior cerebellar artery. (Courtesy of Christopher S. Ogilvy, MD, Massachusetts General Hospital, Boston, MA.)

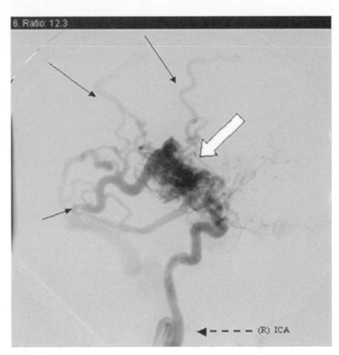

Figure 24-14 • Pretreatment angiogram via right internal carotid artery (ICA, *dashed arrow*) injection. Three *thin arrows* point to draining veins. *Thick arrow* points to nidus of right temporal arteriovenous malformation. (Courtesy of Christopher S. Ogilvy, MD, Massachusetts General Hospital, Boston, MA.)

CLINICAL VIGNETTE: MS is a 44-year-old nurse who works full time and has two daughters, ages 19 and 24. She smokes one pack of cigarettes per day. She had ongoing headaches that prompted her primary care physician to order an MRI. The MRI demonstrated a large right superior temporal gyrus sylvian fissure AVM, approximately 5 cm in length, 2 cm wide, and 3 cm deep with no evidence of prior hemorrhage. A cerebral angiogram was performed in February, which demonstrated the large right temporal AVM with both superficial and deep venous drainage (Fig. 24-14.) A CTA was done in the middle of March to help delineate a focal outpouching of the left anterior choroidal artery (Fig. 24-15). After reviewing her case at the multimodality cerebrovascular meeting, the recommendation was for endovascular treatment and surgery. The surgeon had extensive meetings with the patient and her husband discussing natural history and treatment options, which included continued observation.

The patient, after much research and thought, decided she could not live with the possibility of the AVM hemorrhaging over her lifetime, and agreed to the recommended treatment plan of embolization and surgery. She denied any visual disturbances, dizziness, or any other symptoms. She was told the risks of the procedures, which included the likelihood of a visual field cut due to the proximity of the AVM to the visual cortex.

In the middle of April, she underwent stage I embolization with NBCA glue. She underwent a stage II embolization 2 days later. She presented to the emergency department on May 31, 2005, with headaches and visual disturbance—lines in the left side of her vision. CT scan was reassuring, as no hemorrhage was detected.

A lumbar puncture was also negative, and the patient returned home. She underwent stage III (Fig. 24-16) and IV NBCA embolization on June 14 and 16 without any complication. On June 15, an MRI with gadolinium using the stealth protocol was performed to assist with

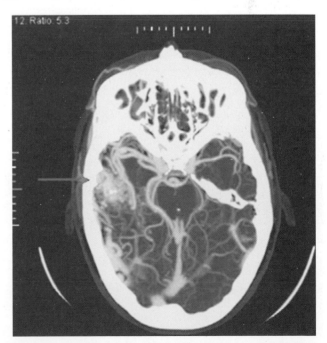

Figure 24-15 • Axial reformatted computed tomography angiogram shows arteriovenous malformation centered in superior right temporal lobe. *Arrow* points to bulk of nidus. (Courtesy of Christopher S. Ogilvy, MD, Massachusetts General Hospital, Boston, MA.)

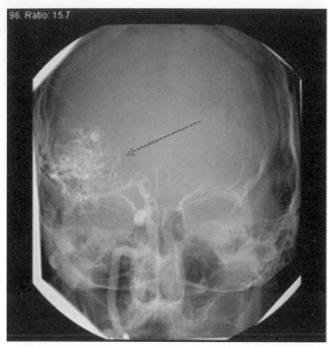

Figure 24-16 • Angiogram shows stage III embolization of right temporal arteriovenous malformation with n-butyl-cyanoacrylate. *Arrow* points to glue cast. (Courtesy of Christopher S. Ogilvy, MD, Massachusetts General Hospital, Boston, MA.)

surgical planning. She was discharged home in mid-June. One week later, she underwent a right temporal craniotomy for resection of the AVM. Postoperative angiogram demonstrated no residual AVM (Fig. 24-17). She awoke with a left-sided hemiparesis and left homonymous hemianopsia. The weakness improved

from a 2/5 to a 5/5 upon discharge to home. She had some generalized weakness, and opted for outpatient therapies. Four months after surgery, she resumed work as a staff nurse on a part-time basis (16 hours/week). She steadily increased her hours, so that 6 months postoperatively she is working three 12-hour shifts. Her major frustration is her inability to drive secondary to the field cut and the state laws that prohibit driving with her specific deficit. She continues to gain strength, and feels her vision has improved since being discharged home. She is determined to drive again. She continues to challenge her vision by working with computerized programs designed to stimulate those with visual impairment.

CLINICAL PEARLS: This Clinical Vignette demonstrates the conscious decision of a nurse to proceed with treatment with known risks of some residual deficit. It demonstrates the complexity of treating AVMs as noted by a number of stage embolizations and ultimately surgery. It is very important when counseling patients who present with unruptured AVMs that they generally present neurologically intact, making them more susceptible to deterioration after elective AVM treatment. Therefore, it is necessary to educate the patient and family of possible risks of postoperative deficits (some oftentimes recoverable), and assist them with the decision-making process based on the overall lifetime risk of hemorrhage. It is critical to remind patients that despite the risks of slight worsening after elective surgery, their final outcome is generally better than the risk of opting for conservative management or having a hemorrhage.[62]

ARTERIOVENOUS MALFORMATIONS AND PREGNANCY

The incidence of hemorrhage from brain AVMs during pregnancy has been a controversial topic over the years. Earlier studies suggested a high incidence of hemorrhage during pregnancy when a patient had a true high-flow AVM.[40,50] The implication is that when the AVM did present in a pregnant woman, it did so in the form of a hemorrhage.

A retrospective study by Horton et al. found the incidence of hemorrhage in pregnant women with unruptured AVMs during the interval of time during and immediately after gestation to be 3.5% annually.[52] These women had no previous history consistent with hemorrhage. In women with a previous clinical history of hemorrhage, the risk was increased to a 5.8% chance of hemorrhage during pregnancy. In nonpregnant patients, the incidence of hemorrhage is 4% per year. It was concluded by the investigators that pregnancy was not a significant risk factor for hemorrhage in women with unruptured AVMs.

Studies have shown that there is no increase in the rate of hemorrhage during labor or the immediate postpartum period. Therefore, when a woman presents during pregnancy with an AVM, the recommendation is that the pregnancy be carried to term. The patient can also be reassured that the risk of hemorrhage during delivery is very small, as is the case throughout the entire pregnancy. Data suggest in most cases that vaginal delivery is safe, but cesarean section may decrease the already low incidence of hemorrhage during delivery. There are no data to support or deny this statement.[50] The patient, neurosurgeon, and obstetrician need to

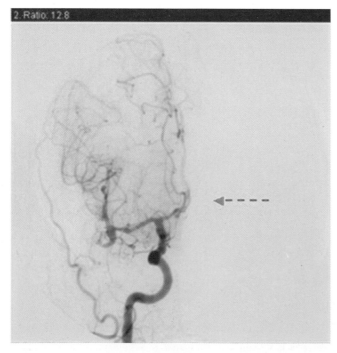

Figure 24-17 • Postoperative angiogram shows no residual arteriovenous malformation (AVM) (*arrow* points to where AVM was located). (Courtesy of Christopher S. Ogilvy, MD, Massachusetts General Hospital, Boston, MA.)

discuss the safety and efficacy of the mode of delivery carefully on a case-by-case basis. All must be comfortable with the decision. According to the statistics, the actual incidence of problems encountered during pregnancy is low.

If the woman presents with a hemorrhage during pregnancy, care should proceed as in the nonpregnant patient. The nurse plays an important role in reassuring the patient while anticipating potential neurological problems. If a hematoma is currently causing significant mass effect, it should be evacuated. Ogilvy and Tatter recommend removal of the clot only and operating on the AVM on an elective basis.[50] Early angiography is often done. This is preferable and is used to define the anatomy of the lesion. If possible, the angiogram should be done during the second or third trimester to avoid added risk to the fetus. As with nonpregnant patients, the treatment modalities of surgery, embolization, radiosurgery, or a combination are selected based on the size, location, and surgical accessibility of the lesion. Women with known AVMs should be carefully counseled before conception. If possible, the lesion should be treated before pregnancy. As previously stated, although the risk of hemorrhage in a pregnant woman with an unruptured AVM is very low, it is not zero. Safe management of pregnant patients with neurological diseases, such as an AVM, requires close collaboration of the health care team, including the neurosurgeon, neurologist, obstetrician, anesthesiologist, and nurses.[50] Reassuring the patient and reinforcing the information given to her by her physicians is an important role of the nurse during this critical time. Providing written information is most helpful.

NURSING MANAGEMENT OF ARTERIOVENOUS MALFORMATIONS

The patient who is suspected of having a cerebral AVM is at risk for hemorrhage. If hemorrhage has not occurred, management is directed toward preventing hemorrhage by controlling hypertension, preventing seizures, and modifying the patient's lifestyle (e.g., avoiding contact sports and lifting) to prevent surges in blood pressure. In the hospital, the nurse can expect to perform the following:

- Conduct a baseline neurological assessment as well as ongoing monitoring of neurological signs
- Monitor vital signs for evidence of hypertension
- Assess and monitor characteristics of headache, if present
- Monitor the patient for evidence of seizure activity
- Administer drug therapy as necessary

If the AVM has ruptured, the patient will be managed in a similar manner to that of other patients who have had a cerebral hemorrhage (see Chap. 23). The severity of the hemorrhage and the patient's clinical presentation will determine the medical treatment selected and the related nursing management. Hemorrhage is usually intracerebral. However, less frequently, subarachnoid hemorrhage, a subdural hematoma, or an intraventricular hematoma may occur. Unlike patients with ruptured aneurysms, vasospasm is not a concern after hemorrhage. There is some risk of rebleeding, and the patient should be monitored for evidence of rapid neurological deterioration. If surgery, embolization, or both are intended, they are usually delayed for about 3 to 6

weeks to allow for planning and for recovery of the brain from hemorrhage.

In addition to carrying out baseline and ongoing monitoring of neurological and vital signs, a major role of the nurse is in providing emotional support and teaching to the patient and family. Most patients with AVMs are young, and the thought of having a serious lesion within the brain is very frightening to them. These patients undergo various diagnostic procedures to collect data about the lesion, and they are given much information, including the advantages and disadvantages of each treatment option. Finally, a decision is made regarding the appropriate course of treatment. The nurse is very much involved in the related patient teaching, as well as in reinforcing the information provided by the physician. Anxiety and fear are common responses of the patient and family. Nursing interventions are directed at alleviating these responses and supporting effective coping strategies. A support group specifically for patients with brain AVMs may help both the patient and family members.

Perioperative Nursing Management

If surgery is planned, the nurse will be responsible for providing basic preoperative teaching (see Chap. 14). Postoperative nursing management for patients with AVMs is similar to that outlined for a craniotomy patient (see Chap. 14). If a large lesion has been resected, there is the concern that normal perfusion pressure breakthrough can occur, as discussed previously. Clinically, there would be evidence of significant neurological deterioration.

The management of the patient after endovascular therapy includes careful monitoring in the neurological intensive care unit. The groin site(s) is/are checked frequently to ensure no arterial "oozing" or bleeding. The patient is kept well hydrated, with tight blood pressure control. Mild systemic hypotension may be helpful in allowing flow changes to occur gradually in the brain tissue surrounding the AVM during the first 24 hours after the procedure. Sometimes, affected patients will complain of headache. This can be attributed to changes in flow dynamics in the brain. The nature of the headache should be documented, and the physician should be notified. If the indication of embolization is adjuvant to surgery, the patient is prepared for surgery 24 to 48 hours after endovascular treatment.[41]

After recovery from surgery, the patient is discharged with orders that often include anticonvulsant therapy. Depending on the presence of neurological deficits, there may be need for rehabilitation. For some patients, a neuropsychological evaluation may be ordered after a few months to evaluate the presence of cognitive deficits. The physician follows the patient's progress. If the lesion has not been obliterated completely, the patient remains at risk for hemorrhage.

Future Trends

Advances in functional imaging, microsurgical technique, neuroanesthesiology, endovascular therapy, and stereotactic radiosurgery have contributed to the ongoing therapeutic care and management of vascular malformations. Also important have been advances in biologic knowledge, which form the foundation for modern success in treatment.[53]

Research continues on various interventional materials, including glue (i.e., NBCA, Onyx), PVA, and other liquid agents that are injected into the feeders of these complex lesions. Fractionated radiation is currently being researched as a mode to treat larger AVMs that were once deemed untreatable. Although technology and knowledge of vascular malformations have increased tremendously over the years, and will continue to do so, one cannot dismiss the importance of characteristics of individual patients, such as age, medical condition, vocation, and psychological factors, in the process of evaluating management options and coming to treatment decisions.

REFERENCES

1. Friedlander, R. M. (2007). Arteriovenous malformations of the brain. *New England Journal of Medicine, 356*(26), 2704–2712.
2. Brown, R. D., Flemming, K. D., Meyers, F. B., Cloft, H. J., Pollock, B.E., & Link, M. L. (2005). Natural history, evaluation, and management of intracranial vascular malformations. *Mayo Clinic Proceedings, 80*(2), 269–281.
3. Mohr, K., Caplan, L., Melski, J. W., et al. (1978). The Harvard Cooperative Stroke Registry: A prospective registry. *Neurology, 28*, 754–762.
4. Guidetti, B., & Delitala, A. (1980). Intracranial arteriovenous malformations: Conservative and surgical treatment. *Journal of Neurosurgery, 53*, 149–152.
5. Sahoo, T., Johnson, E. W., Thomas, J. W., et. al. (1999). Mutations in the gene encoding KRIT1, a Krev-1/rap1a binding protein, cause cerebral cavernous malformations (CCM1). *Human Molecular Genetics, 8*(12), 235–233.
6. Zambramski, J. M., Wascher, T. M., Spetzler, R. F., et al. (1994). The natural history of familial cavernous malformations: results of an ongoing study. *Journal of Neurosurgery, 80*(3), 422–432.
7. Pakzaban, P., & Ogilvy, C. S. (1995). Intracranial dural arteriovenous malformations. In C. W. Mitchell (Ed.). *Surgical management of neurovascular disease* (pp. 387–403). Baltimore: Williams & Wilkins.
8. Lasjaunias, P., Chiu, M., Brugge, K. T., et. al. (1986). Neurological manifestations of intracranial dural arteriovenous malformations. *Journal of Neurosurgery, 64*, 724–730.
9. Awad, I. A., Little, J. R., Akrawi, W. P., et. al. (1990). Intracranial dural arteriovenous malformations: factors predisposing to an aggressive neurological course. *Journal of Neurosurgery, 72*, 839–850.
10. Chandler, H. C., & Friedman, W. A. (1993). Successful radiosurgical management of a dural arteriovenous malformation: a case report. *Neurosurgery, 33*, 139–142.
11. Brown, R. D., Wiebers, D. O., Torner, J. C., & O'Fallon, M. (1996). Frequency of intracranial hemorrhage as a presenting symptom and subtype analysis: A population based study of intracranial vascular malformations in Olmsted County, Minnesota. *Journal of Neurosurgery, 85*, 29–32.
12. Parkinson, D., & Bachers, G. (1980). Arteriovenous malformations: Summary of 100 consecutive supratentorial cases. *Journal of Neurosurgery, 53*, 285–299.
13. Pertuiset, B., Sichez, J. P., Philippon, J., Fohanno, D., & Horn, Y. (1979). Mortality and morbidity after complete surgical removal of 162 intracranial arteriovenous malformations. *Review of Neurology, 135*, 319–327.
14. Ogilvy, C. S., Stieg, P. E., Awad, I., et al. (2001). Recommendations for the management of intracranial arteriovenous malformations: A statement for healthcare professionals from a special writing group of the Stroke Council, American Stroke Association. *Circulation, 103*, 2644–2657.
15. Brown, R. D., Jr., Weibers, D. D., & Forbes, G. S. (1990). Unruptured intracranial aneurysms and arteriovenous malformations: Frequency of intracranial hemorrhage in relation to lesions. *Journal of Neurosurgery, 73*, 859–863.
16. Fults, D., & Kelly, D. L., Jr. (1984). Natural history of arteriovenous malformations of the brain: A clinical study. *Neurosurgery, 15*, 658–662.
17. Kjellberg, R. N., Hanamura, J., Davis, K. R., Lyons, S. L., & Adams, R. D. (1983). Bragg Peak proton-beam therapy for arteriovenous malformations of the brain. *New England Journal of Medicine, 308*, 269–274.
18. Luessenhop, A. J., & Rosa, L. (1984). Cerebral arteriovenous malformations: Indications for and results of surgery, the role of intravascular techniques. *Journal of Neurosurgery, 60*, 14–22.
19. Graf, C. J., Perret, G. E., & Torner, J. C. (1983). Bleeding from cerebral arteriovenous malformations as part of their natural history. *Journal of Neurosurgery, 58*, 331–337.
20. Kondziolka, D., McClaughin, M. R., & Kestle, J.R. (1995). Simple risk predictions for arteriovenous malformation hemorrhage. *Neurosurgery, 37*, 851–855.
21. Brown, R. D., Jr, Wiebers, D. O., Forbes, G., et al. (1988). The natural history of unruptured intracranial arteriovenous malformations. *Journal of Neurosurgery, 16*, 421–430.
22. Wilkins, R. H. (1985). The natural history of intracranial vascular malformations: A review. *Neurosurgery, 16*, 421–430.
23. Ondra, S. L., Troupp, H., George, E. D., & Schwab, K. (1990). The natural history of symptomatic arteriovenous malformations of the brain: A 24-year follow-up assessment. *Journal of Neurosurgery, 73*, 387–391.
24. Forster, D. M., Steiner, L., & Harkanson, S. (1972). Arteriovenous malformations of the brain: A long-term clinical study. *Journal of Neurosurgery, 37*, 562–570.
25. Piepgras, D. G., Sundt, T. M., Jr., Ragoowanse, A. T., & Stevens, L. (1993). Seizure outcome in patients with surgically treated cerebral arteriovenous malformations. *Journal of Neurosurgery, 78*, 5–11.
26. Pollock, B. E., Lunsford, L. D., Kondziolka, D., Maitz, A., & Flickinger, J. C. (1994). Patient outcomes after stereotactic radiosurgery for "operable" arteriovenous malformations. *Neurosurgery, 35*, 1–8.
27. Ogilvy, C. S., Stieg, P. E., Awad, I., et al. (2001). American Heart Association scientific statement: Recommendations for the management of intracranial arteriovenous malformations: A statement from health care professionals from a special writing group of the Stroke Council, American Stroke Association. *Stroke, 32*, 1458–1471.
28. Heros, R. C., & Tu, Y. K. (1986). Unruptured arteriovenous malformations: A dilemma in surgical decision making. *Clinical Neurosurgery, 33*, 187–236.
29. Spetzler, R. F., Hargraves, R. W., McCormick, P. W., et al. (1992). Relationship of perfusion pressure and size to risk of hemorrhage from arteriovenous malformations. *Journal of Neurosurgery, 36*, 918–923.
30. Kondziolka, D., McLaughlin, M. R., & Kestle, J. R. W. (1995). Simple risk predictions for arteriovenous malformation hemorrhage. *Neurosurgery, 37*, 851–855.
31. Greenberg, M. S. (2001). Vascular malformations. In M. S. Greenberg (Ed.). *Handbook of neurosurgery* (5th ed., pp. 804–813). Lakeland, FL: Greenberg Graphics.
32. Spetzler, R. F., & Martin, R. A. (1986). A proposed grading system for arteriovenous malformations. *Journal of Neurosurgery, 65*, 476–483.
33. Harmann, A., Mast, H., Mohr, J. P., et al. (1998). Morbidity of intracranial hemorrhage in patients with cerebral arteriovenous malformation. *Stroke, 29*, 931–934.
34. Duong, D. H., Young, W. L., Vang, M. C., et al. (1998). Feeding artery pressure and venous drainage pattern are primary determinants of hemorrhage from cerebral arteriovenous malformations. *Stroke, 29*, 1167–1176.
35. Nagata, S., Matsushima, T., Takeshita, Il, Fukui, M., & Yasumoori, K. (1991). Lateral ventricular arteriovenous malformations: Natural history and surgical indications. *Acta Neurochirurgica (Wien), 112*, 37–46.

36. Turjman, F., Massoud, T. F., Vinuela, F., Sayre, J. W., Guglielmi, G., & Duckwieler, G. (1995). Correlation of the angioarchitectural features of cerebral arteriovenous malformations with clinical presentation of hemorrhage. *Neurosurgery, 37*, 856–860.

37. Miyasaka, Y., Yada, K., Ohwada, T., Kurata, A., & Irijura, K. (1992). An analysis of the venous drainage system as a factor in hemorrhage from arteriovenous malformation. *Journal of Neurosurgery, 76*, 239–243.

38. Kader, A., Young, W. L., Pile-Spellman, J., et al. (1994). The influence of hemodynamic factors on hemorrhage from cerebral arteriovenous malformations. *Neurosurgery, 34*, 801–807.

39. Purdy, P. D., Batjer, H. H., Risser, R. G., & Samson, D. (1992). Arteriovenous malformation of the brain: Choosing embolic materials to enhance safety and ease of excision. *Journal of Neurosurgery, 77*, 217–222.

40. Robinson, J. L., Hall, C. S., & Sidzimir, C. B. (1972). Subarachnoid hemorrhage in pregnancy. *Journal of Neurosurgery, 36*, 27–33.

41. Hacien-Bey, L., Pile-Spellman, J., & Ogilvy, C. S. (1995). Embolization of brain arteriovenous malformations. In C. W. Mitchell (Ed.). *Surgical management of neurovascular disease* (pp. 404–418). Baltimore: Williams & Wilkins.

42. Fournier, D., TerBrugge, K. G., Willinsky, R., Lasjunias, P., & Montanera, W. (1991). Endovascular treatment of intracerebral arteriovenous malformations: Experience in 49 cases. *Journal of Neurosurgery, 75*, 228–233.

43. Scweitzer, J. S., Chang, B. S., Madsen, P., et al. (1993). Pathology of arteriovenous malformations treated by embolotherapy, part 2: Results of embolization with multiple agents. *Neuroradiology, 35*, 468–474.

44. Wallace, R. C., Flom, R. A., Khayata, M. H., et al. (1995). The safety and effectiveness of brain arteriovenous malformation embolization using acrylic and particles: The experience of a single institution. *Neurosurgery, 37*, 606–618.

45. Jahan, R., Murayama, Y., Gobin, Y. P., Duckwiler, G. R., Vinters, H. V., & Vinuela, F. (2001). Embolization of arteriovenous malformations with onyx: Clinicopathological experience in 23 patients. *Neurosurgery, 48*(5), 984–997.

46. Higashida, R. T. (2001) Comments: Embolization of arteriovenous malformations with onyx: clinicopathological experience in 23 patients. *Neurosurgery, 48*(5), 984–997.

47. Gobin, U. P., Laurent, A., Merriene, L., et al. (1996). Treatment of brain arteriovenous malformations by embolization and radiosurgery. *Journal of Neurosurgery, 85*, 19–28.

48. Dion, J. E., & Mathis, J. M. (1994). Cranial arteriovenous malformations: The role of embolization and stereotactic surgery. *Neurosurgery Clinics of North America, 5*, 459–474.

49. Ondra, J. L., Doty, J. R., Mahla, M. E., & George, E. D. (1988). Surgical excision of a cavernous hemangioma of the rostral brainstem: Case report. *Neurosurgery, 23*, 490–493.

50. Ogilvy, C. S., & Tatter, S. B. (1995). Surgical management of vascular lesions and tumors associated with pregnancy. In H. H. Schmidek & W. H. Sweet (Eds.). *Operative neurosurgical techniques, indications, methods and results* (pp. 1163–1173). Philadelphia: W. B. Saunders.

51. Pollock, B. E., Flickinger, J. C., Lunsford, L. D., Maitz, A., & Kondziolka, D. (1998). Factors associated with successful arteriovenous malformation surgery. *Neurosurgery, 42*(6), 1239–1244.

52. Horton, J. C., Chambers, W. A., Lyons, S. L., et al. (1990). Pregnancy and the risk of hemorrhage from cerebral arteriovenous malformations. *Neurosurgery, 27*, 867–871.

53. Martin, N. A., & Vinters, H. V. (1995). Arteriovenous malformations. In L. P. Carter & R. F. Spetzler (Eds.). *Neurovascular surgery* (pp. 875–903). New York: McGraw-Hill.

54. Kondziolka, D., Humphreys, R. P., Hoffman, H. J., et al. (1992). Arteriovenous malformations of the brain in children: A forty year experience. *Canadian Journal of Neurological Sciences, 19*, 40–45.

55. Hamilton, M. G., Karahalios, D. G., Thompson, B. G., et al. (1994). Pediatric cerebral arteriovenous malformations: A management outcome comparison with an adult cohort. *Neurosurgery, 35*, 564 (Abstract).

56. Hoh, B. L., Ogilvy, C. S., Butler, W. E., et al. (2000). Multimodality treatment in Pediatric Non-Galenic AVMs. *Neurosurgery, 47*, 346–358.

57. Humphreys, R. P., Hoffman, H. J., Drake, J. M. et al. (1996). Choices in the 1990's for the management of pediatric cerebral arteriovenous malformations. *Pediatric Neurosurgery, 25*, 277–285.

58. Kader, A., Goodrich, J. T., Sonstein, W. J., et al. (1996). Recurrent cerebral arteriovenous malformations after negative postoperative angiograms. *Journal of Neurosurgery, 85*, 14–18.

59. Sonstein, W. J., Kader, A., Michelson, W. J., et al. (1996). Expression of vascular endothelial growth factor in pediatric and adult cerebral arteriovenous malformations: An immunocytochemical study. *Journal of Neurosurgery, 85*, 838–845.

60. Morris, P. P., Choi, I. S., Berenstein, A., & Ogilvy, C. S. (1995). Vein of Galen aneurysms. In C. W. Mitchell (Ed.). *Surgical management of neurovascular disease* (pp. 482–488). Baltimore: Williams & Wilkins.

61. Kondziolka, D., McLaughlin, M., & Kestle, J. (1995). Simple risk predictions for arteriovenous malformation hemorrhage. *Neurosurgery, 37*(5), 851–855.

62. Lawton, M., Du, R., Tran, M. N., Achrol, A. S., et al. (2005). Effect of presenting hemorrhage on outcome after microsurgical resection of brain arteriovenous malformations. *Neurosurgery, 56*(3), 485–493.

63. Hoh, B., Ogilvy, C. S., Butler, W. E., et al. (2000). Multimodality treatment of nongalenic arteriovenous malformations in pediatric patients. *Neurosurgery, 47*(2), 346–358.

64. Moriarty, J. L., & Steinberg, G.K. (1994). Surgical obliteration for vein of Galen malformation: A case report. *Surgical Neurology, 44*, 365–370.

RESOURCES

Websites

The following websites provide information on arteriovenous malformations.

http://www.ninds.nih.gov/disorders/avms/detail_avms.htm

http://neurosurgery.mgh.harvard.edu/neurovascular/

http://www.childrenshospital.org/clinicalservices/Site2162/mainpageS2162P4.html

http://www.avmsupport.org.uk/

http://brainavm.uhnres.utoronto.ca/malformations/brain_avm_index.htm

http://www.mayoclinic.org/arteriovenous-malformation/

http://www1.wfubmc.edu/neurosurgery/Brain+Tumor+Center+of+Excellence/(AVM)+Center

http://www.stanfordhospital.com/clinicsmedServices/COE/neuro/vascularMalformations/arteriovenousMalformation.html

http://neuroradiology.rad.jhmi.edu/avm.html

http://neuro.wehealny.org/endo/cond_arteriovenous.asp

http://www.mgh-interventional-neurorad.org/

http://www.snisonline.org

Stroke

Joanne V. Hickey and Ann Quinn Todd

Stroke is the third leading cause of death in the United States, surpassed only by heart disease and cancer. It represents an enormous public health and economic burden, estimated at $62.7 billion for direct and indirect costs.[1] The 2007 update on stroke by the American Heart Association reports the following on an annual basis[2]:

- Each year about 700,000 people experience a new or recurrent stroke (500,000 first attack and 200,000 recurrent); by gender about 46,000 more women than men have a stroke.
- Stroke incidence in men is greater than women at younger ages, but not at older ages. The ratio of male-to-female incidence is 1.25 at ages 55 to 64; 1.50 at ages 65 to 74; 1.07 at ages 75 to 84, and 0.76 at age 85 and older.
- First-time stroke for blacks is almost double that for whites. The age-adjusted stroke incidence rates at ages 45 to 84 are 6.6 per 1000 in black males versus 3.6 in white males, and 4.9 in back females versus 2.3 in white females.
- Over 150,000 deaths (58,660 males, 91,487 females) related to stroke were reported in 2004.
- Eighty-seven percent of all strokes are ischemic and 13% result from intracerebral and subarachnoid hemorrhage.
- In the 45- to 64-year-old age group, 8% to 12% of deaths resulted from ischemic stroke and 37% to 38% from hemorrhagic stroke within 30 days.
- The death rate from stroke in 2004 was reported at 48.1 per 1,000 for white males and 73.9 per 1,000 for black males, and 47.4 per 1,000 for white females and 64.9 per 1,000 for black females.
- The longer life span of women accounts for the fact that more women than men die of stroke each year. In 2004, 61% of U.S. stroke deaths were women.

In the past 15 years, management of stroke has undergone a fundamental transformation as a result of research and technological advances, including improved pathophysiologic models of stroke to understand changes in the biochemical and cellular levels; superior neuroimaging using magnetic resonance imaging (MRI), magnetic resonance angiography (MRA), magnetic resonance with diffusion-weighted and perfusion-weighted imaging, and improved computed tomography (CT) scanning techniques; the introduction of new pharmacologic agents and techniques such as hypothermia; the definitive role of thrombolytic agents in early treatment; advances in radiologic interventional procedures, such as angioplasty, cerebrovascular stenting, and embolic protection; the preventive benefit of carotid endarterectomy in patients with symptomatic high-grade stenosis; neurotransplantation; and other studies and investigative tools that continue to shape and refine patient management.

The term *brain attack* is the preferred term for the lay press to align itself with heart attack, a concept that conveys early identification of symptoms followed by emergent transport for intervention that is often life saving. An appreciation has developed of the stroke timeline associated with the development of neurological deficits and the window of opportunity that exists for reversal of neurological deficits with new interventions. Cardiac resuscitation training programs in basic life support (BLS) and advanced cardiac life support (ACLS) have been revised and now include identification of stroke symptoms and rapid action to save brain tissue as well as save cardiac muscle. Improved emergency medical services' (EMS) recognition of stroke symptoms and triage and the creation of dedicated stroke centers at selected hospitals have significantly enhanced rapid stroke interventions.

A repository of guidelines related to stroke is available at the American Heart Association website. Examples of evidence-based guidelines include primary prevention of ischemic stroke, early management of ischemic stroke, adult stroke rehabilitation care, and other guidelines that address the management of stroke patients along a continuum of care through rehabilitation. They are available at the American Heart Association website and are updated periodically to reflect the latest scientific information to assist health care providers in providing best practices in managing patients.[3,4,5] Other respected groups such as the Veterans Administration have also published evidence-based guidelines that are available at a variety of websites.[6]

Interdisciplinary clinical pathways for stroke management are the norm in practice. The emphasis is on providing coordinated care focused on stabilization through acute care and treatment with early rehabilitation of patients for optimal recovery of function and prevention of recurrent stroke. The processes of care are driven by achievement of identified outcomes that are indicators of quality.

This chapter is based on the most recent guidelines available in mid-2007 and reflects the guidelines posted on the American Heart Association website.

Thanks are extended to Joan Censullo, RN, MSN, CNRN, for contributing "Clinical Pearls" to this chapter.

CLINICAL PEARLS: Name-badge attachments are fast and effective ways to disseminate stroke standards of care to multidisciplinary staff throughout the hospital.

DISEASE-SPECIFIC CERTIFICATION: PRIMARY STROKE CENTER

The Joint Commission offers a program of certification for disease-specific care including stroke.[7] Many institutions are seeking Primary Stroke Certification to distinguish themselves within the community. Whereas some state legislatures and other accrediting organizations have assumed the role of certifying body, the most widely recognized entity for Primary Stroke Certification is the Joint Commission. With more than 50 years of established expertise, the Joint Commission developed the disease-specific certification for Primary Stroke Centers based on the recommendations of the Brain Attack Coalition and the statements and guidelines of the American Stroke Association. Primary Stroke Certification, in which a Certificate of Distinction in Stroke Care is awarded, is valid for 2 years. The initial review, year 1, consists of both off-site and on-site evaluations, and the second-year review is an off-site evaluation of submitted descriptive material.

To be eligible for Primary Stroke Certification, specific requirements must be met. The institution seeking certification must be located within the United States, operated by the U.S. government, or operated under the charter of the U.S. Congress. The stroke program must fit the Joint Commission certified program description and be in operation for a minimum of 4 months. A voluntary process, Primary Stroke Certification Review, is focused on quality and safety within the framework of standards, guidelines, and outcomes. Organized into five domains, the standards are Delivering or Facilitating Clinical Care, Performance Measurement and Improvement, Supporting Self-Management, Program Management, and Clinical Information System. While the Joint Commission does not dictate which clinical practice guidelines are used, the Primary Stroke program must demonstrate the selection, implementation, and integration of the clinical practice guidelines. These guidelines should be based on the same criteria as the National Guidelines Clearinghouse. In regard to Performance Management, the performance measurement and improvement activities must have an organized approach. As of 2007, four measures of the standardized measure set that was agreed upon by the American Stroke Association, the Joint Commission, and a jointly sponsored stroke advisory panel are required for data collection. The performance measures can be found on the Joint Commission website under stroke certification.

PUBLIC AND PROFESSIONAL EDUCATION

Stroke is a preventable health care problem; it is a treatable condition, in most cases, if treatment is prompt and evidence based. A well-developed public education program is critical to have an informed public who can recognize the signs and symptoms of a stroke and know how to respond. In addition, the health care system must be organized to provide evidence-based care provided by stroke-competent health care providers. The following recommendations are made by the American Heart Association[5]:

- Activation of the 911 system by patients and others is strongly supported because it speeds treatment of stroke.
- Public education programs to increase public awareness of stroke is supported to increase the number of patients who can be seen and treated in the first few hours after stroke.
- Education of all health care providers and EMS personnel will increase the number of patients promptly and properly treated.
- Since EMS personnel are often the first responders, education in brief assessment according to an established protocol will facilitate communication of information for decisions about transport to the appropriate health care facility and needed care that alerts health providers.
- It is further recommended that EMS personnel begin the initial management of stroke in the field according to approved protocols.
- The use of a stroke identification algorithm such as the Los Angeles or Cincinnati screens is encouraged.
- Patients should be transported for evaluation and treatment to the closest facility that provides emergency stroke care, even if it means bypassing other health care facilities not prepared to provide emergency stroke care.

DEFINITION AND CLASSIFICATION OF STROKE

Stroke is a heterogeneous, neurological syndrome characterized by gradual or rapid, nonconvulsive onset of neurological deficits that fit a known vascular territory and that last for 24 hours or more. Stroke occurs when oxygen supply to a localized area in the brain is interrupted, resulting in a series of intricate processes that lead to the destruction of neural tissue and consequent brain damage. Stroke includes cerebral infarction (ischemic stroke) and intracerebral hemorrhage and subarachnoid hemorrhage (hemorrhagic stroke). The two categories are further subdivided, as discussed later (Fig. 25-1). The type and severity of neurological deficits encompass a wide range and gradation of signs and symptoms. The severity and permanence of symptoms are the factors that differentiate between so-called minor stroke and major stroke.

Classification of stroke is based on the underlying problem created within the cerebral artery. An analogy to home plumbing pipes can be made. Only two events create problems with household plumbing: plugging of the pipe so that effluence cannot proceed to its destination; and bursting or rupturing of the pipe so that fluid within the pipe flows into the surrounding areas. In the brain, plugging by atherosclerosis or a clot creates a narrow lumen, preventing adequate flow of blood to cerebral tissue. Alternatively, rupture resulting from a weakened vessel causes leakage of blood into the brain or subarachnoid space. Thus, stroke is divided into the

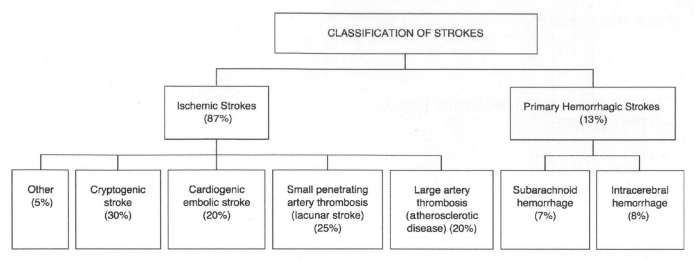

Figure 25-1 • Classification of stroke types.

two major categories of *ischemic stroke* and *hemorrhagic stroke* with subdivisions in each category.

Terms Related to Cerebral Ischemic Events

Transient ischemic attacks (TIAs) are temporary focal brain or retinal deficits, caused by vascular disease, which fit a known vascular territory and clear completely in less than 24 hours. Most TIAs are much shorter, reversing completely within 1 hour. TIAs are classified into TIAs associated with the carotid and TIAs associated with vertebrobasilar vascular territories. One of the most important warning signs of a stroke is a TIA.

TIAs of the carotid (anterior circulation) cause lateralizing signs. When the carotid territory is involved, the symptoms reflect ischemia to the ipsilateral eye or cerebral hemisphere. A common visual deficit is called *amaurosis fugax*, defined as temporary blindness in one eye. Hemispherical ischemia usually causes weakness or numbness of the contralateral face or limb; language deficits and cognitive and behavioral changes may also occur. *TIAs of the vertebrobasilar (posterior) circulation cause diffuse signs.* When the vertebrobasilar territory is involved, the symptoms often include dysarthria, vertigo, dizziness, ataxia, abnormalities of eye movement resulting in diplopia, and unilateral or bilateral motor and sensory deficits (Table 25-1).[8]

A **penumbra** is a zone of compromised neuronal cells that are unable to function but remain viable and are located around an area of lethal injured cells; such a zone is amenable to reversal from ischemia (Fig. 25-2). A **watershed** or **border zone infarction** is an infarcted area that occurs between the terminal distributions of two adjacent cerebral arteries, such as the anterior cerebral and middle cerebral arteries. Because the terminal distributions are at the end of the pipeline, watershed areas are subject to low, marginally adequate arterial pressure under normal circumstances (Fig. 25-3). They are also the first to fail when systemic blood pressure drops further. If systemic hypotension occurs, there is failure to maintain adequate cerebral perfusion.

Ischemic Stroke

Ischemic stroke accounts for 87% of all strokes and is subdivided into thrombotic atherosclerotic large vessel disease (20%); small vessel (penetrating) artery disease, or "lacunae" (25%); cardiogenic embolic (20%); cryptogenic (30%); and other (5%). Note that these percentages are approximate for each category with variations noted depending on resource consulted. Atherosclerosis of large and small cerebral arteries that results in thrombosis is the most common cause of ischemic stroke in North America and Europe and accounts for 45% of strokes in the United States.

TABLE 25-1	COMPARISON OF SIGNS AND SYMPTOMS OF CAROTID AND VERTEBROBASILAR TRANSIENT ISCHEMIC ATTACKS

CAROTID TERRITORY	VERTEBROBASILAR TERRITORY
Related to Ophthalmic Artery	***Related to Posterior Cerebral Artery***
Amaurosis fugax (temporary monocular blindness)	Dysarthria
Transient graying, fogging, or blurred vision	Dysphagia
A "shade" descending over line of vision	Diplopia
	Bilateral blindness
Related to Middle Cerebral Artery	Unilateral or bilateral motor and sensory weakness
	Quadriparesis
Hemiparesis (more arm than leg weakness)	***Related to Cerebellar Arteries***
Hemianesthesia	
Contralateral motor or sensory deficits to face or limbs	Ataxia
	Vertigo
Related to Anterior Cerebral Artery	Dizziness
Hemiparesis (more leg than arm weakness)	

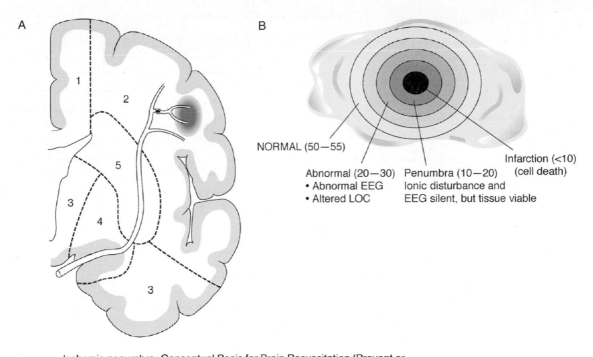

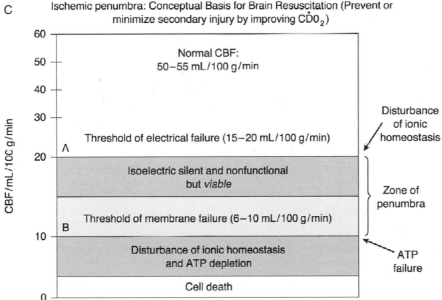

Figure 25-2 • Cerebral blood supply during ischemic events. (*A*) See distribution of middle cerebral artery and occlusion of a branch. Note area of infarction and surrounding penumbra with viable but nonfunctional cells. These cells will either become infarcted or recover, depending on treatment. (*B*) Ischemic penumbra: normal CBF = 50–55 mL/100 g/min. Variations in CBF are noted. Penumbra is the critical area that may be salvageable with appropriate treatment, or cell death will occur if adequate CBF is not restored. (*C*) Ischemic penumbra: conceptual basis for brain resuscitation. ATP = adenosine triphosphate; CBF = cerebral blood flow; EEG = electroencephalogram; LOC = level of consciousness.

Large Artery Atherosclerotic Stroke

The large extracranial and intracranial arteries are subject to atherosclerosis with an associated atheroma plaque that narrows the lumen of the vessel. The *atheroma* can also be the site for thrombus formation. Both conditions can lead to hypoperfusion, ischemia, and ischemic stroke. About 40% of patients have TIAs before a large-vessel ischemic stroke.

The patient typically awakens with neurological deficits or is sedentary when the symptoms occur. During sleep or at rest, blood pressure tends to be lowered, and there is less pressure to push the blood through the narrowed arterial lumen. Systemic hypoperfusion, decreased cerebral perfusion, ischemia, and ischemic stroke can develop. The area of cerebral ischemia depends on the vascular territory involved and the location within the vascular territory (proximal or distal) of the thrombus.

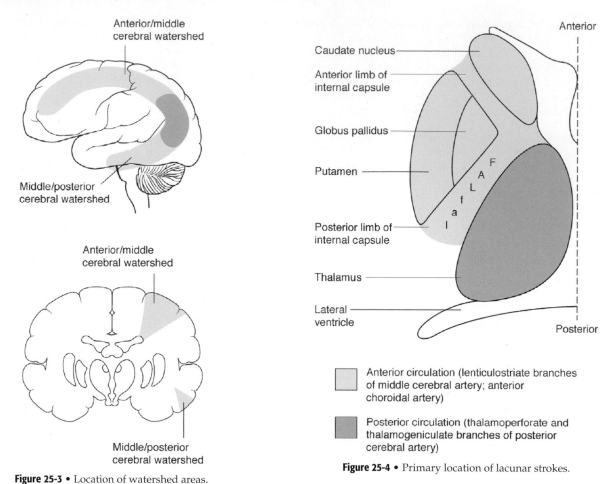

Figure 25-3 • Location of watershed areas.

Figure 25-4 • Primary location of lacunar strokes.

If a major artery is involved, large areas of both gray and white matter become ischemic, infarcted, and necrotic. Neuronal ischemia causes changes in the cell membrane, resulting in intracellular edema and compression of the capillaries, further compromising adequate blood supply. Cerebral edema peaks approximately 2 to 4 days after the stroke. Symptoms of ischemic stroke often develop in a stepwise progression relating to cerebral edema and infarction, reaching a peak in 1 to 3 days before stabilizing.

Small Artery Stroke (Lacunar Stroke)

The term **lacuna** describes the small cavity remaining in the brain tissue that develops after the necrotic tissue of a small, deep infarct has been removed. A **lacunar stroke** is a type of ischemic stroke caused by microatheroma and thrombosis of a small penetrating artery, resulting in a small, softened area in the deep white matter structures of the brain. As the softened tissue sloughs away, a small cavity or lake remains, the lacuna (diameter of 0.5 mm or less). Occlusion occurs in the presence of lipohyalinosis, a condition characterized by pathologic thickening of these small vessels, and leads to a specific clinical stroke syndrome. Hypertension is the principal risk factor for lacunar strokes. Lacunar strokes are seen predominantly in the basal ganglia, especially the putamen, the thalamus, and the white matter of the internal capsule and pons; they occur occasionally in the white matter of the cerebral gyri. They are rare in the gray matter of the cerebral

surface, the corpus callosum, visual radiations, or medulla (Fig. 25-4). Most lacunae occur in the lenticulostriate branches of the anterior cerebral artery and middle cerebral artery, the thalamoperforant branches of the posterior cerebral arteries, and the paramedian branches of the basilar artery.[9]

There are distinct signs and symptoms associated with several recognized lacunar syndromes, including pure motor hemiplegia, pure sensory stroke, homolateral ataxia and leg paresis, dysarthria, clumsy hand syndrome, sensorimotor stroke, and basilar branch syndromes. Even though a lacunar stroke is small, it can cause considerable deficits if a critical area, such as the internal capsule, is involved. Patients may have several lacunae, as evidenced on CT or MRI, and have diffuse white matter changes associated with dementia.

Cardiogenic Embolic Stroke

About 20% of ischemic strokes result from cardiogenic embolism from atrial fibrillation (the most common), patent foramen ovale (PFO), valvular disease, ventricular thrombi, myocardial infarction, congestive heart failure, atrial septal aneurysm, and other cardiac problems. Atherosclerosis and atherogenic plaques of the proximal aorta are another source of cardiac emboli detectable with the use of transesophageal echocardiography (TEE). The atherogenic plaques commonly found in coronary vessels, in the heart, and at the bifurcation of the aorta are precursors for hypertension and atrial fibrillation. Unstable plaques can break off and become microemboli to the brain, causing stroke. Microemboli from the heart are mobilized and enter the cerebral system most often through the carotid arteries, flowing until the vessel is too narrow to allow further passage of the embolus and the vessel becomes occluded. The left middle cerebral artery is affected most often because it is a relatively straight vessel and provides the path of least resistance for the embolus. Cardiogenic strokes associated with PFO occur in approximately 20% to 25% of persons older than 30 years of age and usually occur when the patient is awake and active.[10] The development of the ischemia is very rapid with maximal deficit present within minutes.

Cryptogenic Stroke

About 30% of ischemic strokes are cryptogenic in origin, which means that no cause of the stroke could be found after diagnostic evaluation.

Stroke From Other Causes

About 5% of ischemic strokes result from nonatherosclerotic vasculopathies, hypercoagulable states, hematologic disorders, arteritis, migraine/vasospasm, and cocaine use.[11]

Hemorrhagic Stroke

Intracerebral hemorrhage (ICH), or ICH stroke, represents 13% of all strokes and involves primary rupture of a blood vessel. Although ICH represents a relatively small percentage of total strokes, it is a serious disease, with a 30-day mortality rate threefold to fivefold higher than that for ischemic stroke. The mortality rate in the first 30 days after ICH is 37% to 38%, with more than half of these deaths occurring in the first 2 days and 6% of patients dying before they reach the hospital. The high mortality and morbidity associated with ICH are caused primarily by the blood mass itself and by the mechanical effects it creates.[12]

Hemorrhagic stroke is divided into two categories based on the underlying mechanism. **Intracerebral stroke**, also called **intraparenchymal stroke**, is caused by bleeding into the brain tissue as a result of rupture of a small artery, most often a deep, penetrating vessel. **Subarachnoid hemorrhage** (SAH) is the result of bleeding into the subarachnoid space, most often in relation to a ruptured aneurysm or arteriovenous malformation—in both cases, the result of hemorrhage. In this chapter, only intracerebral hemorrhagic stroke is discussed. Cerebral aneurysms and arteriovenous malformations were addressed in Chapters 23 and 24.

The cause of intracerebral hemorrhagic stroke is a spontaneous hemorrhage related to hypertension and cerebral amyloid angiopathy. The typical profile is that of an older person with a long history of poorly controlled hypertension. At the moment of hemorrhage, the person is active and usually has not experienced any warning signs. A typical situation is one of a patient straining at stool, and then developing a severe headache, decreased consciousness, hemiplegia, and possible focal seizures and vomiting. Subarachnoid hemorrhage is commonly seen in younger people. Hemorrhagic stroke occurs rapidly, with steady development of symptoms over a period of minutes to hours (1 to 24 hours). The most common sites of intracerebral hemorrhage, each of which has distinguishing signs and symptoms, are the following: putamen (part of the basal ganglia) and adjacent internal capsule (50%); thalamus (30%); cerebellum (10%); and pons (10%).

Arterial Dissection

Arterial dissection is an unusual cause of stroke and accounts for 1% to 5% of all strokes, occurring commonly in younger persons (aged between 25 and 45 years), usually in the absence of atherosclerosis. Arterial dissection is typically caused by trauma to a vessel wall (as in the case of iatrogenic trauma associated with catheter passage during an angiographic procedure), vessel abnormality, migraine, and fibromuscular dysplasia. After injury to the vessel wall, hematoma forms in the medial layer and breaks through the intimal wall. Injury to the intimal wall allows blood to dissect through the medial layer, resulting in luminal narrowing; a pseudoaneurysm may result in some cases.

The patient with an arterial dissection is at risk for ischemic stroke due to resulting thrombosis, embolization, or subarachnoid hemorrhage due to vessel rupture. The most common locations for dissection are the cervical carotid, intracranial carotid (usually in the middle cerebral or supraclinoid internal carotid artery), and vertebral artery. Vertebral dissections are often associated with trauma.

The signs and symptoms of an arterial dissection may evolve over hours to days. The patient commonly experiences a severe unilateral headache, scalp throbbing, and/or neck pain. Other presenting signs and symptoms include transient monocular blindness, oculosympathetic paralysis, pulsatile tinnitus, TIAs, or stroke in evolution.

Emergency MRA or cerebral angiography is indicated if an arterial dissection is suspected. After the diagnosis has been established, cautious heparinization is initiated; other measures such as stenting, angioplasty, grafting, and bypass may be undertaken as appropriate. Chronic oral anticoagulation may be necessary in unresolved cases.

ANATOMY, ATHEROGENESIS, AND PATHOPHYSIOLOGY RELATED TO STROKE

Anatomic Basis for and Correlations Related to Stroke

There are four major cerebral arteries that supply the brain: two internal carotid arteries (ICAs) that constitute the anterior circulation, and two vertebral arteries (VAs) that constitute the posterior circulation. The ICAs ascend from the common carotid artery (CCA) bifurcation, enter the cranium at the petrous portion of the temporal bone between the layers of dura, and then begin to branch. The major cerebral arteries arising from the ICAs are the middle cerebral artery (MCA), the anterior cerebral artery (ACA), the anterior communicating artery, and the posterior communicating arteries. The MCA supplies the lateral portion of the cerebral hemisphere (Fig. 25-5). The ACA supplies the frontal pole and medial

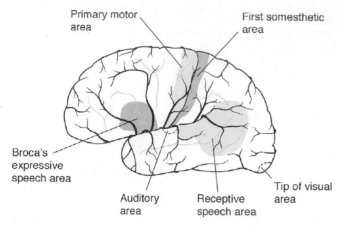

Figure 25-5 • Distribution of the middle cerebral artery (lateral surface of the brain).

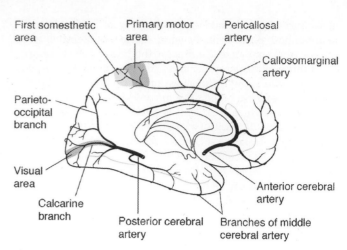

Figure 25-6 • Distribution of the anterior and posterior cerebral arteries on the medial surface of the cerebral hemisphere.

surface of the frontal and parietal lobes (Fig. 25-6). The first major small branch of the ICA after branching from the CCA is the ophthalmic artery, which supplies the eye. Transient ischemia from this vessel results in transitory monocular blindness in one eye, also called *amaurosis fugax*.

The two VAs enter the cranial vault through the foramen magnum, then uniting to form the basilar artery (BA) (Fig. 25-7). The BA then divides to form the two posterior cerebral arteries (PCAs), which supply the medial and inferior surfaces and lateral portions of the temporal and occipital lobes

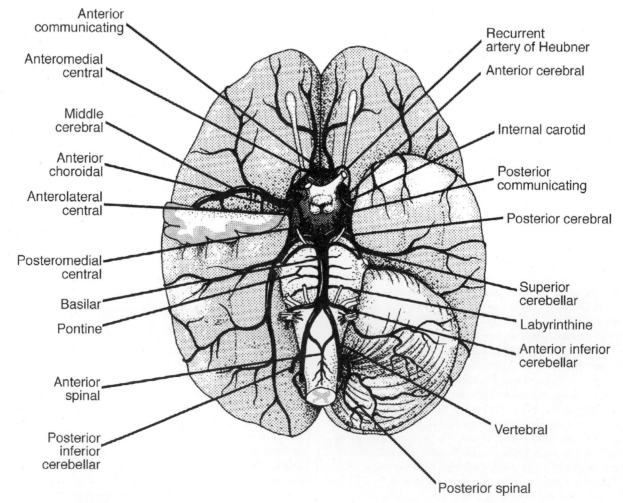

Figure 25-7 • Arteries that supply the brain, as seen from the ventral surface. The right cerebral hemisphere and the tip of the right temporal lobe have been removed.

(see Figs. 25-5 and 25-6). The BA also gives off a number of cerebellar and brainstem arteries. The circle of Willis, at the base of the skull, joins the anterior and posterior circulation. Collateral circulation for an occluded vessel is possible owing to anastomosis between the vessels. However, anomalies of cerebral vessels are common, so it is difficult to predict if a patient will receive collateral circulation to an occluded area. Chapter 7 provides further details regarding cerebral circulation.

Atherogenesis of Ischemic Stroke

Atherogenesis is the pathologic process that results in atherosclerosis. Stroke due to atherosclerosis remains the most common neurological disorder among adults in the United States. There are two dominant theories of atherogenesis, reaction to injury and the lipid hypotheses. Regardless of the specific mechanism of injury, the arterial wall undergoes a series of morphologic changes that result in structural alteration and pathogenesis.

In larger vessels, the earliest lesions of atherosclerosis are seen as yellowish, fatty streaks of the intimal surface of large to medium arteries, which are widely distributed throughout the arterial vasculature and may be seen as early as late childhood or early adolescence. On microscopic examination, the fatty streaks consist of lipid-laden macrophages known as foam cells (some foam cells are smooth muscle cells and some come from circulating monocytes) and extracellular lipid.

Over the course of years the fatty streaks progress, and by middle to older age, fibrosis plaques (atheromas) begin to develop in more localized sites than fatty streaks, typically occurring at arterial branches or opposite arterial bifurcation of extracranial vessels. The maturated fibrous plaque consists of an intact endothelial lining overlaying a fibrous cap (containing foam cells, transformed smooth muscle cells, lymphocytes, a connective tissue matrix, and a central necrotic core of cellular debris, free extracellular lipid, and cholesterol crystals) extruding from the intima and producing varying degrees of alterations in blood flow. As plaques advance, there may be central necrosis and associated changes such as fibrosis, intraplaque hemorrhage, ulceration, and mineralization. Platelet adhesion and aggregation may occur at this later stage, increasing the plaque size. Fibrin and fibrinogen may also be incorporated into the plaque. Small arterioles, commonly observed at the plaque periphery, may be the genesis of possible hemorrhagic transformation in some fibrous plaques that contain hemosiderin, areas of intraplaque calcification, and disruption of the endothelial lining. The plaque destabilization, luminal thrombi, and endothelial injury result in clinical symptoms.[13,14]

Plaque enlargement occurs slowly over decades, and the person is asymptomatic until the plaque intrudes on a substantial percentage of the arterial lumen diameter. Typically, luminal thrombi are associated with luminal surface disruption or ulceration of the endothelial lining, leading to arterial obstruction. Blood within the plaque or intraplaque hemorrhage appears to be secondary to the luminal disruption, with dissection of luminal blood into the plaque.

In **smaller arteries**, the underlying pathologic process for smaller penetrating arteries, such as the lenticulostriate

arteries, basilar penetrating arteries, and medullary arteries that supply deep cerebral white matter, is different than for atherosclerosis found in the larger arteries. The underlying pathologic changes in the small penetrating arteries are attributable to a process called **lipohyalinosis**, in which a hyaline-lipid material coats the small penetrating arteries causing thickening of the walls. Eventually, the vessel thromboses create a lacunar stroke.

Pathophysiology of Ischemic Stroke

The pathophysiology of ischemic stroke due to atheromas, thrombi, or emboli is the same. The lumen of the blood vessel becomes narrowed or occluded, resulting in ischemia in that vascular territory (Fig. 25-8). As shown mainly in animal models, occlusion seldom completely abolishes the delivery of oxygen and glucose to the affected vascular territory because cerebral blood flow (CBF) to the affected vascular territory is usually partly maintained by dense vascular collaterals.

Normally, the rate of CBF to the entire brain is relatively constant, and it does not change in response to alterations in mean systemic blood pressure over a range of 50 to 150 mm Hg. This phenomenon, known as *autoregulation*, protects the brain from possible hypotension or cerebrovascular hemorrhage caused by excessive intravascular pressure. The severity of neuronal injury in ischemic brain tissue is proportional to the reduction of CBF (Table 25-2). In the center of an infarct, blood flow is greatly reduced or absent, whereas at its margin, maximum vasodilation results from the lactic acid formed during anaerobic glycolysis. When CO_2 is inhaled or a cerebral vasodilator is administered to patients with focal infarction, only the vessels in normal areas of the brain dilate, resulting in an intracerebral steal of blood away from the infarcted zone. This same phenomenon can result if hypertension is treated too aggressively during an acute infarct. Judicious use of antihypertensive agents is critical during an acute infarct.

Animal data provide information for the current understanding of the pathogenesis and time course of brain damage. After 5 minutes to 1 hour of severe focal ischemia—that is, ischemia that causes persistent loss of membrane potentials in an animal model—persistent loss of neuronal membrane potentials results in the death of some or all of the selectively vulnerable cells in the affected vascular bed. After

TABLE 25–2   THRESHOLDS OF CEREBRAL ISCHEMIA

Normal range	40–50 mL/100 g/min
Oligemia	30–40 mL/100 g/min
Mild ischemia	30–30 mL/100 g/min Electrical function is affected
Moderate ischemia (penumbra)	10–120 mL/100 g/min Reversible cellular damage
Severe ischemia (lesion core)	0–10 mL/100 g/min Irreversible cellular damage

Hock, N.H. (1999). Brain attack. The stroke continuum. *Nursing Clinics of North America*, 34(3), 697.

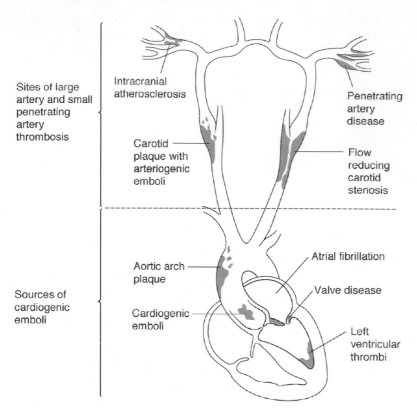

Sites of large
artery and small
penetrating
artery
thrombosis

Intracranial
atherosclerosis

Carotid
plaque with
arteriogenic
emboli

Penetrating
artery
disease

Flow
reducing
carotid
stenosis

Sources of
cardiogenic
emboli

Aortic arch
plaque

Atrial fibrillation

Valve disease

Cardiogenic
emboli

Left
ventricular
thrombi

Figure 25-8 • Major sites and sources related to ischemic stroke.

approximately 1 hour, infarction begins and its volume enlarges progressively.[15]

The time required for progression toward the maximum volume of infarction differs in different species. In nonhuman primates with reversible cerebral artery occlusion, clinical improvement and limited infarct size are observed when occlusion lasts 3 hours or less. When occlusions persist longer, neurological deficits are more pronounced. CBF and metabolic studies in humans provide the basis for determining the treatment window in acute stroke clinical trials and the current thinking on emergent stroke interventions.

Ischemia can cause primary cellular injuries resulting from no blood flow and from secondary cellular injury due to the effects of biochemical and molecular cascades precipitated by ischemia. Ischemia severe enough to cause neuronal death of cerebral cells is called **cerebral infarction**. With infarction, a core of necrotic tissue exists from a lack of adequate oxygen supply and nutrients (e.g., glucose) resulting in rapid depletion of energy stores. However, around the necrotic core is another circumscribed area called the *ischemic penumbra* (see Fig. 25-2). Although the neuronal cells of the penumbra do not function normally due to a decreased blood supply, they remain viable. However, cells in this region die if reperfusion is not re-established.[16] The penumbra is the target for pharmacologic interventions to re-establish adequate perfusion, thus salvaging neuronal cells from infarction. Neuroprotective agents, including the use of mild to moderate brain cooling, are being tested in clinical trials to assess their safety and efficacy in protecting the cells from the secondary injury associated with ischemia. Thus far, there are no drugs tested that provide neuroprotection against ischemia.

The blood supply to the brain can be compromised due to the so-called no-flow phenomenon (e.g., following cardiac arrest resulting in global ischemia) or a low-flow phenomenon (e.g., following stroke resulting in focal ischemia). Low-perfusion states can result in more tissue damage than no-perfusion states because the presence of glucose in an inadequately oxygenated area enhances lactate production.[17] Brain tissue lactate causes severe tissue necrosis and extracellular acidosis that result in infarction. In addition, low-flow states provide a continued supply of both water, which exacerbates edema, and activated white blood cells, platelets, and coagulation factors, which contribute to tissue damage by further impeding the microcirculation.

Secondary cellular injury associated with ischemia occurs in response to deprivation of oxygen and cessation of oxidative metabolism. Complex biochemical and molecular cascades result in ischemic damage to neurons. From 2 and 5 minutes of complete oxygen deprivation is the general benchmark for irreversible neuronal damage. However, extreme hypothermia can significantly increase the viability time, and hypothermia has been used therapeutically to save neurons. Without oxygen, adenosine triphosphate (ATP) energy-dependent cell functions (e.g., the cellular respiratory chain, lipid metabolism, and maintenance of the transmembrane ion channels) rapidly cease. Impairment of the respiratory chain results in anaerobic glycolysis of remaining available glucose. Anaerobic glycolysis proceeds only to pyruvate, which reduces to lactate. Lactic acid and free fatty acid accumulation causes intracellular acidosis, further inhibiting mitochondrial function.

Concurrently, other cell destruction processes occur that include *excitotoxicity, increased intracellular calcium,* and *generation of free radicals.* Hypoxia impairs the reuptake of the excitatory neurotransmitter glutamate at the presynaptic membrane. The excessive extracellular glutamate opens sodium, chloride, and calcium channels, resulting in an influx of sodium and chloride ions with water into the cell, causing acute cellular swelling; the voltage-dependent calcium channels allow influx of calcium into the cytosol and efflux of potassium. (Intracellular calcium is normally maintained at a low level by active transport mechanisms.) The high intracellular calcium activates calcium-dependent degradative enzymes (proteases, phospholipases, and endonucleases) that attack the cell membranes and DNA and further inhibit mitochondrial function. Oxygen free radicals with resultant lipid peroxidation occur in inadequately perfused areas and during reperfusion of previously ischemic areas. Oxygen free radicals, superoxide peroxide, and hydroxyl ions destroy fatty acids and disrupt calcium homeostasis, further contributing to cellular demise. Approximately 8 to 12 hours after the insult, the neuron becomes smaller and more angular. The cytoplasm and nucleus shrink, followed by complete dissolution of the cell and cell death.[18] The ischemic cascade and cellular changes that follow oxygen deprivation are outlined earlier in this chapter.

Reperfusion Injury in Stroke

During ischemia, hypoxic cell injury and death occur distal to the occluded vessel. The injured and dying cells produce proinflammatory mediators that cause inflammation in the area around the infarction. As inflammation subsides, scar tissue develops in the infarcted region. Neurons that have died are replaced by fibrogliotic scar tissue, and neurological function is lost.

Another type of injury to neurons results from reperfusion to previously ischemic areas. The cellular injury due to activated oxygen free radicals that occurs after the blood supply to the ischemic area has been restored is called **reperfusion injury**. Although reperfusion has been shown to be beneficial in experimental systems, evidence suggests that the process of reperfusion may also injure the ischemic brain.[19] This injury involves acute inflammation in the ischemic tissue. During periods of ischemia, endothelial cells secrete many proinflammatory cytokines that attract and activate leukocytes. When reperfusion occurs, neutrophils migrate through the vessel wall into the ischemic brain tissue, potentially releasing various toxic substances, such as oxygen free radicals and proteinases, that may further injure the compromised but viable tissue. Oxygen free radicals, which are partially reduced oxygen molecules that are highly reactive with other molecules, are implicated in postischemic membrane injury. The accumulation of adenosine diphosphate (ADP) and pyruvate during ischemia results in rapid production of electrons when the oxygen supply is re-established. The oxygen free radicals are formed when the electrons are transferred to oxygen. They allegedly injure the cell membrane by stealing hydrogen molecules and by forming abnormal molecular bonds.[20] As a result of reperfusion injury, additional injury to neuronal cells is incurred.

Although reperfusion is best exemplified by the use of thrombolytic therapy, it is also likely to be relevant even without pharmacologic thrombolysis. Advanced imaging studies have demonstrated increased uptake in the brain following a stroke and correlate with neurological outcome.[21] Presumably, circulating leukocytes reach the infarcted area as a result of either spontaneous reperfusion or collateral circulation. It is important to note that when pharmacologic thrombolytic therapy is used, the patient may manifest new or identical stroke symptoms after a successful recanalization. It is therefore critical to observe the patient for reperfusion injury following thrombolytic therapy. Another example of perfusion injury is the natural break-up of an embolic thrombus and the onset of expanded deficits.

Pathophysiology of Hemorrhagic Stroke

The pathophysiology of hemorrhagic stroke is associated with an immediate rise in intracranial pressure (ICP), ischemic cellular responses, cerebral edema, compromised cerebral perfusion pressure, and possible herniation. With ICH, the usual hemorrhage sites are small, deep cortical arteries or subarachnoid hemorrhage due to aneurysmal rupture (see Chap. 23). At the time of ICH, blood is forced into the surrounding cerebral parenchyma, creating a hematoma. The pathology is dynamic and continues to evolve over the first few days after onset. In 20% to 30% of cases, clot volume increases over the first 24 hours. The hematoma displaces and compresses the adjacent cerebral tissue, and ischemic cellular responses and cerebral edema occur, resulting in increased ICP. The final outcome of ICH could also include potential neurotoxicity from the blood degradation products and associated neuronal ischemia. A major ICH can cause midline displacement and herniation syndromes and has a high mortality rate of about 50%.

Hemorrhagic Conversion of an Ischemic Stroke

An embolus that represents all or part of a thrombus has a spontaneous tendency to lysis and dispersion; thrombotic occlusions may also lyse spontaneously. In hemorrhagic infarction, or *hemorrhagic conversion* or *transformation*, varying amounts of red blood cells are found among the necrotic tissues, with hemorrhagic foci ranging from a few scattered petechiae to petechial hemorrhages that merge to form a significant hemorrhagic mass.[22] The timing of hemorrhagic infarction varies from a few hours to as late as 2 weeks or longer after an arterial occlusion. Surges of arterial hypertension or rapid rise of blood pressure might explain hemorrhagic infarction in many cases. Marked hyperglycemia has also been implicated in some cases.[23] Examination of biochemical changes that correlate with hemorrhage into infarcts suggested that marked tissue energy depletion accompanied by acidosis damages brain vessels and renders them penetrable by edema fluid and, ultimately, red blood cell extravasation.

CLINICAL PEARLS: The probability of hemorrhagic conversion after an ischemic event is related to the location and size of the infarct; therefore, it is important to know both the size and location of the infarct.

SIGNS AND SYMPTOMS OF STROKE SYNDROMES ACCORDING TO THE INVOLVED VESSEL

The presenting signs and symptoms of stroke depend on the extent of CBF compromise and the particular cerebral vessel involved. When a cerebral artery is occluded by a thrombus or embolus, classic syndromes are said to develop. The clinical features of stroke are commonly classified as carotid artery (anterior circulation) syndromes and vertebrobasilar (posterior circulation) syndromes. Table 25-3 summarizes the signs and symptoms associated with stroke according the cerebral vessel involved.

Comparison of Left-Sided and Right-Sided Stroke

Some generalizations can be made about the deficits incurred with left-sided and right-sided stroke (Table 25-4). A stroke is a form of cerebral injury. The injury to the brain results from ischemia that develops over time or suddenly, as may be the case in thrombotic or embolic strokes, or from a ruptured blood vessel, in the case of hemorrhagic stroke. In all cases of stroke, areas of the brain are deprived of an adequate oxygen supply. The particular type and degree of neurological deficits incurred depends on the particular area of the brain involved, because the brain is composed of the most highly specialized tissue in the body. If the blood supply is cut off for an extended period, the involved cerebral tissue may become necrotic, resulting in permanent neurological deficits. In instances of ischemia, temporary neurological impairment may result.

CLINICAL PEARLS: For a patient with left middle cerebral artery infarction, expect evidence of aphasia.

Diagnostics for Transient Ischemic Attack or Stroke

A number of diagnostic studies are useful for the investigation of TIA and stroke patients. Diagnostic testing proceeds in a stepwise fashion. When the most common tests fail to uncover the cause of the stroke, other less common tests are ordered. For example, stroke in a young person without the usual stroke risk factors suggests other causes such as PFO or antiphospholipid abnormalities. Table 25-5 describes the commonly recommended diagnostic procedures and laboratory tests.

Initially, the following tests are recommended for all patients: noncontrast brain CT or brain MRI, blood glucose, electrolytes, renal function tests (blood urea nitrogen, creatinine), complete blood count (CBC), platelets, prothrombin time/international normalized ratio (INR), activated partial thromboplastin time, and markers of cardiac ischemia. Oxygen saturation is also monitored. Selected patients may require hepatic function tests, toxicology screen, blood alcohol level, pregnancy test, arterial blood gases, chest x-ray (only if lung disease is suspected), and lumbar puncture

(only if subarachnoid hemorrhage is suspected and a CT scan is negative for blood).

Other tests may be ordered in the course of treatment for special reasons. Besides neuroimaging tests (CT or MRI), blood flow studies (transcranial Doppler) may be ordered. If a vascular anomaly is suspected, a cerebral angiography or MRA may be ordered. Recent reports recommend replacement of CT with MRI as the primary neuroimaging technique for evaluation of acute stroke.[24,25] The multimodal MRI provides more information about brain ischemic pathophysiology, can localize perfusion deficits and ischemic injury including the penumbra within minutes after onset of ischemia, and are useful to guide treatment decisions. Diffusion-weighted imaging (DWI) and perfusion-weighted imaging (PWI) are distinctly different techniques; they are interrelated physiologic parameters, and both are usually performed during the same MRI examination.[26] However, the standard initial diagnostic imaging procedure is an emergency CT scan without contrast medium to differentiate ischemic stroke from hemorrhagic stroke.

CLINICAL PEARLS: TIAs and stroke are not separate diseases. Utilization of the same clinical practice guidelines is appropriate for the work-up of both and saves duplicated effort of developing different unit protocol/guidelines.

Finally, diagnostics associated with cardiovascular risk may be ordered. These tests may include electrocardiogram (ECG) and possibly transthoracic echocardiography (TTE), TEE, or 24-hour ambulatory ECG. If continuing to pursue a cardiogenic source (for silent myocardial ischemia), an exercise ECG or a thallium perfusion may be ordered. The history of the present illness, past medical history including risk factors, and neurological examination are critical for diagnosis (Table 25-6). Although the clinical presentation of TIA/stroke is heterogeneous, the symptoms are dictated by three key variables: affected vascular territory, duration and severity of ischemia, and underlying mechanism of cerebral hypoperfusion. A comparison of signs and symptoms related to carotid and vertebrobasilar TIAs is found in Table 25-1. An understanding of the vascular territories is critical in helping the care provider relate presenting symptoms to vascular territories. Note that a TIA related to a carotid vascular territory results in *lateralizing* signs, that is, hemiparesis or hemiplegia in the contralateral side of the body. By comparison, involvement of vertebrobasilar vascular vessels results in *diffuse* signs and symptoms, that is, bilateral weakness of the lower extremities, dysarthria, vertigo, ataxia, dizziness, or abnormal eye movement.

CLINICAL PEARLS: The anterior cerebral circulation includes the vessels that originate from the carotid arteries and result in lateralizing neurological signs and symptoms. By comparison, the posterior cerebral circulation includes the vessels that originate from the vertebrobasilar arteries and results in diffuse neurological signs and symptoms.

Evidence of neurological deficits does not necessarily mean that the patient has had a TIA or stroke. Deficits may be attributable to other primary conditions. Therefore, a detailed history of onset, signs, symptoms, frequency, progression, and

TABLE 25–3 NAME, DESCRIPTION, AND SIGNS/SYMPTOMS RELATED TO STROKE BY INVOLVED VESSEL

NAME	DESCRIPTION	SIGNS AND SYMPTOMS
Internal carotid artery (ICA) syndrome		• Paralysis of the contralateral face, arm, and leg • Sensory deficits of the contralateral face, arm, and leg • Aphasia, if the dominant hemisphere is involved • Apraxia, agnosia, and unilateral neglect, if the nondominant hemisphere is involved • Homonymous hemianopsia
Middle cerebral artery (MCA) syndrome	• MCA is the most common of all cerebral occlusions • If the main stem of MCA is occluded, a massive infarction of most of the hemisphere results. • Initially, there may be vomiting and a rapid onset of coma, which may last a few weeks. • Cerebral edema is extensive.	• Hemiplegia (involving face and arm on the contralateral side; the leg is spared or has fewer deficits than the arm) • Sensory deficits (same area as hemiplegia) • Aphasia (global aphasia if the dominant hemisphere is involved) • Homonymous hemianopsia
Anterior cerebral artery (ACA) syndrome	• ACA is least often occluded. • If occlusion occurs proximal to a patent anterior communicating artery (ACom), the blood supply may be compromised. • If occlusion is distal or if the ACom artery is inadequate, there will be infarction of the medial aspect of one frontal lobe. • Bilateral medial frontal lobe infarction occurs if one ACA is occluded and the other artery is small and dependent on blood flow.	• Paralysis of contralateral foot and leg (foot drop is a consistent finding) • Impaired gait • Sensory loss over toes, foot, and leg • Abulia (slowness and prolonged delays to perform acts voluntarily or to respond) • Flat affect, lack of spontaneity, slowness, distractibility, and lack of interest in surroundings • Cognitive impairment, such as perseveration and amnesia • Urinary incontinence • Note that aphasia and hemianopsia are not part of the syndrome.
Vertebral artery syndrome	• Occlusion of vessels within the vertebrobasilar system produces unique syndromes. • Vertebral and basilar arteries and their branches supply the brainstem and cerebellum. • Posterior cerebral arteries are the terminal branches of the basilar artery and supply the medial temporal and occipital lobes, as well as part of the corpus callosum.	• Wallenberg's syndrome (lateral medullary syndrome) • Dizziness • Nystagmus • Dysphagia and dysarthria • Pain in face, nose, or eye • Ipsilateral numbness and weakness of face • Staggering gait and ataxia • Clumsiness
Basilar artery (BA) syndrome		• Quadriplegia • Possibly the "locked-in" syndrome • Weakness of facial, lingual, and pharyngeal muscles
Anterior inferior cerebellar artery (AICA) syndrome	Occlusion of the AICA is also known as the lateral inferior pontine syndrome.	• Vertigo • Nausea and vomiting • Tinnitus • Nystagmus *Ipsilateral side* • Paresis of lateral conjugate gaze • Horner's syndrome • Cerebellar signs (ataxia, nystagmus) *Contralateral side* • Impaired pain and temperature sensation in trunk and limbs (may also involve face)
Posterior inferior cerebellar artery (PICA) syndrome (also called Wallenberg's syndrome)	PICA involves the lateral portion of the medulla as a result of the occlusion of the posterior inferior cerebellar artery.	• Nausea and vomiting • Dysphagia and dysarthria • Horizontal nystagmus • Ipsilateral Horner's syndrome • Cerebellar signs (ataxia and vertigo) • Loss of pain and temperature sensation on contralateral side of trunk and limbs
Posterior cerebral artery (PCA) syndrome	• If superficial occlusion (peripheral areas) of a PCA is involved, contralateral homonymous hemianopsia is seen. • If penetrating branches (central areas) are occluded, the cerebral peduncle, thalamus, and upper brainstem are involved.	*Peripheral area* • Homonymous hemianopsia • Memory deficits • Perseveration • Several visual deficits (cortical blindness, lack of depth perception, failure to see objects not centrally located, visual hallucinations)

(continued)

TABLE 25–3   NAME, DESCRIPTION, AND SIGNS/SYMPTOMS RELATED TO STROKE BY INVOLVED VESSEL (*Continued*)

NAME	DESCRIPTION	SIGNS AND SYMPTOMS
	• There is wide variation in the manifestations of the syndrome.	*Central area* • If the thalamus is involved, sensory loss of all modalities, spontaneous pain, intentional tremors, and mild hemiparesis • If the cerebral peduncle is involved, Weber's syndrome (oculomotor nerve palsy with contralateral hemiplegia) • If the brainstem is involved, deficits involving conjugate gaze, nystagmus, and pupillary abnormalities, with other possible symptoms of ataxia and postural tremors
Deep cortical syndromes	• Four syndromes are associated with intracerebral hemorrhagic stroke. • In addition to an altered level of consciousness (confusion to coma), headache, nausea, vomiting nuchal rigidity, hypertension, and bradycardia related to increased intracranial pressure, each syndrome has its own distinguishing characteristics.	*Putamen hemorrhage (often involves the internal capsule)* • Contralateral hemiplegia • Contralateral hemisensory deficits • Hemianopsia • Slurred speech *Thalamic hemorrhage* • Contralateral hemiplegia • Contralateral hemisensory deficits • Deficits of vertical and lateral gaze *Pontine hemorrhage* • "Locked-in" syndrome • Deficits in lateral eye movement *Cerebellar hemorrhage* • Occipital headache • Dizziness • Ataxia • Vertigo

other characteristics is important. A complete medical history and physical and neurological examination begin the collection of data for the database. A National Institutes of Health Stroke Scale (NIHSS) is conducted to determine neurological deficits (Chart 25-1). Every patient with a question of a cerebrovascular problem such as a TIA or stroke requires a cardiovascular examination that includes blood pressure measurement in both arms; cardiac auscultation and rhythm assessment; and auscultation of the neck for bruit, a marker of generalized atherosclerosis, although not all patients with extracranial atherosclerotic disease have a bruit. In the face of neurological deficits that suggest a stroke, time is critical. Some data collection and diagnostics to establish underlying cause may be postponed to begin treatment. The most important piece of information in the history is to determine the exact time that the neurological deficits began. This is important to determine whether a patient is eligible for thrombolytic therapy, if a diagnosis of ischemic stroke is made.

Diagnosis of Transient Ischemic Attacks

By definition, symptoms associated with a TIA clear completely in less than 24 hours; most clear within minutes. The diagnosis of TIA is a clinical diagnosis based on clinical evidence. TIAs are forewarnings of a potential stroke and thus should be investigated aggressively to determine cause *before* a stroke occurs. The focus of care includes diagnosing TIAs versus other problems; determining the cerebral vessel involved based on symptoms if possible, or recognizing whether presenting symptoms are related to the anterior or posterior cerebral circulation; instituting prevention measures for stroke by modification of risk factors; providing antiplatelet drugs; considering surgical intervention if indicated; providing comprehensive patient education including risk modification; and providing ongoing monitoring for change in risk factors or condition.

The American Heart Association has published a number of guidelines and recommendations for the diagnosis and treatment of TIAs.[4,27–30] These guidelines are updated periodically

TABLE 25–4   COMPARISON OF SIGNS AND SYMPTOMS ASSOCIATED WITH RIGHT-SIDED AND LEFT-SIDED HEMIPLEGIA

STROKE SYNDROME ON LEFT SIDE OF BRAIN (RIGHT-SIDED HEMIPLEGIA)	STROKE SYNDROME ON RIGHT SIDE OF BRAIN (LEFT-SIDED HEMIPLEGIA)
• Expressive aphasia *or* • Receptive aphasia *or* • Global aphasia • Intellectual impairment • Slow and cautious behavior • Defects in right visual fields	• Spatial-perceptual deficits • Denial and the deficits of the affected side require special safety considerations • Tendency for distractibility • Impulsive behavior; apparently unaware of deficits • Poor judgment • Defects in left visual fields

TABLE 25–5 DIAGNOSTIC PROCEDURES FOR TRANSIENT ISCHEMIC ATTACKS (TIAs) AND STROKE*

DIAGNOSTIC PROCEDURE	INFORMATION PROVIDED
Computed tomography (CT) scan without contrast	Important immediate diagnostic to differentiate between ischemic and hemorrhagic stroke; if hemorrhagic, antiplatelets or anticoagulants are not given because of the increased risk of more bleeding; important for treatment decisions
CT scan with contrast	Useful to rule out lesions that many mimic a TIA, especially when symptoms are related to hemispheric deficits; hypodense areas on CT scan suggest infarction
Magnetic resonance imaging (MRI)	Offers excellent soft-tissue contrast discrimination with superior demarcation of mass lesion from surrounding structures including areas of ischemia and infarction; good visualization of vascular structures when questioning a vascular lesion; useful for diagnosis of stroke in first 72 h; a diffusion-weighted MRI can show ischemia in first few hours
Magnetic resonance angiography (MRA)	Less available and higher cost; noninvasive imaging of the carotid, vertebral, basilar, and major intracranial and extracranial arteries to determine occlusion; useful for clot visualization
Carotid ultrasonography	Noninvasive imaging; widely used initial diagnostic in patients with carotid territory symptoms for whom carotid endarterectomy (CEA) is considered; cervical carotid artery imaging often required to exclude high-grade stenosis, which is an exclusion for CEA; less sensitive in assessing mild to moderate stenosis
Transcranial Doppler (TCD)	TCDs are now part of standard work-up for stroke, especially when CEA is considered; useful to detect severe intracranial stenosis, evaluate the carotid and vertebrobasilar vessels, assess patterns and extent of collateral circulation in patients with known arterial stenosis or occlusion, and detect microemboli
Cerebral angiography	Ordered for patients considered candidates for CEA to define precisely the percentage of occlusion and in patients with unusual presentation with aneurysm, vasculitis, and high-grade stenosis
Transthoracic echocardiography (TTE)	Helpful in search for cardioemboli sources; TTE is particularly helpful for diagnosing left ventricular thrombi, left atrial myxomas, and thrombi that protrude into the atrial cavity; they are less reliable for small tumors, laminated thrombi, and thrombi limited to the left or right atrium
Transesophageal echocardiography (TEE)	Benefit of TEE is in greater sensitivity for source of cardioemboli (except ventricular disease); TEE provides better visualization of cardiac structures, especially those at greater depth from chest wall and lesions of the atria (atrial appendage thrombi associated with atrial fibrillation), interarterial septum defects (patent foramen ovale, atrial septal defects), mitral valvular vegetation, and atherosclerotic disease of ascending aortic arch
Electrocardiogram (ECG); 12-lead is recommended initially	12-lead ECG recommended immediately because of the high incidence of heart disease in patients with stroke; ECG also useful when cardiogenic embolic stroke or concurrent coronary artery disease is suspected
Ambulatory ECG monitoring	Reserved for patients who have suspicious palpitations, arrhythmias, or enlarged left atrium
Prothrombotic states	Protein C, protein S, antithrombin III, thrombin time, hemoglobin, electrophoresis, anticardiolipin antibody, lupus anticoagulant, and syphilis serology

* Adams, H. P. Jr., del Zoppo, G., Alberts, M. J., Bhatt, D. L; Brass, L., Furlan, A., et al. (2007). Guidelines for the early management of adults with ischemic stroke. *Stroke, 38*, 1655–1711.

to reflect new scientific evidence that is then translated into practice guidelines.

CLINICAL VIGNETTE: A 68-year-old woman has had some episodes of numbness in her right arm and word-finding difficulty, but they don't last long and disappear. Today was different; the episode lasted longer and she could not speak for 10 minutes, but she was able to speak later, although she had difficulty finding words. Her alarmed spouse took her to the emergency department (ED). The physical and neurological examinations were normal. A 12-lead ECG, cardiac enzyme panel, and all other blood work were normal. After questioning the patient about drug allergies, she was placed on 325 mg of aspirin daily. An appointment was made with her primary care physician for the following week.

Diagnosis of Acute Stroke

A patient seen for a possible stroke must be quickly evaluated and treated to save cerebral tissue and for optimal outcomes. Clinically, neurological signs and symptoms are evident and do not resolve. Signs and symptoms will depend on the cerebral vessel that is infarcted and follows the same principle of lateralizing symptoms from carotid vessels and diffuse (bilateral deficits) from vertebrobasilar vessel infarction.

CLINICAL VIGNETTE*:   Forty-seven-year-old Mrs. CS awoke early in the morning, made a visit to the bathroom, and was returning to bed. About halfway back to bed she experienced an abrupt, severe bout of vertigo, requiring her to grab onto the wall and furniture to get back to bed. The vertigo continued, and was soon

TABLE 25–6   MAJOR RISK FACTORS FOR STROKE

Nonmodifiable Risk Factors

• Age	• Race/ethnicity
• Gender	• Heredity

Modifiable Risk Factors	*Goals*
• Hypertension	• <140/90 mm Hg or • <130/80 mm Hg for diabetes mellitus or chronic kidney disease
• Cardiac disease • Coronary artery disease • Atrial fibrillation • Valvular disease	• Antiplatelet agents or anticoagulants (ASA, 75–325 mg/d; if intolerant to ASA use other antiplatelet drugs, clopidogrel 75 mg/d or warfarin) • Beta blockers for all post-MI patients • ACE inhibitors for post-MI patients
• Diabetes mellitus	• HbA$_{1c}$ <7%
• Hypercholesterolemia	• LDL 100 mg/dL • If total cholesterol ≥200 mg/dL, then non-HDL should be <130 mg/dL
• Cigarette smoking	• Complete cessation
• Excessive use of alcohol	• Limit alcohol consumption to one to two drinks per day
• Physical inactivity	• 30–60 min of activity preferably daily
• Obesity	• Body mass index of 18.5–24.9

ACE, angiotensin-converting enzyme; ASA, acetylsalicylic acid; HDL, high-density lipoprotein; LDL, low-density lipoprotein; MI, myocardial infarction.

From Adams, R. J., Chimowitz, M. I., Alpert, J. S., et al. (2003). Coronary risk evaluation in patients with transient ischemic attack and ischemic stroke. *Stroke, 108,* 1278–1290.

CHART 25-1   National Institutes of Health Stroke Scale

1a. Level of consciousness (LOC)	
alert	0
drowsy	1
stuporous	2
coma	3
1b. LOC questions	
answers both correctly	0
answers one correctly	1
answers neither correctly	2
1c. LOC commands	
performs both correctly	0
performs one correctly	1
performs neither correctly	2
2. Best gaze	
normal	0
partial gaze palsy	1
forced deviation	2
3. Visual	
no visual loss	0
partial hemianopsia	1
complete hemianopsia	2
bilateral hemianopsia	3
4. Facial palsy	
normal	0
minor paralysis	1
partial paralysis	2
complete paralysis	3
5. Motor arm	
no drift	0
drift	1
some effort against gravity	2
no effort against gravity	3
no movement	4
amputation, joint fusion (explain)	9
6. Motor leg	
no drift	0
drift	1
some effort against gravity	2
no effort against gravity	3
no movement	4
amputation, joint fusion (explain)	9
7. Limb ataxia	
absent	0
present in one limb	1
present in two limbs	2
8. Sensory	
normal	0
mild to moderate loss	1
severe to total loss	2
9. Best language	
no aphasia	0
mild-to-moderate	1
severe	2
mute	3

Available at www.ninds.nih.gov

---

accompanied by nausea and vomiting. Her husband, recognizing that something was seriously wrong, took her to the nearest ED. In the ED, her initial assessment revealed some mild left upper extremity weakness and dysmetria. A nurse conducted a neurological assessment and checked "neuro status stable" on the assessment form. The vertigo and nausea persisted in spite of antiemetic medications; the patient was admitted to a medical floor and a gastrointestinal (GI) consult ordered. The GI work-up was negative; the vertigo persisted. The ear, nose, and throat (ENT) service was consulted for a possible inner ear problem. This avenue of investigation was also negative. More than 48 hours after presenting to the ED, a neurology consult was ordered. A CT scan of the head revealed a 4.5-cm left cerebellar infarct.

The most commonly recognized signs of stroke involve unilateral weakness and numbness, altered mental status, and speech changes. Strokes can present in atypical presentations and may not fit the stereotype of deficits. Had the ED staff noted the abrupt onset of symptoms and the early neurological signs of left upper extremity weakness along with dysmetria, they may have considered cerebellar stroke as a possible diagnosis in spite of the patient's young age and the unusual presentation of symptoms.

*Jan Flewelling, RN, BSN, CNRN, Stroke Outreach Program Coordinator, The Methodist Hospital, Houston, Texas, provided this Clinical Vignette.

Several diagnostics are helpful in determining the type of stroke, which then determines treatment options (see Table 25-5). Early treatment for ischemic stroke includes thrombolytic therapy and anticoagulation, both of which are contraindicated if hemorrhagic stroke is present. Therefore, differentiating ischemic and hemorrhagic stroke is critical to treatment decisions. The current standard for differentiating ischemic from hemorrhagic stroke is a noncontrast CT scan.

After a patient has been stabilized from acute stroke, further diagnostic investigation may follow to determine primary problems related to the stroke (e.g., cardiac disease, carotid or vertebrobasilar occlusion), which will need to be addressed to prevent future strokes. The American Heart Association has also published guidelines and recommendations for the diagnosis and treatment of ischemic stroke.

MEDICAL MANAGEMENT AND TREATMENT OF ACUTE ISCHEMIC STROKE

For a patient who has had an acute ischemic stroke, the early focus is on physiologic stabilization, selection and evaluation of patients appropriate for thrombolytics, and supportive therapy.[4,31] For patients who meet criteria for thrombolytic therapy, the window of opportunity for administration is within 3 hours of onset of the first neurological symptom. See further discussion in this chapter on thrombolytic therapy. Therefore, the patient must be assessed and screened rapidly within the limited time window.

The following discussion of the early management of ischemic stroke guidelines, including the 2007 updates, provides the context for treatment.[4] CT remains the most widely used neuroimaging technique for the evaluation of suspected acute ischemic stroke. It is recognized that MRI is useful for some patients. The MRI has advantages, which were previously discussed, and also helps to identify patients with previous microhemorrhages that could be markers of high risk for bleeding secondary to thrombolytics.[24,25]

Supportive Care

The major areas of supportive care focus on the following:

- Maintenance of an adequate airway and oxygenation support to prevent hypoxia
- Control of fever
- Ongoing assessment for cardiac arrhythmia and cardiac ischemia/infarction
- Blood pressure management to maximize cerebral perfusion
- Glycemia management to maintain glucose less than 140 mg/dL to decrease risk of cerebral edema and hemorrhage

- Prevention of complications such as aspiration pneumonia, deep vein thrombosis, nosocomial infections, and device-related infections (urinary tract infections, intravascular line infections)

Maintenance of adequate cerebral tissue oxygenation is critical to prevent hypoxia and potential exacerbation or advancement of further neurological injury. A patent airway must be maintained. If the patient cannot maintain patency independently due to a decreased level of consciousness or brainstem stroke, an artificial airway is used along with measures to prevent aspiration. Supplemental oxygen may be provided, and ventilatory support may be necessary for some patients. A pulse oximeter is used for ongoing monitoring of peripheral oxygenation.

Control of fever is associated with better patient outcomes and therefore, aggressive fever control is recommended. Hyperthermia (temperature $>37.5°C$) has been associated with poorer outcome and poorer prognosis following acute stroke. This finding is consistent with experimental studies, which consistently indicate that increased temperature is associated with more severe neuronal injury. Vigilant nursing observation of the patient's temperature and taking active and immediate measures to prevent and control fever are key functions in the care of the stroke patient.

Myocardial infarction and cardiac arrhythmias are potential complications associated with ischemic stroke. The most common arrhythmia is atrial fibrillation. The patient should have continual cardiac monitoring to identify arrhythmias to allow for prompt treatment.

The target level of hypertension at which treatment should be treated with antihypertensives in a stroke patient is not known. However, treatment is generally avoided unless the systolic blood pressure is greater than 220 mm Hg or diastolic blood pressure is greater than 120 mm Hg.[4,31] If it is necessary to administer antihypertensives, short-duration drugs that have little effect on cerebral blood vessels are selected. The blood pressure must be lowered slowly and cautiously. Labetalol is the drug of choice for intravenous treatment because it can be easily titrated and has minimal vasodilator effect on cerebral blood vessels. In some cases sodium nitroprusside may be required for adequate control. Captopril or nicardipine may be administered by the oral route. If a patient is a candidate for thrombolytics, the blood pressure must be carefully managed before and after administration of thrombolytics. Thrombolytics are not given if the systolic blood pressure is greater than 185 mm Hg or diastolic blood pressure is greater than 110 mm Hg at the time of treatment. Treatment with short-acting antihypertensives may be necessary before administering recombinant tissue plasminogen activator (rt-PA).

It is well recognized that glycemia control within a targeted range is important because either hypoglycemia or hyperglycemia can lead to additional cerebral injury. The blood glucose levels can be easily monitored using a fingerstick. According to the guidelines, a judicious approach to management of hyperglycemia is recommended. The data are limited to determine how this statement should be translated into practice.[31] Lowering the blood glucose to targeted levels can be accomplished with saline solution and regular insulin intravenous drip therapy. Many stroke centers have established lower glucose levels and use less than 140 mg/dL as a target.

Preventions of complications related to stroke are clear. Aspiration pneumonia continues to be a serious and mostly preventable problem. Keeping the patient on nothing by mouth (NPO) status until a bedside swallowing screen is conducted and passed is critical to prevent aspiration pneumonia.[32] Removing indwelling devices such as urinary catheters and intravascular devices as soon as possible, and vigilant strict aseptic precautions while in use, decreases the incidence of hospital-acquired infections.

Medical Management

In addition to supportive care, medical management options for ischemic stroke include hypervolemic-hemodilution therapy, thrombolytics, anticoagulants, antiplatelets, neuroprotective drugs, and hypothermia. Although all of these options are not recommended in published guidelines, each category is addressed to briefly discuss the state of the science.

The goal of treatment is to rapidly assess and stabilize the patient to optimize outcomes and to prevent recurrent stroke. Prevention of recurrent stroke includes immediate careful management in the acute phase to prevent complications that will result in cerebral ischemia, hemorrhage, and extension of the stroke or a new stroke. The long-term perspective of secondary prevention is based on risk factor identification and modification to prevent recurrent stroke. This begins in the acute care setting with identification of the patient's risk factors and developing an individualized plan of care based on the most current evidence-based practice recommendations. Guidelines for the prevention of stroke in patients with ischemic stroke or TIAs are found in Table 25-7.

Hypervolemic-Hemodilution Therapy

To support cerebral hemodynamics, hypervolemic-hemodilution therapy has been used (see Chap. 23). This therapy is alleged to help maintain a stable, slightly higher blood pressure, which increases and maintains cerebral perfusion pressure by lowering blood viscosity. According to the 2007 guidelines, at present drug-induced hypertension is not recommended for the treatment of most patients with ischemic stroke.[4,31]

Thrombolytics

Reperfusion drug therapy continues to be a useful option for selected patients with acute ischemic stroke. According to the 2007 guidelines, intravenous administration of rt-PA is the treatment of choice for thrombolytics in acute stroke. Treatment with streptokinase is not recommended, and reteplase, urokinase, and other thrombolytic agents should not be used outside of the setting of a clinical trial. The thrombolytic therapy with rt-PA is used in acute ischemic stroke to restore cerebral blood flow, reduce ischemia, and limit neurological disability. Re-establishing perfusion in an occluded cerebral artery may result in the recovery of ischemic tissue within a brief time span after onset of acute stroke. The major concern with thrombolytic agents is the possibility of hemorrhagic transformation of the infarction.[33] Intravenous rt-PA should be considered for all patients with acute ischemic stroke who meet criteria and who can be treated within 3 hours of stroke symptom onset.[34] Careful selection is imperative in safe drug administration. Chart 25-2 outlines inclusion and exclusion criteria. The recommended dose is 0.9 mg/kg (maximum 90 mg). The initial 10% is given as an intravenous bolus over 1 minute and the remaining rt-PA infused over 60 minutes. Anticoagulants or aspirin should not be given in the first 24 hours after rt-PA treatment.

Thrombolytic therapy with rt-PA is not without risk. Following initiation of therapy, patients must be assessed in an intensive care setting or unit with nurses skilled in monitoring patients. More and more patients are being admitted to non–intensive care units after rt-PA as long as drips that need adjusting or ventilator support is ordered for the patient. Frequent assessment of blood pressure during the first 24 hours, with treatment of blood pressure elevations of more than 185 mm Hg systolic or 110 mm Hg diastolic, helps prevent thrombolysis-related ICH. Frequent neurological assessment can allow early detection of decreased levels of consciousness, headache, nausea and vomiting, or an increase in focal neurological deficits (signs and symptoms that could indicate onset of ICH). Use of rt-PA is not recommended in patients presenting with rapidly improving neurological deficit or minor deficits with an NIHSS score of less than 3 or 4 (see Chart 25-1 for the NIHSS) because they usually have excellent recovery without therapy.

CLINICAL PEARLS: Surgery is not an absolute contraindication for rt-PA administration; intra-arterial doses may be an option for some patients soon after surgery.

Administration of rt-PA requires a setting in which comprehensive stroke services can be provided. This includes ED and neurological expertise for prompt clinical assessment and expert interpretation of the CT brain scan, close monitoring of the patient's vital signs and neurological status for at least 24 hours after treatment, and expertise for management of possible intracranial hemorrhage, including access to neurosurgical care and expertise.

Intra-arterial thrombolytics are an option for treatment of selected patients who have major stroke of less than 6 hours' duration, who have occlusion of the middle cerebral artery, and who are not otherwise candidates for intravenous rt-PA.[4] Treatment requires that the patient be at a recognized stroke center with immediate access to cerebral angiography and qualified interventionists.

Anticoagulants

The most recent evidence does not support the use of early anticoagulation to improve outcomes after acute ischemic stroke.[4,35] The most recent guidelines state that most stroke patients do not need emergency administration of anticoagulants.[4,31,36] Anticoagulation therapy is not recommended in lieu of intravenous thrombolysis and should be withheld in patients with moderate or severe stroke because of an increased risk for intracranial hemorrhage. It is further noted that despite lack of supporting data, anticoagulants are still frequently administered to patients with acute ischemic stroke. More studies are being conducted to determine if there are subgroups of patients who would benefit from

TABLE 25-7 GUIDELINES FOR THE PREVENTION OF STROKE IN PATIENTS WITH ISCHEMIC STROKE OR TRANSIENT ISCHEMIC ATTACKS*

RISK FACTOR	RECOMMENDATION
Hypertension • Normal BP is defined as <120/80 mm Hg by JNC-7[†] • JNC-7 notes that absolute target BP level and reduction are uncertain and should be individualized.	• Maintain blood pressure <140 mm Hg and diastolic blood pressure <90 mm Hg or to individual targeted levels. • Institute lifestyle modifications. • Drug therapy with diuretics and ACEIs should be provided. • Other antihypertensive therapy choices should be individualized.
Diabetes mellitus • ACEIs and ARBs are effective in reducing progression of renal disease. • Near normal glycemic levels reduce microvascular complications.	• More rigorous control of BP and lipids • For people with diabetes mellitus, target blood pressure levels to <130/80 mm Hg[†] • Most patients will require more than one agent to control BP (first-choice medications are ACEIs and ARBs). • Diet and oral hypoglycemics or insulin to keep fasting blood glucose levels <126 mg/dL or to maintain hemoglobin A_{1c} level <7.0%
Lipids • Follow NCEP III guidelines[‡] • Lifestyle modifications • Dietary guidelines • Medications	• AHA step II diet (≤30% of calories derived from fat, <7% from saturated fat, and <200 mg/d cholesterol consumed) • Maintain ideal body weight. • Regular exercise • Target goals for LDL-C is <100 mg/dL, and LDL-C <70 mg/dL for very high-risk persons with multiple risk factors. • Statins are first-line drugs recommended for drug therapy. • If low HDL, consider niacin or gemfibrozil.
Cigarette smoking	• Discontinue smoking. • Counseling, nicotine products, and oral smoking cessation medications are effective. • Avoid environmental smoke.
Excessive alcohol intake	• Eliminate excessive alcohol intake. • Formal alcohol cessation programs are recommended. • Two or fewer drinks per day for men and one drink per day for nonpregnant women may be considered.
Obesity	• Goal is BMI of 18.5–24.9 kg/m² and waist circumference <35 for women and <40 for men • Weight reduction programs that include diet, physical activity, and behavior counseling are encouraged.
Physical activity	• At least 30 min of moderate-intensity physical exercise most days • For those with disabilities after ischemic stroke, a supervised therapeutic exercise program
Coronary artery disease, cardiac dysrhythmias, congestive heart failure, and valvular disease	• Treat disease and underlying cause as appropriate.

ACEI, angiotensin-converting enzyme inhibitors; AHA, American Heart Association; ARBs, angiotensin receptor blockers; BMI, body mass index; BP, blood pressure; HDL, high-density lipoprotein; JNC, Joint National Committee; LDL-C, low-density lipoprotein cholesterol; NCEP, National Cholesterol Education Program.

* Sacco, R. L., Adams, R., Albers, G., et al. (2006). Guidelines for prevention of stroke in patients with ischemic stroke or transient ischemic attack: A statement for healthcare professionals from the American Heart Association/American Stroke Association Council on Stroke: Co-sponsored by the Council on Cardiovascular Radiology and Intervention: The American Academy of Neurology affirms the value of this guideline. *Stroke, 37,* 577–617.

† Chobanian, A. V., Bakris, G. L., Black, H. R., et al. (2004). The seventh report of the Joint National Committee on Prevention, Detection, Evaluation, and Treatment of High Blood Pressure: The JNC 7 Report. *JAMA, 289,* 2560–2571.

‡ US National Heart, Lung, and Blood Institute, National Institutes of Health. (2001). The Third Report of the National Cholesterol Education Program (NCEP) Expert Panel on Detection, Evaluation, and Treatment of High Blood Cholesterol in Adults (Adult Treatment Panel III). NIH Publication No. 01-3670. Bethesda, MD: Author.

early anticoagulation therapy, but currently that information is lacking. In selected cases when anticoagulation therapy is ordered, the INR is used to monitor blood coagulation. The use of prothrombin time (PT) to monitor blood coagulation has also been examined. It is now recommended that use of antifactor Xa replace PT for blood coagulation monitoring.[37]

Antiplatelets

Antiplatelet agents deter the adherence of platelets to the wall of an injured blood vessel or to other platelets. Current antiplatelet drugs include aspirin, ticlopidine, clopidogrel, extended-release dipyridamole, and a combination of dipyridamole and aspirin. A combination of one or two drugs is not uncommon, but this increases the risk of adverse drug responses such as bleeding and thus requires careful monitoring. Current guidelines for antithrombotic therapy are found in Table 25-8.[4] The recommendations include the following: (1) most patients should receive aspirin with 48 hours of acute stroke with the understanding that the effect is modest; and (2) aspirin should not be considered as an alternative to thrombolytic therapy. Research on the possible use of abciximab and other rapid-acting antiplatelet drugs continues;

CHART 25-2 Eligibility Criteria for Thrombolytic Therapy

INCLUSION CRITERIA

1. Symptom onset of <3 hours before beginning treatment
2. Clinical diagnosis of ischemic stroke with measurable deficit on National Institutes of Health Stroke Scale that are neither minor nor are clearing spontaneously
3. Age >18 years
4. Computed tomography scan does not show a multilobar infarction (hypodensity >1/3 cerebral hemisphere); systolic blood pressure (BP) <185 mm Hg and diastolic BP <110 mm Hg
5. If received heparin in previous 48 hours, activated partial thromboplastin time must be in normal range
6. Platelet count ≥100,000 mm^3
7. Blood glucose ≥50 mg/dL (2.7 mmol/L)
8. No seizures with postictal residual neurological impairment

EXCLUSION CRITERIA

1. Stroke or serious cerebral trauma within previous 3 months
2. Myocardial infarction within previous 3 months
3. Gastrointestinal or urinary hemorrhage within previous 21 days
4. Major surgery within previous 14 days
5. Arterial puncture at a noncompressible site within previous 7 days
6. History of previous intracranial hemorrhage
7. Systolic BP >185 mm Hg or diastolic BP >110 mm Hg or BP readings that require aggressive treatment
8. Evidence of active bleeding or acute trauma (fracture) on examination
9. Taking oral anticoagulants or if anticoagulant being taken, international normalized ratio >1.7
10. Woman of childbearing age who has a positive pregnancy test result

From Adams, H. P, Adams, R. J., Brott, T., et al. (2003). Guidelines for the early management of patients with ischemic stroke: A scientific statement from the Stroke Council of the American Stroke Association. *Stroke, 34,* 1056–1083; and Adams, H., Adams, R., Del Zappo, G., & Goldstein, L. B. (2005). Guidelines for the early management of patients with ischemic stroke: 2005 Guidelines update. *Stroke, 36,* 916–921.

currently, there are no recommendations for their use in acute stroke management.

Neuroprotective Agents

A number of potential neuroprotective agents have been considered that represent a broad spectrum of drugs with disparate mechanisms of action: sodium channel blockers, calcium channel antagonists, free radical scavengers, membrane stabilizers, glutamate receptor antagonists, and gamma-aminobutyric acid (GABA) agonists. Currently, new drugs are being investigated. However, no agent has demonstrated clinical benefit, and no drug is currently recommended as a useful neuroprotective agent.[4,31]

TABLE 25-8 USE OF ANTITHROMBOTIC AGENTS FOR PATIENTS WITH ISCHEMIC STROKE OR TIAs (ORAL ANTICOAGULANT AND ANTIPLATELET THERAPIES)

EVENT	RECOMMENDED THERAPY	COMMENT
TIAs or noncardioembolic ischemic stroke	Any of the following are recommended: • ASA 50–325 mg/d • ASA and ER-DP (single formulation) • Clopidogrel 75 mg	• Antiplatelet agents rather than oral anticoagulation are recommended to reduce risk of recurrent stroke or cardiovascular events. • Compared to ASA alone, both the combination of ASA and ER-DP or clopidogrel is safe. • The combination of ASA and ER-DP is suggested over ASA alone. • Selection of an antiplatelet should be individualized based on risk factors, tolerance, and clinical characteristics. • For patients allergic to ASA, clopidogrel is used. • If patient has an ischemic cerebrovascular event while on ASA, there is no evidence supporting benefit from increasing dose.
Patients with ischemic stroke or TIA with persistent or paroxysmal (intermittent) atrial fibrillation	Anticoagulation with adjusted dose of warfarin is recommended: • Warfarin (target 2.5) with a range of 2.0–3.0 INR • For patient unable to take oral anticoagulants, ASA 325 mg/d recommended	• INR must be monitored periodically. • Patient education is important to inform patient about diet, side effects, safety, and adherence to dosage based on INR. • Inform patient of bleeding risk.

ASA, acetylsalicylic acid; ER-DP, extended-release dipyridamole; INR, international normalized ratio; TIA, transient ischemic attack.

From Sacco, R. L., Adams, R., Albers, G., et al. (2006). Guidelines for prevention of stroke in patients with ischemic stroke or transient ischemic attack: A statement for healthcare professionals from the American Heart Association/American Stroke Association Council on Stroke: Co-sponsored by the Council on Cardiovascular Radiology and Intervention: The American Academy of Neurology affirms the value of this guideline. *Stroke, 37,* 577–617.

Hypothermia

In recent years there has been increasing interest in the use of hypothermia in acute stroke patients. Hypothermia (i.e., 32°C to 34°C) has been used in the setting of neurosurgical and cardiothoracic surgery for its neuroprotective benefits, and also in the management of severe brain injury and cardiac arrest. However, hypothermia also carries risks of fatal cardiac dysrhythmias, coagulopathies, electrolyte derangement, and other problems. Although hypothermia research for stroke is promising, the current state of the science is insufficient to recommend its use for the management of stroke patients.[4,31]

Surgical and Endovascular Interventions

Selected patients with extracranial or intracranial atherosclerotic disease located in accessible sites may be good candidates for surgery. The goal of the surgical procedures is to *prevent* TIAs or stroke. Carotid endarterectomy (CEA) and extracranial/intracranial (EC-IC) arterial bypass are designed to improve cerebral perfusion of patients with narrowing of the extracranial artery. EC-IC bypass grafting procedures have been used for a superior temporal artery/middle cerebral artery (STA-MCA) anastomosis. Chart 25-3 provides key points in the acute management of stroke patients after special interventions.

Endovascular therapies encompass interventional radiologic procedures to treat intracranial vascular lesions with high morbidity and mortality. The procedure involves stretching the media of the stenosed vessel and breaking the atherosclerotic plaque by inflating a balloon at the site of the stenosis. Another form of therapy, *intravascular stenting*, is used in conjunction with the angioplasty to maintain vessel patency. Stenting has been proposed as an alternative therapeutic modality for patients with significant carotid, MCA, and vertebrobasilar artery stenosis.[38] Studies are currently under way to evaluate the efficacy.

After review of the current evidence, the 2007 guidelines conclude that the data on the safety and effectiveness of CEA and other operations *for treatment of patients with acute ischemic stroke* are not sufficient to permit a recommendation. Surgical procedures may have serious risks and may not favorably alter the outcome of the patient.[4]

Carotid Endarterectomy

The North American Symptomatic Carotid Endarterectomy Trial (NASCET) clearly demonstrated that CEA is superior to medical therapy alone for *stroke prevention* in patients with 70% or greater symptomatic internal carotid artery stenosis. Patients with 70% or greater carotid stenosis, without major operative risk factors, have a relative reduction of about 60% and absolute risk reduction of 5% to 10% per year within the subsequent 2 years.[39–41] In one study, patients with 50% to 69% stenosis with a recent TIA or minor stroke had a reduced stroke rate with endarterectomy versus medical treatment.[42] However, the absolute benefit of surgery is less than that for patients with higher degrees of stenosis and among women and patients with retinal TIAs. When CEA is indicated, surgery within 2 weeks is suggested rather than delay.[41]

Patients with less than 50% stenosis with recent symptoms do not benefit from CEA. Antiplatelet therapy is recommended for these patients.

The "hot spots" for atheroma build-up are noted in Figure 25-8. A CEA consists of careful removal of the atherosclerotic plaque from the artery after a temporary bypass shunt has been created to provide adequate cerebral perfusion. The plaque is removed after the artery is temporarily occluded both above and below the atheroma. The bypass graft also improves circulation. The major danger during surgery is embolization of atherogenic plaque and thrombi from excessive manipulation of the carotid bifurcation. On completion, a Jackson-Pratt is usually inserted at the operative site to prevent development of a hematoma.

The major postoperative concerns are blood pressure instability, stroke or transient neurological deficits, cranial nerve injury (facial, vagal), wound hematoma, suture line rupture, TIAs, and hyperperfusion syndromes. After surgery, patients experience a period of postoperative blood pressure instability that lasts for approximately 12 to 24 hours, probably as a result of a carotid sinus malfunction and loss of effective baroreceptor action. After blood flow has been restored, maintenance of the systolic pressure at a constant level of approximately 150 mm Hg is critical. The sudden restoration of high flow, especially after removal of a tight stenosis and in the presence of heparin (used during surgery) or antiplatelets, can lead to intracerebral hemorrhage. Hypotensive episodes are just as disastrous and can result in ischemic stroke or TIAs. The potential for cranial nerve injury results from the proximity of these nerves to the operative site.

Hyperperfusion syndromes are related to the marked increase in cerebral blood flow after CEA. Patients often have paralysis of autoregulation ipsilateral to the surgical site so that the profound increase in blood flow is not blunted. When this occurs, blood pressure must be meticulously maintained in the 120 to 130 mm Hg range. Patients may experience vascular headaches or catastrophic intracerebral hemorrhage. Seizures may occur about 7 to 10 days postoperatively. Finally, a leading cause of death after CEA is myocardial infarction, either immediate or delayed. The patient should be monitored carefully for evidence of myocardial ischemia or infarction.

There is no evidence to recommend emergent CEA or other surgical procedures in management of acute ischemic stroke. Currently, CEA is recommended for selected patients who meet criteria as a stroke preventive measure.

Superficial Temporal Artery-Middle Cerebral Artery Anastomosis

EC-IC arterial bypass, most often of the STA to the MCA, is a microsurgical procedure used in the past to allegedly provide collateral circulation to the areas of the brain supplied by the MCA. Currently, this procedure is used infrequently because of the negative results reported in the EC/IC Bypass Trial and other clinical experience.[43,44] National guidelines do not recommended it for acute stroke management.[4,31,41]

Endovascular Procedures

Endovascular treatment of patients with symptomatic extracranial vertebral stenosis may be considered when

CHART 25-3	Key Points in Acute Care Nursing Management of Stroke Patients After Special Interventions

NURSING MANAGEMENT OF PATIENTS WHO HAVE RECEIVED THROMBOLYTIC THERAPY

- Monitor vital signs for evidence of extracranial bleeding (e.g., gastric hemorrhage).
- Monitor neurological signs for evidence of deterioration and increased intracranial pressure (ICP) that may be caused by intracerebral hemorrhage or increasing cerebral edema.
- Monitor for reperfusion injury.*
- Monitor for bleeding at catheter site; bleeding may also be noted in urine or stool, or from mouth.
- Monitor coagulation studies and maintain in therapeutic parameters.
- Protect femoral catheter, which is left in place for as long as 24 hours.

NURSING MANAGEMENT OF PATIENTS WHO HAVE UNDERGONE CEREBRAL ANGIOGRAPHY/STENT PLACEMENT

- Monitor vital signs for hemodynamic instability.
- Monitor for bleeding at catheter site; bleeding may also be noted in urine, stool, GI tract, or mouth.
- Monitor neurological signs for evidence of intracerebral hemorrhage and reperfusion injury.*
- Monitor coagulation studies and maintain in therapeutic range using international normalizing ratio (INR) parameters.

NURSING MANAGEMENT OF PATIENTS WHO HAVE UNDERGONE A CAROTID ENDARTERECTOMY

- Monitor blood pressure and rigorously maintain within set parameters, usually about 150 mm Hg systolic (hypertension predisposes to intracerebral hemorrhage, and hypotension to ischemic stroke); instability of blood pressure is common particularly in the first 12–24 hours postoperatively so expect to monitor and manage blood pressure frequently.
- Monitor for cardiac arrhythmias and evidence of myocardial ischemia (myocardial infarction is not uncommon).
- Monitor neurological signs frequently and observe for early signs of deterioration.
  - Monitor for cranial nerve deficits (especially facial and vagal) as a result of surgery.
  - Monitor for signs of intracerebral hemorrhage (increased ICP, new onset of neurological deficits).
  - Monitor for vascular headache and seizures (hyperperfusion syndrome).
- Monitor for reperfusion injury.*
- Maintain head of bed according to physician orders; because of vascular instability, the head of the bed may be flat for the first 24 hours.
- Observe operative site for hemorrhage, hematoma, or tearing of suture site.

*Reperfusion injury: observe for signs and symptoms of cerebral edema, increased ICP, and recurrence of stroke symptomology or expansion of neurological deficits after successful recanalization.

patients are having symptoms despite medical therapies (e.g. antithrombotics, statins).[41]

Clot Extraction

Mechanical devices have been used to extract thrombi for occluded intracranial arteries.[45] The Mechanical Embolus Removal in Cerebral Embolism (MERCI) device is now recognized as a "reasonable" intervention for extraction of intra-arterial thrombi in carefully selected patients; the panel also recognized that the utility of the device in improving outcomes after stroke is unclear. Further study is recommended to define its role in emergency stroke management.[4]

Acute Management of Intracerebral Hemorrhage Stroke

American Heart Association guidelines have been updated for the management of spontaneous intracerebral hemorrhage in adults and are the basis for current evidence-based practice.[46] The general principles and recommendations include an intensive care unit environment for the monitoring and treatment of patients with ICH stroke because of the emergent nature of the condition and the frequent elevations in ICP and blood pressure, frequent need for intubation and assisted ventilation, and multiple complicating medical problems. The management of the increased ICP is based on a continuum from simple measures such as elevation of the head of the bed 30 degrees to mannitol, ventriculostomy, and hyperventilation based on the clinical condition. Acute management of increased ICP is outlined in Chapter 13. Other recommendations include maintaining normal blood glucose (<300 mg/dL), normothermia (treatment of fever to normal body temperature), management of blood pressure (although it is clear that evidence is incomplete in blood pressure management in ICH), and use of antiepileptic drugs to treat seizures. For management of blood pressure of a systolic pressure greater than 200 mm Hg, intravenous antihypertensive therapy should be considered with a target of 160/90 mm Hg.

Other recommendations focus on management of coagulation and fibrinolysis issues related to ICH. This includes the use of protamine sulfate to reverse heparin-associated ICH; intravenous vitamin K for warfarin-associated ICH; and fresh frozen plasma as an option to address the coagulopathies that occur with ICH. Restarting antithrombotic therapy after ICH depends on the risk of possible arterial or venous thromboembolism and recurrent ICH. Low-molecular-weight

TABLE 25-9   ASSESSMENT OF STROKE PATIENTS

INITIAL BRIEF ASSESSMENT ASSESS FOR:	ASSESSMENT OF REHABILITATION NEEDS INCLUDE:
• Complications and prior and current impairments (e.g., NIHSS for stroke) • Risk factors for recurrent stroke and coronary artery disease • Medical comorbidities • Level of consciousness and cognitive status • Brief swallowing screen (e.g., Massey Swallowing Screen) • Skin integrity and evidence of pressure ulcers • Mobility and need for assistance with movement to maintain safety • Sensory function and impact on safety • Communication skills and need for alternate methods of communication • Risk of DVT	• Prevention of complications (e.g., aspiration, malnutrition, skin breakdown, DVT, bowel/bladder dysfunction) • Assessment of impairments (e.g., communications, motor, cognitive, visual, spatial, sensory, psychological) • Psychosocial assessment and family caregiver support • Functional assessment (e.g., standard forms such as FIM)

DVT, deep vein thrombosis; NIHSS, National Institutes of Health Stroke Scale.

heparin may be considered 3 to 4 days after ICH for prophylaxis. Elastic hose and intermittent pneumatic compression stockings should be provided for patients with hemiparesis or hemiplegia. In treating patients with ICH caused by thrombolytics, urgent therapies are directed at replacing clotting factors and platelets.

Surgical interventions for ICH are also addressed. The following are recommended for possible surgical approaches for patients with cerebellar hemorrhages greater than 3 cm with neurological deterioration or brainstem compression: compression and/or hydrocephalus from ventricular obstruction need evacuation of the hemorrhage as soon as possible; and supratentorial ICH should undergo standard craniotomy for a lobar clot located within 1 cm of the surface. Other combined surgical and direct drug infusion therapies are under investigation, but are not a recommended standard for care currently.

As mentioned above, surgical decompression and stereotactically guided removal of the hematoma may be necessary in certain cases.[12] Care of the postoperative neurosurgical patient is discussed in Chapter 14. Vasospasms are not considered a problem with ICH. Chapter 23 provides guidance for patient management. For patients who survive, rehabilitation is necessary. In addition, identification and modification of risk factors need to be undertaken. Nursing management is outlined in Chapters 13 and 23.

For patients with catastrophic stroke, palliative care may be an option for patients with severe morbidity that will have a significant impact on quality of life and severe disability. Continuation of aggressive treatment may lead to placement in a long-term chronic care facility. Difficult discussions with and decisions by the patient and family may need to occur. Advanced directives help to guide the decision-making process for the family when the patient is unconscious and critically ill.

CLINICAL PEARLS: Palliative care is a legitimate treatment option for patients with severe stroke with a poor prognosis.

There is reason to be hopeful about evidence-based effective ICH treatment for the future, such as recombinant factor VIIa, which is currently being investigated. This is encouraging news because of the high morbidity and mortality rates currently associated with ICH stroke.[46]

CLINICAL PEARLS: Repeated vomiting after an acute mental status decline is highly indicative of intracranial hemorrhage; be prepared for deterioration, possible intubation, or surgery.

Rehabilitation

A recent publication has addressed the evidence for comprehensive rehabilitation after stroke and compiled guidelines. Management of Adult Stroke Rehabilitation Care: A Clinical Practice Guideline provides a comprehensive approach to stroke rehabilitation.[47] The guidelines are organized into the major categories of assessment, inpatient rehabilitation, and community-based rehabilitation. Individual algorithms provide overviews of each step in the overall processes of care. Assessment is further divided into initial brief assessment and assessment of rehabilitation needs (Table 25-9). Table 25-10 lists inpatient rehabilitation focus, and Table 25-11 identifies key issues related to community-based rehabilitation.

Early rehabilitation is critical to making optimal recovery and should be initiated as early as possible, preferably within 24 to 48 hours of the stroke. An individualized rehabilitation plan includes phased interventions along with periodic evaluation of progress toward meeting individual goals. It also includes interventions to prevent a recurrent stroke. Phased interventions relate to implementing deficit-specific interventions along a continuum from simple to complex actions. Usually interdisciplinary collaboration is needed for optimal outcomes. For example, common post-stroke mobility problems include cardiovascular deconditioning, impairment in gait and balance, diminished muscle tone, and weakness. The phasing of interventions often proceeds from range of motion, to muscle strengthening, to gait retraining, to fitness training. Newer treatments based on new motor theory recovery are innovating how physical therapy is provided to patients. Equally important are task-oriented exercises that help the patient regain independence in activities of daily living (see Chap. 13 for rehabilitation content).

TABLE 25–10   INPATIENT REHABILITATION: REASSESSMENT OF REHABILITATION PROGRESS

GENERAL FOCUS	SPECIFIC FOCUS
• Overall medical status • Functional status (FIM and other standardized instruments) • Family support	 • Mobility, ADLs/IADLs, communications, nutrition, cognition, behavior, affect, motivation • Family function • Ability and desire to provide support • Resources • Transportation
• Patient and family adjustment • Reassessment of goals in relation to progress • Risk of another stroke	• Monitoring both patient and family adaptability and adjustment • Refining plan of care based on new information • Prevention of stroke guidelines implemented and monitored

ADLs, activities of daily living; IADLs, instrumental activities of daily living.

GENERAL NURSING MANAGEMENT OF THE STROKE PATIENT

Nursing management of patients with stroke varies according to the specific stroke syndrome and neurological and functional deficits. However, there are several common areas to consider, including primary and secondary prevention of stroke, initial acute care management, early focus on rehabilitation, discharge planning and continuity of care, and patient education. Assessment and nursing diagnosis guide nursing management.

Primary and Secondary Prevention of Stroke

The overall approach to patients with risk factors for stroke—TIAs, stroke, and poststroke—is toward prevention of a first stroke or, in the person who has already had a stroke, prevention of another stroke. Prevention is geared toward identification of all risk factors; modification of modifiable risk factors; drug therapy; surgical interventions, when appropriate; and education of the patient and family. Education is directed at helping the person understand his or her risk factors and the need to make a commitment to lifestyle changes and adherence to treatment plans to prevent stroke. Continued public education to inform all people

that a "brain attack" is a medical emergency that warrants immediate emergency department care must be undertaken. The general public understands that a heart attack is a medical emergency that requires a call to 911 for emergency help to save lives and heart muscle. People need to apply the same sense of urgency to a brain attack. Educating the public about the signs and symptoms of a brain attack and the definitive action to be taken is very cost effective and can save human potential and quality of life. Stroke is now a *treatable* emergency, and timeliness to a stroke center is paramount to achieving the best patient outcomes.

The paradigm shift from treatment to prevention has redefined the nurse's role in identification of risk factors and working with the patient not only to modify risk factors, but also to promote a healthier lifestyle. The major risk factors for stroke are listed in Table 25-6. These major risk factors are the same for stroke and heart disease, the number one and number three causes of death in the United States. Nurses are particularly effective in helping patients think through how they can modify risk factors within the context of their lifestyles. Secondary prevention becomes the focus after a stroke to prevent another stroke, regardless of whether the patient is followed in a stroke prevention clinic or by the primary care provider. Along with education and motivation, the patient must be monitored collaboratively by the nurse and physician. Prevention is cost effective and results in savings.

TABLE 25–11   COMMUNITY-BASED REHABILITATION AND INTEGRATION

ASSESSMENT OF PATIENT READINESS AND DISCHARGE ENVIRONMENT	RELATED ACTIVITIES
• Physiologically stabilized	• All health problems addressed and patient knows plan of care
• Functional deficits identified and plan of care in place	• Interventions implemented and assessed for effectiveness
• Postcare options discussed based on resources and health care plan	• Patient and family involved in selecting the preferred plan
• Home environment assessed for needed alterations to optimize function and safety	• Home environment assessment conducted • Needed equipment in place
• Patient/family education individualized and conducted (e.g., prescriptions, signs and symptoms of recurrent stroke, community resources)	• Educational program completed • Steps in integration into roles and community discussed
• Information provided on what to do if problems occur	• Patient and family have back-up plan for safe recovery
• Follow-up plan in place	• Follow-up plan understood by patient and family.

Possible patient problems and nursing diagnoses related to stroke prevention include Knowledge Deficit, Noncompliance, and Ineffective Management of Therapeutic Regimen.

Initial Acute Care Management

Early treatment of stroke is recognized as a key factor in optimizing outcomes. Care may be rendered in a neurological intensive care unit or special acute care unit. Having been stabilized, the patient may receive therapies to protect the brain from secondary injury related to the ischemic cascade. The current approved window of opportunity to use rt-PA is 0 to 3 hours after onset of ischemic stroke. The acute care management goals for both medical and nursing management are the same, although the interventions and related responsibilities are different.

CLINICAL PEARLS: A diagnosis of stroke does not require a critical care designation. Only stroke patients with immediate or impending critical care needs require intensive care monitoring in a critical care environment.

Patient safety is an additional goal for which nurses assume a major responsibility. These goals include:

- Maintenance of an adequate airway and oxygenation support to prevent hypoxia
- Control of fever
- Ongoing assessment for cardiac arrhythmia and cardiac ischemia/infarction
- Blood pressure management to maximize cerebral perfusion
- Glycemia management to maintain glucose less than 150 mg/dL to decrease risk of cerebral edema and hemorrhage
- Prevention of complications such as aspiration pneumonia, nosocomial infections, and device-related infections (urinary tract infections, intravascular line infections)
- Prevention of deep venous thrombosis and pulmonary embolism
- Fall prevention and patient safety

Many patients will be managed in a stroke unit for close monitoring by nurses with expertise with the stroke population. Some critically ill and unstable patients who require vasoactive intravenous drug therapy or who are on a ventilator will require admission to an intensive care unit. Regardless of the setting, the nurse works collaboratively with the physician and other health professionals to achieve optimal outcomes.

The following patient problems and nursing diagnoses are common in the acute phase of illness: Ineffective Airway Clearance; Risk of Aspiration; Impaired Swallowing; Altered Cerebral Tissue Perfusion; Risk of Infection; Ineffective Breathing Pattern; Sensory Perceptual Alterations; Impaired Physical Mobility; Nutrition Deficits; and Impaired Verbal Communication.

CLINICAL VIGNETTE*:   RJ, a 42-year-old male patient, presents to the ED with new onset right hemiparesis, expressive dysphasia, and dysarthria. Because he had missed the 3-hour window for t-PA, aspirin is ordered. However, he has severe dysarthria, so the physician writes an NPO order. The ED nurse brings him the aspirin but no liquid to facilitate swallowing. When RJ's wife asked for some water, she is told by the nurse that he can't have any water because he is NPO. "How is he supposed to swallow his medicine without water?" inquires RJ's wife. "Maybe he can get let it dissolve in his mouth," says the nurse.

While aspiration is a risk for any patient demonstrating dysarthria, a simple bedside swallow screening would have helped clarify the safety of allowing this patient to take oral medication.

*Jan Flewelling, RN, BSN, CNRN, Stroke Outreach Program Coordinator, The Methodist Hospital, Houston, Texas, provided this Clinical Vignette.

Common collaborative problems include hypoxemia; hypoglycemia or hyperglycemia; increased intracranial pressure; paresis/paresthesia/paralysis; gastrointestinal bleeding; hypertension; reperfusion injury; electrolyte imbalances; dysrhythmias; deep vein thrombosis or pulmonary embolism; anticoagulant therapy adverse effects; and thrombolytic therapy adverse effects.

Frequent neurological, cardiac, hemodynamic, and respiratory monitoring is necessary to determine early changes and the need to adjust management. Cerebral edema generally develops with all ischemic strokes within 24 hours. The larger the stroke, the more edema occurs so that cerebral edema is a major concern with a larger stroke. Severe hypertension increases the risk of hemorrhage or recurrent bleeding. Both cerebral edema and hemorrhage are associated with increased ICP. Increased ICP may result from the original hemorrhage, but hemorrhage can also occur 2 to 4 days after massive infarction of the cerebral hemisphere. The development of edema is heralded by a gradual deterioration in neurological signs, such as drowsiness and sluggish pupillary response. Increased ICP is treated with supportive therapy and depends on the extent of the deficits and complications present. Frequent serial neurological assessment is important in monitoring the patient for onset of complications.

CLINICAL PEARLS: Patients with an NIHSS score of less than 7 have a good chance for complete or near complete recovery. Stroke scores that range from 8 to 17 are highly indicative of the need for some type of long-term assistance. Stroke scores greater than 18 are highly correlated with significant morbidity and mortality.

Careful cardiac monitoring is necessary to determine the need to adjust therapy to maximize hemodynamic parameters and to identify cardiac arrhythmias and myocardial infarction. The level of the head of the bed will depend on stability of hemodynamics and ICP, but it is generally elevated to 30 degrees. Respiratory parameters are also monitored closely for evidence of secondary problems, such as

CHART 25-4   **Summary of Common Patient Problems and Nursing Diagnoses for Acute Stroke Patients**

COMMON PATIENT PROBLEMS AND NURSING DIAGNOSES	NURSING INTERVENTIONS	EXPECTED OUTCOMES
Ineffective Airway Clearance related to (R/T) unconsciousness or ineffective cough reflex	• Position to facilitate drainage of oropharyngeal secretions. • Turn side to side every 2 hours. • Elevate the head of the bed to 30 degrees. • Clear secretions from the airway using suction, as necessary; provide for pulmonary hygiene. • Provide for chest physical therapy.	Patent airway is maintained.
Risk of Aspiration R/T inability to protect airway or unconsciousness	• Maintain on nothing by mouth (NPO) status. • Clear with a swallow assessment before beginning oral intake. • When oral intake is resumed, take precautions to prevent aspiration (elevate head of bed, hold head up, etc.).	There is no evidence of aspiration.
Altered Tissue Perfusion, cerebral, R/T ischemia, cerebral edema, or increased intracranial pressure (ICP)	• Monitor vital and neurological signs. • Maintain cerebral venous outflow by elevating the head of the bed 30 degrees. • Maintain head in neutral position. • Avoid positions that increase intra-abdominal/intrathoracic pressure (hip flexion, prone position, etc.; see Chap. 13). • Maintain normothermia. • Maintain blood pressure within targeted range set for sufficient cerebral perfusion pressure. • Monitor peripheral oxygenation with pulse oximeter.	• Vital signs are maintained within targeted limits. • Cerebral perfusion pressure is supported. • Evidence of neurological deteriorations is quickly noted and action taken.
• Risk of Infection R/T use of invasive devices and hospitalization	• Follow aseptic technique. • If urinary catheter is in place, remove as soon as possible. • Monitor intravascular device sites for infection. • Monitor chest x-ray and blood chemistries for evidence of infection.	Patient is infection free.
Sensory/Perceptual R/T altered consciousness, impaired sensation, or impaired vision	• Assess impact of deficits on function and safety. • Develop compensatory strategies to meet particular patient needs. • Provide for patient safety to prevent burns, injury, or falls. • For double vision, patch one eye. • Approach patient from unaffected side if homonymous hemianopsia is present. • Provide appropriate stimulation to involved areas of sense.	• Optimal sensory input is received and interpreted accurately. • Individualized plan is used to outline compensatory strategies to meet needs. • Safety is maintained.
Impaired Verbal Communication R/T cerebral injury/altered level of consciousness	• Assess type of communication deficit present. • Develop and establish appropriate alternative methods for communication.	• Alternative communication method is developed based on type of deficit. • The patient's attempts to communicate are supported.
Impaired Physical Mobility R/T neurological deficits	• Assess type and degree of impairment. • Provide slings, braces, support shoes, etc., as necessary. • Support alternative methods of mobility. • Collaborate with physical therapist to support exercise and mobility.	• Type and impact on function are established. • Safe compensatory methods are established for motor function.

CHART 25-4 Summary of Common Patient Problems and Nursing Diagnoses for Acute Stroke Patients (Continued)

COMMON PATIENT PROBLEMS AND NURSING DIAGNOSES	NURSING INTERVENTIONS	EXPECTED OUTCOMES
High risk for deep venous thrombosis (DVT) or pulmonary embolism (PE)	• For bedridden patients, apply elastic stockings and compression boots. • SQ heparin or low-molecular-weight heparins are alternatives; be sure some form of prophylaxis is provided. • Monitor for signs and symptoms of DVT and PE.	• Adequate DVT prophylaxis is provided. • Patient is monitored for signs and symptoms of DVT and PE.
Nutrition Deficit R/T swallowing deficits, NPO status, or unconsciousness	• Order nutritional consult. • Order appropriate diet that meets the patient's needs. • Monitor tolerance of diet.	• Nutritional consult is provided within 24 hours. • Adequate nutrition is provided by alternate routes as necessary.

atelectasis and pneumonia. For patients on ventilatory support, weaning should begin as soon as possible. The awake patient is maintained on NPO status until a swallowing study has been conducted and problems of aspiration have been ruled out. In many facilities, an initial swallow screening is conducted in both the ED and stroke center with follow-up with a speech evaluation. Although many screening tools are available, a frequently used assessment tool is the Massey Screening Tool.[32] This is one of the stroke performance measures that may be difficult to ensure because patients in the ED are often given oral medications prior to the swallow screening.

Both hypoglycemia and hyperglycemia are detrimental to the injured brain. Hyperglycemia greater than 140 mg/dL increases infarct size in experimental stroke models and contributes to poorer outcomes. Serum glucose levels should be monitored and kept in the targeted range with regular insulin therapy according to physician orders. In addition, intravenous solutions should be *saline and not glucose*. For patients receiving anticoagulants such as heparin, monitor antifactor Xa and observe for bleeding. Electrolytes, creatinine, and blood urea nitrogen are monitored. Electrolyte imbalance, particularly sodium, is common and should be managed.

Patient safety is always a primary priority in patient care. With the multiple functional deficits common with stroke, fall prevention becomes a major focus of care. There are a number of assessment tools to assist in identifying patients at high risk for falls. However, the correlation of fall prediction and actual falls is not always clear. Stroke patients are all high risk for falls, and a comprehensive fall prevention program must be used.

For details about the key points in acute care nursing management of stroke patients after treatment with special interventions, see Chart 25-3. Chart 25-4 summarizes the common patient problems and nursing diagnoses associated with stroke. Chart 25-5 summarizes the common deficits and emotional reactions related to stroke. See also Chapter 15 for management of the unconscious patient and

Chapter 13 for ICP management. After the patient's condition has stabilized, nursing management is refocused on rehabilitation and prevention of another stroke (Chart 25-6).

Early Focus on Rehabilitation

Rehabilitation begins as soon as the patient is stabilized. The nurse collaborates with other health care professionals to develop a plan of care. The case manager is an integral part of the interdisciplinary team who can facilitate access to rehabilitation resources and community-based rehabilitation services. Nursing responsibilities in the rehabilitation process are outlined in Chart 25-6. See Chapter 11 for information about rehabilitation.

The following patient problems and nursing diagnoses are common in stroke patients and are related to the need for early rehabilitation: Self-Care Deficits; Sensory Perceptual Alterations; Impaired Verbal Communication; Impaired Physical Mobility; Altered Urinary Elimination; Disuse Syndrome; Altered Thought Processes; Impaired Adjustment; Altered Role Performance; and Unilateral Neglect.

Discharge Planning and Continuity of Care

Discharge planning is taken into account early in the rehabilitative program. The plans for discharge are made with the assistance of the case manager, who assists with continuity and facilitates access to the next level of care, whether rehabilitation or home care. The patient and family should be made aware of community resources. A critical point in discharge planning is to be sure that the patient has an appointment for follow-up so that recovery, new problems, and drug therapy can be monitored (see the earlier section on rehabilitation and the *Post-Stroke Rehabilitation* clinical practice guidelines).

CHART 25-5 **Common Deficits and Emotional Reactions to Stroke and Related General Nursing Interventions**

COMMON MOTOR DEFICITS

1. Hemiparesis or hemiplegia (side of the body opposite the cerebral episode)
2. Dysarthria (muscles of speech impaired)
3. Dysphagia (muscles of swallowing impaired)

NURSING INTERVENTIONS

1. Position the patient in proper body alignment; use a splint to keep the hand in a functional position.
   - Provide frequent passive range-of-motion exercises.
   - Reposition the patient every 2 hours.
2. Provide for an alternative method of communication.
3. Test palatal and pharyngeal reflexes before offering nourishment.
   - Keep NPO until swallowing screen completed and oral intake approved by physician.
   - Elevate and turn the head to the unaffected side.
   - If able to manage oral intake, place food on the unaffected side of the patient's mouth.

COMMON SENSORY DEFICITS

1. Visual deficits (common because the visual pathways cut through much of the cerebral hemispheres)
   a. Homonymous hemianopsia (loss of vision in half of each visual field)

   Left    Right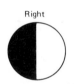

   b. Double vision (diplopia)
   c. Decreased visual acuity
2. Absent or diminished response to superficial sensation (touch, pain, pressure, heat, cold)

3. Absent or diminished response to proprioception (knowledge of position of body parts)
4. Perceptual deficits (disturbance in perceiving and interpreting self and/or environment)
   a. Body scheme disturbance (denial of paralyzed extremities; **unilateral neglect syndrome**)

   b. Disorientation (to time, place, and person)

   c. Apraxia (loss of ability to use objects correctly)

NURSING INTERVENTIONS

1. Be aware that variations of visual deficits may exist and compensate for them.
   a. Approach the patient from the unaffected side; remind the patient to turn the head to compensate for visual deficits.

   b. Apply an eye patch to the affected eye.
   c. Provide good light and assistance as necessary.
2. Increase the amount of touch in administering patient care.
   - Protect the involved areas from injury.
   - Protect the involved areas from burns.
   - Examine the involved areas for signs of skin irritation and injury.
   - Provide patient with opportunity to handle various objects of different weight, texture, and size.
   - If pain is present, assess its location and type, as well as the duration of the pain.
3. Teach patient to check the position of body parts visually.

4. Compensate for patient's perceptual-sensory deficits.

   a. Protect the involved area.
      - Accept patient's self-perception.
      - Position patient to face involved area.
   b. Control amount of changes in patient's schedule.
      - Reorient as necessary.
      - Talk to patient.
      - Provide a calendar, clock, pictures of family, and so forth.
   c. Correct misuse of objects and demonstrate proper use.

| CHART **25-5** | **Common Deficits and Emotional Reactions to Stroke and Related General Nursing Interventions**   (Continued) |

COMMON MOTOR DEFICITS

 d. Agnosia (inability to identify the environment by means of the senses)
 e. Defects in localizing objects in space, estimating their size, and judging distance
 f. Impaired memory for recall of spatial location of objects or places
 g. Right–left disorientation

LANGUAGE DEFICITS

1. Nonfluent aphasia (difficulty in transforming sound into patterns of understandable speech)–can speak using single-word responses
2. Fluent aphasia (impairment of comprehension of the spoken word)–able to speak, but uses words incorrectly and is unaware of these errors
3. Global aphasia (combination of expressive and receptive aphasia)–unable to communicate at any level

4. Alexia (inability to understanding written word)

5. Agraphia (inability to express ideas in writing)

INTELLECTUAL DEFICITS

1. Loss of memory
2. Short attention span
3. Increased distractibility
4. Poor judgment

5. Inability to transfer learning from one situation to another
6. Inability to calculate, reason, or think abstractly

EMOTIONAL DEFICITS

(Recognize that pattern is often inconsistent; patient may have good days and bad days or even good hours and bad hours.)
1. Emotional lability (exhibits reactions easily or inappropriately)

2. Loss of self-control and social inhibitions (may speak inappropriately, swear, expose self, or make sexual advances toward nurse)
3. Reduced tolerance for stress

4. Fear, hostility, frustration, or anger
5. Confusion and despair
6. Withdrawal, isolation
7. Depression

NURSING INTERVENTIONS

 d. Correct misconceptions.

 e. Reduce any stimuli that distract the patient.

 f. Place necessary equipment where the patient will see it, rather than telling the patient "It is in the closet" for example.
 g. Phrase requests carefully, like "Lift this leg." (Point to the leg.)

NURSING INTERVENTIONS

1. Ask patient to repeat individual sounds of the alphabet as a start to retrain.
2. Speak clearly and in simple sentences; use gestures as necessary.

3. Assess for any intact language skills; speak in very simple sentences, ask patient to repeat individual sounds, and use gestures or any other means to communicate.
4. Point to written names of objects and have the patient repeat name of the object.
5. Have patient write words and simple sentences.

NURSING INTERVENTIONS

1. Provide information as necessary.
2. Divide activities into short steps.
3. Control any excessive environmental distractions.
4. Protect patient from injury especially form falls; institute a fall prevention program.
5. Repeat and reinforce instructions as necessary.
6. Do not create unrealistic expectations in the patient; accept patient as he or she is.

NURSING INTERVENTIONS

1. Disregard bursts of emotions; explain that emotional lability is part of the illness.
2. Protect patient as necessary to preserve dignity; recognize involuntary basis of behavior and set limits; anticipate needs.
3. Control environment and maintain routines as much as possible; remove stimuli that upset the patient.
4. Accept behavior; be supportive.
5. Clarify any misconceptions; allow patient to verbalize.
6. Provide stimulation and a safe, comfortable environment.
7. Assess degree of depression; provide a supportive environment; discuss possible pharmacotherapy with physician.

> Explain behavior to family as a manifestation of brain injury. Be supportive.

(continued)

CHART **25-5**	**Common Deficits and Emotional Reactions to Stroke and Related General Nursing Interventions** (Continued)

BOWEL AND BLADDER DYSFUNCTION	**NURSING INTERVENTIONS**

Bladder: Incomplete Upper Motor Neuron Lesion

> Do not suggest insertion of an indwelling catheter immediately after the stroke; intermittent catheterization is better than an indwelling catheter.

1. The unilateral lesion from the stroke results in partial sensation and control of the bladder, so that patient experiences frequency, urgency, and incontinence. (Cognitive deficits affect control.)
2. If stroke lesion is brainstem, there will be bilateral damage, resulting in an upper motor neuron bladder with loss of all control of micturition.

1. Observe patient to identify characteristics of voiding pattern (e.g., frequency, amount, forcefulness of stream, constant dribbling).
2. Maintain an accurate intake and output record.

> *Nursing note:* Incontinence after regaining consciousness is usually attributable to urinary tract infection caused by use of an indwelling urinary catheter.

3. Possibility of establishing normal bladder function is excellent.

3. Try to allow patient to stay catheter-free:
   • Offer bedpan or urinal frequently.
   • Take patient to commode frequently.
   • Assess patient's ability to make need for help with voiding known.
   If a catheter is necessary, remove it as soon as possible and follow a bladder training program (see Chap. 11).

Bowel
1. Altered bowel function in a stroke patient is attributable to:
   • Altered level of consciousness
   • Dehydration
   • Immobility
2. Constipation is the most common problem, along with potential impaction.

1. Develop a bowel training program:
   • Provide high-fiber diet to stimulate defecation (prune juice, roughage).
   • Initiate a suppository and laxative regimen.
2. Institute a bowel program. Enemas are avoided in the presence of increased intracranial pressure.

After the patient has been discharged, integration back into community is important. Rehabilitation continues over time and must be monitored. Depression is common after stroke and is seen in 40% to 50% of patients.[48] Patients and families need to be prepared for this possibility. The patient should be screened for evidence of depression using standardized assessment scales (e.g., Geriatric Depression Scale, Hamilton Rating Scale for Depression). Pharmacotherapy is usually effective in the treatment of depression. Related patient problems and nursing diagnoses are listed in the next section.

Patient Education

Patient and family education takes place within a compressed period of time in the acute care setting. It is unrealistic to expect that all education can be completed during this short period. Patient education must be viewed along a continuum that extends through the next level of care and into the community by the health care provider. Decide what is critical for the patient to know and focus on "just-in-time education." Common patient problems and nursing diagnoses include Knowledge Deficit; Caregiver Role Strain; Altered Family Processes; and Sexual Dysfunction.

CLINICAL PEARLS: Stroke and cardiac risk factors are identical because the vascular system is contiguous. Drawing the correlation between the two can be helpful in patient/family education.

Medications

The most common drug classifications for patients being discharged are antiplatelets and sometimes anticoagulants. Both require special teaching and follow-up. Monitor for obvious and occult bleeding. All patients will need periodic monitoring of coagulation and INR to adjust drug dosage.

CHART 25-6 Rehabilitation Strategies Following Stroke

NURSING RESPONSIBILITIES	RATIONALE
1. Encourage the patient to do as much of self-care as possible.	1. Increases independence.
2. Teach activities of daily living (ADLs) to compensate for functional disability. (ADLs include dressing, toileting, bathing, eating, gait training.)	2. Provides for alternative methods to compensate for disabilities and increases level of independence.
3. Instruct patient on bed exercises, such as quadriceps and gluteal setting.	3. Improves muscle tone and strength.
4. Teach patient transfer techniques (e.g., bed to chair, chair to bed).	4. Increases independence and provides for a greater number of environmental settings for the patient.
5. Provide special skin care to maintain intact healthy skin.	5. Pressure ulcers and skin changes can occur with neurological conditions.
6. Dress patient in own clothes rather than a hospital gown, if possible.	6. Improves the patient's self-image and dispels image of the "sick role."
7. Provide for privacy by screening when the patient is learning new skills (such as relearning to feed self).	7. Preserves self-esteem and decreases embarrassment if "accidents" happen.
8. Provide emotional support and encouragement.	8. Helps to motivate the patient.
9. Encourage the patient to express feelings.	9. Decreases anxiety and allows for correction of misinformation.
10. Be empathetic with the patient's feelings.	10. Increases the nurse's sensitivity to patient needs.
11. Know what physiotherapist is doing with the patient.	11. Activities can be reinforced by the nurse.
12. Encourage the family to participate (e.g., demonstrate range-of-motion exercises to the family).	12. Allows family members to feel that they are "doing something to help."

For patients taking ticlopidine, a complete blood cell count every 2 weeks for 3 months is necessary to monitor for neutropenia. If the patient has not received the drug while in the hospital, he or she needs to be alerted to the possibility of diarrhea or rash. Other medications previously taken before the episode need to be evaluated for continuation such as drugs for hypertension and high cholesterol. In some patients these may be new drugs for which the patient will need education. For example, statins are recommended for patients after ischemic stroke.[49] Giving written instructions about drugs, including time and dosage, side effects to expect, adverse reactions, contacting the health provider, and monitoring the schedule, increases adherence to the plan of care and achievement of expected outcomes.

What to Expect

Both the patient and family need to know what to expect on discharge, community resources such as stroke support groups, and reliable publications and websites. The nurse can provide some anticipatory guidance based on the particular needs of the patient. However, the patient and family cannot be prepared for every contingency. It is helpful to plan a time for the nurse to call to assess adjustment to the community and any special problems or concerns. The nurse can triage some problems and manage others independently.

Recovery

Patients who survive a stroke have potential for recovery of function. The extent of the stroke and pre-existing disease influence the degree of recovery. Most of natural recovery in motor function and speech occurs in the first 3 to 6 months. However, recovery continues at a slower pace up to a year and beyond with therapy.

REFERENCES

1. American Heart Association. (2007). *Heart disease and stroke statistics: 2007 update at a glance.* (p. 37). Dallas, TX: American Heart Association.
2. American Heart Association. (2007). *Heart disease and stroke statistics: 2007 update at a glance* (p. 14). Dallas, TX: American Heart Association.
3. Goldstein, L. B., Adams, R., Alberts, M. J., Appel, L. J., Brass, L. M, Bushnell, C. D., et al. (2006). Primary prevention of ischemic stroke. Retrieved March 18, 2007, from http://www.strokeaha.org
4. Adams, H., Del Zappo, G., Alberts, M. J., Bhatt, D. L., Brass, L., Furlan, A., et al. (2007). Guidelines for the early management of patients with ischemic stroke. A guideline from the American Heart Association/American Stroke association Stroke Council, Clinical Cardiology Council, Cardiovascular Radiology and Intervention Council, and the Atherosclerotic Peripheral Vascular disease and Quality of Care Outcomes in Research Interdisciplinary Working Groups. *Stroke, 38,* 1655–1711.
5. Duncan, P. W., Zorowitz, R., Bates, B., Chow, J. Y., Glasbergy, J. J. Graham, G. D., et al. (2005). Management of adult stroke rehabilitation care: A clinical practice guideline. *Stroke, 36,* e100–e143.
6. Bates, B., Choi, J. Y, Duncan, P. W., Glasberg, J. J., Graham, G. D., Katz, R. C., et al. (2005). Veterans affairs/Department of Defense clinical practice guideline for the management of adult stroke rehabilitation: Executive summary. *Stroke, 36,* 2049–2056.
7. The Joint Commission. (2005). *Joint Commission's disease-specific care certification for primary stroke centers; primary stroke center certification guide.* Oakbrook Terrace, IL: Author.

8. Savitz, S. I., & Caplan, L. R. (2005). Vertebrobasilar disease. *New England Journal of Medicine, 352*, 2618–2626.

9. Mohr, J. P. (1992). Lacunes. In H. J. M. Barnett, J. P. Mohr, B. M. Stein, & F. M. Yatsu (Eds.). *Stroke: Pathophysiology, diagnosis, and management* (2nd ed., pp. 539–541). New York: Churchill Livingstone.

10. Kizer, J. P, & Devereux, R. B. (2005). Patent foramen ovale in young adults with unexplained stroke. *New England Journal of Medicine, 353*, 2361–2372.

11. Adams, R. J., Chimowitz, M. I., Alpert, J. S., et al. (2003). Coronary risk evaluation in patients with transient ischemic attack and ischemic stroke: A scientific statement for healthcare professionals from the Stroke Council on Clinical Cardiology of the American Heart Association/American Stroke Association. *Stroke, 108*, 1278–1290.

12. Manno, E. M., Atkinson, J. L. D., Fulgham, J. R., & Wijdicks, E. F. M. (2005). Emerging medical and surgical management strategies in the evaluation and treatment of intracerebral hemorrhage. *Mayo Clinical Proceedings, 80*(3), 420–433.

13. Biller, J., Feinberg, W. M., Castaldo, J. E., et al. (1998). Guidelines for carotid endarterectomy. *Circulation, 97*, 501–509.

14. Albers, G. W., Hart, R. G., Lutsep, H., Newell, D. W., & Sacco, R. (1999). Supplement to the guidelines for the management of transient ischemic attacks: A statement from the ad hoc committee on guidelines for management of transient ischemic attacks, Stroke Council, American Heart Association. *Stroke, 30*, 2502–2511.

15. Pulsinelli, W. (1992). Pathophysiology of acute ischemic stroke. *Lancet, 339*(8792), 533–536.

16. Back, T. (1998). Pathophysiology of the ischemic penumbra—revision of a concept. *Cellular and Molecular Neurobiology, 18*(6), 621–638.

17. Hossman, K. (1985). Post-ischemic resuscitation of the brain: Selective vulnerability versus global resistance. *Progress in Brain Research, 63*, 3–13.

18. Dutka, A. J., & Hallenbeck, J. M. (1991). Pathophysiology of anoxic-ischemic brain injury. In W. G. Bradley, R. B. Daroff, G. M. Fenichel, & C. D. Marsden (Eds.). *Neurology in clinical practice* (Vol. 2; p. 1354). New York: Butterworth-Heinemann.

19. Hallenbeck, J. M., & Dutka, A. J. (1996). Background review and current concepts of reperfusion injury. *Archives of Neurology, 71*, 281–297.

20. Banasik, J. (1995). Cell injury, aging, and death. In L. C. Copstead (Ed.). *Perspectives on pathophysiology* (p. 66). Philadelphia: W. B. Saunders.

21. Pozilli, C., Lenzi, G., & Argentino, C. (1985). Imaging of leukocyte infiltration in human cerebral infarcts. *Stroke, 16*, 251–255.

22. Martin, N. A., & Saver, J. (1999). Intensive care management of subarachnoid hemorrhage, ischemic stroke and hemorrhagic stroke. *Clinical Neurosurgery, 45*, 101–112.

23. Broderick, J. P., Hagen, T., Brott, T., et al. (1995). Hyperglycemia and hemorrhagic transformation of cerebral infarcts. *Stroke, 26*, 484–487.

24. Kidwell, C. S., Chalela, J. A., Saver, J. L., et al. (2004). Comparison of MRI and CT for detection of acute intracerebral hemorrhage. *JAMA, 292*, 1823–1830.

25. Fiebach, J. B., Schellinger, P. D., Gass, A., et al. (2004). Stroke magnetic resonance imaging is accurate in hyperacute intracerebral hemorrhage: A multicenter study on the validity of stroke imaging. *Stroke, 34*, 502–506.

26. Latchaw, R. E., Yonas, H., Hunter, G. J., Yuh, W. T. C., Ueda, T., Sorensen, A. G., et al. (2003). Guidelines and recommendations for perfusion imaging in cerebral ischemia: A scientific statement for healthcare professionals by the writing groups on perfusion imaging, form the Council on Cardiovascular Radiology of the American Heart Association. *Stroke, 34*, 1084–1104.

27. Feinberg, W. M., Albers, G. W., Barnett, H. J. M., Biller, J., Caplan, L. R., Carter, L. P., et al. (1994). Guidelines for the management of transient ischemic attacks: From the Ad Hoc Committee on Guidelines for the Management of Transient Ischemic Attacks of the Stroke Council of the American Heart Association. *Circulation, 89*, 2950–2965.

28. Albers, G. W., Hart, R. G., Lutsep, H. L., Newell, D. W., & Sacco, R. L. (1999). Supplement to the guidelines for the management of transient ischemic attacks: A statement form the Ad Hoc Committee on Guidelines for the Management of Transient Ischemic Attacks, Stroke Council, American Heart Association. *Stroke, 30*, 2502–2511.

29. Albers, G. W., Hart, R. G., Lutsep, H. L., Newell, D. W., & Sacco, R. L. (2000). Addendum to the supplement to the guidelines for the management of transient ischemic attacks. *Stroke, 31*, 1001.

30. The Stroke Council. (2004). Statins after ischemic stroke and transient ischemic attack: An advisory statement form the Stroke Council, American Heart Association and American Stroke Association. *Stroke, 35*, 1023.

31. Adams, H. P, Adams, R. J., Brott, T., del Zoppp, G. J., Furlan, A., Goldstein, L. B., et al. (2003). Guidelines for the early management of patients with ischemic stroke: A scientific statement from the Stroke Council of the American Stroke Association. *Stroke, 34*, 1056–1083.

32. Massey, R., & Jedlicka, D. (2002). The Massey bedside swallowing screen. *Journal of Neuroscience Nursing, 34*(5), 252–160.

33. Wardlaw, J. M., Zoppo, G., Yamaguchi, T., & Berge, E. (2003). Thrombolytics for acute ischemic stroke. *Cochrane Database Systematic Review*, CD000213.

34. The National Institute of Neurological Disorders and Stroke rt-PA Stroke Study Group. (1995). Tissue plasminogen activator for acute ischemic stroke. *New England Journal of Medicine, 333*, 1581–1587.

35. Adams, H. P., Jr. (2003). Emergent use of anticoagulation for treatment of patients with ischemic stroke. *Stroke, 33*, 856–861.

36. Coull, B. M., Williams, L. S., Goldstein, L. B., Meschia, J. F., Heizman, D., Chaturvedi, S., et al. (2002). American Academy of Neurology, American Stroke Association: Anticoagulations and antiplatelet agents in acute ischemic stroke: Report of the Joint Stroke Guideline Development Committee for the American Academy of Neurology and the American Stroke Association. *Neurology, 59*, 13–22.

37. Hirsh, J., & Raschke, R. (2004). Heparin and low-molecular weight heparin: The seventh ACCP conference on antithrombotic and thrombolytic therapy. *Chest, 126*, 188S–203S.

38. Qureshi, A. I., Luft, A. R., Janardhan, V., et al. (2000). Identification of patients at risk for peri-procedural neurological deficits associated with carotid angioplasty and stenting. *Stroke, 31*, 376–382.

39. North American Symptomatic Carotid Endarterectomy Trial Collaborators. (1991). Beneficial effect of carotid endarterectomy in symptomatic patients with high-grade stenosis. *New England Journal of Medicine, 325*(7), 445–453.

40. Chatuvedi, S., Bruno, A., Feasby, T., Holloway, R., Benavente, O., Cohen, S. N., et al. (2005). Carotid endarterectomy-an evidence-based review: Report of the therapeutic and technology assessment subcommittee of the American Academy of Neurology. *Neurology, 65*, 794–801.

41. Sacco, R. L., Adams, R., Albers, G., Alberts, M. J., Benavente, O., Furie, K., et al. (2006). Guidelines for prevention of stroke in patients with ischemic stroke or transient ischemic attack: A statement for healthcare professionals from the American Heart Association/American Stroke Association Council on Stroke: Co-sponsored by the Council on Cardiovascular Radiology and Intervention: The American Academy of Neurology affirms the value of this guideline. *Stroke, 37*, 577–617.

42. Barnett, H.J., Taylor, D.W., Eliasziw, M., et al. (1998). Benefit of carotid endarterectomy in patients with symptomatic moderate stenosis: North American Symptomatic Carotid Endarterectomy Trial Collaborators. *New England Journal of Medicine, 339*, 1415–1425.

43. Yoshimoto, Y., & Kwak, S. (1995). Superficial temporal artery-middle cerebra artery anastomosis for acute cerebral ischemia: The effect of small augmentation of blood flow. *Acta Neurochirurgica, 137*, 128–137.

44. Kakinumia. K., Ezuka, I., Takai, N., Yamamoto, K., & Saski, O. (1999). The simple indicator for revascularization of acute middle cerebral artery occlusion using angiogram and ultra-early embolectomy. *Surgical Neurology, 51*, 332–341.

45. Smith, W. S., Sung, G., Starkman, S., Saver, J. L., Kidwell, C. S., Gobin, Y., P., et al. (2005). MERCI trial Investigators: Safety and efficacy of mechanical embolectomy in acute ischemic stroke: results of the MERCI trial. *Stroke, 36*, 1432–1438.

46. Broderick, J., Connolly, S., Feldman, E., Hanley, D., Kase, C., Krieger, D., et al. (2007). Guidelines for the management of spontaneous intracerebral hemorrhage in adults. 2007 Update. A guideline from the American Heart Association, American Stroke Association Stroke Council, High Blood Pressure Research Council, and the Quality of Care and Outcomes in Research Interdisciplinary Working Group. *Stroke, 38*, 2001–2003.

47. Duncan, P W., Zorowitz, R., Bates, B., Choi, J. Y., Glasberg, J. J., Graham, G. D., et al. (2005). Management of adult stroke rehabilitation care: A clinical practice guideline. *Stroke, 36*, e100–e143.

48. Farrell, C. (2004). Poststroke depression in elderly patients. *Dimensions of Critical Care Nursing, 23*(6), 264–269.

49. The Stroke Council. (2004). Statins after ischemic stroke and transient ischemic attack: An advisory statement from the Stroke Council, American Heart Association, and American Stroke Association. *Stroke, 35*, 1023.

RESOURCES

Websites

American Stroke Association: www.strokeassociation.org
American Heart Association: www.americanheart.org/
National Stroke Association: www.stroke.org
National Aphasia Association: www.aphasia.org

Other Cerebrovascular Disorders

Joanne V. Hickey

The purpose of this short chapter is to include a few cerebrovascular conditions seen occasionally in neuroscience patient populations that do not easily fit into the previous chapters. Two conditions will be briefly addressed to demonstrate special patient populations and conditions: cerebral venous thrombosis and Moyamoya disease.

CEREBRAL VENOUS THROMBOSIS

Cerebral venous thrombosis (CVT) is a distinct cerebrovascular disorder from arterial stroke that may include thrombosis of the cerebral veins or cerebral venous sinuses or both. In most cases the two processes are seen concurrently. A rare condition, CVT most often affects young women and children. About 75% of patients who have CVT are women. The most common associated risk factors include prothrombotic diseases, dehydration, pregnancy, puerperium, infections (e.g., otitis media, mastoiditis, sinusitis, meningitis), oral contraceptives, and head trauma. A prothrombotic risk factor or a direct cause is identified in about 85% of patients.[1]

Occlusion of cerebral veins can cause localized cerebral edema and venous infarction related to enlarged and swollen veins, edema, ischemic neuronal damage, and petechial hemorrhage. By comparison, occlusion of the major venous sinuses results in increased venous pressure and impaired absorption of cerebrospinal fluid (CSF) that subsequently lead to increased intracranial pressure. The ventricles do not enlarge and dilate because the obstruction to CSF drainage is noted at the end of their transport pathway so that no pressure gradient develops between the subarachnoid spaces at the surface of the brain and the ventricles.[1]

The signs and symptoms of CVT are varied with severe headache the most common symptom, found in 90% of patients. It is described as increasing gradually over the course of a few days, although it can have an abrupt onset such as seen with subarachnoid hemorrhage.[2] Symptoms can be vague and nonspecific and limited to a headache. Those patients who have isolated increased intracranial pressure may have only headache and no neurological findings on examination. Nausea, seizures, focal neurological deficits, and coma are also possible. About 50% of patients develop cerebral lesions and neurological signs. Seizures occur in about 40% of patients and range from focal seizures

to life-threatening status epilepticus.[1] The patient outcome will depend on the degree of neurological involvement and cerebral edema. CVT is a potential lethal condition so that the patient must be carefully managed.

Although the computed tomography (CT) scan of the head lacks sensitivity and specificity needed to identify and evaluate changes related to CVT, it is often the most common first diagnostic. The best diagnostic for CVT is the magnetic resonance venogram (MRV). Cerebral angiography is usually not performed unless magnetic resonance imaging (MRI) and an MRV are not available. If a CT venography or MRI/MRV is still unclear, then a cerebral angiography is performed. The value of a cerebral angiography is that it is the only diagnostic that can evaluate the patency of cortical veins.[3]

The first line of treatment for CVT is anticoagulation with heparin to stop the thrombotic process and to prevent pulmonary embolism.[4] However, the treatment is not without controversy because of the tendency of venous infarctions to convert to a hemorrhagic lesion. About 40% of all patients with CVT have a hemorrhagic infarct even before anticoagulation therapy is begun.[5] The optimal duration of oral anticoagulation therapy after the acute phase is unknown, but a general rule of thumb is 12 months of warfarin at a dose to keep the international normalized ratio at about 2.5. Other treatment options include transvenous clot lysis using injected thrombolytic agents and specialized catheters for clot removal. These options are not without risk, and must be carefully weighed to select the most appropriate treatment. In addition to the specific CVT treatment, general supportive care is also necessary. This includes treatment of increased intracranial pressure with the usual list of component care such as use of osmotic diuretics, airway support, ventricular drainage, and possible decompression hemicraniectomy as outlined in Chapter 13.

Patient acuity will dictate the specific setting within the hospital to which the patient should be admitted. The nurse must frequently assess and monitor trends in neurological sign and symptoms. The responsibility to adjust the rate of heparin drip based on the laboratory reports and targeted therapy ordered by the physician falls to the nurse. If there is an acute change in the neurological assessment while the patient is receiving anticoagulation therapy, the drip should be immediately stopped and the physician notified urgently. The anticoagulant is not resumed until intracranial hemorrhage is ruled out.[3]

In addition, the nurse must provide safe care and use best practices in providing care such as those outlined for increased intracranial pressure management in Chapter 13. Regardless of the acuity of the patient, the nurse assumes responsibility for coordinating the care and preparing the patient from transition along the continuum of care. Because CVT is an uncommon diagnosis, the patient and family will probably need to be educated about the condition. Concurrently, the nursing staff will need information about the condition and treatment to feel comfortable in managing the patient.

Many patients will be discharged home on oral anticoagulation therapy. Patient and family education and follow-up planning become the work of the nurse. Most facilities have printed material on oral anticoagulation education (e.g., bleeding precautions, dietary limitations, need for frequent follow-up blood work). The patient must be well versed in the information and the nurse assured of an adequate knowledge base before the patient is discharged.

MOYAMOYA DISEASE

Moyamoya disease is an uncommon occlusive intracranial vasculopathy of unknown etiology. *Moyamoya* is the Japanese word for a "cloud of smoke," which is descriptive of the appearance of the carotid arteriogram. The carotid arteriogram reveals a network of small anastomotic vessels at the base of the brain around the circle of Willis and segmental stenosis or occlusion of the terminal portions of both internal carotid arteries.[6] There is progressive, bilateral stenosis of the distal internal carotid arteries extending to the circle of Willis. Moyamoya disease peaks in the first and fourth decade of life, thus affecting a much younger age group that usually is seen with the signs and symptoms of transient ischemic attacks (TIAs) and stroke. In children moyamoya disease is characterized by ischemic events, whereas in adults hemorrhagic manifestations are common. The disease may cause TIAs, headaches, seizures, movement disorders, mental deterioration, cerebral infarction, or intracranial hemorrhage.[7] Patients have recurrent strokes over a period of time, which may be years or a compressed time frame. Diagnosis is based on the distinct and characteristic arteriographic appearance. Treatment is not clear, although indirect revascularization techniques have been used to decrease the number of attacks.[8]

SUMMARY

Although both cerebral venous thrombosis and moyamoya disease are uncommon diseases seen most often in large academic medical centers, they do affect atypical patient populations. Both diseases can have devastating consequences. In the case of moyamoya disease, the effects of multiple strokes on young patients reflect the developmental impact and cumulative load of progressive disease on the quality of life of the person. Nurses have an important role in caring for these patients during hospitalization for acute events and being supportive of the patient over time.

REFERENCES

1. Stam, J. (2005). Thrombosis of the cerebral veins and sinuses. *New England Journal of Medicine, 352*(17), 1791–1798.
2. deBruijn, S. F., Stam, S. F., & Kappelle, L. J. (1996). Thunderclap headache as first symptom of cerebral venous sinus thrombosis. *Lancet, 348*, 1623–1625.
3. Lemke, D. M., & Hacien-Bay, L. (2005). Cerebral venous sinus thrombosis. *Journal of Neuroscience Nursing, 37*(5), 258–264.
4. Buccuno, G., Sciditti, U., Pini, M., Menozzi, R., Piazza, P., Zuccoli, P., et al. (2003). Neurological and cognitive long-term outcome in patients with cerebral venous sinus thrombosis. *Acta Neurologica Scandinavica, 107*(5), 330–335.
5. Ferro, J. M., Canhao, P., Stam, J., Bousser, M. G., & Barinagarrementeria, F. (2004). Prognosis of cerebral vein and dural sinus thrombosis: Results of the International Study on Cerebral Vein and dural Sinus Thrombosis (SCVT). *Stroke, 35*, 664–670.
6. Ropper, A. H., & Brown, R. H. (2005). Cerebrovascular disease. In *Adams and Victor's principles of neurology* (8th ed., pp. 706–707). New York: McGraw-Hill.
7. Biller, J., & Love, B. B. (2004). Vascular diseases of the nervous system. In W. G. Bradley, R. B. Daroff, G. M. Fenichel, & J. Jankovic (Eds.). *Neurology in clinical practice* (4th ed., pp. 1217–1218). Philadelphia: Butterworth-Heinemann.
8. Nissim, O., Bakon, M., Men Zeev, B., et al. (2005). Moyamoya disease—diagnosis and treatment: Indirect cerebral revascularization at the Sheba Medical Center. *Israeli Medical Association, 7*(10), 661–666.

Section **8**

Nursing Management of Patients With Pain, Seizures, and CNS Infections

Chronic Pain

Joanne V. Hickey

This chapter provides a brief overview of chronic pain assessment and management with an emphasis on the role of the neuroscience nurse as a member of an interdisciplinary team providing medical and surgical management to people with chronic pain.

Pain is the most universal of all afflictions. It can be described in terms of sensory, emotional, and cognitive components that reflect the transmission and modulation of painful stimuli.[1] Pain can be classified by a biologic mechanism that includes neuropathic, muscular, inflammatory, mechanical/compression, or malignancy or by an acute or chronic designation.[2] **Acute pain** is a response to tissue injury or inflammation and results from the activation of peripheral pain receptors (**nociceptors**) and their specific sensory nerve fibers (A delta fibers and C fibers). It is a complex constellation of unpleasant sensory, perceptual, and emotional experiences and certain associated autonomic, psychological, emotional, and behavioral responses.[3] Acute pain is often associated with an identifiable injury or trauma and resolves as the injury heals.

By comparison, **chronic pain** is persistent pain, continuous or recurrent in nature, and of sufficient duration and intensity to adversely affect a patient's well-being, level of function, and quality of life.[2] Although a strict time frame is not applied, pain that continues after a reasonable time for healing (>6 weeks) suggests the need to assess the patient for presence of chronic pain. The causes of chronic pain are related to continual tissue injury caused by ongoing activation of A delta and C fibers as well as other sensitized pathways. Chronic pain is also a complex multidimensional phenomenon with unclear pathogenesis, continuation of pain after resolution of the initial injury, and an unpredictable course of recovery.[1] Chronic pain is a separate entity from acute pain; it is often a difficult problem to treat.

CLINICAL PEARLS: Pain is a subjective and personal experience; its reality is whatever the patient says it is in terms of description, intensity, and meaning.

Neuropathic pain is a subtype of chronic pain, which is caused by injury or dysfunction of the peripheral nervous system (PNS) or central nervous system (CNS).[4] This includes injury or dysfunction of nerves, the spinal cord, or the brain. Chronic pain can be caused by nociceptive, neuropathic, or a combination of both as a result of injury and other conditions (Chart 27-1). Headache is discussed in Chapter 28, peripheral neuropathies in Chapter 33, and cranial nerve diseases in Chapter 34.

Chronic pain is a significant problem faced by millions of Americans. The economic impact from traditional and non-traditional treatment, over-the-counter drugs, and loss of productivity is estimated at millions of dollars annually. Managing people with chronic pain is one of the greatest challenges in health care today.

DEFINITION OF TERMS

The following are definitions of frequently used terms related to pain[5]:

- **Allodynia:** abnormal perception of pain from a normally nonpainful mechanical or thermal stimulus
- **Anesthesia dolorosa:** pain in an area or region that is anesthetic
- **Central pain:** pain associated with a lesion of the CNS
- **Complex Regional Pain Syndrome Type 1 (CRPS-I)**, previously called *reflex sympathetic dystrophy:* a syndrome of varying patterns that include pain that is out of proportion to injury (if it can even be identified), sensory abnormalities (burning pain and hyperpathia), focal autonomic abnormalities, motor abnormalities, and trophic changes; follows soft-tissue or bone injury most often to the limbs, but *without* discernible nerve injury (Chart 27-2)[6,7,8]
- **CRPS-II**, previously called *causalgia:* has a similar clinical presentation to CRPS-I, but there is related nerve injury
- **Deafferentation pain:** pain due to loss of sensory input into the central nervous system, such as occurs with avulsion of the brachial plexus or other types of lesions of peripheral nerves or due to pathology of the central nervous system
- **Dysesthesia:** an unpleasant abnormal sensation, whether spontaneous or evoked
- **Hyperpathia:** excruciating sensitivity to touch
- **Hyperesthesia:** an increased sensitivity to stimulation, excluding special senses
- **Hypoesthesia:** a diminished sensitivity to stimulation, excluding special senses

CHART 27-1   Common Causes of Chronic Neurogenic Pain

- Spinal cord tumors
- Traumatic spinal injuries
- Intervertebral disc disease/sciatica
- Spinal stenosis with root compression
- Compression of nerve plexuses
- Thalamic pain syndrome
- Metastatic bone pain (e.g., vertebra)
- Cauda equina disease
- Trigeminal neuralgia
- Postherpetic neuralgia
- Peripheral nerve diseases/entrapment syndromes
- Neuropathics: mononeurotherapy, polyneuropathy; diabetic neuropathy
- Complex regional pain syndromes I and II
- Crushing nerve injuries
- Phantom pain

- **Neuralgia:** pain in distribution of a nerve or nerves
- **Neuritis:** inflammation of a nerve or nerves
- **Nociceptor:** a receptor that is preferentially sensitive to a noxious stimulus or to a stimulus that would become noxious if prolonged

CHART 27-2   Complex Regional Pain Syndrome Type I

- Description: severe, deep, burning or lancinating pain that is out of proportion to the injury present and wide variability of symptoms; pathophysiology and treatment are unclear; diagnosis is based on clinical presentation.
- Diagnostic criteria: from the International Association for the Study of Pain:
  - Follows a traumatic event to soft tissue or bone without an apparent nerve lesion (in 10% of patients, no source of trauma can be identified)
  - Spontaneous pain (hyperalgesia and allodynia) disproportionate to the precipitating event
  - From onset of precipitating event there is edema, skin, temperature changes (usually cool), and color changes in distal aspect of affected limb
  - No other explanation for the degree of pain and dysfunction
- In the latter stages look for hair loss, brittle nails, and skin atrophy in affected limb and impaired motor function, including weakness, tremor, and ankylosis.
- Treatment: physical therapy, drug therapy, or spinal cord stimulator (transcutaneous electrical nerve stimulation) or sympathectomy (sympathetic block) in patients who do not respond to physical therapy and drugs used for neuropathic pain. Drug therapy includes tricyclic antidepressants, anticonvulsants, corticosteroids, lidocaine, nonopioids, opioids, adjuvant analgesics, and alendronate.

- **Pain:** an unpleasant sensory and emotional experience associated with actual or potential tissue damage
- **Pain threshold:** the least experience of pain that a person can recognize
- **Paresthesia:** an abnormal sensation, whether spontaneous or evoked
- **Peripheral neurogenic pain:** pain caused by a primary lesion or dysfunction in the PNS
- **Trigger point:** a hypersensitive area or site in muscle or connective tissue, usually associated with myofascial pain syndromes

PAIN THEORIES

Humans have struggled to understand and explain pain since the beginning of time. Some of the earliest pain theories, such as those from ancient Egypt and India, believed that the heart was the center of all sensation and that pain was associated with demons and gods. It was not until the 17th century that Descartes described some of the beginning concepts of pain pathways. According to Descartes, when the foot comes near a fire, the sensation enters the body and travels up threads to the brain (Fig. 27-1).

The 19th century heralded the study of pain physiology, which led to the discovery that the dorsal root of the spinal cord was involved with sensory function and the ventral root with motor function. In 1840, Muller reported that the brain could only receive information about the external

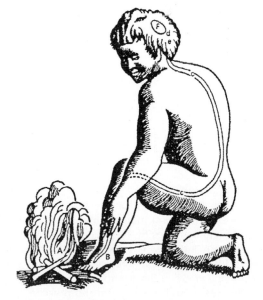

Figure 27-1 • Descartes' (1664) concept of the pain pathway. He writes: "If for example fire **(A)** comes near the foot **(B),** the minute particles of this fire, which as you know move with great velocity, have the power to set in motion this spot of the skin of the foot which they touch, and by this means pulling upon the delicate thread (c.c.) which is attached to the spot of the skin, they open up at the same instant the pore (d.e.) against which the delicate thread ends, just as by pulling at one end of a rope makes to strike at the same instant a bell which hangs at the other end." (From Melzack, R., & Wall, P. D. [1965]. Pain mechanisms: A new theory. *Science,* 150, 971–979.)

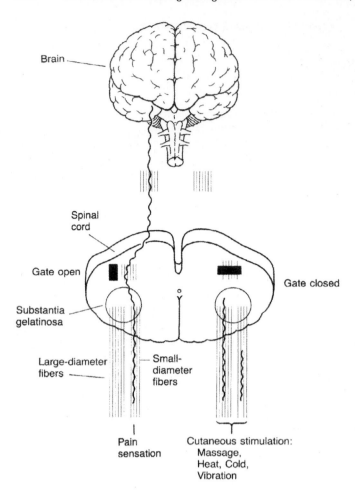

Figure 27-2 • Gate control theory. This shows how thin (tissue damage responding) fibers force open the "gate" into the central nervous system, bringing pain to consciousness. The gate can be pulled shut from the outside, reducing pain, by the activation of large A-beta fibers, rubbing/massage, transcutaneous electrical nerve stimulation, or vibration. The gate can also be pushed shut from inside the central nervous system by various inhibitory systems descending from the brain; some of these inhibitory systems are activated by acupuncture, others by drugs. (From Hudak, C. M., & Gallo, B. M. [1994]. *Critical care nursing: A holistic approach* [6th ed., p. 647]. Philadelphia: J. B. Lippincott.)

environment by way of the sensory nerves. This information, plus discoveries in pain management with morphine, codeine, and regional anesthesia, paved the way for several physiologic pain theories. The *specificity theory* noted that there were different afferent sensory neurons for pain and touch, while the *intensive theory* supported the idea that any sensory stimulus could become painful if it becomes intense enough.

Debate about these theories and development of several new theories continued into the 20th century. One of the most widely accepted theories is *the gate control theory* proposed by Melzack and Wall, which states that the CNS is surrounded by a barrier that can only be entered by a gate (Fig. 27-2).[9] Pain enters through the gate, and increasing noxious stimulation, as well as anxiety and depression, opens the gate wider. The gate can be pulled closed from the outside (peripheral) or pushed closed from the inside (centrally by the brain and spinal cord).

This theory takes into account the effect of the person's motivational, cognitive, and affective state during the pain experience in that the gate can be pushed closed by higher centers of the brain through distraction, relaxation, high levels of endorphins, and enkephalins. Activities such as transcutaneous nerve stimulation can pull the gate closed from the periphery.

ANATOMY AND PHYSIOLOGY OF PAIN

Nociception is the perception of certain afferent signals for sensory noxious receptors. The PNS has specialized nerve fibers with terminal branches in the skin, blood vessels, viscera, and musculoskeletal structures that recognize tissue damage called **nociceptors.** These impulses move from the nociceptors through the cell bodies, which lie in the dorsal root ganglia, and synapse with a secondary neuron in the dorsal horn of the spinal cord, thus entering the CNS. Different types of primary afferent fibers transmit impulses from the PNS to the CNS. The larger (6 to 12 μm diameter) A-beta fibers are myelinated fibers that conduct at higher speed (30 to 70 msec); they transmit impulses for touch, pressure, and vibration. A-delta fibers are also myelinated, but smaller (1 to 6 μm diameter), and conduct impulses at a slower speed (5 to 30 msec). They are associated with mechanical or heat nociceptors and are responsible for pinprick pain. C fibers are the smallest fibers (<1.5 μm diameter) and conduct at the slowest rate of speed (0.5 to 2 msec). They are polymodal unmyelinated fibers that transmit burning sensation and poorly localized aching-type pain (Fig. 27-3).[10] Conduction of the

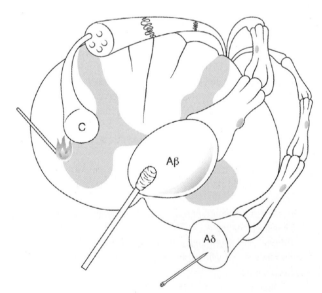

Figure 27-3 • Primary afferent fibers from skin to spinal cord. The largest (Aβ) and most rapidly conducting myelinated fibers are activated by light touch (illustrated by a cotton bud); these are the fibers that are activated by transcutaneous electrical nerve stimulation and vibration. Smaller, more slowly conducting (Aδ) myelinated fibers are activated by pinprick and are involved in acupuncture stimulation. The smallest and slowest fibers (C) are unmyelinated and are excited by tissue damage, here illustrated by a lighted match; they are often called *nociceptors*. (From Carroll, D., & Bowsher, D. [1993]. *Pain management and nursing care* [p. 9]. Boston: Butterworth & Heinemann.)

pain impulse is mediated by activation of voltage-gated sodium channels by excitatory current strong enough to generate an action potential. Pain impulses enter the spinal cord through the dorsal root synapse in lamina I, II, or V and then cross the other side of the spinal cord through the gray matter to the spinothalamic tract. Next, the spinothalamic tract transmits pain impulses to the thalamus and then to the primary sensory cortex, where the discrimination of pain is perceived, and then to the limbic cortical areas for perception of the affective and emotional aspects of pain. The pain impulse activates a reflex withdrawal from the painful stimulus in the spinal cord, and also increases the state of arousal and emotional, autonomic, and neurohumoral responses.[1]

Sensitization is the process by which the action potential threshold is shifted toward less intense stimuli and can be peripheral or central. **Peripheral sensitization** results from a variety of sources such as chemical mediators released as part of the inflammatory response, blood cells (e.g., macrophages, leukocytes, fibroblasts), and other neurons, which are only activated during inflammatory states. Chemical mediators included in the inflammatory response are serotonin, histamine, bradykinins, capsaicin, glutamate, prostaglandins, tumor necrosis factors, and substance P, which activate nociceptors and further contribute to the pain. Neurons can release calcitonin, peptides, somatostatin, neurotrophins, and other substances. **Central sensitization** is the result of increased primary afferent discharges into the spinal cord that maintains a state of excitation, PNS changes, and ongoing tissue damage or inflammation.[10,11] The result of central sensitization is spontaneous discharges, decreased pain threshold, and an increase in the receptivity of the sensory to less intense stimuli.[1,11] Clinically hyperalgesia, allodynia, and dysesthesias are common along with behavioral changes (e.g., hyperactivity, withdrawal, irritability, depression). Because of the "rewiring changes" that can occur in the PNS and CNS from ongoing acute pain, there is good rationale to treat acute pain well before it undergoes changes and becomes chronic pain triggered by a less painful stimulus and diffuse in nature.[1]

CLINICAL PEARLS: The pathophysiology of chronic pain is poorly understood; it is important to treat acute pain early and well so that changes in the nervous system do not occur to create an environment for chronic pain to develop.

ASSESSMENT AND MANAGEMENT OF CHRONIC PAIN

This section examines assessment and management of chronic pain to provide the nurse with an evidence-based practice approach to patient care. There are many published guidelines on the management of chronic pain posted on the National Guideline Clearinghouse website (www.guideline.gov). One of the most comprehensive and current guidelines is from the Institute for Clinical Systems Improvement (ICSI).[12] In this chapter multiple guidelines and other sources of information are included to present best practices for chronic pain management.

Comprehensive Assessment and Development of a Plan of Care

As of 2001, the Joint Commission (JC) required that every patient have his or her pain assessed and treated promptly and adequately.[13] This requirement lends further support to the importance of recognizing and adequately treating pain.

Pain is a subjective and personal phenomenon, which is often challenging to assess. Millions of Americans suffer from chronic pain, most of whom are either managed by their primary health care provider or self-manage. A smaller number of patients with debilitating intractable pain seek care from pain management specialists or pain centers. Interdisciplinary teams provide comprehensive chronic pain care at pain centers. Because of its complexity and the failure to treat pain adequately, chronic pain management is ideal for multidisciplinary teams. In this chapter, chronic pain management is addressed from a center perspective to assist the reader in appreciating a comprehensive view of management.

Chart 27-3 outlines the components of a chronic pain assessment. In addition to a complete medical history and physical examination, a neurological assessment, pain history, and current pain management are collected. A comprehensive initial pain assessment tool or a brief pain inventory form is useful for new or difficult-to-control pain.[14] The following components are included in a pain history:

- **Onset:** collect a historical sequence of the onset of pain such as precipitating injuries; describe the circumstances and mechanism of injury.
- **Characteristics:** what is the pattern of the pain over time? Has it changed over time? Was pain onset gradual or acute? Is it constant or periodic? What triggers onset or resolution? Does it spread? If so, where?

CHART 27-3 Key Components of Assessment for Chronic Pain

- Begin with a general history and physical examination.
- Perform functional assessment to provide baseline data on impact of pain on quality of life and participation in usual life activities (not areas of impairment and disability).
- Use tools (standardized with validity and reliability) that include multidimensional scales to capture the full comprehensive impact of pain on the patient.
- Collect a comprehensive documentation of pain location, intensity, quality, onset, duration, variations, rhythms, pain relief, exacerbating factors, and effects of pain.
- Include a self-assessment tool to document pain intensity, such as the visual analog scale.
- Document all strategies used for pain management, including behavioral, cognitive, pharmacologic, complementary, medical, and others used by the patient.
- Determine how satisfied the patient is with his or her current treatment plan.

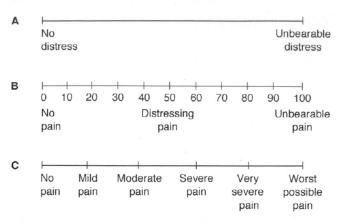

A

No distress — Unbearable distress

B

0 10 20 30 40 50 60 70 80 90 100
No pain — Distressing pain — Unbearable pain

C

No pain — Mild pain — Moderate pain — Severe pain — Very severe pain — Worst possible pain

Figure 27-4 • Pain rating scales. Rating scales for measuring pain: **(A)** Visual analog scale. **(B)** Numeric pain distress scale. **(C)** Simple descriptive pain intensity scale. (From Acute Pain Management Guideline Panel. [1992]. *Acute pain management: Operative or medical procedures and trauma. Clinical practice guideline.* AHCPR Pub. No. 92-0032. Rockville, MD: Agency for Health Care Policy and Research, Public Health Service, U.S. Department of Health and Human Services.)

- **Location:** draw with your finger where the pain is located, or on a printed anterior and posterior anatomic figure, color the body areas affected.
- **Quality:** what does the pain feel like (e.g., stabbing, sharp, dull, "pins and needles," throbbing)?
- **Aggravating circumstances:** what makes the pain worse? What makes it better?
- **Quantity:** how intense is the pain? (Use a standard pain rating scale to quantify the intensity of the pain; see Fig. 27-4.)
- Are **biopsychosocial components** associated with the pain (e.g., nausea, vomiting, dizziness, sensory loss); is there anxiety, depression, or insomnia? How do you feel emotionally in response to the pain (e.g., irritable, teary, stressed, angry)?
- **Functional impact:** how does the pain affect your ability to function (activities of daily living [ADLs], job requirements, roles and responsibilities in the home, family, and community)? How does the pain affect your ability to participate in recreational activities? Instruments such as the SF-36, Oswestry Low Back Disability Index, and others are useful to establish a functional baseline and to monitor the patient over time.
- **Current treatment:** how is your pain treated? Does it work? How much relief do you achieve? What else have you tried in the past? Did it work? If yes, why did you stop using it?

After a complete medical history, physical examination, and pain history have been completed, conduct a psychosocial and physical functional assessment. The examiner is interested in determining if the patient is depressed, is anxious, is under psychiatric care, has a history of substance abuse, or has a history of verbal, physical, or sexual abuse.[12] A detailed history is important to determine how the pain is being treated including all pharmacologic drugs, both prescribed and over the counter, as well as nonpharmacologic treatment options. Assess ability to perform ADLs and ability to participate in work and recreational activities. Accurate diagnosis is important to guide optimal pain management because specific pain syndromes respond to specific treatment modalities.[14] After the necessary data have been collected, the interdisciplinary team can confer and develop a pain control plan with the patient and family.

CLINICAL PEARLS: The visual analogue scale (VAS) is the most commonly used scale to quantify the intensity of pain; it is easy for the patient to understand and can be used for initial assessment and ongoing monitoring.

Pain is a problem requiring a collaborative multidisciplinary team approach. The nurse as a member of the interdisciplinary collaborative team conducts, collects, and analyzes data to identify patient problems and nursing diagnoses to develop the nursing treatment plan of an overall comprehensive plan of care. As part of multidimensional experience of chronic pain, perceptual and sensory alterations are common. Therefore, the coexisting nursing diagnoses of chronic pain and perceptual and sensory alterations are common.

Once comprehensive assessment data are collected, the team meets to review the data, and tries to determine the basic mechanism of pain (e.g., inflammatory, mechanical/compressive, neuropathic, muscle dysfunction). A comprehensive plan of care is then developed. Options must be considered within the context of the individual's life and the effect of pain on the quality of life. Many possible combinations of medical and surgical therapies may be offered to the patient. They are discussed below.

Plan of Care for Chronic Pain Using Biopsychosocial Model

A written comprehensive plan of care is essential to address the many dimensions of chronic pain to optimize successful outcomes. The plan begins with fostering a partnership with the patient around a clear plan of care. The patient is often a person who has seem a number of health providers about his or her pain; has sought information about pain and his or her disease from published materials, friends, and other pain sufferers; and has perused the internet for information. Attempts to control pain have often been unsuccessful or at least unsatisfactory from the patient's perspective. The patient arrives in a very disappointed, often angry, and stressed out state.

The plan of care must be patient centered and agreeable to the patient. Measurement of goals provides data on progress, and if the goals are not being reached, an analysis is undertaken to determine barriers and new strategies for achieving desired outcomes. Include all five of the following major interrelated areas: set personal goals; improve sleep; increase physical activity; manage stress; and decrease pain.[12] Patient education is critical to fostering a therapeutic partnership and setting realistic goals, as are health care providers who are empathetic listeners.

Once the plan is implemented, periodic team meetings and monitoring of the patient will help to measure achievement of goals and patient response. Realizing from the beginning that the plan will probably need fine tuning creates realistic expectations for the patient. Patient monitoring must be multidimensional to provide an accurate assessment of the effect on the treatment.

Overview of Management and Treatment Options for Chronic Pain

Management of chronic pain includes biopsychosocial management, pharmacotherapy, and surgical interventions. The biopsychosocial approach includes *progressive physical activity/physical therapy, psychosocial and cognitive behavioral therapy, and patient education/self-management techniques.*

Physical Activity/Physical Therapy. All patients with chronic pain should engage in a physical exercise program to improve function and fitness. There are many options to consider in creating an individualized treatment program.[15] A physical therapy consult may be necessary to test muscles and prescribe an exercise program that gradually engages the person into increased activity that will lead to strengthening of muscles and improved balance, flexibility, and endurance.[16] Tailor exercise to the needs and preferences, if possible, of the patient in consultation with the provider. Physical therapy uses various therapies, such as cutaneous stimulation and exercises designed to decrease discomfort, promote successful engagement in ADLs, and maintain or restore function. Thermotherapy, cryotherapy, massage, and therapeutic exercise are modalities that may be incorporated into the pain management protocol.

Application of dry or moist heat, called **thermotherapy,** can provide analgesic, antispasmodic, and sedative effects. Increasing the temperature of tissue increases blood flow, relaxes motor tone, and increases local cellular metabolism; therefore, this aids in restoring blood flow to tissues and removing waste products. Stretching and active and passive exercise usually follow heat application; these can lengthen and strengthen muscles and tendons and thereby decrease pain. Use heat application cautiously in patients with loss of sensation, circulatory compromise, acute inflammation, or injury to prevent extension of injury. **Cryotherapy,** the application of cold, has analgesic, anti-inflammatory, and antipyretic effects, and decreases neuromuscular transmission. Initially, cold causes vasoconstriction and decreased nerve conduction, which means fewer noxious stimuli transmissions. The primary physiologic effect of **massage** is stimulation of peripheral receptors through repetitive and irritative movements of the therapist's hands or massage device. This type of stimulation produces impulses that transmit to the higher brain centers, producing sensations of pleasure or well-being.

Psychosocial Support/Cognitive-Behavioral Therapy. Behavioral approaches to the management of chronic pain are well established.[17] The major psychosocial and cognitive-behavioral approaches include emotional support, psychotherapy, counseling, relaxation therapy, meditation, imagery, distraction, reframing, and biofeedback. Patients with chronic pain often have psychosocial problems that extend to psychiatric diagnoses, which often interfere with their ability to work with the team. Depression, anxiety, and maladaptive coping behavior are often related to chronic pain. The health care provider must maintain a high level of vigilance for depression because of the risk of suicide. Therefore, screen the patient and continue to monitor and treat according to guidelines. In some patients, use of antidepressant drugs may be helpful. A short or long course of structured support and peer support groups may be helpful to support the person and develop effective coping strategies.

Cognitive-behavior therapy through a referral to a therapist, counselor, social worker, or psychologist is useful for short-term **psychotherapy,** structured support, and **counseling**; these are helpful to teach techniques such as relaxation, meditation, imagery, distraction, and reframing techniques for pain control. A large body of research supports the effectiveness of these techniques in chronic pain management. **Relaxation therapy** is a strategy used in cognitive-behavioral therapy to decrease stress and pain and regain self-control. It is believed to decrease pain by causing production of endorphins. Physiologically, relaxation lowers blood pressure, respiratory rate, heart rate, and muscle tension and contraction. There are two categories of mental and physical relaxation. The first category involves muscle relaxation, which then facilitates the response of mental relaxation. Examples of this approach are deep breathing, yoga, and progressive muscle relaxation.[18] Relaxation tapes can be purchased in bookstores and health centers for use at home or in health care facilities. The second category of relaxation focuses on mental relaxation to achieve physical relaxation. **Meditation** requires the ability to concentrate and takes practice. **Imagery** is a cognitive-behavioral strategy of focusing on a personalized pleasant mental image to aid in relaxation. Relaxation techniques are most helpful when combined with personalized imagery.[19] **Distraction** is a cognitive strategy of focusing attention on stimuli other than pain or the accompanying negative emotions.[20] Distraction may be internal (e.g., praying) or external (e.g., listening to music, watching television). **Reframing** is a cognitive strategy that teaches the person to monitor and evaluate negative thoughts and images and replace them with more positive ones. For example, if the person is preoccupied with thoughts of being unable to conduct his or her normal business because of pain, substituting self-messages that remind the person that often activities are not negated by pain increases personal control.

Patient Education and Self-Management. Patient education provides the patient and family with comprehensive and accurate information about pain, pain assessment, the use of drugs, other methods of pain control, and community resources with an emphasis on effective self-management. Specifically, self-management includes knowledge about the use of ice, heat, massage, relaxation, and cognitive-behavioral approaches to support self-management. Learning **biofeedback** can be useful. It is a process in which a person learns to influence two types of physiologic responses: those that are not ordinarily under voluntary control and those that are ordinarily regulated, but as a result of disease or trauma, regulation has been interrupted.[19]

Pharmacologic Management: Nonopioids, Opioids, and Adjuvant Analgesics

The pain experience is highly individualized and so drug therapy is also individualized. Analgesics are the pharmacologic mainstay of pain management for both acute and chronic pain. The goal of analgesia in chronic pain management is control of pain to a tolerable level rather than complete elimination of pain.[21] Analgesics can be broadly divided into nonopioids and opioids; nonopioid analgesics are generally used for the treatment of chronic pain. Additionally, adjuvant drugs have properties that enhance the effect of the analgesics. These categories of drugs include antidepressants, anticonvulsants, and anxiolytics. Acetaminophen and nonsteroidal anti-inflammatory drugs (NSAIDs) are the major nonopioid analgesics used and are effective for mild to moderate pain.[22] In addition to their analgesic properties, NSAIDS have antipyretic and anti-inflammatory effects. Acetaminophen should be used cautiously in patients with liver problems because of possible hepatotoxicity. NSAIDs are related to gastrointestinal risks of gastritis and possible gastrointestinal bleeding.

CLINICAL PEARLS: The mainstay pharmacotherapy for chronic pain management is nonopioids. Opioids are useful for some patients who cannot be well controlled by nonopioids.

An **opioid** by definition is any drug, either natural or synthetic, that has similar actions to those of morphine and is effective for moderate to severe pain. Opioids are best suited for acute pain, but under certain conditions opioids can be beneficial for chronic pain.[23] The decision to use opioids is based on a careful risk–benefit analysis and the medical history. The goal of opioid therapy is to provide partial analgesia and maintain or improve function with acceptable side effects.[12] The patient must be well educated about the goals, use, side effects, physical tolerance, and dependency issues. Therefore, opioid therapy requires careful patient selection and close ongoing monitoring for side effects, dependency, and abuse. Neuropathic pain may be less responsive to some opioids, but careful selection of opioids will provide satisfactory pain control.[24]

Adjuvant drugs provide independent analgesia for specific types of pain, enhance the analgesic efficacy of opioids, and treat concurrent symptoms or side effects that exacerbate pain. Classes of drugs used include antidepressants, anticonvulsants, and anxiolytics.[25] Depression and chronic pain go hand in hand, with one reinforcing the other. Lack of sufficient norepinephrine and serotonin may be the cause of depression, and these substances play a role in pain transmission. Therefore, depression enhances the pain experience. Tricyclic antidepressants are the preferred initial therapy for neuropathic pain.[26] Amitriptyline (Elavil), imipramine (Tofranil), nortriptyline (Pamelor), and desipramine (Norpramin) are a few of the widely used antidepressants.

Anticonvulsants stabilize the neuronal membrane, reducing neuronal excitability. These drugs are used most frequently for pain that has a sharp, electrical, shooting quality, such as that of trigeminal neuralgia. Gabapentin (Neurontin) is becoming a first-line drug for neuropathic pain.[27] Carbamazepine (Tegretol) and phenytoin (Dilantin) are other anticonvulsants frequently used. Lamotrigine (Lamictal) is useful for trigeminal neuralgia, neuropathies associated with human immunodeficiency virus (HIV) infection, and poststroke pain.[12,28] Anxiety can increase the perception of pain and can prevent the individual from tolerating pain. The benzodiazepines, such as alprazolam (Xanax), clorazepate (Tranxene), and diazepam (Valium), are common anxiolytic drugs. Baclofen (Lioresal) is a muscle relaxant used to relieve some types of pain associated with spasm and muscle tension.

Topical analgesics are also used for chronic pain management.[29] Capsaicin is a topical cream useful for neuropathic pain that depletes pain mediator substance P from afferent nociceptive neurons. Topical lidocaine cream or a patch is also useful for neuropathic pain.

With chronic pain and long-term pharmacotherapy, the patient must be screened carefully before selecting drug therapy and monitored carefully for the duration of drug use. All drugs have side effects. In addition, side effects from drug therapy must be recognized and treated effectively.[21] The most common side effects of opioids include constipation, sedation, nausea, and itching.[30]

Intervention and Management

The ICSI guidelines divide interventional techniques that are performed to diagnose and treat chronic pain into level I and level II procedures. Level I procedures are commonly performed diagnostic and therapeutic procedures and level II procedures are palliative interventions used for patients who have failed conventional therapy. Examples of level I diagnostic procedures are transforaminal epidural injection and discography. Examples of commonly used level I therapeutic procedures include percutaneous radiofrequency neurotomy, intradiscal electrothermal therapy, epidural, and corticosteroid injections.[12]

Neuropathic pain is described as burning, lancinating, stabbing, stinging, shooting, and sharp.[14] A complete diagnostic work-up of neuropathic pain is necessary to assist the health provider in selecting the best approach for the specific kind of pain based on scientific evidence.[31] One evidence-based algorithm for treatment of neuropathic pain proposes a stepwise approach to treatment.[32] If one applies the ICSI framework to neuropathic pain, several principles emerge. First, eliminate the underlying causes of pain through disease-specific measures such as debulking of a spinal cord tumor compressing nerve roots. Health providers must be able to recognize specific common pain problems that often warrant more specific treatments such as low back pain, spinal cord compression, peripheral neuropathies, fibromyalgia, and others. Second, local or regional interventions can help to control pain. These interventions include nerve blocks, topical agents, physical rehabilitation, and behavioral measures. Drug therapy, as outlined in the previous section, is a mainstay of comprehensive pain management plan and includes nonopioid analgesics and other possible categories such as antidepressants, anticonvulsants, anxiolytics, corticosteroids, and topical creams.

Third, transcutaneous electrical nerve stimulation (TENS) and acupuncture represent counterstimulation techniques designed to activate endogenous pain-modulating pathways by direct stimulation of peripheral nerves.[33,34] TENS is a method of applying controlled, low-voltage electrical stimulation to large, myelinated peripheral nerve fibers through cutaneous electrodes for the purpose of modulating stimulus transmission and relieving pain. Spinal stimulation with an implantable electrode is being used for radicular limb pain. Fourth, for selected patients who have failed other options for neuropathic pain control and who have undergone a complete biopsychosocial reassessment, methadone and tramadol are opioids that may be more useful for improved pain control. Fifth, most pain can be controlled with noninvasive measures. Invasive procedures should be reserved for difficult-to-control pain or for specific pain syndromes likely to respond best to invasive procedures.[14] Surgical interventions alone for chronic pain control have limited scientific evidence for efficacy.[12] Because of the complexity of chronic pain, neurosurgical procedures are not a one-stop solution for pain control. Finally, patients with chronic pain who have failed a pain management program are best managed at a pain management center where an interdisciplinary team approach is available. Evidence confirms positive outcomes for patients with chronic pain who are treated in multidisciplinary pain management centers.[35]

Follow-Up of Patients With Chronic Pain

Patients who are being treated for chronic pain need follow-up at regular intervals. Pain is reassessed after starting a treatment plan, with any change in the pattern or severity of pain symptoms, and after any change in the treatment plan. Assess the qualitative characteristics of pain symptoms and quantitative pain level at each visit. Encourage the patient to keep a pain diary that can be shared at each visit. Be specific on what should be included in the pain diary.

Second, assess the effectiveness of current pain management strategies at each visit. Include an assessment of compliance. If new drugs have been added, verify that they are being taken as ordered. Educate the patient as necessary to expectations of drug effects. For example, some drugs such as Neurontin must be taken for a number of weeks before effectiveness can be evaluated. Encourage the patient to give each therapeutic a reasonable amount of time to judge effectiveness. Monitor each patient for side effects and complications to drug therapy regardless of whether the drug is newly added or a long-standing component of the treatment plan. In addition, any patient who is on opioid therapy must be monitored for inappropriate use of the drugs. Third, recognize that some patients develop maladaptive behavior patterns related to chronic pain. Therefore, ongoing psychosocial assessment is necessary to determine the need for an increased intensity of psychosocial interventions.

NURSING MANAGEMENT OF PATIENTS WITH CHRONIC PAIN

Caring for patients with chronic pain requires a multidimensional approach by the nurse regardless of whether he or she is approaching the patient as an individual practitioner or as a member of a multidisciplinary chronic pain management team. The standards set forth by the Joint Commission are integrated into policies, procedures, and care. Nurses bring a unique comprehensive biopsychosocial approach to the patient with chronic pain through an inclusive understanding of the unique pain experience and the impact on function in the physical, psychological, and social domains. A framework for assessing pain is outlined in Chart 27-3. In addition to data collected in an interview format, use of a number of general and disease-specific instruments helps to assess the impact of pain on ADLs, quality of life, and psychosocial function. Examples of general measure instruments are the SF-36 and the Beck Depression Inventory, while the Oswestry Disability Questionnaire is an example of a specifically focused instrument. Through an interview and ongoing dialogue with the patient, the nurse can better understand the meaning of pain to the patient and how the chronic pain experience affects his or her life, thus providing a context of meaning. Once a comprehensive database has been established, the nurse can provide input to the comprehensive plan of care. In discussions with the patient, the nurse can address the various components of the plan, determine realistic goals and time frame, promote acceptance of the components, and help the patient integrate the plan of care within the context of his or her life. In any chronic illness, education and support are critical to successful adaptation.

The following briefly addresses the major areas of a comprehensive chronic pain treatment plan as it relates to the nurse's role. See also the previous section on follow-up of patients with chronic pain.[36,37]

Progressive Physical Activity/Physical Therapy: In most instances, progressive physical activity is a goal of improved functionality. This may be counterintuitive to a patient who has chronic pain, especially if the pain is initially increased by activity. The patient needs education and support to understand the importance of gradual and progressive physical activity to improve outcomes of pain control. For some patients the progressive activity may be possible within the home environment (i.e., increased walking, stretching exercises). For others, a specific physical therapy program working with a physical therapist may be ordered. Regardless of the approach, the patient must understand the expectations of the patient, process considerations, measures of outcomes, and time frame. Improvement is usually gradual so the patient needs support and encouragement for continued participation.

Psychosocial and Cognitive-Behavioral Therapy: Ongoing assessment of psychosocial response is necessary to identify "red flags" that indicate new or more intensive treatment. Although an important component of the nursing management is ongoing support and encouragement, there are times when onset or escalation of maladaptive behavior triggers new needs. This information is shared with other health providers involved in the patient's care so that the plan of care can be modified. The treatment options are addressed in a previous section and include cognitive-behavioral therapy, pharmacotherapeutics, and other treatment options.

Patient Education/Self-Management Techniques: The backbone of nursing management of a patient with chronic pain is individualized patient education, which includes development of competencies with self-management techniques. Chronic pain is seen through a chronic illness framework in which the patient is helped to manage his or her illness across the phases and transitions of illness. This patient-family empowerment supports managing the chronic pain within the context of the patient's life and within the environment in which he or she lives. The nurse assists the patient to problem solve and to recognize resources to integrate optimal chronic pain management strategies. Establishing and maintaining an open and supportive relationship with the patient provides the context of creating an individualized plan of care that is responsive to the evolution of chronic pain over time.

CLINICAL PEARLS: The approach to chronic pain is comprehensive and multidimensional; nurses play an important role in initial and ongoing assessment and for providing educative and supportive measures for patients.

PAIN MANAGEMENT AND THE FUTURE

Research into the understanding of the pain phenomenon, its human impact, and treatment options continues and is blazing new frontiers of inquiry. The age of molecular biology and neuroimmunology has opened the doors to new understandings about the interplay of the mind on the body and the ability to control pain. These breakthroughs come at a time of a changing health care system and a managed care environment in which treatment options to patients are increasingly controlled by third-party payers. The real challenge is for health care providers to demonstrate the cost effectiveness and improved health outcomes that can be achieved for people who suffer from chronic pain.

REFERENCES

1. Katz, W. A., & Rothenberg, R. (2005). The nature of pain: Physiology. *JCR: Journal of Clinical Rheumatology, 11*(2, Suppl), S11–S12.
2. Institute for Clinical Systems Improvement. (2005). *Assessment and management of chronic pain* (pp. 77–78). Bloomington, MN: Institute for Clinical Systems Improvement. Retrieved February 3, 2007, from http://www.guidlein.gov/summary/summary.aspx?view_id=1&doc_id=8363
3. Bonica, J. J. (1990). *The management of pain* (Vols. I & II, 2nd ed.). Philadelphia: Lea & Febiger.
4. Beers, M. H., Porter, R. S., Jones, T. V., Kaplan, J. L., & Berkwits, M. (Eds.). (2006). Pain: Introduction. In M. H. Beers, R. S. Porter, T. V. Jones, J. L. Kaplan, & M. Berkwits (Eds.). *Merck manual of diagnosis and therapy* (18th ed.). Retrieved February 3, 2007, from http://online.startref.com.ezpoxyhost.library.tmc.edu/Document/DocumentBodyContent.aspx?DocId=717
5. International Association for the Study of Pain. IASP pain terminology. Retrieved February 4, 2007, from http://www.iasp-pain.org/AM/Tempalte.cfm?Section=General_Resoruce_Links&Tempalte=CM/HTMLDi
6. International Association for the Study of Pain. (1993). Complex regional pain syndrome–Type I. In H. Merskey & N. Bogduk (Eds.). *Description of chronic pain syndromes and definitions pain terms* (2nd ed.). Seattle, WA: IASP Press.
7. Greipp, M. E. (2003). Complex regional pain syndrome-type I: Research relevance, practice realities. *Journal of Neuroscience Nursing, 35*(1), 16–20.
8. American College of Physicians. (2007). Reflex sympathetic dystrophy (complex regional pain syndrome). In *PIER: The physicians' information and education resource* (pp. 1–26). Retrieved February 3, 2007, from http://online.statref.com.ezproxyhost
9. Melzack, R., & Wall, P. D. (1965). Pain mechanisms: A new theory. *Science, 150,* 971–979.
10. Rosenow, J. M., & Henderson, J. M. (2003). Anatomy and physiology of chronic pain. *Neurosurgical Clinics of North America, 14,* 445–462.
11. Vanderah, T. W. (2007). Pathophysiology of pain. *Medical Clinics of North America, 91,* 1–12.
12. Institute for Clinical Systems Improvement (ICSI). (2005). *Assessment and management of chronic pain* (pp. 1–47). Bloomington, MN: Institute for Clinical Systems Improvement.
13. Pasero, C., Gordon, D. B., McCaffery, M., & Pasero, C. (1999). JCAHO on assessing and managing pain. *American Journal of Nursing, 99,* 22.
14. American College of Phyisicans. (2007). Pain. In *PIER: The physicians' information and education resource* (pp. 1–16). Retrieved February 3, 2007, from http://online.statref.com.ezproxyhost
15. Stanos, S. P., McLean, J., & Radar, L. (2007). Physical medicine rehabilitation approach to pain. *Medical Clinics of North America, 91,* 57–95.
16. American Geriatric Society. (1998). AGS clinical practice guidelines: The management of chronic pain in older persons. *Geriatrics, 53*(Suppl 3), S6–S7.
17. Okifuji, A., & Ackerlind, S. (2007). Behavioral medicine approaches to pain. *Medical Clinics of North America, 91,* 45–55.
18. Carroll, D., & Bowsher, D. (1993). *Pain management and nursing care* (p. 133). Boston: Butterworth-Heinemann.
19. Jacox, A., Carr, D. B., Payne, R., et al. (1994). *Management of cancer pain. Clinical practice guideline* (p. 82). AHCPR Pub. No. 94-0592. Rockville, MD: Agency for Health Care Policy and Research, Public Health Service, U. S. Department of Health and Human Services.
20. McCaffery, M., & Beebe, A. (1989). *Pain: Clinical manual for nursing practice.* St. Louis, MO: C. V. Mosby.
21. American Pain Society. (1999). *Principles of analgesic use in the treatment of acute pain and chronic pain* (2nd ed.). Skokie, IL: American Pain Society.
22. Munir, M. A., Enany, N., & Zhang, J-M. (2007). Nonopioid analgesics. *Medical Clinics of North America, 91,* 97–111.
23. Eisenberg, E., McNicol, E. D., & Carr, D. B. (2005). Efficacy and safety of opioid agonists in the treatment of neuropathic pain of nonmalignant origin: Systematic review and meta-analysis of randomized controlled trials. *JAMA, 293,* 3043–3252.
24. Ballantyne, J. C., & Mao, J. (2003). Opioid therapy for chronic pain. *New England Journal of Medicine, 349,* 1943–1953.
25. Knotkova, H., & Pappagallo, M. (2007). Adjuvant analgesics. *Medical Clinics of North America, 91,* 113–124.
26. Saarto, T., & Wiffen, P. J. (2005). Antidepressants for neuropathic pain. *Cochrane Database System Review,* CD005454.
27. Wiffen, P. J., McQuary, H. J., Edwards, J. E., & Moore, R. A. (2005). Gabapentin or acute and chronic pain. *Cochrane Database System Review,* CD005452.
28. Simpson, D. M., McArthur, J. C., Olney, R., Clifford, D., So, Y., Ross, D., et al. (2003). Lamotrigine for HIV-associated painful sensory neuropathies: A placebo-controlled trial. *Neurology, 60,* 1508–1514.
29. McCleane, G. (2007). Topical analgesics. *Medical Clinics of North America, 91,* 125–139.
30. Bruera, E., & Watanabe, S. (1994). Psychostimulants as adjuvant analgesics. *Journal of Pain Symptom Management, 9,* 412–415.
31. Horowitz, S. H. (2007). The diagnostic workup of patients with neuropathic pain. *The Medical Clinics of North American, 91,* 21–30.
32. Finnerup, N. B., Otto, J. B., McQuay, H. J., Jensen, T. S., & Sindrup, S. H. (2005). Algorithm for neuropathic pain treatment: An evidence based proposal. *Pain, 118,* 289–305.
33. Gadsby, J. G., & Flowerdew, M. W. (2000). Transcutaneous electrical nerve stimulation and acupuncture-like transcutaneous electrical nerve stimulation for chronic low back pain. *Cochrane Database System Review,* CD000210.
34. Ezzo, J., Berman, B., Hadhazy, V. A., Jadad, A. R., Lao, L., & Singh, B. B. (2000). Is acupuncture effective for the treatment of chronic pain? A systematic review. *Pain, 86,* 217–225.
35. Maruta, T., Swanson, D. W., & McHardy, M. J. (1990). Three year follow-up of patients with chronic pain who were treated in a multidisciplinary pain management center. *Pain, 41,* 47–53.
36. Holm, L. M. (2003). Nursing interventions for patients with chronic conditions. *Journal of Advanced Nursing, 44*(2), 137–153.
37. Goodman, G. R. (2003). Outcomes measurement in pain management: Issues of disease complexity and uncertain outcomes. *Journal of Nursing Care Quality, 18*(2), 105–111.

Headaches

Joanne V. Hickey

Headaches are a common, almost universal experience for about 90% of the population in any given year. New onset of headache or change in the intensity or characteristics of a previous headache pattern may alarm a person sufficiently to seek medical attention. About 9% of adults seek medical attention, while another 83% self-treat.[1] The causes of headaches are exceeding long. Although most headaches are benign, some are serious and even life threatening. This chapter provides a brief overview of headaches in accordance with the most recent headache classification and diagnostic criteria published by the International Headache Society (IHS).[2] Only the most common headaches will be addressed. For a reader who wants information on the less common types of headaches, the IHS publication is the definitive resource.

Within the IHS headache classification system, the major categories of headache are primary and secondary headaches. A **primary headache** is a headache for which no organic structural abnormalities can be identified and accounts for about 90% of headaches. This category includes migraine, tension-type, cluster, and miscellaneous headaches. **Secondary headaches** are associated with various underlying primary organic etiologies that include intracranial, extracranial, and systemic disorders.[3] Assessment and identification of the specific type of headache is key to appropriate treatment and patient education. The impact that a headache has on a person's life varies greatly. In most instances, a headache is an occasional event accompanied by mild discomfort that is relieved by an over-the-counter analgesic. For some, a headache is a frequent and severe event resulting in disability and a decreased quality of life, which often interferes with interpersonal relationships, work productivity, and family life. For others, a headache is a symptom of a serious underlying condition requiring immediate intervention.

PAIN-SENSITIVE CRANIAL STRUCTURES AND PATHOPHYSIOLOGY

Pain-Sensitive Cranial Structures

Not all cranial structures of the head and intracranial space are sensitive to pain. Those structures that do have pain

receptors (nociceptors) and are capable of causing pain include the following:

- Extracranial: skin, subcutaneous tissue, muscles, fascia, extracranial arteries, periosteum, and parts of the eye, ear, nasal cavities, and paranasal sinuses
- Intracranial venous sinuses and their large related vessels including the pericavernous structures
- Meninges: parts of the dura mater at the base of the brain and the arteries within the dural and pia-arachnoid large vessels including parts of the anterior, middle, internal carotid, middle meningeal, and superficial temporal arteries
- Cranial/other nerves: trigeminal, facial, glossopharyngeal, vagus, and second and third cervical nerves

Pain perception may be felt local or referred to different anatomic areas of the head. Pain from supratentorial structures refers to the anterior two thirds of the head, while pain from infratentorial structures refers to the vertex and back of the head and neck.[4]

The pathophysiology of headache begins with traction, pressure, deformation, displacement, inflammation, or dilation of those structures embedded with nociceptors (pain receptors). Pain impulses are transmitted from the periphery by small myelinated fibers and unmyelinated C fibers. These fibers terminate in the dorsal horn of the spinal cord and the trigeminal nucleus caudalis. Secondary neurons from the dorsal horn reach the thalamus through the spinal thalamic pathways. Neurotransmitters play a role in pain. Substance P, a neuropeptide, is a pain neurotransmitter for the primary sensory neurons. Interneurons in the dorsal horn use enkephalins and possibly gamma-aminobutyric acid (GABA) as inhibitory neurotransmitters to block pain transmission.[5]

The **ascending pain pathways** from the supratentorial space (the anterior and middle fossa) carry pain sensation by the trigeminal nerve (cranial nerve [CN] V). Pain sensation from the infratentorial space (posterior fossa) is carried by the glossopharyngeal (CN IX), the vagus (CN X) nerves, and the second and third cervical nerves. The pain pathways ascend through the brainstem to neurons in the midbrain raphe area. From there, they extend to the thalamus, the hypothalamus, and the parietal lobe through the posterior limb of the internal capsule.[6] Serotonin is the primary neurotransmitter in the ascending raphespinal tract. The ascending serotonergic system originates in the midbrain raphe region, innervates the cerebral blood vessels, and is distributed in the thalamus, hypothalamus, and cortex. The major functions of these regions of the brain are cerebral blood flow, sleep, and neuroendocrine control.[3] The **descending pain-modulating pathways** originate in the periaqueductal gray region (PAG) in the midbrain and synapse in the nucleus raphe magnus in the medulla and the dorsal horn. The descending pathways are modulated by norepinephrine, serotonin, and opiates (enkephalins), which produce analgesia by inhibiting pain transmission.

Although there are many theories of chronic headache causation, the precise cause or causes have not been clearly established. The muscle theory hypothesizes that tension-type headaches are secondary to increased muscle contraction of the scalp and cervical muscles and is controversial. The vascular theory implicates vascular changes with migraine and cluster headaches. The neurogenic theory suggests that migraine headache is caused by a primary disturbance of brain function.[5] Perhaps one of the most important considerations in understanding headache is the role of serotonin. The amine neurotransmitter serotonin, which is also called 5-hydroxytryptamine (5-HT), is derived from the amino acid tryptophan. Serotonin, widely distributed in the body, has high concentrations in the gastrointestinal tract, platelets, and brain. Platelets contain all the serotonin normally present in blood.

The relationship between migraine headaches and serotonin is well established. At the onset of a migraine blood serotonin falls, although it is normal between attacks.[5] This is followed by an increase in urinary 5-hydroxyindoleacetic acid, a breakdown product of serotonin that requires platelet aggregation for its release. There are about seven classes of 5-HT receptors in the body, most of which are excitatory. Controversy continues about the pathophysiology of migraines. Some support the notion that abnormal extracranial and intracranial vascular reactions occur in migraine and other vascular bases. Narrowing of the blood vessels supplying the brain and the surrounding tissue results in reduced blood flow. This phase is followed by vasodilation, swelling, and noninfectious inflammation of the blood vessels. Concurrently, platelets clump together during an attack, probably because of exposure to several vasoactive amines, such as serotonin. The role of other vasoactive amines continues to be the subject of research.

CLASSIFICATION OF HEADACHES

Primary Headaches

Primary headaches include migraine headache, tension-type headache, cluster headache, chronic paroxysmal hemicrania, and hemicrania continua all unassociated with structural lesions. Only migraine, tension-type, and cluster headaches will be discussed. A complete description of all of the subtypes of headaches and diagnostic criteria can be found in the IHS document.[2]

Migraine Headaches

Migraine headache is a common, recurring, and disabling primary headache that includes two major clinical presentations of migraine, those with and without an aura. A

> **CHART 28-1   Common Triggers That May Precipitate Migraine Headaches**
>
> The following factors are common triggers that may precipitate migraine headaches in some people:
>
> **FOODS AND BEVERAGES**
> - Caffeine (coffee, tea, cola)
> - Alcoholic beverages, especially red wine and beer (contain tyramine)
> - Chocolate
> - Foods containing tyramine (strong and aged cheeses, pickled foods, canned figs)
> - Nitrites (cured meats)
> - Sulfites
> - Monosodium glutamate
> - Yeast products
> - Dairy products
>
> **OTHER CONDITIONS**
> - Stress (a strong precipitator of headache)
> - Hormonal changes associated with the menstrual cycle and pregnancy
> - Certain drugs such as estrogen and nitroglycerin
> - Weather changes
> - Decreased sleep or sleep deprivation
> - Bright lights
> - Fatigue
> - Fever

---

migraine without aura is the most common. Migraines with and without aura are similar except for the obvious absence of the aura in migraine without aura. For migraine sufferers with aura, focal neurological symptoms either precede or sometimes accompany the headache. The pain is moderate to severe, and is often unilateral, throbbing, and accompanied by autonomic symptoms (e.g., nausea, sometimes vomiting, and sensitivity to light, sound, or odor). Migraines last 4 to 72 hours; those that last longer than 72 hours are called status migrainosus. There is a genetic component to migraines, and migraines are more common in women than in men. The onset is in childhood, adolescents, or early adulthood, and frequently diminishes after age 50.

Several *triggers* are known to precipitate migraine headache, such as psychological stress, sleep deprivation or fatigue, alcohol intake, and environmental factors (bright lights, sunlight, fluorescent lights, and watching television or movies) (Chart 28-1). For women who suffer from migraines, the menstrual cycle is a trigger in about 65% occurring immediately before, during, or immediately after menstruation. For most women with migraines, there is often complete cessation of headaches during pregnancy in 75% to 80%. Patients must be educated to avoid triggers associated with headache.

A migraine attack can be viewed through four possible phases: *prodrome* (premonitory symptoms); *aura*; the *headache*; and the *postdrome*. Patients may experience some or all of the phases in their migraine presentation. About 60% of patients experience a *premonitory phase* that occurs hours or days before the onset of headache.[2] The most common premonitory symptoms include hyperactivity, hypoactivity, depression, craving for particular foods, and repeated yawning. Only about 20% of migraine sufferers have an aura. An **aura** is the constellation of focal neurological symptoms that initiate or accompany an attack. Most auras develop over 5 to 20 minutes and usually last less than 1 hour. Visual disturbances (bright spots, dazzling zigzag lines) or somatosensory phenomena (unilateral or bilateral numbness or tingling of the lips, face, or hand; paresis of an arm or leg; mild aphasia; slight incoordination of gait; confusion; and drowsiness) are common.

The headache phase begins with the onset of a throbbing headache and a decline in serotonin levels. Often unilateral at onset, the headache may be bilateral (40% of patients) either at onset or as the headache intensifies over the next several hours. Simple physical activity or even moving the head can intensify the pain. In addition to the pain, nausea occurs in up to 90% of patients, and vomiting occurs in about one third. Many patients experience heightened sensitivity to light, sound, and smell; they seek a dark, quiet room. Other symptoms that may occur include blurry vision, nasal stuffiness, anorexia, hunger, diarrhea, abdominal cramps, facial pallor, sensation of heat or cold, sweating, scalp tenderness, edema of the temporal artery, and stiffness or tenderness of the neck. Impaired concentration, depression, fatigue, anxiety, and irritability are common. The pain gradually subsides. In the postdromal period there is often scalp or neck tenderness, anorexia, feeling of exhaustion, irritability, listlessness, impaired concentration, and mood change.[7]

Tension-Type Headaches

Tension-type headache (TTH), previously called tension headache, muscle contraction headache, stress headache, and ordinary headache, represents the most common type of primary headaches. The exact mechanism of TTH is not known. TTHs are subdivided into *episodic* and *chronic* TTHs; episodic TTH is further subdivided into *frequent* and *infrequent* TTH (less than one per month).

An **infrequent episodic TTH** is described as a headache that lasts from minutes to days. Pain is bilateral and of mild to moderate intensity with a feeling of tightness and pressure. Unlike migraines, it is not accompanied by nausea, nor does it intensify with routine physical activity. A TTH may be accompanied by sensitivity to light or sound and most often tenderness on palpation in the pericranial area. **Frequent episodic TTHs** are similar to the infrequent TTH except there are at least 10 episodes occurring on a basis of 1 or more but less than 15 days per month for at least 3 months (≥ 12 and < 180 days per year).[2] Frequent TTHs often coexist with migraine headaches without aura. The major difference in the infrequent and frequent TTHs is the impact on the person. Infrequent TTHs have little effect on quality of life, whereas frequent TTHs are disabling and have a major negative impact on quality of life. A **chronic TTH** has the same characteristics as an episodic TTH and evolves from episodic TTH. The difference is the time element. A chronic TTH occurs for 15 or more days a month on average for more than 3 months (≥ 180 days per year).[2] Episodic and chronic TTHs are further classified by whether the headache is accompanied by disorders of muscles around the cranium, such as in the temples and neck. Muscle contractions can be a part of the discomfort experienced in a headache and are further described in the IHS classification.

Cluster Headaches

The third category of primary headaches is the cluster headache and other trigeminal autonomic cephalalgias. A **cluster headache** is a severe, ipsilateral pain located in the orbital, supraorbital, temporal, or any combination of these sites. The headache lasts from 15 to 180 minutes; comes in groups, or "clusters," of one to eight daily, lasting up to several weeks or months; and is followed by a period of remission of months to years. Autonomic phenomena associated with the headache include any one or combination of the following symptoms: tearing, conjunctival congestion, nasal congestion, rhinorrhea, tearing, forehead and facial sweating, miosis, ptosis, and eyelid edema. The headache often awakens the person during the night without prodromal signs or aura. Cluster headaches can be triggered by alcohol, histamine, or nitroglycerin. Cluster headaches are three to four times more prevalent in men, and the onset is usually between 20 and 40 years of age. They are uncommon headaches that occur in about 0.4% of the population.

Paroxysmal hemicrania, short-lasting unilateral neuralgiform headaches, and probable trigeminal autonomic cephalalgia headaches included in the classification are further described in the IHS classification.

Other Primary Headaches

This miscellaneous category includes headaches associated with activity such as coughing, exertion, or sexual activity; environmental factors such as cold; and external compression such as experienced when wearing swimming goggles. These types of headaches are not discussed in this chapter.

Secondary Headaches

Other types of headaches are classified as secondary headaches, some of which are included in Table 28-1. Headache can be a *symptom* of an underlying organic problem. Therefore, the health care provider must determine whether the headache is part of a primary headache disorder or a symptom of another problem. Chronic headaches may be benign or a sign of a serious, life-threatening illness such as a brain tumor, a cerebral hemorrhage, or meningitis. The intensity of headache can be just as great from a benign cause as from a life-threatening illness. Correct diagnosis of the specific headache type is the foundation for selecting appropriate treatment. The diagnostic criteria for secondary headaches are found in Table 28-2.

APPROACH TO MANAGEMENT OF HEADACHES

Patients who seek medical care for their headaches are usually first seen and evaluated by the primary care provider. If

TABLE 28–1   CLASSIFICATION OF SECONDARY HEADACHES FROM THE INTERNATIONAL HEADACHE SOCIETY

CLASSIFICATION OF SECONDARY HEADACHE ATTRIBUTED TO:	SELECTED SUBHEADINGS IN EACH CATEGORY (GROUPED TOGETHER FOR THIS TABLE)
• Head and neck trauma	• Acute and chronic posttraumatic and whiplash headache • Traumatic intracranial hematoma headache • Postcraniotomy headache
• Cranial or cervical vascular disorders	• Ischemic stroke, TIA, intracranial hemorrhage, SAH, cerebral aneurysm, or cerebral arteriovenous malformation • Arteritis, vertebral artery pain, cerebral venous thrombosis, or other intracranial vascular disorders
• Nonvascular intracranial disorder	• High or low CSF pressure; noninfectious inflammatory disease • Intracranial neoplasm; hypothalamic or pituitary hyper- or hyposecretion • Intrathecal injection, epileptic seizure, or Chiari malformation type I
• Substance or its withdrawal	• Acute substance abuse or exposure to nitric oxide, phosphodiesterase inhibitors, carbon monoxide; certain foods and additives; cocaine, cannabis, histamine; calcitonin or other medications • Medication overuse: ergotamine, triptans, analgesics, opioids, or others • Substance withdrawal: caffeine, opioids, estrogen, or other chronically used substances
• Infections	• Intracranial infections (meningitis, encephalitis, brain abscess, subdural empyema • Systemic infections: bacterial, viral, or other • HIV/AIDS • Chronic postbacterial meningitis
• Homeostasis	• Hypoxia and/or hypercapnia (high altitude, diving, sleep apnea) • Dialysis headache • Arterial hypertension (e.g., hypertensive crisis, eclampsia) • Hypothyroidism, fasting, or cardiac cephalalgia
• Disorders of cranium, neck, eyes, ears, nose, sinuses, teeth, mouth, or other facial or cranial structures	• Cranial bone, craniocervical dystonia • Eye: acute glaucoma, refractive error, squinting, or inflammatory disorders • Temporomandibular joint disorder • Other disorders (e.g., sinusitis, tooth decay)
• Psychiatric disorders	• Somatization or psychotic disorders

AIDS, acquired immunodeficiency syndrome; CSF, cerebrospinal fluid; HIV, human immunodeficiency virus; SAH, subarachnoid hemorrhage; TIA, transient ischemic attack.

From Headache Classification Committee of the International Headache Society. (2004). The international classification of headache disorders, 2nd ed. *Cephalalgia*, *24*(1), 1–250.

there is an indication that the headache is secondary to some underlying problem, a referral may be made to a neurologist or possibly a neurosurgeon, depending on the underlying problem. For those with primary headaches such as migraines that are intractable to treatment offered by the primary care provider, a referral may be made to a headache clinic. These patients are sometimes seen in the emergency department for relief from severe, intractable pain. The level and setting of care provided for a patient with headaches depends on underlying cause and available resources.

Diagnosis

Accurate diagnosis of headache type is paramount in selecting the appropriate treatment. There are over 300 differential diagnoses for headache. The primary purpose of the physical examination is to rule out systemic causes for headache. The patient evaluation includes a complete medical history, a family history, a headache history, and a complete physical and neurological examination. The patient's history is the single most important component in diagnosis. From the headache history, the frequency, onset, duration, character, and severity of headache pain guide diagnosis (Chart 28-2). Patients who have difficulty recalling details of their headaches should be encouraged to keep a headache diary (Chart 28-3).

Which diagnostic procedures should be ordered? An exhaustive headache work-up is expensive and most often (99% of cases) identifies no underlying cause for the headache. Clinical judgment and common sense guide the diagnostic work-up. The diagnosis of primary headache is

TABLE 28–2   DIAGNOSTIC CRITERIA FOR SECONDARY HEADACHE

A. Headache with one (or more) of the following (listed) characteristics and fulfills criteria C and D.

B. Another known disorder that can cause headache has been identified.

C. Headache occurs in close temporal proximity to the other disorder and/or there is other evidence of a causal relationship.

D. Headache is greatly reduced or resolved within 3 mo (or less) after successful treatment or spontaneous remission of the causative disorder.

From Headache Classification Committee of the International Headache Society. (2004). The international classification of headache disorders, 2nd ed. *Cephalalgia*, *24*(1), 1–250.

CHART 28-2   Headache History

GENERAL HISTORY

- Were any injuries noted at birth?
- Did you have encephalitis or meningitis, either as a complication of childhood disease or as a separate entity?
- Is there any history of abnormal nervous system development, such as bed-wetting, sleep disturbances, anxiety reactions (nail biting, untoward fear, and so forth), or fainting?
- Have you had middle ear infections, sinusitis, or surgical procedures involving the ears or sinuses?
- Have you had any injuries to the head, neck, or upper spine?
- Is there evidence now or in the past of cardiovascular disease, such as hypertension, heart disease, or orthostatic hypotension?
- Have you ever had kidney disease, pheochromocytoma, tuberculosis, or tropical infections?
- Have you ever had visual problems, such as astigmatism, dysconjugate gaze, or eye strain? Have you had any eye surgery?
- Have you ever had nervous system disease, such as a seizure disorder, vertigo, visual disturbances (diplopia), or psychiatric or emotional problems?
- Do you see the dentist periodically? Have you had any dental problems?
- Have you ever had arthritis or arthropathies of the neck, shoulder, or upper back?
- Do you have any difficulty with chewing?
- Do you use alcohol, tobacco, or any drugs? What kind? How much?
- Do you have any food, drug, or environmental allergies?
- (With women) Are there any particular symptoms associated with menstruation, pregnancy, childbirth, or menopause that are troublesome?

FAMILIAL HISTORY

- Does anyone in your family suffer from headaches? If so, what is their relationship to you? Describe their headaches.
- Is there a history of seizure disorders, allergies, emotional problems, or depression in your family?

OCCUPATIONAL HISTORY

- What kind of work do you do?
- Describe the physical environment in which you work.
- Are chemicals or fumes present? What kind?
- Do your co-workers complain of headaches?

PERSONAL AND FAMILY RELATIONSHIPS

- What about your life concerns you? (Most often anxiety is associated with loss—death, divorce, separation, independence, and so forth.)
- Describe your overall emotional makeup.
- What do you do to relax? Hobbies? Sports?
- Describe how you react to stress. What body signals tell you that you are in a stressful state?
- How do you get along with family members?
- Are you able to discuss problems with family members?
- What would you most like to change about your life?

SPECIFIC HEADACHE HISTORY

- At what age did the headaches start?
- Where is the headache located (generalized, focal, unilateral, bilateral, frontal, occipital)?
- Describe the type of pain (severe, mild, throbbing, aching, constant or intermittent, and so forth).
- How frequent are the attacks?
- How long do they last?
- What factors are associated with the onset of headache (emotions, intoxication, specific foods, temperature, trigger points, menstruation, stress)?
- What relieves the headache?
- What aggravates the headache?
- What is the usual course of events with the headache?
- What symptoms accompany the headache (nausea, vomiting, visual disturbances, vertigo, watering eyes, flushing, sweating, hemiparesis, numbness, fainting, facial tic)?
- How incapacitating is the headache in terms of your normal activities?
- Are all your headaches the same?
- What do you do to treat the headache? Does it help?

---

usually made on clinical grounds (headache history) and negative findings on both the physical and the neurological examinations. No specific diagnostic tests are available to confirm the diagnosis.

Table 28-3 lists "red flags" noted in the headache work-up that suggest the need for further evaluation. Computed tomography or magnetic resonance imaging is the only evidence-based practice imaging studies recommended; an electroencephalogram is not indicated in the routine evaluation of headache.[8] Other laboratory studies such as complete blood cell count, erythrocyte sedimentation rate, antiphospholipids, glucose, electrolytes, creatinine, and thyroid panel may be ordered to rule out other possible causes, depending on findings determined by the history and physical examination. Based on the findings and laboratory data, a referral may be made to other specialists or more diagnostic procedures may be scheduled. After the underlying etiology or type of headache is diagnosed, the appropriate treatment can

be instituted. The specific treatment options are discussed under the specific type of headache.

Treatment

Overview of Management

Treatment of primary headaches involves a combination of nonpharmacologic and pharmacologic therapies. Evidence-based guidelines are available at www.guidelines.gov from the National Headache Foundation.[9] **Nonpharmacologic therapies** include individualized patient teaching, control of risk factors and triggers, and behavioral interventions (stress management, relaxation therapy, biofeedback, and cognitive-behavioral therapy). In migraine and TTHs, stress is a frequently implicated component; thus, causes of stress must be identified and controlled with stress-management

CHART 28-3 Headache Diary

Date	Onset: exact time AM or PM	Ending: exact time AM or PM	Triggers (1)	Prodromal signs (2)	Saverity of headache (3)	Location (4)	Quality of headache (5)	Other symptoms	Medication taken, frequency, and route	Pain relief (6)

A series of codes are listed for each numbers heading, such as Triggers. Include all the codes that apply in that category.

(1) Triggers

1. Emotional stress/family related
2. Emotional stress/work related
3. Fatigue
4. Anxiety
5. Menstruation
6. Sleep deprivation

7. Fasting
8. Missing a meal
9. High altitude
10. Physical illness
11. Major life change
12. None

(1) Triggers: food/beverage

A. Caffeine (coffee, tea, cola)
B. Chocolate
C. Strong/aged cheese
D. Pickled foods
E. Canned figs
F. Yeast products

G. Daily products
H. Cured meats
I. Monosodium glutamate
J. Red wine
K. Beer
L. None

(2) Prodromal signs

1. Depression
2. Irritability
3. Mental slowness
4. Fatigue
5. Sluggishness

6. Yawning
7. Feeling cold
8. Craving special foods
9. Anorexia
10. None

(4) Location of headache (mark location)

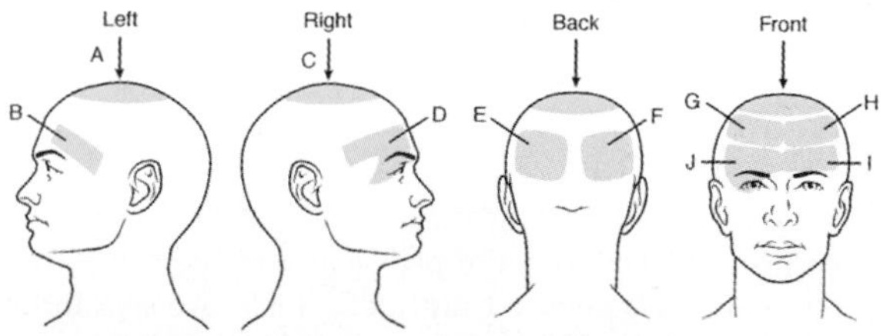

(5) Qualities of headache (include all that apply)

1. Unilateral
2. Bilateral
3. Throbbing
4. Piercing, constant

5. Gradal onset
6. Worse with head movement
7. Worse in lighted room
8. Accompanied by visual changes

(3) Headache severity scale (rate headache)

1	2	3	4	5	6	7	8	9	10

slight   moderate   very severe

(6) Pain relief from drugs scale (rate headache)

1	2	3	4	5	6	7	8	9	10

no relief   moderate   complete relief

TABLE 28-3 HEADACHE "SERIOUS SIGNS" THAT SUGGEST THE NEED FOR FURTHER EVALUATION

- "Worst" headache of my life
- Onset of headache after the age of 45 y
- Onset of a different kind of headache
- Headache with findings on the neurological examination
  - Altered level of consciousness
  - Altered cognition
  - Motor weakness, ataxia, or altered coordination
  - Altered sensation associated with headache such as tingling or numbness
  - Cranial nerve deficits such as asymmetric pupils, extraocular palsies, or decreased hearing
  - Progressive visual deficits
  - Abnormal reflexes
  - Signs of meningeal irritation
  - Abnormal findings on physical examination
    - Fever
    - Hypertension
    - Tenderness or pulsation of temporal arteries

interventions. In addition, identifying postures assumed throughout the day can often uncover sources of prolonged muscle contraction that can lead to TTH. Students, office workers, and those engaged in occupations that require prolonged sitting at a desk or computer are prime targets. Treatment is directed toward using nonpharmacologic interventions such stress management, exercise programs, and ergonomics in workplace design. **Pharmacologic therapies** include both preventive therapies and abortive therapies to promptly relieve the headache and related symptoms such as nausea and vomiting.

Migraine Headaches

Migraine headaches vary in frequency, duration, and disability among patients. The level and intensity of care depend on the level of disability and the severity of pain and accompanying symptoms. Preventive therapy is a first line of treatment. The goals of long-term migraine treatment include reduced headache frequency, intensity, and disability; improved quality of life; comprehensive patient education to support self-management; and reduced headache-related distress and psychological symptoms.

Pharmacologic Basis for Migraine Management. The treatment of migraine headache can be divided into three subtypes: acute (symptomatic), acute nonresponder care (including those with status migrainosus), and prophylaxis.

Acute Therapy. Acute therapy is directed toward alleviating or significantly limiting a headache that is just beginning or is in progress. Several drug options are available. Given that patient response is highly individualized, the health care provider may need to prescribe various drugs before an effective response is achieved. The most common acute therapy drugs are listed in Table 28-4. A few principles guide the approach to the patient with migraine headaches. Treatment of headache when it is in its early stages (e.g., prodromal) and mild is much more effective than treatment initiated later

when the headache intensity is moderate to severe. Frequent use of acute treatment medications can lead to rebound headache; therefore, acute therapy should be restricted to a maximum of 2 to 3 days a week.[1] Treatment must be individualized because patients respond differently to medications across the lifespan of the headaches. A stratified care approach versus a step care approach works best for migraine patients because episodes are different (peak intensity, time to peak intensity, associated symptoms, and disability) and thus require flexible treatment options.[10] For patients with nausea, vomiting, or gastroparesis, nasal, parenteral, or rectal administration routes should be utilized for drug administration.[1]

Treatment of migraine headache has developed rapidly in the last decade. In addition to new drugs and treatment strategies, new routes of administration including nasal spray, self-administered injections, and rapidly dissolving oral tablets are now available.[11] The nonsteroidal anti-inflammatory drugs (NSAIDs) are the most effective drug category for mild to moderate headache; different patients may respond better to a particular drug within the NSAID category.

Once the attack becomes moderate to severe, the triptans (e.g., sumatriptan, zolmitriptan, rizatriptan) and the ergot alkaloids (e.g., ergotamine tartrate and dihydroergotamine) are the most effective forms of treatment and are best administered early in the attack. The triptans are selective serotonin (5-HT) receptor antagonists. The most commonly used drugs within the class are sumatriptan (Imitrex), zolmitriptan (Zomig), naratriptan (Amerge), and rizatriptan (Maxalt and Maxalt-MLT). Each of these drugs is available in oral form. Sumatriptan is also available by injectable subcutaneous and intranasal routes. A single 6-mg dose subcutaneously of sumatriptan is an effective and well-tolerated treatment for migraines; it can be repeated in 1 hour, if necessary.[1] Sumatriptan is available orally in 50- or 100-mg tablets, and takes about 2 hours for full effect. A nasal preparation of the drug is also available, and is particularly useful for patients who have concurrent nausea and vomiting. Rizatriptan is available in wafer form, which allows it to be dissolved on the tongue without the need for water.[12] It is reported to relieve pain at 1 to 2 hours. The triptans are effective for about 70% to 78% of patients, which leaves about 22% to 30% nonresponders. Although a patient may not respond well to one drug in the triptan group, other drugs within the group may be effective. Therefore, the triptans should be fully utilized before withdrawing to another approach.

A second group of drugs used for treatment of migraine is called ergots. Ergotamine tartrate, administered orally, sublingually, rectally, subcutaneously, or intramuscularly at the first sign of a migraine headache, may abort the headache. Rectal suppositories are useful if nausea or vomiting occurs. The ergot preparations are alpha-adrenergic agonists with strong 5-HT receptor affinity and vasoconstriction action. Taken orally in 1- to 2-mg tablets, the drug may be repeated every half-hour until the headache is relieved or up to a cumulative dose of 8 mg. Nausea is a common side effect so that concurrent administration of promethazine or metoclopramide controls nausea and vomiting. The rectal route can be used if nausea persists, or dihydroergotamine (DHE) by nasal spray is also useful.

Acute Severe Migraine Nonresponders. For the approximately 20% to 25% of patients who do not responded to pain relief measures and who arrive in the emergency department,

TABLE 28–4   PHARMACOTHERAPY FOR TREATMENT OF ACUTE MIGRAINE HEADACHES

DRUG	DAILY DOSAGE (DIVIDED)	TYPE/ACTION	MOST COMMON SIDE EFFECTS
Nonnarcotic analgesics		For mild to moderate headache; take early in the attack; monitor for overuse.	Rebound headache with frequent use
• Aspirin (ASA)	• PO: 650–1300 mg	• Analgesic and anti-inflammatory effect	• Bleeding disorder; gastrointestinal (GI) distress
• Acetaminophen	• PO: 650–1300 mg	• Analgesic	• Does not cause GI upset or bleeding; use cautiously with patients with liver or kidney disease
Nonsteroidal anti-inflammatory drugs (NSAIDs)		NSAIDs prevent prostaglandin synthesis by inhibiting cyclooxygenase, a critical element in prostaglandin synthesis; prostaglandin modulates components of inflammation, pain transmission, and platelet aggregation; useful for abortive and preventive therapy.	• Limited by GI, liver, and renal side effects
• Ibuprofen	• PO: 400–800 mg		• Better tolerated than ASA
• Naproxen	• PO: 1000 mg		• Better tolerated than ASA
Triptans: selective serotonin (5-HT) receptor antagonists			
• Sumatriptan	6 mg SC, 50–100 mg PO; take early in the attack; nasal spray helpful if nausea or vomiting present	First-line abortive therapy; causes vasoconstriction of cranial arteries	Contraindicated in pregnancy, coronary artery disease, hypertension, peripheral vascular disease, and stroke; decreases blood pressure and heart rate
• Rizatriptan	10 mg PO	Same as sumatriptan	Same as sumatriptan
• Naratriptan	2.5 mg PO	Same as sumatriptan	Same as sumatriptan
• Zolmitriptan	2.5–5 mg PO or 5 mg nasal spray	Same as sumatriptan	Same as sumatriptan
• Almotriptan	12.5 mg PO	Same as sumatriptan	Same as sumatriptan
Ergots, alpha-adrenergic agonist with strong 5-HT receptor affinity and vasoconstriction			
• Ergotamine tartrate	• PO, SL, PR: 1–4 mg immediately, then 1–2 mg q30 min (total of 6 mg/attack or 10/mg/wk)	• Abortive treatment for headache unresponsive to nonnarcotic treatment	Ergots have a cumulative action so must be taken sparingly and as ordered or ergotism (numbness and tingling of fingers and toes, muscle pain, weakness, gangrene, and blindness) will develop. Nausea is a common side effect; need to premedicate with antiemetics
		• Take usual effective dose at first sign of attack	
		• Causes cerebral vasoconstriction, which decreases pulsation of cranial arteries	
• Dihydroergotamine (DHE)	• .05–1.0 mg IV, or Im; may repeat in 30–45 min; may take up to 3 mg/24 h or 6 mg/wk; 4 mg/mL nasal spray	• Parenteral treatment for an established headache	*Contraindications:* diabetes mellitus, sepsis, hepatorenal disease, peripheral vascular disease, coronary artery disease, hypertension, and pregnancy
			• Nausea and vomiting; premedicate 10–15 min before with prochlorperazine 5–10 mg PO, IM, or IV; or metoclopramide 10–20 mg PO or 10 mg IM/IV
Antiemetics		Administered to control associated nausea/vomiting; taken early in the attack	Drowsiness, dizziness, confusion, hypotension, insomnia, vertigo
• Promethazine	• PO, PR: 25–150 mg	• Adjunct antiemetic therapy	
• Prochlorperazine	• PO, IM 5–20 mg; PR 25 mg	• Adjunct antiemetic therapy	
		• Parenteral treatment for established headache	
• Metoclopramide	• IM: 25–50 mg	• Adjunct antiemetic therapy; give 15–30 min before DHE or meperidine	
	• PO, IM: 10 mg		

TABLE 28–4 PHARMACOTHERAPY FOR TREATMENT OF MIGRAINE HEADACHES *(Continued)*

DRUG	DAILY DOSAGE (DIVIDED)	TYPE/ACTION	MOST COMMON SIDE EFFECTS
Narcotic analgesics • Codeine/ASA • Meperidine • Butorphanol	• PO: 30–60 mg • IM: 75–100 mg • Transnasal: 1 mg followed by 1 mg 1 h later	For severe headache not controlled by nonnarcotics; addictive; use with caution and do not overuse. • Narcotic agonist-antagonist analgesic; very addictive; use cautiously	• Sedation, confusion, and constipation for both codeine and meperidine • Sedation, nausea, sweating, vertigo, lethargy, confusion
Other • Isometheptene (Midrin)	• PO: 2 tabs at onset then q1 h until relief; do not exceed 5/24 h	• Sympathomimetic acts as a vasoconstrictor; mild sedative providing tranquilizing effect	

metoclopramide 10 mg intravenously (IV) followed by 0.5 to 1.0 mg IV of DHE every 8 hours for 48 hours is effective.[13] In addition, oral and IV corticosteroids are useful in some refractory cases and for aborting status migrainosus.[4] Other recommended adjunctive therapy includes prochlorperazine 5 to 10 mg IV; ketorolac 30 to 60 mg intramuscularly (IM); valproate sodium 500 mg in 50 cc's of saline administered over 5 to 10 minutes and repeated every 8 hours; and droperidol 2 to 5 mg IM or IV.[1] All recommended drugs come with cautions.

Migraine Prophylaxis. Consider nonpharmacologic strategies before or concurrent with drug therapy to manage migraine headaches. According to the evidence-based guidelines, the goals of migraine preventive therapy are to reduce attack frequency, severity, and duration; improve responsiveness to treatment of acute attacks; and improve function and reduce disability. The following considerations guide the decision to embark on a prophylaxis program: frequency (four or more per month), disability (interferes with daily routines despite acute treatment), ineffectiveness of current treatment, and presence of uncommon migraine types.

The major drug groups used for prophylactic treatment of migraine headaches are beta-adrenergic blockers, tricyclic antidepressants, and selected anticonvulsants (Table 28-5). Propranolol (Inderal), a beta blocker, is a common first-choice

TABLE 28–5 PHARMACOLOGIC THERAPY FOR PROPHYLAXIS OF MIGRAINE HEADACHES

DRUG	DAILY DOSAGE	TYPE/ACTION	SIDE EFFECTS
Beta blockers • Propranolol • Nadolol • Atenolol • Timolol • Metoprolol	• PO: 20–160 mg • PO: 20–160 mg • PO: 25–100 mg • PO: 5–200 mg • PO: 50–250 mg	• Blocks serotonin receptors; prevents vasodilation; propranolol is first drug of choice for prophylaxis; if it is not tolerated, try others in this class as listed	Bradycardia, fatigue, lethargy, sleep disorders, and depression. Common complaints are gastrointestinal complaints and orthostatic hypotension
Tricyclic antidepressants • Amitriptyline	• PO: 10–100 mg Po at bed side	• Blocks uptake of serotonin and catecholamines centrally and peripherally • Most effective for migraine associated with tension-type headache • Alternative if beta blockers cannot be taken	Causes dry mouth, urinary retention, and sedation *Contraindications:* benign prostatic hypertrophy and glaucoma
Ergotalkaloid • Methysergide	• 4–8 mg with meals; must have a drug-free period q6mo for 3–4 wk	• Blocks serotonin to prevent early ischemic phase and vasodilation • Stabilizes platelets against release of serotonin • Inhibits release of histamine from mast cells • Potentiates norepinephrine to produce vasoconstriction	• Nausea and vomiting; fibrotic changes in the retroperitoneal and pleuropulmonary tissue, although uncommon, are the most serious complications; monitor creatinine • *Contraindications:* peripheral vascular disease, coronary artery disease, and pregnancy
• Valproic acid (divalproex)	• PO: 250–500 mg	• Turns off the firing of serotonin neurons of dorsal raphe, which controls pain; particularly useful for chronic headache	• May alter liver function; may cause sedation, hair loss, tremor, and change in cognitive performance
Calcium channel antagonist • Verapamil	• 240 mg	• Alters calcium flux across smooth muscle • Prevents vasospasm and reactive vasodilation • Drug of choice	*Contraindications:* • Severe left ventricular dysfunction, hypotension, or second- or third-degree heart block • Constipation

drug for prophylaxis because it is effective and inexpensive. However, it may not be well tolerated because of its brady-cardic effect. Other beta blockers can be tried if propranolol is not useful.

Tension-Type Headaches

Pharmacologic management of episodic and chronic TTHs is directed toward rapid treatment to abort the attack. The secondary goal is to prevent or reduce the occurrence of headaches. Most TTHs are thought to be caused by anxiety, stress, and associated muscle tension. Less often, headache can be attributed to the effects of former injury or poor posture. Stress reduction, exercise programs, relaxation techniques, meditation, topical heat or cold packs, ergonomic principles for work environment, biofeedback, and possibly counseling are important non-pharmacologic strategies that should be addressed along with drug therapy.

Drug Therapy. Treatment of the mild to moderate pain of episodic headache includes nonopioid analgesics and muscle relaxants. For symptomatic control of headache the following are commonly used: aspirin, acetaminophen, caffeine, a combination of aspirin and caffeine or aceta-minophen and caffeine (e.g., Excedrin Migraine, Excedrin E. S., Vanquish, Midol), ibuprofen, naproxen, flurbiprofen, cyclooxygenase-2 (COX-2) inhibitors (e.g., Celebrex, Vioxx), Midrin, and Ultram. Some of these drugs are over-the-counter drugs, whereas others require a prescription. Opioids should be avoided because of the concern about addiction.

Preventive therapy may also be considered. Depression, sleep disturbance, and anxiety disorders are often related to patients with frequent TTHs.[3] Amitriptyline, a tricyclic antidepressant, is the most common antidepressant used. Other antidepressants known as the selective serotonin reuptake inhibitors (SSRIs) are also useful for patients with clinical depression. This group includes sertraline (Zoloft) and paroxetine (Paxil). Neurontin (Gabapentin), an anti-convulsant, has been useful for some patients. Combining drug therapy with behavioral and psychological interventions benefits those with frequent headaches. Because pain is interpreted as the presence of a serious problem, headaches may make a person fearful that a life-threatening condition is present. Reassurance helps to relieve such anxiety.

Cluster Headaches

The management of cluster headaches can be divided into three categories: *acute, transitional,* and *preventive care.* Fast-acting treatment is used in the acute (symptomatic) attacks of cluster headache because of the rapid onset, short time to peak intensity, and severity of the headache. The following *acute treatment* options are useful:

- 100% oxygen inhalation using a face mask at 7 to 10 L/min for 15 to 20 minutes with a nonbreathing face mask,[14] preferably at the onset of the attack (effective in about 60% of cases)[1]

CHART 28-4 **Teaching Plan for Persons With Migraine Headaches**

The following list includes the major points of a teaching plan for persons with migraine headaches:

1. Educate the person about what migraine headaches are and what they are not.
2. Help the person to identify triggers for migraine headache and develop a plan to avoid or ameliorate the triggers (see Chart 28–1).
3. Help the person develop a format for a headache diary.
4. Provide a copy of a tyramine-free diet.
5. Teach stress reduction, stress management, behavioral strategies, and lifestyle changes to minimize the number of headaches.
6. Teach the person about his or her medications including action, how to take the drug, side effects, and how to avoid complica-tions of overuse; include a caution about new drugs included for comorbidity and the possibility of interactions.
7. Teach the person about comfort measures during an attack such as lying down in a dark and quiet room with cold compresses to the head.
8. Suggest resources to help the migraine sufferer learn about migraines, such as:

> National Headache Foundation
> 5252 North Western Avenue
> Chicago, IL 60625 (312) 878-7715

- Sumatriptan (subcutaneous or nasal); other triptans may be useful
- DHE by IM, SQ, or nasal routes
- Oral or rectal ergotamine
- Intranasal lidocaine

Transitional treatment is directed at rapid suppression of attacks before a preventive medication takes effect. Transi-tional treatments including a short, tapered course of pred-nisone ergotamine tartrate or DHE are recommended. Note that ergotamine and triptans should not be used within 24 hours of each other.

From a perspective of prevention, a number of drugs are considered effective for *preventive treatment* of cluster headaches. The drugs of choice are the high-dose calcium channel blockers (verapamil 120 to 240 mg three or four times a day), lithium carbonate (300 mg three times a day), methysergide, topiramate (50 to 125 mg daily), divalproex (500 to 2000 mg daily), or baclofen (10 mg tid), or a short-term course of prednisone may be effective.[1,4] In addition to pharmacologic preventive therapy, eliminating triggers known to precipitate the onset of cluster headaches is impor-tant. Triggers are specific for a patient and may include alco-hol consumption, smoking, high altitude, and sleep cycle disturbances (jet lag, shift work).[15]

CHART 28-5	**Common Patient Problems and Nursing Diagnoses Associated With Headache**

PATIENT PROBLEMS/ NURSING DIAGNOSES (ACTUAL OR POTENTIAL)	NURSING INTERVENTIONS	EXPECTED OUTCOMES
Pain related to (R/T) headache	• Document the characteristics and circumstances of the painful experience. • Help the patient identify factors that precipitate headache. • Manipulate the environment to control or prevent headache.	• Pain will be reduced or abolished. • Factors that precipitate headache will be identified and reduced.
Ineffective Individual Coping R/T lifestyle stress	• Develop techniques to identify the causes of ineffective coping. • Establish a therapeutic nurse–patient interpersonal relationship. • Assist the patient to gain insight into the cause–effect relationship of ineffective coping. • Assist the patient in developing adaptive coping skills.	• The causes of ineffective coping will be identified. • The patient will gain insight into the effects of ineffective coping. • Effective adaptive coping skills will be developed.
Fluid Volume Excess (Fluid Retention) R/T premenstrual fluid retention	• Help the patient to understand why fluid retention can contribute to the onset of headaches. • Identify the signs and symptoms of fluid retention. • Identify any dietary patterns that contribute to fluid retention. • Discuss the purpose of any medications and stress the importance of taking the medications as ordered.	• Fluid retention will be eliminated or controlled.
Sensory/Perceptual Alterations R/T paresthesia and visual alterations	• Document the type and characteristics of sensory/perceptual alterations. • Develop strategies to control or eliminate these signs and symptoms, if possible. • Institute measures to prevent injury. • Collaborate with the physician to provide a therapeutic protocol for treating the problem.	• Sensory-perceptual alterations will be identified and controlled or eliminated. • Precautions for the prevention of injury will be implemented.
Sleep Pattern Disturbance R/T stress and serotonin disorder	• Document the sleep-wakefulness pattern. • Identify factors that prevent adequate sleep. • Develop strategies to overcome obstacles to adequate sleep.	• A satisfactory sleep-wakefulness pattern will be established.
Knowledge Deficit R/T lack of understanding of headache dynamics and treatment protocol	• Identify the specific areas of knowledge deficits or misinformation. • Develop a teaching plan to correct these deficits. • Evaluate the acquisition of new knowledge by the patient.	• The patient will demonstrate a knowledge of headache type, precipitating factors, and treatment.
Anxiety R/T the possibility of headache and the disruption of lifestyle routines	• Assess the reason for the anxiety. • Help the patient to set realistic goals. • Develop anxiety and stress-reduction strategies.	• Anxiety related to headache or the potential of headache onset will be reduced or eliminated.

NURSING MANAGEMENT OF THE PATIENT WITH HEADACHE

Patient management for complex, chronic, and hard-to-control headaches is often a collaborative multidisciplinary endeavor. In this section, the nursing management of patients with headache is briefly discussed, with emphasis on the role of the nurse in patient education. More specific detail is included on migraines and TTHs. Cluster headaches are not discussed further because patient education is very similar to that used in migraine headaches.

Nurses care for patients who have various kinds of headaches. Most patients with primary headaches are self-managed in the community setting or by a primary care provider. For those with primary headaches that are difficult to control, a neurologist or a multidisciplinary team at a headache center may be necessary. Occasionally, primary headache sufferers seek relief at an emergency department for a severe intractable headache not controlled by acute drug therapy. These people need to be referred for re-evaluation. The major role of the nurse working with primary headache patients is patient education for self-management, prevention, and adjustment of lifestyle.

In a hospitalized population, secondary headaches are often symptoms associated with other health problems. Nurses caring for these patients manage headache with analgesics administered on an "as necessary" basis. Patients admitted for other problems may also come with a history of primary headache such as migraine or cluster headaches. In these circumstances, consider continuing with any headache prophylactic therapy. In addition, the possibility of drug interactions between headache drugs and drugs ordered to treat other health problems should be considered and clinical decisions made appropriately.

Nursing Assessment

A detailed nursing assessment and nursing history are the foundations for planning care. Chart 28-2 provides a sample headache history. The patient is key to providing a detailed history; take the time to listen and to collect this information. Based on these data, indications for further assessment may be evident. In the hospitalized patient, a headache may be an expected side effect of surgery or an underlying problem. Use of a headache history is not necessary in those situations.

Nursing Intervention

After the diagnosis of a primary headache has been established, the nurse develops a comprehensive patient teaching plan to educate the person about how to limit the number of attacks and treat acute attacks with both nonpharmacologic and pharmacologic methods. Chart 28-4 contains key points to include in a teaching plan for a patient with migraine headache. Depending on the type of primary headache, the nurse individualizes the teaching to the specific needs of the patient.

Regardless of the type of headache, headaches are most apt to occur when the patient is physically ill, overworked, tired, or stressed. Stress is the major trigger in migraines. Therefore, the nurse should encourage proper diet, adequate rest and exercise, and effective stress management techniques. By helping the patient conduct a self-assessment, the nurse and the patient can identify stressors, triggers, and particular circumstances that precipitate headaches. This provides a basis for exploring lifestyle changes to minimize these triggers. Appropriate referrals can be very helpful. Patients should be encouraged to keep a headache diary for reference (see Chart 28-3). The purpose of a headache diary is to identify the individual characteristics and patterns of the headache including duration, intensity, preceding symptoms, triggers, medications, and relief. This information is very helpful to better treat the patient and is enlightening to the patient. For example, the chart may reveal that headaches occur mostly on weekends when the entire family is home, or headaches may be noted to occur around the time of menstruation. It is most important to identify any rhythm or pattern in the occurrence of headaches. The National Headache Foundation provides a headache diary form at their website (www.headaches.org).

For patients who experience fluid retention and weight gain around menstruation, a salt-restricted diet 1 week before menstruation should be encouraged. If this is not helpful, diuretics may be prescribed. Other elimination diets should be encouraged for those patients who have identified relationships between the ingestion of certain foods and beverages and the occurrence of headaches. The major patient problems and nursing diagnoses associated with headaches are found in Chart 28-5.

In summary, headaches are divided into primary headaches and secondary headaches. The most common primary headaches have been briefly addressed, as has treatment for these headaches. There are many variants that have not been addressed in this chapter. The nurse interested in in-depth information is directed to the IHS publications and specific headache websites such the National Headache Foundation. Most nurses will care for patients with secondary headache, that is, a headache that is a symptom of an underlying health problem. For neuroscience nurses, headache is a common symptom in the neuroscience patient population. These nurses must assess the headache and engage in clinical reasoning to determine the significance of the finding in relationship the primary condition such as a brain tumor. The nurse is the direct care provider who recognizes the discomfort of the headache and provides both nonpharmacologic and pharmacologic interventions to support patient comfort. A number of drug options have been outlined. Drugs must be carefully considered for interactions and contraindications. The nurse is critical in patient safety and prevention of adverse drug events.

REFERENCES

1. Evans, R. W. (2007). Headache. *ACP Medicine*. Retrieved February 19, 2007, from http://online.statref.com.ezproxyhost.library
2. Headache Classification Committee of the International Headache Society. (2004). The international classification of headache disorders, 2nd ed. *Cephalalgia, 24*(1), 1–250.
3. *Merck manual of diagnosis and therapy* (18th ed.). (2006). Headache: Introduction. M. H. Beers, R. S. Porter, T. V. Jones, J. L. Kaplan, & M. Berkwitts (Eds.). Retrieved February 19, 2007, from http://online.statref.com/document.aspx?fxid=21&docid=755
4. Ropper, A. H., & Brown, R. H. (2005). Headache and other craniofacial pain. In A. H. Ropper & R. H. Brown (Eds.). *Adams and Victor's principles of neurology* (8th ed., pp. 144–167). New York: McGraw-Hill.
5. Saper, J. R., Silberstein, S., Gordon, C. D., Hamel, R. L., & Swidon, S. (1999). *Handbook of headache management: A practical guide to diagnosis and treatment of head, neck, and facial pain* (2nd ed., pp. 32–41). Philadelphia: Lippincott Williams & Wilkins.
6. Aminoff, M. J., Greenberg, D. A., & Simon, R. P. (1996). *Clinical neurology* (3rd ed., pp. 71–93). Stanford, CT: Appleton & Lange.
7. Silberstein, S. D., & Lipton, R. B. (1994). Overview of diagnosis and treatment of migraine. *Neurology, 44*(Suppl. 7), S6–S16.
8. Silberstein, S. D. (2000). Practice parameter: Evidence-based guidelines for migraine headache (an evidence-based review). Report of the Quality Standards Subcommittee of the American Academy of Neurology. *Neurology, 55*, 754–762.
9. Ruoff, G., & Urban, G. (2004). Treatment of primary headache: Patient education. In National Headache Foundation (Ed.). *Standards of care for headache diagnosis and treatment*. Chicago, IL: National Headache Foundation.
10. Lipton, R. B., Stewart, W. F., Stone, A. M., Lainez, M. J., & Sawyer, J. P. (2000). Stratified care vs. step care strategies for migraine:

The Disability in Strategies of Care (DISC) Study: A randomized trial. *JAMA, 284*(20), 2599–2605.

11. Lin, J. (2001). Overview of migraine. *Journal of Neuroscience Nursing, 33*(1), 6–13.

12. Moriarty-Sheehan, M. (2001). Managing migraine: Strategies for successful patient outcomes. *Nurse Practitioner, 26*(Suppl. 4), 1–13.

13. Raskin, N. H. (1986). Repetitive intravenous dihydroergotamine as therapy for intractable migraine. *Neurology, 36,* 995.

14. May, A. (2005). Cluster headache: Pathogenesis, diagnosis, and management. *Lancet, 366,* 843.

15. Saper, J. R., Silberstein, S., Gordon, C. D., Hamel, R. L., & Swidon, S. (1999). *Handbook of headache management: A practical guide to diagnosis and treatment of head, neck, and facial pain* (2nd ed., pp. 32–41). Philadelphia: Lippincott Williams & Wilkins.

RESOURCES

Websites

National Headache Foundation: www.headaches.org

Seizures and Epilepsy

Joanne V. Hickey

This chapter focuses on adults with epilepsy and the nurse's role in assisting patients to self-manage in the community setting and in assisting hospitalized patients with a seizure disorder. Although seizures and epilepsy are common in children, the special considerations related to children with these conditions are not addressed in this chapter. Other resources should be consulted for specific information on childhood and adolescent epilepsy.

Most people with a seizure disorder are managed in the community by a primary care physician or a neurologist. Patients who are difficult to manage may be referred to an epilepsy center where a neurologist with a practice focused on seizure disorders and a multidisciplinary team can provide comprehensive management. In many geographical areas, advanced practice nurses with a focus on seizure management are available to patients and families or as a consultant to other nurses. Almost all nurses who practice in a hospital environment see patients who have a seizure secondary to a primary condition, such as metabolic imbalance. Other nurses may see people with intractable epilepsy who are admitted for surgical intervention. Regardless of the setting in which care is delivered, nurses play an important role in the management and education of patients and their families.

BACKGROUND AND DEFINITIONS

References to epilepsy date back to ancient times, and mystical explanations about seizures continued until the 1870s when Jackson theorized that seizures originated from a localized, discharging focus in the brain. The introduction of the electroencephalogram (EEG) by Berger in 1929 provided the first recordings of epileptic discharges. This landmark event was followed in the 1930s by the work of Gibbs, who correlated the clinical indicators of epilepsy with EEG patterns. The development of classification systems for both epilepsies and seizures has paved the way to a better understanding of the variations in clinical presentation. Research focused on the clinical and cellular bases for seizures, new drugs, and improved management protocols have all contributed to better outcomes for patients subject to seizures.

The terminology for seizures and epilepsy is imprecise. The following widely accepted definitions have helped overcome imprecise terminology, which created confusion about seizures and epilepsy in the past.

- **Seizure:** a single (finite) event of abnormal discharge in the brain that results in an abrupt and temporary altered state of cerebral function.
- **Epilepsy:** a chronic disorder of abnormal, *recurrent*, excessive, and self-terminating discharge from neurons. Periods between seizures can vary widely and can be measured in minutes, hours, days, weeks, months, or even years. However, there is repetition of seizure activity at some time in the future, regardless of the interval. Clinically, epilepsy is characterized by *recurring seizures* accompanied by a disturbance in some type of behavior (i.e., motor, sensory, autonomic, consciousness, or mentation).
- **Seizure disorder:** a term adopted by some clinicians when referring to epilepsy. Although this has led to some confusion, the terms *epilepsy* and *seizure disorder* are used interchangeably.
- **Epileptic syndrome:** an epileptic disorder characterized by a cluster of signs and symptoms customarily occurring together.

Epidemiology and Risk Factors

Epilepsy is one of the most common neurological conditions representing a heterogeneous collection of disorders that have in common a recurrence of seizures. About 1.25 to 2 million people in the United States have epilepsy. Approximately 30% of all epilepsies and about 60% of all childhood epilepsies may have a significant genetic susceptibility. The risk of epilepsy is about 1% from birth through 20 years and 3% for the 70-year and older age group. The prevalence and cumulative incidence of epilepsy and partial seizures increase in the elderly.[1]

A few basic concepts guide understanding of seizures in individuals. First, anyone can have a seizure, given the right circumstances of central nervous system (CNS) imbalance. However, there are differences among people in their threshold for seizures. Second, there is a high likelihood of a chronic seizure disorder in people with specific conditions such as a penetrating brain injury. Third, seizures are episodic, suggesting that triggers precipitate seizure activity.[2]

The major risk factors for developing seizures can be classified according to age group. In young adults, trauma, alcohol withdrawal, illicit drug use, brain tumor, and other central nervous system conditions are the most common causes. In the 35-year and older age group, cerebrovascular disease, brain tumor, alcohol withdrawal, metabolic disorders (e.g., uremia, electrolyte imbalance), Alzheimer's disease, neurodegenerative diseases, and idiopathic causes rank as the major causes of seizures. The term **idiopathic epilepsy** is used for the 70% of all cases for which no specific cause is identified.

Pathophysiology

Seizures are transient episodes of abrupt and temporary alteration of cerebral function resulting from a paroxysmal high-frequency or synchronous low-frequency, high-voltage electrical discharge.[3] Ropper and Brown note that seizures require three conditions: (1) a population of pathologically excitable neurons; (2) an increase in excitatory glutaminergic activity through recurrent connections to spread the discharge; and (3) a reduction in the activity of the normal inhibitory gamma-aminobutyric acid (GABA) projection.[4] Seizures result from an imbalance between excitation and inhibition within the CNS. Excessive excitation or excessive inhibition may occur in focal areas of the cerebral cortex (focal seizures) or over the entire cerebral cortex (generalized seizures). A focal or generalized *increase in neuronal excitability* may result from energy failure of neurons producing transient depolarization or lack of local inhibition.

Epilepsy can also result from alterations in membrane potentials that predispose certain hyperactive and hypersensitive neurons to respond abnormally to changes in the cellular environment. The hypersensitive neurons have lowered thresholds for firing and can fire excessively, creating an **epileptogenic focus** from which the seizure emanates. The epileptogenic focus generates large numbers of autonomous paroxysmal discharges that can be enhanced or minimized, depending on the neurotransmitter that is active on the postsynaptic membrane. An epileptogenic focus can induce secondary epileptogenic foci in a synaptically related area and also in opposite cerebral hemispheres through connecting pathways between the same anatomic areas.

Precipitating Factors: Triggers

In patients with epilepsy, seizures can be precipitated by various stimuli called *triggers*. Sometimes the trigger is very *specific* for a particular person. Common triggers include particular odors, flashing lights, and certain types of music. If a specific stimulus can be identified, then the pattern is called **reflex epilepsy**. Other *general* triggers include fatigue, sleep deprivation, hypoglycemia, emotional stress, electrical shock, febrile illness, alcohol consumption, certain drugs, drinking too much water, constipation, menstruation, and hyperventilation.

Terminology

A few terms describe the general signs and symptoms of seizures:

- **Aura** is a premonitory sensation or warning experienced at the beginning of a seizure, which the patient remembers. An aura may be a gustatory, visual, auditory, or visceral experience, such as a metallic taste or flashing lights. If a patient has an aura, it usually is the same experience each time.
- **Automatisms** are more or less coordinated, involuntary motor activities that occur during a state of impaired consciousness either in the course of or after an epileptic seizure, for which the person is usually amnesic. Several different types of automatism have been recognized. Examples of automatisms are lip smacking, chewing, fidgeting, and pacing.[5] Automatisms are often associated with temporal lobe seizures but can also occur with complex partial seizures as well as with other types.
- **Autonomic symptoms** are symptoms that occur as a result of stimulation of the autonomic nervous system (e.g., epigastric sensation, pallor, sweating, flushing, piloerection, pupillary dilation).
- **Clonus** is a term used to describe spasms in which a continuous pattern of rigidity and relaxation is repeated. In the second phase of a generalized seizure, called the *clonic phase*, rhythmic movements are followed by muscle relaxation. In the clonic phase, the process repeats again and again.
- **Ictus** refers to an actual seizure; a seizure may be referred to as an *ictal event*.
- **Postictal** refers to the period immediately after a seizure has occurred.
- **Prodromal** refers to symptoms, such as a headache or feeling of depression, that precede a seizure by hours.
- **Tonus** is the degree of tone or contraction present in muscle when it is not undergoing shortening.
- **Todd's paralysis** is a temporary, focal weakness or paralysis following a partial or generalized seizure that can last for up to 24 hours. The deficit can be correlated with an epileptic focus on the motor strip. Temporary neuronal exhaustion is probably the physiologic basis for the deficit.

SEIZURE CLASSIFICATION AND OBSERVATIONS/IDENTIFICATION

Seizures and epilepsy have been classified for clinical and research purposes using several different forms. Most of these are complex and cumbersome to use. In 1981, the International League Against Epilepsy (ILAE) published a modified version of the International Classification of Epileptic Seizures that continues to be a useful classification system (Table 29-1).[6]

The following section briefly discusses partial and generalized seizures. Tonic-clonic seizures, as examples of generalized seizures, are described in greater detail because they are so common. Table 29-2 describes the major subtypes of partial and generalized seizures, and Table 29-3 classifies partial seizures by cerebral lobe involved.

Partial Seizures

Three types of partial seizures are recognized: *simple, complex,* and *evolving into secondary generalized seizures.* Simple

TABLE 29-1   CLASSIFICATION OF SEIZURES

I. Partial (focal, local) seizures
   A. Simple partial seizures (consciousness not impaired)
      1. Focal motor (with and without jacksonian march)
      2. Somatosensory or special sensory symptoms (e.g., simple hallucinations such as tingling, light flashing, buzzing)
      3. With autonomic symptoms (e.g., as epigastric sensation, pallor, flushing)
      4. With psychic symptoms (disturbances of higher cerebral function)
   B. Complex partial seizures (with impairment of consciousness)
      1. Beginning as simple partial seizures and progressing to impairment of consciousness
      2. With no other features
      3. With features as in simple partial seizures
      4. With automatism
   C. With impairment of consciousness at onset
      1. With no other features
      2. With features as in simple partial seizures
      3. With automatism
   D. Partial seizures evolving to secondarily generalized seizures
      1. Simple partial seizures evolving to generalized seizures
      2. Complex partial seizures evolving to generalized seizures
      3. Simple partial seizures evolving to complex partial seizures to generalized seizures
II. Generalized seizures (generalized bilateral without focal onset)
   A. Absence seizures
   B. Myoclonic seizures
   C. Clonic seizures
   D. Tonic seizures
   E. Tonic-clonic seizures
   F. Atonic seizures
III. Unclassified epileptic seizures (including all seizures that cannot be classified due to inadequate or incomplete data and some that defy classification)

From Commission on Classification and Terminology of the International League Against Epilepsy. (1981). Proposal for revised clinical and electroencephalographic classification of epileptic seizures. *Epilepsia, 22,* 489–501.

and complex seizures are distinguished on the sole basis of consciousness. When consciousness is not impaired, the seizure is classified as a **simple partial seizure**; if consciousness is impaired, the seizure is classified as a **complex partial seizure**. The four subcategories of simple partial seizures are named for the areas of their presenting symptoms: *motor, sensory, autonomic,* and *psychic*. Complex partial seizures include both complex symptomatology and impaired consciousness. Another term for complex symptomatology is *automatisms*. These seizures consist of involuntary, but coordinated, motor activity that is purposeless and repetitive. The final category is a partial seizure evolving into a generalized seizure. These seizures are further categorized based on the type of partial seizure that preceded the generalized seizure (i.e., simple partial seizure only, complex partial seizure only, or simple partial seizure evolving into complex partial seizure).[7] On EEG, partial seizures are noted as focal epileptiform discharges with spikes or sharp waves.

Generalized Seizures

There are six categories of generalized seizures: *absence, myoclonic, clonic, tonic, tonic-clonic,* and *atonic*. Each seizure type has characteristic clinical and EEG findings that are outlined in Table 29-2. The absence seizure is subdivided into typical and atypical absence seizures according to the presence of different EEG patterns and clinical presentation. Clinically, atypical absence seizures have a less abrupt onset and termination and are of a longer duration. The most common type of generalized seizure is the **tonic-clonic seizure**, formerly called the *grand mal seizure*.

Description of Generalized Tonic-Clonic Seizures

A tonic-clonic seizure progresses through distinct phases including the prodromal, tonic, clonic, and postictal phases. The **prodromal phase** of irritability and tension may precede the seizure by several hours or days. Some individuals experience an aura, whereas in others the seizure begins without warning. Characteristically, the tonic-clonic seizure begins with a sudden loss of consciousness. Neuronal hyperexcitation spreads to the subcortex, thalamus, and upper brainstem, and consciousness is suddenly lost. In the **tonic phase,** there is a major tonic contraction (increased tonus) of the voluntary muscles so that the body stiffens with legs and arms extended. If standing, the person falls to the ground. The jaw snaps shut and the tongue may be bitten in the process. A shrill cry may be heard because of the forcible exhalation of air through the closed vocal cords as the thoracic muscles initially contract. The bladder and, less often, the bowel may empty. The pupils dilate and are unresponsive to light. Apnea occurs and lasts for only a few seconds, but the patient may appear pale and dusty. The tonic phase lasts less than 1 minute (average of 15 seconds).

The **clonic phase** begins with a gradual transition from the tonicity of the tonic phase. Inhibitory neurons of the cortex, anterior thalamus, and basal ganglion nuclei become active, intermittently interrupting the tonic seizure discharge with clonic activity. The clonic phase is characterized by violent, rhythmic, muscular contractions accompanied by hyperventilation. The face is contorted, the eyes roll, and there is excessive salivation with frothing from the mouth. Profuse sweating and a tachycardia are common.

In the **postictal phase,** the clonic jerking gradually subsides in frequency and amplitude over a period of about 30 seconds, although it may be longer. The involved cells cease firing. The extremities are limp, breathing is quiet, and the pupils, which may be equal or unequal, begin to respond to the light reflex. With awakening, most patients are confused, disoriented, and amnesic for the event. Headache, generalized muscle aching, and fatigue are common. If undisturbed, the patient often falls into a deep sleep for several hours. There may also be temporary paresis, aphasia, or hemianopsia. Following a seizure (i.e., generalized or partial), focal weakness, called **Todd's paralysis,** may occur and last up to 24 hours. If it occurs, the focal deficit is important in localization of a focal epileptogenic site.

Because the seizure frequently occurs without warning, it is possible for injury to be sustained from falls or other accidents related to the seizure. Head injury, fracture of the limbs or vertebral column, and burns are examples of serious injuries that may be sustained. Tonic-clonic seizures may occur at any time of the day or night, whether the patient is awake or asleep. The frequency of recurrence can vary from hours to weeks, months, or years.

TABLE 29-2 MAJOR SUBTYPES OF PARTIAL AND GENERALIZED SEIZURES

TYPE	DESCRIPTION	EEG FINDINGS
Partial Seizures		
Simple partial seizures • Motor	• Symptoms depend on the motor region activated • May remain focal or may spread to other areas on the motor strip, a process called "march"; seizures called jacksonian seizures. For example, the seizure may begin in the fingers of one side, and march to the hand, wrist, forearm, and arm on the same side of the body. The particular sequence of involvement is helpful in locating the epileptic foci on the motor strip in the hemisphere opposite the convulsive movement. • Focal motor attack may cause head to turn to side opposite epileptic foci. • Todd's paralysis may result; last minutes to hours. • Continuous focal motor seizure is called *epilepsia partialis continua.*	*Applies to all simple partial seizures:* may show abnormal discharges in a very limited region; seizures originating from deep structures may not be noted with scalp electrodes
• Sensory	• Arise from cortical sensory strip. • Usually feels like "pins and needles" or numbness; sometimes, spatial disorientation. • May march to other areas or may become a complex partial or generalized tonic-clonic seizure. • Special sensory symptoms may include visual seizures such as flashing lights or visual hallucinations, auditory seizures with various sounds, gustatory sensations such as metallic taste or primary tastes (salty, sweet, sour, or bitter), or vertigo and floating sensations.	
• Autonomic • Psychic	• May occur as simple partial seizures. • Disturbance in a higher-level function (i.e., distortion of memory), distorted time, feeling of déjà vu, illusions, depersonalization, or hallucinations. • Usually occur with impairment of consciousness and become complex partial seizures.	
Complex Partial Seizures		
One category	• Only symptoms may be impaired consciousness or it may progress to include automatisms; note *automatisms* may occur in partial or generalized seizures. • Simple partial seizure followed by impairment of consciousness resulting in a complex seizure with motor, sensory, autonomic, or psychic symptoms as described above.	*All complex seizures:* generalized 2–4-Hz spike waves
Partial Seizures Evolving to Secondary Generalized Seizures		
One category	Includes seizures that may evolve into generalized seizures: simple partial, complex partial, or simple partial evolving into complex and then to generalized seizures.	
Generalized Seizures		
• Absence seizures *Note:* may be seen along with tonic-clonic seizures	*Typical absence seizures:* common in children; characterized by brief interruption in consciousness without loss of postural control. Typically, there is an interruption of activity with a momentary lapse of consciousness lasting 3 to 30 sec. If talking, the speech stops or slows; if eating, the hand and mouth stop, and if patient is called, there is no response. • During an attack, the eyes may appear vacant, stare, or roll upward; the eyelids may twitch. • Seizures occur a few times to hundreds of times per day; person may not be aware of them. • People who have several attacks daily most often experience difficulty in learning or employment because of inattention. *Atypical absence seizures*—the lapse of consciousness is usually of longer duration and less abrupt in onset; more obvious motor signs.	*Typical absences:* 3-Hz spike-wave complexes with abrupt starts and stops *Atypical absences:* ≤2.5 Hz; slower spike-and-wave pattern, and more irregular

(continued)

TABLE 29–2 MAJOR SUBTYPES OF PARTIAL AND GENERALIZED SEIZURES (*Continued*)

TYPE	DESCRIPTION	EEG FINDINGS
• Myoclonic seizures	• Sporadic jerks that are sudden, brief; contractions that are usually symmetric. • When confined to one area, it may be the face and trunk; one or more extremities; an individual muscle; or a muscle group. • Myoclonic jerks are rapidly repetitive or relatively isolated. • Common around time of sleep or awakening; must be differentiated from myoclonic jerks of nonepileptic myoclonus.	Bilateral, generalized epileptiform discharges, typically polyspikes
• Clonic seizures	• Repetitive rhythmic clonic movements that are bilateral and symmetric.	Associated with symmetric spikewave complexes
• Tonic seizures	• Stiffening of the musculature, mostly of the body, but may also involve the arms.	Low-voltage paroxysmal fast activity (10 Hz)
• Atonic seizures	• Abrupt loss of postural muscle tone; last 1–2 sec. • Consciousness is briefly impaired, but usually there is not postictal confusion. • Common in children.	Generalized epileptiform discharges (spikes, spike-wave complexes)
• Tonic-clonic seizures	• Most common of the generalized seizures (see p. 648 for detailed description).	Fast high-voltage spikes seen in all leads

Unclassified Epileptic Seizures

One category	This group includes all seizures that cannot be classified because of inadequate or incomplete data. This self-explanatory category is a catch-all for seizures that do not conform to any of the other headings.

TABLE 29–3 SEIZURE ACTIVITY OF PARTIAL SEIZURES (SIMPLE, COMPLEX, AND SECONDARY GENERALIZED) BY LOBE

CEREBRAL HEMISPHERE LOBE	DESCRIPTION
Frontal lobe epilepsy	• Many overlapping syndromes with frequent brief attacks (<30 sec) • Simple complex seizures • Focal motor seizures (from motor strip) • Supplemental area motor seizures • Tonic and postural signs and symptoms with preserved consciousness; frequent falls • Complex partial seizures • Complex motor activity, vocalization, and gestural automatism (may be sexual) • Common to proceed to secondarily generalized tonic-clonic seizures

Mesial temporal lobe epilepsy	• Most common cause is hippocampal sclerosis
	• Mostly complex partial seizures with automatisms and psychic symptoms
	• Often preceded by an aura in 50%–95% of patients; rising epigastric discomfort is the most common aura
	• Seizure may include:
	  Staring
	  Oral or manual automatisms
	  Olfactory and auditory illusions or hallucinations
	  Unilateral dystonic posturing

Parietal lobe epilepsy	• Usually simple complex and secondarily generalized seizures • >75% have somatosensory auras • May have a distorted body image, visual or auditory hallucinations • Usually proceeds to impaired consciousness and contralateral motor activity
Occipital lobe epilepsy	• Most have visual auras • Elemental visual hallucinations (e.g., flashing lights, colored lights) or sometimes blindness, scotoma, or hemianopsia • Eye blinking, nystagmus, head deviation, tonic and clonic eye movement common • Visual phenomena usually contralateral to side of the seizure • Often progress to complex partial seizures or secondarily generalized seizure depending on pathways stimulated

Status Epilepticus

Although there are many definitions for **status epilepticus**, it is generally defined as *either continuous seizures lasting at least 5 minutes or two or more discrete seizures between which there is incomplete recovery of consciousness.*[8] The most common cause of status epilepticus is an abrupt discontinuation of antiepileptic drugs (AEDs). Other causes include withdrawal from alcohol, sedatives, or fever.

Clinically, status epilepticus can present with obvious tonic, clonic, or tonic-clonic movements; with subtle twitching of the hand or face; or with absence of movement. Absence of observable movement is most commonly seen in hospitalized patients. In this case, the detection of ongoing seizures requires electroencephalography.

With tonic-clonic seizure, the most common type of status epilepticus, the patient is unconscious. Convulsive seizures can be easily observed clinically, but partial seizures are less obvious and more difficult to identify. Subclinical seizures are seizures that do not present with overt clinical signs and symptoms but are apparent on continuous EEG tracing. Suspicion of subclinical seizure should be considered in patients who seem to be improving generally but have not regained consciousness. Continuous EEG monitoring can assist in the recognition of this serious problem. Therefore, an EEG or continuous EEG monitoring is required for any patient with significant alterations in consciousness or when unconsciousness is sustained.

Status epilepticus constitutes a *medical emergency* associated with significant morbidity and mortality (20%). If not treated aggressively, cardiorespiratory dysfunction, hyperthermia, and metabolic imbalances can develop, leading to cerebral ischemia and neuronal death. Treatment of status epilepticus is discussed later in this chapter

Epileptic Versus Nonepileptic Seizures

Seizures may also be classified as either epileptic or nonepileptic. Epileptic seizures include partial and generalized seizures discussed earlier. **Nonepileptic seizures** or **nonepileptic events** account for about 20% of referrals to epilepsy centers. Clinically, the signs and symptoms can look like seizures, but there is no epileptogenic origin. Nonepileptic seizures include physiologic events, psychogenic events, and malingering.[9]

Cardiac, respiratory, metabolic derangement, and drug toxicity can disturb consciousness as a result of decreased oxygen tension to the brain. Perfusion problems as a result of transient ischemic attacks, stroke, or Stokes-Adams syndrome account for underlying cardiac or cerebrovascular problems. Decreased oxygen tension from poor saturation can result from pneumonia, pulmonary emboli, shunting, or coma. Metabolic causes such as hypoglycemia and electrolyte imbalance can cause nonepileptic events. Toxicity resulting from use of street drugs or prescription drugs, including AEDs; alcohol toxicity; and environmental exposures to toxic substances such as lead can also result in nonepileptic seizures.

Differentiation between nonepileptic psychogenic seizures and epileptic seizures can be made only through analysis of simultaneous EEG tracings and audio-video monitoring during a seizure.[10] The audio-video portion records the behaviors of the peri-ictal events, and the EEG demonstrates the presence or absence of abnormal tracings associated with epileptic seizures. The behavior is triggered by psychogenic internal or external factors. The basis for psychogenic nonepileptic events is secondary gains for the individual such as sympathy or relief from unwanted responsibilities.

Observations/Identification

Physiologic causes of nonepileptic seizures must be ruled out with a basic diagnostic work-up of a thorough history, physical examination, and laboratory screening.

With nonepileptic psychogenic seizures, the onset is often dramatic, bizarre, gradual, and in the presence of witnesses. By comparison, epileptic seizures are sudden, paroxysmal, and orderly. Emotional upset usually precipitates nonepileptic seizures, and such an episode lasts longer than a true seizure. The dramatic, violent flinging of the extremities, wiry movements, and inconsistent pattern of development are a sharp contrast to the tonic-clonic, orderly, repetitive movements of true seizures. If a scream is heard during a true seizure, it is at the onset of the event. With nonepileptic seizures, screams are usually heard throughout the course of the episode. Observing the features, development, and finale of seizure activity can be most helpful in differentiating between epileptic and nonepileptic seizures.

DIAGNOSIS

The first step in the evaluation of a patient with possible epilepsy is to determine whether the patient did or did not have a seizure. The diagnostic process requires a past medical history and a careful history of the clinical presentation and events related to the alleged seizure. The history is followed by a general physical and neurological examination and diagnostic testing. A prenatal history and achievement of developmental milestones are very important in infants, children, and adolescents. In adults, a history of trauma, drug use, and toxic environmental exposure are critical. Detailed descriptive information about the seizures is collected, including onset and surrounding events such as fever or withdrawal from alcohol, prodromal or aura experiences, precipitating factors, frequency, loss of consciousness, subjective and objective characteristics of the event, postictal behavior, and any injuries associated with seizures. In addition to the usual baseline blood chemistries, a toxicology screen (e.g., drug levels, barbiturates, street drugs, and lead) may be helpful for some, based on history. Other diagnostic tests that may be ordered include:

- Computed tomography (CT) scan
- Magnetic resonance imaging (MRI) (two to three times more sensitive than CT scan in identifying potential epileptogenic lesions)
- EEG
- Video-EEG monitoring with either noninvasive scalp electrodes or deep invasive electrodes

- Possibly a positron emission tomography (PET) scan (limited availability due to high expense)
- Single proton emission computerized tomography (SPECT) scan (helpful for seizure localization and not diagnosis)

Most patients do not require all diagnostic tests listed, whereas others may require additional studies. The objective of the studies is to identify systemic or CNS processes that are manifested, in part, by seizure activity. For many patients, an extensive search for an underlying etiology will yield negative results. The diagnosis of epilepsy is made after ruling out other possible causes (discussed later). The clinical presentation and EEG findings help classify the particular type of epilepsy. Accurate diagnosis of seizure type is important because selection of appropriate drug therapy is seizure specific in many cases. The EEG is a vital diagnostic procedure because it identifies patterns of abnormal electrical activity that can be correlated with particular types of seizure patterns. An EEG can also aid in lateralization and localization of an epileptogenic trigger focus. However, in about 50% to 60% of patients with confirmed epilepsy, the interictal EEG can be normal.

Several special techniques are useful in augmenting the data from an EEG. A sleep study, in which there is continuous EEG monitoring, is helpful because sleep activates anterior temporal spike discharges and bitemporal discharges in 80% to 90% of persons with complex partial seizures. The increased interictal epileptiform abnormalities are noted most in non–rapid eye movement (non-REM) sleep. Sleep deprivation also increases the frequency of interictal abnormalities. Extra scalp electrodes, nasopharyngeal electrodes, and sphenoid electrodes help to increase the detection of mesial temporal discharges. The ability to detect and localize abnormal ictal discharges in complex partial seizures is greatly enhanced with the use of invasive procedures such as depth, subdural, and cortical electrodes. Surface electrodes often provide false localization.[11] Simultaneous EEG and audiovideo recordings of the patient can distinguish seizure from nonseizure activity and assist in classifying seizure type.

Differential Diagnosis

Given the long list of possible causes of seizure activity, diagnosis can become very difficult. Differentiation between epileptic and nonepileptic seizures (discussed earlier) must be made. Brain tumor, cerebral aneurysm, cerebral arteriovenous malformation, transient ischemic attacks, stroke, migraine headaches, syncope, sleep disorders, myoclonus, cardiac sources, drug and alcohol abuse, drug toxicity, metabolic disorders, breath holding, and psychogenic problems such as anxiety attacks, hysterical responses, and psychosis are some of the possibilities that must be excluded. Nevertheless, accurate classification of seizure type is important to specific treatment choices.

Electroencephalograms and Seizures

The EEG is a diagnostic test during which the amplified electrical potential of the brain is recorded by placing 14 to 21 electrodes on the patient's scalp. Electrodes may also be placed on the cortical surface using an invasive procedure. The tracings reflect the combined electrical activity of several neurons, rather than only one. The basic resting electrical pattern of the brain is altered by opening the eyes, focusing attention on a problem, hyperventilation, photic stimulation, drugs, or sleep. Therefore, recordings are taken at rest, after hyperventilation, during stimulation with a strobe light, and during sleep. The patient must be quiet, relaxed, cooperative, able to follow directions, and seated comfortably in a chair with the eyes closed, although not asleep. The testing room must be shielded from extraneous electrical interference and noise. Often, preparation for the EEG includes keeping the patient awake all night before the recordings. The stress of sleep deprivation is more apt to result in the recording of abnormal EEG tracings.

Even though the EEG is important in diagnosing seizures, these data must be considered in conjunction with other information, including the history, physical examination, and other laboratory studies. Between seizures, normal EEGs are often recorded in patients with epilepsy. In addition, EEGs that are considered to be "borderline" by one interpreter may be read as normal by another, indicating subjectivity in interpretation.

The tracings for the EEG are made with special ink on electromagnetic paper. The recorded tracings signify the electrical potential difference from the scalp to the ear electrodes and from the scalp to the scalp electrodes. The average EEG consists of 150 to 300 or more pages of recordings, with each page accounting for 10 seconds of tracings. In the normal adult, the most characteristic, normal tracings noted at rest are as follows:

Alpha waves: 8 to 12 Hz (Hz = cycles per minute)
Beta waves: 18 to 30 Hz, a faster wave, seen in the anterior areas of the brain

Both alpha and beta waves are bilaterally symmetric. Each has its own characteristic shape and amplitude. Changes occur in the normal EEG pattern with various activities. For example, when the eyes are opened, there is an immediate decrease in the amplitude of the brain waves; in the early stages of sleep, the waves slow (lower voltage); and in the later stages of sleep, "sleep spindles," occurring at a rate of 14 to 16 Hz, develop with subsequent higher voltage and slower waves.

Patients with seizure disorders have abnormal recordings on their EEGs. The most common abnormal findings include:

Delta waves: less than 4 Hz with high amplitude; often associated with destruction of brain tissue, such as occurs with infarction, tumor, or abscess (localized over abnormal area)
Theta waves: 4 to 7 Hz (not always abnormal)
Spikes or **sharp waves:** high-voltage, faster waves; asymmetry of frequency and amplitude from one side to the other

On an abnormal EEG, slow and fast waves may be combined in paroxysmal runs, thereby interrupting the normal pattern. These paroxysmal waves are highly suggestive of epilepsy. Recordings taken between seizures in the epileptic patient often include isolated spikes without evidence of a clinical seizure.

TREATMENT

The approach to a patient with a seizure disorder is multidimensional and comprehensive. It includes:

- Treatment of any underlying condition
- Avoidance of precipitating factors
- Suppression of recurrent seizures by prophylactic therapy with AEDs or surgery
- Comprehensive management of physiologic and social issues related to having seizures

An individual plan of care must be developed for each patient. If there is an underlying problem responsible for seizures, it must be addressed. For example, if the diagnostic work-up revealed a brain tumor as the cause of seizures, the primary problem, the brain tumor, must be treated. Seizures related to the brain tumor can be managed with AEDs. If the diagnosis is epilepsy, identification of the specific type of epilepsy is imperative in developing an effective treatment plan.

After epilepsy has been diagnosed, the patient needs to be made aware of precipitating factors and taught to avoid these situations or conditions. About 75% of patients with epilepsy can be managed satisfactorily with AEDs. Surgery is considered for a small group of patients for whom an epileptogenic focus can be identified or in whom seizures are intractable even with drug therapy. In addition to drug therapy, the management plan must address the behavioral, social, and economic consequences of having epilepsy. For successful adaptation to this chronic problem, it is critical that patients receive education in self-management. Patient counseling and support are also essential components of the management plan.

Medical Management: Drug Therapy

Epilepsy treatment seeks to enable the patient to live as free of the medical and psychosocial complications of seizures as is possible. Pharmacologic therapeutics play a large role in helping to achieve this goal. As with any drug therapy, there is concern about side effects, toxicity, ease of administration, efficacy, and effect on different age groups. Management of epilepsy is complicated by the range of age of patients, the number of categories of drugs, and the psychosocial impacts involved.

Effective drug treatment for epilepsy has two goals: to control or reduce the frequency of seizures, and to minimize side effects. AEDs do not cure epilepsy but provide a chemical means of controlling seizures. As with any drug, side effects, such as sedation, may interfere with activities of daily living. Therefore, effective medical management includes the development of an *individualized* drug program that minimizes side effects and supports compliance.

After a diagnosis has been made, the following principles should guide use of drugs[12]:

- Assess the patient (diagnosis of seizure type and classification, patient characteristics such as age and presence of comorbidity, and insurance drug coverage).
- Select the primary drug that is the most effective for the seizure type; monotherapy is preferred, and about 70% of patients with epilepsy can be maintained on one drug.
- Begin with monotherapy and titrate dosage to achieve appropriate blood concentrations and control.
- Consider the pharmacokinetics of AEDs and free AED concentrations.
- Provide patient education.
- Provide follow-up to assess control, tolerance, and side effects.
- Consider the length of time the patient has been taking AEDs.

Selecting the Primary Drug Most Effective for the Seizure Type

The classifications of epileptic seizures and epilepsies/epileptic syndromes has made easier the selection of the drug of choice for a given seizure problem. Seizure types and drugs of choice plus alternative drug options are outlined in Table 29-4. Table 29-5 outlines the management of status epilepticus.

Some AEDs have a narrow spectrum of action and are effective for only a selected seizure type, whereas other

TABLE 29-4   ANTIEPILEPTIC DRUGS AND RELATED SEIZURE TYPES

	PRIMARY GENERALIZED TONIC-CLONIC	PARTIAL (I.E., SIMPLE, COMPLEX, AND SECONDARY GENERALIZED SEIZURES)	ABSENCE	ATYPICAL ABSENCE, MYOCLONIC, AND ATONIC
First-line drugs	• Valproic acid • Lamotrigine	• Carbamazepine • Valproic acid • Phenytoin • Lamotrigine • Phenobarbital	• Ethosuximide • Valproic acid	• Valproic acid
Alternative drugs	• Primidone • Carbamazepine • Topiramate • Phenobarbital • Felbamate	• Topiramate • Tiagabine • Primidone • Zonisamide • Gabapentin • Tiagabine	• Methsuximide • Lamotrigine • Clonazepam	• Lamotrigine • Clonazepam • Felbamate

Data from Holland, K. D. (2001). Epilepsy: Efficacy, pharmacology, and adverse effects of antiepileptic drugs. *Neurologic Clinics, 19*(2), 313–345; Ropper, A. H., & Brown, R. H. (2005). *Adams and Victor's principles of neurology* (8th ed., pp. 292–293). New York: McGraw-Hill; and Lowenstein, D. H. (2005). Seizures and epilepsy. In D. L. Kasper, E. Braunwald, A. S. Fauci, S. L. Hauser, D. L. Longo, & J. L. Jameson (Eds.). *Harrison's principles of internal medicine* (16th ed., p. 2367). New York: McGraw-Hill.

TABLE 29–5　MANAGEMENT OF STATUS EPILEPTICUS

TIME LINE IN MIN	DRUG THERAPY (PROGRESSION ALONG THIS ALGORITHM ASSUMES THAT THE PREVIOUS DRUG ADMINISTERED DID NOT TERMINATE THE SEIZURES)
0–3	**1. Lorazepam (Ativan):** 0.1 mg/kg IV at 2 mg/min *Note:* additional emergency therapy may not be needed if the seizures terminate *Seizures continue*
4–23	**2. Phenytoin (Dilantin):** 20 mg/kg (about 1 g) in normal saline at a rate of 50 mg/min OR **Fosphenytoin** (20 mg/kg PE (PE = phenytoin equivalent) intravenously at 150 mg/min) *Seizures continue*
22–33	**3. Phenytoin:** (additional) 5–10 mg/kg OR **Fosphenytoin** 5–10 mg/kg PE *Seizures continue* **Proceed immediately to step (6) anesthesia with midazolam or propofol if:** • Patient develops status epilepticus while in the ICU • Patient has severe systemic problems (e.g., extreme hyperthermia) • Patient has seizures that have continued for more than 60–90 min
37–58	**4. Phenobarbital:** 20 mg/kg IV at 50–75 mg/min *Seizures continue*
58–68	**5. Phenobarbital:** additional 5–10 mg/kg *Seizures continue* **6. Anesthesia with midazolam or propofol**

Lowenstein, D. H., & Alldredge, B. K. (1998). Status epilepticus. *New England Journal of Medicine, 338*(14), 970–976.

drugs are broad spectrum and effective against many different types of seizures. Drugs also have different mechanisms of action. Some types of seizures can be exacerbated by AEDs designed to treat another seizure type. For example, carbamazepine, useful for partial seizures, can exacerbate absence seizures. Phenytoin, phenobarbital, and carbamazepine, which are effective in controlling generalized tonic-clonic seizures and partial seizures, are ineffective for absence seizures and may actually precipitate an increase in their incidence. In addition, with a broad-spectrum drug that can be used for various seizure types, the therapeutic range may differ for different seizure types. For example, blood concentrations for complex partial seizures may need to be higher than the concentration for tonic-clonic generalized seizures.

In addition to a particular seizure type, patient characteristics influence drug selection. The plan of care must be individualized to consider age, comorbidity, liver and kidney function, previous drug history for allergies, tolerance of side effects, cost, other drug therapy and potential interactions, and child-bearing potential.

Principles of Drug Therapy: Begin With Monotherapy and Titrate the Dosage to Achieve Appropriate Blood Concentrations

The following are principles recommended for seizure management:

- Begin with a single drug, called monotherapy, which is the drug of choice for the particular seizure type.
- Increase the drug gradually over 3 to 4 weeks until seizure control is achieved, intolerable side effects occur, toxicity develops, or the maximum therapeutic range has been reached.
- Recognize that many AEDs are CNS depressants and that drowsiness, lethargy, and tiredness are common in the beginning of therapy; however, these symptoms will usually subside in 7 to 10 days.
- Because of pharmacokinetics (cited later) and variations in requirements for specific seizure types with the same drug, expect to make individual adjustments in dosage.
- Some patients may need more or less than the recommended average therapeutic range for a particular drug.
- Titrate a single drug until maximum benefit is achieved or intolerance or serious side effects occur. If a therapeutic blood concentration has been achieved and seizure control has not been achieved, a second drug may be added. A second drug may be used in combination with the first or replace the first. With replacement, the first drug should be *gradually tapered* after the second drug has been titrated to the desired dosage. This practice is necessary because the sudden withdrawal of a drug can cause status epilepticus, even though a new drug has been introduced in its place.
- If the patient is seizure free, check drug concentration in blood after 5 to 8 half-lives or a period of 3 to 4 weeks.
- The drug's half-life is important because drugs of long duration (phenytoin, phenobarbital) may be taken once daily in some circumstances.
- Have the patient keep a daily *drug diary* routinely, but especially when a new drug is introduced. The diary should include dosage and side effects. The diary is helpful in evaluating the effectiveness of the drug therapy.

Refractory Epilepsy. About one third of patients with epilepsy do not respond well to treatment with monotherapy. It then becomes necessary to try a combination of drugs to control seizures. Although there are no guidelines for combining drugs, in most instances a combination of two first-line drugs (i.e., carbamazepine, phenytoin, valproic acid, lamotrigine) is tried. If this is not effective, adding one of the newer drugs (i.e., gabapentin or topiramate) is suggested. When seizures cannot be controlled by drug therapy, the condition is called refractory epilepsy and surgery becomes a consideration.

Considering Pharmacokinetics and Free Antiepileptic Drug Concentrations

The pharmacokinetics of AEDs are important to keep in mind. Many AEDs are highly bound to plasma protein. It is the unbound, or "free," concentration that represents the active drug capable of penetrating the blood–brain barrier and interacting with receptor sites. For this reason, patients on high-protein tube feeding will require a higher drug dosage to maintain adequate drug blood levels. Conditions known to alter AEDs' protein-binding capacity are malnutrition, older age, pregnancy, hypoalbuminemia, burns, liver disease, and chronic renal failure. The following are plasma protein-binding capacities for selected AEDs:

- Phenytoin and valproic acid (high protein binding)
- Carbamazepine (variable binding)
- Phenobarbital and primidone (minimal binding)
- Ethosuximide (not bound)

Although therapeutic ranges are cited for each drug, patients vary with regard to pharmacokinetics. Therefore, dosage requirements for individual patients vary. For determining dosage, use the "gold standard" that the patient should become seizure free. The onset of serious side effects or intolerance is a reason to discontinue a drug. Clinical judgment must be used and patient response and blood levels must be monitored to determine the ideal dose and blood concentration for a patient.

Patient Education

Patient education is the cornerstone of drug therapy and promotes a partnership that supports compliance. Patients who understand the purpose of drug therapy and the drugs that they are taking are more compliant. Patient education must be an ongoing process with reinforcement and updates at each appointment. Because many patients are on long-term or life-long therapy, education must also anticipate and prepare patients for developmental changes and changes in normal life routine. If they are to provide comprehensive patient management, health care providers who treat patients with seizures must develop and implement an individualized teaching plan that includes how to initiate and provide ongoing patient education.

Considering Length of Time on Antiepileptic Drug Therapy

Whether AED therapy must be life-long depends on many factors. About 60% of adults who have their seizures completely controlled with AEDs can eventually discontinue therapy. The following conditions are recommended: seizures are controlled for 1 to 5 years; seizures are of a single type (partial or generalized); there is a normal neurological examination; and the patient has a normal EEG.[2] The American Academy of Neurology has noted that after at least a 2-year seizure-free period, health care providers can explore discontinuation of AEDs by gradually tapering them over 2 to 3 months.[13,14] Many individual considerations, such as psychological issues and patient comfort, should be included in the decision. The risk of recurrent seizures is greatest during the first 3 months after discontinuation of AEDs. State laws vary on loss of driving privileges for persons with seizures. In general, most states allow patients to drive after a seizure-free period (on or off medications) of between 3 months and 2 years.[2]

Nursing management associated with a few commonly ordered drugs is discussed below. These drugs include phenytoin, fosphenytoin, carbamazepine, valproic acid, and phenobarbital. More information on drug therapy can be found in Chapter 12.

Phenytoin

Phenytoin (Dilantin), introduced in 1938, is a synthetic drug that is classified as a hydantoin. It is used for the treatment of simple partial, complex partial, and generalized tonic-clonic seizures. It is not effective for absence, myoclonic, or atonic seizures. Phenytoin blocks posttetanic potentiation (PTP) by influencing synaptic transmission through voltage-sensitive sodium channels. Phenytoin is primarily absorbed through the duodenum. There is no first-pass metabolism. Oral absorption is affected by the particle size of the particular brand's formulation so that *there can be variations among brands.* The brand of phenytoin that a patient is receiving should not be switched without careful monitoring. Phenytoin enters the brain quickly and is then redistributed to other body tissues, including breast milk. It crosses the placenta and reaches a state of equilibrium with the mother and fetus. Phenytoin is bound to serum and tissue protein. In the serum, the drug binds primarily to albumin in a predictable, linear fashion provided that the albumin level is normal (see the exceptions in the previous section). Phenytoin is metabolized in the liver and excreted in the urine. At an often unpredictable concentration level, metabolism of phenytoin ceases because of saturation. Any change in dosage at this point will result in significant changes in serum concentrations. In addition, serum concentration does not decline at a predictable linear rate when phenytoin is discontinued. Therefore, serum monitoring is necessary after any dosage change. Because the half-life of phenytoin is 10 to 34 hours (average 22 hours), it may be given once daily.

Administration of phenytoin may be oral or intravenous (IV). Because the pH of phenytoin is about 12, intramuscular (IM) injection should be avoided to prevent tissue irritation. Oral phenytoin comes in three dosage forms. The tablets and suspension contain phenytoin acid, whereas the capsules contain phenytoin sodium. Phenytoin sodium is 92% phenytoin. The parenteral form is phenytoin sodium. If they contain equivalent amounts of phenytoin acid, tablets, capsules, and suspension have the same bioavailability. Phenytoin capsules are designated as immediate release or extended release. Only the extended release should be used for once-daily dosing. The suspension form comes in two strengths; either can settle and thus deliver doses of unequal concentration. To maintain an even blood level, patients on enteral feeding will probably need increased dosage due to the high protein binding of phenytoin. After enteral feeding has been discontinued, the dosage must be decreased. Monitoring phenytoin blood levels provides a guide for adjusting the drug dosage.

If phenytoin is administered IV, it must be administered slowly, at a rate no faster than 50 mg/min in *a solution of normal saline. Maintaining the proper rate is very important because rapid administration depresses the myocardium and can cause cardiac arrhythmias and cardiac arrest.* If given in solution such as 5% dextrose in water, the drug will precipitate into crystals in the solution. If given by IV push, it must be given slowly (no more than 50 mg/min); the effect of rapid administration of phenytoin on the myocardium is dangerous arrhythmias. Patients receiving IV phenytoin should also be observed for the development of phlebitis at the IV site.

Various drugs in common use can interact with phenytoin:

- Drugs that *potentiate* the action of phenytoin include aspirin, cimetidine, chloramphenicol, felbamate, methsuximide, fluconazole, isoniazid, disulfiram (Antabuse), propoxyphene, sulfonamides, and warfarin.
- Drugs that *decrease* the action of phenytoin include antacids, barbiturates, antihistamines, calcium, calcium

gluconate, chronic alcohol, carbamazepine, folic acid, valproic acid, and vigabatrin.

- Phenytoin *decreases* the action of amiodarone, carbamazepine, corticosteroids, cyclosporine, digitalis, dopamine, estrogen, furosemide, haloperidol, oral contraceptives, phenothiazines, quinidine, and sulfonylureas.

There are many potential side effects from phenytoin. Lethargy, fatigue, incoordination, visual blurring, higher cortical dysfunction, and drowsiness are related to CNS depressant effects. When serum concentrations exceed 20 μ/mL, patients may experience nystagmus, ataxia, and slurred speech. A morbilliform rash may occur in some patients 7 to 14 days after beginning the drug. The appearance of such a rash indicates that the drug should be discontinued. A lupus-like syndrome has also been reported and is reversible when phenytoin is withdrawn.

Effects seen with long-term, chronic use include gingival hyperplasia (about 50% of patients), decreased cognitive ability, osteomalacia, hirsutism, hypothyroidism, peripheral neuropathy, megaloblastic anemia, blood dyscrasias, and low serum folate concentrations. Periodic complete blood cell counts (CBCs) are important to monitor the development of anemia or dyscrasias. The low folic acid levels respond to folic acid therapy. There is an increased incidence of malformations in children born of women who are taking AEDs.

Fosphenytoin

Fosphenytoin (Cerebyx) is a water-soluble drug that is rapidly and completely converted to phenytoin after IV or IM administration and has a conversion half-life of 8 to 15 minutes. However, protein binding for fosphenytoin is exceedingly high and nonlinear. Therefore, fosphenytoin displaces phenytoin from albumin, thus increasing the unbound phenytoin concentration. This increase in unbound concentration (pharmacologically active form of phenytoin) offsets the delay in phenytoin formation from the prodrug (i.e., phenytoin), making it bioequivalent to phenytoin at 50 mg/min.

Fosphenytoin is administered IM or IV. Compared with phenytoin, fosphenytoin is rapidly and completely absorbed following IM administration, reaching a peak level in 3 hours. Fosphenytoin is administered in units called phenytoin equivalents (PE, which is the amount of phenytoin to be used) rather than fosphenytoin itself. Fosphenytoin is compatible with standard IV solutions (5% dextrose and water or normal saline [NS]) and can be infused for adults at a rate of 100 to 150 mg PE/kg/min.[22] The most common side effects are nystagmus, ataxia, and sedation. Although fosphenytoin is more expensive than phenytoin, fosphenytoin is safer and can be administered more quickly. IV fosphenytoin is replacing phenytoin in the treatment of status epilepticus.[22] As with phenytoin, continuous electrocardiograms (ECGs), blood pressure, and respiratory status must be monitored when providing a loading dose of fosphenytoin.

Carbamazepine

Carbamazepine (Tegretol, Tegretol-XR) is a relative safe drug used as a first-line agent for the treatment of simple partial, complex partial, and generalized tonic-clonic seizures. Carbamazepine can exacerbate absence and myoclonic seizures. The mechanism of action is depression of transmission via the nucleus ventralis anterior thalamus, which acts to decrease the spread of seizure discharge. In addition, it has some depressive effect on posttetanic potentiation, but to a lesser degree than with phenytoin. Carbamazepine has an absorption rate greater than 75%; the dosage peak is reached in 6 to 24 hours. It has a high affinity for lipids that bind to body fat; it also binds to albumin. Carbamazepine is metabolized by the liver.

Carbamazepine is available only in oral form. It is given in divided doses two to four times daily. Dosage should be adjusted gradually. Because the suspension form of the drug may adhere to the nasogastric tube if not diluted, it is recommended that the suspension form be diluted in an equal amount of diluent before administration with an enteral tube. Some drugs, such as phenytoin and phenobarbital, may interact with carbamazepine by enzyme induction, thus decreasing the concentration of carbamazepine. Other drugs—erythromycin, cimetidine, and isoniazid— interact by enzyme induction; these drugs increase the concentration of carbamazepine. Carbamazepine interacts with other drugs by inducing their metabolism; these drugs include valproic acid, theophylline, warfarin, and ethosuximide. The major dose-dependent side effects are diplopia, nystagmus, ataxia, unsteadiness, dizziness, and headache. Cognitive deficits are minimal, although present. Carbamazepine has been associated with neural tube defects.

Valproic Acid

Valproic acid, which is marketed as both valproic acid (Valproate, Depakene) and divalproex sodium (Depakote), is approved for management of myoclonic, tonic, atonic, absence, and generalized tonic-clonic seizures, and especially for patients with more than one type of generalized seizure. The drug has low toxicity and is well tolerated. Its mechanism of action is unclear. Valproic acid is completely absorbed orally when taken on an empty stomach. Its peak concentration is achieved at between 1 and 3 hours. Food delays the time of absorption but does not interfere with the amount absorbed. Valproic acid distributes widely; it is about 90% bound to albumin. The liver is the site of metabolism. At least 10 metabolites of valproic acid have been identified.

Valproic acid is available in capsule, syrup, and "sprinkle" forms. The tablet form contains divalproex sodium, which must be metabolized in the gut to valproic acid; it is enterically coated to reduce gastrointestinal symptoms. Valproic acid is altered by salicylates, which increase its free concentration. The addition of phenobarbital or phenytoin decreases the concentration of valproic acid.

Mild transient drowsiness and minimal cognitive effects are seen with valproic acid. Hepatic dysfunction, including liver failure, and pancreatitis have been reported. The more common adverse effects include nausea and vomiting, which can be controlled by using enterically coated Depakote or by taking the drug with food. Weight gain, transient hair loss, tremor, and dose-related thrombocytopenia are common. Menstrual disturbances and hyperandrogenism may occur in women. Neural tube defects and congenital abnormalities have been reported in the infants of mothers on the drug.

Phenobarbital

Phenobarbital (Luminal) was introduced in 1912. One of the first drugs available for the control of seizures, it is still widely used as an alternative for generalized seizures, except absence and partial seizures. Other drugs are replacing phenobarbital for treatment of status epilepticus. The drug of choice for seizures in infants, its adverse cognitive and sedative-hypnotic effects make it less than ideal for children and adults. Phenobarbital is a CNS depressant; it elevates the seizure threshold by decreasing postsynaptic excitation, possibly by stimulating postsynaptic GABA inhibitor responses. Phenobarbital is rapidly and completely absorbed by all routes (oral, IM, rectal). The biphasic distribution includes initial penetration of highly perfused organs, including the brain, followed by even distribution to all body tissues, including fat. By the IV route, peak cerebral concentration is achieved in 3 to 20 minutes. Drugs affecting liver enzymes may alter phenobarbital's metabolism. The elimination pattern of phenobarbital is linear. About 20% to 40% of a dose is excreted through the kidneys unchanged. Urinary pH affects tubular absorption of phenobarbital, and the amount of excreted drug can be increased by administering diuretics and urinary alkalizing drugs. The binding of phenobarbital to protein is 50%.

The routes of administration are oral and parenteral. In an emergency, phenobarbital can be given IV as a loading dose. The half-life of phenobarbital is so long that it can be given as a single daily dose. Because it takes about 3 to 4 weeks to reach steady state, changing doses rapidly is not recommended. Phenobarbital decreases the efficacy of oral contraceptives. The chief side effects are sedation, drowsiness, and fatigue. In addition, impairment of higher cortical function and depression of cognitive performance (e.g., learning) are found with the use of phenobarbital.

Summary of Drug Therapy

Any patient receiving long-term drug therapy should be monitored carefully for the development of side effects or toxicity. Most drugs are metabolized by the liver and excreted by the kidneys. Periodic drug blood levels should be monitored. If anemia or blood dyscrasias are common side effects, a CBC should be done routinely. Folic acid deficiency has also been reported with some AEDs; therefore, folic acid levels should be monitored.

Surgical Management

About 20% of patients with epilepsy do not respond well to drug therapy. Those patients who have been given a trial (e.g., 1 year or more) on AEDs and continue to have refractory seizures that impact on their quality of life should be considered for surgical evaluation. Selection criteria are important. Patients who have not responded to medical management of seizure, who have a unilateral focus that will not cause a major neurological deficit if excised, and who have had a significant alteration in their quality of life are good candidates for surgery. Surgery should be preceded by an extensive diagnostic work-up that includes electrophysiology, neuropsychology, and imaging studies. All three should suggest an epileptogenic focus. The purpose of surgery is to locate and excise as much of the epileptogenic area as possible without causing neurological deficits.

The presurgical work-up is comprehensive and directed at identifying the functional and structural basis of the seizure disorder. The work-up includes the following areas[15]:

- In-patient video-EEG monitoring to identify the anatomic location of the seizure site and to correlate behavior patterns with abnormal EEG patterns
- Routine scalp or scalp-sphenoidal recording for localization of lesion
- MRI high resolution with thin slices to localize lesion
- Possible SPECT or PET scans
- Neuropsychological testing
- Possible amobarbital test (Wada's test) to assess language and memory location
- Other tests as necessary

Surgical Procedures

The most common surgical procedure for the treatment of seizures is a cortical excision (lobectomy). A large number of patients with partial complex seizures with a localized focus have that focus in the temporal lobe. With refractory temporal lobe epilepsy, resection of the anteromedial temporal lobe (*mesial temporal lobectomy*) is available. A more limited removal of the underlying hippocampus and amygdala is also available. If scar tissue or other focal epileptogenic area exists, the identified lesion (*lesionectomy*) can be removed. When the cortical region cannot be removed, multiple subpial transection designed to disrupt intracortical connections is sometimes effective in controlling seizures.

A *corpus callosotomy* has been helpful for persons with tonic and atonic seizures. Outcomes vary depending on the type of surgical procedure. For example, outcomes of temporal lobe resections break down as follows: approximately 68% seizure free, 24% improved, and 8% no improvement at all.[15] Outcomes from surgery are superior to prolonged medical therapy for temporal lobe epilepsy.[16] Data on corpus callosotomy surgeries indicate that about 8% became seizure free, 61% had worthwhile improvement, and 31% had no improvement. The best results are reported from centers where large numbers of surgeries for epilepsy are performed.

A *hemispherectomy* is reserved for selected catastrophic infant and early childhood epilepsies. Currently, the practice is to perform a modified radical hemispherectomy leaving the frontal and occipital poles in place although disconnected. The response has been good in that about 67% were seizure free, another 21% had a worthwhile response, and 11% had no improvement.[16]

Local anesthesia is used for adolescents and adults unless they have behavioral problems and need to be sedated. In that case, a light general anesthetic is given. Often, the patient *must* be able to follow commands and answer questions during the EEG and cortical stimulation portion of the lengthy surgical procedure. After surgical exposure of the brain surface and depth, electrodes are applied so that an EEG can be taken to identify the epileptogenic focus. Cortical stimulation is used to identify sensory, motor, and speech areas. After the tissue to be excised has been identified, cortical resection is undertaken. Following excision, the electrodes are reattached to determine the presence of any other epileptogenic activity that would require further resection. If the EEG pattern is satisfactory, the patient is anesthetized so that the incision can be closed. Postoperatively, the patient is managed in the same way as any craniotomy patient (see Chapter 14).

Postoperatively and at discharge, the patient continues on an AED, often carbamazepine. EEG recordings are obtained to determine the presence of seizure activity. The decision to discontinue drug therapy after 2 to 4 years is based on an evaluation of the specific patient.

Complications of Surgery

The mortality from a temporal resection is lower than 1%. The complications of surgery include infection; hydrocephalus; cerebral edema, ischemia, or hematoma; hemiparesis or hemiplegia; aphasia; alexia; or visual field deficits. Higher-level functions of cognition, memory, attention, concentration, or language may be affected. In addition, psychosocial impairment such as family interpersonal dynamics, self-esteem, adverse response to treatment failure, and vocational/education disruption are possible.

Vagus Nerve Stimulation

In 1997, vagus nerve stimulation (VNS) was approved for use in the United States as an adjunctive therapy for adults and adolescents over 12 years of age who have partial-onset seizures that are refractory to AEDs. It consists of:

1. A programmable signal generator that is implanted in the patient's left upper chest
2. A bipolar VNS lead that connects the generator to the left vagus nerve in the neck
3. A programming wand that uses radiofrequency signals to communicate noninvasively with the generator
4. Hand-held magnets used by the patient or health care provider to manually turn the stimulator on or off

The mechanism of action is uncertain. The surgical procedure takes approximately 1 hour and can be done under general or regional anesthesia. The procedure is well tolerated except for hoarseness in some cases. Minimal surgical complications have been reported. Several trials report a decrease in frequency of seizures by 25% or more in patients previously resistant to all AEDs. The role of VNS for intractable seizure management is yet to be established.[17]

MANAGEMENT OF SEIZURES AND STATUS EPILEPTICUS IN AN ACUTE CARE SETTING

Most nurses who practice in an acute care setting manage patients who have seizures, regardless of whether they are assigned to a neuroscience unit or to other types of units. Seizures may also occur in community-based settings where such patients are managed. Nurses need to know how to manage seizures and status epilepticus. The following is designed to provide that information.

Managing the Patient During a Seizure in an Acute Care Setting

When a patient has a seizure, the nurse's role is to protect the patient from injury, care for him or her after the seizure, and document the details of the event. In the hospital environment, persons who are at risk for having a seizure are placed on seizure precautions. This means that (1) the side rails of the bed are up and padded if the patient is at risk for falls, (2) a suction set-up and plastic oral airway are available at the bedside, and (3) the bed is kept in low position.

Management of the patient during a seizure is directed toward preventing injury and observing for complications. The following points should be observed:

Before and During a Seizure

- If the patient is seated when a major seizure occurs, ease him or her to the floor, if possible.
- Provide for privacy by pulling the bed curtains or screen or closing the door.
- If the patient experiences an aura, have him or her lie down to prevent injury that might occur from falling to the floor.
- Remove patient's eyeglasses and loosen any constricting clothing.
- Do not try to force anything into the mouth.
- Guide the movements to prevent injuries; do not try to restrain the patient.
- Stay with the patient throughout the seizure to ensure safety.

After a Seizure

- Position the patient on the side to facilitate drainage of secretions.
- Provide for adequate ventilation by maintaining a patent airway; suctioning may be necessary to prevent aspiration.
- Allow the patient to sleep after the seizure.
- On awakening, orient the patient (he or she will probably be amnesic about the event).

Nursing Assessment and Documentation

Collecting data about the seizure requires well-developed observational skills and an understanding of what to look for and how to document observations. It may be helpful to verbalize the observations as events occur. Verbal reinforcement provides for better recall.

The following are several points to consider when organizing information about a seizure:

- Was the seizure witnessed or not witnessed?
- Were there any warning signs or was there an aura?
- Where did the seizure begin and how did it proceed?
- What type of movement was noted and what parts of the body were involved?
- Were there any changes in the size of the pupils or was there conjugate gaze deviation?

SEIZURE ACTIVITY CHART FOR GENERALIZED TONIC-CLONIC SEIZURES

Patient's Name _____

_____ Age _____

Date	Time	Before		During							After				Nurse's Initials
		Warning Signs	Part of Body Where Seizure Began	General or Localized	Type of Movement	Duration of Each Phase — Tonic	Clonic	Level of Conscious-ness	Pupils	Other	Behav-ior	Paral-ysis	Loca-tion of Paral-ysis	Sleep	

Figure 29-1 • A sample of a seizure activity chart.

- What was the duration of the entire attack and of each phase?
- Was the patient unconscious throughout the seizure?
- Was there urinary or bowel incontinence?
- What was the person's behavior after the seizure?
- Was there any weakness or paralysis of the extremities after the seizure?
- Were there any injuries noted?
- Did the patient sleep after the seizure? How long?

The observations can be recorded in narrative form in the nurse's notes or on a separate seizure activity sheet, which becomes a part of the patient's permanent record. A sample of a seizure activity sheet for generalized tonic-clonic seizures is found in Figure 29-1. Observations are the same for a seizure that was witnessed in a community setting.

Managing a Person During a Seizure in a Community Setting

Seizures may occur in community settings such as ambulatory clinics, work and recreational environments, and the home. The same first aid principles taught to the person and family should be followed by the bystander nurse who comes upon the individual having a seizure. The first aid management of both generalized tonic-clonic seizures and complex partial seizures includes the following[9]:

First aid for *generalized tonic-clonic seizures* that occur in a community setting is similar to the management of this type of seizure in an acute care setting. The seizure may begin abruptly and the person may fall to the ground, become stiff, and demonstrate clonic movements. The following is recommended:

- If the patient is seated, help him or her to lie down.
- Remove eyeglasses and loosen any constricting clothing.
- Do not try to force anything into the mouth.
- Guide the movements to prevent injuries; do not try to restrain the person.
- Stay with the patient throughout the seizure.

After the seizure has stopped, one should position the patient on the side to facilitate drainage of secretions; have someone stay with the patient until he or she is fully awake; and once the patient is awake, orient him or her as necessary.

First aid for a patient with *complex partial seizures* is more subtle. The patient may not seem quite right, engaging in such behaviors as lip smacking or making chewing motions, walking aimlessly, or not responding to questions (symptoms of automatism). Before and during a seizure one should do the following:

- Remove harmful objects from the patient's environment or try to coax the patient away from anything that could be harmful.
- Demonstrate a calm manner that does not agitate the patient.
- Do not try to restrain the patient.
- If alone, do not try to approach an angry or agitated patient.

After the seizure has seized, one should not leave the patient alone, should stay with the patient until consciousness is fully regained, and should reorient him or her.

With any type of seizure activity, a decision may need to be made to call for emergency medical assistance if:

- The person does not begin breathing after the seizure (cardiopulmonary resuscitation should be activated).
- A generalized tonic-clonic seizure lasts for more than 2 minutes.
- The person has one seizure right after another without regaining consciousness.
- The individual is injured.

Status Epilepticus

Status epilepticus is defined as either continuous seizures lasting at least 5 minutes or two or more discrete seizures between which there is incomplete recovery of consciousness.[18] The most common type of status epilepticus is **tonic-clonic status epilepticus.** In over 50% of cases, status epilepticus is the patient's first seizure. Although there are many types of status epilepticus, the following discussion focuses on the management of convulsive status epilepticus because this form is most common and constitutes a medical emergency.

The initial management of a patient with status epilepticus includes the standard ABCs of life support (supporting respirations, maintaining blood pressure, and supporting circulation), administering an AED, finding and treating any underlying cause, and preventing or treating medical complications.

ABCs of Life Support. The ABCs of life support are similar to any other life-threatening situation. Position the patient to avoid aspiration or inadequate oxygenation. A soft, plastic oral airway may be inserted if it is possible to do so without forcing the teeth apart. The airway will need to be suctioned to remain patent. Oxygen is administered at 100% through a nasal cannula. In most instances, patients will breathe on their own as long as the airway is kept patent. Suction the airway to maintain patency. Monitor respiratory function with ongoing pulse oximetry. IV access should be secured, and vital signs and neurological signs should be monitored frequently.

Extreme cerebral hypoxia can result in severe, irreversible neurological deficits. Monitor arterial blood gases because many patients will have a profound metabolic acidosis that corrects itself after seizures are controlled.[18]

Support of adequate oxygenation and cerebral perfusion is critical to preventing these serious problems. Monitor glucose by fingerstick. Hyperglycemia followed by hypoglycemia is common and needs to be treated. Give 50 mL of 50% glucose for hypoglycemia. Hyperthermia occurs often with status epilepticus. If it occurs, it must be treated aggressively with passive cooling to prevent further ischemia to the brain.

Administering Antiepileptic Drugs. The goal of drug therapy is prompt termination of clinical and electrical seizure activity. The best drug treatment protocol for status epilepticus remains under discussion. Table 29-5 outlines a recommended protocol that proceeds along a timeline and assumes that the previous drug administration did not terminate the seizure.[18] If the patient is not already in the intensive care unit, he or she must be moved to that area where intubation, ventilatory support, continuous ECG monitoring, and invasive monitoring can be provided.

Treating the Underlying Cause. The health care provider must try to identify any underlying cause of seizures (e.g., precipitous withdrawal of AEDs, brain tumor) and treat the primary problem. Various possible causative factors are discussed earlier in the chapter.

Preventing or Treating Medical Complications. Adverse physiologic consequences of status epilepticus include hypoxia, hypoglycemia, hypotension, and hyperthermia. Severe metabolic acidosis can occur as a result of loss of base reserve. This change may prevent seizure control with anticonvulsants by increasing the amount of potassium in the extracellular space. It may also contribute to cerebral damage. Blood gases should be monitored. Other medical complications that may develop include cardiac arrhythmias, myocardial infarction, and aspiration pneumonia.

Nursing Management of Status Epilepticus

The nurse works as part of a collaborative team in addressing the medical emergency. Goals and responsibilities include:

- Maintaining a patent airway to ensure adequate ventilation
- Suctioning as necessary to prevent obstruction of the airway and possible aspiration
- Providing oxygen by nasal cannula as ordered
- Protecting the IV site to allow for continuous access for medication
- Protecting the patient from injury
- Providing information to the family

NURSING MANAGEMENT OF PATIENTS WITH EPILEPSY: COMMUNITY-BASED CARE

Most people with epilepsy are managed by their primary care physicians or by a neurologist in the community. In a managed care environment, more patients with epilepsy, who were previously managed by a neurologist, come under the care of the primary care physician. Those with complicated or intractable epilepsy will probably still be managed by a neurologist or in an epilepsy center.

CHART 29-1   Components of a Teaching Plan for Persons With Epilepsy or a Seizure Disorder

DIET/NUTRITION/BEVERAGES

- Eat a well-balanced diet; eat on a routine schedule.
- Avoid excesses of sugar, caffeine, or any other food that may trigger seizures.
- Discuss alcohol consumption with your doctor; if you choose to drink, limit your consumption to whatever your physician recommends. Seizures may be precipitated by alcohol consumption, and even small amounts may trigger a seizure in some people.

GENERAL HEALTH

- Any of the following can trigger seizures in some persons and should be avoided: constipation, excessive fatigue, hyperventilation, and stress.
- Regular exercise is good for general well-being and stress reduction. Avoid overfatigue and hyperventilation. Avoid exercise in hot weather; exercise in a climatecontrolled environment.
- Regular sleep patterns on a regular schedule are important. Insomnia or awakening tired are indications of insufficient sleep. This may be due to stress, poor sleep hygiene, or a side effect of medication. Determine cause of sleep disturbance and correct it or seek assistance from the health care provider.
- Showers, rather than tub baths, should be taken.
- Good oral hygiene and periodic visits to the dentist are important because gingival hyperplasia can occur from some antiepileptic drugs (AEDs) such as phenytoin.

FEVER AND ILLNESS

- Fever can trigger seizures; the fever and underlying cause must be treated.
- Any prescription or over-the-counter drugs should be reviewed for interaction.
- If antibiotics are ordered, interactions with the AEDs should be evaluated.

ENVIRONMENTAL, OCCUPATIONAL, AND RECREATIONAL RISK FACTORS

- Noisy environments should be avoided; control a noisy environment as much as possible.
- Avoid bright, flashing lights or fluorescent lights, strobe lights, discos, a flickering television, and flashing bulbs on signs or Christmas trees. Tinted glass on the windshield and eyeglasses will help to control glare.
- Use a screen filter on the computer screen to control glare.
- Do not use recreational or street drugs.

- Work or recreational activities that could cause injury if a seizure occurred should be avoided.
- Swim with a "buddy"; help should be available if a seizure occurs.
- Contact sports (e.g., football, boxing) that could lead to unconsciousness should be avoided.

STRESS, ANXIETY, AND DEPRESSION

- Emotional stress is a trigger to seizures; measures need to be taken to uncover the basis for the stress and how this can be decreased. Counseling may be helpful.
- Living with a chronic health problem is stressful and can place a varying degree of limitations on lifestyle. Depression may result. Appropriate psychotherapy through counseling and/or drugs should be provided.

WOMEN'S HEALTH

- There may be an increase in seizures around the time of menses. This should be discussed with your health care provider; some adjustment may be made in your medications.
- If the occurrence of seizures increases around the menses, control other triggers for seizures.
- AEDs decrease the effectiveness of oral contraceptives; intrauterine devices or other contraceptive devices may be preferred.
- The seizure pattern often changes during pregnancy; discuss this with your health care provider.
- Some AEDs can cause birth defects. If pregnancy is planned, it should be discussed with the gynecologist and health care provider following the epilepsy.

LEGISLATION TO PROTECT PERSONS WITH EPILEPSY AND SEIZURE DISORDER

The following laws protect persons with epilepsy or seizure disorders from discrimination:

- Americans With Disabilities Act
- Rehabilitation Act
- Individuals With Disabilities Education Act
- Driver's licenses are controlled by individual states; information on the laws governing driving can be obtained from the Division of Motor Vehicles.

OTHER

- Issues related to marriage, child-bearing, and parenting need to be discussed. Risk factors and questions related to children with epilepsy need a frank discussion.

The role of the nurse in managing patients with epilepsy will continue to be important, and in many settings this role will be expanded. In the community, nursing management is initially directed at assisting with the assessment and diagnostic work-up. The components of these activities are discussed in earlier sections. However, the nurse's major role is

to provide patient education and patient monitoring. The next section focuses on this aspect of management. The major patient problem and nursing diagnosis for a newly diagnosed patient with epilepsy is Knowledge Deficit. An individualized teaching plan is developed (Chart 29-1) to educate the patient and family.

Patient Teaching: General Points

Patient teaching requires a comprehensive teaching plan to help the patient adjust to the health problem. Family teaching cannot be excluded because the family needs help to adjust to a chronic condition that is, by its very nature, frightening. The family must be instructed in what to do when a seizure occurs, including first aid. The teaching plan is based on a systematic assessment of patient needs. Physical, social, psychological, and vocational dimensions must be considered along with a drug teaching plan.

Each teaching plan is individual, that is, tailored to the needs of the patient and the problems that arise over time. Major points of information that should be presented to the patient are outlined in Chart 29-1. The plan should expand on these points to include the implications that apply to the patient's individual lifestyle.[19] The plan must be revised periodically to update its relevance. Because nonadherence is a common problem, adherence must be evaluated at each encounter with the health care professional. It is important to reinforce information each time the patient is seen.

Patients may express concerns about how they will cope with certain aspects of their lives. One common concern of most adults is whether they should reveal their condition when applying for a job. Many report discrimination by employers when they reveal their condition. Those who choose to conceal this information often feel guilty and live in fear that they will experience a seizure on the job or that their seizure disorder will become known to the employer. If a seizure did occur on the job, it could endanger the patient and others, depending on the kind of work that is done. Information that is deliberately concealed is cause for immediate dismissal in most places of employment. It is the patient's decision to determine whether to disclose the epileptic condition.

Patient Teaching Related to Drug Therapy

It is imperative to provide detailed information to the patient and/or a responsible family member about epilepsy and drug therapy. Side effects and signs of toxicity should be discussed. The patient must understand that the drug must be taken as ordered *every day*. The most common cause of seizures in patients who have previously been controlled is failure to take the AEDs. The patient should be asked to maintain a drug chart of time, amount taken, and side effects, along with a record of the frequency and characteristics of any seizures.

Because seizures represent a chronic condition (i.e., they are usually not completely arrested), the person must understand the nature of the problem, the precipitating factors, and the adaptations in lifestyle that are required.

The following is an outline of the major points of a drug teaching plan:

- The drug must be taken as ordered to maintain a therapeutic blood level, even if there is no seizure activity.
- AEDs may be necessary for a few years or longer; for some patients, they may be necessary for a lifetime. There are criteria for when and how a trial of drug discontinuation should be managed; discuss this with the health care provider.

- Discontinuation of drugs without the knowledge of the health care provider is the most common cause of seizure activity (e.g., status epilepticus); this should not be done.[20]
- Know the signs of toxicity of the drugs prescribed. Symptoms of toxicity should be reported promptly to the physician.
- Keep drug and seizure charts and bring them with you for your appointment.
- Because there are serious side effects from some drugs, be sure to have blood work done as ordered (e.g., CBC for anemia and blood dyscrasias).
- Because phenytoin is absorbed slowly from the gastrointestinal tract, daily drug schedules can be adjusted for convenience. Missed doses can be "made up" safely.
- Some individuals may be able to take extended-release phenytoin with once-daily dosing; discuss this with your health care provider.
- A Medic Alert bracelet or a card should be carried to indicate a chronic condition. The patient is encouraged to carry a card that indicates that he or she is being treated by a particular physician. If the patient is found unconscious or injured, the physician can be notified.
- Keep follow-up appointments with a health care provider for periodic monitoring and re-evaluation.

Special Populations: Women and the Elderly

Two patient populations that have unique needs when discussing epilepsy and seizure disorders are women and the elderly.

Women

Some of the special needs of women are included in the teaching plan in Chart 29-1. Women who have a seizure disorder need anticipatory guidance about contraception and the implications of child-bearing. The effectiveness of oral contraceptives is decreased by AEDs, which induce liver enzymes and increase the rate of metabolism. A sign of ineffectiveness of the oral contraceptive is breakthrough bleeding; an oral contraceptive with a higher estrogen content needs to be taken or other forms of birth control used.

Women taking AEDs who wish to become pregnant should discuss their particular situation with the physician. Myths need to be dispelled and real risks, including risk of teratogenic effects of many AEDs on a fetus, need to be examined. There is evidence that there is a doubling of the rate of malformations in babies born to mothers taking AEDs. Further, the risk may be dose related.[21] A combination of AEDs, especially carbamazepine, phenytoin, and valproate, causes a much higher risk of neural tube defects. The question arises as to what should be done about AEDs if a woman wants to become pregnant. There is no simple answer. The variables include the particular drugs and dosages involved and the severity of the seizure disorder. For some women, discontinuation of the AEDs may be an option. This is a decision that should be made after careful discussion with the physician. After a woman is pregnant, it does no good to discontinue the AEDs.

During pregnancy, many women notice a change in their seizure pattern, which is unpredictable. The increased risk of complications during pregnancy, delivery, and the postpartum period requires that the neurologist or primary care physician and the obstetrician collaborate closely. If breast-feeding is planned, consideration of the effect of the AED in breast milk on the infant needs to be addressed. For details of management, other sources should be consulted.

The Elderly

A high incidence of new onset of epilepsy is found in persons 65 years old and older. The risk factors associated with the increased incidence in this group include stroke, head trauma, dementia, infection, alcoholism, and aging.[22] Of these, stroke associated with paresis and cortical involvement is the leading risk factor for the development of epilepsy in the elderly. Although generalized tonic-clonic seizures are easily recognizable, simple and complex seizures may pose a more difficult problem because of the subtle symptoms and other competing diagnoses. The differential diagnosis includes transient ischemic attacks, syncope, drop attacks, transient global amnesia, psychiatric disorders, and sleep disorders. To make a diagnosis of a seizure disorder, nurses and physicians first need to recognize it as a possibility when evaluating older patients.[23] With seizure disorder in the differential diagnosis, the health care provider is alerted to collect a detailed history from the person and family member and conduct a complete physical and neurological examination. In addition, MRI and an EEG may be useful. It is noteworthy that a normal EEG does not necessarily exclude the diagnosis of epilepsy. An EEG with stresses such as sleep deprivation increases the possibility of observing epileptiform abnormalities. Focal or diffuse slowing on EEG is not necessarily an indicator of epilepsy in older persons. An EEG finding known as **periodic lateralized epileptiform discharges (PLEDs)** is of particular interest; these are abnormal interictal EEG wave patterns characterized by paroxysmal, sharp wave complexes suggestive of an underlying *focal* seizure disorder.

Management consists of treating the underlying problem and choosing the right AED for the seizure type. In choosing an AED for an elderly person, several points should be considered[24]:

- The pharmacokinetics (absorption, distribution, metabolism, and excretion) are altered in the elderly owing to hematologic, renal, and hepatic function changes. Before ordering any AEDs, CBC, clotting factors, albumin, liver function studies, and creatinine values should be evaluated to determine whether the AED would have an unusual effect given any abnormal values.
- Many older people are taking several drugs for chronic health problems such as cardiac and respiratory problems. Consider drug interactions when choosing an AED.
- Consider the effect of the drug on cognitive function and balance and how it will affect daily living and patient safety.
- Consider cost. If the drug is too expensive for the patient, compliance will not be maintained.

- Begin with AED monotherapy, starting at a low dose, and titrate slowly to monitor seizure control or toxicity. Monitor the patient for side effects such as folate deficiency with phenytoin. Free AED concentrations should be measured in any patient with renal or hepatic dysfunction who has signs of toxicity when within the therapeutic range.

Long-Term Management of Persons With Epilepsy

Long-term management and periodic re-evaluation are necessary with any chronic condition. Because all drugs have side effects and toxicity, patients must be monitored for any signs of toxicity. When adverse reactions occur, medications need to be adjusted or discontinued. Periodic re-evaluation provides the opportunity for assessment of emotional, psychological, social, and vocational problems that are apt to develop as the patient adjusts to living with a seizure disorder.

REFERENCES

1. Browne, T. R., & Holmes, G. L. (2000). *Handbook of epilepsy* (2nd ed., pp. 1–18). Philadelphia: Lippincott Williams & Wilkins.
2. Lowenstein, D. H. (2005). Seizures and epilepsy. In D. L. Kasper, E. Braunwald, A. S. Fauci, S. L. Hauser, D. L. Longo, & J. L. Jameson (Eds.). *Harrison's principles of internal medicine* (16th ed., pp. 2357–2372). New York: McGraw-Hill.
3. Ropper, A. H., & Brown, R. H. (2005). *Adams and Victor's principles of neurology* (8th ed., pp. 271–301). New York: McGraw-Hill.
4. Ropper, A. H., & Brown, R. H. (2005). *Adams and Victor's principles of neurology* (8th ed., p. 281). New York: McGraw-Hill.
5. Kotagal, P. (1997). Complex partial seizures with automatisms In F. Wylie (Ed.). *The treatment of epilepsy: Principles and practice* (2nd ed., pp. 385–400). Baltimore: Williams & Wilkins.
6. Commission of Classification and Terminology of the International League Against Epilepsy. (1981). Proposal for revised clinical and electroencephalographic classification of epileptic seizures. *Epilepsia, 22,* 489–501.
7. Benbadis, S. R. (2001). Epilepsy. *Neurologic Clinics, 19*(2), 251–270
8. Lowenstein, D. H., & Alldredge, B. K. (1998). Status epilepticus. *New England Journal of Medicine, 338*(14), 970–976.
9. Gumnit, R. J. (1995). *The epilepsy handbook: The practical management of seizures* (2nd ed., pp. 124–127). New York: Raven.
10. Schachter, S. C. (2001). Epilepsy. *Neurologic Clinics, 19*(1), 57–78.
11. Trescher, W. H., & Lesser, R. P. (2004). The epilepsies. In W. G. Bradley, R. B. Daroff, G. M. Fenichel, & J. Jankovic (Eds.). *Neurology in clinical practice* (4th ed., pp. 1953–1992). Philadelphia: Butterworth-Heinemann.
12. Graves, N. M., & Garnett, W. R. (1999). Epilepsy. In J. T. DiPiro, R. L. Talbert, G. C. Yee, G. R. Matzke, B. G. Wells, & L. M. Posey (Eds.). *Pharmacotherapy: A pathophysiologic approach* (4th ed., pp. 952–975). Stamford, CT: Appleton & Lange.
13. Quality Standards Committee of AAN. (1996). Practice parameter: A guideline for discontinuing antiepileptic drugs in seizure-free patients–summary statement. *Neurology, 47,* 600–602.
14. French, J. A., & Pedley, T. A. (2008). Initial management of epilepsy. *New England Journal of Medicine, 359*(2), 166–176.
15. Engel, J. (1996). Surgery for seizures. *New England Journal of Medicine, 334*(10), 647–652.
16. Wiebe, S., Blume, W. T., Girvin, J. P., & Eliasziw, M. (2001). A randomized controlled trial of surgery for temporal-lobe epilepsy. *New England Journal of Medicine, 345*(5), 311–318.

17. Wyllie, E. (Ed.). (1997). *The treatment of epilepsy: Principles and practice* (2nd ed.). Baltimore: Williams & Wilkins.

18. Lowenstein, D. H., & Alldredge, B. K. (1998). Status epilepticus. *New England Journal of Medicine, 338*(14), 970–976.

19. Shafer, R. O. (1994). Nursing support of epilepsy self-management. *Clinical Nursing Practice in Epilepsy, 2*(1), 5–6.

20. O'Dell, C., & Shinnar, S. (2001). Epilepsy: Initiation and discontinuation of antiepileptic drugs. *Neurologic Clinics, 19*(2), 289–311.

21. Foldvary, N. (2001). Epilepsy: treatment issues for women with epilepsy. *Neurologic Clinics, 19*(2), 491–515.

22. Collins, N. S., Shapiro, R. A., & Ramsay, R. E. (2006). Elders with epilepsy. *Medical Clinics of North America, 90*(5), 945–966.

23. Nadkarni, S., LaJoie, J., & Devinsky, O. (2005). Current treatments of epilepsy. *Neurology, 64*(12 Suppl), S2–11.

24. Palsalos, P. N., & Perucca, E. (2003). Clinically important drug interactions in epilepsy: Interactions between antiepileptic drugs and other drugs. *Lancet Neurology, 2*(8), 473–481.

RESOURCES

Websites

http://www.efa.org/
http://www.epilepsyfoundation.org/gene

Infections of the Central Nervous System

Joanne V. Hickey

Of the many infectious diseases involving the central nervous system (CNS), only the most common are addressed in this chapter. These include bacterial meningitis, viral encephalitis, and the parameningeal infections, as well as brain abscess and extradural abscess. Features of other selected nervous system infections are presented in tabular format.

MENINGITIS

Bacterial Meningitis

Bacterial meningitis is a pyogenic (purulent or suppurative) infection that involves the pia-arachnoid layers of the meninges and the subarachnoid space (SAS), including cerebrospinal fluid (CSF). Infections can occur when bacteria gain access to the meninges through the blood-borne route or through the spread of nearby infections such as sinusitis, mastoiditis, otitis media, osteomyelitis of the skull or vertebrae, or pneumonia.[1] Other sources of CSF contamination are neurosurgical procedures, lumbar puncture, and penetrating head wounds. Infections of the meninges also result from preexisting connections between the CNS and dural defects, congenital sinuses, or occult encephaloceles.[2]

Common Causative Organisms

The annual incidence is 4 to 6 cases per 100,000 adults (i.e., patients older than 16 years if age).[3] The common causative organisms for bacterial meningitis tend to differ by age group. In older children and adults, *Streptococcus pneumoniae, Neisseria meningitidis, Haemophilus influenzae,* and *Listeria monocytogenes* are the more common causative organisms of meningitis.[4] The first two account for about 80% of meningitis.[5] *L. monocytogenes* is now the fourth most common type of nontraumatic or non–postsurgical bacterial meningitis in adults. *S. pneumoniae* is the most common organism responsible for community-acquired bacterial meningitis. In older adults (50 years of age and older), *S. pneumoniae* is likely to cause meningitis in association with pneumonia or otitis media. In addition, gram-negative bacilli *Enterobacteriaceae* (*Escherichia coli, Klebsiella pneumoniae, Pseudomonas, Enterobacter,* and *Serratia*) are the organisms likely to cause meningitis in association with chronic lung disease, sinusitis, neurosurgical procedures, or chronic urinary tract infection in older patients (Table 30-1). Except during summer when incidence decreases, the rate of cases of meningitis is relatively constant throughout the year.

Pathophysiology

Both *H. influenzae* and *S. pneumoniae* organisms are associated with the respiratory tract and gram-negative rod organisms, *Enterobacteriaceae,* associated with the enteric tract, often inhabit the nasopharynx and are the major organisms causing bacterial meningitis in children and adults. These bacteria attach themselves to mucous epithelium by secreting a substance known as immunoglobin A (IgA) protease, and enter the bloodstream. In the blood, bacteria are inactivated by complement-mediated bactericidal activity and phagocytosis by neutrophils. However, protection from these mechanisms is afforded by a capsular polysaccharide coating. Bacteria that are able to survive in the circulation enter the CSF through the choroid plexus of the lateral ventricles and other areas of the altered blood–brain barrier. The CSF is an area of impaired host defense because of a lack of sufficient numbers of complement components and immunoglobulins for the opsonization (the rendering of bacteria and other cells subject to phagocytosis) of bacteria.[6]

The pathophysiologic events related to meningitis are well described by Roos.[7] Bacteria multiply rapidly in the SAS. Both this multiplication and lysis of bacteria by bactericidal antibiotics cause the release of bacterial cell wall components. These components stimulate the formation of the inflammatory cytokines, interleukin-1 (IL-1) and tumor necrosis factor (TNF), by monocytes, macrophages, brain astrocytes, and microglial cells. Blood–brain barrier permeability is altered; polymorphonuclear leukocytes are recruited. All these events contribute to the formation of purulent exudate in the SAS. Concurrently, IL-1 and TNF induce the formation of molecules that adhere to leukocytes on vascular endothelial cells. This allows neutrophils to traverse the

TABLE 30–1   COMMON CAUSATIVE ORGANISMS OF BACTERIAL MENINGITIS IN ADULTS*

DISEASE	ORGANISM	COMMENTS
Pneumococcal meningitis	*Streptococcus pneumoniae* (gram-positive diplococci)	• Most common type of meningitis with worldwide distribution • Most common in young children and older adults • Occurs mostly in winter and early spring • Predisposing conditions include pneumonia, sinusitis, alcoholism, and head trauma
Haemophilus influenzae meningitis	*H. influenzae* (gram-negative cocci)	• Used to occur most often in infants and children, but occurring more in adults • Incidence has decreased in half due to *H. influenzae* vaccine • Often follows upper respiratory or ear infections
Meningococcal meningitis	*Neisseria meningitidis* (gram-negative diplococci)	• Highest incidence in children and young adults • Presentation includes petechial rash, purpuric lesions, or ecchymosis that develop in 50% of patients • About 10% develop a fulminating infection with overwhelming septicemia (meningococcemia); creates a medical emergency (high fever, circulatory collapse from adrenocortical insufficiency secondary to hemorrhage and necrosis of the adrenals called Waterhouse-Friderichsen syndrome); disseminated intravascular coagulation may also occur • Death can result hours after onset
Listeria monocytogenes meningitis		• Fourth most common cause of meningitis in nonsurgical bacterial meningitis
Less common sources	• *Staphylococcus aureus* • *Streptococcus* group A • *Streptococcus* group B	• Increased incidence of nosocomial infections noted • Often introduced during neurosurgical procedures (craniotomy) or related to brain abscess, epidural abscess, or head trauma
Less common sources	• *Klebsiella* • *Proteus* • *Pseudomonas*	• Related to lumbar puncture, spinal anesthesia, or shunting procedure
Tuberculosis meningitis	• *Myobacterium tuberculosis*	• Secondary infection resulting from bacterial seeding of the meninges from tuberculosis elsewhere in the body • Most common in children • Incidence reflects the rate of tuberculosis in a country (relatively low in the United States)

*The organisms presented here are responsible for 80% to 90% of the cases of bacterial meningitis worldwide; these organisms are normally found in the nasopharynx of a significant portion of the population.

blood–brain barrier. The large numbers of leukocytes in the SAS add to the purulent exudate and obstruction of flow of CSF. Adhesion of leukocytes to the cerebral capillary endothelial cells increases their permeability and allows plasma proteins to leak through open intercellular junctions. This results in vasogenic brain edema and subsequent increased intracranial pressure (ICP).

In the acute phase of meningitis, the cerebral cortex undergoes little change except for perivascular inflammation with some infiltration into the cortex. In subacute cases, there may be diffuse degenerative changes, with necrosis and glial proliferation within the superficial areas of the brain, spinal cord, or cranial nerves. The optic and acoustic nerves are often affected, although the oculomotor, trochlear, abducens, and facial nerves can also be involved.

The resolution of meningitis depends on the extent of the infection and how quickly effective treatment is initiated. If the process is arrested early, resolution may be complete, without major sequelae. However, the arachnoid layer may undergo fibrotic changes and scar tissue formation. Adhesions and effusions can develop in the SAS, thereby interfering with the normal circulation of CSF. Fibrotic changes in the structures responsible for the production and absorption of CSF may result, contributing to the development of hydrocephalus. Some organisms may produce an abscess. Much of the outcome from bacterial meningitis depends on early and aggressive treatment to prevent the development of complications.

Signs and Symptoms

Although many different organisms are capable of producing meningitis, all produce common signs and symptoms. The initial signs and symptoms of bacterial meningitis include headache, fever, stiff neck, lethargy, confusion, coma, nausea, vomiting, and photophobia.

Headache and Fever. The *headache*, which is usually the initial symptom, is described as severe. This symptom is

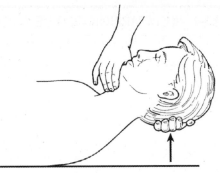

Figure 30-2 • Brudzinski's sign. With the patient lying on his back, place your hand behind the patient's neck and flex the neck toward the sternum. In a patient with meningeal irritation there is neck pain, neck stiffness, and flexion of the hips and knees.

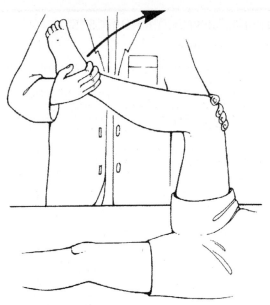

Figure 30-1 • Kernig's sign. With the patient lying on his back, flex one of the patient's legs at the hip and knee. If pain or resistance is elicited as the knee is straightened, this is a positive Kernig's sign, a sign of meningeal irritation.

probably attributable to irritation of the pain-sensitive dura and traction on related vascular structures. *Fever* is the rule with bacterial meningitis, and can vary from 38°C to 39.5°C (101°F to 103°F) or higher. The temperature remains high throughout the course of the illness and can rise to 40.5°C (105°F) and higher in the terminal stages because of decompensation of increased ICP on the brainstem.

Stiff Neck/Nuchal Rigidity, and Other Signs of Meningeal Irritation. A *stiff neck* is an early sign of meningeal irritation. Attempts to flex the neck forward, either actively or passively, prove difficult. This resistance is caused by spasms of the extensor muscles of the neck. Forceful flexion produces severe pain. Two signs of meningeal irritation are Kernig's and Brudzinski's signs. **Kernig's sign** is elicited by flexing the upper leg at the hip to a 90-degree angle and then attempting to extend the knee. In the presence of meningeal irritation, pain and spasm of the hamstrings occur when an attempt is made to extend the knee (Fig. 30-1). The pain is caused by inflammation of the meninges and spinal roots. The spasms are a protective mechanism to deter painful flexion. **Brudzinski's sign** is positive when both the upper leg at the hip and the lower leg at the knee flex in response to passive flexion of the neck and head on the chest (Fig. 30-2). This reflex is caused by irritating exudate around the roots in the lumbar region.

Altered Consciousness. In the very early stages, lethargy and confusion are common. The patient becomes disoriented to time, place, and person; is easily bewildered; has poor memory; and appears to have difficulty following commands. Other patients may become restless, agitated, irritable, and disoriented. Adults may progress rapidly from lethargy to stupor and coma. In the older adult, fever, confusion, stupor, or coma is typical.

Other Signs. *Photophobia* is a common sign of meningeal irritation seen in bacterial meningitis, but the pathophysiology for this symptom is not clear. Other signs and symptoms noted include skin hypersensitivity, hyperalgesia, and muscular hypotonia, although motor function is well preserved. Sensory loss does not occur. Seizures occur in 40% to 50% of patients with bacterial meningitis usually within the first week.[4] Some patients develop hyponatremia or syndrome of inappropriate secretion of antidiuretic hormone (SIADH) from excessive release of antidiuretic hormone. There are signs and symptoms of water retention, along with oliguria and hypervolemia. Nausea and vomiting are common.

Increased ICP accompanies bacterial meningitis because of accumulation of purulent exudate, cerebral edema, and hydrocephalus. Symptoms of brainstem pressure are reflected in Cushing's response of vital sign changes, such as widening of pulse pressure, decreased pulse, and ataxic respirations. Vomiting is a frequent finding and is related to increased ICP. If the infection is not aggressively treated or response to treatment is poor, cerebral herniation can occur.

Meningococcal Meningitis. Some additional differential signs and symptoms are noteworthy with *N. meningitidis* infection. Very rapid development of delirium and stupor, a petechial or purpura rash, or large ecchymotic areas especially of the lower parts of the body are characteristic of meningococcal meningitis. The petechiae may be seen on the conjunctiva and other parts of the skin and mucous membranes. Fulminating meningococcemia, with or without meningitis, has a high mortality rate because of the associated vasomotor collapse and infective shock related to adrenocortical hemorrhage.[8] The adrenal hemorrhage resulting in adrenal insufficiency followed by hypotension, cyanosis, respiratory distress, and circulatory collapse is known as *Waterhouse-Friderichsen syndrome*. If this occurs, immediate administration of adrenal corticosteroids is necessary along with other supportive therapies to treat this life-threatening event.[9]

Isolation Precautions. The need to place a patient on isolation precautions to prevent the spread of disease depends on the type of invading organism and the stage of the illness. For example, in the acute phase of meningococcal meningitis, it is possible to infect others with secretions

TABLE 30-2   COMPARISON OF THE CLASSIC CEREBROSPINAL FLUID (CSF) FINDINGS IN ACUTE BACTERIAL MENINGITIS AND ACUTE ASEPTIC (VIRAL) MENINGITIS

CSF CHARACTERISTICS	ACUTE BACTERIAL MENINGITIS*	ACUTE ASEPTIC (VIRAL) MENINGITIS
Appearance	Turbid, cloudy	Clear; sometimes turbid
Cells	Increased white blood cells (1000–2000 mm^3 or more; mostly polymorphonuclear neutrophils)	Increased white blood cells (300 mm^3; mostly mononuclear)
Protein level	Increased (100–500 mg/dL)	Normal or slightly increased
Glucose level	Decreased (<40 mg/dL or about 40% of blood glucose level)	Normal
Smear and culture	Bacterial present on Gram stain and culture	No bacteria present on Gram stain or culture; the virus may be demonstrated by special techniques
Pressure on lumbar puncture	Elevated (>180 mm of water pressure)	Variable

*All patients do not follow this classic profile; about 30% of patients with bacterial meningitis show some of the findings seen in aseptic meningitis.

from the nasopharynx and droplets from the respiratory tract. Meningococci usually disappear within 24 hours of administration of appropriate antimicrobial drugs. Therefore, respiratory isolation of the patient to protect the nursing and health care personnel, visitors, and other patients should be maintained until cultures are negative. The hospital infection control department is the best source of information regarding type and duration of isolation.

Diagnosis

A diagnosis of bacterial meningitis is often difficult to recognize. The diagnosis of bacterial meningitis relies on a history, a physical examination, and laboratory data.[10] A history of recent infections, such as those involving the ears, sinuses, or respiratory tract, is a risk factor. Examination of CSF is the "gold standard" for the diagnosis of bacterial meningitis. Table 30-2 provides a comparison between the basic CSF criteria for diagnosis of bacterial meningitis and the findings associated with aseptic (viral) meningitis. Collection of CSF requires a lumbar puncture or sample of CSF from a ventriculostomy. The patient must first be assessed for evidence of elevated ICP, which could be a contraindication for lumbar puncture. If an elevated ICP is suspected, a computed tomography (CT) scan may be ordered first to assess for significantly elevated ICP. The CT scan is also useful for detection of abscesses and lesions that erode the skull and provide a route for bacterial invasion (e.g., tumors or sinus wall defects). The classic CSF abnormalities noted in bacterial meningitis include:

- Increased opening pressure on lumbar puncture
- Polymorphonuclear leukocytic pleocytosis
- Decreased glucose concentration
- Increased protein concentration
- Glucose ratio less than 40 mg/dL
- White blood cell (WBC) count of CSF usually more than 100 cells/mm^3 and often more than 1000 WBCs/mm^3
- Protein count higher than 45 mg/dL (most often 100 to 500 mg/dL)

Tests to identify specific causative organisms include Gram stain, smear, and culture. Blood cultures may also be of diagnostic value as they are positive in 40% to 60% of patients with *H. influenzae,* meningococcal, and pneumococcal meningitis.[4] For those patients who have received antibiotics, it is more difficult to establish a diagnosis. Newer laboratory techniques are making it possible to detect bacterial antigen in an hour or two. These options include counterimmunoelectrophoresis (CIE), a sensitive technique that permits the detection of bacterial antigens in the CSF in 30 to 60 minutes; radioimmunoassay (RIA); latex particle agglutination (LPA); enzyme-linked immunosorbent assay (ELISA); and polymerase chain reaction (PCR).[4] Finally, measurements of lactate dehydrogenase (LDH) in CSF appear to be of diagnostic and prognostic value in bacterial meningitis. Elevation of total LDH activity is a consistent finding in bacterial meningitis.

Treatment

Bacterial meningitis is a medical emergency that requires a multidisciplinary approach. Initial treatment is directed at providing general supportive measures, including maintaining blood pressure; maintaining adequate ventilation and a patent airway; treating septic shock; and providing antibacterial drug therapy. Several collaborative problems need to be addressed in the management of these patients:

- Septic shock/sepsis
- Respiratory distress
- Airway patency
- Seizures
- Increased ICP
- Electrolyte imbalance (SIADH, hyponatremia)
- Possibly adrenal insufficiency with meningococcal meningitis
- Hydrocephalus

Recommendations for antimicrobial therapy are changing as a result of the emergence on antimicrobial resistance.[11] Drug therapy is based on the identification of the causative organism from CSF analysis, if possible. Alternatively, the most likely organism is used for drug selection. The drug should be bactericidal for the suspected causative organism, and

TABLE 30-3   EMPIRIC ANTIMICROBIAL THERAPY FOR BACTERIAL MENINGITIS

PATIENT GROUP	MOST LIKELY ORGANISM	ANTIMICROBIAL THERAPY
• Adult: 2–50 yr	*Neisseria meningitides, Streptococcus pneumoniae*	Vancomycin plus a third-generation cephalosporin (ceftriaxone or cefotaxime)
• Adult: >50 yr	*S. pneumoniae, N. meningitides, Listeria monocytogenes,* aerobic gram-negative bacilli	Vancomycin plus ampicillin plus a third-generation cephalosporin (ceftriaxone or cefotaxime)
Immunocompromised patients	Opportunistic organisms	Ceftazidime plus ampicillin
Postneurosurgery	Aerobic gram-negative bacilli (including *Pseudomonas aeruginosa*), *Staphylococcus aureus,* coagulase-negative staphylococci (especial *S. epidermidis*)	Vancomycin plus cefepime, vancomycin plus ceftazidime, or vancomycin plus meropenem
Basal skull fracture	*S. pneumoniae, H. influenzae,* group A beta-hemolytic streptococci	Vancomycin plus a third-generation cephalosporin (ceftriaxone or cefotaxime)
Central nervous system shunts	Coagulase-negative staphylococci (especially *S. epidermidis*), *S. aureus,* aerobic gram-negative bacilli (including *P. aeruginosa*), *Propionibacterium acne*	Vancomycin plus cefepime, vancomycin plus ceftazidime, or vancomycin plus meropenem

From Roos, K. L. (2002). Central nervous system infections. In J. Biller (Ed.), *Practical neurology* (2nd ed., pp. 562–573). Philadelphia: Lippincott-Raven; Ropper, A. H., & Brown, R. H. (2005). *Adams and Victor's principles of neurology* (8th ed., pp. 592–630). New York: McGraw-Hill; Tunkel, A. R., Hartman, B. J., Kaplan, S. L., et al. (2004). Practice guidelines for the management of bacterial meningitis. *Clinical Infectious Diseases, 39*(9), 1267–1284.

treatment should begin while awaiting results of diagnostic tests; treatment should not be postponed until the CSF cultures are available. The empirical drug prescribed can be changed later based on definitive diagnostic findings. Patient age and known drug resistance patterns in a given area of the country should be considered. Table 30-3 outlines empiric antimicrobial therapy, and Table 30-4 lists recommendations for drug therapy based on a known organism. Intravenous drug therapy is usually necessary for a period of 10 to 14 days. *Practice Guidelines for the Management of Bacterial Meningitis* is one of many resources to guide patient management.[12]

TABLE 30-4   RECOMMENDED ANTIMICROBIAL THERAPIES BY ORGANISM FOR BACTERIAL MENINGITIS IN ADULTS

ORGANISM	ANTIMICROBIAL DRUG
Streptococcus pneumoniae	Vancomycin plus a third-generation cephalosporin (ceftriaxone or cefotaxime)
Neisseria meningitidis	Third-generation cephalosporin (ceftriaxone or cefotaxime)
Haemophilus influenzae	Third-generation cephalosporin (ceftriaxone or cefotaxime)
Pseudomonas aeruginosa	Cefepime or ceftazidime
Listeria monocytogenes	Ampicillin or penicillin G
Staphylococcus aureus (methicillin sensitive)	Nafcillin or oxacillin
S. aureus (methicillin resistant)	Vancomycin
Enterobacteriaceae	Third-generation cephalosporin (ceftriaxone or cefotaxime)

Differences of opinion are noted regarding the administration of dexamethasone and phenytoin. Although there is limited evidence to support use of corticosteroids, dexamethasone, a corticosteroid, is recommended for bacterial meningitis to decrease the associated inflammation and edema.[4,6] It should be started immediately after the CSF is collected and *before* antibiotics are begun or at least given with the first dose. The recommended dose of dexamethasone is 0.15 mg/kg intravenously every 6 hours for the first 4 days of therapy.[6] Concurrent use of a histamine-2 receptor antagonist is recommended to prevent gastrointestinal hemorrhage. Prophylactic use of phenytoin is recommended by some to prevent seizures because about 40% of patients will have a seizure. Other physicians choose to begin phenytoin only if the patient has had a seizure.

Complications

Complications of bacterial meningitis relate to the type of causative organism and the severity of the illness. Increased ICP can occur and is managed using the usual increased ICP treatment protocols that include both medical and nursing interventions outlined in Chapter 13. If hyponatremia is present, free water is restricted. Cranial nerve palsies and especially sensorineural hearing loss are common. Meningeal fibrosis around the optic nerve can cause blindness, optic atrophy, or optic neuritis. Hydrocephalus from exudate and meningeal fibrosis can cause dementia, stupor or coma, and paralysis in adults. Other possible complications include personality change, headache, seizure activity, or paresis or paralysis.

Prevention

Bacterial meningitis can often be prevented if the following principles are observed:

• Provide adequate treatment of infections, such as sinusitis, mastoiditis, ear infections, and pneumonias.

- Maintain strict aseptic technique during all intracranial, intraspinal, mastoid, and sinus operations.
- Maintain strict aseptic technique in dressing changes for these procedures.
- Administer prophylactic antibiotics after these procedures.
- Administer prophylactic antibiotics with basal skull fractures, compound skull fractures, dural tears, and injuries causing CSF drainage from the ear or nose.
- Vaccination against *H. influenzae* is effective.

Viral Meningitis

Viral meningitis, also known as *acute benign lymphocytic meningitis* and *acute aseptic meningitis*, occurs sporadically or as small epidemics. Any number of viruses, such as mumps, enteroviruses (Echo, Coxsackie, poliomyelitis), herpes simplex virus type 2, Epstein-Barr virus, and the arboviruses, can be the causative organisms, but no specific organism is identified in most cases. Human immunodeficiency virus (HIV) infection can present as aseptic meningitis, especially at the time of seroconversion. All age groups are susceptible, but children are most often affected.

Signs and Symptoms

Signs and symptoms include those of the meningitis syndrome, such as headache, low-grade fever, stiff neck, and symptoms of a systemic or upper respiratory viral illness. Often, a systemic viral infection can be identified.

Diagnosis and Treatment

The CSF is clear with a WBC count typically in the range of 50 to several hundred cell/mm^3, predominantly mononuclear cells. The glucose level is normal, and protein is in the range of 50 to 100 mg/dL. A CT scan may be ordered if there is evidence of focal neurological signs.

Treatment of viral meningitis is symptomatic and supportive. Mild cases are managed outside the hospital, but patients with extreme discomfort or excessive vomiting may need hospitalization for symptom management. No drug therapy is effective against the virus. Full recovery is usual within 1 to 2 weeks.

Nursing Management of Patients With Meningitis

Various collaborative problems provide the context of care for patients with meningitis. As a member of the collaborative team, the nurse assesses and monitors the patient throughout the course of the illness, recognizing that the patient is at high risk for complications. Regardless of the etiology of the meningitis, nursing management includes providing supportive care, adhering to specific protocols (e.g., ICP and seizure prophylaxis), preventing complications, and enhancing rehabilitation.[13]

Assessment

In the acute stage of meningitis, the patient is seriously ill.

- Assess vital signs frequently and compare with previous results to detect changes and trends. It is not uncommon for the temperature to reach 40.5°C (105°F). The pulse and respiratory rate are also high in response to the fever. If signs and symptoms of increased ICP are present, the pulse may be depressed and systolic blood pressure elevated.
- Monitor neurological signs frequently. The level of consciousness (LOC) characteristically deteriorates from confusion to restlessness, lethargy, stupor, and, finally, coma. As the LOC deteriorates, the nurse should assess the patient's ability to protect his or her airway.
- Note signs and symptoms of meningeal irritation as evidenced by nuchal rigidity such as stiff neck, photophobia, pain upon neck flexion, or positive Kernig's or Brudzinski's signs.
- Monitor for evidence of seizure activity and therapeutic levels of anticonvulsant therapy.
- Maintain an accurate intake and output record. A patient with an elevated temperature can easily become dehydrated from profuse perspiration and insensible loss from the skin. Profuse perspiration, oliguria, and dry skin indicate dehydration that requires intravenous (IV) fluid replacement.
- Monitor serum electrolytes for electrolyte imbalances, such as hyponatremia.

Nursing Management

The key points of nursing management of patients with meningitis and the common patient problems and nursing diagnoses are outlined in Charts 30-1 and 30-2.

Rehabilitation

With meningitis patients, the specific rehabilitative needs depend on the degree of functional disability. Minor functional disabilities may not require any special intervention and improve spontaneously over time with physical activity. Other functional deficits may require an aggressive rehabilitation plan. A comprehensive assessment by the interdisciplinary team is the best means for identifying deficits, determining needed rehabilitation, and setting realistic goals. The nurse works collaboratively with the case manager and other team members to assist in the transition to rehabilitation or home.

ENCEPHALITIS

Encephalitis is an inflammation of the brain caused by viruses, bacteria, fungi, or parasites. Some viruses are endemic to particular geographical areas and to particular seasons of the year. There is a lengthy list of specific viruses known to cause viral encephalitis, but only a few appear with appreciable frequency in the United States. There are about 20,000 cases of acute viral encephalitis reported annually in the United States. Table 30-5 lists and describes the major viruses capable of causing viral encephalitis. Less frequent causes of encephalitis include toxic substances such as lead, arsenic, and carbon monoxide; vaccines for measles,

| CHART **30-1** | **Summary of the Nursing Management of Patients With Acute Meningitis/Encephalitis** |

NURSING RESPONSIBILITIES	**RATIONALE**

ASSESSMENT

- Assess vital signs at frequent intervals.

- Assess neurological signs at frequent intervals.

- Assess for signs of meningeal irritation (nuchal rigidity, hyperirritability, hyperalgesia, photophobia).
- Assess respiratory function (auscultate chest; observe chest movement).

- Establishes a baseline and provides ongoing data to denote stability, improvement, or deterioration in overall conditions
- Establishes a baseline and provides ongoing data for comparison to determine change
- Indicates irritation of the covering of the brain and the need for special nursing intervention
- Alerts the nurse to initiate respiratory support if necessary

BASIC SUPPORTIVE CARE

- Maintain a patent airway.
  - Position the patient to facilitate drainage.
  - Suction as necessary.
- Maintain adequate oxygenation
  - Monitor pulse oximeter.
  - Monitor blood gases.
  - Administer oxygen therapy, as ordered.
  - Assess for signs and symptoms of dyspnea and cyanosis.
- Administer basic hygienic care.
- Provide for mouth care every 2 hours.

- Protect the patient from injury by:
  - Following injury prevention protocol for high-risk patients
  - Raising side rails
  - Keeping the bed low when the patient is left alone
  - Observing frequently
  - Protecting the intravenous site or any tubes
- If the temperature is elevated, follow temperature reduction protocol to control the temperature, including:
  - Administering antipyretic drugs, such as acetaminophen (Tylenol), 650 mg orally or rectally
  - Removing excess bedclothes
  - Maintaining a cool room temperature (68°F or 20°C)
  - Giving tepid baths
- Control headache, if present, by:
  - Elevating the head 30 degrees
  - Applying an ice cap as necessary
  - Maintaining a quiet, darkened room
  - Administering analgesics as necessary (e.g., acetaminophen [Tylenol], 650 mg, or codeine, 15–30 mg q4h)

- Provides for adequate drainage of oral and nasal secretions

- Provides supplemental oxygen to maintain adequate oxygenation

- Keeps patient dry and comfortable, especially when diaphoretic
- Refreshes and moistens the patient's oral cavity, particularly when fever is present
- Prevents physical injury to a patient who has a deteriorated level of consciousness and who is often extremely restless

- An increase in temperature increases the need for oxygen to support increased metabolism. An elevated temperature also increases intracranial pressure.

- Provides for the patient's comfort and removes major source of restlessness

PREVENTION OF COMPLICATIONS

The duration of the acute and chronic phase of meningitis depends on many variables. However, specific nursing protocols are followed to prevent complications.
- Provide skin care every 2 to 4 h.
  - If feverish patient perspires profusely, change bed linens to prevent irritation of the skin.
  - Give special attention to bony prominences.
- If unable to turn independently, turn every 2 h.
  - If the patient can follow instructions, encourage deep breathing exercises every 2 h.
- Apply elastic hose when on bed rest.
- Position in good body alignment.
- Observe for signs of adrenal insufficiency in the patient with meningococcal meningitis (hypotension, respiratory collapse, petechiae).

- Prevents skin breakdown; if unable to change position, lubricate, and inspect the skin.

- Prevents atelectasis and pneumonia

- Improves blood return to the heart and decreases risk of thrombophlebitis
- Prevents development of orthopedic deformities
- Immediate intervention necessary to preserve the patient's life

CHART **30-2**	**Summary of Patient Problems and Nursing Diagnoses Associated With Meningitis/Encephalitis**

PATIENT PROBLEMS/ NURSING DIAGNOSES	NURSING INTERVENTIONS	EXPECTED OUTCOMES
Pain (headache, backache, photophobia, and neck pain) related to (R/T) swelling of intracranial contents and irritation of meninges.	• Assess the location, quality, and severity of pain (cognitively impaired patients may not be able to use the visual analog scale [VAS] to rate severity of pain). • Provide comfort measures, such as positioning, turning, and application of cool, wet cloths to the head. • Control direct light; darken the patient's room. • Assess the need for use of prn analgesics and administer medication as necessary. • Monitor response to pain and analgesics.	• The patient will report relief or amelioration of pain (documented by the VAS, if possible), or will demonstrate signs of enhanced comfort, such as decreased agitation and ability to sleep.
Altered Tissue Perfusion, Cerebral, R/T cerebral edema and increased intracranial pressure (ICP)	• Elevate the head of the bed to a 30-degree angle. • Keep the neck in a neutral position. • Prevent Valsalva's maneuver. • Monitor neurological signs for evidence of neurological deterioration. • If an intracranial pressure (ICP) monitor is in place, monitor cerebral perfusion pressure (CPP). • Monitor blood gas levels. • Use prn measures to support CPP following parameters set by physician.	• If an ICP monitor is in place, CPP will be maintained at >70 mm Hg pressure. • Neurological signs will reflect stability or improvement.
Hyperthermia R/T infection, inflammation, and pressure on the hypothalamus	• Remove excess bedclothes. • Control room temperature at <70°F. • Apply a cool, wet cloth to the head. • Provide tepid water sponge baths as necessary. • Assess the need for use of prn antipyretic drugs and administer drugs as necessary. • Avoid shivering in the patient.	• Temperature will be maintained at 99°F or lower.
Sleep Pattern Disturbance R/T agitation and/or increased sensitivity to environmental stimuli	• Assess sleep-wakefulness pattern. • Manage the environment to control and decrease environmental stimuli at night. • Make the patient comfortable. • Plan nursing care to provide for uninterrupted quiet and rest.	• At least three sleep periods, lasting 2 h each, will be experienced during the night.
High Risk for Injury R/T agitation, seizure potential, altered consciousness, and cognitive impairment	• Maintain seizure precautions. • Provide a safe environment (e.g., keep the bed in a low position). • Observe the patient frequently. • Assess the need for use of prn orders for sedatives and administer as necessary.	• Physical injury will not be sustained while hospitalized.
Risk for Disuse Syndrome R/T prolonged bedrest	• Develop a turning and repositioning schedule to prevent skin breakdown. • Use supportive devices as necessary. • Apply elastic stockings. • Elastic hose and alternating compression air boots may be used. • Institute a bowel care program. • Position to facilitate breathing and airway patency. • Provide a urinary elimination program. • Monitor intake and output, electrolytes, blood gas levels, skin integrity, bowel and bladder elimination pattern, and peripheral tissue perfusion.	• The patient will not develop • Pressure ulcers • Contractures • Deep vein thrombosis • Constipation • Urinary infection • Atelectasis and pneumonia • Dehydration

TABLE 30-5   MAJOR VIRUSES RESPONSIBLE FOR VIRAL ENCEPHALITIS

TYPE OF VIRUS OR DISORDER	SPECIFIC DISORDER OR CAUSATIVE ORGANISM	COMMENTS
Arboviruses (arthropod borne) Altered cycle of infection of mosquito and host Mosquito bites infect host, which subsequently becomes infected Infected mosquito infects host (including humans)	Eastern equine encephalitis* Western equine encephalitis St. Louis encephalitis California virus encephalitis Venezuelan equine encephalitis Japanese B encephalitis Murray Valley (Australian X) encephalitis	Early autumn outbreak in Eastern states; yearround incidence throughout country Late summer outbreak throughout the U.S. except on the West coast Early autumn outbreak in Midwest Year-round incidence in southwestern U.S. South and Central America
Type of virus	von Economo disease, also called encephalitis lethargica and sleeping sickness	Epidemic in U.S. following the influenza epidemic of 1918; has not recurred since 1926
Postviral disease resulting in central nervous system infection	Measles Mumps Chickenpox	
Postvaccination encephalitis	Develops within a week after vaccination for measles, rubella, mumps, or rabies	Appears to be an immune reaction
Other viral infections	Poliomyelitis Rabies Herpes simplex Herpes zoster Infectious mononucleosis	

*Most serious of the arboviruses in the United States; significant mortality rate and serious deficits in many that survive (e.g., retardation, seizures, personality changes, hemiplegia); least frequent arbovirus.

mumps, and rabies, which cause postvaccination encephalitis; and viral infections, such as measles, mumps, infectious mononucleosis, and others. The following section addresses selected encephalitis caused by viruses, the most common cause of encephalitis in the United States.

Signs and Symptoms

The many signs and symptoms of viral encephalitis vary according to the particular invading organisms and the area of the brain involved. The basic encephalitis syndrome is characterized by fever, headache, seizures, stiff neck, and a change in the LOC, which varies from disorientation, agitation, restlessness, and short attention span to lethargy or drowsiness, and finally to coma.[4] In addition to the wide diversity of levels of consciousness, the patient may exhibit any combination of the following symptoms: aphasia or mutism; motor deficits such as hemiparesis, involuntary (myoclonic) movements, ataxia, nystagmus, ocular paralysis, or facial weakness; or generalized seizures.

Diagnosis can be difficult and is based on the clinical picture, rapid serologic assays, and CSF analysis. No specific viral etiology is determined in most cases. CSF findings associated with arboviruses include elevated WBCs (mononuclear cells), increase in protein, and normal glucose. There is no definitive treatment or drug therapy for viral encephalitis. Often, the electroencephalogram (EEG) is characterized by widespread slowing. Serologic diagnosis depends on a fourfold rise in specific antibody titer, which is often not evident in the acute phase. Imaging studies of the brain are often normal, although there may be diffuse edema or enhancement of

the cerebral cortex. In the case of herpes simplex virus (HSV) encephalitis, there is characteristic damage to the inferomedial temporal and frontal lobes.

Although the foregoing description provides the basic clinical picture of acute viral encephalitis, variations in signs and symptoms are noted with specific groupings of viral organisms. The following summarizes cause-specific encephalitis syndromes.

Viral Encephalitis Caused by Arthropod-Borne Viruses

Arthropod-borne viruses, also called arboviruses, causing epidemic encephalitis include Eastern equine, Western equine, St. Louis, California, West Nile, and Japanese encephalitis, all spread by mosquitoes. The Japanese encephalitis (JE) serogroup of genus flavivirus has caused the many cases of encephalitis across the globe; West Nile virus is a member of the JE serogroup.[14] West Nile encephalitis has become endemic in the United States since 1999. There is a wide clinical spectrum that includes aseptic meningitis, meningoencephalitis, or encephalitis with or without flaccid paralysis. The severity of West Nile encephalitis ranges from asymptomatic serum conversion to severe neurologic deficits to death.[15]

The incidence of encephalitis is more prevalent in late summer and early fall. The severity varies by virus type. Eastern equine and JE are severe, and Western equine and St. Louis may be severe. California encephalitis has both mild and severe forms. Western equine and St. Louis encephalitis affect older persons more frequently. HSV encephalitis is the commonest sporadic cause of encephalitis, has no seasonal or geographical predilection, and is seen more often in the 5- to 30-year and over 50-year age groups. The effects of encephalitis on the brain include degenerative changes in the nerve cells, with scattered areas of inflammation and necrosis. There is also some inflammation of the meninges.

Signs and Symptoms

The clinical picture presented by all arboviruses in the United States is essentially the same. In older children and adults, the onset is gradual and is characterized by a febrile illness, headache, listlessness, drowsiness, and several days of nausea and vomiting. Seizures, confusion and stupor, stiff neck, muscle pain, ataxia, photophobia, and tremors are then noted. Reflexes are abnormal, and hemiparesis may be present. Residual effects include mental retardation, epilepsy, personality changes with psychosis, dementia, paresis or paralysis, deafness, and blindness.

Mortality rates and the rates of residual effects associated with viral encephalitis from arboviruses vary greatly. Eastern equine encephalitis (50% mortality rate) and Japanese B encephalitis (most common in the world) have higher mortality rates than the Western variety. Although approximately 80% to 90% of patients with Eastern equine encephalitis develop complications, only 5% to 10% of patients with Western equine infections manifest residual effects. Reported mortality for West Nile encephalitis is 4% to 16%, while the presence of neuropsychiatric sequelae is 50% to 65%.[14]

Diagnosis and Treatment

There is no recognized specific treatment for encephalitis. Treatment is supportive and symptomatic, such as management of increased ICP. Drugs administered may include steroids to control cerebral edema, anticonvulsants to prevent seizures, analgesics for headache, and antipyretics to control hyperthermia.

The nursing management for all patients with viral encephalitis is supportive. The basic points of care are outlined in Charts 30-1 and 30-2.

Herpes Simplex Encephalitis

Herpes simplex encephalitis, caused by herpes simplex virus type 1, is the most common sporadic encephalitis affecting all age groups in the United States. There are two types of herpes simplex virus: type 1, which is associated with the common cold sore and is present in most people in the dormant state, and type 2, which is associated with the sexually transmitted genital disease. Herpes simplex virus type 1 is also capable of producing acute encephalitis in the adult. Although the activating trigger for the latent virus is not known, some believe it is activated by fever, emotional stress, and infectious diseases. It is also unclear how the virus enters the CNS. Possible avenues include the bloodstream and peripheral nerves.

Herpes simplex encephalitis is a severe, life-threatening illness that causes inflammation of the brain parenchyma. The virus attacks the brain and has a particular propensity for the frontal and temporal lobes. The brain or, more specifically, the temporal lobes become edematous, and necrotic areas with or without hemorrhage develop. Once developed, cerebral edema is pronounced with increased ICP and possible temporal lobe herniation. Death occurs in 30% to 70% of patients if treatment is not begun before the onset of coma. The mortality rate is reduced to 28% if treatment with acyclovir (Zovirax) is begun before coma occurs. For those who survive, most are left with serious neurological deficits.

Symptoms evolve over a few days and include fever, nausea and vomiting, headache, memory loss, confusion, stupor, coma, and seizures. Some patients also experience symptoms of temporal lobe-limbic system deficits, such as olfactory and gustatory hallucinations, anosmia, temporal lobe seizures, periodic bizarre behavioral manifestations, and aphasia. Cerebral edema and hemorrhage cause an abrupt increase in ICP. Temporal or brainstem herniation can result. The marked increase in ICP produces coma, causes changes in vital signs, and affects breathing. If the disease is allowed to progress, temporal lobe herniation of one or both lobes occurs, leading to deep coma, respiratory arrest, and death. Death is most apt to occur within the first 72 hours when the cerebral edema is most pronounced.

The diagnosis of herpes simplex encephalitis is difficult to establish in its early stage. By the time a diagnosis is established, it may be too late to benefit the patient; therefore, an aggressive approach to diagnosis is essential. The usual diagnostic work-up includes a history and neurological examination; CSF analysis from lumbar puncture; a CT scan or, preferably, a magnetic resonance imaging (MRI) scan; and an EEG. Pressure during lumbar puncture is markedly elevated. Findings on CSF analysis include increased polymorphonuclear cells (early) and lymphocytes, increased protein, normal glucose (usually), and possible xanthochromia if cerebral hemorrhage has occurred. The EEG is often abnormal, with periodic sharp-wave complexes from one or both temporal regions on a background of low-amplitude activity.

Recent advances in molecular biology now allow very early detection of DNA from the virus in the CSF, and such techniques are routinely used at many centers. Herpes simplex virus itself is difficult to isolate early. Although a fourfold elevation in antibody titer may be seen in the convalescent serum, this is of no help in crucial early diagnosis, and, in fact, may be misleading. For these reasons the detection of viral DNA is an important step in early diagnosis.

Early in the course of the illness, the CT scan may be normal, but the result of the MRI scan is usually abnormal even in the first week of the disease. Hemorrhagic areas in the inferior frontal-temporal region, together with surrounding edema, are usually evident on both studies later in the disease. The EEG may show focal or generalized slowing. Often, there is evidence of seizure activity in the temporal region.

The drug of choice for treatment of herpes simplex encephalitis is acyclovir (Zovirax) 10 mg/kg every 8 hours (30 mg/kg/day) IV for 10 to 14 days. Other drugs that are commonly administered include:

- Dexamethasone (Decadron) in tapering doses to reduce cerebral edema
- Cimetidine (Tagamet) to decrease gastric secretion and prevent development of gastric hemorrhage associated with the use of steroids

- Furosemide (Lasix) or mannitol for diuresis
- Phenytoin (Dilantin) to prevent or control seizures
- Acetaminophen (Tylenol) to control hyperthermia and headache

In addition to drug therapy, treatment is supportive and symptomatic and includes support of respiratory function, an adequate oxygen supply, support of fluid and electrolyte balance, nutrition management, and management of increased ICP.

If the patient survives the acute episode, neurological deficits are common and may include cognitive deficits (e.g., memory, reasoning), personality changes with dementia, seizure disorders, motor deficits, and dysphagia.

Charts 30-1 and 30-2 describe basic principles of management and nursing diagnosis. In some respects management is similar to that of the patient with meningitis. Additional nursing interventions include:

- Monitor neurological signs to detect neurological deterioration; onset of coma indicates a poor prognosis.
- Monitor for evidence of rising ICP; follow treatment protocol to decrease ICP and prevent herniation.
- Isolation is *not necessary*; however, good handwashing technique should be followed.

OTHER VIRAL ORGANISMS THAT ATTACK THE CENTRAL NERVOUS SYSTEM

A few selected, uncommon diseases caused by viruses are presented in Table 30-6. They include poliomyelitis, rabies, tetanus, Lyme disease, cysticercosis, and parameningeal infections. Herpes zoster is seen mostly in older people and thus is seen more in clinical practice because of the increasing numbers of older people in the general population.[16]

Parameningeal Infections

Parameningeal infections are infections that occur in and around the meninges. Three major localized, suppurative lesions in this area are brain abscesses, subdural empyema, and extradural abscesses.

Brain Abscess

A brain abscess is caused by an infection, which extends into the cerebral tissue or by organisms carried from other sites in the body. The major sites of primary infections that extend directly into the brain are infections of the middle ear, mastoid, and sinus. Approximately 40% of all brain abscesses result from middle ear and mastoid infections. Sinus infections (frontal and sphenoid) are responsible for another 10%. A few abscesses occur as a result of intracranial surgery, compound skull fractures, or oral surgery. The remainder of brain abscesses, approximately 50%, are carried by the blood from remote infectious sites. Examples of such sites include generalized lung infection, lung abscess, bronchiectasis, empyema, skin infections, acute bacterial endocarditis, and congenital heart or lung disease with a right-to-left shunt. These abscesses are sometimes called metastatic abscesses.

The location of the brain abscess depends on the source and method of the spread of the infection. Those infections that spread directly from a primary focus create a brain abscess directly adjacent to the primary site. Given that infections around the face spread in retrograde fashion through venous sinuses, an associated brain abscess can be located at some distance from the primary focus.

The pathophysiology is one of initial infected tissue that is soft, edematous, congested, and infiltrated with polymorphonuclear leukocytes. The lesion is poorly delineated and may represent a localized, suppurative encephalitis. Within the next 2 weeks, the necrotic tissue liquefies. The abscess becomes encapsulated by a zone of fibroblasts that surrounds the site and progressively thickens. This wall of granulated tissue is replaced by collagenous connective tissue. The wall is not of uniform thickness and tends to be thinner in its deepest portion. The abscess, which can vary in size and shape, usually lies in the white matter. The deepest thin-walled portion of the abscess lying in the white matter can eventually rupture into the ventricles with catastrophic results. One or more poorly encapsulated daughter abscesses may surround the major abscess, with possible direct communication between them.

Signs and Symptoms. The signs and symptoms of brain abscess can be viewed in two stages: the initial, acute invasion; and the enlarging lesion. The initial invasion corresponds to the initial formation of the abscess. The patient may encounter the following symptoms: headache; chills and fever; malaise; elevated WBCs; and neurological deficits such as confusion and drowsiness, focal or generalized seizures, motor or sensory deficits, and speech disorders. Some patients may be asymptomatic during this period. There may be a history of reactivation of an infectious process in a patient who has had a previous ear, sinus, or lung infection. Symptoms of this earlier recurring infection may be superimposed on the symptoms of brain abscess formation. Symptoms associated with the initial stage may subside temporarily in response to drug therapy.

In the second stage, the formalized abscess behaves as a rapidly growing, space-occupying lesion. Within a few weeks, depending on the size of the abscess, the following signs and symptoms may be observed: flu-like symptoms; recurrent headache that becomes increasingly severe; confusion, drowsiness, and stupor; focal or generalized seizures; focal deficits; signs of increased ICP; and possible herniation syndromes.

Symptoms According to Abscess Location. Abscesses in particular areas have characteristic signs and symptoms. The following are three common areas of abscess formation with a list of related symptoms:

- **Frontal lobe abscess:** contralateral hemiparesis, expressive aphasia (if the dominant hemisphere is involved), focal or jacksonian seizure, and frontal headache
- **Temporal lobe abscess:** localized headache, upper quadrant visual deficit, contralateral facial weakness, and minimal aphasia

TABLE 30-6   OTHER SELECTED NERVOUS SYSTEM INFECTIONS

DISEASE/ORGANISM	DESCRIPTION/COURSE	DIAGNOSIS/TREATMENT
Creutzfeldt-Jakob disease; caused by a prion	• Spongiform encephalopathy characterized by progressive dementia, dysarthria, spastic weakness of the limbs, myoclonic jerks, and seizures • 3 years is the average incubation period • Usually occurs in fifth or sixth decade • Vacuolar or spongelike appearance of brain tissue • Death is the final outcome	• *Diagnosis:* confirmed by brain biopsy • *Treatment:* supportive care
Herpes zoster (shingles) (herpes virus-varicella zoster)	• Latent virus from an attack of chickenpox that remains latent in the sensory ganglia • When the host defenses fail, the virus multiplies within the sensory ganglia and is then transported down the sensory nerve and released to the vesicles at the nerve endings • Involves the dorsal root ganglia; follows the sensory distribution of dermatome • An extremely painful affliction in which a rash (vesicles and large irregular bullae on the erythematous base) develops; rash develops from papules → vesicles → pustules → scabs • Some patients may develop postherpetic neuralgia after an attack; otherwise, it is a self-limiting condition • Herpes zoster can attack the ophthalmic branch of the trigeminal nerve and can cause scarring of the eye	• *Diagnosis:* based on clinical findings (vesicles [occurring 2–5 d after pain]); pain along the peripheral nerve) • *Treatment:* acyclovir, 800 mg 5 times a day for 7–10 d; isolation not required
Poliomyelitis (caused by one of three polioviruses)—type 1, 2, or 3	• Attacks the motor cells of the anterior horn cells of the spinal cord • Severity varies from mild to paralysis, with death from paralysis of respiratory muscle • Enters through gastrointestinal (GI) tract • Spread through contact with feces and pharyngeal secretions from infected persons	• *Diagnosis:* based on clinical findings and isolation of the virus • *Treatment:* supportive care; may need ventilation support; most patients require extensive rehabilitation; isolation precautions are maintained for a period of time. • *Note:* with the advent of the effective Salk vaccine, incidence of this disease has virtually been eliminated because of mass immunization.

Rabies (rhabdovirus) (<10 cases in the U.S./yr)	• An acute encephalomyelitis infection
	• Transmitted to humans from the saliva of infected animals through bite or contact with saliva
	• Spread from the wound to the central nervous system by the peripheral nerves
	• Incubation period varies depending on the distance of the wound from the head
	• Course of disease
	  —*Early phase:* vague flu-like symptoms (headache, malaise, vomiting, fever, drowsiness)
	  —*Second phase:* extreme excitement and salivation, deranged behavior, convulsions, severe and painful spasms of the pharyngeal and laryngeal muscles from slight stimuli or sight of food (lasts 2–7 d)
	  —*Final phase:* onset of coma, followed by cardiac and respiratory arrest
		• *Diagnosis:* based on a history of a bite and isolation of the virus
		• *Treatment:* administration of antitoxin (causes serious side effects); supportive care; isolation required; death may result. Vaccination used even after disease has begun
		• *Note:* vaccination for those traveling to areas of prevalence is encouraged.

Tetanus (*Clostridium tetani*)	• Spread through horse and cattle feces that contaminate soil and objects within the soil • Enters humans from penetrating and crush wounds • Produces three exotoxins that attack the spinal cord and cranial nerves • Causes severe muscle spasms, extreme sensitivity to stimuli, and convulsions • Death may occur from asphyxia	• *Diagnosis:* based on the history and clinical findings • *Treatment:* administration of antitoxin and supportive care • *Note:* immunization is available (tetanus toxoid and tetanus immunoglobulin).

TABLE 30–6 OTHER SELECTED NERVOUS SYSTEM INFECTIONS (Continued)

DISEASE/ORGANISM	DESCRIPTION/COURSE	DIAGNOSIS/TREATMENT

Lyme disease (caused by *Borrelia burgdorferi*)—named for Lyme, Connecticut, where an outbreak first caused attention	• Spirochete transmitted by the bite of an infected tick of the *Ixodes ricinus* complex
	• Carried on white-tail deer and other wild animals
	• Course of disease
	  —*Stage 1:* localized erythema migrans, a rash that resembles a bull's eye; rash fades within 3–4 wk; there may be occurrence of signs of meningitis, radiculitis, and neuritis in an afebrile patient
	  —*Stage 2:* complications may develop—heart block in 10%; Bell's palsy in 10%; other problems may include meningitis, encephalitis, polyradiculitis, or inflammation of the eyes
	  —*Stage 3:* occurs 4 wk to years after the bite; characterized by arthritis symptoms affecting the large joints and chronic joint pain
		• *Diagnosis:* based on a history of bite (which the patient may not recall); elevated titer to Lyme disease after 4 wk
		• *Treatment:*
		  —*Stage 1:* azithromycin, amoxicillin, and doxycycline are recommended for treatment of stage 1 to prevent the development of subsequent stages; ceftriaxone is usually given IV in patients with neurological symptoms and helps to resolve symptoms.
		  —*Stage 2:* IV administration of 20 million U of penicillin; others recommend tetracycline 500 mg qid.
		  —*Stage 3:* controversial; antibiotics are used.

Cysticercosis of central nervous system (CNS) (caused by *Taenia solium*)	• Most common parasite affecting the CNS • In Central and South America, this is the leading cause of epilepsy and neurological disturbances • Humans who consume raw or undercooked meat from infected animals can become contaminated • When ingested, cyst forms that contains larva; the cyst can lodge in the brain, as well as in other areas • May lodge in ventricles	• *Diagnosis:* based on multiple, calcified lesions in the brain noted on computed tomography scan or radiologic studies • *Treatment:* oral praziquantel, for 3 d; symptomatic treatment of cerebral edema with steroids; surgery may be required to remove intracranial cyst.

- **Cerebellar abscess:** postauricular (below the ear) or occipital headache, ipsilateral ataxia and limb paresis, and nystagmus and weakness of gaze to the side of the lesion

Diagnosis and Treatment. The diagnosis of brain abscess is based on the following criteria:

- Identification of a primary infection, such as middle ear, sinus, or lung infection, helps to pinpoint the source of the problem. Chest, skull, and sinus radiographs may be necessary to identify the primary focus of infection.
- On lumbar puncture, the CSF pressure is elevated. Findings on analysis of the CSF include an elevated WBC count from a few to several thousand, with lymphocytes being the predominant cell; elevated protein; and normal glucose. An abrupt onset of coma with a WBC count of 50,000 in the CSF should make one highly suspicious of rupture of an abscess into the ventricles.
- Other laboratory data to localize the lesion include an EEG (area of high voltage over the abscess) and a CT scan.

Early diagnosis and prompt antimicrobial treatment are essential. Because anaerobic *Streptococci* and *Bacteroides* are the predominant causative organisms, penicillin G (20 million U) and chloramphenicol (4 to 6 g daily IV in divided doses) are given. In addition, management of the rapidly rising ICP is achieved with IV mannitol, followed by a course of dexamethasone (Decadron, 6 to 12 mg every 6 hours). If this is not effective, surgery will be necessary to remove or aspirate the abscess. If the abscess is well encapsulated, attempts are made to excise surgically both the abscess and membrane totally. If this is not possible, the abscess is aspirated and drained. Injection of the sac with antimicrobial drugs follows.

It may be necessary at some future time to drain the sac again because of a build-up of suppurative material.

The use of drugs has greatly reduced the mortality rate from brain abscess. The aggressive treatment of infections that can lead to the formation of brain abscesses has also been a prophylactic aid. The cause of death from brain abscess is the massive increase in ICP and rupture of the abscess into the ventricles. Of the patients who survive, approximately 30% develop neurological deficits, of which focal seizures are most common.

Extradural Abscess

Extradural abscesses may be associated with osteomyelitis of a cranial bone; infection of the sinuses or the ear; or a surgical procedure in which the frontal sinus or mastoid has been opened. A pus pocket accumulates between the bone and dura.

Symptoms include localized pain, fever, tenderness, and purulent discharge. Stiffness of the neck is possible. Localized neurological signs are often absent. If they occur, focal seizures, cranial nerve VI palsy, and decreased sensory perception of the face are the most common symptoms. The only abnormalities noted in the CSF are a few lymphocytes and neutrophils and a slightly elevated protein level.

Treatment consists of antibiotics and surgery for removal of the diseased bone at a future date.

Nursing Management of Patients With Parameningeal Infections

The nursing management of the patient with a brain abscess can be viewed in two stages: the acute initial invasion when the infection organizes into an abscess, and the second stage when the abscess behaves like a space-occupying lesion.

During the initial stage, symptoms correspond to a general systemic infection. If neurological symptoms are present, they can be important in localizing the lesion. Often, symptoms are so general that a diagnosis is unclear. Nursing management during this period includes assessing the patient's condition, managing any presenting symptoms, providing supportive care, and administering drug treatment. If signs of increased ICP are present, follow the basic care outlined in Chapter 13. Seizure precautions are maintained to prevent injury. Noting how a seizure progresses is helpful for diagnosis. Neurological assessment, including assessment for signs and symptoms of meningeal irritation, is important. Medications ordered are given through IV. As with meningitis, adherence to the administration timetable is imperative for maintaining therapeutic blood levels. Because the drugs used are potent, the patient must be observed for both drug side effects and the development of secondary infections, which can flourish when antimicrobial therapy is used.

In the second stage, the abscess behaves like a space-occupying lesion. Signs and symptoms of neurological deficit must be investigated to make a diagnosis. After the diagnosis is made, appropriate treatment is begun. If surgery is necessary to remove or drain the abscess, nursing management pertinent to the craniotomy patient should be implemented (see Chap. 14).

SUMMARY

This chapter briefly addressed the most common central nervous systems infections seen in the hospitalized patient. Patients with meningitis or encephalitis are often critically ill and need a multidisciplinary team approach with excellent nursing care to support the patient.

REFERENCES

1. Peltola, H. (1999). Prophylaxis of bacterial meningitis. *Infectious Disease Clinics of North America, 13*(3), 685–710.
2. Guberman, A. (1994). *An introduction to clinical neurology* (pp. 419–452). Boston: Little, Brown.
3. Schuchat, A., Robinson, K., Wenger, J. D., et al. (1997). Bacterial meningitis in the United states in 1995. *New England Journal of Medicine, 337*, 970–976.
4. Ropper, A. H., & Brown, R. H. (2005). *Adams and Victor's principles of neurology* (8th ed., pp. 592–661). New York: McGraw-Hill.
5. Van de Beek, D., de Gauns, J., Spanjaard, L., Weisfelt, M., Reitsma, J. B., & Vermeulen, M. (2004). Clinical features and prormostic factirs in adults with bacterial meningitis. *New England Journal of Medicine, 352*, 950.
6. Roos, K. L. (2002). Central nervous system infections. In J. Biller (Ed.). *Practical neurology* (2nd ed., pp. 562–573). Philadelphia: Lippincott Williams & Wilkins.
7. Roos, K. L. (1999). In C. G. Goetz & E. J. Pappert (Eds.). *Textbook of clinical neurology* (pp. 842–867). Philadelphia: W. B. Saunders.
8. Rosenstein, N. E., Perkis, B. A., Stephens, D. S., Popovic, T., & Hughes, J. M. (2001). Meningococcal disease. *New England Journal of Medicine, 344*(18), 1378–1388.
9. Smillova, A., & Walker, E. (2000). Meningococcemia: A critical care emergency. *Critical Care Nurse, 20*(5), 28–38.
10. Newman, D. H. (2004). Clinical assessment of meningitis in adults. *Annuals of Emergency Medicine 44*(1), 71–73.
11. Van de Beek, D., de gans, J., Tunkel, A. R., & Wijdicks, F. M. (2006). Community-acquired bacterial meningitis in adults. *New England Journal of Medicine, 354*, 44–53.
12. Tunkel, A. R., Hartman, B. J., Kaplan, S. L., et al. (2004). Practice guidelines for the management of bacterial meningitis. *Clinical Infectious Diseases, 39*(9), 1267–1284.
13. Pullen, R. L. (2004). Clinical do's and don'ts. Assessing for signs of meningitis. *Nursing, 34*(5), 18.
14. Solomon, T. (2004). Flavivirus encephalitis. *New England Journal of Medicine, 351*(4), 370–378.
15. Cunha, B. A., Thermidor, M., Mohan, S., & Ly, H. (2005). West Nile viral encephalitis mimicking hepatic encephalopathy. *Heart & Lung, 34*(1), 72–75.
16. Gann, J. W., & Whitley, J. R. (2002). Herpes zoster. *New England Journal of Medicine, 347*(5), 340–346.

RESOURCES

Websites

There are an enormous number of websites available for providers, patients, and family members that can be easily accessed.

Nursing Management of Patients With Neurodegenerative Diseases

Dementias and Alzheimer's Disease

Joanne V. Hickey

DEMENTIA

Dementia is the generic term for a group of disorders that cause irreversible cognitive decline as a result of various pathologic mechanisms that damage brain cells. It is estimated that more than 4% of persons over the age of 65 years have dementia and that approximately 50% to 75% of those people have Alzheimer's disease (AD). The incidence of AD and vascular dementia (VaD) is age related; that is, the older one is, the greater the chance of having either disease. The estimated prevalence of dementia is 20% of people older than 85 years.[1] Considering the demographic projections for the increased number of older people in the United States, health providers must be prepared for the needs of this expanding population.

Definitions of dementia vary and are usually derived from the *Diagnostic and Statistical Manual of Mental Disorders* (4th ed., text revision), known as DSM-IV-TR, and the *International Classification of Diseases* (10th revision), known as ICD-10.[2,3] Currently, to be classified as a type of dementia, the following two criteria are used:[4]

1. Decline is noted in at least two of the four following cognitive functions:
   a. Memory
   b. Ability to generate coherent speech or understand spoken or written language
   c. Capacity to plan, make sound judgments, and carry out complex tasks
   d. Ability to process and interpret visual information
2. Decline is severe enough to interfere with day-to-day life.

The *Diagnostic and Statistical Manual of Mental Disorders*, 4th edition (DSM-IV), defines dementia as "the development of multiple cognitive deficits that include memory impairment and at least one of the following: aphasia, apraxia, agnosia, or a disturbance in executive functioning. These deficits must be sufficiently severe to cause impairment in occupational or social functioning, and must represent a decline from a previously higher level of functioning."[5] Recommended changes to the criteria for the next revision of the DSM-IV include recognition of the acquired nature, progressive loss of functional capacity, and frequent personality and behavior changes.[6]

The causes of dementia are numerous (Table 31-1) and vary by age group. *Alzheimer's disease*, the major cause of dementia accounting for more than half of all dementias

(50% to 70%), is followed by *vascular dementia* (20% to 25%).[7] A classification of dementia is found in Table 31-2. It lists the major categories of dementia including AD, VaD, mixed dementia, Parkinson's disease (PD) with dementia, dementia with Lewy bodies, frontotemporal dementia, and normal pressure hydrocephalus dementia. There has been increased interest in Lewy body causes of dementia. A Lewy body is an intracytoplasmic eosinophilic neuronal body surrounded by a lighter halo seen in some neurodegenerative disease. In PD, Lewy bodies are found in neurons of the degenerating substantia nigra. Lewy bodies can also be found in lesser numbers in other central nervous system (CNS) degenerative conditions, and occasionally in the brains of nonparkinsonian elderly persons.[8]

Some dementias are associated with an underlying primary condition and may be reversible with prompt treatment; these dementias are referred to as the *reversible dementias*. The most important challenge in treating dementia is identifying cases, some of which are uncommon, of *reversible dementia* such as chronic drug intoxication, vitamin deficiencies (B_{12} and folate), subdural hematoma, major depression, normal pressure hydrocephalus, and hypothyroidism.[9] In other instances, dementia is a chronic, irreversible condition, resulting in progressive loss of overall cognitive function. Although the dementia is not curable, it does not mean that symptoms cannot be managed and treated. The symptoms that are treatable include behavioral disorders, sleep disorders, and depression. Some drug therapy is alleged to slow the progression of the neurodegenerative process.

Along with dementias, one other diagnostic category is important to mention. *Mild cognitive impairment* (MCI) is a condition in which a person has a problem with memory, language, or another essential cognitive function serious enough to be noticeable to others and to be documented on tests, but not severe enough to interfere with daily life. It is often difficult to differentiate this problem from normal aging or dementia. Some, but not all, people with MCI develop dementia over time, especially when their primary area of difficulty involves memory.[10]

Diagnosis

There is no standard "work-up" for dementia, although three components guide the diagnostic process: a reliable

TABLE 31-1   COMMON CAUSES OF DEMENTIA

Major Causes of Dementia in U.S. Population

- Alzheimer's disease (>50%) of all cases
- Vascular dementia (20%–25%): also called multi-infarct dementia and poststroke dementia
- Alcoholism
- Parkinson's disease
- Drug/medication toxicity (potentially reversible)*

Other Less Common Causes of Dementia

Degenerative disorders
  Pick's disease, diffuse Lewy body disease; Huntington's disease; cortical basal degeneration; MS; some forms of ALS and PD; and other disorders
Chronic infections
  HIV, Creutzfeldt-Jacob disease, PML, neurosyphilis,* and opportunistic infections (TB, fungal, protozoal);* sarcoidosis*
*Neoplasms**
  Primary and metastatic brain tumors
Toxic
  Heavy metals;* organic toxins
*Vitamin deficiencies**
  Thiamine [B$_1$]—Wernicke's encephalopathy; vitamin B$_{12}$ pernicious anemia
*Endocrine and other system diseases**
  Hypothyroidism; parathyroidism; adrenal insufficiency, and renal, liver, or pulmonary failures
Head trauma and diffuse brain damage
  Chronic subdural hematoma;* normal pressure hydrocephalus;* hypoxic brain syndrome; postencephalitis
*Psychiatric disorders**
  Depression; conversion reaction

*Potentially reversible dementia either by category or specific problem.
 ALS, amyotrophic lateral sclerosis; MS, multiple sclerosis; PD, Parkinson's disease; PML, progressive multifocal leukoencephalopathy; TB, *Mycobacterium tuberculosis.*

history of the illness; physical, neurological, and mental examination; and other supportive investigations such as computed tomograph (CT), magnetic resonance imaging (MRI), electroencephalography (EEG), and laboratory tests.[10,11] Early and accurate diagnosis of dementia is important to avoid overuse of expensive medical resources and waste of precious time during which the patient is cognitively intact to participate in health care, legal, and financial decision making that is reflective of his or her wishes. Early diagnosis separates normal aging from true dementia. Older adults often complain of memory impairment such as difficulty remembering names or appointments or solving complex problems and worry needlessly about AD when normal aging is the operative process. Memory impairment is also a hallmark of AD as well as aging. The difference between the two causes is degree of memory loss and the impact on activities of daily living (ADLs). Multiple variables, including age, native intelligence, education, normal cognitive demand of work and daily living, nutrition, and psychological well-being, make normal age-related cognitive decline difficult to differentiate from AD.

The diagnosis of age-related cognitive decline should not be made without screening the patient for dementia. Table 31-3 lists signs and symptoms that suggest the need for a dementia evaluation, including a careful history, a general physical examination and neurological examination, and diagnostics tailored to the differential diagnoses suggested by the history and physical examination.[11] Figure 31-1 provides a flow chart for the recognition and initial assessment for dementias.

History of Present Illness and a Physical/Neurological Examination

Some patients fearful of dementia seek medical attention for reassurance. Other undiagnosed patients with dementia may visit the health care provider reluctantly, coming at the insistence of family members. Often a frightening event has triggered the decision to seek medical evaluation. Common triggers often involve a threat to safety such as leaving a stove on or becoming lost in familiar surroundings. The patient may try to provide a plausible explanation to downplay the event and show little insight into the concerns expressed by the family.

Screening begins with a complete medical history and detailed description of the current illness that includes impairments of function, behavior, and cognition. Conversation with the patient is useful to determine the presence of a progressive decline in memory, personality or behavioral changes, psychiatric problems, or functional deterioration in the ability to conduct ADLs and instrumental ADLs, to participate in hobbies and social functions, or to conduct work-related activities. Friends or family members can often provide a perspective about troubling events that have occurred as well as functional and behavioral changes such as forgetfulness. Although the clinical presentation of dementia may vary, depending on the etiology, the diagnostic criteria are consistent.[12] The criteria are well outlined in the DSM-IV. In addition to the interview, various reliable and valid rating scales are available to screen for dementia in the office setting. A commonly used scale that screens for dementia is the Mini-Mental Status Examination (see Table 6-1), which can be completed in 5 minutes in any setting. A score of 24 or higher (range 0 to 30) is generally considered normal, although performance varies depending on age and education.[13] It is important to take a careful medical and drug history to rule out reversible causes of cognitive dysfunction.

The physical examination should include a general systems examination as well as a detailed neurological examination *to detect any focal or generalized neurological signs (e.g., monoplegia, ataxia, myoclonic jerking).* A detailed mental status and cognitive function examination is also conducted. Evaluation of orientation, recent and remote memory, calculation, serial 7s, naming of objects, spelling a word forward and backward, and following simple and complex commands can reveal cognitive deficits. Attention should be given to screening for aphasia (i.e., expressive or receptive deficits), apraxia (e.g., drawing a clock, performing a skilled act on command such as combing the hair), agnosia (e.g., identification of objects), and executive functioning.

Diagnostic Testing

There is no definitive test for dementia or the multiple subcategories of dementia. The use of multiple laboratory tests in the evaluation of dementia is controversial. The health care provider does not want to miss reversible conditions, but sensitivity to cost must be a consideration. When the history and physical examination suggest the need for further

TABLE 31–2   CLASSIFICATION OF MAJOR TYPES OF DEMENTIAS

TYPE	DESCRIPTION	PRESENTATION
Alzheimer's disease (AD)	• Most common dementia accounting for 50%–70% of cases • Hallmarks are plaques of β-amyloid deposits and tangles of protein	• Begins with loss of short-term memory • Progresses to personality changes, global cognitive dysfunction, and functional impairments
Vascular dementia (VaD)	• Second most common dementia • Also called multi-infarct dementia or poststroke dementia • Caused by reduced blood flow to the parts of the brain; related to multiple tiny strokes that block small cerebral arteries called lacunae • Infarcts on cerebral imaging	• Cognitive deficits associated with stroke • Abrupt onset following stroke • Findings on neurological exam consistent with prior stroke
Mixed dementia	• A combination of abnormalities characteristic of both AD and VaD • Thought to be very common	• Dementia profile that combines both AD and VaD symptoms
Parkinson's disease (PD) with dementia	• Large number of patients with PD develop dementia in later stages of disease • PD is associated with Lewy bodies (see below) in the areas of the brain that control movement	• Gradual progressive dementia
Dementia with Lewy bodies (DLB)	• Lewy bodies are deposits of a protein called α-synuclein in various areas of the brain • Lewy bodies occur in regions of the brain related to cognitive function and cause dementia	• A gradual progressive dementia • Fluctuations in cognitive function • Motor features of parkinsonism
Frontotemporal dementia	• Cellular deterioration/atrophy is primarily concentrated in the frontal and temporal lobes of the brain • Heterogeneous entity that includes diseases such as Pick's disease	• Presentation includes gradual changes in personality and behavior and gradual and progressive language dysfunction
Normal pressure hydrocephalus dementia	• Etiology is unknown • An accumulation of cerebrospinal fluid (CSF)	• Memory loss, difficulty walking, and urinary incontinence • If diagnosed *early*, a shunt may be surgically implanted to drain CSF and reverse symptoms

TABLE 31–3   CHANGES SUGGESTIVE OF NEED FOR A DEMENTIA WORK-UP

Cognitive Changes

Impaired memory (forgets address, phone number); forgetfulness; confusion; difficulty understanding the written or spoken word; word-finding difficulty; lack of knowledge about current activities and events; poor concentration; difficulty recognizing faces and common objects

Change in Daily Function

Self-care and grooming neglect; getting lost in previously familiar surroundings or routes; difficulty managing finances and completing home activities (e.g., cooking, cleaning); difficulty with shopping, using the telephone, or simple problem solving; making mistakes in usual work or volunteer activities

Personality Changes

Social withdrawal; mood swings; loss of appropriate social behavior; loss of self-control; easily frustrated; explosive spells; crying spells

Problematic and Psychiatric Behaviors

Agitation; restlessness; boisterousness; demanding; uncooperative; wandering; sleeplessness; outburst; sexual aggressiveness; verbal/physical abusiveness; safety concerns such as forgetting to turn off stove; losing things such as keys; apathy; depression; suspiciousness; anxiety; fearfulness; paranoia; hallucinations; insomnia

evaluation, laboratory tests, brain imaging (e.g., CT, MRI), EEG, neuropsychological testing, and other tests are available. In addition to the history and physical examination data, laboratory investigation may include tests such as thyroid function, vitamin B_{12}, complete blood count, electrolytes, and Venereal Disease Research Laboratories' (VDRL) testing. Depending on clues uncovered in the history and physical examination, other optional tests may be ordered such as liver function, renal function, human immunodeficiency virus (HIV), chest x-ray, lumbar puncture, urine toxin screen, and neuropsychological testing.[7]

The main purpose of neuroimaging (CT or MRI) of the brain is to exclude a focal or generalized structural and potentially reversible cause of dementia. CT or MRI is widely used to exclude brain tumors, hydrocephalus, cerebrovascular disease, or subdural hematoma. Imaging may suggest the presence of opportunistic infections in patients at risk for HIV. MRI is preferred to detect infarction, small lesions, white matter changes, normal pressure hydrocephalus, focal atrophy or generalized atrophy, and pathologic changes poorly visualized by CT (e.g., base of the temporal lobe and posterior fossa).

Neuropsychological testing can make an important contribution to identification of mild dementia and can suggest productive avenues for treatment and management of behavior problems. A battery of tests addressing multiple domains of cognitive function measures the functional level

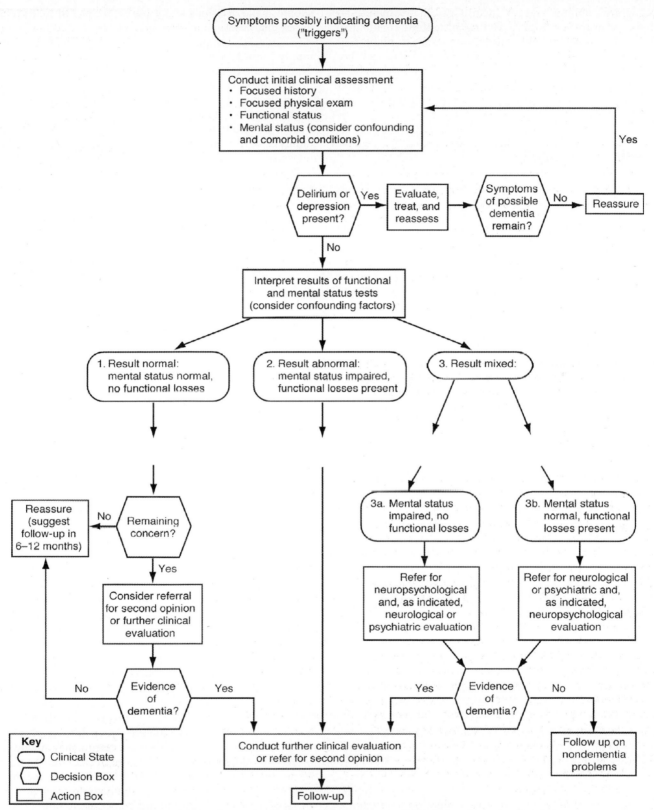

Figure 31-1 • Flow chart for the recognition and initial assessment of Alzheimer's disease and related dementias. (Costa, P. T., Jr., Williams, T. F., Somerfield, M., et al. [1996]. *Early identification of Alzheimer's disease and related dementias. Clinical practice guideline: Quick reference for clinicians, No. 19.* Rockville, MD: U.S. Department of Health and Human Services, Public Health Service, Agency for Health Care Policy and Research. AHCPR Publication No. 97-0703.)

of cognitive abilities and can identify psychiatric manifestations. Neuropsychological testing is helpful to identify dementia among people with high premorbid intellectual dysfunction.[14] In a patient with dementia, the neuropsychological battery can establish a baseline to monitor disease progression and the effectiveness of treatment. Neuropsychological testing takes several hours to complete and requires the cooperation of the patient.

Treatment and Management

There are a number of major goals that guide the treatment and management of dementia. Treat any underlying causes of dementia that could reverse the dementia. Conditions such as a B_{12} deficiency, hypothyroidism, drug toxicity, and brain tumor are treatable, and the treatment may reverse or improve the dementia. Next, problematic behaviors (e.g., agitation, sleep disorder, wandering) that often present safety concerns must be managed. For example, if agitation and wandering behaviors are present, interventions designed to address the underlying cause of these problems must be implemented. Interventions may include cognitive therapy, drug therapy, or a combination of both.

Identify and treat depression. Although depression is the most common psychiatric illness in older people, it is often underdiagnosed, especially when concurrent physical illness is present. The diagnosis may be complicated because depression may be mistaken for dementia or vice versa or dementia and depression may coexist. There are serious implications for the misdiagnosis of dementia as depression. Inappropriate treatment for nonexistent depression in a person with progressive dementia may exacerbate dementia because antidepressants that have anticholinergic properties may exacerbate confusion or memory impairment.[14] A change in sleep pattern or appetite, fatigue, behavioral slowing or agitation, complaints of diminished ability to think or concentrate, and apathy are symptoms of major depression and also symptoms of AD. In persons with coexisting depression and AD, failure to diagnose and treat depression may cause unnecessary emotional, physical, and social discomfort for both the patient and family. Therefore, assessment for depression is an important component of the initial evaluation.

There are a number of standardized scales to detect depression, such as the Geriatric Depression Scale (GDS) and the Center for Epidemiological Studies Depression Scale (CES-D). The GDS uses a 30-item questionnaire with a simple yes/no format. It was developed especially for older people and takes 8 to 10 minutes to administer. The CES-D uses a 20-item questionnaire and takes 5 to 8 minutes to administer. Antidepressant drugs such as selective serotonin reuptake inhibitors (e.g., sertraline [Zoloft]) and tricyclics (e.g., nortriptyline) are examples of drugs commonly ordered. In addition, a stable controlled environment helps minimize disorientation, confusion, frustration, agitation, and combative behavior. Too many environmental stimuli, tasks beyond the patient's ability, or unfamiliar surroundings are examples of situations that may precipitate behavioral problems.

Prepare the patient and family for the future in a supportive, sensitive manner. The type and extent of preparation depends on the diagnosis. Generally, a patient with dementia should make decisions about his or her health care preferences, finances, legal matters, and advanced directives while decision-making capabilities remain intact. The patient and family should receive anticipatory guidance about what to expect in the future and rate of decline that is geared to the underlying cause of the dementia.

Finally, help the patient maintain the highest quality of life possible for as long as possible. Monitoring should be conducted every 3 to 6 months to re-evaluate the patient's and family caregivers' functional levels and to identify new problems that can be addressed to support the patient and family.

The primary health care provider must decide whether he or she will manage the patient alone or whether referral to a specialist such as a neurologist is useful. This decision is based on the complexity of the patient, provider comfort, and patient/family wishes. A collaborative interdisciplinary team approach is important to assist both the patient and family over the trajectory of the illness. The role of the nurse is particularly important in providing care for the patient and supporting the family caregiver. In summary, the prevalence of dementia, an enormous problem in the United States, is expected to increase as baby boomers age. AD is the most common cause of dementia and is discussed in the next section.

ALZHEIMER'S DISEASE

Alzheimer's disease is the most common cause of progressive dementia in the elderly population. It is a chronic neurodegenerative disorder that leads to progressive disturbances of cognitive functions including memory, judgment, decision making, awareness of physical surrounding, and language.[15] Characteristic neuropathological findings include some neuronal and synaptic losses, extracellular neuritic plaques containing the β-amyloid peptide, and neurofibrillary tangles composed of hyperphosphorylated forms of the tau protein.[16] AD was first described by the German psychiatrist Alois Alzheimer in 1907 while treating a 55-year-old woman. The condition was initially thought to represent an uncommon form of presenile dementia, but it has become evident that adults of any age can develop AD, although it most often affects older people.

The Alzheimer's Association has released a number of facts and figures about AD, which are described in this section.[17] In 2007, it was estimated that the prevalence of AD was more than 5 million people in the United States. This includes 4.9 million people over the age of 65 and another 200,000 to 500,000 people who are under the age of 65 with early onset AD and other dementias. One out of eight people 65 years or older has AD, and one out of two over the age of 85 has it. About 70% of people with AD live at home in the community and are cared for by family and friends. AD is the seventh leading cause of death for people in the United States, and the fifth leading cause of death for people over the age of 65 years. The direct and indirect cost of AD and other dementias is more than $148 billion annually. In 2005, Medicare spent $91 billion on AD and other dementias, and that number is projected to more than double to $189 billion by 2015. About 10 million Americans are caring for a person with AD or another dementia; approximately one out of three of those caregivers is over the age of 60 years. It is clear that the national scope of the problem is tremendous and will only increase in the future.

Signs and Symptoms

Clinically, progressive impairment of short- and long-term memory and cognitive functions is the major feature of AD. Because AD begins with forgetfulness that can be subtle, it can be dismissed easily by the patient and the family. The patient may try to conceal the forgetfulness with excuses, compensating with notes and reminders. Difficulty with new learning, language, and visuospatial function, as well as apraxias and agnosias are features of the deterioration. There is a deterioration in ADLs and instrumental ADLs as noted in work performance and ability to deal with everyday family living and social situations. As AD progresses, some patients have psychiatric manifestations such as paranoia, delusions, agitation, and depression. Focal motor or sensory deficits are uncommon. About 8% of patients have seizures. The progressive course continues until there is loss of global cognitive function that includes impaired abstract thinking, impaired judgment, and personality change. In the end stage, the patient is bedridden, emaciated, aphasic, and apraxic and lacks bodily control, including sphincters. All cognitive functions and emotional responses are lost. Death is usually caused by an infection, such as aspiration pneumonia.[18]

The DSM-IV outlines the diagnostic criteria for dementia of the Alzheimer type. The average course of AD is 8 to 10 years, although the range is 1 to 25 years.[7] The course of AD is often divided into early, middle, and end stages based on the clinical presentation. Chart 31-1 describes the typical behaviors seen in each stage. Various probable and possible risk factors have been identified for AD. They include older age, familial history, genetic factors, perhaps female gender, lower educational level, head trauma with loss of consciousness, myocardial infarction, diabetes mellitus, hypothyroidism, exposure to organic solvents, PD, and Down's syndrome.[18] Protective factors include greater educational achievement, estrogen replacement in women, and use of anti-inflammatory drugs.

Diagnosis

Diagnosis of AD is by exclusion of other causes and is based on a clinical and neuropathological pattern. The definitive diagnosis of AD is made based on meeting the clinical criteria and histologic evidence based on examination of brain tissue obtained from biopsy or autopsy. The histologic changes associated with AD include gross, diffuse atrophy of the cerebral cortex with secondary enlargement of the ventricular system. On microscopic examination, there are extracellular neuritic plaques containing $A\beta$ amyloid, silver-staining neurofibrillary tangles in neuronal cytoplasm, and accumulation of $A\beta$ amyloid in arterial walls of cerebral blood vessels.[7] The neurofibrillary tangles and amyloidal plaque deposits are found chiefly in the temporoparietal and anterior frontal regions. The degenerative changes in the basal frontal-temporal region profoundly reduce the content of acetylcholine and the activity of choline acetyltransferase.[19] Other neurotransmitters can be involved, but the loss of acetylcholine occurs early and correlates with the impairment of memory. Symptomatic treatment of AD has focused on augmenting cholinergic neurotransmission.[16,20]

CHART 31-1   Stages of Alzheimer's Disease

The stages of Alzheimer's disease vary from patient to patient, but a few time approximations, as well as characteristic behaviors, can be identified.

STAGE 1: EARLY STAGE—2 TO 4 YR

- Forgetful—may be subtle, may try to cover up by using lists and notes
- Exhibits a declining interest in environment, people, and present affairs
- Demonstrates vague uncertainty and hesitancy in initiating actions
- Performs poorly at work, may be dismissed from job

STAGE 2: MIDDLE STAGE—2 TO 12 YR

- Exhibits progressive memory loss
- Hesitates in response to questions; shows signs of aphasia
- Has difficulty following simple instructions or doing simple calculations
- Has episodic bouts of irritability
- Becomes evasive, anxious, and physically active
- Becomes more active at night owing to sleepwakefulness cycle disturbance
- Wanders, particularly at night

- Becomes apraxic for many basic activities
- Loses important papers
- Loses way home in familiar surroundings or loses way in own home
- Forgets to pay bills; lets household chores slip and newspapers pile up; does not dispose of garbage; does not take medications
- Loses possessions and then claims that they were stolen
- Neglects personal hygiene (bathing, shaving, dressing)
- Loses social graces; can cause embarrassment to family and friends, which usually results in social isolation of the family and patient

STAGE 3: FINAL STAGE

- Loses much weight because of lack of eating; becomes emaciated
- Is unable to communicate verbally or in writing
- Does not recognize family
- Is incontinent of urine and feces
- Has a predisposition for major seizures
- Grasping, snout, and sucking reflexes are readily elicited
- Finally loses the ability to stand and walk and becomes bedridden
- Death is usually caused by aspiration pneumonia

As previously discussed, the differential diagnosis is problematic in dementias. Some of the difficulty in distinguishing the dementia of AD from dementias associated with other conditions is the lack of clarity of definitions. For example, both delirium and depression can resemble dementia and must therefore be excluded. **Delirium** is a *transient and potentially reversible condition* in which there is fluctuation in levels of awareness (agitation to stupor), hallucinations, and cognitive impairment, particularly memory. The key defining characteristic of delirium is the pattern of *rapid fluctuation of symptoms over a short period of time*. **Depression**, which has many symptoms common to AD (e.g., behavioral slowing or agitation, complaints of diminished ability to think or concentrate, fatigue, changes in sleep pattern or appetite), must be ruled out. It is a common problem seen in older people and is treatable.

CT and MRI are not specific for AD and may produce normal findings in the early course of the disease. As AD progresses, diffuse cortical atrophy is noted and the MRI shows significant atrophy of the hippocampus, an anatomic area associated with memory. Enlarged ventricles are also noted. Imaging is useful to rule out treatable causes of dementia such as a brain tumor or CNS infection. A positron emission tomography (PET) scan, although sometimes ordered, is controversial and not readily available in all facilities. The use of single proton emission computed tomography (SPECT) perfusion imaging has shown promise as a means of earlier diagnosis of AD.[21] Further investigation is needed to determine its use in practice. In the later stages of AD, there is diffuse slowing of the waves on EEG. Other laboratory tests are ordered to rule out treatable conditions (see discussion in section on dementia).

Pathophysiology

The cause of AD is unknown. Four susceptibility genes for AD have been identified, which are important to the understanding of the biologic basis of AD. Familial AD has an autosomal dominant pattern of inheritance[22] and can be caused by a mutation in the genes for amyloid precursor protein (APP), presenilin-1, or presenilin-2.[23] Presenilin-1 and presenilin-2 form complexes with at least one other protein, nicastrin, a transmembrane neuronal glycoprotein. These complexes may contribute to the production of $A\beta$.[24] In both the sporadic and familial forms of AD, the age of onset is modulated by allelic variants of apolipoprotein E (Apo E).[16,25] Apo E has three alleles: $\varepsilon2$, $\varepsilon3$, and $\varepsilon4$. The $\varepsilon4$ allele shows a strong association with AD in the general population, including sporadic and late-onset familial cases. In many people with two $\varepsilon4$ alleles, AD develops at least a decade before it does in those with two copies of $\varepsilon2$, and $\varepsilon3$, a condition associated with an onset of disease at an intermediate age.[25] Intensive research continues on the genetics of AD, with much interest focused on development of an early diagnostic test to identify AD, preventive therapy for those at risk, and cure rather than temporary symptomatic treatment of AD.

Treatment

Unfortunately, there is no cure for AD. Currently, the goal of treatment is to improve or slow the loss of memory and cognition and to maintain independent function for as long as possible. A multidisciplinary approach meets the changing needs of the patient and the family over the course of the illness. Working collaboratively, the multidisciplinary team (i.e., physician, nurse, social worker, case manager, rehabilitation specialist, neuropsychologist) provides sensitive support and counseling, education, and strategies to control the behavioral manifestations of the disease. Providing support, counseling, and education is an ongoing process to which all team members contribute. Anticipatory guidance to the family helps prepare them for the cognitive and physical decline and for planning ways of managing the patient. There are many patients with AD who do not have family support. They come to the attention of health providers when worried neighbors contact the police to express concern about the patient's safety or behavior. Most patients do not have the opportunity to be treated by a multidisciplinary team in a center dedicated to the comprehensive care of AD. Patients are managed by a primary care provider who monitors the patient (e.g., 3 to 6 months), manages symptoms, and provides support. Management options include drug therapy and psycho-education and counseling.

Drug Therapy to Slow the Progression of Alzheimer's Disease

A group of drugs classified as cholinesterase inhibitors (anticholinesterases) have shown encouraging results for the symptomatic treatment of impairment in memory and cognitive function for persons with mild to moderate AD. These drugs act to increase cholinergic synaptic transmission by inhibiting acetylcholinesterase in the synaptic cleft, resulting in a decrease in the hydrolysis of acetylcholine released from presynaptic neurons. There were four drugs approved by the Food and Drug Administration (FDA) drugs in this class, of which tacrine has fallen out of favor because of hepatotoxicity (Table 31-4). The drugs within the class differ from one another in inhibitor action of acetylcholinesterase activity and in side effects. Treatment with cholinesterase inhibitors can begin at any time after diagnosis. Higher doses have the greater benefits and also the more adverse effects. The recommendation is to increase the dose to the maximum tolerable level gradually. Cholinesterase inhibitor therapy is only effective in mild to moderate AD.

Another class of drugs, N-methyl-D-aspartate (NMDA) antagonists, which target the glutamatergic system, is approved for the treatment of moderate to severe AD. The drug that has demonstrated most benefit is memantine. Adding this drug has been shown to have better outcomes on measures of cognition, ADLs, behavior, and clinical global status. Other drugs such as antioxidants, anti-inflammatory drugs, vitamins, and others have not proven to be helpful after initial excitement of usefulness.

Management of Behavioral Manifestations

Management of the behavioral manifestations of AD is important. Major depression occurs in 5% to 8% of patients with AD, and up to 25% of patients have some depressive symptoms at the time of onset of memory impairment.[9] The tricyclic antidepressants (e.g., amitriptyline, imipramine) have not been effective in AD. In addition, some tricyclics

TABLE 31-4   DRUGS FOR TREATMENT OF ALZHEIMER'S DISEASE (AD)

DRUG	ACTION	DOSE/FREQUENCY	COMMON SIDE EFFECTS
Cholinesterase Inhibitors: Used for Mild to Moderate AD			
Donepezil (Aricept)	Inhibits formation of enzyme–acetylcholine complex	5–10 mg daily	Nausea, diarrhea, vomiting
Rivastigmine (Exelon)	Inhibits action of enzyme–acetylcholine complex	1.5–6 mg bid	Nausea, vomiting
Galantamine (Reminyl)	Acts on nicotinic acetylcholine receptors	4–12 mg bid	Nausea, vomiting, dizziness, diarrhea, anorexia, weight loss
N-methyl-D-aspartate (NMDA) Antagonists: Used for Moderate to Severe AD			
Memantine (Namenda)	Glutamate antagonist controls action of glutamate, the key excitatory neurotransmitter in the brain	5–10 mg bid	Dizziness, agitation, confusion, headache, and constipation

like amitriptyline have anticholinergic actions and can cause confusion or orthostatic hypotension. The selective serotonin reuptake inhibitors (e.g., citalopram, fluoxetine, paroxetine) showed improvement in depression scores on standard depression scales. The side effects noted were insomnia, anorexia, nausea, and diarrhea.

Delusions and psychosis are common and increase with the progression of AD. Use of neuroleptic drugs such as haloperidol and risperidone may be helpful. However, extrapyramidal signs are common side effects. Agitation, another common problem, is treated with benzodiazepines and carbamazepine. Side effects include sedation and ataxia, and both are risk factors for falls. Other nonpharmacologic strategies have been developed to assist with problematic behaviors such as wandering and "sundowning."

When compared with family care for other chronic illnesses of older persons, the progressive dementia of AD is more disruptive to family life, more likely to have negative mental health outcomes for family caregivers, and more of a deterrent to the patient living alone. Research has shown that programs for family education and counseling can decrease the burden of caring and delay nursing home placement of the AD patient.

Nursing Management

Patients with AD are generally managed in the home with the assistance of family, home services, and health care providers. Patient needs vary depending on the stage of disease and individual differences, but the AD trajectory is one of progressive decline to total loss of personality, cognitive function, and independence. Thus, symptoms and management problems vary over the course of the illness. For example, in the middle stage of AD, wandering is a common problem. The person may wander aimlessly within or outside the home or facility, becoming a danger to self. Low-cost, low-tech interventions, such as altering the physical environment so that doors are not readily visible, have had some success in limiting wandering. In addition, use of movement alarms has been helpful in alerting the staff to patients wandering into unsafe or unsupervised areas. Many nursing studies have contributed to better and safer ways of providing sensitive care to patients with AD.

Management of patients with AD is a collaborative multidisciplinary problem directed at providing care for patients with progressive dementia. With the number of patients diagnosed with AD rising, nurses will provide care for AD patients in a variety of facilities and community-based settings. Nurses employed in hospitals have contact with AD patients admitted for other problems such as a fractured hip related to a fall. Nurses based in clinics or community-based care will see patients in nursing homes, day care, and long-term care facilities. Although there is no specific treatment for AD, there are many palliative interventions available directed at maintaining function and independence for as long as possible to provide the highest quality of life possible. Common patient problems and nursing diagnoses are based on manifestations of the progressing dementia and include:

- High Risk for Injury (e.g., falls, burns) related to poor memory, judgment, and self-control
- Altered Thought Processes related to cognitive decline
- Self-Care and Self-Management Deficits related to losses of abilities for decision making, assuming responsibility for self, and independence
- Sleep Pattern Disturbance related to agitation and daytime sleeping
- Altered Communications related to cognitive decline
- Social Isolation related to withdrawal and inability to interact with others and the environment
- Caregiver Stress related to ongoing responsibility for the 24-hour care of a family member with progressive dementia
- Knowledge Deficit related to course of AD and management strategies for symptoms

It falls to the nurse to provide support for the patient and family and assist them to deal with the painful decisions that will need attention as the disease progresses. Patients with progressive dementia need to be approached with sensitivity to the ongoing losses incurred with the disease. In mild AD, patients are resourceful and learn to write lists and use other methods for reminders. As the disease progresses, health care providers and family caregivers gradually assume responsibility for structuring the environment and meeting basic and maintenance needs for the patient. Communication skills gradually decline, and the caregiver must learn to anticipate needs and interpret nonverbal cues. Sleep-pattern disturbance is particularly disruptive to other members of the family. Appropriate use of drugs, exercise during the day, and preventing daytime sleeping are helpful strategies in resetting circadian clocks. Agitation and aggressiveness make it difficult to manage the patient and increase the threat to safety for the patient and family members. When this occurs, it can become difficult to manage the patient at home. Again, drug therapy and structured activities are useful interventions to ameliorate these problems.

As the disease progresses, loss of social skills, withdrawal, and impulsive behavior further isolate the patient from interaction with others and the environment. At this stage, the patient will need close supervision, which limits the family's opportunities for social interaction. Finally, keeping the patient safe from injury to self and others is an ongoing concern. Because the patient often lacks insight and good judgment, high-risk situations are not recognized. For example, there will come a point in the illness when a patient should cease to drive. This is often viewed as a major unwelcome loss to independence that is protested by the patient. The health care provider can assist by assuming some responsibility and supporting the family's decision.

The patient and family need support and anticipatory education during the course of this devastating illness. Often, the nurse is called on to provide patient/family education and assist with symptom management issues. The nurse can:

- Encourage the patient to participate in ADLs, hobbies, and community activities for as long as possible to maintain independence
- Encourage the patient to take his or her medications as ordered and monitor for side effects
- Provide the patient and family with specific information about AD in both oral and written forms
- Help the family develop strategies to adequately monitor, supervise, and protect the patient from injury, humiliation, or becoming lost
- Help the family develop strategies to deal with the specific problems of patient management such as insomnia and wandering
- Make the patient and family aware of available community resources and support services, such as the Alzheimer's Disease Association and other support groups
- Encourage the patient and family to make decisions regarding financial matters, advanced directives, end-of-life care, and other matters while the patient still has decision-making abilities intact
- Encourage the patient and family to develop realistic short- and long-term plans
- Help the family understand caregiver stress and options for coping and minimizing stress
- Support the family in decision making regarding the need for institutionalization
- Make referrals to social services and community resources to assist the patient and family in planning for the future

REFERENCES

1. Short, R. A., & Graff-Radford, N. R. (2002). Approach to the patient with dementia. In J. Biller (Ed.). *Practical neurology* (2nd ed., pp. 19–26). Philadelphia: Lippincott Williams & Wilkins.
2. American Psychiatric Association. (2000). *Diagnostic and statistical manual of mental disorders* (4th ed., text revision, pp. 135–180). Washington, DC: Author.
3. World Health Organization. (1992). *International classification of diseases* (10th revision). Geneva: Author.
4. Alzheimer's Association. (2007). *Alzheimer's disease facts and figures*. Washington, DC: Author.
5. American Psychiatric Association. (1994). *Diagnostic and statistical manual of mental disorders* (4th ed., pp. 123–163). Washington, DC: Author.
6. Reisberg, B. (2006). Diagnostic criteria in dementia: A comparison of current criteria, research challenges, and implications for DSM-V. *Journal of Geriatric Psychiatry and Neurology, 19,* 137–146.
7. Bird. T. D., & Miller, B. L. (2005). Alzheimer's disease and other dementias. In D. L. Kasper, E. Braunwald, A. S Fauci., S. L. Hauser, D. L. Longo, & J. L. Jameson (Eds.). *Harrison's principles of internal medicine* (16th ed., pp. 2393–2406). New York: McGraw-Hill.
8. Rodnitzky, R. L. (1995). Clinical correlation: Parkinson's disease. In P. M. Conn (Ed.). *Neuroscience in medicine* (pp. 427–430). Philadelphia: J. B. Lippincott.
9. Sucholeiki, R., & Caselli, R. J. (2006). Dementia: Overview of pharmacotherapy. Retrieved May 2, 2007, from http://www.emedicien.com/neuro/topic597.htm
10. Ropper, A. W., & Brown, R H. (2005). *Adams and Victor's Principles of neurology* (8th ed., pp. 367–384). New York: McGraw-Hill.
11. Devinsky, O., Feldman, E., & Weinreb, H. I. (2000). *Neurological pearls* (pp. 115–125). Philadelphia: F. A. Davis.
12. Santacruz, K. S., & Swagerty, D. (2001). Early diagnosis of dementia. *American Family Physician, 63*(4), 703–713.
13. Crum, R. M., Anthonym J. C., Bassett, S. S., & Folstein, M. F. (1993). Population-based norms for the Mini-Mental State Examination by age and educational levels. *Journal of the American Medical Association, 18,* 2386–2392.
14. Costa, P. T., Jr., Williams, T. F., Somerfield, M., et al. (1996). Early identification of Alzheimer's disease and related dementias. Clinical practice guideline: Quick reference for clinicians, No. 19. AHCPR Publication No. 97-0703. Rockville, MD: U.S. Department of Health and Human Services, Public Health Service, Agency for Health Care Policy and Research.
15. Nussbaum, R. I., & Elliss, C. E (2003). Alzheimer's disease and Parkinson's disease. *New England Journal of Medicine, 348,* 1356–1364.
16. Klafki, H. W., Staufenbiel, M., Kornhuber, J., & Wiltfang, J. (2006). Therapeutic approaches to Alzheimer's disease. *Brain, 129,* 2840–2855.
17. Alzheimer's Association. (2007). *Alzheimer's Association Report: 2007 Alzheimer's disease facts and figures*. Washington, DC: Author.
18. Kukull, W. A., & Ganguli, M. (2000). Epidemiology of dementia. *Neurologic Clinics, 18*(4), 923–950.
19. Mayeux, R., & Sano, M. (1999). Treatment of Alzheimer's disease. *New England Journal of Medicine, 341*(22), 1670–1679.
20. Francis, P. T., Palmer, A. M., Snape, M., & Wilcock, G. K. (1999). The cholinergic hypothesis of Alzheimer's disease: A review of progress. *Journal of Neurology, Neurosurgery, & Psychiatry, 66,* 137–147.
21. Jagust, W., Thisted, R., Devous, M. D., et al. (2001). SPECT perfusion imaging in the diagnosis of Alzheimer's disease. *Neurology, 56,* 950–956.
22. Prusiner, S. B. (2001). Shattuck lecture—Neurodegenerative diseases and prions. *New England Journal of Medicine, 344*(20), 1516–1526.

23. St. George-Hyslop, P. H. (1999). Molecular genetics of Alzheimer disease. In R. D. Terry, R. Katzman, K. L. Bick, & S. S. Sisodia (Eds.). *Alzheimer disease* (2nd ed., pp. 311–326). Philadelphia: Lippincott Williams & Wilkins.

24. Yu, G., Nishimura, M., Arawaka, S., et al. ((2000). Nicastrin modulates presenilin-mediated notch/glp-1 signal transduction and βAPP processing. *Nature, 407,* 48–54.

25. Martin, J. B. (1999). Molecular basis of the neurodegenerative disorders. *New England Journal of Medicine, 340*(25), 1979–1980.

RESOURCE

The following is a resource for patients and families (there are many resources available on the Internet):

Alzheimer's Association (there are chapters nationwide)
National Office
225 North Michigan Ave
Chicago, IL 60601-7633
1-800-272-3900, http://www.alz.org

Neurodegenerative Diseases

Joanne V. Hickey

This chapter addresses the four most common neurodegenerative diseases: Parkinson's disease, multiple sclerosis, amyotrophic lateral sclerosis, and myasthenia gravis. All are chronic conditions with varying patterns of progression over time. The epidemic of chronic illness creates strains, stresses, and challenges for the patient and family as well as for the health care system. This chapter begins with a brief discussion of chronic illness and chronic illness management and how these general principles apply to neurodegenerative conditions.

A *chronic illness* is any physical or mental condition that requires long-term (over 6 months) monitoring and/or management to control symptoms and to shape the course of the disease.[1] It has also been defined as the irreversible presence, accumulation, or latency of disease states or impairments, which involve the total human environment to provide supportive care and self-care, to maintain function, and to prevent further disability.[2] Chronic illness is the epidemic of the 21st century. By 2020, it is expected that 157 million Americans will have one or more chronic conditions. Of that number, 42 million will have activity limitations restricting their ability to work and live independently.[3] Advances in medical science, especially in molecular and genetic research, have greatly increased our understanding of many of the neurodegenerative diseases. Although cures remain elusive, breakthroughs have been made in treatments directed at symptom management.

Several characteristics of chronic illness are important when considering neurodegenerative disorders. A chronic illness tends to include multiple diseases as a result of the impact of the primary disease on other body systems. As chronic illnesses follow uncertain and changing courses, they greatly intrude on the life of the patient and family over a long period (i.e., years). The level of disability waxes and wanes with the course of the illness, which creates a sense of uncertainty. Because of its changing nature, effective management of a chronic illness requires a variety of primary and ancillary services. Chronic illness is expensive to treat and manage, and often third-party reimbursement is lacking or very limited. The quality of chronic illness management varies significantly, especially when compared to the high-tech, protocol-driven, hospital-based care that is the hallmark of acute care.

Chronic illness management usually involves home-based care with little use of technology. Day-to-day care is provided by family members in the home setting. Hospitalization, if necessary, is usually short term and limited to serious relapses or complications related to the disease. Ongoing patient and family education, counseling, and empowerment for self-management are cornerstones of a patient-focused approach. Care focuses on symptom management and interventions to stabilize the disease process and prevent complications. The ultimate goal with chronic disease is adapting to the illness and promoting an acceptable quality of life. This means that care is directed at keeping the patient as independent and functional as possible for as long as possible within the context of his or her lifestyle.

The needs of the patient are best provided for through a collaborative, multidisciplinary, integrated, holistic model with the patient and family as the centerpiece of care. Nurses are an integral part of the health care team and provide comprehensive care and support to both the patient and the family. Unfortunately, much of what nurses do as part of chronic illness care is invisible because outcomes are difficult to measure and attribute to the nurse. Nurses make a major contribution through teaching patients how to integrate their treatment regimens into their lives and how to recognize signs of complications.[1] The nurse's role involves assessing, communicating, teaching, coaching, counseling, role-modeling, comforting, advising, advocating, and coordinating activities and care. Because nurses are attuned to subtle signs that indicate changes in the status of an illness, they can advise the patient when to seek medical assistance. They provide the knowledge and support, both prerequisites to successful adaptation, that assist the patient and family to understand and accept the illness. Assuming a major role for communicating with other team members and community services, the nurse provides for coordination of care through case management and advocacy.

MODELS FOR CHRONIC ILLNESS MANAGEMENT

Several models or frameworks for chronic illness management are available to guide nursing practice. Although acute care is often structured around a medical model based on pathophysiology, diagnosis, and treatment, chronic illness is best structured around a psychosocial adaptation model. The trajectory of illness model provides a framework to guide care for chronic illnesses.[4] A *trajectory* is defined as a course of illness over time, plus the actions taken by patients, families, and health care professionals to manage or shape the course of the illness. To encompass the dynamic and changing character of chronic illness, the concept of *phasing* has been added to trajectory.[1] Nine different trajectory phases, identified by Corbin and Strauss, are briefly described with application to neurodegenerative diseases.[4]

The **pretrajectory phase** includes identification of lifestyle and genetic risk factors that predispose a person to develop a chronic illness (i.e., neurodegenerative disease). It is the ultimate goal of neuroscience research to identify genetic markers and lifestyle characteristics that can be modified before a disease develops. Currently, neuroscience has not developed to this level of knowledge. The next phase is the **trajectory onset**. During this phase, onset of symptoms, seeking medical attention, diagnostic work-up, and finally diagnoses occur. The patient begins to learn about the disease and begins to cope with the implications of the illness. In neurological patients, symptoms that cannot be ignored lead to diagnosis, often a frightening term that has no meaning to the patient. The patient begins to learn about what it means to have multiple sclerosis or Parkinson's disease, and what might lie ahead. The **stable phase** is one in which the illness and symptoms are under control and everyday life is being managed within the limitations of the illness. Care is centered in the home. For example, a patient with Alzheimer's disease (AD) is functional and has routines and strategies such as a notepad with activities for the day that keep him or her involved in home activities.

The next phase is the **unstable phase**. The symptoms are not under control, and there is an exacerbation of the illness. This is disruptive to carrying out the usual routines at home that have been effective previously. Adjustments are made to return to the normal, stable phase. For example, a previously effective drug schedule for a patient with myasthenia gravis is no longer effective. The patient feels weak and cannot accomplish the home or work activities usually completed. This leads to a search for the cause of this change in status such as an infection, too much of an anticholinesterase drug, or emotional stress. The **acute phase** is described as the development of severe and unrelieved symptoms or complications that require bed rest or hospitalization. Normal activity abruptly ceases, and the patient wonders whether he or she will ever recover. For example, a patient with amyotrophic lateral sclerosis develops aspiration pneumonia. A decision regarding a gastrostomy tube placement may need to be made, and the possibility of mechanical ventilatory support may be discussed. A **crisis phase** is a critical or life-threatening situation requiring emergency treatment or care. Everyday life is placed indefinitely on hold. Myasthenic crisis requiring intubation and use of mechanical ventilation is an example with a neurological patient population. The **comeback phase** is a gradual return to an acceptable way of life within the limits imposed by the recovery process and any irreversible losses incurred during the crisis. This phase involves the physical healing, rehabilitation procedures, and psychosocial coming to terms with the events. It also includes a re-entry and adjustment to everyday life and any new limitations.

The **downward phase** is characterized by a gradual or rapid physical deterioration and difficulty with symptom control. It requires alterations in everyday life and loss of some functional abilities. For example, a patient with Alzheimer's disease may now become confined to bed. The final phase is the **dying phase** and includes the final days or weeks before death. The body gradually or rapidly shuts down; the person disengages and comes to closure. In patients with neurodegenerative diseases, often cognitive function has been compromised so that psychological disengagement may have occurred in a previous phase. In other neurodegenerative conditions, the patient is cognitively aware of approaching death and has made decisions for a peaceful death.

The trajectory of illness offers an excellent model to assist the neuroscience nurse in providing care to the patient with neurodegenerative disease. It suggests need for the nurse to provide education, support, and care in each phase of the trajectory. The very nature of a degenerative disease indicates a process of losses. How quickly functional deterioration occurs depends on the particular disease and the individual course. Successful adaptation to chronic illness with an acceptable quality of life is characterized by psychosocial adjustment and an ability to cope with losses while positively reforming intact function. For there to be successful adjustment and adaptation to the illness, each phase of the trajectory requires special work for the patient and family. The nurse can provide the knowledge and skill for this process to occur.

PARKINSON'S DISEASE

Parkinson's disease is the second most common neurodegenerative disease after AD, affecting 1% of people over the age of 65 years. Typically beginning in middle or late life, PD is more common in the 65 and older age group. Approximately 1 million people live with PD in the United States, and with current demographic trends, the number of cases of PD is expected to increase significantly in the next three decades.[5,6] Early-onset PD affecting persons as early as their 20s is being recognized with greater frequency. More than 10 autosomal dominant and recessive genes or gene loci have been linked to PD.[7] PD is a chronic, slow, progressive disorder caused by loss of dopaminergic neurons in the substantia nigra of the basal ganglia. The major signs and symptoms include tremors, rigidity, akinesia/bradykinesia, and postural deformity (thus the mnemonic *TRAP*), although postural deformity is usually a later finding. PD causes significant disability and decreased quality of life.[8]

Neuroanatomy

The **basal ganglia** is a collective term for the subcortical motor nuclei of the cerebrum. The structures that compose the basal ganglia include the substantia nigra, striatum, globus pallidus, subthalamic nucleus, and red nucleus. Symptoms of PD are caused by loss of nerve cells in the pigmented substantia nigra pars compacta, including the locus ceruleus in the midbrain. Cell loss also occurs in the globus pallidus and putamen.[9] Depletion of the dopaminergic neurons (pars compacta) of the substantia nigra results in reduction of dopamine, the main biochemical abnormality in PD. Normally, the pars compacta neurons of the substantia nigra provide dopaminergic input to the striatum, a part of the basal ganglia. In PD, loss of pars compacta neurons leads to striatal dopamine depletion and reduced thalamic excitation of the motor cortex.[9]

Pathogenesis

The etiology of PD is unknown. PD is defined by the presence of Lewy bodies and nerve cell loss in the substantia nigra. In the laboratory, parkinsonism has been induced by exposing animals to 1-methyl-4-phenyl-1,2,3,6-tetrahydropyridine (MPTP), a potent neurotoxin that has been sometimes accidentally taken by heroin users. It is this connection that supports a hypothesis that exposures to pesticides and other toxins containing MPTP may be one cause of PD.

Both inherited and sporadic forms of PD have been identified. In both cases, Lewy bodies (eosinophilic intraneural inclusion granules) are widespread within neurons and occur especially in the substantia nigra of the basal ganglia. In PD, Lewy bodies contain α-synuclein. Mutations in the gene for α-synuclein have been found in patients with familial PD.[10] Much about the pathogenesis of PD remains unknown.

Signs and Symptoms

Because symptoms develop insidiously, diagnosis is often delayed, with symptoms sometimes attributed to aging. The disease is progressive, so that eventually the patient's ability to perform activities of daily living (ADLs) and other independent functions is reduced. The major signs and symptoms of PD include the following:

- Tremors (resting tremors)
- Rigidity of muscles
- Akinesia/bradykinesia
- Postural disturbance and loss of postural reflexes

The secondary manifestations include the following:

- Difficulty with fine motor function such as writing and eating
- Soft monotone voice
- Mask-like face
- General weakness and muscle fatigue
- Cognitive impairments/dementia
- Sleep disturbances
- Autonomic manifestations

Major Manifestations

Tremors. The classic tremor of PD is a resting tremor in a limb, most commonly one hand, which disappears with voluntary movement.[8] Tremors occur most often in the distal portions of extremities and especially in the hands. A so-called *pill-rolling* motion of the fingers is characteristic. Other areas where tremors are seen include the foot, lip, tongue, and jaw. Tremors are present when the hand is

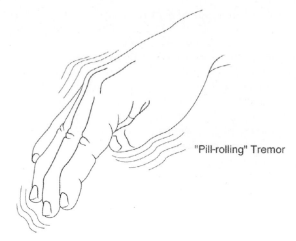

"Pill-rolling" Tremor

Figure 32-1 • The tremor in Parkinson's disease is exaggerated by the resting posture, is often relieved by movement, and usually disappears during sleep. The movement of the thumb across the palm gives it a "pill-rolling" character.

motionless and thus are termed *resting tremors* (Fig. 32-1). Tremors are absent during sleep.

Rigidity of Muscles. Muscle rigidity is associated with slowness of voluntary movement (bradykinesia or akinesia); it may be felt as stiffness associated with vague aching and discomfort of a limb. The muscle feels stiff and requires much effort to move. The patient has difficulty in initiating movement. Because PD patients move minimally when sitting, edema can develop in the feet, legs, hands, and arms. **Cogwheel rigidity** is characterized by ratchet-like, rhythmic contractions, especially in the hand, on passive muscle stretching.

Akinesia/Bradykinesia. Initiating a movement is difficult and movement is slow. Gait is slowed with dragging of the foot and decreased arm swing on the affected side. As a result, difficulty in rising from a chair, getting into a car, and performing ADLs is common. Slow or absent movement renders the patient at high risk for pneumonia, deep vein thrombosis, constipation, and pressure ulcers.

Postural Disturbance, Loss of Postural Reflexes. Patients walk in a stooped-over position with small, shuffling steps and often a broad base on turns. The forearms are semiflexed, and the fingers are flexed at the metacarpophalangeal joints. The characteristic appearance and posture of the patient with PD are illustrated in Figure 32-2. After movement is initiated, it frequently accelerates almost to a trot. The patient may fall forward (propulsion) or backward (retropulsion). If pushed, he or she makes no attempt to brace or to reach out and protect himself or herself. As a result, the patient is at high risk for injury, especially from falls. Patients have difficulty in maintaining balance and sitting erect.

Secondary Manifestations

Fine Motor Deficits. Difficulty with fine motor control is seen early in the disease. Handwriting becomes progressively smaller and more difficult to read. Clumsiness and difficulty with ADLs, such as buttoning clothing, is evident.

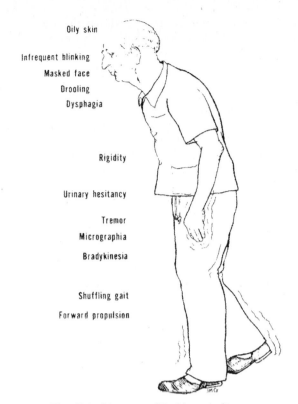

Oily skin

Infrequent blinking

Masked face

Drooling

Dysphagia

Rigidity

Urinary hesitancy

Tremor

Micrographia

Bradykinesia

Shuffling gait

Forward propulsion

Figure 32-2 • The clinical features of Parkinson's disease.

Monotonic Voice. The voice gradually becomes soft to whisper-like, monotonic, and muffled. These changes result in impaired verbal communications

Mask-like Face. The face becomes expressionless and the eyes stare straight ahead; blinking is less frequent than normal—5 to 10 times per minute rather than the normal 15 to 20 times.

General Weakness and Muscle Fatigue. Initiation of purposeful movement is slow. During movement, the patient may become momentarily frozen. Fatigue is a common complaint, especially when ADLs are attempted. Muscle cramps of the legs, neck, and trunk are common.

Cognitive Changes/Dementia and Psychiatric Symptoms. Incidence of cognitive impairment in PD increases with age from 2.7% per year at ages 55 to 64 to 13.7 per year at ages 70 to 79; dementia is noted in 20% to 40% of patients.[11] Cognitive impairments to visuospatial function, executive functions, and memory are common in many patients over the course of the illness. Depression (very common) is seen in over 50% of persons with PD and may even occur before classic symptoms of PD are noted. Hallucinations (especially of people and animals), delusions, anxiety, and apathy are also seen.

Other Common Manifestations. Additional signs and symptoms, many associated with autonomic dysfunction, include the following:

- Drooling: secondary to decreased frequency of swallowing. When the patient awakens, the pillow is wet.
- Seborrhea (oily, greasy skin): probably attributable to hypothalamic dysfunction, which causes release of an increased amount of sebotrophic hormone.

- Dysphagia: secondary to the neuromuscular incoordination of the hypopharyngeal musculature. This problem can interfere with normal fluid and dietary intake.
- Excessive perspiration: probably the result of a disorder of the hypothalamic heat regulator mechanism, as well as impairment of perspiration controls. The patient may be diaphoretic even in cold weather and may have a fever in warm weather.
- Constipation: secondary to hypomotility of the gastrointestinal tract and associated with prolonged gastric emptying time. Decreased fluid intake, lack of roughage, and decreased activity contribute to the development of constipation.
- Orthostatic hypotension: probably the result of peripheral autonomic failure noted in parkinsonism. It is also a side effect of levodopa therapy.
- Urinary hesitation and frequency: secondary to autonomic dysfunction. A catheter is rarely necessary.
- Erectile dysfunction and impotence.

Scales developed to rate the severity of signs and symptoms of PD objectively are useful clinically and in drug trials for staging the disease and for monitoring deterioration. The categorical, nonlinear scale described by Hoehn and Yahr is frequently used to characterize the severity of illness (Table 32-1).[12] The United Parkinson's Disease Rating Scale (UPDRS) is a standard rating scale used for evaluation of all patients. It is a comprehensive clinical rating instrument that measures the patient's and physician's assessment of neurological disability initially and over time. It has four subscales: cognitive, ADLs, motor examination, and complications of treatment. Items include speech, salivation, swallowing, handwriting, cutting of food and handling utensils, dressing, hygiene, turning in bed, falling, freezing, walking, tremor, and sensory symptoms. Each item is scored on a scale from 0 to 4 (0 = normal to 4 = most severe).[13] The scores on the subscales are added to yield a total score (higher scores indicate a higher degree of disability). The scale has good interrater reliability. In addition, other standardized scales, such as the Beck Depression Inventory for depression are helpful for assessing and monitoring other symptoms common in PD.

TABLE 32-1	MODIFIED HOEHN AND YAHR SCALE FOR PARKINSON'S DISEASE
STAGE OF DISEASE	**DESCRIPTION**
Stage 0	No signs of disease
Stage 1	Unilateral disease
Stage 1.5	Unilateral plus axial involvement
Stage 2	Bilateral disease, without impairment of balance
Stage 2.5	Mild bilateral disease, with recovery on pull test
Stage 3	Mild to moderate bilateral disease; some postural instability; physically independent
Stage 4	Severe disability; able to walk or stand unassisted
Stage 5	Wheelchair-bound or bedridden unless aided

Diagnosis

The diagnosis of PD is based on a careful history and physical examination. There are no laboratory tests or imaging tests currently available to confirm the diagnosis of PD.[14] Magnetic resonance imaging (MRI) is usually normal. Single photon emission computed tomography (SPECT) imaging has demonstrated promise in supporting the diagnosis of PD, but it is not commonly used at this time. Electroencephalography (EEG) is not helpful. The diagnosis of PD is made based on history and clinical findings.

Medical Management

The American Academy of Neurology has issued clinical practice guidelines for the initial therapy in Parkinson's disease,[15,16] and the Movement Disorder Society has published evidence-based recommendations for PD therapy.[17,18] Patients with PD require two types of management: symptomatic therapies and preventive or protective therapies. Symptomatic therapies are directed toward ameliorating the symptoms of PD but do not affect the progression of the disease. They include both nonpharmacologic and pharmacologic interventions. Neuroprotective therapies are directed at halting or slowing the course of PD. Drug therapy plays an important role in both categories of PD management, although drugs that have been shown to be protective have been generally disappointing. Several drug groups are represented in the symptomatic drug category. Selegiline was the first drug marketed as a neuroprotective drug, that is, a drug that slowed the course of PD. However, prospective long-term studies found no difference between selegiline and placebo. According to recent guidelines, selegiline has mild symptomatic benefit. There is no convincing clinical evidence for a neuroprotective benefit with selegiline.[16]

Symptomatic Supportive Approach

Long-term studies of a multidisciplinary clinical program in the management of PD have shown that the vast majority of patients maintain or even improve their motor function for up to 3 years after initiation of the program.[19] Multidisciplinary teams are most helpful in chronic conditions such as PD. Symptomatic, nonpharmacologic, supportive therapy is directed toward managing symptoms that are common in PD, such as movement disorders, constipation, perspiration, and urinary dysfunction. Advising on adjustments of lifestyle and preventing complications and injuries are critically important. Speech therapy may be recommended for some patients with deficits in speaking. A comprehensive physiotherapy program that may include gait retraining, balance maintenance, and exercise can be most helpful in keeping the patient functional. Occupational therapy is helpful in teaching patients alternate ways of achieving ADLs and instrumental ADLs to overcome motor and perceptual deficits. Patient and family education is an integral part of management.

Most patients can be managed at home with varying degrees of family support. Whether home health care or community services are needed depends on the associated disabilities and the availability of family assistance. An effective pharmacologic program often allows the individual to optimize function depending on the degree of disability. In the advanced stages, management in a nursing home may be necessary if adequate arrangements cannot be made at home. Admission to an acute care facility is necessary only for special problems such as surgery or treatment of complications. Individuals with PD are at high risk for injury because of incoordination, loss of postural reflexes, and rigidity. Injuries, such as a fractured hip, head injury, or spinal fracture, can result from a fall and are often the reason for hospitalization.

Some nondrug therapies that should be incorporated into the overall management of patients include the following recommendations[20]:

- Encourage regular exercise to maintain physical and mental function. Patients whose health is otherwise good should engage in activities that emphasize aerobic conditioning and stretching such as tai chi, stretching classes, and pool therapy. Stretching alleviates the symptoms of PD such as rigidity and bradykinesia.[21–23]
- A low-protein diet to optimize the effect of levodopa in some patients with *advanced* PD is helpful. High-protein meals block the effect of levodopa when given alone or in combination. Therefore, restrict protein at the noon meal in patients whose response to levodopa has decreased. Recommend protein consumption at the evening meal when physical activity is decreased.[24]
- Dietary supplements according to risk to prevent osteoporosis should be addressed.
  - Recommend a daily calcium intake of 1200 mg for men and premenopausal women and 1500 mg for postmenopausal women.
  - Recommend a daily vitamin D intake of 400 to 600 IU.
- A regular balanced diet with adequate water and fiber is helpful to combat constipation.[24]
- Wearing elastic stockings will help to avoid orthostatic hypotension.

Symptomatic Pharmacologic Treatment

The diagnosis of PD is not necessarily cause to begin drug therapy. Drug therapy is recommended when the patient is sufficiently bothered by symptoms to desire treatment or when the disease is cause of disability.[8] The decision to begin drug therapy is a combined decision of the patient and provider. Although PD cannot be cured or arrested, symptoms can often be controlled with drug therapy. Consideration must be given to timing of drug introduction, selecting the right drug, monitoring and managing side effects, and adjusting the drug schedule for optimal results. The patient and family must be educated about the drugs used, side effects, and precautions to be observed while taking the drugs.

There are five drug classes used in the management of PD: *levodopa, dopamine agonists, anticholinergics, antivirals,* and *selective monamine oxidase B inhibitors.* These drugs are summarized in Table 12-10. A few additional comments are provided to expand the understanding of drug management. Once the diagnosis of PD has been made, the severity of symptoms must be assessed and an appropriate management plan developed with the age, lifestyle, and degree of disability kept in mind. The patient and family need to be involved in decision making and educated about the disease and the drugs used. According to the American Academy of Neurology guidelines, initiation of selegiline in order to confer mild, symptomatic benefit prior to the institution of dopaminergic therapy may be considered.

An important decision is when to begin levodopa therapy, especially in younger patients. In patients with PD who require the initiation of dopaminergic treatment, either levodopa or a dopamine agonist may be used. The selected drug depends on the relative impact of improving motor disability (better with levodopa) compared with the lessening of motor complications (better with dopamine agonists) for each individual patient with PD.[16] Although levodopa is the mainstay of drug treatment for PD, it has many side effects and a limited time span for effectiveness. Patients with severe cerebral or cardiovascular disease, psychosis, or severe medical problems need to be carefully evaluated for use of levodopa. If levodopa therapy is begun, either an immediate-release levodopa or sustained-release levodopa may be used. Long-term use of levodopa can result in toxicity and unpredictable responses to other drug therapy. The "on-off" phenomenon, a side effect, is described as a fluctuation in motor function from being ambulatory and active one moment ("on" phase) to being unable to rise from a chair ("off" phase), all within a few minutes.

One might wonder why dopamine is not given rather than its precursor, levodopa. If dopamine were given orally, it would be metabolized before reaching the brain. Levodopa, however, is able to cross the blood–brain barrier and, once there, become converted into dopamine. For this chemical reaction to take place, the enzyme dopa decarboxylase must be present. In its presence, levodopa converts to dopamine and carbon dioxide, both in peripheral tissue and in the brain.

For the symptoms of PD to be controlled, levodopa must be converted to dopamine within the brain. If the reaction occurs in peripheral tissue, side effects of nausea and other symptoms occur. Inhibitors are given to prevent the conversion of levodopa to dopamine in peripheral tissue. The inhibitors selected to block the dopa decarboxylase enzyme do not cross the blood–brain barrier and thus allow dopamine production in the brain. By using levodopa in combination with **dopa decarboxylase inhibitors**, the dosage of levodopa can be reduced and side effects can be eliminated or greatly diminished. The inhibitor most often used is carbidopa (Sinemet). When given in combination, the dosage often used is carbidopa, 10 to 25 mg, and levodopa, 100 to 250 mg, three or four times daily. A combination of levodopa, carbidopa, and entacapone is available, called Stalevo. The addition of entacapone prolongs the half-life of a given dose of levodopa by 1.3 to 2.4 hours.

Anticholinergic drugs are used in conjunction with levodopa or singularly if the patient cannot tolerate levodopa or if symptoms are mild. The drugs most often used are trihexyphenidyl hydrochloride (Artane) (2 to 5 mg three or four times daily) and benztropine mesylate (Cogentin) (0.5 to 6.0 mg daily).

In summary, the drugs currently available provide only symptom relief. Protective drugs that alter the underlying progressive disease are still to be developed. In the early stages of PD, when only mild resting tremors are present, anticholinergic drugs are helpful for about 6 to 18 months. As the disease progresses, the patient will need drugs that provide dopaminergic stimulation. Levodopa is the mainstay of drug therapy. The addition of peripheral dopa decarboxylase inhibitors has helped to control its many side effects (e.g., anorexia, nausea, vomiting). Sinemet combines levodopa and carbidopa in one medication. Treatment of drug toxicity and unresponsiveness to drugs is problematic. Drug therapy may be changed or dosages altered. So-called "drug holidays" of a few days have been suggested, with hospital supervision. The effect of such an approach may improve clinical function, which lasts weeks to months.

Surgery

Surgical treatment of PD has a role for patients with long-standing severe disease who have become refractory to drug therapy or who have inadequate symptom control (e.g., fluctuations or "on-off" phenomena).[25] For highly selected patients with advanced PD, subthalamic stimulation is a consideration.

Over the last 5 years high-frequency subthalamic stimulation using an implanted electrode and pulse generator has gained favor for control of tremors by targeting the subthalamus.[26] A quadripolar deep brain stimulator is implanted in the subthalamus, which is a small structure deep in the subcortical area. It is connected to a neurostimulator implantable pulse generator (IPG), which is placed in the subcutaneous infraclavicular area. The generator has four contacts that can be programmed in a few ways. An external programming device is used to adjust the stimulus parameters and to turn the stimulator on or off.

Careful selection of patients based on type of PD (e.g., idiopathic), age, and intact cognitive status is important. Cognitive function in a patient who is cognitively impaired can become worse with deep brain stimulation. In addition, the patient needs education about the procedure and the realistic outcomes that can be expected. Preoperatively, all PD medication is stopped the evening before surgery to minimize medication-induced dyskinesia, which can interfere with intraoperative microelectrode recordings and with intraoperative microelectrode recordings.[26] At the time of surgery, the head is shaved and placed in a head frame, anatomic landmarks identified, and mapping techniques used to located the subthalamus. Stereotactic coordinates are calculated from MRI or computed tomography (CT) images. To prevent seizures, a dose of intravenous fosphenytoin is administered. Extracellular microelectrode recordings are taken to determine appropriate location. The patient's limbs are monitored for tremors that are noted when the subthalamic nucleus (STN) is stimulated. Once the precise location of the STN is verified, the microelectrode is removed and replaced with the quadripolar deep brain stimulator (DBS) lead.[26] Doing bilateral placement of DBSs at one time is controversial. Some surgeons prefer to stage the surgery by implanting bilateral DBS electrodes at the same time and the neurostimulators about 3 weeks later under general anesthesia. If the placement of the electrodes is planned for insertion during one procedure, a second quadripolar DBS lead is placed on the other side of the brain.

In the immediate postoperative period the patient must be carefully monitored for neurological complications as evidenced by weakness, paresthesia, confusion, decreased level of consciousness, arrhythmias, or seizures. Intracranial hemorrhage is a possible complication that requires early identification and intervention.[25] In addition, infection and technology malfunction are possible. Subthalamic nucleus DBS has been shown to be effective for the various symptoms of advanced PD and is more effective than medical management alone.[27]

Investigational Work

Interest in transplantation of fetal and stem cells to be implanted into the caudate nucleus to decrease the debilitating effects of PD are investigational and controversial. Embryonic stem cell transplantation, adult stem cell transplantation, human fetal cell transplantation, and porcine fetal cell transplantation are not approved by the Food and Drug Administration (FDA). The controversy about the ethical implications regarding the use of tissue from aborted fetuses continues.

Nursing Management

People with PD are usually managed in the community or in long-term facilities. Placement into a long-term care facility may be necessary for end-stage disease when confinement to bed is necessary or dementia makes home management impossible. Nurses provide direct care, support, education, and monitoring of patients over the course of illness, with the goal of helping the patient stay independent for as long as possible. Drug therapy and effective methods of dealing with the symptoms of PD can prolong independence. However, the complications of supportive drug therapy are many and the responses to drugs vary over the course of the illness.[28]

During the long course of the illness, patients need assistance from multidisciplinary professionals to manage symptoms and treatment complications related to PD. Therefore, a collaborative interdisciplinary model of care provides the best outcomes and quality of life for the patient.[19] The nurse is an important member of the team and may be the contact person for the patient and family. Their concerns can often be addressed by the nurse, but there may also be a need for referral to other members of the health team.

The following are major patient problems and nursing diagnoses related to the care of patients with PD:

- Impaired Physical Mobility related to rigidity, bradykinesia, and weakness
- High Risk for Injury from falls related to rigidity, bradykinesia, and weakness
- Impaired Communications related to change in voice (monotone, soft) and difficulty with writing
- Body Image Disturbance related to signs and symptoms of the illness
- Cognitive Deficits related to impaired memory and executive functions secondary to dementia
- Knowledge Deficit related to the disease process and treatment (especially drug therapy)

As the disease progresses, impairment of *physical mobility* is gradual, making it difficult or impossible for the patient to be independent in ADLs and other home and work environment activities. Keeping the patient active and functional for as long as possible is helpful. The physical therapist can recommend an exercise program, and the occupational therapist can identify assistive devices that can be used to assist with the accomplishment of tasks. Use of a walker, cane, or other ambulatory assistive device can promote safe ambulation. Integral in working with the patient and family is the concern for injury. As the rigidity, bradykinesia, weakness, and loss of postural reflexes develop, the *risk of falls* in particular is high.[29] A number of nursing interventions can assist in keeping the patient safe. Because most patients live at home, the awareness of the patient and family of risk factors in the home must be heightened.

Both *verbal and written communications* become impaired as the disease progresses. A consultation with a speech therapist can provide strategies to maintain function for as long as possible. Bradykinesia, a mask-like face, drooling, lack of eye blinking, and other symptoms can cause a *body image disturbance*. The patient may withdraw from social interactions and activities that would bring him or her in contact with other people. The change in body image should be explored with the patient. Patients need to be encouraged to interact with others.

Dementia, cognitive deficits, depression, and psychiatric manifestations such as hallucinations are commonly seen with PD. The nurse needs to monitor for evidence of these problems. Depression, for example, can be treated with drug therapy if it is recognized. Discussion with the family may also suggest behavioral or cognitive deficits that can benefit from treatment.

Patient and family education is key to management. The teaching needs of the patient will depend on the stage of the illness and the symptoms at that time. The following are general considerations that should be addressed by the teaching plan:

- Provide a clear explanation of PD and what to expect.
- Give an explanation of the drugs being used, including side effects, toxicity, and precautions (see earlier discussion of patient teaching precautions for levodopa).
- Discuss the high risk for injury (e.g., falls, spilling hot liquids).
- Help the patient and family evaluate the home environment for potential dangers (e.g., scatter rugs, poor lighting, need for hand rails in the bathroom).
- Advise the patient to maintain a weight chart. Weight loss can occur as a result of inadequate nutrition secondary to nausea, vomiting, and dysphagia. Dietary alterations for dysphagia should include soft, ground-up foods and small feedings with limitation of protein.
- Constipation can be managed with the use of stool softeners.
- Urinary problems should be evaluated carefully. Incontinence may be caused by an inability to get to the bathroom fast enough; suggest use of a bedside urinal at night.
- Orthostatic hypotension can be helped by wearing elastic stockings and changing position slowly.
- A bedridden person should change position every 2 hours to prevent skin breakdown, contractures, and pulmonary complications. Deep breathing should be encouraged to avoid lung congestion and pneumonia.

- Range-of-motion exercises prevent stiffness and contractures and are encouraged three to four times daily.
- Speech can be improved by reading aloud, singing, and raising the voice. (Consult with a speech therapist, as necessary.)
- Intolerance to heat is common; temperature control is needed for comfort.
- Using a wide-based (12 to 15 inches) stance improves balance and walking.
- Make the patient and family aware of community resources for PD that can provide educational material, referrals, and community activities such as exercise programs for PD patients. There are often support groups for patients and family members available locally. The following are recognized organizations that are good resources:
  - National Parkinson Foundation, Inc., (800) 327-4545, http://www.parkinson.org
  - The Parkinson's Disease Foundation, (800) 457-6676, http://www.pdf.org
  - Michael J. Fox Foundation, www.michaeljfox.org

MULTIPLE SCLEROSIS

Multiple sclerosis (MS) or disseminated sclerosis is characterized by chronic inflammation, demyelination, and scarring (gliosis) of the myelin sheath of the central nervous system (CNS). The manifestations of the disease vary from a benign disease to a rapidly progressive and disabling illness that has a profound effect on physical function and quality of life. The classification of MS is based on its variable clinical courses (Table 32-2). The etiology of MS is unknown, although it is hypothesized that a virus may precipitate an autoimmune response in a genetically susceptible individual. MS has been called the disease of young adults because the highest rate of incidence is between the ages of 20 and 40 years, followed by a gradual decline. The age at onset in men is slightly older than in women.

There are approximately 350,000 cases of MS in the United States,[30] with women being affected about twice as frequently as men. Whites are affected more frequently than any other racial group. Epidemiologic studies report that MS is more prevalent in the colder northern latitudes, such as the northern Atlantic states, the Great Lakes region, and the Pacific Northwest, than in southern parts of the United States. In Europe, high-incidence areas include Scandinavia, northern Germany, and Great Britain. Moving to a warmer climate after diagnosis does not arrest the disease.

Pathogenesis and Pathophysiology

The pathologic hallmark of chronic MS is the demyelinated lesions or plaques, which are sharply demarcated areas easily distinguishable from surrounding white matter.[31] The composition of a lesion varies depending on its age. In an acute lesion, there is partial or complete damage to the myelin, called *vesicular demyelination*. The damage consists of a breakdown of the myelin sheath that surrounds axon cylinders. As the lesion evolves, there is a proliferation of astrocytes and oligodendrocytes (myelin-producing cells), although many oligodendrocytes are destroyed by the cellular infiltrates of T cells and macrophages. The surviving oligodendrocytes may partially remyelinate affected areas. Long-standing lesions are composed of thick, matted, relatively acellular fibroglia tissue. The axon cylinders of the nerves are relatively spared, preventing wallerian degeneration. Lesions have an affinity for the optic nerves, periventricular white matter, brainstem, cerebellum, and spinal cord white matter. The plaques vary in diameter from 1 to 2 mm to several centimeters.[32]

MS affects primarily the white matter of the brain and spinal cord by causing scattered, demyelinated lesions, preventing or impeding conduction of normal nerve impulse through the demyelinated zone. Conduction blocks occur when the nerve impulse is unable to move across a demyelinated segment. This is caused by a resting axon membrane that becomes hyperpolarized due to the exposure of voltage-dependent potassium channels (normally located under the myelin sheath). A temporary conduction block often follows a demyelinating event before the sodium channels (originally concentrated at the nodes) have undergone a redistribution that allows the continuous propagation of nerve action potentials through the demyelinated segment. However, the leakage currents are too large for the nerve impulse to jump the internode distance, and conduction fails.[30] These variations in conduction help to explain the variations in symptoms that occur with MS throughout a day or a week and in relationship to activity (fever and exercise may exacerbate symptoms).

TABLE 32-2   FOUR CATEGORIES OF MULTIPLE SCLEROSIS (MS) BASED ON CLINICAL COURSE

TYPE	DESCRIPTION
Relapsing-remitting MS (RRMS) (80% of all cases)	Characterized by recurrent attacks of neurological dysfunction that evolve over days to weeks and may be followed by complete, partial, or no recovery; there is no progression of symptoms between attacks; this pattern is often seen in the early course of the disease and is the most common form seen
Secondary progressive MS	Gradual neurological deterioration with or without acute relapses, minor remissions, and plateaus in a patient who previously had RRMS
Progressive-relapsing MS	From the onset, there is gradual progression of disability; unlike RRMS, there is continuing disease progression without stabilization of the disease
Primary progressive MS	A pattern of gradual neurological deterioration from the onset of symptoms, but with superimposed relapses noted

Remission or improvement of symptoms may occur with MS as the result of healing or in response to the conclusion of an acute inflammatory event. Eventually, the axis cylinder of the neuron may become affected, so that disabilities increase and become permanent. At autopsy, multiple sclerotic plaques are scattered throughout the white matter of the brain and cord. The scattering differs from patient to patient, accounting for the variety of presenting symptoms experienced by patients. Some cases of MS are clinically silent, and the presence of the disease process is identified incidentally at autopsy.

Signs and Symptoms

The signs and symptoms of MS vary greatly from patient to patient and can vary over time in the same patient. The most common initial symptoms are sensory loss (37%), optic neuritis (36%), weakness (35%), paresthesias (24%), diplopia (15%), ataxia (11%), and vertigo (6%).[33] There are other sundry symptoms, mentioned below, that occur in 1% to 4% of patients. The multiple signs and symptoms of MS may include the following:

- Sensory symptoms: numbness or sensory loss; paresthesia (burning, prickling, tingling); pain; decreased proprioception and perception of temperature, depth, and vibration
- Motor symptoms: paresis, paralysis, dragging of foot; spasticity; diplopia; bladder and bowel dysfunction (incontinence or retention)
- Cerebellar symptoms: ataxia; loss of balance and coordination; nystagmus; speech disturbances (dysarthria, dystonia, scanning speech, slurred speech); tremors (intentional tremors, described as tremors that increase when a purposeful act is initiated); vertigo
- Other symptoms: fatigue; optic neuritis; impotence or decreased genital sensation and sexual dysfunction; neurobehavioral disorders such as depression or euphoria. Fewer than 4% of patients experience paroxysmal attacks, visual loss, trigeminal neuralgia, facial palsy, and impotence.

Sensory Symptoms

Sensory loss and tingling on the face or involved extremities are common. Loss of proprioception and joint sensation is frequently accompanied by edema of the limb or feelings of constriction. Fifty percent of patients develop objective sensory loss (position, vibration, shape, texture). Pain is uncommon except with flexor spasms of the limbs. **Lhermitte's sign** is described as an electric or shock-like sensation that extends down the arms, back, or lower trunk bilaterally upon flexion of the neck. The sensation probably results from the buckling effect on the dorsal roots of the posterior columns from sclerotic plaques. (Unilateral Lhermitte's sign has been noted in such conditions as cervical spondylosis and narrowing of the cervical spinal canal.)

Motor Symptoms

Motor symptoms often begin with weakness in the lower extremities and complaint of a feeling of heaviness or uselessness of the involved limb. Although complaints initially center on one limb, both limbs are usually involved to varying degrees. Spasticity, with its usual concurrent hyperreflexia, is common. Presence of spasticity often interferes with ambulation and ADLs. The decline in motor function may last from minutes to hours and is, therefore, not always observed by the physician. Motor function can worsen spontaneously after strenuous exercise, fever, or a hot shower or hot tub bath. This response is called **Uhthoff's sign**.

Incoordination is another frequent symptom. Intentional tremors are noted in the upper extremities. An **intentional tremor** is defined as a tremor occurring when a voluntary act is initiated. The finer the required movement, the greater the tremor will be. In the lower extremities, the incoordination appears as ataxia. Head tremors are not evident until the terminal stages, when the cerebellum is involved. Spastic weakness or ataxia of the muscles of speech is responsible for the dysarthria common in MS. Speech, in the early stages, is often slurred. Later, it becomes explosive or staccato and unintelligible. **Scanning speech**—slow and measured with pauses between syllables—is seen sometimes with late-stage bulbar involvement if cerebellar ataxia is prominent.

Ocular, Vestibular, and Auditory Symptoms

Optic neuritis, a common early symptom, is evidenced by visual clouding, visual field (often central) deficits, and pain with eye movement; pallor of the optic discs is noted. Diplopia and nystagmus are common. Internuclear ophthalmoplegia of lateral gaze, when noted, strongly suggests MS. The Marcus Gunn phenomenon, related to reduced light perception in the affected eye, is seen with retrobulbar neuritis. Vertigo is a common early symptom usually noted as a mild instability. Vomiting and nystagmus can accompany the vertigo. Deafness is a rare finding.

Paroxysmal Symptoms

Paroxysmal symptoms, which are less common but can occur in MS, include focal or generalized epilepsy, tonic seizures, trigeminal neuralgia, and occasionally, paroxysmal spasms (tetanus-like spasms). The spasms are described as contractions of the hands or feet into a dystonic, sustained, abnormal position and can be very painful.

Neurobehavioral Disorders

Neurobehavioral disorders associated with MS include emotional lability, irritability, apathy, inattentiveness, poor judgment, euphoria, dementia, and cognitive impairment. Depression is very common, occurring in 30% to 50% of patients. Less common are extreme anxiety, bipolar disease, and psychosis.

Other Symptoms

Fatigue is a very common symptom in MS and can range from mild to severely disabling. The basis for fatigue is unknown. Bladder and bowel dysfunction and impotence are common. Bladder retention or reflex emptying is often seen in later stages of MS. Impotence in men and genital numbness in women are also reported.

Course of the Illness

The course of MS is varied and unpredictable, as outlined earlier. Symptom clusters have been noted when a particular area of the brain is involved. For example, **Charcot's triad**, which includes nystagmus, intentional tremors, and staccato speech, occurs with brainstem involvement. Events that may precipitate relapses are menstruation; emotional stress; cold or humid, hot weather; hot baths; overheating; fever; and fatigue. Many relapses last a few days to a few weeks, after which there is complete or incomplete reversal of symptoms. Deficits present after 3 months are usually permanent. Prediction of when the next episode will occur is impossible. Some patients may experience another attack in a few weeks, whereas others may be spared for many years.

Diagnosis

The neurological history and examination are cornerstones for diagnosis along with imaging studies. The MRI, especially with gadolinium enhancement, has revolutionized the diagnosis of MS. The diagnostic shows plaque lesions and inflammation, and is useful not only for initial diagnosis, but also for monitoring changes during treatment. The Schumacher criteria and revised McDonald criteria are commonly used criteria for diagnosis of MS.[34,35] The Schumacher criteria is based on the neurological history and examination. It includes the following:

- Neurological examination that reveals objective abnormalities attributable to the CNS
- White matter involvement
- Two or more sites of CNS involvement
- Relapsing-remitting or chronic (>6 months) progressive course each lasting 24 hours and at least 1 month apart, or a gradual or stepwise progression over at least 6 months
- Age at onset of 10 to 50 years
- No better explanation of symptoms

The McDonald criteria include the number of clinical attacks, the number of objective lesions noted on MRI, and, in some categories, additional required evidence to make a diagnosis. Cerebrospinal fluid (CSF) findings are used in the criteria in some categories.

Magnetic Resonance Imaging and Evoked Potentials

The MRI is a sensitive diagnostic test and has greatly improved the ability to make an accurate diagnosis of MS. Multiple hyperintense lesions, which are best seen on the T2-weighted images, reveal multiple foci in MS (Fig. 32-3). Evoked potential assesses function in afferent (visual, auditory, and somatosensory) or efferent (motor) CNS pathways. In MS, evoked potentials are characterized as slow or abnormal conduction patterns on visual, auditory, somatosensory, or motor pathways.

Laboratory Studies

Laboratory tests may help to establish the diagnosis of MS. Three CSF abnormalities may be noted: mononuclear cell

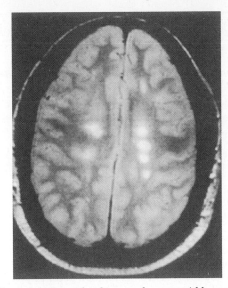

Figure 32-3 • Axial T2-weighted image shows ovoid hyperintense lesions in both hemispheres.

pleocytosis, an elevation in the total immunoglobulin (Ig), and presence of oligoclonal Ig. The *mononuclear cell pleocytosis* is usually less than 50 cells/mm³. In rapid progressive MS, the level may reach 100 cells/mm³. The proportion of gamma-globulin (mostly IgG) is increased to values greater than 12% of total protein in about two thirds of patients. The *IgG synthesis rate* represents a calculation of the level of IgG within the intrathecal space. It is increased to more than 3 mg/d in 80% to 90% of MS patients. This rate is a reflection of MRI plaque burden. The *IgG index* indicates the proportion of IgG in the intrathecal space. It is increased to a value greater than 0.7 in 86% to 94% of MS patients.[36]

Oligoclonal bands are discrete electrophoretic bands that are frequently found in the CSF of almost all (90% to 97%) of MS patients. The bands of MS are found only in the CSF when concurrent CSF and serum samples are evaluated simultaneously, and differ from the pattern seen in other inflammatory neuropathies, neoplasms, and systemic immune responses.

Treatment

In the last few years, development in drug therapy options for MS patients has been significant, and research continues on other possible avenues of treatment. The Kurtzke Expanded Disability Status Score, the most widely accepted measure of neurological impairment in MS,[37] is used to compare the clinical effect of current and proposed drugs for treatment of MS. There are two categories of treatment for MS: treatment to arrest the disease process and treatment for symptom management.

Treatment to Arrest the Disease Process

In the United States, three FDA-approved drugs, called the ABCs, are used to modify or arrest the MS disease process for relapsing-remitting MS (RRMS): interferon beta-1a (Avonex), interferon beta-1b (Betaseron), and glatiramer acetate (Copaxone). Ninety percent of MS patients receive one of the

TABLE 32–3   DRUG TREATMENT OPTIONS FOR MULTIPLE SCLEROSIS

DRUG	DOSE	SIDE EFFECTS
For Relapsing-Remitting Multiple Sclerosis (RRMS): Reduces Rate of Clinical Relapse; Reduces the Development of New Lesions on MRI		
Interferon beta-1b (Betaseron) FDA approved in 1993	8 million IU S. qid	Flu-like symptoms following injection, which lessen over time for many patients; injection site reactions, of which 5% need treatment; rarer findings: elevated liver enzymes, low white blood count; can cause abortion in pregnant woman
Interferon beta-1a (Avonex) FDA approved in 1996	30 mcg IM q/wk	Flu-like symptoms of muscle ache, fever, and chills; pain, weakness; rarely, mild anemia, elevated liver enzymes
Glatiramer acetate (Copaxone) FDA approved in 1996	20 mcg S. q/d	Injection site reaction; rarer, an immediate postinjection reaction of anxiety, chest tightness, shortness of breath, and flushing that lasts 15–30 min
High-dose interferon beta-1a (Rebif) Not FDA approved; available in Canada and Europe	Possible dose-related benefit in patients with more severe disabilities	Injection site reactions and flu-like symptoms most common adverse effects; elevated liver enzymes
For Secondary Progressive MS (SPMS): Same as for RRMS but Also Delays Progression of Disability		
Interferon beta-1b (Betaseron)	8 million IU S. qid	As above
Mitoxantrone (sometimes listed as an "off-label" treatment option)	Several administration schedules reported in the literature; one example is 5–12 mg/m² of body surface IV q/3/mo for 2 yr	Amenorrhea, alopecia, nausea/diarrhea, respiratory and urinary infections, anemia, and decreased white blood count
For Primary Progressive MS (PPMS)		
None; offer symptom management therapy		
Therapy for Acute Exacerbations and Relapses: Severity and Duration Reduced With the Use of Glucocorticosteroids		
Methylprednisolone	Various drugs and schedules reported; one example is 1000 mg IV daily for 3 d followed by prednisone 60 mg daily for 5 d then taper to 10 mg daily	Fluid retention, loss of potassium, gastric irritation, weight gain, and emotional lability

FDA, U.S. Food and Drug Administration; MRI, magnetic resonance imaging.

interferons as first-line therapy; the other 10% receive glatiramer acetate.[62] Through incompletely understood immune-mediated activities, all three drugs reduce the rate of clinical relapse and the development of new lesions seen on MRI.[38] Table 32-3 summarizes drug therapy options.

Each of these drugs is also used for patients with secondary progressive MS (SPMS) who have frequent exacerbations. There is no standard time to begin using these drugs. This decision is tempered by the knowledge that formation of neutralizing antibodies may render interferons inactive, leaving the patient without this treatment option in the future.[39] Approximately 35% of patients receiving Betaseron and 24% of patients receiving Avonex develop neutralizing antibodies.[40] A knowledgeable physician is the best person to make these treatment decisions. Careful patient selection and monitoring are critical to patient management.

Drug Therapy for Acute Relapses/Exacerbations

A short course of corticosteroids may be given to treat acute relapses and accelerate recovery. The determining factor is the presence of functionally disabling symptoms with objective evidence of neurological impairment. The preferred treatment is a short course of methylprednisolone, 1 g intravenously daily for 3 days, followed by a short prednisone taper. A prednisone taper may begin with 60 mg every day for 3 days followed by decreases in dosage by increments of 10 mg/d. Selection of appropriate drug therapy depends on the severity of the relapse and the resources available to treat the patient with intravenous therapy.

Symptom Management

The management of symptoms associated with MS often requires a collaborative multidisciplinary approach. The major problems requiring management include spasticity, sensory symptoms, urinary problems, tremors, pain, fatigue, and depression. Table 12-9 briefly outlines drugs useful to treat management symptoms. Drug management begins with an initial dose and is titrated to symptom control and tolerance of side effects. Therefore, close management and follow-up is necessary to achieve optimal results. In addition, patient and family education is very important to manage symptoms and to maintain a reasonable quality of life.

Both nonpharmacologic and pharmacologic strategies are cornerstones of symptom management. The goal of care is to keep the patient as independent and functional for as long as possible. Although lost motor function usually is not regained, range-of-motion and muscle-strengthening exercises are important to maintain intact function. A physiotherapy program using exercise and ambulatory assistive devices should be designed to maintain function. The physiotherapist can prescribe a brace or support device (e.g., cane, walker), as necessary, to maintain ambulation and independence. If leg spasticity develops, gait retraining designed to develop alternative muscles may be helpful. Stretching exercises are effective for both spastic arms and legs. With severe spasticity, drugs such as baclofen (Lioresal), diazepam (Valium), and dantrolene sodium (Dantrium) may be beneficial in improving motor function. Baclofen may be given intrathecally using an infusion pump with very good effect. Surgical procedures may be necessary for some patients. To prevent muscle shortening and joint contractures, passive range-of-motion exercises must be a daily part of any patient activity. The patient who is ataxic may be helped by means of gait retraining or by use of a weighted cane or walker to widen the base of support. Weighted bracelets on either extremity are also of value. Occupational therapy provides education and therapy in maintaining ADLs and other instrumental activities of living. Speech therapy is helpful for difficulty in articulation or staccato speech.

Patients with sensory loss must be taught to protect themselves from injury by using their eyes to locate the extremities. The body must also be protected from trauma, heat, cold, and pressure. For patients with paresthesias (abnormal sensations such as burning or prickling), drug therapy may be helpful. Limb pain may be managed with exercise and pharmacologic agents. Finally, fatigue and depression are very common. Fatigue is particularly disabling. It contributes to social isolation and depression. Exploration for contributing factors to fatigue helps to identify patterns that may be ameliorated. Risk modification, along with drug therapy, is useful to decrease fatigue. Depression is very common in MS, and the patient, family, and health care providers must be vigilant for signs and symptoms. Approximately 25% to 55% of patients with MS are depressed, and the suicide rate is significantly higher than in the healthy population. The use of standardized depression scales plus monitoring of the patient provides the means for early identification and treatment. Selective serotonin reuptake inhibitors are recommended for treatment.

Nursing Management

Most patients with MS live normal lives between periods of relapses. When relapses occur, most patients are managed in the community by a primary care physician or a neurologist in a clinic. When the physical environment of the home has been adequately adapted, patients with permanent disabilities often live independently with the aid of family members. Some patients with advanced disease are managed in nursing homes. When severe relapses or complications occur, patients are seen in the acute care setting where stays are usually short. Regardless of the setting in which the nurse

---

CHART 32-1   Exacerbating Factors in Multiple Sclerosis

The following factors are known to exacerbate symptoms and should be avoided:
- Undue fatigue or excessive exertion
- Overheating or excessive chilling or exposure to cold
- Infections
- Hot baths
- Fever
- Emotional stress
- Pregnancy (should be discussed with the physician to weigh the problems before a decision is made to become pregnant)

---

comes in contact with the patient, it is important for the nurse to assess the patient's understanding of the illness, the factors related to relapse (Chart 32-1), and the need for lifestyle adaptation to live as independently and normally as possible. A teaching plan should be individualized according to the patient's needs.

The significant degree of psychosocial adaptation required of MS patients means that major adjustments must be made over the course of the illness. If permanent disabilities develop, the amount of support necessary from the nurse and other health care professionals increases. Many patients will note a decreased energy level, urinary tract problems, motor deficits, sexual dysfunction, changes in their social and recreational activities, and concerns about roles and employment. Most patients need support in their adjustment process. Some patients need counseling and psychotherapy to deal with behavioral and cognitive deficits. Cognitive-behavioral programs have improved outcomes for many patients, especially women.[41]

The nurse, as a member of the multidisciplinary team, plays a key role in patient/family education, symptom management, and support. The major patient problems and nursing diagnoses include:

- Knowledge Deficits related to lack of knowledge about MS, treatment options, course of illness, and available resources
- Impaired Physical Mobility related to muscle weakness and ataxia
- Self-Care Deficits related to muscle weakness, incoordination, sensory/perceptual deficits, and fatigue
- High Risk for Injury related to weakness, incoordination, and sensory/perceptual deficits
- Self-Concept Disturbance related to physical disabilities, altered role performance, and altered self-esteem
- Impaired Home Maintenance related to weakness, incoordination, sensory/perceptual deficits, and fatigue

For the patient with advanced disease, the use of braces and canes and, finally, confinement to a wheelchair may become a reality. These patients need instruction and help in modifying their lifestyles to maintain the greatest level of independence possible. In some instances, the patient will become bedridden. The nurse should modify care depending on the needs of the patient.

Local and national resources are available to assist patients, families, and health care providers through the following:

- The National Multiple Sclerosis Society, (800) 344-4867, http://www.nmss.org
- The Multiple Sclerosis Association of America, (800) 833-4MSA, http://www.msaa.com

AMYOTROPHIC LATERAL SCLEROSIS

Amyotrophic lateral sclerosis (ALS) is a progressive motor neuron disease that involves both the upper and lower motor neurons. It is characterized by wasting of the muscles of the body as a result of destruction of motor neurons in the brainstem and the anterior gray horns of the spinal cord, along with degeneration of the pyramidal tracts. Sensory changes are not a part of the disease. Some muscles become weak and atrophy, whereas spasticity and hyperreflexia are noted in others. Various patterns of involvement can develop, but the classic pattern begins with a combination of weakness with increased tone, atrophy, and fasciculations of the limbs.

The etiology of ALS is unknown, although there is a genetic component in some families. Most cases of ALS are sporadic, although 5% to 10% of cases are inherited as an autosomal dominant trait. In the United States, the incidence of ALS is 3 to 5 per 100,000 people. Men are affected more frequently than women. The most common age group affected is the 40- to 60-year group. African Americans, Asians, and Hispanics have a lower rate than Caucasians.[42] ALS is a progressive disease that leads to death from respiratory arrest. The median survival is 3 to 5 years.[43]

Pathophysiology

There are marked degenerative changes in the following structures: anterior horn cells of the spinal cord; motor nuclei of the brainstem (especially nuclei of cranial nerves VII [facial] and XII [hypoglossal]); corticospinal tracts; and Betz's and precentral cells of the frontal cortex. Involvement of the upper motor neurons results in spasticity and reduced muscle strength, whereas lower motor neuron involvement results in flaccidity, paralysis, and muscle atrophy. Functions that are not affected include intellectual ability, sensory function, vision, and hearing. The bowel and bladder are usually spared until very late in the disease.

Signs and Symptoms

The signs and symptoms of ALS can vary from patient to patient. The initial symptoms are usually weakness and wasting of the limbs. A summary of the signs and symptoms follows:

- Muscle weakness, wasting, and atrophy: the muscles most commonly affected are the intrinsic muscles of the hand, as evidenced by clumsiness. The next most commonly affected muscles are the shoulder and upper arm muscles. The lower limbs are affected last; they characteristically feel heavy and are subject to fatigue and easy cramping.
- Muscle spasticity and hyperreflexia
- Fasciculations
- Brainstem signs evidenced by atrophy of the tongue causing dysarthria. The muscles of speech, chewing, and swallowing are affected so that dysarthria and dysphagia occur.
- Dyspnea that progresses to respiratory paralysis
- Fatigue

Diagnosis

The diagnosis of ALS is made primarily based on the history and a neurological examination that demonstrates upper and lower motor neuron disease. An electromyogram (EMG) is helpful because it will demonstrate fibrillations, which are signs of denervation, muscle wasting, and atrophy. The blood creatine phosphokinase (CPK) level is often elevated. A myelogram may be ordered to rule out other diseases.

Treatment and Management

There is no known treatment to cure this fatal disease. The first drug to slow the deterioration from ALS is riluzole, which was approved by the FDA in late 1995. Riluzole is generally well tolerated. Although the effectiveness of riluzole is not clear, no other treatment is currently available. Patients must be managed with a multidisciplinary approach that includes the following:

- Physical therapy: range-of-motion exercises to control or improve the weakness or spasticity. Support devices, such as a cervical collar, foot brace, foot drop and finger extension splints, or slings, are useful. A cane, walker, gait training, or wheelchair may be prescribed to assist the patient in ambulation. Although the disease is progressive, therapy optimizes independence for as long as possible.
- Occupational therapy: useful in selecting equipment, such as special eating utensils, and electronic equipment for alternative ways of accomplishing ADLs
- Speech therapy: helpful in giving the patient instruction on projection of the voice; also, speech synthesizers and computer technology provide a means to maintain communications.
- Gastrostomy tube: if ability to chew and swallow is limited, a gastrostomy tube may be inserted to facilitate nutrition and prevent aspiration.
- Nutrition assessment: to assess caloric needs and modify diet to meet nutrition goals and patient's nutritional needs as they change; educate to prevent aspiration.
- Periodic assessment of respiratory function and monitoring of pulmonary function studies including vital capacity; use of respiratory therapy, incentive spirometry, intermittent positive pressure breathing, and suctioning, as necessary
- Respiratory support with a ventilator can be life sustaining; long-term assistive ventilation, when necessary and if desired

- Ongoing counseling, support, and patient/family teaching: the patient and family need support and help in coping with the problems associated with this debilitating, fatal disease.
- Home health referral and assistance with home equipment and community services
- Management of any other health problems or complications precipitated by the disease
- Drug therapy for spasticity: diazepam (Valium) or dantrolene sodium (Dantrium)
- Frank discussion for planning and decision making for the future, including end-of-life care, advance directives, hospice care, and financial, estate, and other issues

Course of Illness

Because the onset of ALS is insidious, the early signs and symptoms may be overlooked. Diverse muscle groups gradually become involved. The degree of weakness, atrophy, muscle wasting, and fasciculations increases. As the disease progresses, the arms and legs become severely impaired, and spasticity and hyperreflexia are noted. If the frontal lobe cells are involved, emotional lability may be apparent even though intellectual function is not affected. In the advanced stages, when the brainstem is involved, the muscles of speech and swallowing are affected. Speech is thick and hard to understand, and chewing, swallowing, and managing secretions become very difficult. At the terminal stage, the patient has dyspnea and shortness of breath. Speaking may no longer be possible. Death usually occurs as a result of aspiration, infection, or respiratory failure. ALS is a rapidly progressing disease in which 50% of victims die within 3 years of onset.

Collaborative Problems

No treatment can currently arrest ALS. A collaborative multidisciplinary approach is necessary to meet the needs of the patient and family. The major collaborative problems addressed by the multidisciplinary team include high risk for aspiration pneumonia, loss of ability to speak, muscle spasticity and wasting, malnutrition, respiratory insufficiency, ventilator dependency, depression, and preparation for disease progression and death. The focus of care is palliation and comfort. As a team member, the nurse participates in achieving the following goals:

- Developing and implementing an individualized teaching plan
- Providing information about support groups
- Assisting the patient to be as independent and comfortable as possible for as long as possible through symptom management
- Limiting the development of complications
- Providing ongoing emotional and psychological support for the patient and family
- Making appropriate referrals to other health care professionals and community resources
- Making decisions on desire for a gastrostomy tube and mechanical ventilation, when needed

- Helping the patient to make decisions about end-of life care, advance directives, hospice care, and settling personal affairs
- Preparing the patient for a peaceful death; reassurance of comfort at the time of death

End-of-Life Issues

Key decision points in management must be discussed in advance of a crisis.[44] Two key decisions involve insertion of a gastrostomy tube and mechanical ventilation. There comes a time when the patient cannot chew or swallow and protect his or her airway because of disease progression. Because insertion of a temporary feeding tube is inappropriate for long-term management, a surgically placed gastrostomy tube is recommended. Since this is a permanent artificial route for nutrition, the patient must decide whether he or she chooses to accept this approach. Not to accept a gastrostomy will lead to aspiration pneumonia and probable death. The second, more difficult, decision point is related to mechanical ventilation. As the disease progresses, respiratory function is affected. At that point, the decision will be made for tracheostomy and chronic ventilatory support. Unlike other situations in which mechanical ventilator support is temporary, in ALS there will be no reversal of mechanical ventilation. For many patients, permanent mechanical ventilatory support represents an unacceptable quality of life, and they choose not to accept it. Unless these decisions are made proactively, a patient may receive a standard of care that he or she would not have chosen, given an option. Therefore, it is important to address these issues and other end-of-life issues before an emergency arises.

Nursing Management

The nurse's role in managing an ALS patient mirrors the overall needs of the patient and family. Patient problems are numerous in the rapidly developing trajectory of ALS. The major patient problems and nursing diagnoses relate to the functional losses associated with disease progression and include the following:

- Impaired Physical Mobility related to muscle wasting, weakness, and spasticity
- Impaired Self-Care related to muscle wasting, weakness, and spasticity
- Impaired Communications related to impairment of muscles of speech
- High Risk for Aspiration related to impaired muscles of swallowing
- Ineffective Breathing Pattern related to impairment of respiratory muscles
- Altered Nutrition, Less Than Required, related to inability to swallow

The nurse has special skills and knowledge to assist the patient in finding ways to ameliorate these symptoms in light of a rapidly progressive disease process with continued deterioration of neurological function and increasing disabilities. Psychological and emotional support is very important as the patient adapts to loss of function and approaching death.

Preparation of the Hospitalized Patient for Discharge and Crisis

The patient and family are central to planning for discharge from the hospital. They need to know what lies ahead so that plans can be made to deal with the inevitable. If home discharge is chosen, plans must be made that include the following:

- Patient and family education about treatment protocols and treatment routines
- Home care services and equipment (e.g., suction, oxygen, ventilator, walker)
- Adjustment in household routines and environment
- Arrangement for outpatient services and community resources
- Special therapeutic regimens, such as physical therapy, speech therapy, and occupational therapy
- Spiritual support and counseling
- What to do in an emergency (i.e., aspiration or respiratory insufficiency)
- Continued follow-up and monitoring
- Awareness of the services offered by the National Amyotrophic Lateral Sclerosis Foundation and community support groups
  - Amyotrophic Lateral Sclerosis Association, (800) 782-4747, http://www.alsa.org

Patient and Family Emotional and Psychological Support

The stresses of coping with a diagnosis of ALS and its effects are overwhelming. ALS radically alters roles, relationships, self-concept, self-esteem, body image, finances, and independence. The patient and family need a tremendous amount of support. Depression is commonly seen and needs to be treated. A multidisciplinary collaborative approach is mandatory, and the nurse can contribute to meeting this need as a collaborative group member.

MYASTHENIA GRAVIS

Myasthenia gravis (MG) is a chronic disease of the neuromuscular junction in which an autoimmune process destroys a variable number of acetylcholine (ACh) receptors at the postsynaptic muscle membrane. The hallmarks of the disease are fatigability and fluctuating muscle weakness of selected voluntary muscle distribution, particularly those innervated by motor nuclei of the brainstem (i.e., extraocular, mastication, facial, swallowing, and speech).[45] The weakness tends to increase with repeated activity and improves with rest. MG used to have a fatal outcome for many people, but treatment now available is highly effective, although there is no cure. MG is classified as an autoimmune disease, and persons with MG may have other autoimmune conditions. Some patients with MG have a thymoma, which affects the symptoms of the disease.

The prevalence of MG is about 1 per 7500 people. The National Myasthenia Gravis Foundation estimates that there are approximately 100,000 patients in the United States with the disease. It affects people of all ages, and women are affected more frequently than men by a 3:2 ratio. The highest incidence noted is in women in their 20s and 30s and men in their 50s and 60s.

Pathophysiology

Muscle weakness and fatigability are due to a reduction in the number of acetylcholine receptor (AChR) sites. This reduction is caused by antibody-mediated autoimmune attacks directed against the sites at the neuromuscular junctions. Which factors trigger and maintain the autoimmune response in MG is still unknown. Studies of muscle biopsy specimens of the neuromuscular junctions of myasthenia patients demonstrate only about one third as many AChRs as in unaffected people. The degree of severity of MG correlates with the number of AChRs. In MG, there is loss of postsynaptic membrane folds and an increase in the gap between the nerve terminal and the postsynaptic membrane.

Muscle contraction is controlled by effective neuromuscular impulse transmission. The effectiveness of transmission depends on the number of interactions between ACh molecules and AChRs. When ACh binds to the AChR, the receptor's cation channel opens transiently, producing a localized electrical end-plate potential. If the amplitude of this potential is sufficient, it generates an action potential that spreads along the length of the muscle fiber and triggers the release of calcium from internal stores, leading to muscle contraction. At normal neuromuscular junctions, the end-plate potentials are adequate for generation of action potentials consistently. However, at myasthenia junctions, the decreased number of AChRs results in end-plate potentials of decreased amplitude and a failure to trigger action potentials in some fibers. The strength of a muscle contraction decreases given a sufficient number of junctional failures, and muscle weakness is observed. With repeated stimuli, there is a reduction in the amount of ACh and the muscle becomes fatigued. This is compounded by a concurrent decrease in the number of AChRs, resulting in an ACh "run-down" phenomenon.[46]

Signs and Symptoms

The onset of MG is usually gradual, although rapid onsets have been reported in association with respiratory infections or emotional upset. The course of the illness is extremely variable. In some patients, the disease is unchanged for months and may or may not progress, whereas in others, there is rapid involvement of other muscle groups. The muscle groups affected have a characteristic pattern. Table 32-4 provides a widely adopted classification for the staging of MG. Early findings in most patients are ptosis and diplopia, which involve the levator palpebrae and extraocular muscles. Ptosis may be unilateral or bilateral and becomes intensified when the patient attempts to look upward. Pupillary response to light and accommodation remain normal. Chart 32-2 provides a clinical classification of MG based on the degree of disability it causes.

TABLE 32-4 STAGES OF MYASTHENIA GRAVIS

STAGE	DESCRIPTION OF STAGE	CASES (%)
I	Ocular myasthenia	15–20
II-A	• Mild generalized myasthenia with slow progression • No crises • Responsive to drug treatment	30
II-B	• Moderately severe generalized myasthenia • Severe skeletal and bulbar involvement, but no crisis • Drug response is less than satisfactory	25
III	• Acute fulminating myasthenia • Rapid progression of severe symptoms with respiratory crises and poor drug response • High incidence of thymoma • High mortality rate	15
IV	• Late, severe myasthenia • Symptoms same as stage III, but result from steady progression over 2 yr from class I to class II	10

CHART 32-2 Global Clinical Classification of Myasthenic Severity

Class 0	No complaints, no signs after exertion or at special testing.
Class 1	No disability. Minor complaints, minor signs. The patient knows that he or she (still) has myasthenia gravis (MG), but family members or outsiders do not perceive it. The experienced doctor may find minor signs at appropriate testing (e.g., diminished eye closure, some weakness of the foot extensors or triceps muscles, the arms cannot be held extended for 3 minutes). The patient may have complaints such as heavy eyelids or diplopia only when fatigued, as well as inability to perform heavy work.
Class 2	Slight disability, clear signs after exertion. The patient has some restrictions in daily life (e.g., he or she cannot lift heavy loads, cannot walk for more than half an hour, has intermittent diplopia). Bulbar signs are not pronounced. Family members are aware of the signs but outsiders (inexperienced doctors included) are not. Weakness is obvious at appropriate testing.
Class 3	Moderate disability, clear signs at rest. The patient is restricted in domestic activities, needs some help in dressing, and meals have to be adapted. Bulbar signs are more pronounced. Signs of MG can be observed by any outsider.
Class 4	Severe disability. The patient needs constant support in daily activities. Bulbar signs are pronounced. Respiratory function is decreased.
Class 5	Respiratory support is needed.

From Oosterhuis, H. J. G. H. (1984). *Myasthenia gravis.* Edinburgh: Churchill Livingstone.

The next muscles to be affected are the facial, masticator, speech, and neck muscles. When chewing food, the patient becomes tired and must rest. After a few moments of rest, chewing can be resumed, but muscles fatigue quickly again. Because the facial muscle is affected, the mobility and expression of the face are altered. Any attempt to smile looks like a snarl, and there is flattening of the nasolabial fold. The voice is often nasal and weak and fades after talking. There may be problems in managing saliva because of difficulty with swallowing. Food must be eaten very slowly to prevent aspiration.

Generalized weakness develops in a large percentage of patients. The limb muscles and, often, the proximal muscles, as well as the diaphragm and the neck extensor muscles, are affected. Weakness of the neck extensors causes the head to fall forward. If the shoulder girdle is involved, patients have difficulty keeping their arms above the head when reaching for an object, and with hair grooming. When the intercostal muscles or the diaphragm is involved and breathlessness and dyspnea are present, a condition called *myasthenia crisis* exists. Intubation and mechanical ventilation are necessary. In summary, the muscle groups affected tend to be weaker after use or toward the end of the day when the patient is fatigued. As the disease progresses, muscle fatigue is noted with less exertion and earlier in the day.

Diagnosis

The diagnosis of MG is based on history, physical examination, and confirmatory laboratory testing. The patient usually reports that selected muscles become weak with activity and that a period of rest improves the motor function. However, the muscle becomes fatigued again quickly. On physical examination, there is muscle weakness. MG does not affect reflexes, coordination, or sensory perception. Confirmation of MG is based on results of the following tests: anticholinesterase test; antibody titer for AChRs, repetitive nerve stimulation; and single-fiber EMG.

- **Anticholinesterase testing:** the drug commonly used is edrophonium (Tensilon) because it has a rapid onset of 30 seconds and a short duration of about 5 minutes. The test is performed by drawing 10 mg of Tensilon into a syringe and administering 2 mg intravenously. If no adverse symptoms appear, the remaining 8 mg is injected. If there is improvement in the muscle strength of a previously weak muscle that lasts 5 to 10 minutes, the test result is considered positive.
- **Antibody titer for AChR:** this is conducted by assay of blood. In 80% to 90% of patients with generalized myasthenia, the level of AChR antibody titer is elevated.
- **Repetitive muscle stimulation:** while electrical shocks are delivered to a nerve at the rate of 3 per second, surface electrodes over the muscle record electrical potentials. A rapid reduction of the amplitude of the muscle potential is considered positive.
- **Single-fiber electromyography:** this test can detect delay or failure of neuromuscular transmission in pairs of muscle fibers supplied by branches of a single nerve fiber.[20] It is about 99% sensitive in confirming MG.

- **Mediastinal MRI:** an MRI of the mediastinal cavity may be ordered to determine whether the thymus gland is enlarged because many people with MG have a thymoma.

Treatment

Four options are useful for the treatment of MG: anticholinesterase drugs, immunosuppressive therapy, plasmapheresis or intravenous (IV) Ig, and thymectomy.[46] After the diagnosis of MG has been established, an *individualized* management plan is developed because no single treatment plan is effective for all patients. The goal of treatment is to achieve a quality of life that is as symptom free as possible.

Anticholinesterase Drugs

Anticholinesterase drugs are the first-line approach for the management of symptoms of MG, although they do not treat the underlying disease. Anticholinesterase drugs enhance the neuromuscular transmission of an impulse by preventing the degradation of ACh by the enzyme cholinesterase (ChE). The ACh inhibitor drug that is the mainstay in managing symptoms of MG is pyridostigmine (Mestinon). Neostigmine (Prostigmin), formerly prescribed, is used much less frequently, and most experts do not include it in their discussions of management. Muscarinic- and nicotinic-type side effects (discussed later) occur with both drugs. Atropine is the antidote for ChE inhibitor drugs and must be available for any patient receiving anticholinesterase therapy. There is no standard dosage of Mestinon because there are great variations among patients and in the same patient from time to time.

Pyridostigmine (Mestinon). Mestinon, the drug of choice, is available in tablet, syrup, time-release, and IV forms. Its effects begin within 30 to 45 minutes, peak in about 2 hours, and last 3 to 6 hours. The daily dosage and time interval are carefully adjusted, using an affected muscle group to gauge effect. The goal is to produce maximal muscle strength with minimal side effects. For example, if the oropharyngeal muscles are weak, then dosage should be timed to enhance muscle strength optimally at mealtime.[81] The dosage prescribed for most patients falls within the range of 30 to 120 mg every 4 hours orally during daytime hours. Pyridostigmine in 180-mg time-release tablets is sometimes advisable at bedtime for patients who have nocturnal weakness or weakness on arising in the morning.

If ChE inhibitors become ineffective in treating symptoms, then other forms of therapy may be indicated.

The following are common drug-related side effects:

Muscarinic-Type Side Effects (On Smooth Muscle and Glands)

- Gastrointestinal tract: heartburn, belching, epigastric distress, abdominal cramps, increased peristalsis, diarrhea, nausea, and vomiting
- Genitourinary tract: involuntary micturition, increased tone and motility of uterus
- Cardiovascular: bradycardia
- Vision: blurred vision, constricted pupils

- Respiratory tract: bronchoconstriction/bronchospasm, increased bronchial secretions, wheezing cough
- Other: profuse sweating and increased salivation

Nicotinic-Type Side Effect (On Skeletal Muscle)

- Skeletal muscle fasciculations (twitching) and spasms followed by fatigue and weakness

Immunosuppression: Glucocorticosteroid Therapy and Other Agents

For those who do not respond well to anticholinesterase drugs, long-term corticosteroid therapy may be tried (Table 32-5). Prednisone is the drug of choice, producing marked improvement or remission in about 70% to 80% of cases. The choice of drugs depends on an assessment of risks and benefits to the patient and the urgency of treatment.[47] Azathioprine (Imuran) is frequently used with success to treat symptoms of MG. It is the second-line choice after prednisone and a good choice if prednisone is contraindicated. After 1 to 2 years of improvement, the drug can be gradually discontinued. Cyclophosphamide (Cytoxan) is rarely used for treatment of MG because of its high toxicity.

Plasmapheresis and Intravenous Immunoglobulin

Plasmapheresis removes antibodies from the blood. In the case of MG, plasmapheresis removes the anti-AChR antibodies, resulting in short-term clinical improvement. The indications for plasmapheresis are to stabilize a patient in myasthenic crisis or to serve as a short-term treatment for a patient undergoing thymectomy. The plasmapheresis is done at the bedside with a blood cell separator machine and albumin as the plasma exchanger. An antecubital shunt provides access. The procedure takes 3 to 5 hours, depending on the weight of the patient. Five exchanges over a 2-week period are the usual regimen. An improvement in muscle strength is usually noted in about 1 to 5 days after the first exchange, but it is temporary.

The indications for the use of **IV Ig** are the same as for plasmapheresis: short-term treatment for a serious relapse of MG. IV Ig is useful for immunodeficiency and autoimmune conditions and has been used with success in MG. As with plasmapheresis, improvement occurs in a few days.

Thymectomy

Some MG patients have a thymoma, and a thymectomy is indicated. About 85% of patients experience improvement in their MG after surgery, and about 35% have a drug-free remission after the thymectomy. Surgery is planned collaboratively by the surgeon and anesthesiologist because the MG patient is prone to have unpredictable responses to drugs, and the possibility of respiratory failure is always present. Therefore, a thymectomy should only be performed at a designated center with a surgical and anesthesia staff experienced in the perioperative management of the patient.

Cholinergic Crisis Versus Myasthenic Crisis

Two situations can precipitate a crisis that requires respiratory support and intensive care: myasthenic crisis and

TABLE 32–5 IMMUNOSUPPRESSION IN MYASTHENIA GRAVIS

DRUG	DESCRIPTION	SIDE EFFECTS
Immediate Response		
Intravenous immunoglobulin (IV Ig)	• 2 g/kg administered over 5 d	• Headache • Fluid overload • Rarely, renal failure
Intermediate: 1–3 Mo		
Glucocorticoids (prednisone)	• Begin low (15–25 mg/d) and increase stepwise up to maximum improvement or 50 mg/d • Optimal dose is maintained for 1–3 mo • Next an alternate-day schedule is begun • Most patients need some form of chronic therapy	• Peptic ulcer • Hyperglycemia • Fluid retention
Cyclophosphamide (Cytoxan) may be used with glucocorticoids	• Rarely used except if unresponsive to other drugs • 4–5 mg/kg/d in 2 divided doses	• Hypertension • Nephrotoxicity
Response: Long-Term (Months to 1 Yr)		
Azathioprine (Imuran) may be used with glucocorticoids	• Used frequently after prednisone • Range: 2–3 mg/kg total body weight • Monitor white and red blood count • Works in 3–6 mo	• Flu-like symptoms (fever, malaise) • Bone marrow depression • Hepatotoxicity • Anorexia, nausea, vomiting
Mycophenolate mofetil	• 1 g bid • Inhibits purine synthesis	• Side effects rare • Diarrhea and leukopenia

cholinergic crisis. **Myasthenic crisis** is a sudden relapse of myasthenic symptoms in a patient with moderate to severe myasthenia or generalized myasthenia. A common precipitating event for crisis is infection, although in some instances there is no apparent cause. Even with an increase in medication, the patient can rapidly develop swallowing and respiratory difficulties that may require intubation and ventilation support. Vital capacity and blood gases are often monitored, and many physicians set a predetermined value, such as a vital capacity of less than 1000, for an elective intubation. By following such a protocol, an emergency intubation is avoided. These patients require intensive medical and nursing management. It is important to be attuned to the warning signs of imminent respiratory failure in neurological patients.[48]

There are many drugs that may compromise transmission of impulses across the neuromuscular junction and exacerbate myasthenic muscle weakness. They include neuromuscular blocking drugs such as curare-like drugs; local anesthetics, and antiarrhythmics (quinine, quinidine, procainamide); aminoglycoside antibiotics (gentamicin, kanamycin, neomycin, streptomycin); clindamycin and lincomycin; trimethadione; morphine; chloroquine; beta blockers; calcium channel blockers; and D-penicillamine. Many other drugs intensify myasthenic weakness. As a rule, MG patients should be observed for deterioration after any new medication is begun. Patient education is critical.

In myasthenic crisis, anticholinesterase drugs are usually ineffective and are therefore discontinued. After the patient is stabilized, drug therapy is reintroduced, and the patient is re-evaluated for response. At this time, the best dosage and combination of drugs must again be determined. Concurrently, as motor strength and respiratory function improve, the patient is weaned from the ventilator.

Cholinergic crisis is an event precipitated by toxic effects of ChE-inhibitor drugs and the subsequent muscarinic and nicotinic effects described earlier. It is essentially a problem of overmedication. Muscarinic effects develop slowly. Abdominal cramping and diarrhea are often present for some time before the onset of nicotinic effects, which is rapid. Clinical examination reveals profound, generalized weakness; excessive pulmonary secretions; and impaired respiratory function. Management is similar to that for myasthenic crisis—that is, monitoring of respiratory function for difficulty, possible elective intubation, ventilatory support, and temporary withholding of ChE-inhibitor drugs.

The Tensilon test can be used to differentiate myasthenic crisis from cholinergic crisis. An improvement in muscle strength on injection of the drug suggests myasthenic crisis. If there is no improvement or if there is deterioration in muscle strength, the patient is probably in cholinergic crisis.

Collaborative Problems

The myasthenic patient is usually managed in the community by a neurologist, unless a myasthenic or cholinergic crisis occurs. At that time, admission to an intensive care unit may be necessary, where a multidisciplinary team cares for the patient. In addition, hospitalization is required for a thymectomy. During these times, an endotracheal tube may be necessary and may be used in conjunction with ventilatory support. Management of the myasthenic patient during complications depends on the specific presenting complications. However, assessment and management of muscle weakness, respiratory pattern, airway protection, and drug therapy are major concerns. The nurse provides care for the patient as a member of the multidisciplinary team.[49]

Nursing Management

Careful assessment and monitoring of the *hospitalized patient* is focused on the following areas:

- Assess respiratory function by auscultation and observation and by evaluating respiratory tests for vital capacity and tidal volume.
- Observe for unpredictable responses to drugs used (e.g., excessive sedation, decreased respirations, or agitation).
- Assess the strength of all muscles involved:
  - Respirations: rate, rhythm, quality (labored or smooth), abdominal breathing
  - Voice: quality of voice (whisper, monotone, normal intensity)
  - Hand strength and equality: ability to hold or pick up objects
  - Leg movement: ability to move legs freely in bed
  - Extraocular muscles: full range of extraocular movement; presence of eyelid ptosis
  - Head: ability to hold head up

The major patient problems and nursing diagnoses associated with the management of MG patients include:

- Knowledge Deficit related to the disease process and treatment
- Fatigue related to muscle weakness
- High Risk for Aspiration related to muscle weakness and difficulty managing own secretions
- High Risk for Falls related to muscle weakness and clumsiness
- Activity Intolerance related to muscle weakness and fatigue

Patient Teaching

While the patient is undergoing diagnostic testing or making adjustments in lifestyle or drug schedule, a comprehensive teaching plan should be developed as an important part of nursing management. Encourage living as normal a life as possible. The patient and a responsible family member should be familiar with all drugs being taken, as well as the prescribed dosage and potential side effects. They should also know the signs, symptoms, and differences between cholinergic and myasthenic crises. An Ambu bag and portable suction device should be available at home for patients who are prone to crisis. Provide information about the Myasthenia Gravis Foundation (MGF) and other available resources. The MGF is an excellent resource for educational material and referral information for patients, their families, and health professionals. Educated patients are the powerful and effective means of disease and illness management.

- Myasthenia Gravis Foundation of America, Inc., (800) 541-5454, myastheniagravis@msn.com

The following points should be included in the patient teaching plan:

- Wear a Medic Alert bracelet to identify yourself as having MG, and carry a card stating the name of your primary care physician.
- Take medication with bread or a cracker to reduce the risk of nausea and gastric irritation.
- Take the medication long enough before eating to optimize maximal strength of muscles for chewing and swallowing.
- Do not take any over-the-counter medication without your doctor's permission.
- Eat slowly and select a soft diet if you have difficulty in swallowing.
- Relapses of symptoms can be caused by menstruation, infections, extremes in temperature, extensive exposure to sunlight (or ultraviolet light), and emotional stress.
- Provide for adequate rest periods during the day.
- Set priorities and plan ahead so that undue fatigue will not develop. Pace yourself.
- Wear sensible shoes to minimize weakness and loss of balance.

SUMMARY

The most common neurological degenerative diseases and their management have been discussed in this chapter. There are many other disorders too numerous to cover within the limits of this text. However, a common thread for all chronic degenerative conditions is that patient and family education and support are vital to successful adjustment and adaptation. This is true regardless of the course of the chronic illness. Although there may be no cure, the nurse, along with other health care team members, can help the patient maintain the highest level of independence at each stage of the illness. As skills and functions are lost, the nurse can help the patient adapt and compensate for these deficits. Along with the physical adjustment, there is the need for psychological adjustment and mobilization of effective coping skills. The desired outcome of the comprehensive plan of care is to maintain an optimal quality of life for the patient and family.

REFERENCES

1. Corbin, J. M. (2001). Introduction and overview: Chronic illness and nursing. In R. B. Hyman & J. M. Corbin (Eds.). *Chronic illness: Research and theory for nursing practice* (pp. 1–15). New York: Springer.
2. Lubkin, I. M., & Larsen, P. D. (2006). *Chronic illness: Impact and interventions* (6th ed.). Boston: Jones & Bartlett.
3. The Institute for Health & Aging, University of California, San Francisco. (1996). *Chronic care in America: A 21st century challenge.* Princeton, NJ: Robert Wood Johnson Foundation.
4. Corbin, J. M., & Strauss, A. (1988). *Unending work and care: Managing chronic illness at home.* San Francisco: Jossey-Bass.
5. De Rijk, M. C., Breteler, M. M., Graveland, G. A., et al. (1995). Prevalence of Parkinson's disease in the elderly: The Rotterdam Study. *Neurology, 45,* 2143–2146.
6. Marras, C., & Tanner, C. M. (2004). Epidemiology of Parkinson's disease. In R. I. Watts, & W. C. Koller (Eds.). *Movement disorders: Neurologic principles & practice* (2nd ed., pp. 177–195). New York: McGraw-Hill.
7. Healy, D. G., Abou-Sleiman, P. M., & Wood, N. W. (2004). PINK, PANK, or PAEK? A clinicians' guide to familial parkinsonism. *Lancet Neurology, 3,* 652–662.
8. Nutt, J. G., & Wooten, G. F. (2005). Diagnosis and initial management of Parkinson's disease. *New England Journal of Medicine, 353,* 1021–1027.
9. DeLong, M. R., & Juncos, J. L. (2005). Parkinson's disease and other movement disorders. In D. L. Kasper, E. Braunwald, A. S. Fauci, S. L. Hauser, D. L. Longo, & J. L. Jameson (Eds.). *Harrison's principles of internal medicine* (16th ed., pp. 2406–2418). New York: McGraw-Hill.

10. Dawson, T. M., & Dawson, V. L. (2003). Molecular pathways of neurodegeneration in Parkinson's disease. *Science, 302,* 819.

11. Galvin, J. E. (2006). Cognitive change in Parkinson disease. *Alzheimer Disease Association Disorders, 20,* 302–310.

12. Hoehn, M. M., & Yahr, M. D. (1967). Parkinsonism: Onset, progression, and mortality. *Neurology, 17,* 427–442.

13. Fahn, S., Marsdin, C. D., Caine, D. B., & Goldstein, M. (Eds.). (1987). *Recent developments in Parkinson's disease* (Vol. 2, pp. 153–163, 293–304). Fiorha Park, NJ: Macmillan Health Care Information.

14. Colcher, A. (1999). Clinical manifestations of Parkinson's disease. *Medical Clinics of North America, 83*(2), 327–347.

15. Quality Standards Subcommittee of the American Academy of neurology. (1993). Practice parameters: Initial therapy of Parkinson's disease. *Neurology, 43,* 1296–1297.

16. Miyaski, J. M., Martin, W., Suchowersky, O., Weiner, W. J., & Lang, A. E. (2002). Practice parameter: Initiation of treatment for Parkinson's disease: An evidence-based review: Report of the Quality Standards Subcommittee of the American Academy of Neurology. *Neurology, 58,* 11–17.

17. Goetz, C. G., Koller, W. C., Poewe, W., Rascol, O., & Sampaio, C. (2002). Management of Parkinson's disease: An evidence-based review. *Movement Disorders, 17* (Suppl 4), S1–S166.

18. Goetz, C. G., Poewe, W., Rascol, O., & Sampaio, C. (2005). Evidence-based medical review update: Pharmacological and surgical treatments of Parkinson's disease: 2001 to 2004. *Movement Disorders, 20,* 523–539.

19. Carne, W., Cifu, D. X., Marcinko, P., Baron, M., Picket, T., Qutubuddin, A., et al. (2005). Efficacy of multidisciplinary treatment program on long-term outcomes of individuals with Parkinson's disease. *Journal of Rehabilitation Research & Development, 42*(6), 779–786.

20. American College of Physicians. (2007). Parkinson's disease. In *PIER: The physicians' information and education resource.* Retrieved May 12, 2007, from http://online.statref.com.ezproxyhost.library.tmc.edu/document/DocumentBodyContent.aspx?Docld=232

21. Miya, I., Fujimoto, Y., Ueda, Y., Yarnamoto, H., Nozaki, S., Saito, T., et al. (2000). Treadmill training with body weight support: Its effect on Parkinson's disease. *Archives of Physical and Medical Rehabilitation, 81,* 849–852.

22. Wright, J. N. (1999). Nonpharmacological management strategies. *Medical Clinics of North American, 83,* 499–508.

23. Suchowersky, O., Gronseth, G., Perlmutter, J., Reich, S., Zesiewicz, T., & Weiner, W. J. (2006). Practice parameter: Neuroprotective strategies and alternative therapies for Parkinson's disease: Report of the Quality Standards subcommittee of the American Academy of Neurology. *Neurology, 66,* 976–982.

24. O'Sulleanbhain, P. E., & Murphy, S. M. (2000). Adjunctive therapies in Parkinson's disease: Diet, physical therapy, and networking. In C. H. Adler & J. E. Ahiskog (Eds.). *Parkinson's disease and movement disorders: Diagnosis and treatment guidelines for the practicing physician* (pp. 197–208). Totawa, NJ: Humana Press.

25. Aminoff, M. J. (2001). Neurological treatment: Parkinson's disease. *Neurologic Clinics, 19*(1), 119–128.

26. Sanghera, M., Desaloms, J. M., & Stewart, R. M. (2004). High-frequency stimulation of the subthalamic nucleus for the treatment of Parkinson's disease-A team perspective. *Journal of Neuroscience Nursing, 36*(6), 301–311.

27. Deuschi, G., Schade-Brittinger, C., Krack, P., Volkmann, J., Schafer, H., Botzel, K., et al. (2006). A randomized trial of deep-brain stimulation for Parkinson's disease. *New England Journal of Medicine, 355*(9), 896–908.

28. Herndon, C. M., Young, K., Herndon, A. D., & Dole, E. J. (2000). Parkinson's disease revisited. *Journal of Neuroscience Nursing, 32*(4), 216–221.

29. Gray, P., & Hildebrand, K. (2000). Fall risk factors in Parkinson's disease. *Journal of Neuroscience Nursing, 32*(4), 222–228.

30. Hauser, S. L, & Goodin, D. S. (2005). Multiple sclerosis and other demyelinating diseases. In D. L. Kasper, E. Braunwald, A. S. Fauci, S. L. Hauser, D. L. Longo, & J. L. Jameson (Eds.). *Harrison's principles of internal medicine* (16th ed., pp. 2461–2471). New York: McGraw-Hill.

31. Noseworthy, J. H., Lucchinetti, C., Rodriquez, M., & Weinshenker, B. G. (2000). Multiple sclerosis. *New England Journal of Medicine, 343*(13), 938–952.

32. Ropper, A. H., & Brown, R. H. (2005). *Adams and Victor's principles of neurology* (8th ed., pp. 771–790). New York: McGraw-Hill.

33. Compston, A., Ebers, G., Lassmann, H., McDonald, I., Matthews, B., & Wekerle, H. (1998). *McAlpine's multiple sclerosis* (3rd ed.). New York: Churchill Livingstone.

34. Olek, M. J., & Dawson, D. M. (2000). Multiple sclerosis and other inflammatory demyelinating diseases of the central nervous system. In W. G. Bradley, R. B. Daroff, G. M. Fenichel, & C. D. Marsden (Eds.). *Neurology in clinical practice: The neurological disorders* (3rd ed., pp. 1431–1465). Boston: Butterworth-Heinemann.

35. Polman, C. H., Reingold, S. C., Edan, G., Filippi, M., Hartung, H. P., Kappos, L., et al. (2005). Diagnostic criteria for multiple sclerosis: 2005 revisions to the "McDonald Criteria." *Annals of Neurology, 58,* 840–846.

36. Leary, S. M., & Thompson, A. J. (2004). Multiple sclerosis: Diagnosis and the management of acute relapses. *Postgraduate Medical Journal, 81,* 302–308.

37. Kurtzke, J. F. (1983). Rating neurologic impairment in multiple sclerosis: An expanded disability status scale. *Neurology, 33,* 1444–1452.

38. Noseworthy, J. H., Lucchinetti, C., Rodriquez, M., & Weinshenker, B. G. (2000). Multiple sclerosis. *New England Journal of Medicine, 343*(13), 938–952.

39. Van Oosten, B. W., Truyen, L., Barkhof, F., & Polman, C. H. (2000). Choosing drug therapy for multiple sclerosis. In A. Wagstaff (Ed.). *Drug treatment of multiple sclerosis* (pp. 1–16). Auckland: Adis International.

40. National Multiple Sclerosis Society. (1999). *Comparing the A, B, and C drugs.* New York: Author.

41. Sinclair, V. G., & Scroggie, J. (2005). Effects of a cognitive-behavioral program for women with multiple sclerosis. *Journal of Neuroscience Nursing, 37*(5), 249–258.

42. Cronin, S., Hardiman, O., & Trayor, B. J. (2007). Ethnic variation in the incidence of ALS: A systematic review. *Neurology, 68*(13), 1002–1007.

43. Brown, R. H., Jr. (2005). Amyotrophic lateral sclerosis and other motor neuron disease. In D. L. Kasper, E. Braunwald, A. S. Fauci, S. L. Hauser, D. L. Longo, & J. L. Jameson (Eds.). *Harrison's principles of internal medicine* (16th ed., pp. 2424–2428). New York: McGraw-Hill.

44. Rowland, L. P., & Shineider, N. L. (2001). Amyotrophic lateral sclerosis. *New England Journal of Medicine, 344*(22), 1688–1700.

45. Ropper, A. H., & Brown, R. H. (2005). *Adams and Victor's principles of neurology* (8th ed., pp. 1250–1259). New York: McGraw-Hill.

46. Drachman, D. B. (1994). Myasthenia gravis. *New England Journal of Medicine, 339*(25), 1797–1810.

47. Drachman, D. B. (2005). Myasthenia gravis and other diseases of the neuromuscular junction. In D. L. Kasper, E. Braunwald, A. S. Fauci, S. L. Hauser, D. L. Longo, & J. L. Jameson (Eds.). *Harrison's principles of internal medicine* (16th ed., pp. 2518–2523). New York: McGraw-Hill.

48. Rabinstein, A. A., & Wijdicks, E. F. M. (2003). Warning signs of imminent respiratory failure in neurological patients. *Seminars in Neurology, 23*(1), 97–104.

49. Donohoe, K. M. (1994). Nursing care of the patient with myasthenia gravis. *Neurologic Clinics of North America, 12*(2), 370–385.

Nursing Management of Patients With Peripheral Nerve Diseases

Peripheral Neuropathies

Joanne V. Hickey

This chapter discusses selected peripheral neuropathies commonly seen by nurses in clinical practice. Peripheral neuropathies related to chronic disease such as diabetes mellitus, entrapment syndromes, and Guillain-Barré syndrome (GBS) are included. **Peripheral neuropathy** is defined as a condition in which there is alteration in function and structure of the motor, sensory, or autonomic components of a peripheral nerve. By comparison, *radiculopathy* refers to pathology affecting the nerve root, resulting in signs and symptoms in the corresponding dermatome and myotome.[1] As a group, peripheral neuropathies are common, especially among people over the age of 55 years, affecting 3% to 4% of people in this group.

Neuropathies can be classified according to:

- *Anatomic involvement or distribution:* single or multiple peripheral nerves, symmetric or asymmetric, proximal or distal involvement
- *Cause:* infections, inflammation, vascular compromise, entrapment, diseases (e.g., diabetes mellitus), alcohol abuse, vitamin deficiency, immune system disorders, toxic substances, and others
- *Pathologic process:* wallerian degeneration, segmental demyelination, distal axonal degeneration
- *Time frame of development:* acute, subacute, chronic
- *Clinical presentation:* presenting signs and symptoms including functional losses related to motor, sensory, autonomic, or mixed nerve changes
- *Genetic inheritance or mutations*

PATHOPHYSIOLOGY

The peripheral nervous system includes cranial nerves, spinal nerves that divide into peripheral nerves, and the autonomic innervation (e.g., sympathetic and parasympathetic nervous system). Peripheral nerves are the major nerves in the extremities and are derived from associated plexuses (e.g., brachial, lumbosacral). Each peripheral nerve has a well-defined anatomic course (dermatome) within an extremity, supplies a specific area of skin, and often provides innervation to specific muscles. The neural vasculature, which nourishes peripheral nerve tissues, is called the *vasa nervorum*. When it is damaged, it ultimately results in nerve ischemia. Most peripheral nerves have both motor and sensory

components, although a few are only one or the other. The motor fibers that compose the cranial and peripheral nerves have their origin in the lower motor neurons. A disturbance of function at any point in the peripheral nervous system (i.e., anterior horn cell, nerve root, limb plexus, peripheral nerve, or neuromuscular junction) can disrupt motor function. Disease that primarily affects the muscles can also disrupt function. In some cases, the proximity of some nerves to bony structures makes them particularly vulnerable to injury.

Although there are several etiologies of peripheral neuropathy, the pathophysiologic processes can generally be grouped into four categories: (1) wallerian degeneration, (2) axonal degeneration, (3) primary neuronal degeneration or neuronopathy, and (4) segmental demyelination.[2] An injury that causes degeneration of the axon and myelin sheaths, as in a transection of a nerve, results in *wallerian degeneration* distal to the injury site. The myelin and axon degeneration result in a loss of electrical conduction. Regrowth may occur proximal to the transection, but it is slow and often incomplete, and recovery of the nerve is limited. *Axonal degeneration* refers to distal axonal breakdown resembling wallerian degeneration. However, the degeneration is caused from metabolic changes within neurons (e.g., diabetes mellitus, toxins). The myelin sheath and axon break down in a process that begins at the most distal part of the nerve fiber and progresses toward the nerve cell body; this process is called *dying-back neuropathy*. *Neuronopathy* is a primary loss or destruction of nerve cell bodies with degeneration of their entire peripheral and central axons. *Segmental demyelination* (e.g., GBS) results from an injury to the myelin sheath or the myelin-producing Schwann cells. Although the myelin breaks down, there is relative sparing of axons.[2]

DISTRIBUTION PATTERNS OF PERIPHERAL NEUROPATHIES

Peripheral neuropathies are classified based on the distribution of peripheral nerves involved and the *pattern* of involvement. The classification includes three categories:

- **Mononeuropathy simplex** or **mononeuropathy** involves a single peripheral nerve (e.g., median nerve in carpal tunnel syndrome).

TABLE 33–1   CATEGORIES AND ETIOLOGIES OF PERIPHERAL NEUROPATHIES

Metabolic/nutritional	Common chronic conditions: diabetes mellitus, hypothyroidism, acromegaly, uremia, liver disease, vitamin B_{12} deficiency
Drug induced	*Antineoplastics:* cisplatinum, vincristine *Antimicrobials:* chloroquine, dapsone, isoniazid, metronidazole, nitrofursantoin *Cardiovascular:* amiodarone, hydralazine *Central nervous system:* alcohol, lithium, phenytoin *Other:* cimetidine, colchicine, disulfiram, gold, pyridoxine
Industrial/environmental toxins	*Organic and industrial compounds:* acrylamide, carbon disulfide, dimethylaminoproprionitrile, ethylene oxide, hexacarbons, organophosphates, thallium, trichlorethylene *Heavy metals:* arsenic, lead, mercury, gold, platinum
Connective tissue processes/ vasculitis	Polyarteritis nodosa, rheumatoid arthritis, systemic lupus erythematosus, scleroderma, ischemic neuropathies, critical care polyneuropathy, systemic necrotizing vasculitis, giant cell arteritis, Wegener's granulomatosis
Infections/infectious processes	Leprosy, human immunodeficiency virus, diphtheria, Epstein-Barr virus, rabies, sarcoidosis
Inflammatory processes	Acute idiopathic polyneuropathy (Guillain-Barré syndrome); chronic inflammatory demyelinating polyneuropathy
Neoplasms	Compression and infiltration by tumor, multiple myeloma, nonhereditary amyloidosis
Trauma/compression	Severance, contusion, stretching, compression, crushing, ischemia, electrical, thermal, and radiation injuries and drug injection; stretch injuries from orthopedic traction; compression from prolonged pressure, herniated discs, osteophytes, or fractures
Entrapment syndromes	*Lower extremities:* sciatic and peroneal entrapment syndromes *Upper extremities:* carpal tunnel syndrome, ulnar entrapment syndrome, radial nerve entrapment, thoracic outlet syndrome
Hereditary disorders	Hereditary motor and sensory neuropathies; hereditary sensory and autonomic neuropathies types I–IV, Friedereich's ataxia, porphyria, hereditary amyloidosis

- **Mononeuropathy multiplex** involves several, isolated, unilateral nerves often widely separated by location (multifocal). Mononeuropathy multiplex usually results from disseminated vasculitis, such as seen in association with diabetes mellitus or polyarteritis.
- **Polyneuropathy** describes impairment of multiple peripheral nerves simultaneously, resulting in a symmetric, bilateral pattern of functional loss, usually occurring distally before proximally. Polyneuropathy is seen with many systemic processes. The presentation may be mainly sensory (e.g., amyloidosis, leprosy) or mainly motor (e.g., GBS, porphyria).

DEVELOPMENT AND CAUSES

The development of signs and symptoms of neuropathy can be acute, subacute, or chronic. The general time frames for the development of neuropathies are acute, less than 4 weeks; subacute, 1 to 3 months; and chronic, greater than 3 months.[3] GBS is an example of an acute-onset polyneuropathy. Subacute onset can be seen in drug-induced (e.g., isoniazid, metronidazole, cisplatin, vincristine, intramuscular injection), environmental toxin–induced (e.g., lead, hexacarbons, organophosphates), and nutritionally induced (e.g., vitamin B_{12} deficiency) neuropathies. Malignant diseases (carcinoma, lymphoma), connective tissue diseases (systemic lupus erythematosus, polyarteritis nodosa, scleroderma), and metabolic disorders (diabetes mellitus, uremia, hypothyroidism) are examples of chronic time frames for development. Various causes of peripheral neuropathies are outlined

in Table 33-1. Note that an entrapment syndrome refers to a single peripheral nerve. Most of the other categories of peripheral neuropathies present as polyneuropathies.

The categories of etiology for peripheral neuropathy are many and include metabolic/nutritional, drug induced, environmental toxins, idiopathic inflammatory neuropathies, neoplasms, infections, and entrapment syndromes (see Table 33-1).

SIGNS, SYMPTOMS, AND CLINICAL PRESENTATIONS

Disorders of one or more peripheral nerves cause various signs and symptoms that correspond to the anatomic distribution and normal function of the nerve. Some peripheral nerves are purely motor, some are purely sensory, and others are mixed. Diagnostic accuracy depends on a thorough knowledge of specific sensory dermatomes, muscle innervation, reflexes, and autonomic function related to a particular peripheral nerve. The signs and symptoms of a peripheral nerve disorder include *pain, paresthesia, sensory loss, weakness, unstable balance, and autonomic or trophic changes.*[4,5] They may occur in any combination depending on the peripheral nerves involved.

When *sensory* nerves or components are affected, there is decrease or loss of light touch and pinprick sensation along the involved dermatome. Clinically, tingling, numbness, paresthesias, and dysesthesias are common. *Paresthesias* are sensations such as "pins and needles," whereas *dysesthesias* are unpleasant sensations such as burning. Neuropathic pain is a feature of some neuropathies, especially if small fibers within the nerves are affected. The sensation of pain can take

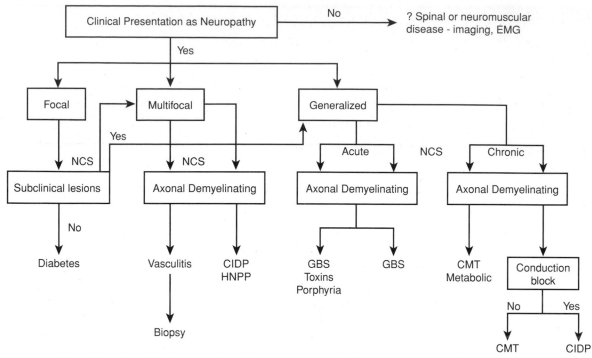

Figure 33-1 • Algorithm for stepwise approach to assessing and investigating a possible neuropathy. CIDP = chronic inflammatory demyelinating polyneuropathy; CMT = Charcot-Marie-Tooth disease; EMG = electromyography; GBS = Guillain-Barré syndrome; NCS = nerve conduction study; HNPP = hereditary neuropathy with liability to pressure palsies. (From Figure 1 from Willison, H. J., & Winer, J. B. [2003]. Clinical evaluation and investigation of neuropathy. *Journal of Neurology, Neurosurgery, & Psychiatry, 74*[Suppl II], ii3–ii8.)

on many forms including burning, jabbing, hypersensitivity to nonnoxious stimuli (called *allodynia*), or tight band-like pressure pain. Pain may be *hyperalgesic,* which is an increased pain response to noxious stimuli. Examples of polyneuropathies associated with pain include those related to diabetes, alcoholism, porphyria, rheumatoid arthritis, and acquired immune deficiency syndrome (AIDS). Pain is also a common finding with many entrapment neuropathies such as carpal tunnel syndrome. Finally, sensory loss is described as a "dead" feeling in an extremity.

Involvement of the *motor* fibers of a purely motor nerve or a mixed nerve results in lower motor neuron weakness or paralysis of the muscles innervated by the involved peripheral nerve. Atrophy of the specific muscle groups and related deformities follow. Fasciculations may also be noted. Deep tendon *reflexes* of the involved muscles are decreased or absent. The weakness may be described as unilateral or symmetric; a proximal or distal distinction may also be made. *Autonomic and trophic changes* are noted in the affected area. Skin may become dry, thin, scaly, inelastic, and cold and cease to sweat. The nails may become curved and brittle; nail and hair growth is stunted.

ASSESSMENT, INVESTIGATION, AND DIAGNOSIS OF NEUROPATHIES

One of the most common consultations with neurologists is for a possible neuropathy, although many patients never receive this detail of evaluation. An organized approach

guides questions and clinical reasoning to narrow an exceptionally long list of possibilities to a few possibilities where pattern recognition of symptoms guides the neurologist to the final diagnosis. See Figure 33-1 for an algorithm for assessing and investigating a possible neuropathy.

The following questions guide the clinical reasoning and diagnostic process[3]:

- Does the history/physical exam suggest localized peripheral nerve involvement?
- Have detailed past, family, occupational, and drug histories been collected?
- Have all symptoms been fully described and accounted for?
- Is the neuropathy focal, multifocal, or generalized?
- What is the involvement of motor, sensory, and autonomic involvement?
- What diagnostics might be helpful?
- What pattern of signs and symptoms has unfolded?

Diagnostics ordered to investigate neuropathies include sensory nerve action potentials to determine if there is evidence of demyelination and to determine the pattern of deficits (e.g., focal, multifocal, asymmetric, symmetric).[2] A nerve biopsy may be considered in selected cases. Selected serum autoantibody studies and genetic testing may also be considered.

SELECTED PERIPHERAL NEUROPATHIES

The following section addresses selected neuropathies related to chronic illnesses, entrapment syndromes, and GBS.

Neuropathies Related to Chronic Conditions

Neuropathies related to diabetes mellitus, vasculitis, human immunodeficiency virus (HIV), vitamin deficiency, toxic exposures, alcohol abuse, and metastatic lesions, as commonly encountered in clinical practice, are briefly discussed. In addition, chronic inflammatory demyelinating polyneuropathy is discussed.

Diabetic Neuropathy

Diabetic neuropathy, the most common polyneuropathy seen in general clinical practice, is a consequence of poor long-term glucose control in patients with diabetes mellitus (DM), especially in insulin-dependent diabetics. Ropper and Brown outline several distinct neuropathic clinical syndromes related to DM[6]:

- Distal, symmetric, mostly sensory polyneuropathy affecting feet and legs greater than hands that progresses slowly (most common)
- Acute diabetic ophthalmoplegia (affects third and sometimes sixth cranial nerve)
- Acute mononeuropathy of limbs or trunk including a painful thoracolumbar radiculopathy
- Rapidly evolving, painful asymmetric, mostly motor neuropathy that affects the upper lumbar roots and proximal leg muscles
- Symmetric proximal motor weakness and wasting often without pain and with variable sensory loss pursuing a subacute or chronic course
- Autonomic neuropathy with bowel, bladder, and circulatory reflexes
- Painful thoracoabdominal radiculopathy

These syndromes may be seen individually or in any combination. Neuropathies often occur in combination with vascular complications, such as retinopathy and nephropathy.

Prevention of neuropathies through tight glucose control is the best approach to patients with diabetes.[6,7] Daily glucose levels by self-monitoring and periodic glycosylated hemoglobin (A_{1C}) are useful indicators of short- and long-term glucose control. Most of the current treatment of diabetic neuropathy is focused on treatment of pain. No therapeutic modality aside from tight glucose control by whatever means necessary is recommended. The treatment of neuropathic pain associated with DM includes amitriptyline, nortriptyline, carbamazepine, phenytoin, or gabapentin. Amitriptyline is particularly effective for the treatment of painful diabetic neuropathy and postherpetic neuralgia.[8] Capsaicin cream applied to the affected area three times daily may provide temporary relief for some patients. Patient education is required with the use of capsaicin that includes washing the hands carefully after use and avoiding the eyes, open areas, and some other parts of the body with the cream. The patient should also be informed that transient burning or stinging occurs with application, but will subside after several days with continued use.[9] Nonopioid drugs are also used for neuropathic pain. Patients who fail nonopioid therapy may be offered methadone.[10]

Vasculitic Neuropathy

Vasculitis is described as a clinicopathologic process characterized by inflammation of the vasa nervorum, which provides blood supply to the peripheral nerve.[4] This process can cause ischemia. The vasculitis is usually a component of a systemic disease such as polyarteritis nodosa. In rare cases, it may be limited to the vessels of the peripheral nerve. The clinical presentations of vasculitic neuropathies are varied and may include any of the following patterns:

- Overlapping multifocal neuropathies (mononeuropathy multiplex) of varying degrees of asymmetry; differences in sensory and motor deficits between limbs may be subtle over days or weeks.
- Multifocal neuropathies occurring simultaneously in different limbs that evolve over days to years
- Distal symmetric, sensorimotor stocking-glove polyneuropathy

A careful medical history is conducted to uncover underlying processes such as malignancy, infection, or connective tissue disease. Because several laboratory studies are useful in ruling out underlying disease processes, the diagnostic net is cast wide. To look for a nonspecific, systemic inflammatory process, erythrocyte sedimentation rate, and C-reactive protein, a complete blood count, blood urea nitrogen, creatinine, liver enzymes, and urinalysis are ordered. In addition, the antineutrophilic cytoplasmic antibody (ANCA) test is ordered for polyarteritis nodosa, and the Anti Hu test for paraneoplastic, small-vessel vasculitis and sensory neuropathy.[11] In addition, nerve conduction studies (NCSs), needle electromyography (EMG), and possibly nerve biopsy may be ordered. Treatment depends on the underlying cause, but immunosuppressive drugs such as prednisone and cyclophosphamide may produce remission.[12]

Human Immunodeficiency Virus–Associated Neuropathies

Neuropathies are common in HIV-infected patients who may present with neuropathy or develop neuropathy during the course of their illness. The exact pathogenesis of HIV/AIDS neuropathies remains unclear, although factors such as concurrent infection, use of neurotoxic medications, nutritional deficiencies, and metabolic disorders may contribute to the process. Other possible mechanisms are direct viral infection or cell-mediated immune attack on various components of peripheral nerves.[13]

Distal sensory polyneuropathy (DSP) and antiretroviral toxic neuropathy are the most common of the neuropathies seen in patients with HIV/AIDS. The primary symptom of DSP is symmetric burning pain in the soles of the feet, which is exacerbated by touch or pressure. Stocking and glove sensory loss, distal weakness, and muscle atrophy may occur later in the course. Physical examination of the lower extremities demonstrates a distal to proximal decrease in sensation to pinprick, cold, and vibration, along with hypoactive Achilles tendon reflexes. Nerve conduction studies show mild slowing of maximal conduction velocity with low-amplitude sensory nerve action potentials and minimal denervation on needle EMG. Cerebrospinal fluid (CSF) is usually normal, although a lymphocytic pleocytosis and increased protein may be seen. Treatment is symptomatic with tricyclic antidepressants (amitriptyline, nortriptyline), carbamazepine, phenytoin, and topical capsaicin cream or topical lidocaine.[13]

Inflammatory demyelinating polyneuropathy (IDP) is an acute monophasic, relapsing, or chronic progressive process that tends to occur early in the course of HIV infection. Symptoms resemble those of GBS. Patients present with progressive weakness, areflexia, and mild sensory changes. The CSF generally shows pleocytosis. Electrophysiologic studies generally indicate features of primary demyelination. Nerve biopsy in IDP reveals segmental demyelination and perivascular lymphocytic infiltrates. The pathogenesis has not been proved but may be autoimmune. The clinical course is variable. Patients with acute onset and rapid progression generally do poorly irrespective of therapy and have more residual disability. Chronic IDP is more common in asymptomatic patients with immune systems that are still partially intact. Steroid therapy, plasmapheresis, or both may be effective in restoring motor function. High-dose intravenous immunoglobulin may also be effective.[11] Treatment with zidovudine (ZDV) has been reported to produce improvement in symptoms in some patients, supporting the hypothesis of an infectious cause.

Mononeuropathy multiplex may be noted in the cranial, peripheral, or spinal nerves. Asymmetric multifocal peripheral and cranial nerve deficits may occur, along with fever, generalized wasting, and CSF pleocytosis. When individual nerve lesions become diffuse or confluent, the course of the disease may resemble that of IDP. Electrophysiologic studies may assist in distinguishing the axonal lesions of mononeuropathy multiplex from primary demyelinating pathology. Treatable etiologies of mononeuropathy such as infections related to herpes zoster virus and cytomegalovirus (CMV) must be ruled out. No specific therapy has been identified.[14]

Treatment-associated neuropathies occur in as many as 22% of patients on didanosine (ddI) and 45% of patients on dideoxycytidine (ddC). The specific mechanism by which these two nucleotide analogs cause neuropathy is unclear. This specific toxicity is not associated with the use of ZDV, the other commonly used antiretroviral. Patients complain of painful neuropathy characterized by tingling, burning, or aching, primarily in their feet. Physical examination shows mild sensory loss and diminished ankle reflexes. The degree of neuropathy appears to be dose related and may continue to intensify for 6 to 8 weeks after discontinuing the drug.

Nutritional and Alcohol-Related Neuropathies

The neuropathies associated with malnutrition and alcohol abuse are clinically the same. The most common presentation is sensory or sensorimotor distal polyneuropathy. The insidious course begins in the toes and soles of the feet and progresses in a proximal and symmetric pattern. The neuropathy may be discovered incidentally while evaluating the patient for another problem such as liver disease, or in response to complaints of neuropathic pain. Sharp or burning pain or aching of the legs and feet may be early complaints progressing to sensory loss.

On examination, the sensory examination is diminished (i.e., light touch, pinprick, temperature, vibration), with greater loss noted in the feet. The legs appear weaker than the arms. Atrophy of distal foot muscles is common. The ankle tendon reflexes are absent. Autonomic disturbances and trophic skin changes are common. Diagnosis is made based on a history of alcohol abuse or malnutrition. In the case of alcohol-related neuropathy, cessation of alcohol consumption

is recommended, but this usually requires a comprehensive rehabilitation program. If the neuropathy is due to malnutrition, nutritional support with vitamins is necessary. For example, beriberi is caused by thiamine deficiency and thus requires thiamine. With treatment, slow improvement over weeks and months is possible.

Metastatic Lesions

Sensory and mixed sensorimotor neuropathy may be seen with malignancy, particularly with small-cell lung carcinoma. Neuropathy has also been associated with Hodgkin's disease and lymphomas. On laboratory examination, the presence of anti-Hu antibodies is found in the serum. Neuropathy may precede clinical evidence of a malignancy by months and possibly years.[15] With *sensory neuropathy*, there is progressive sensory loss, paresthesia, "burning" dysesthesia, and sensory ataxia. By comparison, a *sensorimotor neuropathy* includes a distal sensory loss and mild motor weakness of gradual onset. A less common acute severe neuropathy can resemble GBS. Treatment for the neuropathy is primarily with immunosuppressive drugs.

Chronic Inflammatory Demyelinating Polyneuropathy

Chronic inflammatory demyelinating polyneuropathy (CIDP) is an acquired neuropathy believed to be of immunologic origin. The clinical presentation and course are variable; typically there is progression of relapsing-remitting motor and sensory deficits, or exclusively motor or sensory deficits. The neurological manifestations include the following frequency: motor weakness, sensory deficits, and sensory-motor deficits.[16] CIDP is one of the few neuropathies that responds well to treatment. Treatment includes corticosteroids, intravenous immunoglobulins, plasma exchanges, and immunosuppressive drugs.[17]

Nursing Management of the Patient With Neuropathy

Neuropathy is common with a number of conditions and, therefore, will be encountered by nurses caring for patients in various settings. The pain associated with neuropathy is a major focus of care provided by the nurse. Pain management is difficult and is compounded by the presence of paresthesias and dysesthesias. In addition, motor deficits interfere with ambulation and other activities of daily living. A careful neurological examination with emphasis on sensory and motor function is essential in determining the degree of discomfort and functional loss present. Education, support, and assistance in modifying any risk factors that contribute to the neuropathy are also important. A focus for ongoing management is helping the patient optimize relief of pain and other sensory discomfort by effective titration of drug therapy. See Chapter 27 for management of pain.

Entrapment Syndromes

In **entrapment syndromes** or **entrapment neuropathies,** a nerve is compressed by the anatomic structure through

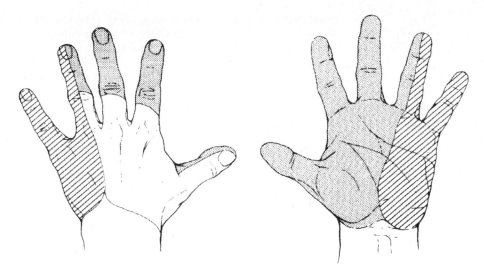

Figure 33-2 • Cutaneous innervation of the hand by the radial (*clear section*), median (*stippled section*), and ulnar (*diagonal lines*) nerves.

which it passes. This can occur in areas where peripheral nerves are encased by bone or rigid material, as when cranial and spinal nerves pass through narrow foramina or channels. For example, the median nerve passes between the carpal ligament and tendon sheath of the flexor arm muscles of the forearm and is involved in carpal tunnel syndrome. The narrowness of the foramina and channels, combined with edema from nearby soft-tissue trauma or pressure from a vascular lesion (hematoma or aneurysm), can easily produce a peripheral nerve entrapment syndrome. Ischemia as a cause of peripheral nerve injury is closely associated with compression injuries because compression eventually deprives a nerve of an adequate blood supply. In such circumstances, the etiology of nerve injury is most accurately attributed to the compression-ischemia mechanism. Occlusion of a major artery of a limb can lead to nerve injury because of ischemia. Generally, chronic entrapment syndromes require surgical intervention, whereas the neuropathies associated with exposure to toxins, drug therapy, and chronic diseases are managed medically by a neurologist. Carpal tunnel syndrome, ulnar entrapment syndrome (cubital tunnel), and radial nerve entrapment are the entrapment syndromes discussed in this chapter.

Carpal Tunnel Syndrome

In carpal tunnel syndrome, the median nerve is compressed by edema of tissue in and around the carpal tunnel. The median nerve is most frequently entrapped at the wrist because of its vulnerable anatomic position. It lies between the tendons of the flexor carpi radialis and palmaris longus. The flexor pollicis longus and the flexor digitorum profundus separate the median nerve from the radius. The nerve crosses the wrist level and enters the carpal tunnel, located beneath the transverse carpal ligament. The carpal tunnel is a narrow tunnel through which the median nerve passes. It is bound superiorly by the transverse carpal ligaments and laterally and inferiorly by the carpal bones, including fibrous coverings and interosseous ligaments. If the lumen of this channel is narrowed, the movement of the nerve and muscles is compromised. The result is the development of carpal tunnel symptoms.

Occupation-related activities that require forceful and repetitive movements of the wrists or keeping the wrists in abnormal positions for prolonged periods appear to predispose people to carpal tunnel syndrome. Such occupational categories include press operators, construction workers who use vibrating equipment, hairdressers, typists, computer keyboarders, and pianists. Women are more commonly affected than men. Several endocrine conditions (e.g., myxedema or acromegaly, pregnancy, and use of oral contraceptives) are also related to this syndrome.

Symptoms of carpal tunnel syndrome include:

- *Sensory loss* in the palmar aspect of the first three and a half fingers and the dorsal aspect of the terminal phalanges of the second, third, and half of the fourth fingers (Fig. 33-2)
- *Pain or paresthesias* in the wrist and hand especially during the night, often awakening the person; although these symptoms are usually confined to the wrist or median-innervated fingers, they may spread upward into the forearm; pain worse on wrist flexion
- *Paresis* of the abductor pollicis brevis and opponens pollicis muscles (difficulty in abducting and opposing the thumb)
- *Wasting* of the thenar hand muscles

Severe pain and paresthesias accompany the use of the hand during daytime hours as the disease progresses. Pain becomes constant, with motor weakness and atrophy. Vasomotor changes are intermittent.

On physical examination, Tinel's and Phalen's signs are positive. **Tinel's sign** is positive if pain and tingling are elicited by tapping over the median nerve at the wrist on the affected side. **Phalen's sign** is positive if tingling and pain occur in the wrists when they are flexed at right angles for at least 1 minute (Fig. 33-3). There may be evidence of atrophy of the hand muscles. EMG and nerve conduction studies confirm the diagnosis.

Carpal tunnel syndrome is treated with a variety of options including nonsteroidal anti-inflammatory drugs, injection of corticosteroids, immobilization of the wrist with splints, rehabilitation modalities (e.g., ultrasound, stretching and strengthening exercises), and surgery to free the median

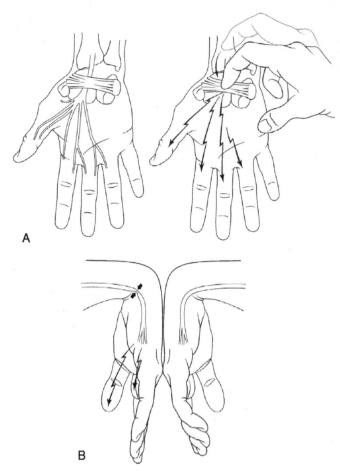

Figure 33-3 • Carpal tunnel syndrome: (*A*) Tinel's sign and (*B*) Phalen's sign.

nerve of compression.[18] Most patients do well with surgical decompression.

Ulnar Nerve Entrapment Syndrome

Entrapment of the ulnar nerve in the elbow region is most commonly caused by compression in the *cubital tunnel* that narrows during movement, especially elbow flexion. The roof of the tunnel is formed by the aponeurosis of the flexor carpi ulnaris muscle and the floor formed by the medial ligament of the elbow. The ulna nerve runs through this space and then underneath the flexor carpi ulnaris muscle. Repeated leaning on the elbows, fractures, or bony spurs cause the compression. The signs and symptoms include[19]:

- *Paresthesias and sensory loss* in the fifth finger and medial half of the fourth finger and ulnar part of the hand below the wrist
- *Weakness* of the abductor digiti minimi, adductor pollicis, and sometimes flexor carpi ulnaris
- *Wasting* of the interossei and hypothenar eminence (claw-hand deformity may develop)
- *Pain* in the medial forearm and elbow

The diagnosis is made based on a history and the presenting clinical picture. On physical examination, a taut, palpable,

enlarged nerve is noted in the ulnar groove. EMG and nerve conduction studies will localize the lesion to the cubital tunnel. Surgery is indicated to release the nerve.

Radial Nerve Entrapment Syndrome

The radial nerve may be compressed against the humerus by external pressure in the axilla or the spiral groove. Axillary compression can be caused by improper use of crutches. Compression of the spiral groove can occur if a person falls asleep with an arm hanging over a chair. Compression can also occur in a sleeping person under the influence of alcohol who has someone's head against the arm. This prevents the paresthesias from awakening the individual. The radial nerve may also be injured if an arm tourniquet is left on for a prolonged period of time such as during surgery. Signs and symptoms seen with radial nerve injury include:

- *Sensory loss* on the dorsal aspects of the hand, thumb, index, and middle fingers; if the axilla portion is involved, there will be sensory loss on the entire extensor surface of the arm and forearm.
- *Paresis* of the triceps with axillary compression only; wrist drop, weakness of finger extensors, and brachioradialis for forearm flexion
- *Wasting* of the triceps and posterior surface of the forearm[19]

The diagnosis is made based on a history and presenting clinical picture. EMG and nerve conduction studies localize the lesion to the radial nerve. Surgical exploration may be indicated for pain control and progressive motor weakness.

Nursing Management of the Patient with an Entrapment Syndrome

Nurses should be familiar with the selected entrapment syndromes discussed in this chapter because they are commonly seen in practice and because nurses have some influence for preventing them. Such is the case with radial compression from improper use of crutches. There are several other entrapment syndromes, including those of the lower extremities, which can be found in medical texts. As with the neuropathies previously mentioned, recognition of the patient who is at high risk for entrapment neuropathies is the first step toward prevention. Pain control and motor weakness are the major problems experienced by the patient. Patient education provides the patient with information on symptom management and corrective interventions to treat the underlying problem.

Guillain-Barré Syndrome

Guillain-Barré syndrome is an acute inflammatory polyneuropathy that is the most common cause of acute or subacute generalized paralysis.[20] It is caused by an autoimmune response to a viral infection. Most patients give a history of a recent (i.e., 1 to 3 weeks) acute infection, such as an upper respiratory infection, viral pneumonia, or gastrointestinal (GI) infection. A *Campylobacter jejuni* infection is often an antecedent to GBS. In a few instances, the patient reports receiving a vaccination prior to the onset of GBS. As a result of improved respiratory management, most patients survive. Most patients (75% to 85%) make a good recovery from GBS, although 2% to 12% succumb to complications.[21]

GBS is a rapidly evolving areflexic motor paralysis with or without sensory disturbance.

Pathophysiology

GBS is an immune-mediated cellular and humoral response that triggers antibody production against specific gangliosides and glycolipids that cause destruction of the myelin sheath surrounding the cranial and spinal nerves. The demyelination process is accompanied by edema and inflammation of the peripheral nerves. Collections of lymphocytes and macrophages are responsible for the demyelination of axons resulting in loss of saltatory conduction. In addition, the inflammatory process may result in varying degrees of axonal injury, which is related to a reduction in amplitude of muscle potential. The remyelination process in the recovery phase occurs slowly.

Subtypes of Guillain-Barré Syndrome

Several subtypes of GBS are recognized reflecting differences in the pattern and symptoms of peripheral nerve involvement. The most common are acute inflammatory demyelinating polyneuropathy (AIDP), acute motor axonal neuropathy (AMAN), acute motor sensory axonal neuropathy (AMSAN), and Miller-Fisher syndrome (MFS).

Acute Inflammatory Demyelinating Polyneuropathy

- Most common presentation
- Weakness and numbness begin in the legs, then progress upward to the trunk, arms, and cranial nerves
- Motor: paresis to quadriplegia; deficits are symmetric
- Sensory: mild numbness, which is worse in toes
- Reflexes: diminished or absent
- Respiratory: respiratory insufficiency occurs in about 50% of patients
- Electrophysiologic diagnosis: demyelinating disease

Acute Motor Axonal Neuropathy

- Affects children and young adults
- Identical to ascending GBS, except sensory signs and symptoms are absent
- May be a mild form of ascending GBS
- Muscle pain is generally not present
- Electrophysiologic diagnosis: axonal involvement

Acute Motor Sensory Axonal Neuropathy

- Affects mostly adults
- Motor: initial weakness in the brainstem cranial nerves (facial, glossopharyngeal, vagus, and hypoglossal nerves); then weakness progresses downward
- Sensory: numbness occurs distally, more often in the hands than in the feet
- Often rapid respiratory involvement
- Electrophysiologic diagnosis: axonal involvement

Miller-Fisher Syndrome

- Rare (5% of patients with GBS)
- Affects adults and children
- Seen as a triad of ophthalmoplegia, ataxia, and areflexia
- Usually no sensory loss
- Electrophysiologic diagnosis: demyelinating disease

Pharyngeal-Cervical-Brachial Variant[20]

- Rare
- Isolated facial, oropharyngeal, cervical, and upper limb weakness without lower limb involvement
- Occurs with or without ptosis

Clinical Presentation

In general, GBS is characterized by motor weakness, flaccid paralysis, and areflexia. Motor weakness tends to be symmetric, beginning in the legs and progressing to the trunk and arms. Respiratory failure is attributable to mechanical failure and fatigue of the intercostals and diaphragm. If the cranial nerves (CNs) are involved, the facial (CN VII) nerve is most often affected. Other cranial nerves that are less often affected are the glossopharyngeal (CN IX), vagus (CN X), spinal accessory (CN XI), and hypoglossal (CN XII). Signs and symptoms of facial nerve dysfunction include an inability to smile, frown, whistle, or drink with a straw. Dysphagia and laryngeal paralysis can develop as a result of paralysis of cranial nerves IX and X. Vagus nerve deficit, if present, is thought to be responsible for the autonomic dysfunction noted in some patients.

When sensory changes are present, paresthesias and pain may be noted. The paresthesia is frequent and temporary and is described as a tingling, "pins and needles" feeling, a heightened sensitivity to touch, or numbness. Sensory changes are often noted in the hands and feet (glove and stocking distribution). About 25% of patients experience pain. Pain is underrated in terms of frequency and intensity. The pain may begin as cramping and progress to frank pain in the arms, legs, back, or buttock. Pain is often worse at night and often interferes with sleep. Analgesics are often necessary to keep the patient comfortable. The pain may be so severe that a morphine drip is necessary.

Autonomic dysfunction is much more common than once thought. The signs and symptoms may include any of the following: cardiac arrhythmias, paroxysmal hypertension, orthostatic hypotension, paralytic ileus, urinary retention, or syndrome of inappropriate secretion of antidiuretic hormone (SIADH). GBS does not affect the level of consciousness, cognitive function, or pupillary signs.

Clinical Course

The progression of GBS is viewed in three stages: acute, plateau, and recovery. The acute stage begins with the onset of definitive symptoms and ends when no additional symptoms or deterioration are noted (lasts from 1 to 3 weeks). In the plateau stage, the clinical presentation remains constant; the time frame is a few days to a few weeks. In the recovery stage, there is gradual improvement of signs and symptoms over time. The recovery phase is synonymous with the remyelination and axonal regeneration process. In patients who have sustained secondary axonal injury, maximal improvement may take up to 2 years and permanent deficits may result.[22]

Diagnosis

Diagnosis is based on the clinical presentation and diagnostic criteria. The required diagnostic criteria for GBS includes progressive weakness of two or more limbs due to neuropathy (excluding Miller-Fisher Syndrome); areflexia; disease course less than 4 weeks; and exclusion of other causes of the symptoms.[23,24] A history of a recent viral infection, elevated CSF protein levels with a normal cell count, and abnormal EMG studies are seen. Nerve conduction velocities are slowed soon after paralysis develops. If denerved potentials (fibrillations) develop, they will occur later in the illness.

Medical Treatment

Patients with GBS require comprehensive supportive therapy that includes respiratory and cardiovascular monitoring and management as well as prevention of electrolyte imbalance, gastrointestinal hemorrhage, and pulmonary embolism.[20] Specific therapy with immunotherapy using either high-dose intravenous immunoglobulin (IV Ig) or plasmapheresis is effective in most patients. The IV Ig is usually given on 5 sequential days for an overall dose of 2 g/kg of body weight.[21] If the choice of therapy is plasmapheresis, 40 to 50 mL/kg plasma exchange daily for 4 to 5 days is provided. Some patients require a second course of treatments because of relapse. Patients with GBS need to be hospitalized and observed carefully for deterioration and respiratory compromise. If this occurs, therapy in an intensive care unit will be necessary.

Respiratory Support. Respiratory mechanical failure secondary to neuromuscular weakness is common in GBS. Vital capacity decreases, the cough weakens, and ineffective airway clearance results. Peripheral alveoli collapse for longer portions of the respiratory cycle, lose their surfactant coating, and remain collapsed. This creates pulmonary tissue that is unventilated but perfused. Pulmonary vascular shunting develops as the vital capacity declines, causing a diminished CO_2 level. The consequences of a lowered vital capacity are atelectasis and probable hypoxemia. Concurrently, the intercostal muscles and diaphragm become fatigued, and tachycardia, dyspnea, and diaphoresis develop rapidly. Some patients will need to be intubated and supported temporarily on a ventilator. To avoid emergency intubation and the increased risk of aspiration, vital capacity is monitored and compared with a predetermined optimal level for the patient (approximately 12 to 15 mL/kg). In a 160-pound person, the target vital capacity is about 1000 to 1200 mL. When the patient's vital capacity falls below this level, elective intubation and mechanical ventilation may be indicated.[23] Pneumonia related to mechanical respiratory failure is a common complication in these patients.

Some patients require ventilatory support for a short time (<2 weeks). However, for those who require extended ventilation, a tracheotomy is necessary. After the patient's illness has stabilized and respiratory function has improved (as evidenced by a vital capacity of 8 to 10 mL/kg), weaning from the ventilator is begun.

The mainstay of treatment is supportive care. Recovery from GBS is usual but takes time. Hospitalization in the intensive care unit usually continues for approximately 2 to 3 months. Supportive care is directed toward preventing complications and maintaining the patient in the best condition possible. In addition to respiratory problems, other complications may include **autonomic dysfunction** (i.e., hypotension, hypertension, cardiac arrhythmias, paralytic ileus, bladder retention, and SIADH), **sleep dysfunction**, possible **pain, nutrition,** and **psychological responses** (i.e., fear, depression).

Management of Complications

Autonomic Dysfunction. Monitoring of autonomic cardiac responses is required so that tachycardia and arrhythmias can be detected early and treatment instituted as necessary. Placing the patient on a cardiac monitor is helpful in identifying cardiac arrhythmias. If paralytic ileus occurs, a nasogastric tube is inserted for gastric decompression. An intermittent catheterization program is instituted to relieve urinary retention. Fluid and electrolytes are monitored for imbalance caused by SIADH.

Sleep Dysfunction. A disturbed sleep-wakefulness cycle leads to sleep deprivation. The basis for this problem is unclear, but it contributes to the psychological stress experienced by the patient.

Pain. Pain, the quality of which is described as a "severe charley horse," can be underrated in those 25% of patients who have pain. The pain appears to be worse at night and is not relieved by nonsteroidal anti-inflammatory agents or by nonnarcotic agents. Narcotic agents may be indicated for some patients. Administering narcotics with a slow IV drip has yielded good results. Pain can interfere with sleep, although the altered sleep patterns common to GBS patients may also have an autonomic basis.

Nutrition. Patients rapidly lose weight and muscle mass, leading to weakness, fatigue, and failure to wean from a ventilator. Nutritional support is aimed at beginning feeding as soon as is appropriate for the patient.

Immobility. The nursing staff must address problems related to immobility collaboratively. Emphasis should be on such nursing interventions as proper nutrition and maintenance of skin integrity. Minidoses of heparin are administered to prevent deep vein thrombosis (DVT) and pulmonary emboli. The use of compression boots for the prevention of DVTs is controversial, because the boots themselves may apply undue pressure to the sensitive demyelinated peripheral nerves of the leg (e.g., peroneal), leading to palsies. On this basis, heparin is usually chosen rather than compression boots for patients with GBS. Careful positioning and very gradual introduction of limited physical therapy also help to prevent palsies.

Respiratory rehabilitation may take some time and may limit the progress of a rehabilitation program, which includes extensive physical therapy and occupational therapy. Many patients fatigue easily and have a limited tolerance to activity. After respiratory function has been well established, the rehabilitation program can be managed either in a rehabilitation facility or on an outpatient basis.

Nursing Management

Nursing management in the acute phase of GBS includes a comprehensive baseline neurological and respiratory assessment and ongoing monitoring for early recognition of change. Assessment and ongoing monitoring include the following:

Respiratory Focus

- Assess respiratory rate and quality frequently.
- Assess vital capacity frequently; know the predetermined value for intubation.
- Monitor the patient for respiratory insufficiency (e.g., air hunger, abdominal breathing, cyanosis, diaphoresis, dyspnea, confusion, and anxiety).
- Monitor perfusion with pulse oximetry.
- Administer oxygen as ordered.
- Be prepared for the possibility of intubation.

Neurological Focus

- Assess motor and sensory function frequently.
- Assess cranial nerve function.

Other

- Autonomic dysfunction: monitor for cardiac arrhythmias; vital signs indicating hypotension or hypertension; and urinary retention.

Initially, neurological assessment is the area of focus in the acute phase. As the signs and symptoms of GBS develop, concern shifts to respiratory insufficiency, and the top priority is providing appropriate support. Many patients will require intubation and ventilatory support. Nursing interventions are directed toward maintaining adequate respirations, maintaining a patent airway, and preventing pulmonary infections.

The patient is maintained on bed rest for an extended period and is, therefore, at high risk for the multiple problems associated with immobility. A major concern is the development of DVTs and pulmonary emboli. As discussed earlier, the physician will probably order minidoses of heparin, rather than compression boots, to prevent DVTs. Special attention to positioning and turning is important to avoid pressure on vulnerable peripheral nerves and to prevent nerve palsies. Other areas of concern include managing paralytic ileus and urinary retention and providing range-of-motion exercises and nutritional support.

The quality and quantity of the pain and fear associated with the acute phase of GBS are unique to this illness. As discussed earlier, those patients who have pain can have such severe pain that only a continuous titration of IV narcotics can give relief. The pain, described as worse at night, interferes with sleep. There may also be some autonomic changes that alter the sleep cycle. The patient experiences sleep deprivation, which also influences the ability to cope with immobility and the powerlessness associated with the illness.

Most patients with GBS are very fearful, often fearing that they are dying. It is often difficult to convince a patient that recovery from GBS is possible. These patients need continued reinforcement that the outcome is optimistic. To be fully conscious and cognitively intact and yet on ventilatory support is an overwhelmingly frightening experience. Because some patients are maintained on a ventilator for a few months before weaning is completed, continued support and information are very important throughout the long months of recovery.

As patients move into the plateau and rehabilitation phases of GBS, the nursing focus changes to meet the altered needs of the patient. Many patients require rehabilitation that extends beyond acute care in the hospital. Multidisciplinary management and planning assist the patient toward an optimal recovery. The major patient problems and nursing diagnoses related to the nursing management of patients with GBS include the following:

- Risk for Ineffective Breathing Pattern related to neuromuscular weakness of the respiratory muscles (diaphragm and intercostals)
- Ineffective Airway Clearance related to weakness of the cough reflex and the respiratory muscles (diaphragm and intercostals)
- Knowledge Deficit related to acute illness and hospitalization
- Risk for Disuse Syndrome related to immobility secondary to paralysis and confinement of ventilator
- Impaired Verbal Communication related to paralysis of the muscles of speech or intubation
- Pain related to peripheral nerve injury
- Sleep Pattern Disturbance related to altered autonomic function and pain
- Fear related to illness, hospitalization, treatment protocols, and death

Although patients with GBS who are admitted to the intensive care unit are critically ill, they are conscious and acutely aware of the critical nature of their illnesses. With potential or actual respiratory insufficiency, it is understandable why they are fearful. Maintaining a patent airway and providing respiratory support as needed are the first priorities of care. For those who are intubated, developing a method for communication helps to alleviate fear. The autonomic effects of GBS can be significant. Cardiac arrhythmias and variations in blood pressure are common and continuous electrocardiography and frequent vital sign monitoring is necessary. Patients and families need education and support throughout the illness.

As the patient reaches a plateau and begins to recover, severe pain is common. The pain can be so severe that a continuous morphine drip is necessary to keep the patient comfortable. The morphine also serves to reduce anxiety. An aggressive rehabilitation program is required to help the patient reach optimal recovery. Therefore, a multidisciplinary approach is necessary to provide care throughout the illness trajectory. Patients and families may receive information from a number of websites.

REFERENCES

1. Briemberg, H. R., & Amato, A. A. (2005). Approach to the patient with sensory loss. UpToDate online. Retrieved July 7, 2005, from http://www.uptodateonline.com/applicaiton/topic/preint.asp?file=genneuro/5436&type=A7s

2. Bosch, E. P., & Smith, B. E. (2004). Disorders of peripheral nerves. In W. G. Bradley, R. B. Daroff, G. M. Fenichel, & J. Jonkovic (Eds.). *Neurology in clinical practice* (4th ed., pp. 2299–2401). New York: Butterworth-Heinemann.

3. Willson, H. J., & Winer, J. B. (2003). Clinical evaluation and investigation of neuropathy. *Journal of Neurology, Neurosurgery, & Psychiatry, 74*(Suppl II), ii3–ii8.

4. Kincaid, J. C. (2002). Neuropathy. In J. Biller (Ed.). *Practical neurology* (2nd ed., pp. 614–622). Philadelphia: Lippincott Williams & Wilkins.

5. Mendell, J. R., & Sahenk, Z. (2003). Painful sensory neuropathy. *New England Journal of Medicine, 348*(13), 1243–1255.

6. Ropper, A. H., & Brown, R. H. (2005). Diseases of the peripheral nerves. In A. H. Ropper & R. H. Brown (Eds.). *Adams and Victor's principles of neurology* (8th ed., pp. 1110–1177). New York: McGraw-Hill.

7. Boulton, A. J. M., Kirsner, R. S., & Vileikyte, L. (2004). Neuropathic diabetic foot ulcers. *New England Journal of Medicine, 351*, 48–55.

8. Cayley, W. E. (2006, June). Antidepressants for the treatment of neuropathic pain. *American Family Physician, 73*(11). Retrieved January 6, 2007, from http://www.aafp.org/afp/20060601/cochrane.html#c1

9. Pearson, L. J. (2000). *Nurse practitioner's drug handbook* (3rd ed., pp. 159–160). Springhouse, PA: Springhouse Corporation.

10. Hays, L., Doran, M., Reid, C., & Geary, K. (2005). Use of methadone for the treatment of diabetic neuropathy. *Diabetic Care, 28*, 485–487.

11. Younger, D. S., Dalmu, J., Inghirami, G., et al. (1994). Anti-Hu-associated peripheral nerve and muscle microvasculitis. *Neurology, 44*, 181–183.

12. Chad, D. A., Smith, T. W., & Lacomis, D. (2001). Vasculitic neuropathy: Classification, evaluation, and treatment. In D. Cros (Ed.). *Peripheral neuropathy: A practical approach to diagnosis and management* (pp. 160–176). Philadelphia: Lippincott Williams & Wilkins.

13. McArthur, J. C., & Nath, B. A. (2005). Neurological complications of HIV infection. *Lancet Neurology, 4*, 543–555.

14. Newton, H. B. (1995). Common neurologic complications of HIV-1 infection and AIDS. *American Family Physician, 51*(2), 387–398.

15. Lindsay, K. W., Bone, I., & Callander, R. (1999). *Neurology and neurosurgery illustrated* (3rd ed., pp. 414–447). Edinburgh: Churchill Livingstone.

16. Koller, H., Kieseier, B., Jander, S., & Hartung, H-P. (2005). Chronic inflammatory demyelinating polyneuropathy. *New England Journal of Medicine, 352*(13), 1345–1356.

17. Said, G. (2006). Chronic inflammatory demyelinating polyneuropathy. *Neuromuscular Disorders, 16*, 293–303.

18. Wilson, J. K., & Sevier, T. L. (2003). A review of treatment for carpal tunnel syndrome. *Disability and Rehabilitation, 25*(3), 113–119.

19. Ross, M. A. (2002). Approach to the patient with upper extremity pain and paresthesias and entrapment neuropathies. In J. Biller (Ed.). *Practical neurology* (2nd ed., pp. 289–304). Philadelphia: Lippincott Williams & Wilkins.

20. Ropper, A. H., & Brown, R. H. (2005). Diseases of the peripheral nerves. In A. H. Ropper & R. H. Brown (Eds.). *Adams and Victor's principles of neurology* (8th ed., pp. 1117–1127). New York: McGraw-Hill.

21. Davids, H. R. (2006). Guillain-Barre syndrome. Retrieved January 6, 2007, from http://www.emedicien.com/pmr/topic48.htm

22. Sulton, L. L. (2002, July). Meeting the challenge of Guillain-Barre syndrome. *Nursing Management, 33*, 25–30.

23. Hauser, S. L., & Asbury, A. K. (2005). Guillain-Barre syndrome and other immune-mediated neuropathies. In D. L. Kasper, E. Braunwald, A. S. Fauci, S. L. Hauser, D. L. Longo, & J. L. Jameson (Eds.). *Harrison's principles of internal medicine* (16th ed., pp. 2513–2516). New York: McGraw-Hill.

24. Ashbury, A. K., & Cornblath, D. R. (1990). Assessment o current diagnostic criteria for Guillain-Barre syndrome. *Annals of Neurology, 27*(suppl), S21–S24.

Cranial Nerve Diseases

Joanne V. Hickey

Certain cranial nerves (CNs) are especially vulnerable to injury because of their location within the cranial vault. Other cranial nerves, namely, the trigeminal (CN V), the facial (CN VII), the glossopharyngeal (CN IX), and the vagus (CN X), are subject to specific disease processes. Four major cranial nerve diseases are discussed in this chapter: trigeminal neuralgia, Bell's palsy, Ménière's disease, and glossopharyngeal neuralgia.

TRIGEMINAL NEURALGIA

Trigeminal neuralgia (TN), formerly known as *tic douloureux*, is characterized by severe, unilateral, brief, stabbing, recurrent pain in the distribution to one or more branches of CN V. The pain is abrupt in onset, is unilateral, and lasts for a few seconds. No motor or sensory deficits are found with TN. Terms commonly used to describe the pain are paroxysmal, sharp, piercing, lancing, shooting, burning, and lightning-like jabs. *Status trigeminus*, a rapid succession of tic-like spasms triggered by almost any stimuli, is a rare manifestation of the disease.

Most patients can identify trigger zones, which are small areas on the cheek, lip, gum, or forehead that initiate a bout of pain when stimulated. These trigger zones are sensitive to the most minimal of stimuli, such as touch, cold, pressure, or a blast of air. Chewing, talking, smiling, shaving, brushing the teeth, or going out of doors on a breezy day are common activities that may result in acute pain. TN may occur at any age, although it is most common in middle and later life. Women are affected more frequently than men by a ratio of 3:2.

Although the etiology of TN is unclear, it is generally accepted that classic TN is a consequence of vascular compression and demyelination of the trigeminal nerve.[1] Trauma, infection of the teeth or jaw, and flu-like illnesses have also been suggested as contributing to TN. An elongated, usually atherosclerotic artery adjacent to the trigeminal nerve can cause pressure on the nerve as it exits the brainstem. This pressure seems to be the etiology in most patients. Compression by an aneurysm or neoplasm, arachnoiditis, or multiple sclerosis can also produce the symptoms of TN. In making a diagnosis, other etiologies such as dental disease or temporomandibular joint dysfunction must be ruled out in order to initiate appropriate treatment.

The trigeminal nerve emerges from the pons, passing across the petrous ridge to become the gasserian ganglion, which, in turn, separates into the ophthalmic, maxillary, and mandibular divisions (Fig. 34-1). It is the largest of the cranial nerves, with both motor and sensory components. The sensory fibers relay touch, pain, and temperature sensations, whereas the motor component innervates the temporal and masseter muscles used for chewing, jaw clenching, and lateral movement. The three branches of the nerve include:

- *Ophthalmic:* forehead, eyes (including the cornea), nose, temples, meninges, paranasal sinuses, and part of the nasal mucosa
- *Maxillary:* upper jaw, teeth, lip, cheeks, hard palate, maxillary sinus, and part of the nasal mucosa
- *Mandibular:* lower jaw, teeth, lip, buccal mucosa, tongue, part of the external ear, auditory meatus, and meninges

In TN, the second and third branches of the trigeminal nerve are about equally affected. Fortunately, involvement of the first branch is rare, occurring in only about 10% of patients. When the ophthalmic branch is involved, the corneal reflex, a very important protective mechanism, may be lost.

The diagnosis of TN is based on the history and exclusion of other etiologies.[2] The neurological examination is entirely normal except in the patient who has multiple sclerosis (MS) or a tumor that compresses the trigeminal nerve. TN is common in MS. Some physicians find a magnetic resonance imaging (MRI) study useful before beginning pharmacologic therapy, while others recommend an MRI only in patients in whom pharmacotherapy was unsuccessful.[3] Regardless, the MRI is the imaging study of choice.

Course of the Disease

Many individuals with TN experience bouts of pain for several weeks or months, followed by spontaneous remission. The length of remission varies from days to years. TN usually has an exacerbating and remitting course, and patients experience shorter periods of remission as they age. The pain can cause much suffering and limitation of the activities of daily living (ADLs). Because of the fear of pain, patients may not want to talk, eat, or attend to personal hygiene, such as washing the face, brushing the teeth, or shaving.[4] Some people

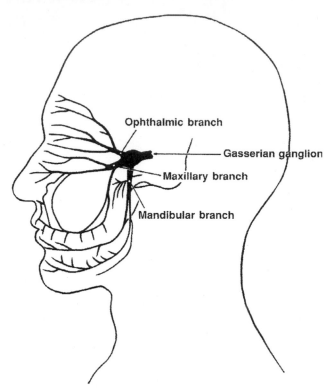

Figure 34-1 • The main divisions of the trigeminal nerve are the ophthalmic, maxillary, and mandibular. Sensory root fibers arise in the gasserian ganglion.

have become emaciated from not eating in their attempt to keep the face immobilized to prevent triggering pain.

Treatment

Both medical and surgical treatments are available with drug therapy, injection with glycerol, and surgery. Carbamazepine is the drug most commonly used to suppress or shorten the bouts of paroxysmal pain. Because carbamazepine can cause myelosuppression and liver damage, patients must be closely monitored with periodic complete blood counts (CBCs), liver enzymes, and liver function tests. If carbamazepine is not successful or is poorly tolerated, baclofen, phenytoin, and gabapentin alone or in combination are good choices. Other choices include lamotrigine, zolpidem, and tizanidine.[5] Glycerol injection into the Meckel's cave causes destruction to the myelinated fibers of the trigeminal nerve. Pain control is not immediate and may take up to 21 days. It does not cause sensory loss or facial numbness.[6,7]

Surgical Procedures

For some, medical therapy gradually becomes less effective because of the progressive nature of the disease. Surgical options are then considered. The patient with severe pain may be considered for surgery. One possible approach is a percutaneous trigeminal rhizotomy (PTR).[8,9] This is a common, well-established technique that involves controlled thermal ablation of trigeminal nerve fibers in the trigeminal

ganglion using radiofrequency energy with relative preservation of the sense of tough and facial sensations.[10] PTR provides lasting relief of pain with limited destruction of the trigeminal nerve. The basic principle is that small, poorly myelinated fibers that carry pain impulses are more sensitive to thermal lesions. With a heat-controlled electrocoagulation instrument, the sensory fibers are sufficiently destroyed to relieve pain without compromising touch or motor function.

During the procedure, a state of sedation and analgesia is achieved by administering small doses of intravenous diazepam and fentanyl during the procedure. The patient is comfortable but still able to respond verbally to questions. After each lesion is made, the corneal and ciliary reflexes, as well as facial sensation, are checked. Access to the foramen ovale, an opening from which the third branch of the trigeminal emerges, is gained through the cheek. The needle is advanced until cerebrospinal fluid is obtained. Radiographic verification of the location within the foramen ovale follows. The electrode is inserted so that the selective electrocoagulation can proceed. The advantages of the procedure are many and include long-term, if not permanent, relief of pain; shorter-term hospitalization (the patient may be discharged the day of the procedure); good toleration by the elderly; no facial paralysis; and intact sensation. Disadvantages include the possibility of puncturing the internal carotid artery and the occurrence of anesthesia dolorosa.

Other options include peripheral nerve ablation or neurectomy, percutaneous retrogasserian glycerol rhizotomy (PRGR), microvascular decompression (MVD) of the trigeminal root, and stereotactic radiosurgery.[8] In the microvascular decompression a posterior fossa craniectomy is conducted. Any blood vessel that appears to be compressing the trigeminal nerve is padded away from the nerve. If no vessel is seen that appears to be compressing the nerve, the trigeminal nerve may be partially dissected to provide pain relief. If the nerve is resected at surgery, some sensory loss to the face may be expected postoperatively.

Nursing Management

TN can be very disabling and painful. Fear of triggering spasms may prevent an individual from engaging in ADLs, social and recreational activities, and eating. Nursing management includes identifying trigger points, assessing the frequency of spasms, assessing the effectiveness of drug therapy, providing emotional support, and educating the individual in the ways to avoid triggering spasms. The major patient problems/nursing diagnoses related to TN include the following:

- Pain related to spasms
- Knowledge Deficit related to understanding the disease and triggers of spasms
- Self-Care Deficit related to fear of triggering pain by touching the face
- Altered Nutrition, Less Than required, related to fear of triggering spasms by chewing or putting food into the mouth
- Social Isolation related to fear of triggering spasm with activity

Postoperative Care

Postoperatively, periodic neurological assessments are conducted. Areas of special focus include the corneal reflex, extraocular movement, and symmetric facial movement. The sense of taste on the anterior two thirds of the tongue should also be assessed. The motor component of the trigeminal nerve is evaluated by asking the patient to clench the teeth. The contracted masseter and temporal muscles are then palpated to feel the bulk and tightness of the contracted muscles. To test the pterygoid muscles, the patient is directed to open the mouth slightly and press the examiner's finger laterally with the jaw. Weakness of the muscle will result in deviation of the jaw toward the weaker side.

After surgery that has resulted in dissection of some sensory tracts, the affected side of the face may be insensitive to pain. The patient is cautioned against rubbing the eye because the protective mechanism of pain, which warns of injury, is absent. The eye is inspected for redness and conjunctival erythema. Because of altered pain sensation on the affected side, routine visits to the dentist are recommended. Artificial tears are instilled into the eyes on the affected side, and the eye is protected from injury. Chewing is prohibited on the operative side until the paresthesia has diminished. A soft diet is ordered.

BELL'S PALSY

Bell's palsy is characterized by an abrupt onset of unilateral facial weakness now thought to be caused mainly by a herpes simplex virus type 1 and herpes zoster virus.[11] It is also seen with other diseases, such as Guillain-Barré syndrome or the mass effect of a tumor. The most common causes of abrupt onset of unilateral facial weakness or paralysis is attributable to stroke and Bell's palsy. The clinician must first determine if the facial weakness is due to a central nervous system problem (i.e., stroke) or of the peripheral nervous system (Bell's palsy). This determination is based on clinical examination. Central lesions, such as stroke, cause upper motor neuron disease, while peripheral lesions, such as Bell's palsy, result in lower motor neuron disease.

Pathophysiology

A central nervous system lesion causes *lower* facial weakness, as seen in stroke. It is due to a lesion above the level of the facial nucleus in the pons of the contralateral hemisphere. The cells of the facial nucleus that innervate the lower face receive corticobulbar fibers primarily from the contralateral cerebral hemisphere. By comparison, cells of the facial nucleus that innervate the upper face receive corticobulbar fibers that originate from both cerebral hemispheres. Therefore, a unilateral cortical lesion (such as a stroke) or one in the underlying corticobulbar fibers will produce contralateral voluntary central-type facial paralysis and a contralateral hemiplegia, but does not affect the salivary or lacrimal secretions or the sense of taste. In Bell's palsy there is weakness or paralysis of all of the muscles of facial expression. This is due primarily to a lesion of the ipsilateral facial nerve.[12]

Diagnosis

The diagnosis of Bell's palsy is made by clinical examination. Ask the patient to show his or her teeth and to smile. Note if there is weakness of just the lower face (i.e., central) such as in stroke or if there is weakness of the upper and lower face (i.e., peripheral) as in Bell's palsy. Bell's palsy may be preceded by symptoms of pain behind the ear or on the face for a few hours or days before onset of weakness/paralysis. In Bell's palsy, all deficits are on the ipsilateral side to the lesion. The eye does not close and the forehead does not wrinkle (Fig. 34-2). The patient cannot smile, whistle, or grimace. The affected side of the face is mask-like and sags, with constant tearing of the eye and possible drooling. The sense of taste for the anterior two thirds of the tongue may also be affected. The diagnosis is based on the history and clinical picture of unilateral CN VII deficits.

Bell's palsy can occur at any age but is most frequent in the 20- to 60-year-old age group. Both genders are affected about equally. Weakness or paralysis may gradually evolve over 24 to 36 hours, or it may be abrupt. Eighty percent

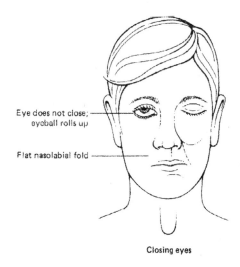

Eye does not close; eyeball rolls up

Flat nasolabial fold

Closing eyes

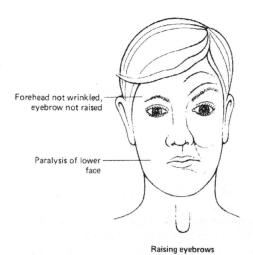

Forehead not wrinkled, eyebrow not raised

Paralysis of lower face

Raising eyebrows

Figure 34-2 • Presentation of Bell's palsy.

recover completely within a few weeks or a few months. Electromyography studies of denervation conducted 10 days after the onset indicate a prolonged or incomplete recovery. Recovery depends on nerve regeneration.

Treatment

A course of glucocorticoid therapy (e.g., a tapering dose of prednisone) is often ordered, although some studies have not shown efficacy. In addition, analgesics are given to relieve pain. Gentle massage, moist heat, and electrical stimulation of the nerve are sometimes ordered. Recovery is usual. As muscle tone improves, grimacing, wrinkling the brow, forcing the eyes closed, whistling, and blowing air out of the cheeks should be practiced three or four times daily for 5 minutes in front of a mirror. Surgical decompression may be useful in some patients if it is believed that the facial nerve is compressed.[12]

Nursing Management

Nursing management for patients with Bell's palsy focuses on prevention of injury and the need to provide psychological and emotional support. Because the eye does not close, the cornea must be protected from injury and from drying to prevent corneal ulceration and blindness. Instruct the patient to close the eyelid manually. Artificial tears are instilled into the eyes four times daily for lubrication. The eyelids may be taped closed, or an eye patch may be worn for protection. Eyestrain and sunlight are other stressors that may be avoided by wearing sunglasses.

Eating is problematic because the patient is unable to sip through a straw, chew, or control saliva on the affected side. Frequent, small feedings of soft food can be managed. The problems associated with eating are major sources of anxiety and embarrassment. Mealtime, a time of relaxation and socialization for many, becomes overwhelming unless the patient is helped to cope and adapt to the situation.

The simple techniques of moist heat application, massage, and facial exercise can easily be taught to the patient at home. A patient who develops Bell's palsy without other disorders is treated in the community. If electrostimulation therapy is ordered, it will be provided on an outpatient basis or with a home unit. Patient education for home care outlines eye care and protection, mechanical adjustments of the diet, and a simple physiotherapy and exercise program.

Patients with Bell's palsy need much emotional support to cope with the radical change in self-concept and body image. Fortunately, most patients (80%) recover completely, but this is of little comfort when a patient views his or her distorted reflection in the mirror.

MÉNIÈRE'S DISEASE

Ménière's disease (MD) is characterized by a triad of symptoms that includes tinnitus, fluctuant or permanently impaired hearing, and episodes of vertigo.[13] Tinnitus may be replaced or supplemented by aural fullness or pressure.

Tinnitus and hearing loss may not be evident initially but will gradually increase in severity as the attacks continue. MD is thought to result from dilation and periodic rupture of the endolymphatic compartment on the inner ear.[13]

The vertigo of MD is rotational or whirling in nature, lasting from minutes to a few hours and becoming so severe that the patient is unable to stand or walk. Other accompanying symptoms include nausea and vomiting and rotational or horizontal nystagmus followed by a fast component in the opposite direction. In most patients, vertigo ceases with complete hearing loss, although there are exceptions. The attacks vary in frequency and severity, with remission between bouts. Patients with recurrent attacks are often anxious.

The hearing loss associated with MD may begin early, even before the onset of vertigo. Hearing loss occurs gradually until there is complete unilateral deafness. Both genders are affected with equal frequency. The onset is most often between the ages of 40 and 60 years and usually involves one ear. In 10% of patients, the disorder is bilateral.

Diagnosis

The diagnosis of MD is based on the patient's history, neurological examination, and clinical findings of fluctuating, progressive hearing loss; episodes of vertigo; and significant tinnitus. The disease is usually unilateral and is characterized by periods of remission and exacerbation. Diagnostic testing includes audiography and electrocochleography (ECOG), a variation of brainstem auditory evoked responses. Electrodes are positioned in the external ear canal. Abnormal ECOG findings suggest MD.[13] Magnetic resonance imaging may be used to rule out other structural lesions outside the labyrinth that may require specific treatment.

Treatment

Limitation of sodium intake to 2000 mg daily and caffeine is recommended. Use of the diuretic acetazolamide (Diamox) is useful to decrease ear fullness. Meclizine (Antivert) is used for vertigo. Promethazine (Phenergan) or trimethobenzamide (Tigan) given in 200-mg suppositories is helpful for nausea and vomiting. Mild sedatives and hypnotics control anxiety. If medical treatments have failed and the condition is incapacitating, surgical options include an endolymphatic shunting procedure, direct application of corticosteroid to the inner ear, nonselective vestibular ablation (surgical labyrinthectomy, middle ear perfusion with gentamicin, translabyrinthine section of the eighth cranial nerve), and selective vestibular neurectomy.[14]

Nursing Management

Most patients with MD are treated at home unless admitted for surgery or for other conditions. A major concern is the prevention of accidents from falls because of the vertigo. The nurse should assist the patient in evaluating the efficacy of the prescribed drugs in controlling symptoms, and should educate the patient about salt and caffeine restriction.

GLOSSOPHARYNGEAL NEURALGIA

Glossopharyngeal neuralgia (GN) is a much rarer syndrome than trigeminal neuralgia. The two syndromes resemble each other in some respects. Similar aspects include attacks of intense, paroxysmal pain; certain activities triggering bouts of pain; no sensory or motor loss of the cranial nerve; and unclear etiology. In GN, the paroxysmal pain is located at the base of the tongue and the throat. Pain may also be localized in the ear or may radiate to the ear from the throat. The paroxysmal pain may be initiated by swallowing, talking, chewing, yawning, laughing, sneezing, coughing, or pressure on the tragus of the ear. The diagnosis of GN is based on the patient's history.

Treatment

The same drugs used to treat TN are used in GN. For a patient who is not responsive to medical management, there are surgical options that include microvascular decompression or nerve division of the glossopharyngeal nerve and upper rootlets of the vagus nerve near the medulla.

Nursing Management

Nursing management for GN is directed toward evaluating the patient's response to drug therapy in terms of pain control and development of side effects. If drug therapy is unsuccessful and the symptoms incapacitating (interfering with activities of daily living), surgery is an option. If surgery is performed, nursing management follows the principles outlined for posterior fossa surgery (see Chap. 14).

REFERENCES

1. Brown, C. Surgical treatment of trigeminal neuralgia. *AORN, 78*(5), 744–758.
2. Hentschel, K., Capoblanco, K. J., & Dodick, D. W. (2005). Facial pain. *Neurologist, 11*(4), 244–249.
3. Bagheri, S. C., Farhidvash, F., & Perciaccante, V. J. (2004). Diagnosis and treatment of patients with trigeminal neuralgia. *Journal of the American Dental Association, 135*, 1713–1717.
4. Dufour, S. K. An unusual case of stabbing eye pain: A case report and review of trigeminal neuralgia. *Optometry, 73*(10), 626–634.
5. Sarlani, E., Grace, E. G., Balciumas, B. A., & Schwartz, A. H. (2005). Trigeminal neuralgia in a patient with multiple sclerosis and chronic inflammatory demyelinating polyneuropathy. *Journal of the American Dental Association, 136*, 469–476.
6. Filipchuk, D. (2003). Classic trigeminal neuralgia: A surgical perspective. *Journal of Neuroscience Nursing, 35*(2), 82–85.
7. Tekkok, I., & Brown, J. A. (1996). The neurosurgical management of trigeminal neuralgia. *Neurosurgery Quarterly, 6*(2), 89–107.
8. Greenberg, M. S. (2006). *Handbook of neurosurgery* (6th ed., pp. 378–386). New York: Thieme.
9. Apfelbaum, R. I. (1999). In R. G. Grossman & C. M. Loftus (Eds.). Trigeminal and glossopharyngeal neuralgia and hemifacial spasm. *Principles of neurosurgery* (2nd ed., pp. 407–419). Philadelphia: Lippincott-Raven.
10. Tew, J. M., & Taha, J. M. (1995). Percutaneous rhizotomy in the treatment of intractable facial pain (trigeminal, glossopharyngeal and vagal). In H. H. Schmidek & W. H. Sweet (Eds.). *Operative neurosurgical technique: Indications, methods, and results.* Philadelphia: Saunders.
11. Holland, N. J., & Weiner, G. M. (2004). Recent developments in Bell's palsy. *British Medical Journal, 329*, 533–557.
12. Gilden, D. H. (2004). Bell's palsy. *New England Journal of Medicine, 351*(13), 1323–1331.
13. Hain, T. C., & Uddin, M. K. (2002). Approach to the patient with dizziness and vertigo. In J. Biller (Ed.). *Practical neurology* (2nd ed., pp. 189–205). Philadelphia: Lippincott Williams and Wilkins.
14. Greenberg, M. S. (2006). *Handbook of neurosurgery* (6th ed., pp. 591–593). New York: Thieme.

Index

Page numbers followed by *f* indicate figures; those followed by *t* indicate tables; those followed by *c* indicate charts; those followed by *b* indicate boxes.

A

A-beta fibers, 626
A-delta fibers, 626
A (plateau) waves, 299, 301
Abciximab, 605–606
ABCs of life support, 660
Abducens nerve (CN VI)
  anatomy, 86
  assessment of, 164*t*
  extraocular movement and, 168
  eye movement and, 85*t*
  location of, 57*f*
  nucleus, 86
    location of, 66
  testing of, 124–128
Abductor digiti quinti muscle, 134*t*
Abrasions, 374
Abscesses, 675. *See also* Infections
  diagnosis, 677
  signs and symptoms, 675–677
  treatment, 677
Absence seizures, 649*t*, 653*t*
Abstract thinking skills, 117
Abstraction, evaluation of, 109
ACA. *See* Anterior cerebral artery
    (ACA)
Acceleration-deceleration injuries,
    371–372, 372*f*, 412
Access to care, managed care and, 11
Accommodation, of lens, 86, 128
Acetaminophen (Tylenol)
  after lumbar puncture, 99
  in HSV encephalitis, 675
  for hyperthermia, 292, 358, 397–398
  in management of chronic pain, 630
  for migraine headache, 640*t*
  for tension-type headaches, 642
Acetazolamide (Diamox), 303
Acetylcholine (ACh), 46*t*
Acetylcholine (ACh) receptors, 704,
    705
Achilles tendon reflex
  assessment of, 146*f*
  hypoactive, 715
  nerve root involved in, 462*t*
Acidosis, 596

Acomm. *See* Anterior communicating
    artery (Acom)
Acoustic nerve (CN VIII)
  assessment of, 129–130, 164*t*
  nucleus, 66
Acoustic neuromas, 163, 504*t*
Action potentials, 43
Activities of daily living (ADLs)
  assessment of
    in peripheral nerve injury, 493
    rehabilitation goals and, 216
  in chronic illness, 13
  chronic pain and, 631
  cognitive rehabilitation and, 237
  dementia screening and, 681
  dementia work-up and, 682*t*
  instrumental, 216
  in Parkinson's disease, 696
  personal, 216
  postoperative period, 325
  skilled nursing facilities and, 16
Activity intolerance, 218
Acupuncture, 630
Acute care hospitals, focus of, 14–16
Acute care units, transfers to, 319–320
Acute cord compression, 474
Acute-critical care, 13, 15*t*
Acute disability, 214
Acute inflammatory demyelinating
    polyneuropathy (AIDP), 719
Acute inpatient rehabilitation facilities,
    14–15
Acute motor axonal neuropathy, 719
Acute motor sensory axonal neuropa-
    thy, 719
Acute pain, 624
Acute-phase responses, to stress, 184
Acute phases, in chronic illness, 691
Acute respiratory distress syndrome
    (ARDS), 396–397
Acyclovir, 251*t*, 253
Adaptation, 207
  chronic care and, 13
Adaptive behaviors, 207
Adaptive-phase responses, 184
Addiction, fears of, 30–31
Adductor brevis muscle, 138*t*

Adductor longus muscle, 138*t*
Adductor magnus muscle, 138*t*
ADH. *See* Antidiuretic hormone
    (ADH)
Adie pupils, 128*t*
Adjustment, rehabilitation and,
    214
ADLs. *See* Activities of daily living
    (ADLs)
Adrenal glands, autonomic effects on,
    79*t*
Adrenocorticotropic hormone (ACTH).
    See also Corticotropin
  function of, 64
  replacement, 329
ADS. *See* Autonomic dysfunction
    syndrome (ADS)
Advance directives, 26–28
Advanced practice nurses (APNs), 7,
    352–353
Advanced Trauma Life Support
    (ATLS), 385
AEIOU mnemonic, 157
Affect, mental state and, 114
Afferent fibers
  general somatic, 70
  general visceral, 70
  sensory, 64, 80
  special somatic, 83
  special visceral, 83
  to spinal cord, 626*f*
Age/aging
  cerebral aneurysms and, 536
  degenerative changes in, 454
  dementias and, 680–681
  demographic trends, 4
  ethical decision making and, 4
Agency for Health Care Policy and
    Research (AHCPR), 215
Agency for Healthcare Research and
    Quality, 6
Agitation
  in Alzheimer's disease, 687
  of ICU patients, 361
Agnosia, 227*t*, 681
AICA. *See* Anterior inferior cerebellar
    artery (AICA)

of upper extremities, 133, 173
of urinary bladder function, 231–232, 234c
of the vagus nerve, 130–132, 131, 131f, 164t
of wrist extension, 137f
Assisted suicide, 31–32
Assistive devices, for ambulation, 225f
Association areas, brain, 60
Association fibers, anatomy, 60
Association of Rehabilitation Nurses, 217
Astereognosis, 138, 227t
Astrocytes, 40, 497
Astrocytomas
  characterization of, 502t, 504t
  development of, 497
  low-grade
    MRI of, 507f
    treatments for, 514
Ataxic breathing, 177t
Atelectasis, assessment of, 404–405
Atenolol
  function of, 241
  in migraine prophylaxis, 641t
Atherogenesis, 595
Atheromas, 595
  carotid endarterectomy for, 329–330
  hot spots for buildup of, 607
  thrombus formation and, 591
Atherosclerosis, 595
  carotid endarterectomy for, 329–330
Atethis, 144t
Athletes, head injuries in, 401
Athletoid gait, 143t
Atlantoaxial subluxation, 417–418
Atlas, spinal, 48, 50f
Atlas fractures, 417–418
Atlectasis, 342
Atonic bladder, 439
Atonic seizures, 650t, 653t
Atracurium, 392
Atropine sulfate, 103
Attention, evaluation of, 109, 115, 615c
Audiometric studies, 108
Auditory agnosia, 227t
Auditory association areas, 63
Auditory stimuli, 157
Auditory system, 87
Auerbach's plexus, 76
Auras
  migraine, 634, 635
  seizures and, 647
Automatisms, 647, 648
Autonomic dysfunction syndrome (ADS)
  laboratory investigations, 399
  signs and symptoms, 399
  in traumatic brain injury, 398–399
  treatment of, 399
Autonomic dysreflexia, 443–445
Autonomic hyperreflexia, 447f
Autonomic nervous system (ANS)
  anatomy, 76–82
  components, 72f
  diagram of, 78f
  dysfunction
    in Guillain-Barré syndrome, 720
    in traumatic brain injury, 398–399

Autonomic seizures, 649t
Autonomic storming, 398–399
Autonomic symptoms, 647
Autonomy, concept of, 22
Autoregulation, 273
AVE coronary stent, 557
AVMs. See Arteriovenous malformations
Avulsion fractures, 418
Avulsions, peripheral nerves, 486
Awareness. See also Cognitive function; Consciousness
  concept of, 161
  consciousness and, 155
  level of, 114
Axial loading injuries, 412, 414f
Axis, spinal, 48, 50f
Axis cylinder, 41
Axonal transport, 486
Axonotmesis, 488
Axons, 42–43, 42f, 486–487
  A-beta fibers, 626
  A-delta fibers, 626
  C fibers, 626
Axotomy, 380, 381
Azathioprine (Imuran), 263, 706

B

B-mode (brightness-modulated) imaging, 101
B waves, 299, 301
Babinski response, 448, 465f
Babinski sign, anatomy of, 80
Babinski's reflex, 144, 149f
Back pain. See also Low back pain; Spine, pain
  conditions related to, 454–460
  initial management, 455–461, 458
    patient education in, 455, 458
  problems related to, 455
  "red flags," 455t
Baclofen (Lioresal)
  in cluster headache prophylaxis, 642
  in management of chronic pain, 630
  in multiple sclerosis, 701
  in spasticity management, 448
  in trigeminal neuralgia, 724
Bacteremia, in TBI patients, 397
BAERs. See Brain-stem auditory evoked responses (BAERs)
Balance
  assessment of, 138
  rehabilitation exercises, 221
Ballism, 144t
Balloon angioplasty, 560
Balloon remodeling techniques, 555–556
  microballoons, 577
Barbiturate-induced coma, 293
Barbiturate therapy, 393
Barbiturates, 243t
Baroreceptors, 174, 196
Basal caloric requirement, 186–187
Basal ganglia
  development of, 41t
  general functions of, 63

lower motor neurons and, 72–73
Parkinson's disease and, 691
Basal skull fractures, 374–375
  meningitis in, 669t
  nursing management of, 405
Basal sulcus, anatomy, 66
Basilar artery
  area supplied by, 57f
  distribution of, 594f
  formation of, 594
  location of, 56f
Basilar artery syndrome, 599t
Basilar penetrating arteries, 595
Basilar sutures, 48
Basilar tip aneurysms, 554f, 555f
Basis pedunculi, 65
Basis pontis, 66
Battle's sign, 403
BBB. See Blood-brain barrier (BBB)
Beck Depression Inventory, 631
Becker intraventricular external drainage, 290f, 297
Bed rest
  deconditioning during, 220
  fatigue and, 218
  in herniated intervertebral discs, 468, 470
  orthostatic hypotension and, 220–221
  prolonged, effects of, 458
  transfer activities, 221–223
Beds. See also Head of beds
  selection of, 438
  specialty types, 340–341
  transfer activities, 221–223, 222f, 223f
Bedside assessments, 162–163, 171c
Behavior
  in Alzheimer's disease patients, 686–697
  dementia work-up and, 682t
  disorders, in multiple sclerosis, 698
  general evaluation of, 114
  stress responses and, 206–212
Bell's palsy, 725
  diagnosis, 725–726
  lesions, 129
  middle fossa fractures and, 375
  nursing management, 726
  pathophysiology, 725
  presentation, 725f
  treatment, 726
Beneficence, concept of, 22
Benign intracranial hypertension, 303
Benign paroxysmal positional vertigo (BPPV), 130
Benzodiazepines, 247
  for agitation, 687
  in increased ICPs, 390
  in management of chronic pain, 630
Benztropine (Cogentin), 265t, 266
Bereavement, patient response to, 210–211
Berry aneurysms, 540
Best practices, process model, 8–9
Beta blockers, 241
  adverse effects, 242t
  for migraine prophylaxis, 641t
Beta-lactam antibiotics, 249–251
Beta-lactamase inhibitors, 250t–251t